Diseases of the Liver

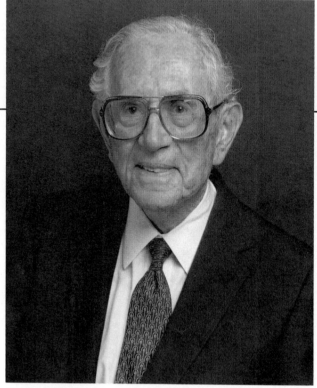

Leon Schiff

Seventh Edition

Diseases

of the **Liver**

Volume 2

Edited by

LEON SCHIFF, MD, PhD

Emeritus Professor of Medicine
University of Cincinnati College of Medicine
Cincinnati, Ohio
Clinical Professor of Medicine
University of Miami School of Medicine
Consultant in Hepatology
Department of Veterans Affairs Medical Center
Miami, Florida

EUGENE R. SCHIFF, MD

Professor of Medicine
Chief, Division of Hepatology
Director, Center for Liver Diseases
University of Miami School of Medicine
Chief, Hepatology Section
Department of Veterans Affairs Medical Center
Miami, Florida

97 Contributors

 J.B. Lippincott Company   PHILADELPHIA

Acquisitions Editor: Charles McCormick, Jr
Associate Editor: Kimberley Cox
Associate Managing Editor: Grace R. Caputo
Production Manager: Caren Erlichman
Senior Production Coordinator: Kevin P. Johnson
Design Coordinator: Kathy Kelley-Luedtke
Interior Designer: Arlene Putterman
Indexer: Alexandra Weir Nickerson
Compositor: Compset Inc
Printer/Binder: R.R. Donnelley & Sons Company

7th Edition

Library of Congress Cataloging-in-Publication Data

Diseases of the liver.—7th ed./edited by Leon Schiff, Eugene R.
  Schiff; 97 contributors.
        p.   cm.
    Includes bibliographical references and index.
    ISBN 0-397-51127-2 (two-volume set)
    ISBN 0-397-51362-3 (volume 1)
    ISBN 0-397-51363-1 (volume 2)
    1. Liver—Diseases.   I. Schiff, Leon.   II. Schiff,
  Eugene R.
    [DNLM: 1. Liver Diseases.   WI 700 D615]
  RC845.D53   1993
  616.3'62—dc20
  DNLM/DLC
  for Library of Congress   92-48245
                                                        CIP

Dedicated to the memory of
Hugh Edmonson and Robert Peters,
distinguished pathologists
and devoted friends,
for their important contributions
to the field of liver pathology

David H. Alpers, MD
Professor of Medicine
Chief, Division of Gastroenterology
Washington University School of Medicine
Attending Physician
Barnes Hospital
St Louis, Missouri

James M. Anderson, MD, PhD
Associate Professor of Internal Medicine and Cell Biology
Attending Physician
Yale–New Haven Hospital
New Haven, Connecticut

Colin E. Atterbury, MD
Professor of Medicine
Associate Dean for Veterans Affairs
Yale University School of Medicine
New Haven, Connecticut
Chief of Staff
Department of Veterans Affairs Medical Center
West Haven, Connecticut

William F. Balistreri, MD
Dorothy M.M. Kersten Professor of Pediatrics
University of Cincinnati College of Medicine
Director, Division of Pediatric Gastroenterology
 and Nutrition
Children's Hospital Medical Center
Cincinnati, Ohio

Hope Barkoukis, MS, RD, LD
Department of Nutrition
Case Western Reserve University School of Medicine
Cleveland, Ohio

Jean-Pierre Benhamou, MD
Professor of Hepatology and Gastroenterology
University of Paris
Head, Department of Hepatology
Hopital Beaujon
Clichy, France

George Berci, MD
Clinical Professor Emeritus of Surgery
University of California, Los Angeles, UCLA School
 of Medicine
Senior Consulting Surgery
Former Director, Surgical Endoscopy
Cedars-Sinai Medical Center
Los Angeles, California

Joseph R. Bloomer, MD
Professor of Medicine
Director, Division of Gastroenterology, Hepatology,
 and Nutrition
University of Minnesota Medical School—Minneapolis
Attending Physician
University of Minnesota Hospital and Clinic
Minneapolis, Minnesota

H. Worth Boyce, Jr, MD
Professor of Medicine
University of South Florida College of Medicine
Tampa, Florida

James L. Boyer, MD
Professor of Medicine
Director, Liver Center
Chief, Division of Digestive Diseases
Yale University School of Medicine
Attending Physician
Yale–New Haven Hospital
New Haven, Connecticut

Justine Meehan Carr, MD
Instructor in Pathology
Harvard Medical School
Medical Director, Hematology Laboratory
Beth Israel Hospital
Boston, Massachusetts

Peter L. Chiodini, PhD, FRCP
Consultant Parasitologist
Hospital for Tropical Diseases
London, England

Alan S. Cohen, MD
Conrad Wesselhoeft Professor of Medicine
Director, Arthritis Center
Boston University School of Medicine
Chief of Medicine
Director, Thorndike Memorial Laboratory
Boston City Hospital
Boston, Massachusetts

Harold O. Conn, MD
Professor (Emeritus) of Medicine
Yale University School of Medicine
Attending Physician
Yale–New Haven Medical Center
New Haven, Connecticut
Attending Physician
Department of Veterans Affairs Medical Center
West Haven, Connecticut

James M. Crawford, MD, PhD
Assistant Professor of Pathology
Harvard Medical School
Associate Pathologist
Brigham and Women's Hospital
Boston, Massachusetts

Horacio B. D'Agostino, MD
Assistant Professor of Radiology
University of California, San Diego, School of Medicine
Staff Physician
UCSD Medical Center
San Diego, California

Kevin M. DeCock, MD, MRCP(UK), DTM&H
Director, Project RETRO-CI
Abidjan, Cote d'Ivoire
West Africa
Medical Epidemiologist
Division of HIV/AIDS
National Center for Infectious Diseases
Centers for Disease Control
Atlanta, Georgia

Murray Epstein, MD
Professor of Medicine
Attending Physician
Department of Veterans Affairs Medical Center
Jackson Memorial Medical Center
Miami, Florida

Serge Erlinger, MD
Professor of Hepatology and Gastroenterology
Faculty of Medicine Xavier Bichat
University of Paris
Hospital Beaujon
Director, Unite de Recherches de
    Physiopathologie Hepatique
Clichy, France

Michael B. Fallon, MD
Assistant Professor of Medicine
Liver Center and Department of Medicine
Yale University School of Medicine
New Haven, Connecticut

Zoheir Farid, MB, BCh, DTM&H
Special Assistant to the Commanding Officer for
    Clinical Medicine
US Naval Research Unit
Consulting Physician
Abbassia Fever Hospital
Egyptian Ministry of Health
Cairo, Egypt

Philip Feliciano, MD
Assistant Professor of Surgery
Oregon Health Sciences University School of Medicine
Medical Director, Surgical Intensive Care Unit
University Hospital
Portland, Oregon

Joseph E. Geenen, MD
Clinical Professor of Medicine
Medical College of Wisconsin
Milwaukee, Wisconsin

Paul Genecin, MD
Assistant Clinical Professor of Medicine
Division of Digestive Diseases
Yale University School of Medicine
Chief, Internal Medicine
Yale University Health Services
Attending Physician
Yale–New Haven Hospital
New Haven, Connecticut
Attending Physician
Department of Veterans Affairs Medical Center
West Haven, Connecticut

John L. Gollan, MD, PhD, FRACP, FRCP
Associate Professor of Medicine
Harvard Medical School
Director, Gastroenterology Division
Senior Physician
Brigham and Women's Hospital
Boston, Massachusetts

Robert D. Gordon, MD
Professor of Surgery
Emory University School of Medicine
Chief, Liver Transplant Service
Emory University Hospital
Atlanta, Georgia

Roberto J. Groszmann, MD
Professor of Medicine
Yale University School of Medicine
New Haven, Connecticut
Chief, Digestive Disease Section
Department of Veterans Affairs Medical Center
West Haven, Connecticut

J. Michael Henderson, MD, ChB, FRCS
Chairman, Department of General Surgery
The Cleveland Clinic Foundation
Cleveland, Ohio

Anastacio M. Hoyumpa, MD
Professor of Medicine
University of Texas Health Science Center
Staff Physician
Audie L. Murphy Memorial Veterans Affairs Hospital
San Antonio, Texas

Kamal G. Ishak, MD, PhD
Clinical Professor of Pathology
Uniformed Services University of the Health Sciences
Medical Care Consultant
National Institutes of Health
Bethesda, Maryland
Chairman, Department of Hepatic and
    Gastrointestinal Pathology
Armed Forces Institute of Pathology
Washington, DC
Professorial Lecturer
Mount Sinai School of Medicine
New York, New York

D. Geraint James, MA, MD, FRCP FACP(Hon), LID(Hon)
Adjunct Professor of Medicine
Royal Free Hospital School of Medicine
University of London
London, England
Adjunct Professor of Medicine
University of Miami School of Medicine
Miami, Florida

Lennox J. Jeffers, MD
Associate Professor of Medicine
Division of Hepatology
Center for Liver Diseases
University of Miami School of Medicine
Hepatology Section
Department of Veterans Affairs Medical Center
Miami, Florida

Marshall M. Kaplan, MD
Professor of Medicine
Tufts University School of Medicine
Chief, Division of Gastroenterology
New England Medical Center Hospital
Boston, Massachusetts

Reuben Kier, MD
Clinical Assistant Professor of Radiology
Yale University School of Medicine
New Haven, Connecticut
Director, Body MR Imaging
Bridgeport Hospital
Bridgeport, Connecticut

Michael E. Kilpatrick, MD
Executive Officer
Naval Hospital
Orlando, Florida

Samuel Klein, MD
Associate Professor of Medicine
Division of Gastroenterology
Director, Clinical Nutrition Center
University of Texas Medical Branch at Galveston
Galveston, Texas

Raymond S. Koff, MD
Professor of Medicine
University of Massachusetts Medical School
Worcester, Massachusetts
Chairman, Department of Medicine
Metrowest Medical Center
Framingham, Massachusetts

Masamichi Kojiro, MD
Professor and Chairman
The First Department of Pathology
Kurume University School of Medicine
Kurume-Shi, Japan

Nicholas F. LaRusso, MD
Professor of Medicine and Biochemistry and
    Molecular Biology
Chairman, Division of Gastroenterology
Director, Center for Basic Research in Digestive Diseases
Mayo Medical School
Consultant
Mayo Foundation and Hospitals
Rochester, Minnesota

Patricia S. Latham, MD
Assistant Professor
George Washington University School of Medicine and
    Health Sciences
Washington, DC

Jurgen Ludwig, MD
Professor of Pathology
Mayo Medical School
Mayo Clinic and Mayo Foundation
Rochester, Minnesota

Willis C. Maddrey, MD
Professor of Internal Medicine
Vice President for Clinical Affairs
University of Texas Southwestern Medical Center at Dallas
Dallas, Texas

Jay W. Marks, MD
Associate Professor of Medicine
University of California, Los Angeles, UCLA School
    of Medicine
Associate Director, Division of Gastroenterology
Cedars-Sinai Medical Center
Los Angeles, California

Arthur J. McCullough, MD
Associate Professor of Medicine
Case Western Reserve University School of Medicine
Director of Gastroenterology
Metro Health Medical Center
Cleveland, Ohio

Charles L. Mendenhall, MD, PhD
Professor of Medicine
University of Cincinnati Medical Center
Director of Hepatic Research
Department of Veterans Affairs Medical Center
Cincinnati, Ohio

Frank G. Moody, MD
Denton A. Cooley Professor and Chairman
Department of Surgery
University of Texas Medical School at Houston
Chief of Surgery
The Hermann Hospital
Houston, Texas

Kevin D. Mullen, MD, FRCPI
Assistant Professor of Medicine
Case Western Reserve University School of Medicine
Consultant Gastroenterologist
Metro Health Medical Center
Cleveland, Ohio

Ronald Neuman, MD
Chief, Nuclear Medicine Department
Clinical Center
National Institutes of Health
Bethesda, Maryland

Michael A. Nissenbaum, MD
Fellow, Department of Radiology
University of California, San Diego, School of Medicine
San Diego, California
Deputy Director
Magnetic Resonance Imaging
Beth Israel Hospital
Harvard Medical School
Boston, Massachusetts

John G. O'Grady, MD, MRCPI
Consultant Hepatologist
St James's University Hospital
Leeds, United Kingdom

Hiroaki Okuda, MD
Assistant Professor
Institute of Gastroenterology
Tokyo Women's Medical College
Tokyo, Japan

Kunio Okuda, MD, ScD, PhD
Emeritus Professor of Medicine
Chiba University School of Medicine
Chiba, Japan

M. James Phillips, MD, CM, FRCP(C)
Professor and Vice-Chairman
Department of Pathology
University of Toronto
Pathologist-in-Chief
The Hospital for Sick Children
Toronto, Ontario, Canada

Michael K. Porayko, MD
Assistant Professor of Medicine
Mayo Medical School
Mayo Clinic and Mayo Foundation
Rochester, Minnesota

Bernard Portmann, MD, FRCPath
Honorary Senior Lecturer and Consultant Pathologist
Institute of Liver Studies
King's College School of Medicine and Dentistry
London, England

John R. Potts III, MD
Associate Professor of Surgery
University of Texas Medical School at Houston
Chief, Orange Surgery Service
The Hermann Hospital
Houston, Texas

Siria Poucell-Hatton, MD
Visiting Scholar, Gastroenterology Division
University of California, San Diego, School of Medicine
Department of Medicine
Department of Veterans Affairs Medical Center
San Diego, California

Jeffrey M. Rank, MD
Assistant Professor of Medicine
University of Minnesota Medical School—Minneapolis
Gastroenterologist
Section of Gastroenterology, Hepatology, and Nutrition
University of Minnesota Hospital and Clinic
Minneapolis, Minnesota

Aron M. Rappaport, MD, PhD†
Professor Emeritus of Physiology
University of Toronto Faculty of Medicine
Toronto, Ontario, Canada

K. Rajender Reddy, MD
Associate Professor of Medicine
Division of Hepatology
University of Miami School of Medicine
University of Miami Hospital and Clinic
Jackson Memorial Hospital
Cedars Medical Center
Miami, Florida

Caroline A. Riely, MD
Professor of Medicine and Pediatrics
University of Tennessee, Memphis, College of Medicine
Attending Physician
William F. Bowld Hospital
Memphis, Tennessee

Adrian Reuben, BSc, MBBS, FRCP
Associate Professor of Medicine
Section of Digestive Diseases
Yale University School of Medicine
Attending Physician
Yale–New Haven Hospital
New Haven, Connecticut

Telfer B. Reynolds, MD
Clayton G. Loosli Professor of Medicine
University of Southern California School of Medicine
Los Angeles, California

Bruce A. Runyon, MD
Associate Professor
University of Iowa College of Medicine
University of Iowa Hospitals and Clinics
Iowa City, Iowa

Seymour M. Sabesin, MD
Josephine Dyrenforth Professor of Medicine
Rush Medical College of Rush University
Director, Section of Digestive Diseases
Presbyterian–St Luke's Medical Center
Chicago, Illinois

Philip Sandblom, MD, PhD
Professor (Emeritus) of Surgery
Former President
University of Lund
Lund, Sweden

†Deceased.

Jay P. Sanford, MD
Clinical Professor of Medicine
University of Texas Southwestern Medical School at Dallas
Dean Emeritus
Uniformed Services University of the Health Sciences
Attending Physician
Parkland Memorial Hospital
Consultant
Department of Veterans Affairs Medical Center
Dallas, Texas

I. Herbert Scheinberg, MD
Professor (Emeritus) of Medicine
Albert Einstein College of Medicine of Yeshiva University
Bronx, New York
Senior Research Associate
St Luke's–Roosevelt Hospital Center
Senior Lecturer
College of Physicians and Surgeons
New York, New York

Steven Schenker, MD
Professor of Medicine and Pharmacology
Division Chief, Division of Gastroenterology and Nutrition
University of Texas Health Science Center at San Antonio
Staff Physician
Audie L. Murphy Memorial Veterans Hospital
San Antonio, Texas

Eugene R. Schiff, MD
Professor of Medicine
Chief, Division of Hepatology
Director, Center for Liver Diseases
University of Miami School of Medicine
Chief, Hepatology Section
Department of Veterans Affairs Medical Center
Miami, Florida

Gilbert M. Schiff, MD
Professor of Medicine
University of Cincinnati College of Medicine
President
James N. Gamble Institute of Medical Research
Cincinnati, Ohio

Leon Schiff, MD, PhD, MACP
Emeritus Professor of Medicine
University of Cincinnati College of Medicine
Cincinnati, Ohio
Clinical Professor of Medicine
University of Miami School of Medicine
Consultant in Hepatology
Department of Veterans Affairs Medical Center
Miami, Florida

Leslie J. Schoenfield, MD, PhD
Professor of Medicine
University of California, Los Angeles, UCLA School
   of Medicine
Director of Gastroenterology
Cedars-Sinai Medical Center
Los Angeles, California

William K. Schubert, MD
Professor and Chairman
Department of Pediatrics
University of Cincinnati College of Medicine
President and Chief Executive Officer
Children's Hospital Medical Center
Cincinnati, Ohio

Sarah Jane Schwarzenberg, MD
Associate Professor of Pediatrics
University of Minnesota Medical School—Minneapolis
Minneapolis, Minnesota

Harvey L. Sharp, MD
Professor of Pediatrics
University of Minnesota Medical School—Minneapolis
Section Head of Pediatrics, Gastroenterology, and Nutrition
University of Minnesota Hospital and Clinic
Minneapolis, Minnesota

Sheila Sherlock, MD, DBE
Professor and Chairman Emeritus
Department of Medicine
The Royal Free Hospital
School of Medicine
University of London
London, England

Jerome H. Siegel, MD
Associate Clinical Professor of Medicine
Mount Sinai School of Medicine of the City University of
   New York
Chief of Endoscopy
Beth Israel Medical Center, North Division
New York, New York

Martha Skinner, MD
Professor of Medicine
Boston University School of Medicine
Director of Research, Arthritis Center
Boston, Massachusetts

Elizabeth J. Smanik, MD, PhD
Assistant Professor of Medicine
Case Western Reserve University School of Medicine
Staff Gastroenterologist
Metro Health Medical Center
Cleveland, Ohio

Thomas E. Starzl, MD, PhD
Professor of Surgery
University of Pittsburgh School of Medicine
Director
Transplantation Institute
Pittsburgh, Pennsylvania

Irmin Sternlieb, MD
Professor of Medicine and Associate Director
Marion Bassin Liver Research Center
Albert Einstein College of Medicine of Yeshiva University
Attending Physician
Bronx Municipal Hospital Center and Montefiore Hospital
   and Medical Center
Bronx, New York

James G. Straka, PhD
Research Associate
University of Minnesota Medical School—Minneapolis
Minneapolis, Minnesota

Paul H. Sugarbaker, MD
Medical Director
The Cancer Institute
Washington Hospital Center
Washington, DC

Eric G.C. Tan, MD
Department of Surgery
University of Camberra
Camberra, Australia

Anthony S. Tavill, MD
Professor of Medicine
Case Western Reserve University School of Medicine
Director, Friedman Center for Digestive and
   Liver Disorders
Mount Sinai Medical Center
Cleveland, Ohio

Kenneth J.W. Taylor, MD, PhD
Professor of Radiology
Director, Experimental Laboratory
Director, Vascular Laboratory
Yale University Medical School
New Haven, Connecticut

Howard C. Thomas, BSc, MBBS, PhD, FRCP, FRCPath
Professor and Chairman of Medicine
St Mary's Hospital Medical School
Imperial College, University of London
Paddington
London, England

Donald Trunkey, MD
Professor and Chairman
Department of Surgery
Oregon Health Sciences University School of Medicine
Chief of Surgery
University Hospital
Portland, Oregon

David H. Van Thiel, MD
Professor of Medicine, Surgery, and Psychiatry
Medical Director of Transplantation
University of Pittsburgh School of Medicine
Pittsburgh, Pennsylvania

Eric vanSonnenberg, MD
Professor of Radiology and Medicine
Director of Interventional Radiology
University of California, San Diego, School of Medicine
San Diego, California

Annamalai Veerappan, MD
Department of Gastroenterology
Washington Hospital
Fremont, California
Valleycare Medical Center
Pleasanton, California
Livermore, California

Rama P. Venu, MD
Associate Clinical Professor of Medicine
Medical College of Wisconsin
Milwaukee, Wisconsin

Ian R. Wanless, MD
Associate Professor of Pathology
University of Toronto Faculty of Medicine
Director, Canadian Liver Pathology Reference Centre
Staff Pathologist
The Toronto Hospital
Toronto, Ontario, Canada

Kenneth W. Warren, MD
Honorary Member
Department of Surgery
New England Baptist Hospital
Former Chairman
Department of Surgery
Lahey Clinic Foundation
Emeritus Clinical Instructor in Surgery
Harvard Medical School
Boston, Massachusetts

Heather M. White, MD
Assistant Professor of Medicine
Division of Gastroenterology
Washington University School of Medicine
St Louis, Missouri

Russell H. Wiesner, MD
Professor of Medicine
Mayo Medical School
Medical Director of Liver Transplantation
Rochester, Minnesota

Roger Williams, MD, FRCP, FRCS, FRCPE, FRACP
Consultant Physician and Director
Institute of Liver Studies
Kings College Hospital
Kings College School of Medicine and Dentistry
London, England

Hyman J. Zimmerman, MD
Professor of Medicine (Emeritus)
George Washington University School of Medicine and
    Health Sciences
Distinguished Scientist (Emeritus)
Armed Forces Institute of Pathology
Washington, DC
Clinical Professor of Medicine
Uniformed Services University of the Health Sciences
Bethesda, Maryland

The field of liver disease continues its rapid growth. The number of liver-oriented societies and their publications, journals, and texts are increasing throughout the world. Attendance at the annual meetings of the American Association for the Study of Liver Diseases has grown from two dozen at the initial gathering at Hektoen Institute in Chicago to more than 1750. The number of pages in *Diseases of the Liver* has grown from 718 in the first edition to 1516 in the current one.

It is always difficult to include every development up to the time of each new edition. Regardless, the field of hepatology is exploding with new knowledge. Examples of such advances and observations described in this edition of *Diseases of the Liver* include the following:

1. There has been a large increase in the number of drugs that produce liver injury, as there has in the mechanisms by which cytochrome P-450 produces such damage.
2. A striking advance in gallbladder surgery has been the introduction of laparoscopic cholecystectomy, which may largely replace the conventional surgical approach. The advantages include less operative pain, less discomfort from transitional ileus, earlier hospital discharge, and earlier resumption of full physical activities.
3. The number of liver transplant centers in this country and abroad has greatly increased, as have transplantations in cases of cirrhosis and fulminant hepatitis. What a thrill it has been to witness the rescue of a patient with fulminant Wilson's disease.
4. Using animal models, Grossman and colleagues have precisely defined the pathophysiologic factors in portal hypertension.
5. There has been more resort to segmental hepatectomy in focal neoplastic invasions of the liver.
6. Beneficial effects from the use of ursodeoxycholic acid are being seen in primary biliary cirrhosis and sclerosing cholangitis.

7. Intensive research, both clinical and biomedical, continues in the field of viral hepatitis. The discovery of hepatitis C and E has clarified the epidemiology of viral hepatitis. The ability to measure HCV RNA and HBV DNA helps in assessing the efficacy of antiviral therapy in chronic hepatitis C and B, respectively.
8. Ultrasound Doppler methodology has proved to be safe and effective in studying the hepatic vasculature. Dynamic computed tomographic scanning and positron emission tomographic techniques are being investigated to identify metabolic changes perhaps prior to anatomic defects.
9. Despite the advances contributed by hepatobiliary imagery, the images are often nonspecific. For example, a blood clot in the common bile duct may stimulate a gallstone, as may a ductal neoplasm. Iatrogenic stenosis of the junction of the hepatic ducts may be indistinguishable from Klatskin's tumor. Carcinoma of the gallbladder enveloping the hepatic duct may mimic a bile duct tumor.

On the 36th anniversary of *Diseases of the Liver*, the editors extend their gratitude to contributors past and present. We trust that the seventh edition will be viewed as voiced by Franz Ingelfinger of a previous edition: "not too much oriented toward basic science nor too clinical, but the perfect blend of the fundamental and practical."

We wish to thank Charles McCormick, Jr, Kimberley Cox, and Grace Caputo of the J.B. Lippincott Company for their untiring cooperation in the publication of this edition. We also thank Patricia Villacorta, Sabrina Des Rosiers, and Mari Sweney for their editorial assistance, as well as Marcus Rothschild for his helpful suggestions.

Leon Schiff, MD, PhD
Eugene R. Schiff, MD

In the recent words of Himsworth, the present time seems to be particularly opportune for reviewing our knowledge of liver disease. A partial list of reasons would include the advances made in the fundamental sciences as they pertain to liver structure and function; the advances in the experimental approach to liver disease; the increased knowledge in the field of viral hepatitis; the newer clinical criteria and concept of hepatic coma, with attention focused on disturbance in the metabolism of ammonia; a better understanding of the pathogenesis and the treatment of cirrhosis; a clearer concept of the metabolic defect in hemochromatosis and the apparent effectiveness of depleting iron stores in the treatment of this disorder; the implication of disturbed copper metabolism in hepatolenticular degeneration; the increasing experience with needle biopsy of the liver; and the surgical attack on portal hypertension.

This book is not intended to be encyclopedic in nature but rather the expression of present-day information pertaining to various aspects of liver disease by a group of authors particularly qualified by their experience, interest, and scientific contributions. The reader may discover certain omissions, but he usually will find these to be matters of lesser importance. They will be more than compensated by the quality of the information contained, which deals with those aspects of hepatic disease that are much more apt to concern him, including the description of the principles of treatment, both medical and surgical, by experts in the field. Furthermore, he will frequently find it unnecessary to consult other books, particulary on points dealing with basic concepts.

To various contributors the editor expresses his deep gratitude for their excellent and willing cooperation. He has considered it good fortune indeed to have been associated with them in this undertaking. He wishes to express his thanks to Cecil J. Waston, Arthur J. Patek, Jr, and to his colleague, Edward A. Gall, for their helpful suggestions. He is particularly indebted to Miss Olive Mills, without whose tireless and able secretarial and editorial assistance he would not have been able to accomplish his task.

In some instances individual authors have appended acknowledgments of assistance to their respective chapters. To those concerned the editor wishes to express his apologies for not having included these expressions of gratitude for the sake of uniformity of composition and conservation of space.

Leon Schiff

Contents

50   The Liver and Its Effect on Endocrine Function in Health and Disease   1373

ELIZABETH J. SMANIK
HOPE BARKOUKIS
KEVIN D. MULLEN
ARTHUR J. McCULLOUGH

51   The Liver in Pregnancy   1411

CAROLINE A. RIELY

52   The Liver in Circulatory Failure   1431

SHEILA SHERLOCK

53   The Porphyrias   1438

JOSEPH R. BLOOMER
JAMES G. STRAKA
JEFFREY M. RANK

54   Amyloidosis of the Liver   1465

ALAN S. COHEN
MARTHA SKINNER

55   Trauma to the Liver, Gallbladder, and Bile Ducts   1480

PHILIP FELICIANO
DONALD TRUNKEY

Diseases of the Liver, Seventh Edition, edited by
Leon Schiff and Eugene R. Schiff. J.B. Lippincott Company, Philadelphia © 1993.

Fatty Liver: Biochemical and Clinical Aspects

David H. Alpers

Seymour M. Sabesin

Heather M. White

Clinical Presentation

Fatty liver results from the accumulation of lipid exceeding the normal 5% of liver weight (normal liver is composed of triglycerides, fatty acids, phospholipids, cholesterol, and cholesterol esters). When fat accumulates, the lipid is stored primarily as triglyceride but may also be phospholipid. The clinical importance of fatty liver is highly variable. For example, steatosis during prednisone therapy may have minimal consequences, but fatty liver of pregnancy may be life-threatening. The liver serves a pivotal biochemical role in lipoprotein metabolism and in neutral lipid clearance, especially free fatty acids, triglycerides, cholesterol, and cholesterol esters. Disease states or medications may alter these biochemical processes, resulting in clinical expression of fatty liver. The spectrum of disease includes steatosis, steatohepatitis, and cirrhosis.

SIGNS AND SYMPTOMS

Most patients with fatty liver have no symptoms, and fatty liver is usually suggested by abnormal laboratory tests or radiologic findings. Of the patients with symptoms, right upper quadrant fullness or discomfort is the most common complaint.[205,226] Individual causes of fatty liver, however, characteristic of the underlying disease may be associated with systemic symptoms. These signs and symptoms are covered separately under each disorder. Physical findings include palpable hepatomegaly in 90% of cases.[205]

LABORATORY FINDINGS

Laboratory abnormalities in fatty liver are typically mild. Elevated serum transaminase, γ-glutamyl transferase, alkaline phosphatase, and bilirubin are most common; these are helpful as screening parameters in identifying the presence of some liver disease but do not identify fatty liver as the cause. The degree of the biochemical abnormality does not correlate with the extent or severity of fatty liver.[2,68] The frequency of specific laboratory abnormalities are discussed with each clinical setting.

IMAGING STUDIES

Fatty infiltration may be detected by a number of imaging techniques that offer noninvasive methods for assessing hepatic lipid content and thus provide an explanation for hepatomegaly. Fatty infiltration may be focal or diffuse. In most disease states, the process is diffuse; however, focal fatty change has been reported in a variety of disorders. These lesions may be several centimeters in diameter[16] and may be mistaken for space-occupying lesions. In patients with focal fatty infiltration, diffuse fatty infiltration may or may not be present in the rest of the liver. Because of its lower density, intrahepatic lipid alters the density of the hepatic parenchyma analyzed by computed tomography (CT). The portal venous system then appears as higher-density linear structures within a background of lower-density parenchyma.[218] Ultrasound can also distinguish fatty infiltration by differences in echogenicity. The radiographic diagnosis can be made, however, with an 80% probability of being correct only when there is macrovesicular change in at least half of the liver cells within the imaged region. When fatty change affects less than 30% of cells, the infiltration is barely detectable.[226]

Hepatic steatosis can also be detected by the degree of hepatic xenon-133 retention as measured during pulmonary ventilation studies.[3] Furthermore, the degree of hepatic xenon retention correlates with the degree of steatosis found histologically. Magnetic resonance imaging has been performed using a modified spin-echo technique (simple proton spectroscopic imaging) that is designed to exploit the difference in the rate of procession between the protons in water and fatty acid molecules.[116] In the conventional spin-echo technique, the image intensity is the sum of the signal produced by water and fat protons. With proton spectroscopic imaging, the opposed image intensity is the difference between the water and fat signals. It seems likely that this method will be quantitatively useful in the near future. Additionally, the technique can distinguish hepatic metastases from focal fatty infiltration.[117]

When should imaging studies be obtained, and which one should be chosen? If a focal of diffuse lesion is noted by any modality and fatty liver can be strongly suggested, further imaging is not necessary if the presence of fatty liver is the answer that ends the diagnostic pursuit. If the imaging study identifies a lesion (focal or diffuse), but its nature is uncertain, and one would be satisfied with the finding of fatty liver, another imaging technique chosen to identify fat can be used. If, on the other hand, it is deemed that biopsy or angiography is necessary (eg, to exclude neoplasm or evaluate for concurrent pathology), further imaging is not helpful except to direct the biopsy needle.

DIFFERENTIAL DIAGNOSES

Numerous disease states are associated with fatty liver. Table 30-1 delineates these various states with the major subgroupings of alcoholic and nonalcoholic fatty liver disease as well as with a number of systemic diseases associated with fatty liver. Each entity is discussed separately later in this chapter. Although fatty infiltration may be suspected by noninvasive techniques, definitive diagnosis usually requires a liver biopsy. The decision to pursue biopsy when fatty liver is the expected result thus becomes part of a complex paradigm whenever the diagnosis is considered important and will modify physician behavior.

WHEN TO PERFORM BIOPSY

Deciding when to pursue a liver biopsy in fatty infiltration can be difficult. The clinical status of the patient is paramount in deciding the timing and necessity of liver biopsy. Incidental imaging detection of diffuse or focal fatty infiltration with normal enzymes probably does not warrant percutaneous biopsy. Because fatty infiltration frequently exists in the presence of concurrent hepatic pathology, in the setting of abnormalities in serum biochemistries, a biopsy may be warranted to determine the presence or absence of inflammation, fibrosis, and cirrhosis, particularly when medical management will be affected (eg, distinction from focal metastases, reversal of jejunoileal bypass, continuation of drug therapy such as amiodarone). Fatty infiltration may exist in the absence of concurrent hepatic pathology. In this setting (eg, during total parenteral nutrition or ketoacidosis in diabetes), biopsy is not needed unless warranted by lack of resolution of the hepatic abnormality.

Pathology

MACROSCOPIC

Macroscopically, the liver is usually large and may weigh up to 6000 g. The bulk of fat is triglyceride and may comprise up to one fourth of the liver wet weight. A notable exception is found in acute fatty liver of pregnancy (AFLP), where the liver is frequently small, weighing from 800 to 1200 g.[192] On cut section, the fatty liver is yellow as a result of the accumulation of carotenes and other lipochromes.

MICROSCOPIC

Microscopically, a variety of pathologic lesions can be seen, including lipid, Mallory's bodies, cellular inflammatory infiltrates, fibrosis, and cirrhosis. This chapter focuses on diseases that manifest hepatic lipid as a primary pathologic process. By the nature of differences among concurrent disorders, however, other diagnostic or associated processes may be seen histologically. When examining liver biopsy specimens by light microscopy, it is important to consider the

TABLE 30-1 *Differential Diagnosis of Conditions Associated With Fatty Liver*

Alcoholic Liver Disease
Alcoholic fatty liver
Alcoholic fatty liver with cholestasis
Alcoholic hepatitis
Alcoholic cirrhosis

Nonalcoholic Fatty Liver Disease
Protein-calorie malnutrition
    Starvation
    Jejunoileal bypass
    Gastric partitioning
Obesity
Diabetes mellitus
Acute fatty liver of pregnancy
Drugs
    Triglyceride accumulation
        Corticosteroids
        Methotrexate
        Tetracycline
        Valproic acid
        Salicylates
    Phospholipid accumulation
        Amiodarone
        Perhexiline maleate
Toxins
    Jamaican vomiting sickness
    Phosphorus
    Chlorinated hydrocarbons
Systemic diseases with fatty liver
    Primary liver disease
        Non-A, Non-B hepatitis
        Wilson's disease
    Inflammatory bowel disease
    Human immunodeficiency virus
    Hepatic resection
    Primary nonfunction of hepatic allografts
    Diseases of infancy and childhood
        Weber-Christian disease
        Reye's syndrome
        Galactosemia
        Fructose intolerance
        Abetalipoproteinemia
        Wolman's disease
        Cholesterol ester storage disease

architectural integrity of the hepatic lobule and portal triads, the presence and type of inflammatory infiltrate, the presence of fibrosis or cirrhosis, and the presence of hepatocyte inclusions, such as lipid. For disorders associated with fatty liver, the presence of steatosis is required, but the presence or absence of other lesions may help to make a more specific diagnosis in the appropriate clinical setting. This section is designed to describe the major pathologic findings in the spectrum of diseases associated with fatty liver.

Lipid

Hepatic lipid or steatosis is present primarily as small (microvesicular) or large (macrovesicular) droplets (Color Fig. 26). Although both patterns can coexist, the predominance of one form over the other suggests a differential diagnostic list (Table 30-2). The affected cells look foamy (microvesicular) or ballooned (macrovesicular) depending on the size and num-

TABLE 30-2 *Classification of Fatty Liver According to Microscopic Pattern of Lipid*

Cause	Macrovesicular	Microvesicular
Nutritional	Starvation Obesity Diabetes mellitus Jejunoileal bypass Gastroplasty Parenteral alimentation	
Metabolic	Wilson's disease Weber-Christian disease Galactosemia Hereditary fructose intolerance Abetalipoproteinemia	
Toxin induced	Alcohol Phosphorus Chlorinated hydrocarbons	Alcohol Jamaican vomiting sickness
Drug induced	Corticosteroids Methotrexate	Tetracycline Valproic acid Salicylates
Infectious	Acquired immunodeficiency syndrome	Viral hepatitis non-A, non-B
Unknown	Hepatic resection Primary allograft nonfunction	Acute fatty liver of pregnancy Reye's syndrome

ber of fat droplets. Microvesicular steatosis usually is associated with more serious illness than macrovesicular fat. Initially, the droplets are small and surrounded by membranes of the endoplasmic reticulum. As the droplets enlarge and merge, the membranes become difficult to see. When large droplets are present, the hepatocytes look like adipocytes with flattened peripheral nuclei. This pattern can often be seen in metabolic disorders or after administration of ethanol or steroids. Although alcoholic steatosis is characteristically centrilobular (zone 3 of Rappaport's acinus), the distribution of fat as pericentral or diffuse is not usually helpful in assigning an etiology. Small droplets with centrally placed nuclei are seen in some drug reactions (eg, tetracycline, valproic acid) or in AFLP. Reye's syndrome and Jamaican vomiting sickness demonstrate small droplets of fat in hepatocytes as well.

Foamy degeneration is an unusual pathologic finding described in alcoholic liver disease in patients with clinical features of alcoholic hepatitis. This entity was first described in an autopsy series in 1983[231] in 4% of subjects who had alcohol-associated hepatic failure. The lesion was characterized as occurring in the first episode of hepatic decompensation. The biopsy specimens showed swelling of the perivenular hepatocytes, with microvesicular steatosis producing a foamy appearance. Some macrovesicular steatosis was also present, and individual cells demonstrated both large and small fat globules.

In addition to fatty hepatocytes, there may be an accumulation of lipid- and lipofuscin-containing macrophages in fatty liver. These macrophages may be included in lipogranulomas along with lymphocytes and eosinophils.[30] When the severe fatty accumulation subsides, the lipid droplets in the macrophages diminish, and the lipogranulomas may be difficult to distinguish from other granulomas. Usually, how-

ever, the fat in these periportal granulomas persists long after the hepatocellular steatosis and may raise the suspicion of preceding steatosis.

Mallory's Hyalin

Mallory's hyalin (also called Mallory's bodies), sometimes referred to as alcoholic hyalin, is often seen in fatty liver. Mallory's hyalin is most commonly seen in alcoholic liver disease but is not specific for that condition, with or without fat. By light microscopy, the bodies are eosinophilic, coarsely granular, usually perinuclear, and always intracellular (Color Fig. 27). The loss of Mallory's bodies typically takes 6 to 12 weeks if the precipitating substance (eg, alcohol) is removed.[205] Mallory's bodies may be highly variable in size and number in various disease states but are more numerous in alcoholic liver disease than in other conditions.[48] They may be found in 49% to 100% of liver biopsy specimens from patients with nonalcoholic steatohepatitis.[48,98,118,131] Mallory's hyalin has been described in the livers of malnourished children in India,[214] jejunoileal bypass,[170] prolonged cholestatic jaundice, cirrhosis, hepatoma,[158] and Wilson's disease.

Cellular Infiltrate

Cellular inflammatory infiltrate accompanying steatosis may consist of neutrophils or lymphocytes. The presence of inflammatory infiltrate is required for the diagnosis of alcoholic hepatitis, alcoholic steatohepatitis, or nonalcoholic steatohepatitis. In alcoholic hepatitis, the predominant cellular infiltrates are neutrophils, typically present within sinusoids and around foci of liver cell necrosis,[133] usually in zone 3 (Color Fig. 28). Alcoholic and nonalcoholic steatohepatitis are characterized by the presence of fat and inflammatory infiltrate, which may be mixed neutrophils and lymphocytes (again predominantly in zone 3) but also present within the lobule in a patchy distribution. Portal tracts are relatively spared from inflammation except in advanced disease when central–portal bridges have formed.[133] In several series, no histologic cellular features clearly distinguished the patients with alcoholic or nonalcoholic steatohepatitis.[48,98,118,131]

Fibrosis and Cirrhosis

Important histologic consequences of alcoholic and nonalcoholic fatty liver disease are fibrosis and cirrhosis. The severity of fatty infiltration alone, in the absence of alcoholic hepatitis, on initial biopsy does not appear to influence the progression of fibrosis.[137] The fibrous tissue is first laid down in the pericellular distribution in zone 3, entrapping individual liver cells or groups of cells and producing a chicken-wire appearance on reticulin stains.[48,118,133] Eventually, the fibrosis increases, and the central-to-portal bridging that results leads to cirrhosis, usually of the micronodular type. Occasionally, a mixed micronodular or macronodular cirrhosis can occur, but cirrhosis of a predominantly macronodular pattern is uncommon.[133] Previously, nonalcoholic steatohepatitis was not believed to progress to cirrhosis, but several studies clearly document the presence of cirrhosis at initial biopsy,[48,98,118,131] and the progression to cirrhosis has been reported in patients followed up serially over 1 to 7 years.[118] The estimated incidence of cirrhosis in alcoholic liver disease is 10% to 20% and, in nonalcoholic liver disease, is 8%.[205] Using specific antibodies, increases in procollagen, type IV collagen, fibronectin, and laminin have been demonstrated in the space of Disse in alcoholic fatty liver and hepatitis.[133]

Other Histologic Lesions

Other histologic findings described in association with alcoholic liver disease with steatosis include hepatocellular carcinoma, hepatic siderosis, and coexistent liver diseases, such as hepatitis C. Hepatocellular carcinoma may develop in 5% to 15% of these patients, usually in association with cirrhosis; however, tumors may arise in alcoholics in the absence of cirrhosis.[133] Hepatic siderosis is typically mild in alcoholic liver disease, with iron deposition in hepatocytes and Kupffer's cells. A portion of the liver biopsy specimen should be reserved for determination of quantitative iron if massive siderosis is suspected on visual examination or found on histologic examination.[133] Hepatitis C antibody has been detected with increased frequency in alcoholics, and concurrent viral hepatitis should be considered in patients with predominantly portal involvement or portal-to-portal bridging fibrosis or cirrhosis.

Ultrastructural Aspects of Fatty Liver

Electron microscopic studies of human or experimental fatty liver reveal a monotonous engorgement of the cytoplasm with triglyceride droplets that are intensely stained with the osmium tetroxide used for fixation (Fig. 30-1). Because the triglycerides and apoproteins are synthesized in relation to the membranes of smooth and rough endoplasmic reticula, and since the secretory particle is transported within the channels formed by these tubular organelles, an accumulation of triglyceride, due either to an imbalance between synthesis and secretion or to inhibition of secretion, results in vesiculation of the endoplasmic reticulum (see Fig. 30-1). The vesiculation is caused by the gradual coalescence of triglyceride molecules into larger and larger lipid droplets. At higher magnification with the electron microscope, it is obvious that the retained triglyceride is surrounded by membranes of the smooth or the rough endoplasmic reticulum (Fig. 30-2).[194]

In certain clinical conditions, fat accumulation appears, by light microscopy, as small discrete microvesicular fat droplets (eg, tetracycline fatty liver, Reye's syndrome, AFLP) whereas other disorders (eg, alcoholic fatty liver) may be characterized by massive cytoplasmic fat droplets (macrovesicular fat droplets). With prolonged steatosis, there is progressive aggregation of triglyceride into large droplets. These droplets eventually assume enormous proportions and impinge on the barriers imposed by the endoplasmic reticulum membranes, resulting in the formation of massive lipid aggregates. Ultrastructural studies of several experimental models of fatty liver have provided some insight into the mechanism by which certain toxins or drugs may interfere with lipoprotein synthesis, intracellular transport, or secretion and thus produce fatty liver.[70] Therefore, experimental alcoholic fatty liver is characterized initially by excessive triglyceride synthesis, engorgement of the Golgi complexes with very-low-density lipoprotein (VLDL), and active secre-

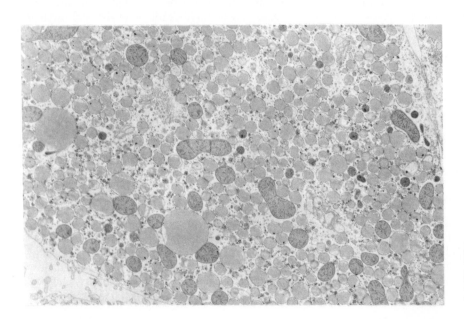

FIGURE 30-1 Electron micrograph of rat liver obtained 10 days after rat was fed a semisynthetic diet containing 1% orotic acid. The hepatocyte contains a massive accumulation of triglyceride droplets ($\times$ 5865).

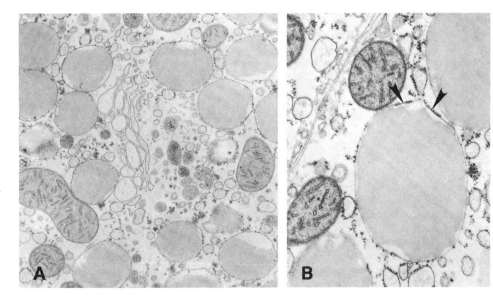

FIGURE 30-2 Higher magnification electron micrographs of orotic acid-induced fatty liver illustrating the vesiculation of the smooth endoplasmic reticulum (**A**) and the rough endoplasmic reticulum (**B**). In **B**, arrows point to ribosomes with retained triglyceride (**A**, × 10,780; **B**, × 16,800).

tion. In toxic states associated with inhibition of protein and presumably apoprotein synthesis (eg, tetracycline), there is extreme accumulation of triglyceride droplets in the vesiculated endoplasmic reticulum but no evidence of VLDL secretion.

Abnormalities in other steps in the pathway leading to VLDL secretion have also been described for other experimental models of fatty liver. Feeding 1% orotic acid, incorporated into a semisynthetic diet, produces a profound accumulation of triglycerides in rat liver, associated with a specific defect in VLDL secretion.[191,243] Because orotic acid does not interfere specifically with protein or lipoprotein synthesis, it has been suggested that it may prevent the assembly or secretion of lipoproteins by the liver.[243] Apparently, the hepatic synthesis of the apoproteins involved in VLDL formation is not prevented after orotic acid feeding; however, there is a marked decrease in plasma triglyceride, cholesterol, and low-density lipoprotein (LDL) concentration. The isolated, perfused rat liver, obtained from animals treated with orotic acid, cannot release lipoproteins containing Apo B (VLDL, LDL) but can secrete high-density lipoprotein (HDL), albumin, and other plasma proteins.[191]

Mechanisms for Production of Fatty Liver

The liver subserves many important functions in plasma lipoprotein metabolism, including the biosynthesis of VLDL.[99] VLDL formation is related directly to the availability of free fatty acids. Free fatty acids bound to albumin or chylomicron remnants are transported to the liver and then taken up by hepatocytes, where they are used for triglyceride synthesis. Next, the triglycerides are combined with specific proteins (apoproteins), forming lipoprotein particles that are secreted into the circulation. There they undergo extensive alterations in composition during their metabolism.

The availability of free fatty acids for hepatic triglyceride synthesis is dependent on many factors, including nutritional status (ie, type and quantity of diet), hormonal influences (ie, insulin availability and pituitary and adrenocortical hor-

mones), and exogenous factors, such as alcohol. Within the hepatocyte, the availability of free fatty acids for triglyceride synthesis is also dependent on the status of complex regulatory mechanisms, such as mitochondrial fatty acid oxidation, ketone body formation, endogenous fatty acid synthesis, and availability of precursors for glycerol synthesis. VLDL synthesis and secretion are also regulated precisely by the availability of Apo B; the assembly of Apo B with triglyceride, phospholipid, and cholesterol; the glycosylation of the apoproteins; and the transport of the nascent (newly formed) VLDL particles sequentially through several subcellular compartments, culminating in secretory vesicle formation and exocytosis of nascent VLDL into the perisinusoidal space of Disse.[199]

It is apparent that derangements in one or more of the metabolic regulatory steps leading to hepatic triglyceride synthesis, alterations in nutritional or hormonal status, and toxic influences on hepatocyte function could lead to imbalances in the biosynthesis, assembly, intracellular transport, or secretion of VLDL. Put another way, the constant cycling of fatty acids between liver and adipose tissue is easily distorted and in the direction of hepatic deposition. There are limits to the rate of oxidation but not of esterification, and there is relatively limited triglyceride secreted as VLDL. The net result of such derangements leads to an excessive accumulation of triglyceride within hepatocytes.

Ultrastructural analysis of the alterations in rat hepatic subcellular organelles after orotic acid feeding strongly suggests that orotic acid induces a VLDL secretory block within the Golgi apparatus.[194] This interpretation is based on the distention of Golgi cisternae and vesicles with lipid droplets at various phases during the development of fatty liver. The presence of VLDL-size droplets within elements of the Golgi apparatus is accompanied by a progressive distention of the endoplasmic reticulum, owing to the presence of triglyceride droplets that presumably cannot be transported into the already lipid-filled Golgi stacks. The retention of triglycerides within endoplasmic reticulum cisternae causes vesiculation of the cisternae as the small droplets aggregate into increasingly large triglyceride-rich droplets.

These ultrastructural observations of the orotic acid–induced fatty liver suggest that the primary defect in lipoprotein transport may be related to interference with normal Golgi function. In the early phases of orotic acid–induced fatty liver, the Golgi cisternae are distended with lipid, secretory vesicles do not form, and there is no evidence of VLDL exocytosis.[194] After 10 or more days of orotic acid feeding, the Golgi complexes appear flattened and somewhat devoid of lipoprotein particles, suggesting secondary effects that prevent entrance of nascent VLDL into the Golgi apparatus.[159]

Ultrastructural studies of the effects of colchicine and other microtubular inhibitory agents on VLDL secretion indicate a role for microtubules in the secretory process.[219a] The administration of colchicine is associated with a marked defect in VLDL secretion, disappearance of hepatocyte microtubules, diminished secretory vesicle formation, and vesiculation of the endoplasmic reticulum, as a result of triglyceride retention. Although colchicine has many effects on the cell, its inhibition of microtubule formation may be of major importance in the pathogenesis of fatty liver caused by this drug. In this regard, microtubules may subserve an essential function in guiding the movement of secretory vesicles that contain nascent VLDL to the plasma membrane for exocytosis (Fig. 30-3, step 8).

Although many chemicals, pharmacologic agents, and hormonal imbalances may cause fatty liver, usually the accumulation of fat is only one facet of a broader metabolic derangement, which often includes significant hepatocellular necrosis. In fact, the severity of the clinical manifestations resulting from deranged hepatic function is dependent more on the extent of hepatocellular injury than on the presence of fat. Even when excessive, necrosis and fatty infiltration are separate processes with differing pathogenesis and the ability to develop and resolve independently. Thus, fatty liver can occur before necrosis and then resolve while hepatocellular necrosis persists.

In this chapter, the description of the pathogeneses of fatty liver is based on knowledge of peripheral and hepatic fatty acid metabolism and hepatic lipoprotein synthesis, secretion, and metabolism. Because hepatic lipoprotein formation is so important for triglyceride secretion (and animal studies indicate a critical role for deranged lipoprotein metabolism in many types of drug- or toxin-induced fatty liver), composi-

tion and metabolism of plasma lipoproteins and subcellular aspects of lipoprotein synthesis and secretion are emphasized.

LIPID SOURCES

Fatty Acid Metabolism

In fatty liver, the major lipid fractions that increase in amount are the fatty acids and triglycerides. Phospholipids, cholesterol, and cholesterol esters usually increase to a limited extent. It is important to consider the physiology of fatty acid and triglyceride metabolism within the hepatocyte since the pathogenesis of fatty liver is intimately related to derangements in the regulation of these metabolic processes. Figure 30-4 is a schema of hepatic fatty acid and triglyceride metabolism emphasizing the sources of hepatic fatty acids and their fate in the liver.

The triglyceride-rich lipoproteins of exogenous (dietary) origin, chylomicrons, are metabolized in the capillary bed of tissues throughout the body where lipoprotein lipase (LPL) is located on vascular endothelial surfaces. The fatty acids formed during chylomicron triglyceride lipolysis can be used directly as a source of energy (ie, muscle), can be taken up by adipocytes where they are esterified again to triglycerides and stored, or can be transported to the liver where they enter various biochemical pathways. The stored triglyceride in adipose tissue is an important potential source of energy that can be mobilized at time of need by once again undergoing hydrolysis, releasing fatty acids into the blood. The control of triglyceride lipolysis in adipose tissue is under exquisite hormonal regulation and provides a prime source of fatty acid influx into the liver under various changes in nutritional and hormonal status.[187] Thus, fatty acids entering the liver, in the fasting state, are derived from the hydrolysis of adipose tissue triglyceride. In the postprandial state, the fatty acids are derived mostly from the hydrolysis of dietary triglycerides, either from peripheral degradation of chylomicron triglyceride by LPL or by the direct uptake of chylomicron remnants with subsequent hydrolysis by hepatic triglyceride lipase. Within the hepatocyte, the fatty acids then may be oxidized and used for energy, converted to phospholipids, used for the formation of cholesterol esters, or used for triglyceride syn-

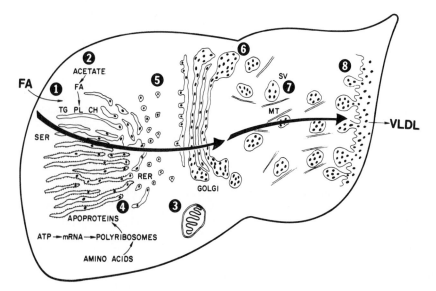

FIGURE 30-3 Postulated mechanisms by which alterations in triglyceride synthesis and derangements in VLDL assembly, intracellular transport, and secretion can lead to fatty liver. The numbers refer to possible sites of such abnormalities.

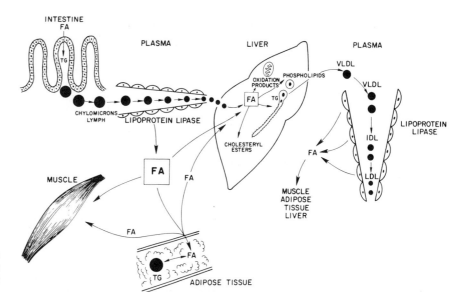

FIGURE 30-4 Sources and metabolism of plasma fatty acids (FA) emphasizing the role of the liver in FA uptake and triglyceride synthesis and secretion.

thesis. The release of triglyceride as newly synthesized VLDL provides another source of fatty acids that can be oxidized in muscle, stored as triglyceride in adipose tissue, or returned once again to the liver (see Fig. 30-4).

Plasma Lipoproteins

The lipoproteins isolated from fasting plasma are the end products of the metabolism of lipoproteins secreted by the liver and intestine.[14,39,70,99,134,198] The most commonly used separation procedure involves the sequential ultracentrifugation of plasma at increasing solution densities and isolation of each fraction within a predetermined density range (Table 30-3).

Composition. The main function of lipoproteins is the transport of lipids in the plasma. Except for the intestinal synthesis of chylomicrons after a fatty meal, the liver is the major source of plasma lipoproteins. Electrophoresis has been used for the separation and identification of lipoproteins in whole plasma, leading to a nomenclature used widely in clinical applications. Chylomicrons do not move electrophoretically, whereas LDL migrates with β-globulins, VLDL migrates with pre–β-globulins, and HDL migrates with α_1-globulins. Each of these lipoprotein classes has a characteristic lipid and apoprotein composition (see Table 30-3).

The apoproteins subserve several critical functions in lipoprotein metabolism[204] (Table 30-4). Structurally, they comprise the surface layer of the spherical lipoprotein parti-

TABLE 30-3 *Properties of Plasma Lipoproteins*

	Chylomicrons	*VLDL*	*LDL*	*HDL*
Source	Intestine	Liver	Plasma	Intestine, liver
Diameter (Å)	800–5000	280–800	200–250	50–150
Density (g/mL)	<0.95	<1.006	<1.063	<1.21
Electrophoretic mobility	Origin	Pre-β	β	
Lipid content	≈98%	≈90%	≈75%	≈50%
Lipid classes (% of total lipid)	≈90% TG ≈ 8% PL ≈ 5% CH	≈60% TG ≈20% PL ≈17% CH	≈60% CH ≈30% PL ≈10% TG	≈50% PL ≈32% CH ≈10% TG
Protein content	0.5%–2.5%	10%–13%	20%–25%	45%–55%
Major apoproteins	B-48, C-I, C-II, C-III	B-100, C-III, E	B-100	A-I, A-II
Minor apoproteins	A-I, A-II, A-IV, E	A-I, A-II, C-I, C-II	C-I, C-II, C-III, E	C, E
Function	Exogenous TG transport*	Exogenous TG transport	CH transport to peripheral cells; regulation of cholesterol biosynthesis	LCAT substrate; CH transport from peripheral cells to liver

TG, triglycerides; PL, phospholipids; CH, cholesterol.
*Chylomicron remnants are formed in the plasma compartment. They contain mostly cholesterol esters and Apo B-48 and E.

TABLE 30-4   *Source and Function of Plasma Apoproteins*

Apoprotein	Source	Lipoprotein	Function*
A-I	Intestine, liver	CM, HDL	LCAT activator
A-II	Intestine, liver	CM, HDL	Hepatic lipase activator
A-IV	Intestine	CM, HDL	Unknown
B-48	Intestine	CM	Secretion of VLDL receptor; ligand for LDL
B-100	Liver	VLDL, IDL, LDL	Secretion of CM
C-I	Liver	CM, VLDL, IDL, HDL	LCAT activator
C-II	Liver	CM, VLDL, IDL, HDL	LPL activator
C-III	Liver	CM, VLDL, IDL, HDL	TG-rich lipoprotein removal
E-2-3-4	Liver, peripheral tissues	CM, VLDL, IDL, HDL	Ligand for LDL receptor; ? CM remnant receptor

CM, chylomicrons; LPL, lipoprotein lipase; LCAT, lecithin:cholesterol acyltransferase; IDL, intermediate-density lipoprotein; TG, triglycerides.
*In addition to the physiologic functions listed, the apoproteins are integral structural components of the lipoprotein molecule and are essential for stabilizing the surface coat of the lipoprotein particle.

cles, allowing the hydrophobic lipids (triglycerides, cholesterol esters) to occupy the core.[115] This spatial arrangement permits the transport of lipids in the aqueous environment of the blood. Specific apoproteins are also critical for various aspects of lipoprotein metabolism, functioning as cofactors for enzymes involved in triglyceride hydrolysis (Apo C-II) and in cholesterol esterification (Apo A-I) and functioning as ligands for receptor-mediated uptake of lipoproteins by various tissues (Apo B, Apo E; see Table 30-4).

The isolated lipoproteins have a characteristic particle diameter. A rather broad range exists within each density class, however, reflecting, in part, different stages of catabolism at the time of their isolation (see Table 30-3). The particles can be visualized directly by negative staining techniques. By electron microscopy, the lipoproteins in each density class appear as dense spherical particles without any obvious substructure (Fig. 30-5). Although lipoprotein classes can be segregated because of their average composition or physical properties, the particles within a class are somewhat heterogeneous, reflecting the state of metabolic transformations occurring in the circulation.

In addition to classification based on criteria of density or electrophoretic mobility, it is useful to classify lipoproteins on the basis of their probable function. Three major functions are believed to be provided by plasma lipoproteins:

- Transport of a prime energy source, triglyceride, from biosynthetic sites in the intestine and liver to peripheral cells (chylomicrons and VLDL)
- Transport of cholesterol required for cell membrane and steroid hormone synthesis from the liver to peripheral cells (LDL)
- Transport of excess tissue cholesterol from peripheral cells to the liver for disposition into the bile or reutilization (HDL)

Sources. Chylomicrons synthesized by the small intestinal absorptive cells, in response to the absorption of dietary lipid, are large triglyceride-rich particles that are secreted directly into the lymph.[14,197] The newly secreted (nascent) chylomicrons undergo rapid metabolic transformations and are cleared from the circulation within a few minutes (Fig. 30-6). Thus, chylomicrons are not detected normally in fasting plasma. When first secreted into lymph, the chylomicrons contain a low-molecular-weight form of Apo B—Apo B-48[178]—as well as other Apo A-1, A peptides. Subsequently, chylomicrons acquire Apo E and Apo C proteins by transfer from HDL. The A, C, and E apoproteins subserve important

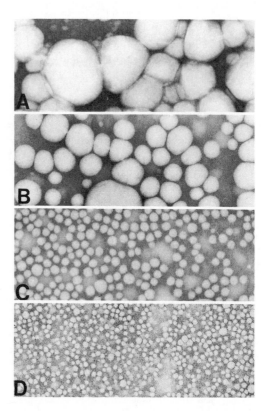

FIGURE 30-5 Electron microscopic appearance of human plasma lipoproteins isolated by ultracentrifugation. **(A)** Chylomicrons, **(B)** VLDL, **(C)** LDL, **(D)** HDL (**A,** × 72,000; **B** to **D,** × 95,000).

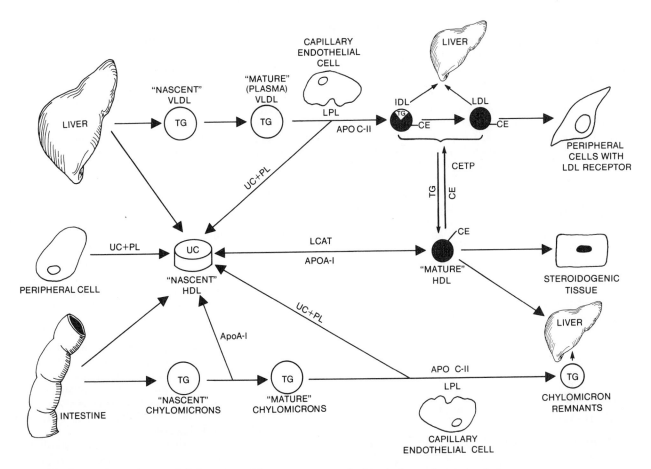

FIGURE 30-6 Somewhat simplified versions of the major steps involved in the biosynthesis, metabolic conversions, and catabolism of chylomicrons, VLDL, LDL, and HDL. These schemas emphasize the transfer of apoproteins and lipids between lipoprotein particles and the activity of lipoprotein lipase and lecithin:cholesterol acyltransferase (LCAT). *Chylomicron metabolism.* Chylomicrons are synthesized in the intestine after a fatty meal. They undergo rapid metabolic transformations in the lymph and plasma, resulting in the formation of chylomicron remnants, which are removed by the liver by a receptor-mediated process. *VLDL metabolism.* The VLDL are synthesized by the liver, acquire certain apoproteins and cholesterol ester (CE) by transfer from HDL, and are converted to remnants by LPL. The VLDL either are taken up directly by the liver or are converted, in the plasma, to LDL. *VLDL remnant metabolism.* Those VLDL remnants not taken up directly by the liver are further metabolized by H-TGL to LDL. The lipolytic activity of H-TGL removes residual TG, and with loss of apo-C and apo-E, the VLDL remnant is converted into an LDL particle containing only CE and apo B-100. *LDL metabolism.* LDL are taken up by the liver or by peripheral cells. In the liver, 25% of the LDL are removed by non–receptor-mediated pathways; and in peripheral cells, about one third of LDL is removed by non–receptor-mediated pathways. *HDL metabolism.* HDL are synthesized as nascent discoidal particles by the liver and intestine. The nascent particle is acted on by LCAT, converting the discoidal to spherical particles as CE are formed. The CE in HDL can be transferred by CE transfer protein to the VLDL → IDL → LDL pathway. HDL can be removed directly by the liver or its CE used by various tissues for biosynthetic processes (eg, cell membrane formation, steroid hormone synthesis).

functions in lipoprotein metabolism, but the availability of Apo B is essential for the secretion of chylomicrons from the intestinal absorptive cells and of VLDL from hepatocytes. Apo B deficiency due perhaps to enhanced degradation (abetalipoproteinemia)[70a] or to decreased synthesis because of drug or toxic inhibition (tetracycline, carbon tetrachloride) is associated with severe impairment of chylomicron and VLDL secretion and thus intracellular triglyceride accumulation. There is evidence that the liver and intestine synthesize separate B apoproteins, which differ in molecular weight; however, their physiologic functions appear to be similar (see Table 30-4).

In the absence of dietary lipid, the intestinal absorptive cells also synthesize some VLDL-size particles. Studies in the rat indicate the intestinal production of lipoprotein particles with the characteristics of nascent HDL.[14,76] In support of the production of nascent HDL by the intestine is the observation that most of the intestinal Apo A-I is not associated with the HDL particle until it reaches the lamina propria, after the secretion from the enterocyte.[5] Most of the endogenously formed triglycerides in plasma are present in the VLDL, synthesized primarily in the liver. Studies using liver perfusion indicate that nascent VLDL is different in composition from circulating plasma VLDL. The apoprotein content of circulating VLDL includes Apo C, peptides Apo B (Apo B-100), and Apo E, whereas nascent VLDL consists almost entirely of Apo B.[204] Thus, it appears that most of the Apo C and most of the Apo E are acquired by transfer from HDL after the nascent VLDL is secreted from the hepatocyte.

The major lipoprotein of human plasma, LDL, is not synthesized by the liver but is formed in plasma as a product of VLDL catabolism[39] (see Fig. 30-6). The principal lipid component of LDL is esterified cholesterol, and it contains only Apo B. The other lipoprotein synthesized and secreted by the liver is nascent HDL, which is strikingly different in structure and composition from the HDL found in fasting plasma (see Fig. 30-6). Evidence for the synthesis of nascent HDL is the isolation, from rat liver perfusates,[83] of a discoidal particle enriched in Apo E, phospholipid, and unesterified cholesterol. Further evidence supporting the hepatic formation of nascent HDL is the accumulation of a similar discoidal particle in patients with severe alcoholic hepatitis,[182,202,240] in whom cholesterol esters are greatly decreased in plasma because of deficiency of the cholesterol-esterifying enzyme lecithin cholesterol acyltransferase (LCAT).[181] In these patients, the HDL fractions contain considerable Apo E and relatively little Apo A-I, which is normally the major apoprotein (85%) of circulating HDL.

LIPID METABOLISM

Fatty Acids

Adipose Tissue. Both exogenous and endogenous sources contribute free fatty acids for triglyceride synthesis by the liver; however, the relative contribution from each source varies under different physiologic and hormonal conditions. In the fasting state, most free fatty acids used in hepatic triglyceride production are derived from peripheral adipose tissue.[70] These free fatty acids are the products of triglyceride hydrolysis within adipose tissue cells. This reaction, under the influence of a hormone-sensitive lipase, results in the liberation of free fatty acids and glycerol in the adipose cells. The uptake or release of free fatty acids by adipose tissue is regulated by neural and hormonal stimuli. This process is enhanced by the rich vascular supply of adipose tissue and its direct contiguity with autonomic nerve endings.

In the fed state, when caloric intake exceeds the immediate metabolic needs of the animal, chylomicrons supply free fatty acids to the liver. The amount of free fatty acids extracted by the liver is proportional to the free fatty acid concentration in portal venous blood. An increase in exogenous triglyceride intake increases the quantity of fatty acids available for immediate energy needs and for uptake by the liver or adipocytes.

Free fatty acids entering the adipose tissue cells can be used directly for triglyceride synthesis, provided that glucose is available for glycerol formation. Glucose is essential in many respects for fat formation in adipose tissue. Glucose forms α-glycerol phosphate and thus regulates the use of free fatty acids for triglyceride synthesis. Free fatty acids may also be synthesized directly from glucose using acetyl coenzyme A (CoA) as an intermediate. Via the pentose phosphate shunt, glucose generates NADPH, which enhances fatty acid synthesis. Thus, despite an adequate supply of free fatty acids, fat synthesis in adipose tissue does not occur unless glucose is available. This has implications both for the disposition of free fatty acids arriving from peripheral triglyceride lipolysis as well as of those resulting from adipocyte lipolysis by hormone-sensitive lipase.

Insulin is crucial in the regulation of adipose tissue triglyceride synthesis by promoting glucose entry into adipocytes and by inhibiting cyclic adenosine monophosphate (cAMP) formation, which regulates the activity of the hormone-sensitive lipase. Thus, the insulin response to alterations in blood glucose concentration determines whether fat synthesis and storage occur or whether triglyceride lipolysis is dominant in adipose tissue. Insulin deficiency, by promoting lipolysis, is an important cause of fatty liver in patients with poorly controlled diabetes mellitus. In that situation, massive lipolysis results in an enormous mobilization of free fatty acids, which are taken up by the liver and used, in part, for triglyceride synthesis.

Mobilization. Mobilization of fatty acids from adipose tissue is subject to numerous regulatory mechanisms that determine the rate at which free fatty acids enter the blood.[187] The hormone-sensitive lipase is responsive to hormonal, nutritional, chemical, or nervous factors, thereby providing a means of increasing the plasma free fatty acid concentration to satisfy energy requirements in various tissues (Table 30-5). Epinephrine, norepinephrine, adrenocorticotropic hormone, thyroid-stimulating hormone, adrenocortical steroids, thyroxine, and glucagon all stimulate activation of cAMP. Because cAMP activates hormone-sensitive lipase, the hormonal activation of cAMP provides a mechanism promoting triglyceride lipolysis.

Hormonal factors that increase lipid mobilization may act on adipose tissue by stimulation of the lipolytic process (catecholamines and glucagon). Thyroid hormones appear to sensitize adipose tissue to the stimulatory action of catecholamines on lipolysis. Adrenocortical hormones potentiate the lipolytic action of catecholamines by inhibiting carbohydrate metabolism in adipose tissue.

Low glucose availability is thought to increase lipid mobilization indirectly as the body seeks alternative means of energy. Additionally, fasting hypoglycemia is characterized by low insulin levels. Thus, the inhibition of adipose tissue lipolysis exerted by insulin is removed, and an increase in free fatty acid mobilization occurs. Conversely, in states of high glucose availability and increased insulin levels, inhibition of adipose tissue lipolysis occurs, and free fatty acid mobilization is decreased.

The mode of action of the sympathetic nervous system in lipid mobilization relates to release of catecholamines (epinephrine), which stimulate adipose tissue lipolysis, regulate hepatic glycolysis, impair peripheral glucose uptake, and suppress insulin release. Cordotomy or administration of sympathetic or adrenergic-blocking agents would, by direct interference with catecholamines, be expected to reduce peripheral fat mobilization. Prostaglandins have an inhibitory effect on catecholamine-stimulated lipid mobilization in animals. Certain nucleotides also exert a similar inhibitory effect. Whether these effects are important in physiologic situations is unknown.

Other chemicals, notably adenosine triphosphate (ATP), appear to decrease the fat accumulation produced by agents such as ethionine, carbon tetrachloride, and ethanol[96] (see Table 30-5). Administration of ATP leads to a decrease in circulating free fatty acids, which appears to be secondary to the relative hypothermia that follows ATP injections.

TABLE 30-5   *Factors Affecting Mobilization of Fatty Acids From Adipose Tissue*

Factor	Increased Mobilization	Decreased Mobilization
Nutritional	Low glucose availability	High glucose availability
Hormonal	Adrenocorticotropic hormone	Insulin
	Thyroid-stimulating hormone	
	Growth hormone	
	Corticosteroids	
	Thyroid hormone	
	Glucagon	
Nervous	Sympathetic stimulation	Cordotomy
		Sympathetic blocking agents
		Hypophysectomy
		Adrenalectomy
Chemical	Epinephrine	Prostaglandins
	Norepinephrine	Nucleotides
		Nicotinic acid
		Salicylates
		Tranquilizers
		Adenosine triphosphate
		Chlorphenoxyisobutyrate (Atromid)

Numerous other chemicals, including salicylates, propranolol,[65] and tranquilizers, decrease fatty acid mobilization.[25] Whether these drugs can improve liver histology in humans by reducing fatty infiltration is not known.

Uptake and Use.   Fatty acids liberated from adipose tissue are carried in the bloodstream bound to albumin (see Fig. 30-4). About one third of the circulating fatty acids are removed by the liver, one third by skeletal muscle, and the rest by other tissues, especially myocardium.[180,210] Hepatic triglyceride formation or accumulation is greatly affected by the rate at which fatty acids are presented to the liver. Fatty acids released from adipose tissue have a short half-life in the plasma, about 2 minutes. Normal levels of plasma free fatty acids are less than 500 mEq/L, and the liver can extract 30% of circulating free fatty acids in a single cycle.

After uptake of exogenously or endogenously derived fatty acids, hepatic triglyceride esterification occurs rapidly. The rate of esterification may be measured by the administration of radiolabeled fatty acids into the blood and measurement of labeled fatty acids in hepatic tissue. Within 2 minutes after the injection of radiolabeled fatty acids, most fatty acids recovered from the liver are in esterified form. Electron microscopy reveals lipid droplets within rough and smooth endoplasmic reticulum soon after injection of fatty acids, and radiolabeled fatty acids may be found in the endoplasmic reticulum.

The esterification process is closely linked to hepatic oxidative phosphorylation and is dependent on a ready supply of α-glycerophosphate, the precursor of glycerol, supplied almost exclusively from glucose, and the availability of fatty acyl CoA. As with adipose tissue, glucose and insulin are extremely important in the regulation of hepatic fat formation, but the liver is considerably more active than adipose tissue in triglyceride synthesis. The liver is the major site of glucose removal. This is controlled in part by insulin; but, in addition, a major effect of insulin is the inhibition of hepatic glucose release. Insulin also determines the fate of glucose in

the hepatocyte by regulating the activity of glucokinase essential for glucose phosphorylation, by increasing fatty acid synthesis from glucose, and by promoting hepatic triglyceride secretion.[156]

In addition to triglyceride synthesis, other fates exist for fatty acids in the hepatocyte.[10] In the fasting state, or when metabolic demands are great, fatty acids are oxidized to acetoacetate and other ketone bodies, which then may be used for energy. Fatty acid oxidation is important in removing excess lipid from the liver so that accumulation within the organ does not occur ordinarily. Finally, fatty acids may be incorporated into phospholipids and other lipids within the hepatocyte. They are thus stored in the formed membrane lipids or in the exchangeable phospholipid pools.

The rate of hepatic triglyceride synthesis is usually regulated by about equal hepatic secretion of triglyceride, but acute stresses of the system, such as mobilization of fatty acid from adipose tissue or a rapid and prolonged increase in dietary chylomicron triglyceride, can result in increased hepatic triglyceride synthesis. Hepatic triglyceride formation or accumulation is greatly affected by the rate at which fatty acids are presented to the liver,[217] but undoubtedly, other factors affect this also.[220]

The liver may respond to an increased fatty acid influx by increasing the rate of lipoprotein and ketone body synthesis, but there is a limit to the extent to which the activity of these pathways may increase. When the rate at which fatty acids are brought to the liver exceeds the ability of the liver to metabolize or resecrete the fatty acids into the circulation as lipoproteins, storage of fat within the hepatocyte ensues. Although fatty acids are incorporated into phospholipids and cholesterol esters, when a fatty liver is produced, the predominant lipid that accumulates is triglyceride.

Lipoproteins

Biosynthesis and Secretion by the Liver.   Studies using in vitro techniques, or isolated hepatic perfusion, have shown that the liver is the major site of VLDL synthesis.[39,70]

The sequential steps involved in hepatic VLDL formation and intracellular transport and secretion, emphasizing the translocation of nascent particles through subcellular compartments, is shown schematically in Figure 30-7, whereas actual electron micrographs are illustrated in Figure 30-8. After uptake by the hepatocyte, fatty acids are reesterified to triglycerides, used for cholesterol or phospholipid synthesis, or oxidized. Acetate may also serve as a fatty acid precursor. Specific genes code for each individual apoprotein.[28,72,204,245] After formation on the polyribosomes of the rough endoplasmic reticulum, the nascent apoproteins are translocated into the cisternae of the rough endoplasmic reticulum, where they commence a vectorial transport through the endoplasmic reticulum channels toward their assembly with the lipid moieties.[32]

The enzymes involved in triglyceride, cholesterol, and phospholipid synthesis are located in the smooth endoplasmic reticulum, and presumably, the newly formed lipids are then directed into the cisternae of the smooth endoplasmic reticulum. Assembly of the lipid and the apoprotein moieties probably occurs at the junction of the smooth and rough endoplasmic reticula (see Fig. 30-8A), with the final assembly, concentration, and glycosylation of lipoproteins occurring within the Golgi apparatus.

The exact structural relation between the transport of nascent proteins from the endoplasmic reticulum and the Golgi apparatus components is not known. One concept suggests continuous connections between endoplasmic reticulum and the Golgi components, with passage of nascent particles directly into the Golgi cisternae. Alternatively, it has been suggested that nascent proteins may be transported in so-called shuttling vesicles derived from transitional elements of the smooth-surfaced extensions of the endoplasmic reticulum[93] (see Fig. 30-8B). After final assembly of nascent VLDL in the Golgi apparatus (see Fig. 30-8C), smooth-surfaced secretory vesicles derived from the Golgi apparatus and containing nascent VLDL migrate through the cytoplasm, where they merge with the lateral plasmalemma of the hepatocyte (see Fig. 30-8D) and secrete the VLDL into the space of Disse by exocytosis (see Fig. 30-8E). Biochemical evidence for this sequence of assembly and transport to the Golgi complex re-

sides in subcellular fractionation studies in which Golgi vesicles have been isolated and their contents purified, demonstrating lipoprotein particles strikingly similar to VLDL in size and composition.[94]

Metabolism.   Lipoproteins should be thought of as dynamic particles that are constantly in a state of synthesis, degradation, and removal from the plasma compartment, rather than as static transport vehicles whose lipid and apoprotein composition is uniform and unvarying.[20,39,70,71,99,134] During the process of lipoprotein catabolism, the nascent (secretory) particles of intestinal or hepatic origin undergo triglyceride hydrolysis, acquire new apoproteins (which subserve physiologic functions), lose apoproteins of endogenous origin, and thus alter drastically in size and composition. The end products of these complex transformations also perform important functions. For example, LDL is a major source of cholesterol for peripheral cells, transports cholesterol to the liver and other tissues for excretion (in bile), degradation, or reutilization and regulates plasma cholesterol levels by influencing the formation of hepatic LDL receptors.

CHYLOMICRON METABOLISM.   Chylomicrons (see Fig. 30-6) are synthesized by the intestinal mucosal absorptive cells in response to the uptake of the lipolytic products of dietary fat absorption. When formed in the enterocyte, the nascent chylomicron particle contains mostly triglycerides and a small amount of cholesterol esters. Nascent chylomicrons contain Apo B-48, required for their intracellular assembly, transport, and secretion and Apo A-I, -II, and -IV. After secretion into the lymph and entry into the plasma compartment, the chylomicrons become enriched rapidly with Apo C and Apo E. The acquisition of Apo C-II is critical for chylomicron catabolism since Apo C-II activates LPL, which hydrolyzes chylomicron triglycerides. The chylomicron particles encounter LPL at the surface of vascular endothelial cells, and the result of the hydrolytic process is the release of free fatty acids and Apo A and C peptides. Repetitive cycles of lipolysis reduce the chylomicron particle to a much smaller residual particle, the chylomicron remnant. The cessation of chylomicron triglyceride hydrolysis may be related to the loss of Apo C-II.

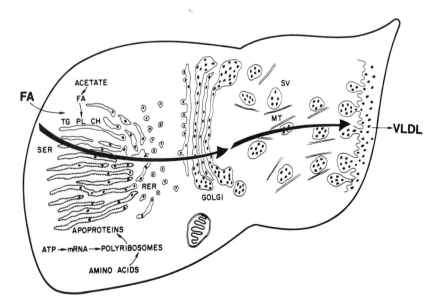

FIGURE 30-7   Steps in the hepatic synthesis, intracellular transport, and secretion of VLDL. SER, smooth endoplasmic reticulum; RER, rough endoplasmic reticulum; SV, secretory vesicle; MT, microtubule.

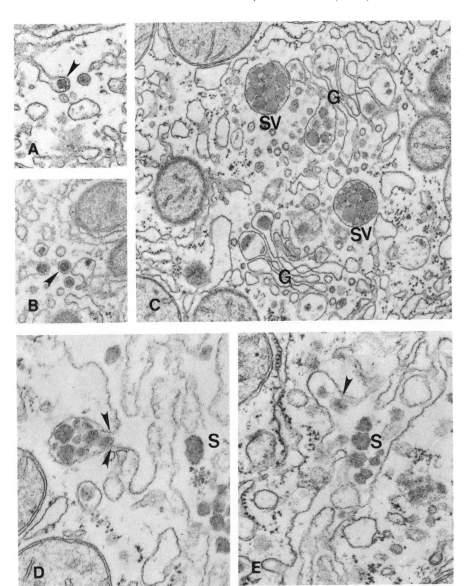

FIGURE 30-8 Electron micrographs illustrating various aspects of the assembly, intracellular transport, and secretion of VLDL by rat liver. (**A**) Formation of nascent VLDL in the endoplasmic reticulum (*arrow*). (**B**) Vesicular transport of nascent VLDL (*arrow*) from the endoplasmic reticulum to the Golgi complex. (**C**) VLDL in Golgi cisternae (G) and in secretory vesicles (SV). (**D**) Exocytosis of VLDL. The arrows point to areas of fusion of a secretory vesicle, containing VLDL, with the hepatocyte sinusoidal membrane. Note the presence of VLDL in the perisinusoidal space of Disse (S). (**E**) Secretion of VLDL (*arrow*) into the space of Disse (S) (**A**, × 44,000; **B**, × 40,800; **C**, × 30,000; **D**, × 50,490; **E**, × 50,400).

The chylomicron remnants, depleted of triglycerides and enriched in cholesterol esters, are removed by the liver as intact particles by a receptor-mediated process.[39,40] The cholesterol contained in chylomicron remnants regulates (decreases) the activity of 3-hydroxy-3-methylglutaryl-CoA (HMG-CoA) reductase, the rate-limiting enzyme of cholesterol synthesis.[134] Only a small amount of chylomicron Apo B appears to become LDL Apo B[56]; therefore, it appears that most of chylomicron remnants are removed by the liver, whereas some of the end products of VLDL metabolism circulate longer as LDL.

The mechanism by which chylomicron remnants are removed by the liver and their remaining triglyceride hydrolyzed is unclear. A lipolytic enzyme, hepatic triglyceride lipase (H-TGL), which has activity against monoglycerides, diglycerides, and triglycerides, has been postulated to have a role in both processes.[39,110] It has been suggested that H-TGL resides on hepatocytes near a lipoprotein remnant receptor and that it is interiorized during remnant endocytosis, where it can function in lysosomal triglyceride hydrolysis.[27]

A study of chylomicron cholesterol ester hydrolysis comparing the activities of different cholesterol ester hydrolases in liver cells led to the conclusion that hydrolysis of chylomicron cholesterol esters was not required before their uptake by hepatocytes.[64] Furthermore, it appears that cholesterol esters could be hydrolyzed without prior triglyceride hydrolysis and that lysosomal enzymes could degrade both the cholesterol esters and triglycerides of chylomicron remnants taken up by endocytosis.

During chylomicron catabolism in plasma, the surface lipids, phospholipids, and unesterified cholesterol are removed and replenish nascent HDL (see Fig. 30-6), while the Apo A-I of the fresh chylomicrons in lymph are also removed and transferred to HDL. Apo C peptides are probably exchanged back and forth between HDL and chylomicrons.

The replenishment of nascent HDL during chylomicron (and VLDL) catabolism is extremely important for other aspects of lipoprotein metabolism.[54] Because nascent HDL is the substrate for LCAT, the replenishment of HDL provides a means by which additional cholesterol can be esterified and then shunted into the pathway leading to LDL formation. Alternatively, cholesterol esters in HDL can be removed from the plasma as HDL is taken up by the liver, or other tissues, and catabolized (see Fig. 30-6). At the same time, the transfer of Apo A-I from chylomicrons to nascent HDL provides the cofactor for LCAT activity, while transfer of Apo C-II between HDL and the triglyceride-rich lipoproteins ensures LPL activation.

The chylomicron remnants are removed rapidly by hepatocytes by a process involving high-affinity receptor-mediated binding to an apoprotein constituent of the chylomicron remnant as well as to receptor-independent sites.[154] There is still debate about whether the hepatocyte chylomicron receptor recognizes both Apo B and Apo E on the chylomicron remnant, but recent studies suggest that the receptor is specific for Apo E.

The intracellular metabolism of chylomicron remnants has important implications for the effects of dietary cholesterol on plasma cholesterol levels. As indicated earlier, the free cholesterol released by the hydrolysis of cholesterol esters inhibits the activity of HMG-CoA reductase and thus suppresses hepatocyte cholesterol synthesis; however, the increase in hepatocyte cholesterol concentration down-regulates LDL-receptor synthesis, resulting in a decrease in hepatocyte LDL uptake and a subsequent tendency for plasma cholesterol elevation. In this way, dietary cholesterol transported in chylomicron remnants, in part, regulates plasma cholesterol levels.

VERY-LOW-DENSITY LIPOPROTEIN METABOLISM. The early steps in VLDL metabolism (see Fig. 30-6) are similar to those described for chylomicrons. The VLDL are secreted as nascent triglyceride-rich particles by the liver and enter the plasma compartment containing Apo B-100 and some Apo E. They rapidly become enriched in Apo C-II, C-III, and E and in cholesterol esters by transfer from HDL. The triglycerides in mature VLDL are hydrolyzed by LPL, using Apo C-II as an activator. The degradation of VLDL to VLDL remnants is accompanied by release of fatty acids and phospholipids and the transfer of Apo E, C-II, and C-III to HDL. The VLDL remnants, now greatly depleted in triglyceride content and enriched in cholesterol esters, undergo two catabolic pathways. The VLDL remnants can be taken up directly by the liver by a receptor-mediated process that recognizes Apo B on the VLDL remnant particles, or the VLDL remnants can be metabolized further to LDL.

Most evidence suggests that the hepatocyte receptor (the LDL receptor) binds Apo B-100 on the VLDL remnant, but some receptor-mediated uptake may be related to the recognition by the LDL receptor of Apo E also located on the surface of the VLDL remnant particle. About 60% to 70% of the VLDL remnants are removed by this receptor-mediated pathway. The remaining VLDL (about 30% to 40%) is converted into LDL, this catabolic pathway involves hepatic triglyceride lipase, which hydrolyzes the residual triglyceride in the remnant particle. The loss of triglycerides (as fatty acids) is accompanied by depletion of Apo C and E, resulting in an LDL particle composed almost exclusively of cholesterol esters and Apo B-100.

As in chylomicron catabolism, concurrent with depletion of the triglyceride core is loss of VLDL surface constituents, which replenish HDL. It appears most likely that cholesterol esters are acquired by VLDL by transfer from HDL, perhaps in conjunction with Apo E. Apo E, a major constituent of VLDL, is not present in plasma HDL; however, nascent HDL is enriched in Apo E, whereas nascent VLDL does not contain Apo E.[139]

LOW-DENSITY LIPOPROTEIN METABOLISM. LDL (see Fig. 30-6), the product of VLDL catabolism, is the major cholesterol-transporting lipoprotein. Containing almost exclusively cholesterol esters and Apo B-100, LDL particles are removed from the plasma by receptor-mediated or non–receptor-mediated pathways in the liver or extrahepatic tissues.[19] The liver is responsible for most LDL removal (75%), of which about 75% is receptor-mediated.

In extrahepatic tissues, receptor-mediated uptake of LDL accounts for about two thirds of LDL removal. The binding and subsequent internalization of LDL are critical for the intracellular regulation of cholesterol synthesis and for the control of plasma cholesterol concentration.[20,134] The LDL receptor has high-affinity binding to Apo B-100 and results in rapid internalization of the LDL particles, which are then catabolized within the lysosomal compartment. The cholesterol esters of LDL are hydrolyzed, and then the unesterified cholesterol can be either reesterified and stored in the hepatocyte, secreted, or used for cell membrane synthesis. The intracellular pool of unesterified cholesterol is critical for regulating the activity of HMG-CoA reductase and the synthesis of LDL receptors.

HDL METABOLISM. HDL synthesis and metabolism (see Fig. 30-6) involve a complex and extremely important process since the esterification of cholesterol by LCAT in the nascent HDL particle is the major source of plasma cholesterol esters. Nascent HDL is synthesized by the liver and intestine as a discoidal particle composed of unesterified cholesterol and phospholipids. Nascent HDL is also formed in the plasma compartment subsequent to the catabolism of chylomicrons and VLDL, a process that depletes these lipoproteins of their surface components, unesterified cholesterol and phospholipids. The nascent discoidal HDL contains Apo A-I, A-II, and some E. The discoidal particle becomes enriched in unesterified cholesterol by transfer from cell membranes or other lipoproteins, and then, in the presence of LCAT and Apo A-I (the LCAT activator), cholesterol esters are formed, converting the discoidal into a spherical particle. The initial spherical HDL particle, called HDL$_3$, is converted into a larger particle, HDL$_2$, as a more unesterified cholesterol is acquired and cholesterol esters synthesized.[29] Complex interconversions occur between the various HDL particles, and cholesterol esters are also transferred to the VLDL catabolic pathway by a cholesterol ester transfer protein, thereby providing the main source of cholesterol esters in VLDL and LDL. HDL may provide the most important pathway for the removal of excess cholesterol from peripheral tissues, its subsequent transport to the liver, and its excretion in the bile. The process of so-called reverse cholesterol transport is a key factor in cholesterol metabolism since the liver is the only organ involved in cholesterol degradation and excretion.

POTENTIAL MECHANISMS OF FATTY LIVER

The numerous theories proposed for the pathogenesis of fatty liver are based on derangements of the normal physiology of hepatic triglyceride synthesis and secretion.[70,195] These theories include not only abnormalities of physiologic and biochemical regulation but also derangements in the series of steps by which the VLDL lipid and apoproteins are synthesized, assembled into nascent particles, transported sequentially through subcellular compartments, and finally secreted. Singly or in combination, derangements of these events can be involved in the pathogenesis of fatty liver, as illustrated in the representation of VLDL synthesis and secretion in Figure 30-3. Thus, an increased supply of fatty acids leading to an imbalance between triglyceride synthesis and secretion could result from enhanced fatty acid mobilization from adipose tissue or diet, increased fatty acid synthesis, or decreased mitochondrial fatty acid oxidation. The secretion of triglycerides might be impaired secondary to inhibition of apoprotein synthesis or to inadequate apoprotein synthesis when a large triglyceride load is available for lipoprotein formation.

Defects in one or more of the steps involved in the assembly, intracellular transport, or secretion of nascent VLDL can also lead to fatty liver. These include inhibition of nascent VLDL transport from the endoplasmic reticulum to the Golgi complex; impaired Golgi function, preventing the final glycosylation of nascent VLDL apoproteins or decreased secretory vesicle formation; interference with the migration of secretory vesicles to the plasmalemma membrane, possibly secondary to microtubule dysfunction; and impaired exocytosis of nascent VLDL.

Although there are no definitive data concerning the relative importance of these mechanisms, some are undoubtedly more important than others, depending on the agent directly responsible for the production of a fatty liver. Some of the pharmacologic or toxic agents for which a mechanism has been suggested in animals are discussed next.

Increased Fatty Acid Supply and Enhanced Triglyceride Synthesis

The data on fatty livers produced acutely by a number of agents suggest that much of the lipid that accumulates in the liver is derived from adipose tissue.[10] This is not surprising since most acute studies have been performed on fasting animals, and under these conditions, the plasma free fatty acids are predominantly those released from peripheral lipid depots. Many of the hormonal and experimental manipulations that interfere with the mobilization of fatty acids from adipose tissue are also effective in blocking development of fatty liver. By varying the supply of fatty acids to the liver, one can influence directly the amount of fat that accumulates in the liver. Thus, if the rate of fatty acid influx in the liver is reduced, less fat accumulates.

It is likely that the hepatic steatosis that develops under conditions of enhanced supply of free fatty acids reflects an imbalance between triglyceride synthesis and the assembly and secretion of VLDL. This imbalance may be due to an inability of the hepatocyte to synthesize Apo B rapidly enough to accommodate the increase in triglyceride awaiting assembly into lipoproteins or to a relative deficiency in the secretory process. The latter could involve the final formation of nascent VLDL in the Golgi complex, inadequate secretory vesicle formation or movement, or the exocytotic process itself. In many conditions characterized by fatty liver, secondary to increased supply of free fatty acids, there is concomitant hypertriglyceridemia, indicating active VLDL secretion even while fat accumulates in the liver. The secreted VLDL are larger and enriched in triglyceride compared with VLDL isolated from plasma under basal conditions.[196,200] The secretion of large, triglyceride-rich particles implies an adaptive response by the hepatocyte, enabling the secretion of more triglyceride with less apoprotein.

Decreased Synthesis or Release of Lipoproteins

In earlier studies, the inhibitory effect of certain drugs and hepatotoxins on hepatic VLDL secretion provided reasonable support for the hypothesis that hepatic triglycerides accumulate secondary to a lipoprotein secretory defect.[58,189] This concept was supported by many studies of hepatic lipoprotein synthesis that showed that the apoprotein moiety of VLDL is actually synthesized within the hepatocytes and that the final secretory product is assembled within the liver.[70]

The demonstration that inhibitors of protein synthesis can interfere with VLDL biosynthesis led to the conclusion that a lipoprotein secretory defect is the main cause of fatty liver. Despite the fact that some protein synthesis inhibitors produce fatty liver, it is evident that many of these agents cause only a moderate increase in hepatic triglyceride content. Thus, the hepatic triglyceride concentration after ethionine[58] or puromycin[189] administration is slight when compared with the massive fatty liver induced by orotic acid.[194,243] The discrepancy between protein synthesis inhibition and extent of fat accumulation in the liver is even more striking in the case of cycloheximide[100,233] and acetoxycycloheximide,[201] which produce only a two-fold increase in hepatic triglyceride content despite their ability to inhibit protein synthesis almost completely. Ethionine and D-galactosamine also both induce hypoglycemia and a secondary elevation of plasma free fatty acids.[202] Many of the hepatotoxic effects of ethionine can be prevented by glucose infusions or by feeding the animals throughout the experiment.[23,147] Thus, despite the inhibition of secretion produced by ethionine or D-galactosamine,[200] fatty liver does not occur unless there is a stimulus for fatty acid influx into the liver.

It is tempting to speculate that the orotic acid–induced secretory block may be related to a defect in the glycosylation of certain VLDL apoproteins within the Golgi apparatus. Because it has been shown that the B and C apoproteins of VLDL are present within hepatic triglyceride droplets after orotic acid feeding, it is conceivable that certain sugar moieties cannot be added to these apoproteins after the nascent VLDL enter the Golgi apparatus.[174] Orotic acid is known to produce an imbalance in hepatic nucleotide levels, causing an increase in uridine and a decrease in adenine and cytidine nucleotides.[138] The decreased availability of specific sugars for transfer to incompletely glycosylated apoproteins within the Golgi apparatus might conceivably cause the secretory block. In this regard, there is some evidence that a defect in glycoprotein formation may be important in the pathogenesis of the orotic acid–induced effect in VLDL secretion. Thus, liposomes isolated from the orotic acid fatty liver contain three of the four VLDL apoproteins normally found in plasma VLDL, and the missing VLDL band is defective in its carbohydrate moiety but not in its peptide content.[175] Orotic acid might regulate synthesis of the enzyme required to glycosylate this apoprotein, or the enzyme may be inhibited by uridine diphosphate N-acetylglucosamine, which accumulates in the liver of the orotic acid–fed rats. It has also been shown that the VLDL apoproteins, derived from the orotic acid liver liposomes, are deficient in N-acetylglycosamines, galactose, and N-acetylneuraminic acid, perhaps owing to a lack of exposure of the apoproteins to glycosylating enzymes in the Golgi apparatus.

In considering the mechanisms by which orotic acid might alter normal glycosylation reactions, it is noteworthy that orotic acid produces a decrease in hepatic levels of adenine and cytidine nucleotides.[138] The decrease in cytidine nucleotides may have important implications for the pathogenesis of fatty liver since the hepatic Golgi complexes contain a sialyltransferase that catalyzes the incorporation of sialic acid from cytidine monophosphate N-acetylneuraminic acid into a sialidase-treated Apo C peptide isolated from VLDL.[292] A decrease in the availability of this sugar nucleotide might prevent adequate sialylation of C peptides in the Golgi apparatus and could explain the observations discussed previously. If one assumes that VLDL secretion is dependent on the presence of the sugar moieties of the VLDL apoproteins, then defective sialylation of the C peptides could cause the secretory block.

Fatty liver has been produced by a variety of agents that bring about decreased hepatic ATP concentration, inhibition of protein synthesis, and impaired lipoprotein formation. Ethionine is a prototypic agent in this respect.[58] The administration of ATP or an ATP precursor, such as adenine, completely protects against ethionine-induced fatty liver in rats and reverses the ethionine-induced inhibition of protein synthesis. In other models (eg, azaserine and carbon tetrachloride), administration of ATP also reverses the hepatic triglyceride accumulation. Fatty liver production by these two models, however, is not specifically dependent on inhibition of protein synthesis since ATP repletion does not alter the inhibition of protein synthesis evoked by these agents. The effects may be due to inhibition of fatty acid mobilization.

In the case of carbon tetrachloride, one of the earliest lesions noted microscopically is at the level of the endoplasmic reticulum, and biochemically, protein synthesis is dramatically decreased.[186] This is associated with a breakdown of polyribosomes (needed for protein synthesis) to single ribosomes. The exact mechanisms by which this occurs are unknown. Peroxidation of lipids, including microsomal lipids, is increased after ingestion of carbon tetrachloride, and it is possible that microsomal membrane function is affected by this process.[185] Peroxidation is the oxidative degradation of unsaturated fatty acids in the presence of oxygen. None of the many agents used to prevent carbon tetrachloride–induced fatty liver or necrosis in animals (adrenergic-blocking agents, antihistamines, antioxidants) has proved useful clinically since they must all be given before the toxin is administered. Increased lipid peroxidation has been found in human liver at autopsy after carbon tetrachloride ingestion, but its pathogenetic significance is still unclear.

Nutritional deficiencies or imbalances of various types have led to fatty liver in animals, presumably related to a decrease in packaging or secretion of lipoproteins. The best studied of the deficiencies is that of choline.[130] Choline deficiency is characterized by growth failure, weakness, hemorrhagic lesions, myocardial and renal lesions, as well as fatty liver and cirrhosis. Choline is a precursor of phosphoryl choline and is therefore important in lipoprotein production; however, its effect is nonspecific—methionine and cysteine can replace choline. Moreover, choline is metabolized poorly in humans, owing to the almost total absence of choline oxidase.

Fatty Liver Disease

ALCOHOLIC LIVER DISEASE

Mechanisms

Fatty liver can follow either acute or chronic administration of alcohol in laboratory animals and in humans. It is clear that alcohol alters a number of processes that affect triglyceride accumulation in the liver. Many of the mechanisms postulated in Figure 30-8 have at some time been proposed for the alcoholic fatty liver by various investigators. Alcohol apparently does not affect intestinal absorption of lipids, hepatic chylomicron uptake, hepatic protein synthesis, or lipoprotein formation. It does, however, increase adipose tissue lipolysis and thus influx of fatty acids to the liver (step 1), increase hepatic synthesis (step 2) and decrease oxidation of fatty acids (step 3), and increase triglyceride formation and decrease release of lipoproteins from the liver (steps 5 through 8).[128] Ethanol decreases the intracellular NAD/NADH ratio.[157] The change in this ratio, however, is unlikely to be the only factor in the production of fatty liver. First, the NAD/NADH ratio decreases early after ingestion of ethanol and returns to normal when fat is still accumulating. Second, sorbitol changes the ratio but does not cause fatty liver.[184] Finally antioxidant treatment reduces the fatty liver but does not alter the NAD/NADH ratio.[193] Moreover, the metabolism of ethanol itself produces metabolites (eg, acetate) that can be used as precursors for fatty acid synthesis.

In reviewing the many studies on the effect of alcohol on lipid metabolism, numerous reports on first inspection appear to give conflicting results and to be contradictory. Many of the discrepancies, however, are perhaps explained by the fact that the effects of alcohol may differ within a variety of experimental or clinical conditions. In vitro preparations, perfused livers, intact animals, and normal alcoholic human subjects have all been used for study. Different sampling times have been used. Because a high-fat diet suppresses hepatic fatty acid synthesis, the nutritional state of the subjects is another important variable. The dose of ethanol is significant because, at high doses, nonspecific neural or hormonally mediated responses may be evoked. Most authors accept as a major factor a direct toxic effect of ethanol at moderate doses on hepatic triglyceride metabolism.[128]

Results of acute experiments performed with large doses of alcohol differ from those of chronic experiments when alcohol is given in smaller amounts and other dietary nutrients are provided. Gender is also important because the female animal is much more susceptible to hepatic fat accumulation than the male. It is clear that fatty liver in humans can develop at or above the blood alcohol level that is defined as legal intoxication. Dietary deficiencies are not required for the production of such an acute fatty liver but clearly play a modifying role in the more chronic syndromes associated with ethanol ingestion.[127,171] In humans, the degree of fatty liver appears to correlate with the severity of overall dietary deficiency.[120] For example, patients with the lowest protein intake have the most hepatic steatosis. On the other hand, prospective studies in male volunteers with initially normal livers showed that ingestion of 150 to 200 g of ethanol per day for 10 to 12 days produced fatty livers, regardless of the content of the rest of the diet.[124] In addition to the variations in dose and time of ingestion and nutritional status, other factors, such as genetic and metabolic differences, may account for the presence or absence of hepatic fat.[174]

Fatty Acid Mobilization. Animal experiments show that the fatty acids present in hepatic triglycerides after acute alcohol administration are of extrahepatic origin and reach the liver in the blood. Under fasting conditions during acute alcohol intoxication, most of the plasma fatty acids that reach the liver are derived from adipose tissue. Mobilization of fatty acids is greatly potentiated in the presence of adrenocortical and pituitary hormones. In acute experiments with single, large doses of alcohol, the fatty acid composition of the liver suggests that much of the lipid is derived from extrahepatic sources.[124,207] The fatty acid derives from increased lipolysis, probably related to activation of adenyl cyclase. Epinephrine, norepinephrine, cortisol, adrenocorticotropic hormone, and prostaglandins, among other hormones, can mediate this enhanced enzyme activity and lead to increased cAMP concentrations in adipocytes. When mobilization of fatty acids from adipose tissues is interfered with, as by adrenalectomy, cordotomy, hypophysectomy, and adrenergic-blocking agents, the amount of fat that accumulates in the liver after alcohol is markedly reduced.[184] Thus, with acute intoxication, the fatty acid mobilization may be a nonspecific result of a stress reaction.

On the other hand, when alcohol and food are administered chronically to rats, the fatty acids in the plasma reflect the fatty acids present in the triglycerides absorbed from the intestinal tract.[126] In chronic experiments in rats and humans, in which alcohol plus food was administered, the fatty acids in the liver tended to reflect the lipids in the diet.[124,126] These acute and chronic experiments are not contradictory but simply reflect the importance of hepatic influx of fatty acids and the relation of hepatic lipid to the plasma composition. The latter is in turn influenced by whether the animal or subject is fasting or is ingesting fat. Therefore, while increased peripheral mobilization of free fatty acids may increase only with high blood-alcohol levels, influx of fatty acids to the liver is usually normal when significant hepatic fat accumulation occurs.

When alcohol is highly concentrated in the blood (ie, greater than 250 mg/dL), the free fatty acids in the serum increase markedly.[206] At lower blood-alcohol levels (80 to 100 mg/dL), no significant changes in serum free fatty acids are detected.[123] Hepatic uptake is proportional to the plasma free fatty acid concentration. Because a fatty liver may develop with prolonged alcohol administration and normal serum fatty acid concentrations, hepatic steatosis may result from an increased plasma flux of fatty acids or from altered synthesis or oxidation of fatty acids in the hepatocyte.

Increased Hepatic Fatty Acid Synthesis. Ethanol inhibits the tricarboxylic acid cycle in hepatocytes, in part by damaging mitochondria, by increasing the NADH/NAD ratio, and by shuttling NADH into mitochondria for oxidation. By decreasing the condensation of maleate to oxaloacetate, the production of pyruvate (and acetate) is increased, and the acetate is available for fatty acid synthesis. High levels of acetate also inhibit fatty acid oxidation.

The hydrogen ion used to reduce NAD comes from ethanol rather than from fatty acids by means of the citric acid cycle. Thus, fatty acids that normally serve as an energy source are replaced. In fasted animals with lower energy needs, ethanol does not increase fatty acid synthesis,[163] whereas in the fed state, lipogenesis increases.[73] The changes in hepatic redox become attenuated with time, and fat does not continue to accumulate.[40]

Ethanol stimulates hepatic fatty acid synthesis in vivo and in vitro.[125] Ethanol is largely metabolized in the liver (90% to 98%), and hepatic alcohol dehydrogenase converts NAD to NADH as ethanol is metabolized to acetaldehyde. In the de novo synthesis of fatty acids, from acetate, however, NADPH rather than NADH is required. Some fatty acids are produced by elongation, and the NADH, as well as NADPH, may serve as a hydrogen donor in the elongation of fatty acid chain lengths and in the conversion of saturated to unsaturated fatty acids.[92] Thus, there may be a nonspecific effect of altered NADH/NAD ratios on fatty acid synthesis, other than supplying increased acetate as substrate.[184]

Glucose and sorbitol increase fatty acid synthesis without the concomitant formation of a fatty liver. In cordotomized rats, ethanol increases hepatic fatty acid synthesis but does not produce a fatty liver. Thus, while the acute administration of ethanol may, under certain conditions, increase hepatic fatty acid synthesis, it is unclear whether this is a major factor in the production of the alcohol-induced fatty liver. Few data are available on the effects of chronic alcohol administration on hepatic fatty acid synthesis.

Decreased Fatty Acid Oxidation. In humans, ingestion of alcohol decreases oxidation of lipids under conditions that do not affect carbohydrate or protein metabolism. Oxidation of long-chain fatty acids after ethanol ingestion is impaired to a greater extent than that of medium-chain fatty acids, perhaps accounting for the greater accumulation of long-chain fatty acids after ethanol ingestion.[122]

Acetaldehyde, the major metabolic product of ethanol, increases in concentration after ethanol ingestion in humans.[145] In rats, acetaldehyde metabolism is decreased in the presence of acetaldehyde administration. Acetaldehyde raises serum free fatty acids and triglyceride levels. Thus, the production of acetaldehyde may provide a vicious cycle in which damage to mitochondria further increases acetaldehyde and free fatty acid levels. Other hepatotoxins (carbon tetrachloride, phosphorus, ethionine, and choline) cause mitochondrial damage, which contributes to maintenance of high triglyceride levels in the liver but probably does not alone explain the onset of fat accumulation.[47]

The evidence that decreased oxidation is a major factor in the alcoholic fatty liver must be examined further. In vitro, ethanol can decrease oxidation of lipids, but so can other substances (glucose, sorbitol, xylitol, and nicotinamide) that do not lead to the development of a fatty liver.[184] In fact, ethanol has been reported to increase the oxidation of some lipids by the mechanism of peroxidation.[38]

Increased Esterification of Fatty Acids to Triglycerides. When fatty acids are presented to the liver, they are esterified to triglycerides, phospholipids, and cholesterol esters. Alcohol could lead to increased conversion of fatty acids to triglycerides either directly or indirectly by inhibiting their incorporation into phospholipids and cholesterol esters. Acute alcohol administration to rats alters the esterifying system in liver microsomes. Microsomes isolated from rats 16 hours after an acute alcohol load show a fourfold increase in the conversion of ^{14}C-palmitate to triglyceride.[207] Enhanced esterification of fatty acids has been associated with an increased hepatic level of α-glycerophosphate, a substrate for triglyceride formation.[241] α-Glycerophosphate production is increased by NADH and the ethanol-induced activity of the microsomal enzyme α-glycerophosphate transferase, which catalyzes the first step of triglyceride formation.[145] Few studies have been performed with chronic alcohol administration.

Decreased Hepatic Release or Secretion of Triglycerides.   There has been no demonstrated effect of alcohol on protein synthesis or on the interaction of lipid and apoprotein to form lipoprotein, as has been demonstrated in orotic acid fatty liver. Many other toxic agents leading to fatty liver cause a decreased synthesis of protein and lipoprotein and, as a consequence, decreased release of lipid into the blood. When alcohol is administered to humans, plasma triglycerides initially increase.[206] This increased release of lipoproteins from the liver, however, is not sufficient to compensate for increased triglyceride production, so that fatty liver develops. When blood alcohol reaches high levels (ie, over 250 mg/dL), plasma triglycerides decrease, accompanied by an increase in plasma free fatty acids. Because hepatic lipid first accumulates at lower levels of blood alcohol, and because at these levels decreased hepatic lipid release has not been demonstrated, one must assume that this mechanism is not a primary one but possibly a contributory factor.

In summary, alcohol administration both acutely and chronically affects many aspects of lipid metabolism. Some of these actions may be primary or major in regard to production of fatty liver. Others may be minor or serve only to contribute to or affect the extent of the fatty liver.

Clinical Considerations

The diagnosis of alcoholic liver disease is often suspected by a recent or excessive exposure to alcohol, even in the absence of signs or symptoms of acute liver disease. One should be careful, however, not to rely too heavily on such a history. The chance of chronic liver disease being related to alcohol is never 100%, even with excessive alcohol ingestion (more than 150 g/d for men, more than 120 g/d for women). Moreover, other liver diseases can occur in patients who also ingest alcohol. The spectrum of alcoholic liver disease includes fatty liver, alcoholic hepatitis (with or without steatosis), and alcoholic cirrhosis. In each case, one must assume that the damage from alcohol is chronic, even if the presentation is acute. Each entity is discussed separately, although they may all be present to varying degrees simultaneously or may progress over time from less serious to more extensive lesions.

Alcoholic Fatty Liver.   Fatty liver is the most common response to alcohol ingestion[155] and may occur within a few days or weeks.[226] Up to one third of asymptomatic alcoholics have fatty liver.[21] A small group of patients may have jaundice, ascites, peripheral edema, or signs of vitamin deficiency. The more severe the hepatic fat accumulation, the more likely is vitamin deficiency. Splenomegaly is uncommon unless hepatic fibrosis or frank cirrhosis is present.[120] If alcohol is withheld, splenomegaly and early fibrotic changes may be reversible. When the patient presents with hepatic decompensation, the prevalence of fatty liver is much lower.[13] The two clinical syndromes associated with the ethanol-induced fatty liver are the asymptomatic enlarged liver and alcoholic hepatitis with or without cirrhosis. This second group more often presents with pain and tenderness in the right upper quadrant, but pain and tenderness are present in some patients with fatty liver alone.[120]

Fatty liver is a major pathologic condition reported by medical examiners.[46,111] Most of the fatal cases of fatty liver have no cirrhosis or other obvious cause of death. In a study of 268 autopsies of chronic alcoholics, 78% of these patients with fatty liver had fat embolism, especially in the lungs.[132]

Thus, fat embolism may be a more important complication than was previously recognized. Sudden death in alcoholics with fatty liver may also occur as a result of hypoglycemia, adrenergic hypersensitivity, or alcohol withdrawal.[183] A different cause of death is found in patients with huge livers (up to 4 kg in weight) who die after an acute illness with jaundice, usually in association with nutritional deficiency. Centrilobular necrosis and alcoholic hyalin, with only scattered focal leukocyte infiltration and intact lobular architecture, is seen.[173] Obese women, aged 30 to 40 years, are most often affected.

Laboratory features in alcoholic fatty liver are variable and may be normal. The serum albumin is often normal, and the globulin value may be elevated. Hyperbilirubinemia up to 8 mg/dL is seen in about one fourth of cases. The serum aminotransferases may be elevated; serum aspartate aminotransferase (AST) is usually less than 300 IU/L but is frequently higher than the serum alanine aminotransferase (ALT) by a factor of two or more.[34] Prothrombin time is prolonged by 2 seconds in about half of patients. The alkaline phosphatase level is elevated up to 200 IU/L in 15% of cases. The leukocyte count is usually normal, but rarely, a leukemoid reaction may be seen.[35] The laboratory findings and clinical features depend on whether fatty liver alone predominates or whether there is also some degree of necrosis or intrahepatic cholestasis. The amount of fat does not correlate well with the degree of abnormality of liver function tests.[95] The presence of fat alone does not appear to be associated with progression to fibrosis and cirrhosis, and no relation between the degree or progression of fibrosis and the extent of fatty infiltration in the absence of alcoholic hepatitis has been shown.[137] Most likely, it is the degree of accompanying inflammation that is crucial. The syndrome of alcoholic fatty liver is probably a variant of alcoholic hepatitis since nearly all cases show some inflammatory response. Fatty liver is reversible if the patient abstains from alcohol. Reversal may take several weeks to months, depending on the extent and severity of fatty infiltration and accompanying inflammatory response.

Alcoholic Fatty Liver With Cholestasis.   Rarely, alcoholic fatty liver presents as obstructive jaundice.[9,150] Typically, these patients have a history of marked alcohol ingestion for years, with an increase in intake before hospitalization. The presenting symptoms are frequently identical to those seen in alcoholic hepatitis: in fact, acute inflammatory changes in the liver can often accompany this form of fatty liver. Acute right upper quadrant pain can be seen with a rigid epigastrium. Over half of patients are febrile (higher than 38°C [101°F]), and one third have leukocytosis. About 10% have splenomegaly and ascites. The liver is characteristically large and tender, and liver function tests indicate the presence of cholestasis. Alkaline phosphatase is two to eight times normal. Serum cholesterol may be above 400 mg/dL, and about half of patients have jaundice. AST is more than 100 IU/L in most cases.

Grossly, the liver is large and yellow; and microscopically, practically every liver cell is filled with microvesicular fat. Cholestasis may be difficult to detect because of the severe fatty changes. Central zones often show necrosis. The syndrome of increased alkaline phosphatase (greater than four times normal) and a clinical picture of extrahepatic biliary obstruction may also occur without a fatty liver or even hepatomegaly.[166] Hepatic failure and death have been described.[150]

These patients are often thought to have biliary tract disease because of fever, right upper quadrant pain, and obstructive liver chemistries. A large, tender liver and radiologic confirmation of a normal biliary tract by ultrasound or CT may be clues to the correct diagnosis. Other causes of cholestasis in alcoholic patients include severe alcoholic hepatitis and superimposed drug-induced or viral hepatitis, in none of which does ductal dilation occur. Of course, gallstones and pancreatitis or pancreatic tumors may produce ductal dilation. When surgical intervention is contemplated, the possibility of alcoholic liver disease, with or without fat, must be considered beforehand.

Alcoholic Hepatitis. Alcoholic hepatitis is not a syndrome separate from alcoholic fatty liver. Inflammatory infiltrate and necrosis are merely another manifestation of hepatic injury related to alcohol. Alcoholic hepatitis is also covered in Chapter 31. In liver biopsy specimens, one usually sees much fat, but fat may also be almost totally absent. The characteristic lesions seen include alcoholic hyalin (Mallory's bodies) and polymorphonuclear leukocytes associated with cell necrosis (see Color Fig. 28). Sharply focal involvement of cells in the centrilobular regions, with or without sclerosis of terminal hepatic veins, is common.[53] The lesions are usually diffuse. In rare cases of alcoholic hepatitis, periportal hepatocytes are affected primarily.

Patients present with hepatomegaly and abdominal pain just as they do with uncomplicated fatty liver alone.[67,100] However, anorexia, nausea, vomiting, fever, and jaundice tend to be more frequent. Anemia and leukocytosis are usually present, and the alkaline phosphatase level is more frequently elevated—but in most cases, only up to 200 IU/L. This syndrome is most commonly seen after a prolonged bout of drinking.

Most reported patients have had a history or past evidence of chronic liver disease. Hepatomegaly is found in about 80% of patients, with splenomegaly, jaundice, abdominal pain, and fever in one third to one half.[67] AST levels are elevated in most but not all patients. Typically, the AST value is double the ALT level.[34] Despite the necrosis seen in liver biopsy specimens, the transaminase level is usually not above 500 IU/L. Alkaline phosphatase is elevated in 60% to 80% of patients but need not correlate with the degree of cholestasis on biopsy.[75] This condition is a frequent cause of undiagnosed fever in alcoholic liver disease. Although the fatty liver of the alcoholic may be associated with a variable degree of necrosis, necrosis in alcoholic hepatitis is invariable and is sometimes seen in the absence of fat. The degree of necrosis does not correlate well with the amount of fat or with the liver function tests. The more severe the necrosis, the more serious the clinical course.

Alcoholic Cirrhosis. Alcoholic cirrhosis is found in association with variable amounts of fatty infiltration. The cirrhosis is most commonly micronodular, but occasionally a mixed micronodular or macronodular cirrhosis can be seen.[133] Features of alcoholic fatty liver and alcoholic hepatitis may be present as well; however, in more advanced stages, when inactive cirrhosis is present, it may be difficult to identify characteristics of alcoholic cirrhosis.[133] The incidence of alcoholic cirrhosis in patients with long-standing alcohol abuse varies from 10% to 20%.[137] Several reports demonstrate an increased susceptibility of women to the development of alcoholic cirrhosis.[112,137,149,230]

Clinical presentation of these patients is similar to other patients with cirrhosis. The major complications include encephalopathy, coagulopathy, ascites, and portal hypertension associated with variceal bleeding. Synthetic function is frequently abnormal, with hypoalbuminemia and prolonged prothrombin time. Patients may have normal synthetic function and transaminase levels.

Treatment

All the syndromes presenting with acute manifestations that are induced by ethanol (fatty liver, acute fatty liver with cholestasis, and alcoholic hepatitis) are potentially reversible. This is because these syndromes occur relatively early in the natural history of chronic alcohol-induced liver injury. The diagnosis of these syndromes can be suspected clinically or by imaging techniques but is best made by needle biopsy of the liver. The mainstay of therapy is abstinence from alcohol, with supportive care and supplementation of diet and vitamins. Although these lesions can be reversible, the change may occur slowly. In fact, patients present when they begin to have increased symptoms, but their condition may worsen after being admitted to the hospital. It is not unusual for recovery to begin after 2 to 3 weeks of hospitalization and for total recovery to require months. Recently, steroid therapy has once again demonstrated some efficacy in severe alcoholic hepatitis,[24] but whether long-term survival is favorably affected requires further study.

Alcoholic cirrhosis is not reversible, and complications require specific management. Alcoholic hepatitis is a risk factor for the development of alcoholic cirrhosis.[137] Although abstinence from alcohol improves the prognosis of alcoholic liver disease, it has been shown that progression to cirrhosis may occur even after total alcohol abstinence.[67] Ultimately, these patients may require liver transplantation. Recent reviews suggest that livers of alcoholic patients can be transplanted successfully, and long-term survival is no different than for hepatic transplantation patients with other diseases.[113,219]

NONALCOHOLIC FATTY LIVER DISEASE

Although alcohol is the most common agent associated with fatty liver disease, patients may have a similar clinical presentation and the histologic features of alcoholic liver disease but either no antecedent alcohol history or a history of alcohol ingestion that only accompanies another diagnosis. A variety of terms have been used to describe this entity, including *fatty liver hepatitis,*[2] *nonalcoholic steatohepatitis,*[98,131] *nonalcoholic Laënnec's disease,*[229] *diabetic hepatitis,*[11] and *alcohol-like liver disease.*[48] The entity, however, should further distinguish fatty infiltration (steatosis) from fatty infiltration associated with inflammation (steatohepatitis). The clinical entities associated with steatosis and steatohepatitis include malnutrition (eg, starvation), jejunoileal bypass, gastric partitioning, obesity, and diabetes mellitus. Other conditions associated with fatty infiltration and variable degrees of inflammation, but not with the histologic features characteristic of alcoholic liver disease, include AFLP, administration of certain drugs (eg, corticosteroids, methotrexate, tetracycline, valproic acid, salicylates, amiodarone, perhexiline maleate), and toxin exposure (eg, Jamaican vomiting sickness, phosphorus, carbon tetrachloride).

Patients with nonalcoholic steatohepatitis are more often women and obese (defined as over 110% of ideal body weight).[48,131] A variable incidence of diabetes has been reported in a series of patients with nonalcoholic steatohepatitis[48,98] but diabetes appears to be more frequent in nonalcoholic steatohepatitis than in alcoholic steatohepatitis. Nonalcoholic steatohepatitis patients more frequently have coexistent medical problems and take more medications (particularly estrogens, oral hypoglycemics, diuretics, thyroid supplements, and cardiac and antihypertensive medications) than alcoholic patients.[48] Recently, investigators have attempted to clarify risk factors for nonalcoholic steatohepatitis and determine the frequency of progression to fibrosis and cirrhosis.[48,98,118] These studies identify the risk factors of female gender, obesity, and diabetes mellitus and conclude that a subset of patients will progress to cirrhosis.

Malnutrition

Protein-Calorie Malnutrition.

Most workers recognize two distinct syndromes, kwashiorkor and marasmus, and believe that the former is related to a relative deficiency of protein and the latter to deficiency of both protein and calories. Dietary history, however, is of little help in distinguishing these two syndromes. If one defines kwashiorkor by gross edema, hepatomegaly, and depigmentation of skin, 11% of cases of malnutrition can be so classified.[237] When marasmus is defined as body weight less than half of expected, with no edema or skin changes, 21% of the cases fall into this category. Lipid changes in marasmic children are much less striking, and fatty liver does not occur in this syndrome. The remainder are mixed cases clinically. For this reason, many workers prefer the comprehensive term of *protein-calorie malnutrition*. This group of disorders is worldwide in distribution but occurs uncommonly in the United States in its overt clinical form. Liver function is only mildly impaired; AST values are usually less than 100 IU/L but may be over 500 IU/L, possibly related to secondary changes from marked steatosis.[239]

Fatty liver is only one aspect of the syndrome. The liver is enlarged and yellow, and there is a striking degree of fatty infiltration. The earliest deposition of fat is in the cells at the periphery of the lobules, but as the condition progresses, the cells of the middle and central areas of the lobules become involved.[143] When a high-protein diet is administered, fat disappears first from the center of the liver lobule and last from the peripheral cells.[144] The condition does not progress to cirrhosis, which suggests that fat alone is an insufficient stimulus for the formation of fibrosis.

The hepatic concentration of palmitic acid is increased, and that of linoleic acid is decreased.[142] Because these findings resembled those in animals fed a high-carbohydrate diet, it seemed that the fat was originally synthesized from carbohydrate since the fat intake of these children is so low.[143] In rodents, it is clear that glucose administration triggers hepatic lipid synthesis, but the sugar acts indirectly by lactate or glycogen as the precursor.[108] When fatty liver is severe, the serum triglyceride and VLDL levels are low. The serum free fatty acids are increased, which suggests that increased mobilization of fat is also important. The rate of albumin synthesis is diminished, and it has been suggested that lipo-

protein synthesis is also affected, impairing the release of triglyceride from the liver. No evidence for lipotroph deficiency exists. With ingestion of dietary protein, there is a marked rise in VLDL, accompanied by a rise in triglyceride, phospholipid, and cholesterol in that fraction.[64]

Starvation.

During starvation, serum free fatty acids increase, and the plasma flux of these fatty acids is enhanced.[25] This can be associated with a moderate increase in liver fat. The mechanism appears to be related to the lack of availability of glucose, increase in growth hormone, and heightened sympathetic nervous activity, all of which mobilize free fatty acids from adipose tissue. Liver function tests are usually normal, except for bromosulfophthalein retention, which has been reported to be as high as 44% during starvation. Prolonged fasting, however, can also reduce fat within the liver.[43] This apparent paradox can be explained by the following mechanism.[22] During prolonged fasting, the brain, which usually requires glucose, uses ketone bodies resulting from fatty acid oxidation. Other tissues adapt likewise, so that fat supplies 95% of body energy needs. Hepatic gluconeogenesis is markedly decreased, essential amino acids are conserved, and fat does not accumulate in the liver. If small amounts of carbohydrate are ingested, this adaptation does not occur, lipids are mobilized but not oxidized, and fatty liver results. Thus, the development of hepatic steatosis depends on the completeness of starvation.

Jejunoileal Bypass.

Jejunoileal bypass is a surgical technique for the control of morbid obesity in which 30 to 35 cm of jejunum is anastomosed to the distal 10 to 15 cm of ileum, resulting in a bypass of about 90% of the small intestine. Although the procedure is effective for weight reduction, it is associated with a large number of postoperative complications, including liver disease, kidney disease, cholelithiasis, arthritis, dermatitis, and bone disease.[1] For these reasons, it is no longer recommended for treatment of obesity. Jejunoileal bypass for obesity leads to a variety of pathologic changes in the liver, including increased steatosis and fibrosis, inflammation, granulomas, and cirrhosis.[81] The most consistent change after bypass is increasing steatosis. No relation has been detected between the amount of prebypass hepatic lipid or fibrosis and the subsequent development of cirrhosis or hepatic failure.[168] Perivenular sclerosis has been suggested as a prognostic indicator of cirrhosis.[79,140] In a retrospective analysis of 34 patients with prebypass and postbypass biopsies, pericellular fibrosis was present in all patients with progressive liver injury, and the histologic features closely resembled alcoholic liver disease.[235]

The clinical features may range from only abnormal liver test results to frank hepatic failure in 2% to 5% of cases.[81] If results of hepatic tests fail to return to preoperative levels (see section on obesity), one should look for serious hepatic disease. Elevated AST and alkaline phosphatase levels are most commonly present, but leukocytosis, hypoalbuminemia, and prolonged prothrombin times may also be noted.[170]

Nearly all patients demonstrate increasing hepatic fat for the first 6 months after bypass.[172] After 6 months, the degree of steatosis diminishes until it reaches prebypass amounts, usually at 2 or 3 years after operation.[203] These changes in hepatic fat are not associated with predictable changes in liver function test results. In fact, the only certain means of following the hepatic disease is by repeated liver biopsies.[68] Increased mobilization of adipose tissue fat is partially responsible for the increased steatosis after bypass. More than this explanation is involved since morbidly obese patients who lose weight by dieting or by gastric bypass operations (see section on gastric partitioning) do not usually deposit increased fat in the liver. While fat is accumulating in the liver, serum essential amino acid levels fall.[153] This is similar to the situation seen in protein-calorie malnutrition, but the distribution of fat in kwashiorkor is periportal, a pattern seen rarely after bypass surgery. Bacterial toxins or toxic bile acids (lithocholic acid) may also play a role in the production of post-bypass liver disease.[57] Tetracycline prevented steatosis in dogs,[161] and removal of the excluded loop in rats decreased liver toxicity.[232] In humans, treatment with metronidazole resulted in clinical and histologic improvement independent of protein-calorie malnutrition effects.[52] Bacterial overgrowth in the bypass segment could help to explain the hepatic necrosis and fibrosis that sometimes develop.

Patients with progressive liver disease after bypass surgery have morphologic changes beyond fatty liver. The most consistent other feature is increased fibrosis with foamy degeneration of hepatocytes (see Fig. 30-7). This change appears to varying degrees (27% to 49% of cases)[84,170] but becomes almost universal when frank cirrhosis occurs.[170] Alcoholic hyalin has been found, with severe progressive hepatic disease[170] and neutrophil infiltration. When progressive hepatic disease develops, reversal of the bypass is necessary.[82] Criteria for reversal include the onset of icterus and prolongation of prothrombin time. Oral amino acid supplementation[129] or parenteral alimentation[6,8] is probably advisable before reanastomosis is performed, especially if the patient is severely ill. Although most hepatic failure develops in the first 24 months after bypass, occasionally patients present at a later time with a change in hepatic function. The finding of steatosis at that time, by itself, does not imply progressive fibrosis or impending hepatic failure. If the patient is otherwise doing well, continued surveillance with periodic biopsy is indicated.

Gastric Partitioning. Gastric partitioning is the process of altering the stomach by either complete partitioning in gastric bypass or by partial partitioning in gastroplasty. Gastric bypass was first performed in 1969[141] as an alternative to jejunoileal bypass. The procedure is a modification of the Billroth II procedure, leaving a small functional residual pouch, about 10% of the stomach, connected to the jejunum by a gastroenterostomy. Gastric bypass is associated with significant postoperative complications, but weight loss results are similar to jejunoileal bypass, and the long-term complications are less serious than with jejunoileal bypass.[1] The long-term sequelae of this procedure have not been evaluated, but there have been no reports of hepatic failure.[1]

Gastroplasty is similar to gastric bypass, but the partitioning is achieved by partial stapling of the upper portion of the stomach, which allows food to pass through at a much slower rate to the distal stomach, and no gastroenterostomy is performed. The most common complications are staple-line disruption and emesis.[1] Most gastroplasty patients do not have hepatic complications, but severe hepatic damage resembling alcoholic hepatitis complicated by ascites and coagulopathy has been reported.[83] This patient was administered hyperalimentation, and reversal of gastroplasty was performed,

resulting in normalization of liver tests and resolution of ascites.

Obesity

The frequency of fatty liver in obese patients is well recognized and ranges from 66% to 99% of cases.[42,95] In general, steatosis and steatohepatitis are more frequent in obese women than obese men, but it is unclear if this is related to a hormonal effect or because women are more often obese than men in study populations.[236] Enhanced fatty acid synthesis and altered partition of fatty acids between oxidation and esterification are the major causes of hypersecretion of triglyceride-rich lipoprotein in genetically obese rats.[7] Presumably, hepatic accumulation of triglyceride exceeds secretion rate. Fatty liver may also be related to an increase in free fatty acid supply from the peripheral fat depots. As the mass of adipose tissue increases, free fatty acid release increases. These substrates diminish glucose utilization and increase serum glucose concentrations. Insulin secretion is stimulated and thus tends to lower free fatty acid levels. Although insulin decreases the rate of release of free fatty acids per kilogram of adipose tissue, the increased mass of adipose tissue overcomes this regulatory effect. Thus, insulin resistance and increased supply of free fatty acids may be secondary to the increased adipose tissue mass.[61]

Most obese patients with fatty liver have abnormal glucose tolerance tests but are not severely diabetic (see section on diabetes mellitus). Mildly elevated AST and alkaline phosphatase levels are the most frequent abnormal result of liver function tests.[136] Liver biopsy has revealed, in addition to fat, periportal inflammation and fibrosis and occasional areas of necrosis[2] (see Fig. 30-6). In obese patients, the frequency of fibrosis may be as high as 10% to 30%,[31] and the frequency of cirrhosis is 1% to 3%.[236] In most cases, the fat is diffusely distributed, but in milder cases, it is centrilobular.[224] In early studies, no clear correlation between the degree of obesity and the amount of hepatic fat[224] was apparent. Recent data suggest there is a correlation between obesity and steatosis and that the degree of obesity correlated with the degree of steatosis.[236] Although one long-term follow-up of nonalcoholic, nondiabetic patients revealed no progression from fatty liver to cirrhosis,[88] a larger, more recent study suggests that obese patients have an increased incidence of fibrosis and cirrhosis.[236]

Diabetes Mellitus

Fatty liver occurs in diabetic patients, but the etiology and the importance attached to the observation remain unclear. Most of the diabetic patients with fatty liver are obese women with adult onset diabetes. Hepatomegaly occurs frequently in untreated diabetic patients (both type I and II) but does not always mean fatty infiltration. Diabetes mellitus occurs in 4% to 46% of patients with fatty liver, with an average of 25%.[42] It does not matter whether the diabetes is chemical or overt. On the other hand, about half of patients with diabetes have fatty liver.[42,106,119] In addition, 50% to 80% of adult-onset diabetic patients are obese, and fatty liver was found at autopsy in 51% of patients with diabetic ketoacidosis. It appears that obesity is the major factor in the fatty infiltration seen in adult-onset diabetes and not the diabetes mellitus itself. Fatty liver is uncommon (4.5% of patients) in insulin-deficient juvenile diabetic patients.[225] The incidence of fatty liver in diabetic patients over age 60 is about 45%.[225]

No correlation exists between the degree of control or duration of the diabetes and the fatty infiltration. In about 75% of cases, the fat is either centrilobular or diffuse in distribution.[85]

It is possible that decreased glucose tolerance in some patients with fatty liver is a consequence of the hepatic involvement. After alcohol withdrawal, abnormal glucose tolerance and fatty liver have both been seen to disappear. Other primary liver diseases can also be associated with abnormal glucose tolerance. Certainly, if fat in the liver is significant in a stable, adult diabetic patient, causes other than the diabetes should be sought.

The presence of hepatic steatosis has little effect on the prognosis of the diabetes mellitus. Treatment should include weight reduction with a low-carbohydrate, high-protein diet. Insulin therapy alone is of little value in the steatosis of adult-onset diabetes.

Acute Fatty Liver of Pregnancy

Acute fatty liver of pregnancy is a serious hepatocellular dysfunction of unknown etiology that typically occurs in the third trimester or puerperium, with an estimated incidence of 1 in 10,000 pregnancies. The major differential diagnoses are preeclampsia or eclampsia and fulminant viral hepatitis. The laboratory and pathologic features clearly distinguish these syndromes. AFLP has been diagnosed with increasing frequency during the past 20 years, probably related to the recognition of less severe cases. About half of cases are nulliparous, and 20% have associated preeclampsia. The disorder occurs with increased frequency in twin gestations and with male fetuses.[192] Previously, intravenous tetracycline was associated with the disorder, but the cause of most cases are unknown.[114] Typically, patients present with nonspecific complaints of nausea, anorexia, headache, and right upper quadrant pain; however, pruritus is distinctly unusual and should raise suspicion of the more common gestational disorder of intrahepatic cholestasis of pregnancy.[238] Hematemesis may result from mucosal ulcerations of the esophagus or stomach and is aggravated by coagulation defects. The liver is frequently not palpable.

Laboratory features include moderate transaminitis with AST and ALT levels ranging from 300 to 500 IU/L, hyperbilirubinemia, leukocytosis, hyperuricemia, and hypoglycemia.[192] CT and ultrasound may demonstrate increased echogenicity of the liver, but no study is diagnostic, and normal studies do not exclude the diagnosis.[238] Grossly, the liver is small and yellow. The pathologic examination shows microvesicular steatosis deposited first centrally, then spreading through the entire lobule. The fat is best demonstrated by oil red O stain. Other microscopic features include intrahepatic cholestasis and cytoplasmic ballooning; electron microscopy shows enlarged, needle-shaped mitochondria that contain crystalline inclusions and dilated smooth endoplasmic reticulum.[192] Multiple organ systems may be involved (pancreas, kidney, intestine), and fat may be found in these organs. The mechanism of AFLP is unknown.

Patient management is supportive and requires prompt delivery of the fetus, although the disease may progress for 2 to 5 days after delivery.[215] In earlier times, most infants were stillborn,[104] and maternal mortality was high; since 1980, maternal mortality rates have dropped to near 20%,[107] and fetal survival has also improved. Fetal distress is common, possibly because of uteroplacental insufficiency associated with the administration of fresh frozen plasma and platelets to manage disseminated intravascular coagulopathy.[148] Liver transplantation for AFLP has been reported.[162] Before 1991, no well-documented case of recurrent AFLP had been described. The disorder was not believed to occur in successive pregnancies, and a review of 21 patients with prior AFLP had a total of 25 subsequent uncomplicated pregnancies.[238] In 1991, however, a case was described of two successive pregnancies complicated by AFLP, and both infants succumbed to an ill-defined disorder of fatty acid oxidation.[209]

Drugs

Triglyceride Accumulation

CORTICOSTEROIDS. In Cushing's syndrome, moderate to severe fatty infiltration of the liver is reported commonly.[216] Moreover, fatty liver has been reported in patients receiving high doses of exogenous steroids over a period of weeks. In animals, plasma free fatty acids increase when high doses of cortisol are given,[89] suggesting that increased mobilization of fatty acid is involved. In one study using low doses of steroids, however, all the increase in fatty acids can be accounted for by a decreased esterification of fatty acids in the liver.[101] Clinically, fatty liver occurs only with high doses of steroids. Systemic fat embolism has been reported after abrupt cessation of steroid therapy,[90,103] and fatty liver has been implicated as a possible source. Despite this rare association, corticosteroids can usually be continued in the face of fatty liver. A common clinical dilemma is the finding of fatty liver in a patient receiving corticosteroids for an underlying disorder that ordinarily does not cause fatty liver (eg, for autoimmune chronic active hepatitis). In such a setting, factors other than corticosteroids are often considered as part of the differential diagnosis when corticosteroids are an adequate explanation for the steatosis.

METHOTREXATE. Methotrexate is a folic acid antagonist used in the management of many oncologic, dermatologic, and rheumatologic diseases. Side effects may include minor gastrointestinal and mucocutaneous toxic effects, idiosyncratic pulmonary hypersensitivity, and hepatic fibrosis. Appreciation of its hepatic toxicity was complicated by the high incidence of pretreatment for liver lesions, especially among those consuming excess alcohol. The mechanisms of methotrexate hepatotoxicity include its action as an indirect cytotoxic hepatotoxin due to reversible inhibition of dihydrofolate reductase; the steatogenic effect is attributed to its interference with the synthesis of methionine and choline.[121] Clinically, patients frequently have no specific symptoms. The histologic pattern is one of macrovesicular steatosis and hepatocellular necrosis in a portal and periportal distribution. The fibrosis may progress to cirrhosis.[121] Prospective studies in psoriatic patients demonstrated significant fibrosis and cirrhosis in one quarter of patients receiving cumulative doses greater than 2 g over a period of more than 5 years.[121] The effects are dose-related and can be minimized if the drug dose is adjusted to the lowest effective level.[44]

Factors associated with methotrexate toxicity include preexisting liver disease, daily methotrexate dosing, renal insufficiency or failure, and active or recent alcohol abuse. No clear association with injury has been found for age, gender, human leukocyte antigen status, extent of psoriasis, previous or concurrent steroids, obesity alone, or diabetes alone. Factors that may be associated with toxicity but that have not been adequately evaluated include patients with both obesity and diabetes mellitus, prior treatment with arsenicals, hypoalbuminemia, and the duration of treatment greater than 2 years or cumulative dose greater than 1500 mg.[121]

Liver function tests are not sensitive enough to detect hepatotoxicity. Hypoalbuminemia is the best predictor of hepatic fibrosis.[222] Unfortunately, ultrasonographic evaluation is not usually helpful and cannot be used to distinguish fatty change and fibrosis.[41] Therefore, liver biopsy is recommended to reliably diagnose hepatotoxicity. The American Academy of Dermatology[190] recommends premethotrexate liver biopsy and repeat biopsy after 1500 mg, with subsequent biopsies after every 1000 to 1500 mg. In patients with rheumatoid arthritis, the Health and Public Policy Committee of the American College of Physicians[87] recommends methotrexate only for those refractory to other agents and no known risk factors for toxicity. Further, pretreatment biopsies are recommended only for those patients with known or suspected preexisting liver disease with monthly liver enzymes during therapy. Biopsies during treatment should be considered at 2- to 3-year intervals or after every 1500 mg.

Development of hepatotoxicity, as manifest by inflammation, fibrosis, or cirrhosis, should be a relative contraindication to continued use of the drug. Liver enzyme abnormalities may improve after discontinuation of methotrexate, but this can take several weeks.[121] The reported histologic course after withdrawal of methotrexate has been variable, so it is not always evident that the drug must be stopped if the clinical benefit to continued use is great.

VALPROIC ACID. Valproic acid is a branched medium-chain fatty acid that is used in the treatment of petit mal epilepsy. Although overt liver damage is uncommon, fatal hepatotoxicity does occur[223,246] and is estimated at 0.01% of newly treated patients.[74] Children are more frequently affected than adults.[244] The incidence of hepatic abnormalities peaks at 2 to 4 months after the onset of therapy but may occur within weeks or after more than 4 months.[246] Many patients with reported toxicity were taking other anticonvulsants as well. Clinical symptoms in severe cases commonly include lethargy, anorexia, nausea, generalized edema with facial puffiness; less commonly, fever, ascites, or jaundice may be noted. Laboratory abnormalities may include elevations in serum transaminases; bilirubin; alkaline phosphatase; leukocytosis with neutrophilia, but not eosinophilia; and in severe cases, hypoglycemia, hypoalbuminemia, and prolonged prothrombin time indicative of hepatic failure.[246] Liver histology characteristically shows centrilobular necrosis with microvesicular steatosis,[223,246] but bile duct injury and submassive necrosis have been seen.[223] Recovery is usually spontaneous when the drug is withdrawn, but in severe cases of advanced liver failure, hepatic transplantation may be indicated. Because the liver disease associated with valproic acid is so severe, the drug is usually stopped when evidence of liver injury is detected.

The rare occurrence of severe hepatic disease in proportion to the number of patients taking valproic acid suggests idiosyncratic susceptibility rather than intrinsic toxicity.[246] Clinical features typically associated with hypersensitivity, including rash and eosinophilia, are absent in this disease. The etiology of the liver damage is unknown. The drug might be converted into an analogue of 4-pentanoic acid, an agent that causes derangements similar to hypoglycin A (ie, impaired fatty acid oxidation and decreased available CoA and carnitine, along with fine droplets of fat in hepatocytes). A hypoglycin metabolite is the cause of Jamaican vomiting sickness, another disorder associated with small droplets of hepatocyte lipid.

TETRACYCLINE. The administration of large intravenous doses (more than 2 g/d) of tetracycline and its derivatives is associated with a fine, fatty vacuolization of the liver. This injury has also been seen with oral administration and in any setting in which the blood levels of tetracycline are unusually high.[169] A few cases have been reported using parenteral doses of only 1 g/d, so that during pregnancy, an upper limit of 1 g/d should be used. The dose-related aspect of tetracycline is important because the fear of fatty liver should not prevent the indicated use of tetracycline or its derivatives in lower doses. Many early cases occurred when tetracycline, which is excreted primarily in the urine, was given to patients with renal dysfunction. This condition usually has been seen in pregnant women but has been reported in nonpregnant females and males. In either case, the pathology is similar to that seen in fatty metamorphosis of pregnancy. A number of cases of fatty liver have been reported in association with tetracycline administration during pregnancy.[51] The fatty liver was reversible when tetracycline was discontinued.

Tetracycline inhibits protein synthesis and impairs triglyceride secretion when used in large doses, but mechanisms other than impaired hepatic VLDL output probably are also responsible for tetracycline-induced fatty liver.[17] The drug inhibits mitochondrial β-oxidation, and this increases substrate concentration for triglyceride synthesis.[66] Moreover, tetracycline appears to interfere with the association of triglycerides and apoproteins to form lipoproteins.[45]

Pathologically, the fatty accumulation is localized to the central and mid-zonal areas, with fine, foamy infiltration of the cell, and to the nucleus of the hepatocyte in the center,[37] not pushed to the edge as is seen with alcoholic fatty liver. Necrosis is uncommon.

About 75% of the reported patients have died, but it is important to recognize that death was probably the reason for the case report. In a typical case, 3 to 12 days after tetracycline has been given, there is an abrupt onset of jaundice, nausea, and vomiting, spontaneous delivery, renal failure, gastrointestinal bleeding, coma, and finally death 1 to 2 weeks after the first dose of tetracycline. The laboratory findings and pathology in tetracycline-induced fatty liver are similar to those in fatty metamorphosis of pregnancy, except that jaundice is not so common. Leukocytosis, lactic acidosis, and rising blood urea nitrogen, bilirubin, and AST usually occur. Fewer than half of patients develop a high AST of more than 400 IU/L.[37] Some patients have recovered, but only when the tetracycline administration was stopped.

SALICYLATES. Salicylate intoxication (more than 120 mg/kg) can cause a variety of toxicities, including respiratory alkalosis with metabolic acidosis, hypoglycemia, hyperglycemia, cerebral edema, coma, and death.[164] Hepatotoxicity is primarily manifested as nausea, vomiting, anorexia, and abdominal pain; however, patients are usually asymptomatic. Most salicylate toxicity has been reported with aspirin, but other salicylate agents have also been implicated. Additionally, salicylates have been implicated in the pathogenesis of Reye's syndrome (see section on Reye's syndrome). Hepatic fat predominantly has been described in salicylate-associated cases of Reye's syndrome. In the adult population, however, the association of salicylate hepatotoxicity and rheumatologic disorders, such as rheumatoid arthritis, has been made. Fat is not usually a prominent feature of salicylate hepatotoxicity in this population.[26] Laboratory abnormalities include AST elevations (from normal to more than 2000 IU/L) in most patients, slight prolongation of prothrombin time in about 10% of patients, and only rarely is hyperbilirubinemia seen with only 3% of patients with bilirubin levels higher than 2.5 mg/dL. In most cases, enzymes return to normal with cessation of therapy, but recurrence has been shown after rechallenge. Hepatic damage has been correlated with salicylate levels, which are over 15 mg/dL in 90% of patients with evidence of hepatic injury. The damage typically occurs between 5 and 60 days after initiation of therapy and is believed to be the result of the formation of a salicylate moiety that is an intrinsic hepatotoxin. Pathologic examination shows focal cellular necrosis, inflammatory infiltrate, and rarely, chronic active hepatitis.[26]

Phospholipid Accumulation

AMIODARONE. Amiodarone is an iodinated benzofuran derivative prescribed in the treatment of angina and cardiac arrhythmia refractory to other medications. Several side effects have been reported, including pulmonary fibrosis, peripheral neuropathy, thyroid dysfunction, ocular and cutaneous manifestations, as well as hepatotoxicity. Hepatotoxicity may range from mild transaminitis, occurring in 3% to 50% of patients,[151] acute hepatitis, and most commonly, chronic lesions resembling alcoholic liver disease.[78] Marked cholestasis and hyperbilirubinemia occur occasionally.[151]

By light microscopy, liver biopsy specimens usually resemble alcoholic hepatitis, with macrovesicular steatosis, Mallory's bodies with surrounding polymorphonuclear leukocytes, and a mixed inflammatory infiltrate surrounding bile ducts. Micronodular cirrhosis has been described.[176] By electron microscopy, prominent round to oval, irregularly shaped lysosomal inclusions are seen that show lamellar myelin figures consistent with high phospholipid content.[176] Some patients have phospholipidosis without pseudoalcoholic liver disease changes, suggesting the two may be independent phenomena.[78] Additionally, pleomorphic mitochondria have been observed.[176]

Amiodarone and its major metabolite, N-desethylamiodarone, may be detectable in tissues months after discontinuing therapy. It is unclear if the injury is dose related, and variable reversibility has been reported. Patients on amiodarone should have transaminases monitored, and liver biopsy should be considered in those patients with persistent abnormalities.[151,176,213] Patients on therapy who have liver biopsies consistent with amiodarone toxicity should have the drug discontinued. Because amiodarone is generally prescribed in refractory cardiac cases, however, patients and clinicians may be faced with balancing malignant arrhythmia and angina against the risk of liver disease.

PERHEXILINE MALEATE. Perhexiline maleate is an antianginal drug not presently available in the United States that has been reported to produce elevated transaminase levels in 24% to 50% of treated patients.[167] Symptoms may include jaundice, encephalopathy, ascites, and a peripheral neuropathy. Liver biopsy shows lesions similar to alcoholic hepatitis, including fat, necrosis, and alcoholic hyalin.[177] Electron microscopy demonstrates enlarged lysosomes containing myeloid figures[167] consistent with phospholipid. Despite discontinuing medication in patients, unresolved inflammation or inactive cirrhosis was demonstrated months

later.[167] Because the drug causes changes in total liver gangliosides, its effects may be related to a drug-induced defect in glycolipid metabolism.[91]

Toxins

Jamaican Vomiting Sickness. Jamaican vomiting sickness results from the ingestion of unripe fruit from the ackee tree. The ingestion produces symptoms within 2 to 3 hours associated with profound hypoglycemia, vomiting, coma, and, biochemically, a depletion of hepatic glycogen, increased plasma free fatty acids, and an accumulation of triglyceride in the liver. The primary mechanism of action of hypoglycin, the toxic component of the ackee fruit, is the inhibition of branched-chain fatty acid oxidation and gluconeogenesis. Several antidotes have been used for this poisoning, including glucose, carnitine, riboflavin, glycine, and clofibrate.[212]

Phosphorus. Of the three forms of elemental phosphorus, only yellow phosphorus is appreciably toxic to the liver. It is a common component of many roach and rat poisons. After ingestion, frequently a burning sensation is felt in the mouth and throat. Abdominal pain and vomiting of violent nature follow. Within 1 or 2 days, jaundice appears, and death can occur fairly rapidly. A fatal dose for humans is about 60 mg. Most patients recover in 1 to 3 days or progress to a syndrome of generalized toxicity, involving liver, kidney, heart, and central nervous system.[62]

The mechanism of action of phosphorus and halogenated hydrocarbons is similar.[47] Hepatic protein (and apolipoprotein) synthesis is impaired, leading to decreases protein secretion. This can lead to a bleeding tendency and may account for the only moderate serum transaminase levels in some cases. In addition, these substances are potent generalized toxins and produce cellular damage and inflammatory lesions. If recovery occurs, liver histology and function return to normal.

Pathologically, the liver shows periportal necrosis and fat at early times, with the center of the lobule relatively spared. With severe poisoning, the entire liver is rapidly involved. Gastric lavage within 6 hours of ingestion is the treatment of choice.

Chlorinated Hydrocarbons. The chlorinated hydrocarbons are an infrequent cause of hepatotoxicity in the United States, but their potential toxicity is a significant environmental and industrial concern. Although the chlorinated hydrocarbons can cause hepatotoxicity and fatty liver, it is important to remember the confounding variables of diabetes mellitus, obesity, and alcohol (as well as other potential causes of abnormal liver tests) in patients being evaluated for accidental or occupational exposure to these agents.

Carbon tetrachloride has attracted more attention in recent years as an experimental hepatotoxin than as a course of fatty liver in humans. Its former presence in fire extinguishers and cleaning fluids made it available for toxicity in humans. In recent years, most commercial preparations that once contained carbon tetrachloride now contain another chlorinated hydrocarbon, trichloroethylene, which also has excellent solvent properties. Hepatotoxicity due to this solvent is much rarer than with carbon tetrachloride.[33,234] Chronic use has been reported to result in hepatitis, renal failure, myocarditis, or cranial nerve palsies. Ethanol potentiates the hepatic effects. Chronic liver disease due to these compounds has never been reported in the absence of ethanol use.

Trichloroethylene is usually inhaled but may be ingested accidentally. Clinically, trichloroethylene often produces dizziness, nausea, vomiting, and headache as early symptoms. The time of onset depends on the dose. A burning sensation in the mouth, esophagus, and stomach is often present soon after ingestion. Subsequently, abdominal cramps, confusion, decreased consciousness, delirium, restlessness, choreiform movements, muscle pain, diarrhea, vasomotor collapse, and even coma may ensue. Neither jaundice nor hepatomegaly need occur, even after ingestion, and deaths have been reported without much evidence of liver failure. When death occurs, it is usually the result of respiratory muscle paralysis, pulmonary edema, or cardiac or renal involvement.

Laboratory data usually reveal elevated transaminases, prolongation of the prothrombin time, and normal or slightly elevated alkaline phosphatase levels. Hepatic pathology shows mild fatty change, often mid-zonal, with centrilobular necrosis. Many acute inflammatory cells are present, especially in the centrilobular areas. The fat may be present in cells as fine vacuoles or large cysts. Treatment is only supportive.

Systemic Diseases With Fatty Liver

TRIGLYCERIDE

As stated previously, fatty liver is commonly found on liver biopsy in patients with and without intrinsic liver disease. This results from the fact that fatty acid flux from adipose tissue to liver is constantly changing, and the hepatic uptake depends on their rate of delivery. Because the capacity of the liver to oxidize, esterify, and secrete fatty acid in the form of VLDL is limited, accumulation often occurs. The presence of conditions such as diabetes mellitus or corticosteroid or alcohol ingestion may be superimposed on systemic illnesses that produce hepatic fat accumulation. By itself, fatty liver tells nothing of the other functional capacities of the liver.

Primary Liver Disease

In distinction from other forms of viral hepatitis, non-A, non-B hepatitis[49] can produce microvesicular steatosis. The steatosis is not the most prominent histologic feature, however, and other findings of inflammatory infiltrate and cellular necrosis associated with viral hepatitis are also present. Moderate microvesicular fat can also be seen in Wilson's disease (see Chap. 25), especially in the early stages of the hepatic dysfunction.[221] In these stages, the cells can appear pleomorphic, but no other distinctive biopsy changes may be seen, so that microvesicular fat in young people without obvious cause should raise the suspicion of Wilson's disease. Definitive diagnosis may require quantitative copper measurement on biopsy specimens.

Inflammatory Bowel Disease

Fat accumulation has been found in livers from patients with both ulcerative colitis and Crohn's disease, with a prevalence ranging from 0% to 80%. The fat is primarily macrovesicular with a diffuse distribution. The cause of the fatty liver is multifactorial. Many patients are malnourished and chronically ill. The incidence in livers seen at autopsy is higher than at biopsy but is also higher than in patients dying from other diseases.[152] Thus, malnutrition probably is not the sole cause.

Many patients are taking corticosteroids, but other patients have had fatty liver while not receiving corticosteroids. Alcohol ingestion remains a possible factor, and no study has addressed this issue. The possibility of some absorbed bacterial toxin has been suggested; however, the frequency of fatty liver was the same after colectomy for ulcerative colitis as before resection. Generally, patients are asymptomatic from fatty liver itself, but fatty liver may occur with other hepatic lesions. Thus, abnormal laboratory tests and symptoms usually cannot be attributed to fatty liver alone. (See Chapter 44 for further discussion and references.) Total parenteral nutrition, if used, can also lead to fatty liver (see section on parenteral alimentation).

Parenteral Alimentation

Elevated serum AST, alkaline phosphatase, and bilirubin levels have been observed along with occasional pathologic evidence of fatty liver during intravenous alimentation.[102] Cholestasis and periportal inflammation have been found along with fatty changes.[211] Cholestasis with mild fibrosis has also been seen in children. In adult patients, fatty metamorphosis is associated most commonly with excessive caloric infusion (4000 to 6000 kcal) for over 6 weeks.[135] In this case, the calorie/nitrogen ratio may be excessive, and hepatic fatty acid synthesis may outstrip the ability of the liver to secrete lipids (see section on protein-calorie malnutrition). In animals, parenteral feeding causes steatosis by enhanced hepatic synthesis of fatty acid and reduced triglyceride secretion.[80] Rarely, essential fatty acid deficiency secondary to prolonged intravenous feeding may cause fatty metamorphosis. In children, steatosis is found commonly with premature infants or in the presence of infection or intrinsic liver disease. When protein malnutrition is the cause of the steatosis, as in obese patients after bypass surgery, treatment with parenteral nutrition actually causes a decrease in hepatic fat.

Human Immunodeficiency Virus

Up to 80% of liver biopsy specimens from patients with acquired immunodeficiency syndrome (AIDS) demonstrate a spectrum of histopathologic abnormalities.[59] Among the common nonspecific hepatic abnormalities is macrovesicular steatosis, which may be present in up to half of all specimens.[105,208] Serum alkaline phosphatase is typically elevated[139] but does not help to distinguish fatty infiltration or steatohepatitis from many other hepatic disorders that may affect AIDS patients. Factors that may contribute to the steatosis include malnutrition, profound weight loss, total parenteral nutrition, or alcohol abuse.[139] Proposed mechanisms of fatty liver in AIDS patients relate to these factors and well as to increased activity of cachectin and tissue necrosis factor.[77]

Hepatic Resection

After a two-thirds hepatic resection in animals, steatosis develops almost immediately.[12] Hepatic lipid increases two-fold within 10 hours, the majority being triglyceride. In humans, the serum triglyceride, phospholipid, and cholesterol levels all fall acutely after resection and recover within 2 to 3 weeks.[4] The marked decrease is presumably due to impaired synthesis and release of lipoproteins by the liver. Although jaundice often occurs postoperatively, there is no indication of any functional impairment due to steatosis. Moreover, the steatosis has been more apparent in experimental animals than in humans, in whom its demonstration has been limited by the availability of biopsy material within the immediate postoperative period.

Primary Nonfunction of Hepatic Allografts

With the expanding number of patients with acute and chronic liver failure, hepatic transplantation has become an effective therapy. Unfortunately, waiting recipients exceed the donor liver supply. Primary nonfunction of hepatic allografts is a relatively infrequent occurrence, but requires re-transplantation. Although the major causes of primary nonfunction are believed to be intraoperative injury of the allograft, ischemic injury, or humoral rejection, recent reports suggest preexisting fatty infiltration may be responsible for a proportion of primary nonfunction cases.[179,227] In these cases, livers were grossly yellow, enlarged, and greasy. Microscopically, macrovesicular steatosis was present, but no evidence of inflammatory infiltrate or vascular thrombosis was evident. The proposed mechanism of primary nonfunction was the rupture of hepatocytes with the release of globules into the hepatic microcirculation, leading to destruction and malfunction of hepatocytes.[227]

Diseases of Infancy and Childhood

Weber-Christian Disease.   Weber-Christian disease is a panniculitis of unknown etiology that predominantly affects females. It is associated with relapsing fevers, crops of subcutaneous nodules, and in some cases, hepatic pathology. Fatty change, portal fibrosis, and Mallory's bodies have been described[109]; however, normal hepatic parenchyma with extrahepatic portal hypertension and bleeding varices also have been noted.[18]

Reye's Syndrome.   Reye's syndrome was originally described in 1963 by Reye as a condition of unknown etiology occurring in children and characterized by a viral prodrome, vomiting, and progressive hepatic failure.[188] Although unusual in adulthood, 2% of reported cases of Reye's syndrome are patients over 20 years of age. Clinically, 90% of patients have an antecedent viral infection, and 95% of patients have ingested aspirin. The viral prodrome is followed by vomiting and the onset of encephalopathy, frequently within 72 hours. Patients may have hepatomegaly but are rarely jaundiced. Laboratory abnormalities are typical of acute hepatic failure with transaminitis, hypoglycemia, and prolonged prothrombin time. Histologically, there is a microvesicular steatosis due to triglycerides with glycogen depletion. Endoplasmic reticulum may be proliferated, and mitochondria are swollen. Mitochondrial enzyme abnormalities are characteristic, while cytosolic enzyme function is preserved. In those patients with spontaneous recovery, liver abnormalities resolve completely within 2 weeks.[164]

Galactosemia.   Galactosemia is an inborn error of metabolism resulting from either complete loss of galactose-1-phosphate uridyl transferase enzyme activity or variants of enzyme with variable activity. Clinically, infants exhibit failure to thrive, hepatosplenomegaly, and cataracts with retarded psychomotor and mental development. Galactose-free diets can prevent symptoms, but even small amounts of galactose can lead to cirrhosis, which has been associated with the development of hepatocellular carcinoma.[165]

Fructose Intolerance.   Hereditary fructose intolerance results from a deficiency of fructose-1 phosphate aldolase. This deficiency produces fatty metamorphosis, variable fibrosis, and can lead to cirrhosis. In the early stages, fatty change is typical and may be associated with cholestasis and pseudogland formation.[97]

Abetalipoproteinemia.   Abetalipoproteinemia is an autosomal recessive disorder characterized by severe hypolipemia due to a lack of plasmatic Apo B. Serum chemistries demonstrate low levels of chylomicrons, LDL, and VLDL, which in turn results in the clinical malabsorption of fat and fat-soluble vitamins.[222] Abnormalities in hepatic histology may include predominantly macrovesicular and some microvesicular steatosis, fibrosis, micronodular cirrhosis, and abnormal hepatic peroxisomes.[36]

PHOSPHOLIPID OR CHOLESTEROL

Wolman's Disease

Wolman's disease is a rare lipidosis of infancy inherited in an autosomal recessive pattern that is frequently fatal in the first year of life. Wolman's disease is caused by a deficiency in lysosomal acid lipase, which catalyzes the hydrolysis of triglycerides and cholesterol. This deficiency results in the abnormal storage of cholesterol esters and triglycerides in the histiocytes of various organs. Clinically, infants present with failure to thrive, hepatosplenomegaly, and abdominal distention. Histologically, lipid-laden histiocytes are seen.[146]

Cholesterol Ester Storage Disease

Cholesterol ester storage disease is a milder form of lysosomal acid lipase deficiency (see section on Wolman's disease). The clinical course is more benign, and patients survive to adulthood.[146] An association exists between cholesterol ester storage disease and type II hyperlipidemia. Because of a variable clinical presentation in adults, liver biopsy is usually needed for diagnosis.[55]

References

1. Adibi SA, Stanko RT. Perspectives on gastrointestinal surgery for treatment of morbid obesity: the lesson learned. Gastroenterology 87:1381, 1984
2. Adler M, Schaffner F. Fatty liver hepatitis and cirrhosis in obese patients. Am J Med 67:811, 1979
3. Ahmad M, et al. Xenon-133 retention in hepatic steatosis: correlation with liver biopsy in 45 patients. J Nucl Med 20:397, 1979
4. Almersjo O, et al. Serum lipids after extensive liver resection in man. Acta Hepatosplen 15:1, 1968
5. Alpers DH, et al. Distribution of apolipoproteins A-I and B among intestinal lipoproteins. J Lipid Res 26:1, 1985
6. Ames FC, Copeland E, Leib D, et al. Liver dysfunction following small bowel bypass for obesity. JAMA 235:1249, 1976
7. Azain MJ, Fukuda N, Chai FF, et al. Contributions of fatty acid and sterol synthesis to triglyceride and cholesterol secretion by the perfused rat liver in genetic hyperlipidemia and obesity. J Biol Chem 260:174, 1985
8. Baker AL, Elson CO, Gaspan J, et al. Liver failure with steatonecrosis after jejunoileal bypass. Arch Intern Med 239:239, 1979
9. Ballard H, et al. Fatty liver presenting as obstructive jaundice. Am J Med 30:196, 1961

10. Baraona E, et al. Effects of ethanol on lipid metabolism. J Lipid Res 20:289, 1979

11. Batman PA, Scheuer PJ. Diabetic hepatitis preceding the onset of glucose intolerance. Histopathology 9:237, 1985

12. Bengmark S. Liver steatosis and liver resection. Digestion 2:304, 1969

13. Bhathal PS, et al. The spectrum of liver disease in an Australian teaching hospital: a prospective study of 205 patients. Med J Aust 2:1085, 1973

14. Bisgaeir CL, Glickman RM. Intestinal secretion and transport of lipoproteins. Ann Rev Physiol 45:625, 1983

15. Blaufuss MC, Gordon JI, Scholfeld G, et al. Biosynthesis of apolipoprotein C-III in rat liver and small intestinal mucosa. J Biol Chem 259:2452, 1984

16. Brawer MK, Austin GE, Lauren KJ. Focal fatty change of the liver: a hitherto poorly recognized entity. Gastroenterology 78:247, 1980

17. Brean KJ, et al. Fatty liver induced by tetracycline in the rat. Gastroenterology 69:714, 1975

18. Broe PJ, Kelly CJ, Bouchier-Hayes DJ. Systemic Weber-Christian disease with portal hypertension and oesophageal varices. J R Soc Med 81:669, 1988

19. Brown MS, Goldstein JL. A receptor-mediated pathway for cholesterol homeostasis. Science 232:34, 1986

20. Brown MS, Goldstein JL. Lipoprotein receptors in the liver: control signals for plasma cholesterol traffic. J Clin Invest 72:743, 1983

21. Brugerera M, Borda JM, Rodes J. Asymptomatic liver disease in alcoholics. Arch Pathol Lab Med 101:644, 1977

22. Cahill GF Jr. Starvation in man. N Engl J Med 282:668, 1970

23. Campagnari-Visconti L, et al. Inhibition by glucose of the ethionine-induced fatty liver. Proc Soc Exp Biol Med 111:479, 1962

24. Carithers RL, Herlong HF, Diehl AM, et al. Methylprednisolone therapy in patients with severe alcoholic hepatitis. Ann Intern Med 110:685, 1989

25. Carlson LA, et al. Some physiological and clinical implications of lipid mobilization from adipose tissue. In: Renold AE, Cahill GR Jr, eds. American Physiologic Society handbook of physiology. 5. Adipose tissue. Baltmore, Williams & Wilkins, 1965, p 625

26. Cersosimo RJ, Matthew SJ. Hepatotoxicity associated with choline magnesium trisalicylate: case report and review of salicylate-induced hepatotoxicity. Drug Intell Clin Pharm 21:621, 1987

27. Chajek R, et al. Effect of colchicine, cycloheximide, and chloroquine on the hepatic triacylglycerol hydrolase in the intact rat and perfused liver. Biochim Biophys Acta 488:270, 1977

28. Chan L. Hormonal control of gene expression. In: Arias IM, Schacter D, Shafritz DA, eds. The liver: biology and pathobiology. New York, Raven Press, 1982, pp 143–167

29. Chang L, Clifton P, Barter P, et al. High density lipoprotein subpopulations in chronic liver disease. Hepatology 6:46, 1986

30. Christofferson P, Braerstrup O, Juhl E, et al. Lipogranulomas in human liver biopsies with fatty change: a morphological, biochemical and clinical investigation. Acta Pathol Microbiol Scand 79:150, 1971

31. Clain DJ, Lefkowitch, JH. Fatty liver disease in morbid obesity. Gastroenterol Clin North Am 16:239, 1987

32. Claude A. Growth and differentiation of cytoplasmic membranes in the course of lipoprotein granule synthesis in the hepatic cell. I. Elaboration of elements of the Golgi complex. J Cell Biol 47:745, 1970

33. Clearfield HR. Hepatorenal toxicity from sniffing spot remover (trichloroethylene). Am J Dig Dis 15:851, 1970

34. Cohen JA, Kaplan MM. The SGOT/SGPT ratio: an indicator of alcoholic liver disease. Dig Dis Sci 24:835, 1979

35. Coleman RW, Shein HM. Leukemoid reaction, hyperuricemia, and severe hyperpyrexia complicating a fatal case of acute fatty liver of the alcoholic. Ann Intern Med 57:110, 1962

36. Collins JC, Scheinber IH, Giblin DR, et al. Hepatic peroxisomal abnormalities in abetalipoproteinemia. Gastroenterology 97:766, 1989

37. Combes B, et al. Tetracycline and the liver. Prog Liver Dis 4:589, 1972

38. Composti M, et al. Studies on in vitro peroxidation of liver lipids in ethanol-treated rats. Lipids 8:498, 1973

39. Cooper A. Role of the liver in the degradation of lipoproteins. Gastroenterology 88:192, 1985

40. Cooper AD. The metabolism of chylomicron remnants by isolated perfused rat liver. Biochim Biophys Acta 488:464, 1977

41. Coulson IH, McKenzie J, Neild VS, et al. A comparison of liver ultrasound with liver biopsy histology in psoriatics receiving long-term methotrexate therapy. Br J Dermatol 116:491, 1987

42. Creutzfeldt W, et al. Liver diseases and diabetes mellitus. Prog Liver Dis 3:371, 1970

43. Czernobilsky B, Bergnes MA. Acute fatty metamorphosis of the liver in pregnancy with associated liver cell necrosis. Obstet Gynecol 26:792, 1965

44. Dahl MGC, Gregory MM, Scheuer PJ. Methotrexate hepatotoxicity in psoriasis: comparison of different dosage regimens. Br Med J 1:654, 1972

45. Deboyser D, Goethals F, Krack G, et al. Investigation into the mechanism of tetracycline-induced steatosis: study in isolated hepatocytes. Toxicol Appl Pharmacol 97:473, 1989

46. DeLint J, Schmidt W. Mortality from liver cirrhosis and other causes in alcoholics: a follow-up study of patients with and without a history of enlarged fatty liver. Q J Stud Alcohol 31:705, 1970

47. Dianzani MU. Biochemical aspects of fatty liver. In: Slater TF, ed. Biochemical mechanisms of liver injury. New York, Academic Press, 1978, pp 45–96

48. Diehl AM, Goodman Z, Ishak KG. Alcohol-like liver disease in nonalcoholics. Gastroenterology 95:1056, 1988

49. Dienes HP, Popper H, Arnold W, et al. Histologic observations in human hepatitis non A-non B. Hepatology 2:562, 1982

50. Domschke S, Domschke W, Lieber CS. Hepatic redox state: attenuation of the acute effects of ethanol induced by chronic ethanol consumption. Life Sci 15:1327, 1974

51. Dowling HF, Lepper MH. Hepatic reactions to tetracycline. JAMA 188:307, 1970

52. Drenick EJ, Fisler J, Johnson D. Hepatic steatosis after intestinal bypass: prevention and reversal by metronidazole, irrespective of protein-calorie malnutrition. Gastroenterology 82:535, 1982

53. Edmondson HA, et al. Sclerosing hyaline necrosis of the liver in the chronic alcoholic: a recognizable clinical syndrome. Ann Intern Med 59:656, 1963

54. Eisenberg S. High density lipoprotein metabolism. J Lipid Res 25:1017, 1984

55. Elleder M, Ledvinova J, Cieslar P, et al. Subclinical course of cholesterol ester storage disease (CESD) diagnosed in adulthood. Virchows Arch [A] 416:357, 1990

56. Faergeman O, et al. Metabolism of apoprotein B of plasma very low density lipoproteins in the rat. J Clin Invest 56:1396, 1975

57. Faloon WW, et al. Lithogenic and hepatotoxic potential in intestinal bypass. Gastroenterology 68:1073, 1975

58. Farber E, et al. Biochemical pathology of acute hepatic adenosine triphosphate deficit. Nature 203:34, 1964

59. Ferrell LD. Gastrointestinal pathology of AIDS. Semin Gastrointest Dis 2:37, 1991

60. Fielding PE, et al. Lipoprotein lipase: properties of the enzyme isolated from post-heparin plasma. Biochemistry 13:4318, 1977

61. Flatt JP. Role of the increased adipose tissue mass in the ap-

parent insulin insensitivity of obesity. Am J Clin Nutr 25:1189, 1972

62. Fletcher FG, Galambos JT. Phosphorus poisoning in humans. Arch Intern Med 112:846, 1963
63. Floren CH, et al. Binding, interiorization and degradation of cholesteryl ester–labelled chylomicron-remnant particles by rat hepatocyte monolayers. Biochem J 168:483, 1977
64. Flores H, et al. Lipid transport in kwashiokor. Br J Nutr 24:1005, 1970
65. Fredholm B, Russell S. Effect of adrenergic blocking agents on lipid mobilization from canine subcutaneous adipose tissue after sympathetic nerve stimulation. J Pharmacaol Exp Ther 159:1, 1968
66. Freneaux E, Labbe G, Letteron P, et al. Inhibition of the mitochondrial oxidation of fatty acids by tetracycline in mice and in man: possible role in microvesicular steatosis induced by this antibiotic. Hepatology 8:1056, 1988
67. Galambos J. Alcoholic hepatitis: its therapy and prognoses. Prog Liver Dis 4:567, 1972
68. Galambos JT, Wills CE. Relationship between 505 paired liver tests and biopsies in 242 obese patients. Gastroenterology 74:1191, 1978
69. Glickman RM, et al. The intestine as a source of apolipoprotein A1. Proc Natl Acad Sci USA 74:1569, 1977
70. Gibbons GF. Assembly and secretion of hepatic very-low-density lipoprotein. Biochem J 268:1, 1990
70a. Glickman RM, Glickman JN, Magun A, Brin M. Apolipoprotein synthesis in normal and abetalipoproteinemic intestinal mucosa. Gastroenterology 101:749, 1991
71. Goldstein JL, Kita T, Brown MS. Defective lipoprotein receptors and atherosclerosis. N Engl J Med 309:288, 1983
72. Gordon JI, Smith DP, Alpers DH, et al. Proteolytic processing of the primary translation product of rat intestinal apolipoprotein A-IV mRNA. J Biol Chem 257:8418, 1982
73. Graham M, Taketomi S, Fumno K, et al. Metabolic studies on the development of ethanol induced fatty liver in KK-A4 mice. J Nutr 105:1500, 1975
74. Granneman GR, Wan SI, Kesterson JW, et al. The hepatotoxicity of valproic acid and its metabolites in rats. II. Intermediary and valproic acid metabolism. Hepatology 4:1153, 1984
75. Green J, et al. Acute alcoholic hepatitis: a clinical study of 50 cases. Arch Intern Med 11:67, 1963
76. Green PHR, et al. Rat intestine secretes discoid high density lipoproteins. J Clin Invest 61:528, 1978
77. Grunfeld C, Kotler DP. The wasting syndrome and nutritional support in AIDS. Semin Gastrointest Dis 2:26, 1991
78. Guigue B, Perrot S, Berry JP, et al. Amiodarone-induced hepatic phospholipidosis: a morphological alteration independent of pseudoalcoholic liver disease. Hepatology 8:1063, 1988
79. Haines NW, Baker AL, Boyer JL, et al. Prognostic indicators of hepatic injury following jejunoileal bypass performed for refractory obesity: a prospective study. Hepatology 1:161, 1981
80. Hall RI, Grant JP, Ross LH, et al. Pathogenesis of hepatic steatosis in the parenterally fed rat. J Clin Invest 74:1658, 1984
81. Halverson JD, et al. Jejunoileal bypass for morbid obesity: a critical appraisal. Am J Med 65:561, 1978
82. Halverson JD, et al. Reanastomosis after jejunoileal bypass. Surgery 84:241, 1976
83. Hamilton RL, Vest TK, Brown BS, et al. Liver injury with alcoholiclike hyalin after gastroplasty for morbid obesity. Gastroenterology 85:722, 1983
84. Hamilton RL, et al. Discoidal bilayer structure of nascent high density lipoproteins from perfused rat liver. J Clin Invest 58:667, 1976
85. Hano T. Pathohistological study on the liver cirrhosis in diabetes mellitus. Kobe J Med Sci 14:87, 1968
86. Harinasuta U, et al. Steatonecrosis: Mallory body type. Medicine 46:161, 1967

87. Health and Public Policy Committee, American College of Physicians. Methotrexate in rheumatoid arthritis. Ann Intern Med 107:418, 1987
88. Hilden M, et al. Fatty liver persisting for up to 33 years: a follow-up of the Iverson-Roholm liver biopsy material. Acta Med Scand 194:485, 1973
89. Hill RB Jr, et al. Hepatic lipid metabolism in the cortisone treated rat. Exp Mol Pathol 4:320, 1965
90. Hill RB Jr. Fatal fat embolism from steroid-induced fatty liver. N Engl J Med 265:318, 1961
91. Hoenig N, Warner F. Effect of perhexilene maleate on lipid metabolism in the rat. Pharmacol Res Commun 12:29, 1980
92. Holloway PW, et al. On the biosynthesis of dienoic fatty acids by animal tissues. Biochem Biophys Res Commun 12:300, 1963
93. Hornick CA, Hamilton RL, Spaziani E, et al. Isolation and characterization of multivesicular bodies from rat hepatocytes: an organelle distinct from secretory vesicles of the Golgi apparatus. J Cell Biol 100:1558, 1985
94. Howell KE, Palade GE. Heterogeneity of lipoprotein particles in hepatic Golgi fractions. J Cell Biol 92:833, 1982
95. Hoyumpa AM, et al. Fatty liver: biochemical and clinical considerations. Am J Dig Dis 20:1142, 1975
96. Hyams DE, et al. The prevention of fatty liver by administration of adenosine triphosphate. Lab Invest 16:604, 1967
97. Ishak KG. Hepatic morphology in the inherited metabolic diseases. Semin Liver Dis 6:246, 1986
98. Itoh S, Yougei T, Kawagoe K. Comparison between nonalcoholic steatohepatitis and alcoholic hepatitis. Am J Gastroenterol 82:650, 1987
99. Jackson RL, et al. Lipoprotein structure and metabolism. Physiol Rev 56:259, 1976
100. Jazcilevich S, et al. Induction of fatty liver in the rat after cycloheximide administration. Lab Invest 23:590, 1970
101. Jeanrenaud B. Effect of glucocorticoid hormones on fatty acid mobilization and reesterification in rat adipose tissue. Biochem J 103:627, 1967
102. Jeejeebhoy KN, et al. Total parenteral nutrition at home: studies in patients surviving four months in five years. Gastroenterology 71:943, 1976
103. Jones JP Jr, et al. Systemic fat embolism after renal homotransplantation and treatment with corticosteroids. N Engl J Med 273:1453, 1965
104. Joske RA, et al. Acute fatty liver of pregnancy. Gut 9:489, 1968
105. Kahn SA, Saltzman BR, Klein RS, et al. Hepatic disorders in the acquired immune deficiency syndrome: a clinical and pathological study. Am J Gastroenterol 81:1145, 1986
106. Kalk H. The relationship between fatty liver and diabetes mellitus. Germ Med Monthly 5:81, 1960
107. Kaplan MM. Acute fatty liver of pregnancy. N Engl J Med 313:367, 1985
108. Katz J, McGarry JD. The glucose paradox: is glucose a substrate for liver metabolism? J Clin Invest 74:1901, 1984
109. Kimura H, Kako M, Yo K. Alcoholic hyalins (Mallory bodies) in a case of Weber-Christian disease: electron microscopic observations of liver involvement. Gastroenterology 78:807, 1980
110. Komaromy MC, Schotz MD. Cloning of rat hepatic lipase cDNA: evidence for a lipase gene family. Proc Natl Acad Sci USA 84:1526, 1987
111. Kramer K, et al. The increasing mortality attributed to cirrhosis and fatty liver in Baltimore (1957–1966). Ann Intern Med 69:273, 1968
112. Krasner N, Davis M, Portmann B, Williams R. Changing pattern of alcoholic liver disease in Great Britain: relation to sex and signs of autoimmunity. Br J Med 1:1497, 1977
113. Kumar S, Stauber RE, Gavaler JS. Orthotopic liver transplantation for alcoholic liver disease. Hepatology 11:159, 1989
114. Kunelis CT, Peter JL, Edmondson HA. Fatty liver of preg-

nancy and its relationship to tetracycline therapy. Am J Med 38:359, 1965

115. Law SW, Lackner KJ, Fojo SS, et al. The molecular biology of human apo-A-I, apo-A-II, apo-C-II and apo-B. Adv Exp Med Biol 151:162, 1986

116. Lee JKT, et al. Fatty infiltration of the liver: demonstration by proton spectroscopic imaging. Radiology 153:195, 1984

117. Lee JKT, Heiken SP, Dixon WT. Detection of hepatic metastases by proton spectroscopic imaging: work in progress. Radiology 156:428, 1985

118. Lee RG. Nonalcoholic steatohepatitis: a study of 49 patients. Hum Pathol 20:594, 1989

119. Leevy CM. Diabetes mellitus and liver dysfunction. Am J Med 8:290, 1950

120. Leevy CM. Fatty liver: a study of 270 patients with biopsy proven fatty liver and the pathogenesis of fatty liver. Am J Clin Nutr 15:161, 1964

121. Lewis JH, Schiff E. Methotrexate-induced chronic liver injury: guidelines for detection and prevention. Am J Gastroenterol 88:1337, 1988

122. Lieber CS, et al. Difference in hepatic metabolism of long and medium chain fatty acids. J Clin Invest 146:1451, 1967

123. Lieber CS, et al. Effect of ethanol on plasma free fatty acids in man. J Lab Clin Med 59:826, 1962

124. Lieber CS, et al. Effects of prolonged ethanol intake: production of fatty liver despite adequate diets. J Clin Invest 44:1009, 1965

125. Lieber CS, Schmid R. The effect of ethanol on fatty acid metabolism: stimulation of hepatic fatty acid synthesis in vitro. J Clin Invest 40:394, 1961

126. Lieber CS, Spritz N. Effects of prolonged ethanol intake in man: role of dietary, adipose, and endogenously synthesized fatty acids in the pathogenesis of the alcoholic fatty liver. J Clin Invest 45:1400, 1966

127. Lieber CS. Alcohol–nutrition interaction: 1984 update. Alcoholism 1:151, 1984

128. Lieber CS. Metabolism and metabolic effects of ethanol. Semin Liver Dis 1:189, 1981

129. Lockwood DH, et al. Effect of oral amino acid supplementation on liver disease after jejunoileal bypass for morbid obesity. Am J Clin Nutr 30:58, 1977

130. Lucas CL, Ridout JH. Fatty liver and lipotropic phenomena. Prog Chem Fats Other Lipids 10:1, 1967

131. Ludwig J, Viggiano TR, McGill DB, Ott BJ. Nonalcoholic steatohepatitis: Mayo Clinic experiences with a hitherto unnamed disease. Mayo Clin Proc 55:434, 1980

132. Lynch MJC, et al. Fat embolism in chronic alcoholism. Arch Pathol 67:68, 1959

133. MacSween RNM, Burt AD. Histologic spectrum of alcoholic liver disease. Semin Liver Dis 6:221, 1986

134. Mahley RW, Innerarity TL. Lipoprotein receptors and cholesterol homeostasis. Biochim Biophys Acta 737:197, 1983

135. Maini P, et al. Cyclic hyperalimentation: an optimal technique for preservation of visceral protein. J Surg Res 20:515, 1976

136. Manes JL, et al. Relationship between hepatic morphology and clinical and biochemical findings in morbidly obese patients. J Clin Pathol 26:776, 1973

137. Marbet UA, Bianch L, Meury U, Stalder GA. Long-term histological evaluation of the natural history and prognostic factors of alcoholic liver disease. J Hepatol 4:364, 1987

138. Marchetti M, et al. Metabolic aspects of orotic acid fatty liver: nucleotide control mechanisms of lipid metabolism. Biochem J 92:46, 1964

139. Margulis SJ, Jacobson IM. Hepatobiliary and pancreatic manifestations of AIDS. Semin Gastrointest Dis 2:49, 1991

140. Marubio A, Buchwald H, Schwartz MZ, et al. Hepatic lesions of central protocellular fibrosis in morbid obesity and after jejunoileal bypass. Am J Clin Pathol 66:684, 1976

141. Mason EE, Printen KJ, Blommers TJ, et al. Gastric bypass in morbid obesity. Am J Clin Nutr 33:395, 1980

142. McDonald I, et al. Liver depot and serum lipids during early recovery from kwashiorkor. Clin Sci 24:55, 1963

143. McLaren DS, et al. Protein calorie malnutrition and the liver. Prog Liver Dis 4:527, 1972

144. McLaren DS, et al. The liver during recovery from protein calorie malnutrition. J Trop Med Hyg 71:271, 1978

145. Mezey E. Metabolic effects of ethanol. Fed Proc 44:134, 1985

146. Mitsudo S, Zucker P. Wolman's disease. Pediatr Pathol 9:193, 1989

147. Miyai K, et al. Effects of glucose on the subcellular structure of the rat liver cells in acute ethionine intoxication. Lab Invest 23:268, 1970

148. Moise KJ, Shah DM. Acute fatty liver of pregnancy: etiology of fetal distress and fetal wastage. Obstet Gynecol 69:482, 1987

149. Morgan MY, Sherlock S. Sex related differences among 100 patients with alcoholic liver disease. Br J Med 1:939, 1977

150. Morgan NY, Sherlock S, Scheuer PJ. Acute cholestasis, hepatic failure, and fatty liver in the alcoholic. Scand J Gastroenterol 313:299, 1978

151. Morse RM, Valenzuela GA, Greenwald TP, et al. Amiodarone-induced liver toxicity. Ann Intern Med 109:838, 1988

152. Mouto AS. The liver in ulcerative colitis of the intestinal tract: functional and anatomic changes. Ann Intern Med 50:1385, 1959

153. Moxley RT, et al. Protein nutrition and liver disease after jejunoileal bypass for morbid obesity. N Engl J Med 290:921, 1974

154. Nagata Y, Chen J, Cooper A. Role of LDL receptor–dependent and –independent sites in binding and uptake of chylomicron remnants by rat liver. J Biol Chem 263:15151, 1988

155. Nanji AA, Tsukamoto H, French SW. Relationship between fatty liver and subsequent development of necrosis, inflammation and fibrosis in experimental alcoholic liver disease. Exp Mol Pathol 51:141, 1989

156. Newsholme EA. Role of the liver in integration of fat and carbohydrate metabolism and clinical implications in patients with liver disease. Prog Liver Dis 5:125, 1976

157. Nikkila EA, Ojala K. Role of hepatic L-glycerophosphate and triglyceride synthesis in production of fatty liver by ethanol. Proc Soc Exp Biol Med 113:814, 1963

158. Norkin SA, Compagna-Pinto D. Cytoplasmic hyaline inclusions in hepatoma. Arch Pathol 86:25, 1968

159. Novikoff PM, et al. Production and prevention of fatty liver in rats fed clofibrate and orotic acid diets containing sucrose. Lab Invest 30:732, 1974

160. Novikoff PM. Intracellular organelles and lipoprotein metabolism in normal and fatty livers. In: Arias IM, Popper H, Schacter D, et al, eds. The liver: biology and pathobiology. New York, Raven Press, 1982, pp 143–167

161. O'Leary JP, et al. Pathogenesis of hepatic failure following jejunoileal bypass. Gastroenterology 66:859, 1974

162. Ockner SA, Brunt EM, Cohn SM, et al. Fulminant hepatic failure due to acute fatty liver of pregnancy treated by orthotopic liver transplantation. Hepatology 11:59, 1990

163. Olivecrona T, Hernall O, Johnson O, et al. Effect of ethanol on some enzymes inducible by free refeeding J Stud Alcohol 33:1, 1972

164. Osterloh J, Cunningham W, Dixon A, et al. Biochemical relationships between Reye's and Reye's-like metabolic and toxicological syndromes. Med Toxicol Adv Drug Exp 4:272, 1989

165. Otto G, Herfarth C, Senninger N, et al. Hepatic transplantation in galactosemia. Transplantation 47:902, 1989

166. Perrillo RP, et al. Alcoholic liver disease presenting with marked elevation of serum alkaline phosphatase. Am J Dig Dis 23:1061, 1978

167. Pessayre D, Bichara M, Feldmann G, et al. Perhexiline maleate–induced cirrhosis. Gastroenterology 76:170, 1979

168. Peters RL, et al. Postjejunal bypass hepatic disease: its simi-

larity to alcoholic hepatic disease. Am J Clin Pathol 63:318, 1975

169. Peters RL, Edmondson HA, Mikkelsen WP, et al. Tetracycline-induced fatty liver in nonpregnant patients: a report of six cases. Am J Surg 113:622, 1967

170. Peters RL. Hepatic morphologic changes after jejunoileal bypass. Prog Liver Dis 6:581, 1979

171. Phillips GB. Acute hepatic insufficiency of the chronic alcoholic: revisited. Am J Med 75:1, 1983

172. Pie P, et al. Fatty metamorphosis of the liver following small intestinal bypass for obesity. Arch Pathol Lab Med 101:411, 1977

173. Popper H, Thung SN, Gerber MA. Pathology of alcoholic liver disease. Semin Liver Dis 1:203, 1981

174. Porta EA. Nutrition and diseases of the liver and gallbladder. Prog Food Nutr Sci 1:289, 1975

175. Pottenger LA, et al. Carbohydrate composition of lipoprotein apoproteins isolated from rat plasma and from livers of rats fed orotic acid. Biochem Biophys Res Commun 54:770, 1973

176. Poucell S, Ireton J, Valencia-Mayoral P, et al. Amiodarone-associated phospholipidosis and fibrosis of the liver. Gastroenterology 86:926, 1984

177. Poupon R, Rosensztajn C, de Saint-Maur RD, et al. Perhexilene maleate-associated hepatic injury: prevalence and characteristics. Digestion 20:145, 1980

178. Powell LM, Wallis SC, Pease RJ, et al. A novel form of tissue-specific RNA processing produces apoliporotein-B48 in intestine. Cell 50:831, 1987

179. Protmann B, Wight DGD. Pathology of liver transplantation (excluding rejection). In: Calne R, ed. Liver transplantation: the King's College Hospital experience. Orlando, Grune and Stratton, 1987, p 437

180. Quarfordt SH, Goodman DWS. Metabolism of doubly-labelled chylomicron cholesteryl esters in rat. J Lipid Res 8:264, 1967

181. Ragland JB, et al. Identification of nascent high density lipoprotein containing arginine-rich protein in human plasma. Biochem Biophys Res Commun 80:81, 1978

182. Ragland JB, et al. The role of LCAT deficiency in the apoprotein metabolism of alcoholic hepatitis. Scand J Clin Lab Invest 38:208, 1978

183. Randall B. Sudden death and hepatic fatty metamorphosis. JAMA 293:1723, 1980

184. Reboucas G, Isselbacher JJ. Studies on pathogenesis of ethanol-induced fatty liver. I. Synthesis and oxidation of fatty acids by liver. J Clin Invest 40:1355, 1961

185. Recknagel RO, et al. Lipoperoxidation as a vector in carbon tetrachloride hepatotoxicity. Lab Invest 15:132, 1966

186. Recknagel RO, et al. Carbon tetrachloride hepatotoxicity. Pharmacol Rev 19:145, 1967

187. Renold AR, et al. Metabolism of isolated adipose tissue: a summary. In: Renold AE, Cahill GR Jr, eds. American Physiologic Society handbook of physiology: 5. adipose tissue. Baltimore, Williams & Wilkins, 1965, p 483

188. Reye RDK, Morgan G, Baral J. Encephalopathy and fatty degeneration of the viscera: a disease entity in childhood. Lancet 2:749, 1963

189. Robinson DS, et al. The development in the rat of fatty livers associated with reduced plasma-lipoprotein synthesis. Biochim Biophys Acta 62:163, 1962

190. Roenigk HH Jr, Auerbach R, Maibach HI, et al. Methotrexate guidelines: revised. J Am Acad Dermatol 6:145, 1982

191. Roheim PS, et al. Alterations of lipoprotein metabolism in orotic acid-induced fatty liver. Lab Invest 15:21, 1966

192. Rolfes DB, Ishak KG. Acute fatty liver of pregnancy: a clinicopathologic study of 35 cases. Hepatology 5:1149, 1985

193. Rossiter P, Slater TF. The effects of antioxidants on the concentrations of reduced and oxidized nicotinamide-adenine dinucleotide and of triglyceride in rat liver after the administration of ethanol. Biochem Soc Trans 1:933, 1973

194. Sabesin SM, et al. Accumulation of nascent lipoproteins in rat hepatic Golgi during induction of fatty liver by orotic acid. Lab Invest 37:127, 1977

195. Sabesin SM. Biogenesis of rat hepatocyte Golgi during the induction of lipoprotein secretion by sucrose feeding. Gastroenterolgy 75:985, 1978

196. Sabesin SM, et al. D-Galactosamine hepatotoxicity. V. Role of free fatty acids in the pathogenesis of fatty liver. Exp Mol Pathol 29:82, 1978

197. Sabesin SM, et al. Electron microscopic studies of the assembly, intracellular transport and secretion of chylomicrons by rat intestine. J Lipid Res 18:496, 1977

198. Sabesin SM, et al. Lipoprotein disturbances in liver disease. Prog Liver Dis 6:243, 1979

199. Sabesin SM, et al. Lipoprotein metabolism in liver disease. In: Stollerman C, ed. Advances in internal medicine, vol 25. Chicago, Year Book Medical Publishers, 1980, pp 117–146

200. Sabesin SM, et al. D-Galactosamine hepatotoxicity. IV. Further studies of the pathogenesis of fatty liver. Exp Mol Pathol 24:424, 1976

201. Sabesin SM. Effects of acetoxycycloheximide on the metabolism of hepatic triglycerides in the rat. Exp Mol Pathol 25:227, 1976

202. Sabesin SM. Lipid and lipoprotein abnormalities in alcoholic liver disease. Circulation 64:72, 1981

203. Salmon PA, Reedy KL. Fatty metamorphosis in patients with jejunoileal bypass. Surg Gynecol Obstet 141:75, 1975

204. Scanu AM, Edelstein C, Gordon JI. Apolipoproteins of human plasma high density lipoproteins: biology, biochemistry and clinical significance. Clin Physiol Biochem 2:111, 1984

205. Schaffner F, Thaler H. Nonalcoholic fatty liver disease. Prog Liver Dis, 8:283–298, 1986

206. Schapiro RH, et al. Effect of prolonged ethanol ingestion on the transport and metabolism of lipids in man. N Engl J Med 272:610, 1965

207. Scheig R, Isselbacher KHJ. Pathogenesis of ethanol-induced fatty liver. III. In vivo and in vitro effects of ethanol on hepatic fatty acid metabolism in rat. J Lipid Res 6:269, 1965

208. Schneiderman DJ, Arenson DM, Cello JP, et al. Hepatic disease in patients with the acquired immune deficiency syndrome (AIDS). Hepatology 7:925, 1987

209. Schoeman MN, Batey RG, Wilcken B. Recurrent acute fatty liver of pregnancy associated with a fatty-acid oxidation defect in the offspring. Gastroenterology 100:544, 1991

210. Shapiro B. Lipid metabolism. Annu Rev Biochem 36:247, 1967

211. Sheldon GF, Peterson SR, Sanders R. Hepatic dysfunction during hyperalimentation. Arch Surg 113:504, 1978

212. Sherratt HSA. Hypoglycin, the famous toxin of the unripe Jamaican ackee fruit. Trends Pharmacol 7:186, 1986

213. Simon JB, Manley PN, Brien JF, et al. Amiodarone hepatotoxicity simulating alcoholic liver disease. N Engl J Med 311:167, 1984

214. Smetana HG, et al. Infantile cirrhosis: an analytical review of the literature and a report of 50 cases. Pediatrics 23:107, 1961

215. Snyder RR, Hankins GD. Etiology and management of acute fatty liver of pregnancy. Clin Perinatol 13:813, 1986

216. Soffer LJ, et al. Cushing's syndrome: a study of 50 patients. Am J Med 30:129, 1961

217. Spitzer JJ, McElroy WT Jr. Some hormonal effects on uptake of free fatty acids by the liver. Am J Physiol 199:876, 1960

218. Stanley RJ, et al. Computed tomography of the liver. Radiol Clin North Am 5:331, 1978

219. Starzl TE, Van Thiel D, Tzakis AG, et al. Orthotopic liver transplantation for alcoholic cirrhosis. JAMA 260:2542, 1988

219a. Stein O, et al. Colchicine-induced inhibition of lipoprotein and protein secretion into the serum and lack of interference with secretion of biliary phospholipids and cholesterol by rat liver in vivo. J Cell Biol 62:90, 1974

220. Steinberg D, Vaughan M. Release of free fatty acids from adipose tissue in vitro in relation to rates of triglyceride synthesis and degradation. In: Renold AE, Cahill GR Jr, eds. American

Physiologic Society handbook of physiology. 5. Adipose tissue. Baltimore, Williams & Wilkins, 1965, p 335

221. Sternlieb I: Mitochondrial and fatty change in hepatocytes of patients with Wilson's disease. Gastroenterology 55:354, 1980

222. Suarez L, Valbuena ML, Moreno A, et al. Abetalipoproteinemia associated with hepatic and atypical neurological disorders. Pediatr Gastrointest Nutr 6:799, 1987

223. Suchy FJ, Balistreri WF, Buchino JJ, et al. Acute hepatic failure associated with the use of sodium valproate. N Engl J Med 300:962, 1979

224. Szilagyi A, Le Compte P, Goosens J, et al. Comparison of liver injury and alcoholism and post jejunoileal bypass surgery. In: Bank PD, Chalmers TC, eds. Frontiers in liver disease. New York, Thieme-Stratton, 1981, pp 156–166

225. Takac A, et al. Leberverfettung bei diabetes mellitus. Michen Med Wochenschr 107:1148, 1965

226. Thaler H. Fatty change. Baillieres Clin Gastroenterol 2:453–462, 1988

227. Todo S, Demetris AJ, Makowka L, et al. Primary nonfunction of hepatic allografts with preexisting fatty infiltration. Transplantation 47:903, 1989

228. Tolman JG, Clegg DO, Lee RG, et al. Methotrexate and the liver. J Rheumatol 12(suppl 12):29, 1985

229. Torosis JD, Barwick KW, Miller DJ, et al. Nonalcoholic Laennec's: clinical characteristics and long term follow-up. (Abstract) Hepatology 6:1170, 1986

230. Tuyns AJ, Pequignot G. Greater risk of ascitic cirrhosis in females in relation to alcohol consumption. Int J Epidemiol 13:53, 1984

231. Uchida T, Kao H, Quispe-Sjogren M, Peters RL. Alcoholic foamy degeneration: a pattern of acute alcoholic injury of the liver. Gastroenterology 84:683, 1983

232. Vander Hoof JA, Tuma DJ, Sorrell MF. Role of defunctionalized bowel in jejunoileal bypass–induced liver disease in rats. Dig Dis Sci 24:916, 1979

233. Verbin RS, et al. The biochemical pathology of inhibition of protein synthesis in vivo. Lab Invest 20:529, 1969

234. Von Oettingen WF. The halogenated hydrocarbons of industrial and toxicological importance. Amsterdam, Elsevier, 1964, p 107

235. Vyberg M, Ravn V, Andersen B, et al. Pattern of progression in liver injury following jejunoileal bypass for morbid obesity. Liver 7:271, 1987

236. Wanless IR, Lentz JS. Fatty liver hepatitis (steatohepatitis) and obesity: an autopsy study with analysis of risk factors. Hepatology 12:1106, 1990

237. Waterlow JC, Alleyne GAD. Protein malnutrition in children: advances in knowledge in the last 10 years. Adv Protein Chem 25:117, 1971

238. Watson WJ, Seeds JW. Acute fatty liver of pregnancy. Obstet Gynecol Surv 45:585, 1990

239. Webber BL, Freiman L. The liver in kwashiorkor. Arch Pathol 98:400, 1974

240. Weidman SW, Ragland JB, Sabesin SM. Plasma lipoprotein composition in alcoholic hepatitis: accumulation of apolipoprotein E-rich high density lipoprotein and preferential reappearance of HDL_2 during recovery. J Lipid Res 23:556, 1982

241. Wene JD, et al. The development of essential fatty acid deficiency in healthy man fed fat-free diets intravenously and orally. J Clin Invest 56:127, 1975

242. Wetmore S, et al. Incorporation of sialic acid into sialidase-treated apolipoprotein of human very low density lipoprotein by pork liver sialyltransferase. Can J Biochem 52:655, 1974

243. Windmueller HG, Levy RI. Total inhibition of hepatic-lipoprotein production in the rat by orotic acid. J Biol Chem 242:2246, 1967

244. Zafrani ES, Berthelot P. Sodium valproate in the induction of unusual hepatotoxicity. Hepatology 2:648, 1982

245. Zannis VI, Kurmit DM, Breslow JL. Hepatic apo A-I and apo E and intestinal apo A-I are synthesized in precursor isoprotein forms by organ cultures of human fetal tissues. J Biol Chem 257:536, 1982

246. Zimmerman HJ, Ishak KG. Valproate-induced hepatic injury: analyses of 23 fatal cases. Hepatology 2:591, 1982

Diseases of the Liver, Seventh Edition, edited by Leon Schiff and Eugene R. Schiff. J.B. Lippincott Company, Philadelphia © 1993.

31

Alcoholic Hepatitis

Charles L. Mendenhall

Simply stated, alcoholic hepatitis is a form of toxic liver injury associated with chronic excess ethanol consumption. Reports of clinical jaundice after excessive ethanol consumption were not unusual in the early literature. As far back as 1892,[220] Osler attributed "acute necrosis of the liver" to excessive alcohol consumption. These reports most likely represented instances of alcoholic hepatitis. *Progressive alcoholic cirrhosis, subacute alcoholic cirrhosis,*[107,108] *florid cirrhosis,*[241] *sclerosing hyalin necrosis,*[69] *fatty liver with hepatic failure,*[240] *acute hepatic insufficiency of the chronic alcoholic,*[233] and *steatonecrosis*[113,115] all were terms used to describe the severe form of toxic alcoholic liver disease. Note that these early names all attempted to show the association of this form of alcoholic injury with various histologic and clinical manifestations of the disease, such as cirrhosis, necrosis, fatty liver (steatosis), and liver failure. The term *alcoholic hepatitis* was first used in 1961 by Beckett and coworkers,[14] who described the clinical features of the disease in seven jaundiced patients with moderate disease (mean bilirubin, 10.5 mg/dL). The following year, Beckett and coworkers[15] described an additional five cases. This time, the patients all had mild disease, were anicteric, and had the diagnosis made by liver biopsy. Thus, the full clinical spectrum of alcoholic hepatitis was recognized, ranging from anicteric to deep jaundice and fulminant hepatic failure. In the anicteric cases, the authors point out that misdiagnosis was frequent in the absence of distinguishing histologic features. This fact has not changed in the more than 30 years since then.

Pathology and Pathogenesis

The pathologic spectrum associated with chronic alcoholism ranges from no abnormalities to far-advanced cirrhosis. Characterization of the pathologic changes of alcoholic hepatitis preceded the clinical definition of the disease by about 50 years. Mallory, in 1911,[169] first described in detail the changes in the liver that preceded the late end stages of cirrhosis in the alcoholic.

The four most important alcohol-induced liver lesions are fatty liver, alcoholic hepatitis, cirrhosis, and perhaps hepatocellular carcinoma.[127] By itself, alcoholic hepatitis represents a serious (frequently life-threatening) but often reversible stage in the disease process. Association with some degree of fatty liver and cirrhosis is present in over half the cases, however.[44]

Three obligatory features have been defined as essential for the histologic diagnosis of alcoholic hepatitis[127]:

- Liver cell damage, typically ballooning degeneration with areas of necrosis
- Inflammatory cell infiltration, predominantly polymorphonuclear leukocytes
- Fibrosis, both pericellular, producing a lattice-like or chicken-wire appearance, and perivenular (centrolobular)

The area of earliest pathologic process and most severe injury is the centrolobular area (zone three of Rappaport). Ballooning degeneration begins in this region and is characterized by large, swollen hepatocytes with a pale granular-appearing cytoplasm. In some instances, finely dispersed particles are entrapped among cobweb-like strands. Within such cells, alcoholic hyalin or Mallory's bodies often can be seen.[88,127] The incidence of Mallory body formation varies with the acumen of the pathologist and the severity of the disease. It is reported in up to 86% of the cases.[44] Histologically, Mallory's bodies appear as irregular aggregates of purplish red material (as seen with hematoxylin–eosin stain), which typically are intracytoplasmic and perinuclear in location. In the centrolobular area, they are characteristic but not pathognomonic of alcoholic hepatitis.[96] When the process has progressed to alcoholic cirrhosis with fibrotic distortion of the centrolobular areas, Mallory's bodies are found at the periphery of the cirrhotic nodules. Although less common, Mallory's bodies, along with the other features typical of alcoholic hepatitis, have been observed in a nonalcoholic liver pathologic condition (Table 31-1). In this instance, the condition usually is referred to as *nonalcoholic steatohepatitis*[152]. In the absence of alcohol, steatohepatitis has been reported with most forms of cirrhosis, nutritional abnormalities, metabolic dysfunction, and drug toxicity. The exact prevalence is unknown, but in one large series of 543 cases of histologic alcoholic hepatitis, 49 cases (9%) were not clinically related to alcoholism.[153]

In the alcoholic, the pathogenesis of the swollen balloon-like hepatocytes is believed to be related to an ethanol-induced impairment in the microtubular transport and release into the serum of lipoproteins and serum proteins by the hepatocytes. Retention of these transport proteins and lipids results in cellular swelling.[10,83] The net result of these changes is the hydropic degenerative appearance of the cytoplasm,[10,69,70] which eventually progresses to the disintegration of the hepatocytes.

The antimicrotubular action of ethanol results in failure of the microtubular secretory apparatus of the cell. It appears likely that alcoholic hyalin or Mallory's bodies are formed from intermediate filaments of this secretory apparatus.[81] The

TABLE 31-1 *Conditions Associated With Nonalcoholic Steatohepatitis*

Cirrhosis Related
Indian childhood cirrhosis[203,258]
Postnecrotic cirrhosis[95]
Primary biliary cirrhosis[95,196]
Chronic obstructive biliary cirrhosis[95]
Wilson's disease[238,270]
Hepatoma[68,227]

Nutrition Related
Morbid obesity[3,165,202]
Bulimia and anorexia nervosa[61]
Jejunoileal bypass surgery[172,228]
Gastroplasty for obesity[111]
Extensive small bowel resection[60,235]
Small bowel diverticulosis[204]

Metabolic Diseases
Diabetes mellitus[13,85,152]
Weber-Christian disease (recurrent panniculitis)[143]

Therapeutic Drug Toxicity
Amiodarone[243,280]
Perhexiline maleate[226]
Glucocorticoids[132]
Synthetic estrogens[275]

appearance of these Mallory's bodies originally was classified as a form of hyalin degeneration occurring with hepatocyte damage,[115,127] associated with more severe clinical, biochemical, and histologic abnormalities,[113] and carrying a more serious prognosis[141,150,251]; however, survival does not appear to be adversely affected by their presence.[44,89,113,257] Furthermore, in tissue culture experiments[24] in which Mallory's bodies were produced by hepatocytes, there was no association between Mallory's bodies and degenerative changes in the hepatocyte. French and Burbige[80] have suggested that the appearance of Mallory's bodies in alcoholic hepatitis may result from the expression of a gene normally repressed in the adult that regulates the formation of intermediate filaments in the fetus (gene derepression phenomena). Activation of such a suppressed fetal gene would result in excessive intermediate filament formation and afford the appropriate conditions for Mallory body formation. This is not to say that Mallory's bodies are without adverse biologic effects. Like intermediate filaments,[219] they bind nonspecifically to immunoglobulins.[229,281] Mallory's bodies, extruded from dead or dying liver cells and complexed with serum and tissue carbohydrates and immunoglobulins, possess strong chemotactic properties,[158] which may account for part of the polymorphonuclear inflammatory response seen in alcoholic hepatitis. Indeed, inflammatory cells frequently are seen in proximity to necrotic and Mallory's body–containing liver cells.[127] Mallory's body complexes also have been implicated in fibrogenesis by activating lymphocytes to secrete fibrogenic lymphokines.[307] Specific antibodies to Mallory's bodies have been reported in the serum of patients with alcoholic hepatitis, and immune complexes have been found in their livers.[135] This raises the possibility that they may act as a neoantigen[283] for an autoimmune-type liver injury.

The centrolobular location of the early injury may be re-

lated to hypoxia. This area of the liver lobule has the lowest oxygen content. Furthermore, animal studies[130,215] have shown that during the early phase of ethanol withdrawal, a decrease in hepatic venous oxygen content is associated with a significant increase in oxygen consumption by the liver. Thus, the centrolobular area becomes more susceptible to hypoxic injury and necrosis.[130] The extensive loss of hepatocytes in this perivenular area is replaced by a relatively acellular confluent sclerotic area. This pathologic change has been termed *sclerosing hyalin necrosis*[69] and is believed by some to be an obligatory step in the natural evolution of alcoholic liver injury into cirrhosis.[136] In the Department of Veterans Affairs cooperative study,[44] such changes were observed in 68% of the 106 patients with alcoholic hepatitis before the development of cirrhosis.

Although the sclerotic process may be sharply outlined in the pericentral area, necrosis and inflammation (active alcoholic hepatitis) frequently extend into the surrounding areas. In the more advanced cases, fibrosis and necrosis develop in the portal areas (perhaps by another mechanism to be discussed) so that they join to form central–central and central–portal bridging necrosis and fibrosis, which may lead rapidly to the development of cirrhosis.[74,272] The time required for the completion of the cirrhotic process is not well established and appears to be variable. In Galambos' series of 23 patients[86] in whom serial biopsies were performed at 3- to 4-month intervals, progression to cirrhosis was observed to have occurred before the initial follow-up biopsy in 61% (14 of 23).

Other mechanisms, in addition to anoxia and autoimmune injury, also may be operational in the alcoholic to explain the development of liver cell necrosis. Considerable indirect experimental evidence exists that suggests free radical formation is a contributing factor.[54,55,65,146,247] Using in vitro microsomal preparations, reactive hydroxyl radicals can be generated from ethanol.[37,52] These radicals have not been detected in vivo, however.[67] Acetaldehyde, the first oxidation product of ethanol, also may result in the formation of destructive, high-energy free radicals. In the presence of molecular oxygen, such radicals attack unsaturated fatty acids in membranes and organelles to produce lipid epoxides and peroxides. These unstable intermediates then undergo peroxidative degradation with loss of membrane permeability, changes in membrane fluidity, altered enzyme function, and, ultimately, cellular death and necrosis. Unfortunately, high-energy free radicals are short-lived and are present in low concentration, so that evidence for their existence is mainly indirect. Studies from a number of different laboratories[54,55,146] observed increases in peroxidative lipid degradation products, principally malonaldehyde, after ethanol consumption. These products were markedly reduced when ethanol metabolism was blocked by pyrazole, which diminishes acetaldehyde formation, and were increased by disulfiram, an inhibitor that promotes acetaldehyde accumulation.[67] These studies suggest that acetaldehyde-generated free radicals are responsible for the injury. If lipid peroxidation is occurring after ethanol consumption, then a reduction in tissue antioxidants would be anticipated. When antioxidants were measured after ethanol treatment, mitochondrial concentrations were significantly reduced.[66] Furthermore, when a technique to quantify peroxidative degradation (diene conjugation absorption spectroscopy) was used,[23] ethanol treatment resulted in selective enhanced diene absorption in the mitochondria.[65] Such an organelle localization of injury might be anticipated, since acetaldehyde is metabolized primarily in the mitochondria.[106,170] Pathologically, mitochondrial abnormalities are known to occur frequently in alcoholic liver injury.[19] In one large study,[43] 44 (20%) of 220 patients with alcoholic hepatitis had swollen, deformed mitochondria (giant mitochondria). These are not unique to alcoholic hepatitis but have been reported in other forms of liver injury.[28,32,145,149,231] In the alcoholic, they appear to be more common in milder forms of alcoholic hepatitis before the progression to cirrhosis.[43] They frequently are observed in the peripheral regions of the liver lobules without marked inflammatory cell infiltration. They may appear as rounded hyalin bodies or as cigar-shaped structures. It is theorized that they represent a series of degenerative changes of mitochondria as well as of other cytoplasmic organelles.[126]

The inflammatory changes in alcoholic hepatitis are predominantly polymorphonuclear and may be focal or diffuse in distribution, depending on the severity of the disease and usually in relation to areas of necrosis and Mallory's bodies, with their heaviest infiltration in the centrolobular areas. Other cell types (lymphocytes and plasma cells) also infiltrate and may have clinical importance. Although they too may be present in the centrolobular areas,[83] more often they are seen in the portal areas located at the limiting plate and in association with piecemeal necrosis. In the VA Cooperative Study on Alcoholic Hepatitis,[44] piecemeal necrosis and limiting plate erosion were present in 89% of the biopsy specimens. These findings suggest a cytotoxic role for lymphocytes, similar to that in chronic active hepatitis[137] or in orthotopic liver homograft rejection.[59] Phenotype identification of the lymphocytes has shown them to be T cells.[82,124,263] Because T lymphocytes tend to be decreased in the peripheral blood of alcoholic hepatitis patients,[84,124,263] sequestration into the liver has been postulated.[17,278,304] Lymphocytes with cytotoxic effects on hepatocytes have been found in the blood of baboons chronically fed ethanol,[222] as well as in patients with alcoholic hepatitis,[134] suggesting that chronic ethanol ingestion leads to sensitization of lymphocytes to liver cell antigens.[135,158,263,307] Sensitized lymphocytes with cytotoxic potential adhere to target cells in vitro,[306] producing cell death. In the case of alcoholic hepatitis, such sensitized lymphocytes bind to hepatocytes and lead to hepatocellular destruction. Immunohistochemical analyses of liver in patients with alcoholic hepatitis have demonstrated such potentially cytotoxic T lymphocytes in proximity to portal areas of necrosis,[278] similar to observations in chronic active hepatitis or rejection of liver allografts.[279] These observations may explain in part the chronicity associated with alcoholic hepatitis,[87] and suggest the possibility of more than one mechanism operating concomitantly to produce injury.

Hepatic fibrosis associated with alcohol injury begins early and is an integral part of the pathologic process. Pericentral venous sclerosis has been observed to occur in the absence of the inflammatory changes of alcoholic injury. Such lesions were observed in the alcoholic fatty livers of both baboons and alcoholic patients.[294] This has suggested to some that cirrhosis may develop in the alcoholic without going through the alcoholic hepatitis phase.[239,294] This question is not yet resolved. In the VA Cooperative Study on Alcoholic Hepatitis,[44] 100% of the 220 livers on which biopsy or autopsy had been performed had increased fibrosis, ranging from focal scarring (16%) to bridging fibrosis (28%) and established cirrhosis (56%). The overall incidence of established cirrhosis was most likely higher than the observed 56%, because histologic studies were not available for 46% (200/435) of the patients, predominantly in the group of severely ill patients in whom the prevalence of cirrhosis would be expected to be highest.

Mallory, in 1911,[169] postulated that fibrosis in alcoholic liver disease resulted from the inflammatory exudate, which produced mechanical injury followed by proliferation of fibroblasts and the deposition of connective tissue. The mechanism for increased collagen formation and deposition in the liver of the alcoholic appears to be much more complex than merely a response to inflammation. In part, this may be related to Mallory's body–activated secretion of lymphokines. Ethanol, however, does have a direct effect on the biochemistry of collagen-stimulating hepatocyte proline uptake[179] and collagen synthesis in the absence of inflammation and alcoholic hepatitis.[74,191,192,225] This may account for the early appearance of fibrosis in alcohol-induced liver injury.

Other pathologic changes common in alcoholic hepatitis, but not obligatory for its diagnosis, include fatty metamorphosis, intrahepatic cholestasis, and iron deposition.

Fatty metamorphosis is present, to some degree, in over 95% of the cases.[44] (The pathogenesis and clinical significance of fatty liver are discussed in detail in Chapter 30.) It is sufficient to note here that fatty infiltration is not a totally benign condition; it is associated with some morbidity and mortality[101,140,154] and, perhaps, predisposes to cirrhosis.[56,282]

Intrahepatic cholestasis may occur in a significant number of patients. Thirty-eight percent in the VA series had histologic evidence of cholestasis. In some patients, this may be attributed to large bile duct obstruction associated with sclerosing pancreatitis. In most, the cholestatic picture represents a part of the alcohol-induced injury and is associated with bile stasis, bile plugs, periportal necrosis, mixed inflammatory exudate, and destruction of intralobular bile ducts.[4] This has long-term prognostic significance because the presence of moderate to severe tissue cholestasis was associated with more severe jaundice, coagulopathy, and a 2.5-fold increase in mortality.[209]

Excessive iron deposits occur both in parenchymal cells and in Kupffer's cells of livers of patients with alcoholic liver injury. In one series of 329 alcoholic patients studied histologically by liver biopsy, hemosiderosis was observed in 168 (51%) of patients.[51] It is said to be most commonly associated with cirrhosis[127]; however, in this series,[51] no difference in prevalence was observed between cirrhotic and noncirrhotic patients. Iron overload may result through a variety of mechanisms, possibly as a result of increased iron absorption,[303] increased iron content in alcoholic beverages (especially wine), hemolytic episodes, or secondary to repeated episodes of liver cell necrosis. This has clinical significance in that blood loss anemia may complicate the course of the disease and may require iron therapy. Prolonged use of such medications, however, may result in iron overload.

Incidence

The true incidence of alcoholic hepatitis, especially of the milder forms, is unknown, since the people may be asymptomatic and the diagnosis usually requires biopsy confirmation. Again, the incidence appears to differ among countries.

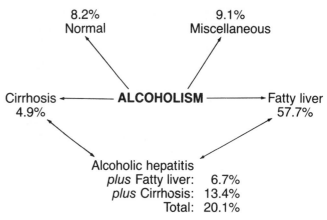

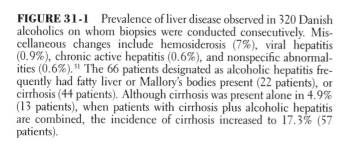

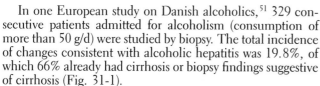

FIGURE 31-1 Prevalence of liver disease observed in 320 Danish alcoholics on whom biopsies were conducted consecutively. Miscellaneous changes include hemosiderosis (7%), viral hepatitis (0.9%), chronic active hepatitis (0.6%), and nonspecific abnormalities (0.6%).[51] The 66 patients designated as alcoholic hepatitis frequently had fatty liver or Mallory's bodies present (22 patients), or cirrhosis (44 patients). Although cirrhosis was present alone in 4.9% (13 patients), when patients with cirrhosis plus alcoholic hepatitis are combined, the incidence of cirrhosis increased to 17.3% (57 patients).

In one European study on Danish alcoholics,[51] 329 consecutive patients admitted for alcoholism (consumption of more than 50 g/d) were studied by biopsy. The total incidence of changes consistent with alcoholic hepatitis was 19.8%, of which 66% already had cirrhosis or biopsy findings suggestive of cirrhosis (Fig. 31-1).

The spectrum of liver disease in the alcoholics of Japan is somewhat different.[211] In several large series of hepatitis B surface antigen (HBsAg)–negative alcoholics, the incidence of chronic inflammatory liver disease (chronic persistent and chronic active hepatitis) was much higher (10% to 61%), as was the incidence of cirrhosis or hepatic fibrosis (16% to 59%) and hepatocellular carcinoma in cirrhosis (16%). Fatty liver and alcoholic hepatitis were less frequent (1% to 15% and 6% to 11%, respectively). The incidence seemed to depend on the patient population (medical service versus psychiatric service), with the higher incidence of inflammatory disease in the psychiatric patients. Although no evidence of hepatitis B viral infections could be detected, the possibility of hepatitis non-A, non-B infection was not excluded. The high prevalence of these changes in alcoholic persons with liver disease in the absence of clinical or laboratory evidence of viral infection has suggested to some that chronic lymphocytic inflammatory changes may be one of the pathologic changes induced by alcohol injury to the liver.[103]

In an epidemiologic study in the United States[90,93] based on discharge diagnoses (nongovernment hospitals), 136.5 hospitalizations for alcoholic hepatitis were observed per 100,000 population (0.14%). The ratio of alcoholic fatty liver to alcoholic hepatitis to alcoholic cirrhosis was 1.0:5.3:3.8. The high prevalence of alcoholic hepatitis and the low prevalence of fatty liver may reflect the more severe, sometimes life-threatening range of symptoms in acute alcoholic hepatitis, which requires hospitalization more readily. It does not necessarily reflect the prevalence among all alcoholics.

These data suggest that the prevalence of acute alcoholic hepatitis in the United States is much higher than that reported in Denmark and Japan. In a prospective study of six Department of Veterans Affairs Medical Centers,[178] of the initial 995 alcoholics with liver disease who were screened, 33.8% of those studied by biopsy had alcoholic hepatitis. These observations reflect only the prevalence of alcoholic hepatitis among patients with existing liver disease severe enough to require hospitalization. The mild or asymptomatic disease would not be reflected in these studies; thus, the total

prevalence is probably even higher. Fifty-five percent of these patients already had established cirrhosis.

CONTRIBUTING ETIOLOGIC FACTORS

Excess alcohol consumption is the essential element in the etiology of alcoholic hepatitis; however, the amount of ethanol consumed necessary to produce clinically significant liver lesions varies markedly among individuals. For most patients, this represents an excess of 80 g/d for 15 years or more.[159] When this quantity is converted to volumes of alcoholic beverages consumed, it represents more than eight 12-ounce 6% beers, a liter of 12% wine, or 1 cup of 80 proof whiskey per day. For some, the susceptibility to alcohol injury may be considerably less.[261] In the VA cooperative study,[102,180] mean consumption even for clinically mild disease was 234 g/d for a mean duration of 22 years. A pathologic condition of a lesser nature may have been present for some time, however, before the clinical diagnosis was made.

This relation between alcoholism and alcoholic liver injury appears to be confounded by other factors. Although alcoholism is a worldwide problem, the world incidence of alcohol-induced liver injury varies considerably among countries. In general, a significant correlation between alcohol consumption and deaths from cirrhosis has been reported within a given country,[159] but comparisons among countries show much more variation and suggest interactions with other local factors. For example, Austria ranks 1st on the list for reported deaths while ranking 10th for alcohol consumption. Similarly, Japan ranks 12th for deaths but only 24th for alcohol consumption. Figure 31-2 shows the correlation between these two variables. These differences have been attributed to genetic predisposition,[8,175,277] malnutrition,[116,234] and concomitant viral hepatitis infections.[25,94,230]

Genetic

Some evidence for genetic predisposition has been reported based on ethnic differences in disease severity and survival.[186] Among 437 patients studied, more severe disease occurred in Native Americans and Hispanics, with a significantly higher mortality. In this study, African Americans tended to have a better prognosis. The authors admit that other factors than ethnicity (ie, environmental cultural factors, socioeconomic status, and dietary practices) could have confounded the observations. Further support for a genetic predisposition to al-

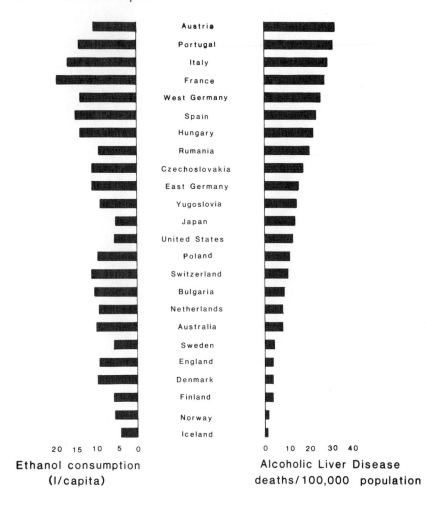

FIGURE 31-2 Incidence of deaths from alcoholic liver disease in various countries, with their corresponding consumption of ethanol. Countries are arranged in order of decreasing mortality.[90,160,211]

coholic liver disease can be found in the surveys of major histocompatibility antigens. Unfortunately, the results have not been unanimous or consistent. Most have reported some significant alterations in human leukocyte antigen (HLA) distributions, namely, a disproportional prevalence of HLA-B8,[8,198,264,265] B13,[175] BW40,[16] and DR3.[264] Scott and coworkers,[274] however, in a small group (18 patients with alcoholic cirrhosis), could find no selective distribution. Thus, the genetic contribution to the disease process remains unclear.

Nutritional

Considerable data in the literature suggest a relation between nutritional deficiency and alcoholic liver injury.[232] The mechanism for the deficiency state is multifaceted. In some instances, chronic alcoholism may induce pancreatitis, cause malabsorption and diarrhea, and alter biochemical processes essential for nutrient use.[7,9,42,100,110,129,155,157,163,164,188-190] Of more importance is the poor nutrient value of ethanol, providing mainly empty calories that are wasted as heat.[237] Thus, although total caloric intake may seem adequate or marginal, when ethanol constitutes 40% to 60% of these calories, a catabolic state can develop. When this is combined with a low dietary protein intake, inadequate cell repair after injury may occur. Although additional calories are needed to meet metabolic needs, the alcoholic experiences anorexia, which results in decreased caloric intake.[182] It should not be surprising, then, that all of the initial 363 patients enrolled in

the VA cooperative study[180] had some evidence of protein-calorie malnutrition. Fat stores, creatinine height index, responsiveness to skin tests, and visceral protein depletions were the most commonly observed abnormalities in patients with severe disease (Fig. 31-3). Furthermore, if one considers the nutritional parameters collectively as a percentage of normal, a highly significant correlation ($P < .0001$) between the degree of nutritional deficiency and acute 30-day mortality was observed.[184] Although its frequent association is irrefutable, a cause-and-effect relation is more difficult to establish. The mere presence of the malnutrition does not prove that it initiated or even potentiated the associated liver injury. This will be discussed more in association with therapy.

Viral Hepatitis

A contributing role for concomitant hepatitis virus B (HBV) or C (HCV) infections in the pathogenesis of alcoholic liver injury has been proposed. Numerous serologic surveys have established an increased prevalence of positive markers for HBV, increased lymphocyte transformation in the presence of HBsAg as well as HBV DNA, and the identification of HBcAg within liver tissue of alcoholic cirrhosis.[11,22,25,30,49,78,104,120,167,194,195,213,214,221,230,285,295] One investigation[297] even was able to document an increase in toxicity after the ingestion of quantities of ethanol (under 80 g/d) that in their noncarrier controls were harmless. Unfortunately, an almost equal number of reports have failed to confirm these observations with HBV and alcoholic liver in-

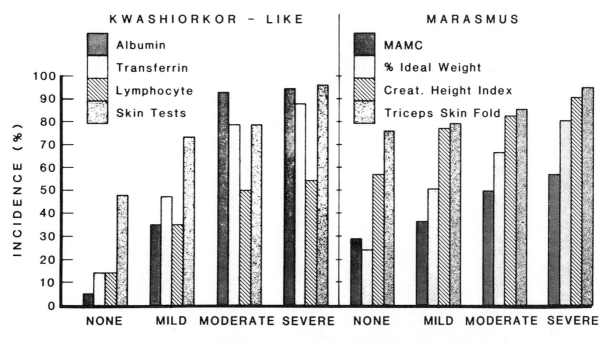

FIGURE 31-3 Prevalence of abnormalities for each of the parameters used to diagnose protein–calorie malnutrition in 373 alcoholic patients with varying degrees of alcoholic hepatitis. MAMC, midarm muscle circumference. (Mendenhall CL, et al. Protein–calorie malnutrition associated with alcoholic hepatitis: Veterans Administration Cooperative Study on Alcoholic Hepatitis. Am J Med 76:211, 1984)

jury.[12,40,79,98,99,114,118,121,266,291,305] The case for HCV is much less extensively studied because of lack of available serologic testing techniques. Using the enzyme-linked immunosorbent assay as a screening test for antibodies to a nonstructural protein of the HCV, several investigators have observed an increased prevalence of positive reactivity, ranging from 28% to 35% of those patients tested.[27,187] This has been associated with a significantly poorer prognosis with histologic changes of both viral injury and alcoholic hepatitis, and a high prevalence of cirrhosis. Unlike posttransfusion hepatitis patients, however, the reactive patients tended to have few clinical or laboratory changes suggestive of viral injury, have higher immunoglobulins, and in many instances could not be confirmed by recombinant immunoblot assay. Hence, the possibility of false-positives could not be ruled out.

Immune Dysfunction

The evidence that immune abnormalities contribute to pathogenesis of the liver injury still is controversial. More than 100 reports have been published describing immune alterations. Yet, despite the large number of publications, many still doubt the role of alcohol as an immune modulator and the immunologic contribution to the pathogenesis of the liver injury. To quote from a 1988 text of pathology[259] relating to alcoholism and immune dysfunction: "Despite tantalizing clinical anecdotes and a substantial number of serious investigations, no consistent effect of alcohol on humoral or cell-mediated immunity has yet been conclusively established." Clinically, an alcoholic person has a two- to three-fold increase in infections[33,35,39,41,123,151,197,210,250,273] and responds

poorly to immunization,[185] and over 60% of the patients are anergic.[180] Furthermore, once initiated, the liver injury can progress for months or even years after ethanol consumption has been stopped,[29,86] supporting the possibility that an autoimmune component is operative.

The T-lymphocyte system seems to be the more extensively involved. Animal studies indicate thymic atrophy, small spleens, and delayed formation of T-cell–initiated antibody production to various antigens after chronic alcohol consumption.[105] In humans, circulating peripheral T cells are depressed.[17,166,255] Quantification of T-cell subsets by monoclonal antibody tagging reveals a decrease in total numbers, with maximal involvement with helper cells resulting in a significant depression in the helper-to-suppressor cell ratio.[112] Function also is affected by ethanol consumption. DNA synthesis of T cells after phytohemagglutinin (PHA) or concanavalin A simulation (in vitro) is universally depressed.[47,166,293] Selective suppressor cell activity after concanavalin A stimulation has been variously observed to be decreased,[139,244,300] whereas killer cell cytotoxicity to Chang's cells, autologous hepatocytes,[134] or xenogenic hepatocytes[199] was increased. T lymphocytes of patients with alcoholic liver injury, particularly those with alcoholic hepatitis, are sensitized to liver extract,[193,283] alcoholic hyalin,[138,308] liver-specific antigen,[138,193] as well as ethanol and its metabolite, acetaldehyde.[2,138] These examples of T-cell sensitization could account for the increased resting levels of soluble mediators that occur even in the absence of infection and in the presence of decreased lymphocyte numbers and function.

Indeed, although lymphocyte numbers are decreased,

their secretory products, interleukin-1 (IL-1) and tumor necrosis factor (TNF) have been reported to be increased in the alcoholic.[6,75,173,174] McClain and Cohen[174] reported on TNF activity in 16 patients with alcoholic hepatitis. Basal release of TNF from peripheral monocytes was elevated in 50% of the patients and in only 12.5% of the healthy controls. In vitro stimulation of their mononuclear cells with lipopolysaccharide resulted in more striking differences (25.3 U/mL in patients with alcoholic hepatitis versus 10.9 U/mL in healthy controls; $P < .005$). Similar findings in vitro of increased cytotoxicity were observed by Wickramasinghe[302]; however, Nelson and associates[205] reported in alcoholic rats decreased activity after both lipopolysaccharide stimulation and after infection with *Klebsiella pneumoniae*.[206] In addition to the obvious species and organ differences in these reports, the diverse observations also may represent differences in dose response, nutritional status, and other uncontrolled variables, including the bioassay system used. In support of McClain and Cohen's finding, Allen and Khoruts,[6] Felver and coworkers,[75] and Bird and colleagues[20] observed increased concentrations of TNFα. Of more significance, TNFα but not IL-1 in the latter two reports correlated significantly with survival ($P = .002$)[75] and disease severity ($P = .0009$).[20] The consensus appears to be an increase for both IL-1 and TNFα. Studies with IL-2 also appear conflicting. At low-dose ethanol in rodents, IL-2–mediated killer cell activity was increased[267]; Ericasson and colleagues,[73] in well nourished chronic alcoholics, saw no changes. Most of the studies using higher ethanol intake, however, reported diminished IL-2–mediated natural killer activity.[1,252,268,284,287,299] These in vitro differences in immune response associated with differences in ethanol intake (low-dose stimulatory versus high-dose depressive) are similar to in vivo responses reported[62] using skin test changes as a measure of immune activity.

The pathologic condition of the liver provides perhaps the strongest evidence that immune dysfunction contributes to liver injury. Histologically, lymphocyte numbers increased in the liver in association with alcoholic liver pathologic process.[31,263] Using monoclonal antibody tagging, clusters of helper–inducer cells have been observed in areas of fibrosis, whereas suppressor–cytotoxic cells were seen in areas of necrosis,[278] suggesting an active and specific contribution to the liver injury. Surprisingly, with all these T-cell changes, the B cells appear to be minimally involved. They are neither decreased in peripheral blood[38] nor increased in liver tissue,[45,46] and the observed functional changes in antibody production appear to be related to helper T or suppressor T cell changes.[185]

Symptomatology

The spectrum of clinical signs and symptoms varies from mild with minimal or no complaints to that of severe, life-threatening liver failure. At the mild end of the spectrum, one of the earliest signs is the presence of some degree of liver enlargement. In the VA study,[178] a liver greater than 12 cm in the right midclavicular line was present in more than 85% of patients with even the mild symptoms. The presence of cirrhosis in combination with alcoholic hepatitis is a frequent occurrence seen in 55% (126/228) of all patients for whom histologic studies were available.[44] Typically, patients with cirrhosis are said to have a small, shrunken liver. Hepatomegaly was observed in nearly every patient regardless of clinical severity, however, and was not helpful in differentiating the presence or absence of cirrhosis. In mild cases, only the liver biopsy can establish the diagnosis and differentiate it from pure fatty liver, chronic persistent hepatitis, malignancy, or a variety of other liver lesions. The presenting signs and symptoms depend to a great extent on the severity of injury. Shown graphically in Fig. 31-4 is the prevalence of

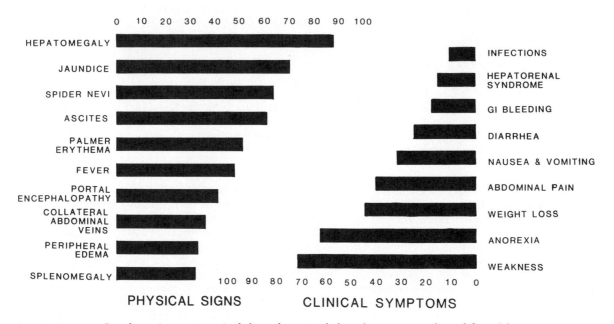

FIGURE 31-4   Prevalence (in percentage) of physical signs and clinical symptoms is derived from 16 reported series of 1108 patients with alcoholic hepatitis.[14,15,21,34,63,133,115,117,161,168,182,216,233,239,242,292]

observed findings in 16 reported studies on 1108 patients. [14,15,21,34,63,113,115,117,161,168,181,216,233,241,292]

When certain of these symptoms occur in combination, pitfalls in the diagnosis may result and are worthy of comment. Alcoholic liver disease in general, and alcoholic hepatitis in particular, produce laboratory changes that are cholestatic in nature. (These will be discussed later in the section on laboratory findings.) In a small but significant number of patients, symptoms of anorexia, nausea, vomiting, and right upper quadrant pain are associated with fever, jaundice, leukocytosis, and liver biochemistries consistent with cholestasis. In these instances, a false diagnosis of cholelithiasis or an acute abdomen may result. This may be disastrous for these patients, because surgery is poorly tolerated and may be associated with a high morbidity and mortality. [15,177,178]

In some, signs and symptoms of liver failure predominate, with ascites, portal hypertension, and hepatic encephalopathy. The range of symptoms may not correlate well with histologic findings, so that an incorrect diagnosis of irreversible cirrhosis results, when in fact the condition is reversible. Portal hypertension with bleeding esophageal varices has been described with perivenular fibrosis, inflammation, and necrosis, but without cirrhosis. [69] Ascites and encephalopathy have been observed with minimal or no clinical jaundice and without cirrhosis. In the VA cooperative study, [44] ascites was observed in 39% of cases in which, histologically, only alcoholic hepatitis was present and cirrhosis was absent. In these cases, even tense ascites was observed in 5%. Changes consistent with portal systemic encephalopathy were reported in 33% of these cases. These changes typically were grade 1; however, 10% had clinical and physical findings of grades 2 to 4.

Laboratory Findings

The laboratory changes shown in Table 31-2 are taken from the initial data on the 363 patients in the VA Cooperative Study on Alcoholic Hepatitis. [102,179,180] The laboratory changes in these patients reflect the multisystem involvement by alcohol as well as the dysfunction present in the liver. Frequently, several pathologic processes interact so that a variety of laboratory results may be seen, depending on which process predominates. Hematologic changes demonstrate this diversity of response. Leukocytosis was present in 41% of the patients, with the frequency increasing as the severity of the liver disease increased. Leukopenia, however, was observed in 8%, presumably as a result of direct bone marrow suppression by ethanol. A normal white cell count was observed in 51% of the cases. Chronic liver disease and malnutrition may result in anemia. Indeed, anemia was seen in over 90% of patients with severe alcoholic hepatitis. Typically, this is a macrocytic type resulting from membrane alterations by ethanol. Folate deficiency may further complicate the picture and represents one of the most frequent vitamin deficiencies in the alcoholic. This has been reported to be present in 78% of alcoholics. [156] Less frequently, vitamin B_{12} deficiency may occur (25%) and contribute to the macrocytosis. More often, serum vitamin B_{12} levels are elevated in alcoholic hepatitis, reflecting acute liver cell injury and release from liver stores. [183] As a result of these two processes (direct toxicity of ethanol on red cells and vitamin deficiency), the mean corpuscular volume (MCV) typically is

increased. Mean value in the VA cooperative study was 102.4/mL. Gastrointestinal tract blood loss is frequent in the alcoholic as a result of increased peptic ulcer disease, alcoholic gastritis, esophagitis, and esophageal varices. When this blood loss occurs with sufficient severity, iron deficiency anemia results, with a decrease in MCV. This phenomenon was seen in 2% of the VA patients. Associated with severe liver disease, renal functional impairment was a frequent observation. Blood urea nitrogen (BUN) and serum creatinine levels both tended to be higher, whereas urine volume tended to be lower. A low BUN (under 5 mg/dL) is said to occur in severe liver disease because of decreased liver synthesis of urea by the failing liver. This was not observed in any of the 435 VA patients. Although 6% (25 of 435) did have values below 5 mg/dL, these typically were patients with mild disease, good renal function, and reasonably good liver function (mean bilirubin, 6.9 ± 1.7), rather than end-stage liver disease. None of those critically ill patients who died of their disease in the initial 30 days of hospitalization had a low BUN.

Abnormalities in the biochemical tests related to liver injury usually were diffusely abnormal. A pattern of change, however, can be detected. Typically, the serum glutamic-oxaloacetic transaminase (asparate aminotransferase [AST]) level is less than five times the upper limits of normal (depending on the laboratory, this usually is less than 200 IU/L). Only 5% of the VA patients had AST levels greater than 200 IU/L, and most of these were terminal patients. Even in this seriously ill group, none of the levels were above 300 IU/L. In other series of patients, scattered observations of high values have been observed, but they are infrequent, [115,262] so that in the presence of a high level of AST the diagnosis of alcoholic hepatitis should be suspect unless proven histologically. The serum glutamic-pyruvic transaminase (alanine aminotransferase [ALT]) level reflects even less the degree of alcohol injury, and its levels typically are less than half those of the AST. Because of this relation, a ratio (AST/ALT) of greater than 2.0 has been suggested as a diagnostic test for this disease. [53] Results of the VA study suggest that although 93% of the patients had an AST level higher than that of the ALT, the ratio exceeded 2.0 in only 58%. This was almost exclusively in the more severely ill patients, especially those with cirrhosis. [103] The explanation for the low levels of AST and ALT in the face of cellular injury and necrosis is not proven. Certainly, the magnitude of the changes does not parallel the degree of injury. [117] Vitamin—particularly pyridoxine—deficiency has been implicated, [208] but remains to be proven. γ-Glutamyltransferase levels almost invariably are elevated in alcoholic hepatitis; however, increases may reflect microsomal enzyme induction rather than liver injury. [254,290] For that reason, this enzyme is less useful for diagnosis and management of this disease. Typically, alcoholic hepatitis may be considered a cholestatic type of liver disease. The most commonly used laboratory tests for cholestasis are the serum alkaline phosphatase and bilirubin. Usually these tend to parallel each other and were observed to be abnormal in 82% (over 120 IU/L) and 78% (over 1.1 mg/dL), respectively. Cholestatic laboratory changes in which AST and ALT levels were normal or only minimally elevated relative to a disproportionately elevated alkaline phosphatase or bilirubin level were observed in 46% of the patients (mean bilirubin 18 mg/dL; mean alkaline phosphatase 253 IU/mL). The prognostic significance of these changes will be discussed later.

Prothrombin time and albumin concentration both are

TABLE 31-2 *Laboratory Changes Associated With Alcoholic Hepatitis* *

Laboratory Tests	Severity of Alcoholic Hepatitis[†]			
	Mild (113)	Moderate (124)	Severe (126)	Combined (363)
Hematology				
Hemoglobin (14–18 g/dL)	12.7 ± 0.2	11.7 ± 0.2	11.2 ± 0.2	11.8 ± 0.1
Abnormal	63%	90%	91%	80%
Hematocrit (47% ± 5%)	38.0 ± 0.5	35.1 ± 0.5	33.1 ± 0.5	35.3 ± 0.3
Abnormal	65%	91%	94%	82%
MCV (80–94 µL)	100.1 ± 0.7	103.4 ± 0.8	103.4 ± 0.8	102.4 ± 0.5
Increased	64%	86%	85%	77%
Decreased	2%	4%	1%	2%
WBC (5–10 × 10⁹)	8.7 ± 0.3	11.2 ± 0.5	12.3 ± 0.6	10.8 ± 0.3
Increased	23%	51%	53%	41%
Decreased	8%	7%	9%	8%
General Chemistry				
Blood glucose (75–120 mg/dL)	108 ± 3	108 ± 3	107 ± 3	107 ± 2
Increased	22%	20%	27%	23%
Decreased	0%	0%	1%	<1%
Amylase (60–160 Su/dL)	125 ± 8	157 ± 37	111 ± 9	131 ± 13
Abnormal	19%	19%	21%	20%
BUN (4–20 mg/dL)	10 ± 1	16 ± 1	23 ± 2	16 ± 1
Increased	6%	20%	37%	20%
Decreased	4%	3%	0%	2%
Creatinine (0.6–1.7 mg/dL)	1.0 ± 0	1.5 ± 0.2	1.9 ± 0.2	1.5 ± 0.1
Abnormal	3%	19%	31%	17%
Immunoglobulins				
IgA (70–312 mg/dL)	556 ± 26	797 ± 33	1065 ± 44	802 ± 23
Abnormal	89%	98%	97%	94%
IgG (639–1349 mg/dL)	1582 ± 65	1758 ± 67	2123 ± 73	1815 ± 41
Abnormal	53%	71%	87%	70%
IgM (56–352 mg/dL)	229 ± 13	276 ± 15	312 ± 15	272 ± 9
Abnormal	13%	25%	33%	23%
Chemistries Related to Liver Injury				
AST (10–40 mIU/mL)	82 ± 5	109 ± 5	115 ± 6	103 ± 3
Abnormal	55%	97%	96%	80%
ALT (10–30 mIU/mL)	51 ± 5	45 ± 3	48 ± 5	48 ± 3
Abnormal	45%	62%	64%	56%
AST/ALT ratio	2.33 ± 0.15	3.27 ± 0.20	3.13 ± 0.16	2.93 ± 0.10
>2.0	35%	67%	74%	57%
<1.0	23%	2%	2%	10%
Total bilirubin (0.1–1 mg/dL)	1.5 ± 0.1	14.6 ± 0.8	17.1 ± 1.0	11.3 ± 0.6
Abnormal	37%	100%	100%	76%
Prothrombin time (0 second above control)	1.0 ± 0.1	2.6 ± 0.2	5.8 ± 0.2	3.2 ± 0.1
Abnormal	69%	95%	100%	87%
Alkaline phosphatase (40–120 IU/L)	165.8 ± 8.5	276.3 ± 14.5	224.9 ± 14.2	224.9 ± 14.2
Abnormal	67%	100%	88%	88%
Albumin (3.5–5 g/dL)	3.7 ± 0.1	2.7 ± 0.1	2.4 ± 0.1	2.9 ± 0.0
Abnormal	29%	93%	98%	70%
Cholyl glycine (0–60 µg/dL)	413 ± 48	1595 ± 86	1758 ± 97	1269 ± 58
Abnormal	75%	100%	100%	91%

MCV, mean corpuscular volume; WBC, white blood cell count; BUN, blood urea nitrogen; AST, aspartate aminotransferase; ALT, alanine aminotransferase.
* Data derived from 363 patients in the Veterans Administration cooperative study.[102,181]
† The numbers in parentheses indicate the number of patients in each severity group.
(Mendenhall CL. The Department of Veterans Affairs Cooperative Study Group on Alcoholic Hepatitis: unpublished observations)

used as a measure of the liver's capacity to synthesize proteins; however, both may be altered during malnutrition. Abnormalities in these two parameters are observed frequently; thus, they are of little use in the initial diagnosis. Alterations in the liver function (protein synthesis) tend to develop more slowly, however, with normal or near normal values observed with clinically mild disease, whereas severe alterations are common with far advanced illness. Similar observations on the magnitude of the serum bilirubin also have been observed such that these parameters have been used to predict severity of disease.[48,168,181,217] Their accuracy in this regard will be discussed in the section on prognosis.

Course and Prognosis

It is not unusual for the illness to increase in severity during the initial 10 days to 2 weeks after hospitalization, at a time when alcohol consumption has been stopped and essential nutrients are restored to the diet.[171] This increased severity is manifest primarily by a 10% to 20% increase in serum bilirubin and AST levels. The apparent increasing severity may persist for as long as 3 weeks before improvement begins or the patient succumbs to his or her disease. Acute 30-day mortality varies considerably and depends on the severity of the disease at the time of admission. In the Department of Veterans Affairs study,[102,181] the overall acute 30-day mortality rate for all degrees of severity was 15% (55 of 358). This increased progressively to 39% (114 of 291) by 1 year.

Three major attempts have been made to assess disease severity on the basis of clinical and laboratory findings. To be useful, such an assessment must be simple to apply and give a reasonable estimate of prognosis. Child and Turcotte[48] used five parameters (ascites, encephalopathy, nutritional state, albumin, and bilirubin) to evaluate the ability of alcoholic patients to tolerate shunt surgery. This subsequently has been modified to assess survival in alcoholic cirrhosis[50] by assigning numeric values from 1 to 3 for each of the five parameters, with a maximum score of 15. Orrego and coworkers[217] have done more complex analyses consisting of 14 parameters, each weighted a variable amount from 1 to 3 so that the maximum score is 25. Maddrey and colleagues,[168] using discriminant analysis, observed the bilirubin concentration and prothrombin time to be the two best indicators of survival, where the discriminant function = 4.6 (prothrombin time) + bilirubin.

When these three estimates of disease severity were applied to the VA cooperative study patients (using 30-day mortality as the gold standard for severity), all correlated significantly with survival. The Maddrey formula gave the best correlation. In addition, the Orrego and Child-Turcotte criteria suffered from their complexity, since they used 5 and 14 variables, respectively, versus 2 for Maddrey's. When one wishes to identify 90% of those who will die in 30 days with the fewest number of false-positives (patients who by the various criteria are severely ill enough to die but who survive), then again Maddrey's discriminant function is superior, with 32% false-positive versus 34% and 41% for Orrego and Child-Turcotte, respectively.

Two individual parameters, bilirubin and creatinine alone, without applying any formula such as Maddrey's, gave a reasonable prediction. For bilirubin and creatinine, a 90% accuracy for mortality was associated with a 39% and 37% incidence of false-positives, respectively (superior to the Child-Turcotte criteria,[50] and only slightly less precise than Orrego's[217]). Figure 31-5 shows the values for Maddrey's dis-

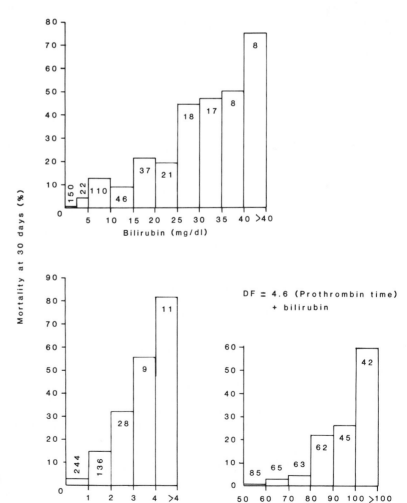

FIGURE 31-5 Correlation between acute 30-day mortality and admission serum bilirubin, serum creatinine, and Maddrey's discriminant function.[168] Observations on mortality taken from the VA cooperative study.[102,180] The numbers within the graphs indicate the number of patients in each group.

criminant function, bilirubin alone, and creatinine alone, and corresponding mortality percentage. Other parameters that correlated with survival included encephalopathy, age, prothrombin time, and albumin. None, however, were as accurate as Maddrey's discriminant function, bilirubin, or creatinine. The enzymatic biochemical tests of liver injury, AST, and ALT did not correlate significantly. Although bilirubin and alkaline phosphatase levels typically are elevated together, in those patients with a high acute mortality, only the bilirubin level was markedly elevated. The alkaline phosphatase changes did not correlate significantly with survival.

Most of the early mortality from alcoholic hepatitis occurs in the initial 2 weeks after admission.[178] Clinical features of liver failure and portal hypertension (hepatic encephalopathy, ascites, and bleeding esophageal varices) were present in 91%, 63%, and 37% of the fatal cases, respectively. These features were not useful as prognostic indicators, however, because they were observed so frequently in surviving patients (false-positives).

Beyond the initial acute mortality, few studies have been performed in which serial liver biopsies have established the natural course of the disease. In the Emory series,[86] complete recovery established by serial biopsy appeared to be unpredictable. If alcohol consumption continued, no patient recovered from his or her disease and a persistent alcoholic hepatitis resulted, with 38% progressing to cirrhosis within 18 months. Even abstinence from ethanol did not guarantee recovery. Only 27% of abstainers returned to normal by the seventh month, and 18% had progressed to cirrhosis. The remaining 55% still had active persistent alcoholic hepatitis that had neither returned to normal nor progressed to cirrhosis by 12 to 14 months. These observations suggest that alcoholic hepatitis, once initiated, is slow to resolve and that other factors capable of causing continuation and progression are present even after ethanol consumption has ceased.

Treatment

The essential role of ethanol in the initiation and potentiation of the morbidity, mortality, and progression of the alcoholic liver injury is undeniable.[29,162,178,269] Hence, abstinence should be the mainstay for any treatment program. Although there is no evidence that occasional drinking of small amounts is harmful, the psychodynamics of the chronic alcoholic make complete abstinence the more desirable goal. Achieving total abstinence is a difficult task. In one large study of patients with alcoholic hepatitis[218] in which morning urine alcohol levels were collected and measured daily, 35% to 40% of the samples were positive throughout the study, whereas less than 10% of the patients maintained sobriety for the entire duration (2 years) of the study. Thus, although total sobriety is the desired goal for most patients for a long period of time, it rarely is achieved. In the VA Cooperative Study on Alcoholic Hepatitis,[102,181] after 1 year of monthly visits, more than 80% of the patients gave a history of consuming less than 35 g/d ethanol at one or more of their interviews; 39% denied any drinking, with only 12% continuing at their initial excessive level of consumption. Although these were soft data obtained by interviewing, the information was consistent with the overall improvements in the clinical and laboratory variables as well as the low observed incidence (16%, 40 of 253) of relapses over the 4.4-year study period.

More specific therapy has been directed at a variety of specific clinical and pathologic features associated with alcoholic hepatitis that contribute to its morbidity and mortality. Malnutrition is a prominent feature of hepatitis. Hence, diet therapy represents the second most important mainstay for treatment. As indicated earlier, nutritional deficits almost invariably are present. Experimental evidence suggests that nutrition therapy results in improved nutritional status,[182] and that repletion of the malnutrition is essential for improvement of the liver disease.[232–234] When alcohol consumption was stopped but malnutrition allowed to persist, only minimal improvement in the liver disease occurred. Conversely, alcohol administration did not prevent or delay improvement in the liver disease so long as nutritional support was adequate.[72,223,249,286,298]

In the VA study,[44,178,180–184,209] patients were hospitalized for 30 days of treatment, thus preventing (in most instances) ethanol consumption. Although multivitamins and minerals were provided along with a well balanced, 2500-kcal diet, the anorexia associated with the disease impaired adequate intake such that only 63% of the estimated energy requirements were consumed by the moderately ill patients and 53% of the estimated energy requirements by the severely ill patients. It is not surprising that after 1 month of hospitalization, 19% showed some deterioration. This was not the case for those receiving active nutritional supplementation.[182] Older studies have reported on the therapeutic use of diets rich in protein and B-complex vitamins,[223,224] in which significant improvement in 5-year survival was observed. Unfortunately, the comparison control group was obtained retrospectively from a different hospital. More recently, several reports from Galambos and associates[91,201] have noted significant improvement in survival after more vigorous parenteral hyperalimentation with amino acid therapy. Although the number of patients evaluated under appropriate controlled conditions was small, these results strongly attest to the importance of nutritional therapy in this disease. It is suggested that when malnutrition is observed to be severe,[184] the prognosis is grave and vigorous replacement therapy should be provided. In the absence of hepatic encephalopathy, this therapy may consist of any high-calorie, high-protein nutrient. When encephalopathy is present, however, protein intake should be maintained using high branch chain amino acid types of nutrients, since these are well tolerated[182] and may be therapeutic for the encephalopathy.[122] Every effort should be made to meet the estimated energy requirements and produce a positive nitrogen balance.

Vitamin and mineral deficiencies in this population are frequent and typically multiple.[9,156,183] Because serum levels do not correlate well with the deficiency present in the tissues, replacement therapy usually is given empirically. A high-potency multivitamin preparation that includes B_{12}, folic acid, thiamine, pyridoxine, vitamin A, vitamin D, and such minerals as zinc, magnesium, calcium, and phosphorus should be provided. Unless iron loss is present, replacement of iron should be given with caution in view of the increased iron absorption seen in cirrhosis[303] and the high prevalence of hemosiderosis in alcoholic hepatitis.[51] Assessment of the efficacy of specific therapy is considerably more controversial, producing in many instances contradictory results. Adrenal corticosteroids are one such group of drugs. Because alcoholic hepatitis is characterized by inflammation and necrosis, one theoretic approach to therapy is with an antiinflammatory agent such as glucocorticosteroids. These agents, in addition to their antiinflammatory effects, also are immunosuppressive. Hence, to whatever degree an autoimmune component operates in alcoholic hepatitis, these steroids might be of further benefit. Of the 11 major studies published since 1971, encompassing 515 patients,[21,34,36,57,63,117,161,168,181,242,292] the acute 30-day mortality was unaffected by these corticosteroids in 34% treated versus 33% placebo controls. Furthermore, of the 11 studies, only 3 observed beneficial improvement in survival.

Some have suggested a beneficial effect in a select population of severely ill patients with encephalopathy.[117,161] In the VA study,[181] 70 patients met this criteria (severely ill with encephalopathy); unfortunately, no improvement in survival was effected by corticosteroid treatment. It appears that although corticosteroids did not increase the incidence of complications, they did little to improve survival.

In 1990, Imperiale and McCullough[125] used metaanalysis to evaluate corticosteroid effects on survival. Metaanalysis is a statistical tool in which data from multiple studies with comparable patient populations treated in a similar manner are pooled to detect a difference. Although no significant improvement in survival was observed for the entire patient population, they described a subpopulation who appeared to benefit from such treatment, namely, those patients with spontaneous hepatic encephalopathy, but without gastrointestinal bleeding. In this select group, one of three patients had improved survival. It is necessary to confirm these findings in a prospective randomized study. In an effort to stimulate protein synthesis and cell repair, androgenic anabolic steroids have been used as therapy. With this form of treatment, liver fat is mobilized rapidly so that fatty liver rapidly undergoes restoration to a normal histologic condition, and results of biochemical tests for liver injury return to normal.[176] In more severe disease, improvement in defective synthesis of coagulation factors has been reported after treatment with large doses.[288]

Of the 11 published reports on the use of anabolic steroids in alcoholic liver disease, 9 reported clinical improvement.[58,76,77,97,119,128,144,177,200,256,301] Unfortunately, only the VA study[181] was performed on sufficient numbers of patients with a randomized double-blind experimental design. For reasons not well understood, perhaps related to differences in binding affinity at the target organ level,[26] a therapeutic effect after 80 mg of oxandrolone daily for 30 days was delayed so that no improvement in survival was observed in the initial 30 days during treatment. Long-term effects on survival in the 6-month posttreatment period were observed, however. This was especially true for the moderately ill patients. In this group, the 6-month conditional death rate for those patients treated with oxandrolone was 3.5%, compared to a 19.7% mortality in the controls. By 12 months (11 months after treatment had been stopped), only 24% of the treated patients had died versus 55% of the controls ($P < .02$). Although these results are impressive, additional studies are needed to confirm efficacy and establish the optimum dose and duration of treatment. In addition, since anabolic steroids increase protein use,[147,245] the combination of anabolic steroids and vigorous nutrition therapy needs evaluation. Because chronic alcoholism can induce a hypermetabolic state in the liver,[18,296] and because the centrolobular area of the liver, with the lowest oxygen tension, also suffers the most severe pathologic processes,[260] an effort to depress this hypermeta-

bolic state with propylthiouracil has been suggested as therapy.[131,215,216] Using the Orrego clinical severity index,[217] a more rapid normalization was observed. Subsequently, in a larger study,[218] improvement in mortality also was observed. Of the six published reports using propylthiouracil,[109,215,216,218,236,276] only three from Orrego's group observed significant improvement. The efficacy of this form of therapy for alcoholic hepatitis remains to be established, and is not widely used by hepatologists.

Because cirrhosis and hepatic fibrosis are frequent and early pathologic changes associated with alcoholic hepatitis, agents that inhibit collagen synthesis have been used for therapy. D-Penicillamine, a drug that retards the cross-linking of collagen, has been recommended.[248] Unfortunately, D-penicillamine has numerous undesirable side effects, including nausea, vomiting, urticaria, skin eruptions, renal toxicity, and bone marrow suppression. Another, less toxic agent is colchicine, which interferes with the transcellular movement and transport of collagen from the cytoplasm to the extracellular space.[64,71,212] In a preliminary 4-year study involving 43 cirrhotic patients,[142] mortality improved from 40% with placebo to 17% with colchicine, 1 mg/d, 5 days per week. Clinical symptomatology (ascites, encephalopathy, splenomegaly) improved significantly ($P < .05$). Because of the small number of patients in each treatment group and the slow rate at which histologic improvement in fibrosis occurred (only 3 of 20 improved), statistical significance was not obtained histologically.

Since this initial report, six additional studies have appeared, making a total of seven. Of the seven published reports on the use of colchicine,[5,84,92,142,207,246,253,289] four reported significant improvement and two observed a tendency toward improvement. These are encouraging results for a stage in the alcoholic liver pathologic process previously considered irreversible. Many still are skeptical about its efficacy, however, and it remains to be established when colchicine treatment should be initiated and to what extent established cirrhosis can be reversed. Additional, well controlled studies are needed.

The final approach to therapy is the application of orthotopic liver transplants to alcoholic liver disease. The results from the largest series have been reported,[148] describing experiences in 73 patients treated by orthotopic liver transplants. Their response to therapy was comparable to that seen in patients with other forms of terminal liver disease (ie, 71% were alive 25 months after transplantation). Perhaps most surprising was the fact that only about 11% returned to alcoholism, with 54% returning to some gainful employment. The decision to undertake such extreme therapy, in addition to the patient's medical status, must include consideration of the danger of recidivism back to alcoholism by the patient, the availability of donor livers, and finally the economic issue of payment for the procedure.[271] These considerations make the application of this mode of therapy more arbitrary and less dependent on objective medical judgment.

References

1. Abdallah RM, Starkey JR, Meadows GG. Toxicity of chronic high alcohol intake on mouse natural killer cell activity. Res Commun Chem Pathol Pharmacol 59:245–258, 1988
2. Actis GC, Ponzetto A, Rizzetto M, Verme G. Cell-mediated

immunity to acetaldehyde in alcoholic liver disease demonstrated by leukocyte migration test. Dig Dis 23:883–886, 1978

3. Adler M, Schaffner F. Fatty liver and cirrhosis in obese patients. Am J Med 67:811, 1979
4. Afshani MD, et al. Significance of microscopic cholangitis in alcoholic liver disease. Gastroenterology 75:1045, 1978
5. Akriviadis E, Steindel H, Pinto P, Fong TL, Kenel G, Reynolds TB, Gupta S. Failure of colchicine to improve short-term survival in patients with severe alcoholic hepatitis. Hepatology 8:1239, 1988
6. Allen JI, Khoruts A. Increased plasma tumor necrosis factor and interleukin-1 in patients with alcoholic liver disease. Hepatology 10:649, 1989
7. Arky RA. The effect of alcohol on carbohydrate metabolism: carbohydrate metabolism in alcoholics. In: Kissin B, Begleiter H, eds. The biology of alcoholism, vol 1. New York, Plenum Press, 1977, p 197
8. Bailey RJ, et al. Histocompatibility antigens, autoantibodies, and immunoglobulins in alcoholic liver disease. Br Med J 2:727, 1976
9. Baker H, et al. Effect of hepatic disease on liver B-complex vitamin titers. Am J Clin Nutr 14:1, 1964
10. Baraona E, et al. Alcoholic hepatomegaly: accumulation of protein in the liver. Science 190:794, 1975
11. Basile A, Vitale G, Macor C. Hepatitis B virus infection in alcoholic cirrhosis. Br Med J 282:1705, 1981
12. Bassendine MF, Della Seta L, Salmern J, Thomas HC, Sherlock S. Incidence of hepatitis B virus infection in alcoholic liver disease, HBsAg negative chronic active liver disease and primary liver cancer in Britain. Liver 3:69–70, 1983
13. Batman PA, Scheuer PJ. Diabetic hepatitis preceding the onset of glucose intolerance. Histopathology 9:237–243, 1985
14. Beckett AG, et al. Acute alcoholic hepatitis. Br Med J 2:1113, 1961
15. Beckett AG, et al. Acute alcoholic hepatitis without jaundice. Br Med J 2:580, 1962
16. Bell H, Nordhager R. Association between HLA-BW40 and alcoholic liver disease with cirrhosis. Br Med J 2:822, 1978
17. Bernstein IM, et al. Reduction in circulating T-lymphocytes in alcoholic liver disease. Lancet 2:488, 1974
18. Bernstein J, et al. Metabolic alterations produced in the liver by chronic ethanol administration: changes related to energetic parameters of the cell. Biochem J 134:515, 1973
19. Bianchi L, Winckler K, Mihatsh M,, et al. Mallory bodies and giant mitochondria: two different structures in liver biopsies from alcoholics. Beitr Pathol 150:298–310, 1978
20. Bird GLA, Shernon N, Goka AKJ, Alexander GJ, Williams RS. Increased plasma tumor necrosis factor in severe alcoholic hepatitis. Ann Intern Med 112:917–920, 1990
21. Blitzer BL, et al. Adrenocorticosteroid therapy in alcoholic hepatitis: a prospective double-blind randomized study. Dig Dis Sci 22:477, 1977
22. Blum HE, Offensperger WB, Walter E, Offensperger S, Zeschnigk C, Wahl A, Gerok W. Hepatitis B virus DNA in chronic liver disease. N Engl J Med 317:116–117, 1987
23. Bolland JL, Koch HP. The course of autoxidation reactions in polyisoprenes and allied compounds: IX. the primary thermal oxidation product of ethyl linoleate. J Chemical Soc 19:445, 1945
24. Borenfreund E, et al. In vivo initiated rat liver cell carcinogenesis studies in vitro: formation of alcoholic hyalin-type bodies. Cancer Lett 3:145, 1977
25. Brechot C, Degos F, Lugassy C, et al. Hepatitis B virus DNA in patients with chronic liver disease and negative tests for hepatitis B surface antigen. N Engl J Med 312:270–276, 1985
26. Breuer CB, Florini JR. Amino acid incorporation into protein by cell-free systems from rat skeletal muscle. IV. Effects of animal age, androgens, and anabolic agents on activity of muscle ribosomes. Biochemistry 4:1544, 1965
27. Brillanti S, Barbara L, Miglioli M, Bonino F. Hepatitis C virus: a possible cause of chronic hepatitis in alcoholics. Lancet 2:1390–1391, 1989
28. Bruguera M, et al. Giant mitochondria in hepatocytes: a diagnostic hint for alcoholic liver disease. Gastroenterology 73:1383, 1977
29. Brunt PW, et al. Studies in alcoholic liver disease in Britain. Gut 15:52, 1974
30. Buffet C, Attali P, Papoz, Chaput JC, Etienne JP. Evidence for previous hepatitis B virus infection in alcoholic cirrhosis. (Letter) Dig Dis Sci 27:473–474, 1982
31. Burbige EJ, Tarder G, Denton T, Harkin C, Luehro D, Bourke E, French SW. Predominantly T cell infiltrate in the liver in alcoholic hepatitis. Gastroenterology 71:900, 1976
32. Burns WA, et al. Cytoplasmic crystalline regions in hepatocytes of liver biopsy specimens. Arch Pathol 97:43, 1974
33. Busch LA. Human listeriosis in the United States. J Infect Dis 123:328, 1971
34. Campra JL, et al. Prednisone therapy of acute alcoholic hepatitis: report of a controlled trial. Ann Intern Med 79:625, 1973
35. Capps JA, Coleman GH. Influence of alcohol on prognosis of pneumonia in Cook County Hospital. JAMA 80:750–752, 1923
36. Carithers RI Jr, Herlong HF, Diehl AM, et al. Methylprednisolone therapy in patients with severe alcoholic hepatitis: a randomized multicenter trial. Ann Intern Med. 110:685–690, 1989
37. Cederbaum AI, et al. The effect of dimethylsulfoxide and other hydroxyl radical scavengers on the oxidation of ethanol by rat liver microsomes. Biochem Biophys Res Commun 78:1254, 1977
38. Chadha KC, Whitney RB, Cummings MK, Norman M, Windle M, Stadler I. Evaluation of interferon systems among chronic alcoholics. Prog Clin Biol Res 325:123–133, 1990
39. Chafetz ME. Alcoholism: a multilevel problem. Department of Health Education and Welfare publication no. (ADM) 75-137, 1974
40. Chalmers DM, Bullen AW. Evidence for previous hepatitis B virus infection in alcoholic cirrhosis. Br Med J 282:219, 1981
41. Chaves AD, Robins AB, Abeles H. Tuberculosis-case finding among homeless men in New York City. Am Rev Respir Dis 84:900, 1961
42. Chang T, et al. Effect of ethanol and other alcohols on the transport of amino acids and glucose by everted sacs of rat small intestine. Biochim Biophys Acta 135:1000, 1967
43. Chedid A, et al. The significance of megamitochondria in alcoholic liver disease. Gastroenterology 10:279, 1986
44. Chedid A, Mendenhall CL, Gartside P, French SW, Chen T, Rabin L, the Veterans Administration Cooperative Study Group. Prognostic factors in alcoholic liver disease. Gastroenterology 86:210, 1991
45. Chedid A, Mendenhall CL. The Veterans Administration Cooperative Study #275. Hepatology 8:1285, 1988
46. Chedid A, Mendenhall CL. The Veterans Administration Cooperative Study #275. Submitted to the Biennial Meeting of the International Association of Liver Study, Queensland, Australia, September, 1990
47. Chen T, Leevy CM. Lymphocyte proliferation inhibitory factor (PIF) in alcoholic liver disease. Clin Exp Immunol 26:42–45, 1976
48. Child CG, Turcotte JG. Surgery and portal hypertension. In: Child CG, ed. The liver and portal hypertension. Philadelphia, WB Saunders, 1964, p 50
49. Chevilotte G, Durbee JP, Gerolami A, Bethezner P, Bidart JM, Camatte R. Interaction between hepatitis B virus and alcohol consumption in liver cirrhosis: an epidemiologic study. Gastroenterology 85:141–145, 1983
50. Christensen E, et al. Prognostic value of Child-Turcotte criteria in medically treated cirrhosis. Hepatology 3:430, 1984
51. Christoffersen P, Nielsen K. Histologic changes in human

liver biopsies from chronic alcoholics. Acta Pathol Microbiol Scand [A] 80:557, 1972

52. Cohen G, Cederbaum AI. Chemical evidence for production of hydroxyl radicals during microsomal electron transfer. Science 204:66, 1979

53. Cohen JA, Kaplan MM. The SGOT/SGPT ratio: an indicator of alcoholic liver disease. Dig Dis Sci 24:835, 1979

54. Comporti M, et al. Effect of in vivo and in vitro ethanol administration on liver lipid peroxidation. Lab Invest 16:616, 1967

55. Comporti M, et al. Studies on the in vitro peroxidation of liver lipids in ethanol-treated rats. Lipids 8:498, 1973

56. Connor CL. Fatty infiltration of the liver and the development of cirrhosis in diabetes and chronic alcoholism. Am J Pathol 14:347, 1938

57. Copenhagen Study Group for Liver Diseases. Effect of prednisone on the survival of patients with cirrhosis of the liver. Lancet 1:119, 1969

58. The Copenhagen Study Group for Liver Diseases. Testosterone treatment of men with alcoholic cirrhosis: a double-blind study. Hepatology 6:807–813, 1986

59. Cossel L, et al. "Killer" lymphocytes in action: light and electron microscopical findings in orthotopic liver homografts. Virchows Arch [A] 364:179, 1974

60. Craig Rm, Neumann T, Jeejeebhoy KN,, et al. Severe hepatocellular reaction resembling alcoholic hepatitis with cirrhosis after massive small bowel resection and prolonged parenteral nutrition. Gastroenterology 79:131–137, 1980

61. Cuellar RE, Tarter R, Hays A, Van Thiel DH. The possible occurrence of alcoholic hepatitis: in a patient with bulimia in the absence of diagnosable alcoholism. Hepatology 7:878–883, 1987

62. Dehne NE, Mendenhall CL, Roselle GA, Grossman CJ. Cell mediated immune responses associated with sort-term alcohol intake: time course and dose dependency. Alcohol Clin Exp Res 13:201–205, 1989

63. Depew W, et al. Double-blind controlled trial of prednisolone therapy in patients with severe acute alcoholic hepatitis and spontaneous encephalopathy. Gastroenterology 78:524, 1980

64. Digelman RF, Peterkofsky B. Inhibition of collagen secretion from bone and cultured fibroblasts by microtubular disruptive drugs. Proc Natl Acad Sci USA 69:892, 1972

65. DiLuzio NR. Antioxidants, lipid peroxidation and chemical-induced liver injury. Fed Proc 32:1875, 1973

66. DiLuzio NR, Hartman AD. The effect of ethanol and carbon tetrachloride administration on hepatic lipid-soluble antioxidant activity. Exp Mol Pathol 11:38, 1969

67. DiLuzio NR, Stege NR. The role of ethanol metabolites in hepatic lipid peroxidation. In: Fisher MM, Rankin JG, eds. Hepatology: research and clinical issues, vol 3. Alcohol and the liver. New York, Plenum Press, 1977, p 45

68. Edmondson HA. Tumors of the liver and intrahepatic bile ducts. Armed Forces Institute of Pathology, section 7, part 25, 1958, p 49

69. Edmondson HA, et al. Sclerosing hyalin necrosis of the liver in the chronic alcoholic. Ann Intern Med 59:646, 1963

70. Edmondson HA, et al. The early stage of liver injury in the alcoholic. Medicine 46:119, 1967

71. Ehrlich HR, Bornstein P. Microtubules in transcellular movement of procollagen. Nature 238:257, 1972

72. Erenoglu E, et al. Observations on patients with Laennec's cirrhosis receiving alcohol while on controlled diets. Ann Intern Med 60:814, 1964

73. Ericasson CD, Kohl S, Pickering LK, Davis J, Glass GS, Fallace LA. Mechanisms of host defense in well nourished patients with chronic alcoholism. Alcohol Clin Exp Res 4:261–265, 1980

74. Feinman L, Lieber CS. Hepatic collagen metabolism: effect of alcohol consumption in rats and baboons. Science 176:795, 1972

75. Felver FE, Mezey E, McGuire M, Mitchell MC, Herlong HF, Veech GA, Veech RL. Plasma tumor necrosis factor a predicts decreased long-term survival in severe alcoholic hepatitis. Alcohol Clin Exp Res 14:225–259, 1990

76. Fenster LF. The nonefficacy of short-term anabolic steroid therapy in alcoholic liver disease. Ann Intern Med 65:738, 1966

77. Figueroa RB. Mesterolone in steatosis and cirrhosis of the liver. Acta Hepatogastroenterol 20:282, 1973

78. Figus A, Blum HE, Vyas GN, Virgilis S, Cao A, Lippi M, Lai E, Balistrieri A. Hepatitis B viral nucleotide sequences in non-A, non-B, or hepatitis B virus–related chronic liver disease. Hepatology 3:364–368, 1984

79. Fong TL, Govindarajan S, Valinluck B, Redeker AG. Status of hepatitis B virus DNA in alcoholic liver disease: a study of a large urban population in the United States. Hepatology 8:1602–1604, 1988

80. French SW, Burbige EJ. Alcoholic hepatitis: clinical, morphologic, pathogenic, and therapeutic aspects. In: Popper H, Schaffner F, eds. Progress in liver disease, vol 6. New York, Grune & Stratton, 1979, p 557

81. French SW, Davies PL. The Mallory body in the pathogenesis of alcoholic liver disease. In: Khanna JM, Israel Y, Kalant H, eds. Alcoholic liver pathology. Toronto, Addiction Research Foundation of Ontario, 1975, p 113

82. French SW, et al. Percent T and B cells in the liver in alcoholic hepatitis. (Abstract) Am J Pathol 86:20, 1977

83. French SW, et al. Alcoholic hepatitis. In: Fisher MM, Rankin JG, eds. Alcohol and the liver. New York, Plenum Press, 1977, p 261

84. Frysak Z, Matouskova I, Barborik J. Vliv podavini kolchicinu na biochemicky obraz jaterni cirhozy. Vnitr Lek 31:862–869, 1985

85. Fulchuk KR, et al. Pericentral hepatic fibrosis in diabetes mellitus. Gastroenterology 78:535, 1980

86. Galambos JT. Natural history of alcoholic hepatitis. III. Histologic changes. Gastroenterology 63:1026, 1972

87. Galambos JT. Alcoholic hepatitis: its therapy and prognosis. In: Popper H, Schaffner F, eds. Progress in liver disease, vol 6. New York, Grune & Stratton, 1972, p 567

88. Galambos JT. Alcoholic hepatitis. In: Schaffner F, Sherlock S, Leevy CM, eds. The liver and its diseases. New York, Intercontinental Medical Book Corporation, 1974, p 255

89. Galambos JT. The course of alcoholic hepatitis. In: Khanna JM, Israel Y, eds. Alcoholic liver pathology. Toronto, Addiction Research Foundation of Ontario, 1975, p 97

90. Galambos JT. Epidemiology of alcoholic liver disease: United States of America. In: Hall P, ed. Alcoholic liver disease: pathobiology, epidemiology, and clinical aspects, p 230. New York, John Wiley & Sons, 1985

91. Galambos JT, et al. Hyperalimentation in alcoholic hepatitis. Am J Gastroenterol 72:535, 1979

92. Galambos JT, Riepe SP. Use of colchicine and steroids in the treatment of alcoholic liver disease. Recent Dev Alcohol 2:181–194, 1984

93. Garagliano CF, et al. Incidence rates of liver cirrhosis and related diseases in Baltimore and selected areas of the United States. J Chronic Dis 32:543, 1979

94. Gerber MA, et al. Hepatitis virus B and chronic alcoholic liver disease. Lancet 2:1034, 1972

95. Gerber MA, et al. Hepatocellular hyalin in cholestasis and cirrhosis: its diagnostic significance. Gastroenterology 64: 89, 1973

96. Gerber MA, et al. Hepatocellular hyalin in cholestasis and cirrhosis: its diagnostic significance. Gastroenterology 64:89, 1973

97. Girolami M. Treatment of ascitic atrophic cirrhosis of the liver with high dosages of testosterone propionate. J Am Geriatr Soc 6:306, 1958

98. Gluud C, Aldershvile J, Henrikson J, Kryger P, Mathiesen L.

Hepatitis B and A virus antibodies in alcoholic steatosis and cirrhosis. J Clin Pathol 35:693, 1982

99. Gluud C, Gluud B, Aldershvile J, Jacobsen A, Dietrichson O. Prevalence of hepatitis B virus infection in out-patient alcoholics. Infection 12:72–74, 1984

100. Goidsnohoven van EG, et al. Pancreatic function in cirrhosis of the liver. Am J Dig Dis 8:160, 1963

101. Goldberg M, Thompson CM. Acute fatty metamorphosis of the liver. Ann Intern Med 55:116, 1961

102. Goldberg SJ, et al. Veterans Administration Cooperative Study on Alcoholic Hepatitis. IV. The significance of clinically mild alcoholic hepatitis: describing the population with minimal hyperbilirubinemia. Am J Gastroenterol 11:1029–1034, 1986

103. Goldberg SJ, et al. "Non-alcoholic" chronic hepatitis in the alcoholic. Gastroenterology, 72:598, 1977

104. Goudeau A Maupas P, Dubois F, Coursaget P, Bougnoux P. Hepatitis B infection in alcoholic liver disease and primary hepatocellular carcinoma in France. Prog Med Virol 27:26–34, 1981

105. Grossman CJ, Rosselle GA, Sholiton LJ, Mendenhall CL. The effect of chronic ethanol (E) on rat thymus: a possible mechanism for the altered immune response of the alcoholic. (Abstract) Gastroenterology 77:A14, 1979

106. Grunnet N. Oxidation of acetaldehyde by rat liver mitochondria in relation to ethanol oxidation and the transport of reducing equivalents across the mitochondrial membrane. Eur J Biochem 35:236, 1973

107. Hall EM, Morgan WA. Progressive alcoholic cirrhosis: a clinical and pathologic study of 68 cases. Arch Pathol 27:672, 1930

108. Hall EM, Ophuls W. Progressive alcoholic cirrhosis: report of 4 cases. Am J Pathol 1:477, 1925

109. Halle P, Pare P, Kaptein E, Kanel G, Redeker AG, Reynolds TB. Double-blind controlled trial of propylthiouracil in patients with severe acute alcoholic hepatitis. Gastroenterology 82:925–931, 1982

110. Halsted CH, et al. Intestinal malabsorption in folate-deficient alcoholics. Gastroenterology 64:526, 1973

111. Hamilton DL, Vest TK, Brown BS, et al. Liver injury with alcoholic like hyalin after gastroplasty for morbid obesity. Gastroenterology 85:722–726, 1983

112. Haranaka K, Satomi N, Sakurai A. Antitumor activity of murine tumor necrosis factor (TNF) against transplanted murine tumors and heterotransplanted human tumors in nude mice. Int J Cancer 34:263–267, 1984

113. Harinasuta U, Zimmerman HJ. Alcoholic steatonecrosis: Relationship between severity of hepatic disease and presence of Mallory bodies in the liver. Gastroenterology 60:1036, 1971

114. Harrison TJ, Anderson MG, Murray-Lyon IM, Zuckerman AJ. Hepatitis B virus DNA in the hepatocyte: a series of 106 biopsies. J Hepatol 2:1–10, 1986

115. Harinasuta U, et al. Steatonecrosis: Mallory body type. Medicine 46:141, 1967

116. Hartroft WS. On the etiology of alcoholic liver cirrhosis. In: Khanna JM Israel Y, Kalani H, eds. Alcoholic liver pathology. Toronto, Addiction Research Foundation of Ontario, 1975, p 189

117. Helman RA, et al. Alcoholic hepatitis: natural history and evaluation of prednisolone therapy. Ann Intern Med 74:311, 1971

118. Hino O, Kitagawa T, Koike K, et al. Detection of hepatitis B virus DNA in hepatocellular carcinomas in Japan. Hepatology 4:90–95, 1984

119. Hirayama C, et al. Anabolic steroid effect on hepatic protein synthesis in patients with liver cirrhosis. Digestion 3:41, 1970

120. Hislop WS, Follett EAC, Bouchier IAD, MacSween RNM. Serological markers of hepatitis B in patients with alcoholic liver disease: a multi-center study. J Clin Pathol 34:1017–1019, 1981

121. Horiike N, Michitaka K, Onji M, Murota T, Ohta Y. HBV-DNA hybridization in hepatocellular carcinoma associated with alcohol in Japan. J Med Virol 28:189–192, 1989

122. Horst D, et al. Comparison of dietary protein with an oral, branched-chain enriched amino acid supplement in chronic portal-systemic encephalopathy: a randomized controlled trial. Hepatology 4:279, 1984

123. Hudolin V. Tuberculosis and alcoholism. Ann NY Acad Sci Hepatol 252:353, 1975

124. Husby G, et al. Localization of T and B cells and alpha-fetoprotein in hepatic biopsies from patients with liver disease. J Clin Invest 56:1198, 1975

125. Imperiale TF, McCullough AJ. Do corticosteroids reduce mortality from alcoholic hepatitis?: a meta-analysis of the randomized trials. Ann Intern Med 113:299–307, 1990

126. Inagaki T, Koike M, Ituka K, Kobayashi S, Suziki M, Kato K, Kato K. Ultrastructural identification and clinical significance of light microscopic giant mitochondria in alcoholic liver injuries. Gastroenterol Jpn 24:46–53, 1989

127. International Group. Review of alcoholic liver disease morphologic manifestations. Lancet 1:707, 1981

128. Islam N, Islam A. Testosterone propionate in cirrhosis of the liver. Br J Clin Pract 27:125. 1973

129. Israel Y, et al. Inhibitory effects of alcohol on intestinal acid transport in vivo and in vitro. J Nutr 96:499, 1968

130. Israel Y, et al. Experimental alcohol-induced hepatic necrosis suppression by propylthiouracil. Proc Natl Acad Sci USA 72:1137, 1975

131. Israel Y, et al. Liver hypermetabolic state after chronic ethanol consumption: hormonal interrelationships and pathogenic implications. Fed Proc 34:2052, 1975

132. Itoh S, Igrashi M, Tsukada Y, et al. Nonalcoholic fatty liver with alcoholic hyalin after long-term glucocorticoid therapy. Acta Hepatogastroenterol 24:415–418, 1977

133. John WJ, Phillips R, Ott L, Adams LS, McClain CJ. Resting energy expenditure in patients with alcoholic hepatitis. JPEN J Parenter Enteral Nutr 13:124–127, 1989

134. Kakumu S, Leevy CM. Lymphocyte cytotoxicity in alcoholic hepatitis. Gastroenterology 72:594, 1977

135. Kanagasundaram N, et al. Alcoholic hyalin antigen (AHAg) and antibody (AHAb) in alcoholic hepatitis. Gastroenterology 73:1368, 1977

136. Karasawa T, Chedid A. Sclerosis hyalin necrosis in non-cirrhotic chronic alcoholic hepatitis. Am J Clin Pathol 66:802, 1976

137. Kawanishi H. Morphologic association of lymphocytes with hepatocytes in chronic liver disease. Arch Pathol Lab Med 101:286, 1977

138. Kawanish H, Ibrahim M, Wong KM, MacDermott RP, Sheagren JN. Stimulation of lymphotoxin production in vitro by liver specific protein in patients with active alcoholic and chronic active liver disease. Gastroenterology 76:1166, 1979

139. Kawanishi H, Travassolie H, MacDermott P, Sheagren JN. Impaired concanavalin A inducible suppressor T cell activity in alcoholic liver disease. Gastroenterology 80:510–517, 1981

140. Keffer CCS, Fries ED. Fatty liver: its diagnosis and clinical course. Trans Assoc Am Physicians 57:283–289, 1942

141. Kern WH, et al. The significance of hyalin necrosis in liver biopsies. Surg Gynecol Obstet 128:749, 1969

142. Kershenobich D, et al. Treatment of cirrhosis with colchicine: a double-blind randomized trial. Gastroenterology 77:532, 1979

143. Kimura H, Kaka M, Yo K, et al. Alcoholic hyalins (Mallory bodies) in a case of Weber-Christian disease: electron microscopic observations of liver involvement. Gastroenterology 78:807–812, 1980

144. Kinsell LW. Factors affecting protein balance in the presence of chronic viral liver damage. Gastroenterology 11:672, 1948

145. Koch OR, et al. Ultrastructural and biochemical aspects of liver mitochondria during recovery from ethanol-induced alterations. Am J Pathol 90:325, 1977

146. Koes M, et al. Lipid peroxidation in chronic ethanol treated rats: in vitro uncoupling of peroxidation from reduced nicotine adenosine dinucleotide phosphate oxidation. Lipids 9:899, 1974
147. Kruskemper HL. Clinical application of anabolic steroids: exogenous protein deficiency. In: Kruskemper HL, ed. Anabolic steroids. New York, Academic Press, 1968, p 126
148. Kumar S, Stauber RE, Gavaler JS, Basista MH, Dindzvans VJ, Schade RR, Rabinovitz M, Tarter RE, Gordon R, Starzl TE, et al. Orthotopic liver transplantation for alcoholic liver disease. Hepatology 11:159–164, 1990
149. Lane BP, lieber CS. Ultrastructural alterations in human hepatocytes following ingestion of ethanol with adequate diets. Am J Pathol 49:595, 1966
150. Lang AP, et al. Preoperative liver biopsy and the prognosis of portosystemic shunt surgery. (Abstract) Lab Invest 38:353, 1978
151. Lavetter A, Leedom J, Matheis A, Ivlerand D, Wehrke P. Meningitis due to *Listeria monocytogenes*. N Engl J Med 285:598, 1971
152. Ledwig J, et al. Nonalcoholic steato-hepatitis: Mayo Clinic experiences with a hitherto unnamed disease. Mayo Clin Proc 55:434, 1980
153. Lee RG. Nonalcoholic steatohepatitis: a study of 49 patients. Hum Pathol 20:594–598, 1989
154. Leevy CM. Fatty liver: a study of 240 patients with biopsy proven fatty liver and a review of the literature. Medicine 41:249, 1962
155. Leevy CM, Zetterman RK: Malnutrition and alcoholism: an overview. In: Rothschild MA, Orztz M, Schreiber SS, eds. Alcohol and abnormal protein biosynthesis: biochemical and clinical, vol 1. New York, Pergamon Press, 1975, p 3
156. Leevy CM, et al. Vitamins and liver injury. Am J Clin Nutr 23:493, 1970
157. Leevy CM, et al. Alcoholism, drug addiction, and nutrition. Med Clin North Am 54:1567, 1970
158. Leevy CM, et al. Liver disease of the alcoholic: role of immunologic abnormalities in pathogenesis recognition and treatment. In: Popper H, Schaffner F, eds. Progress in liver disease, vol 5. New York, Grune & Stratton, 1976, p 516
159. Lelbach WK. Epidemiology of alcoholic liver disease. In: Popper H, Schaffner F, eds. Progress in liver disease, vol 5. New York, Grune and Stratton, 1976, p 494
160. Lelbach WK. Epidemiology of alcoholic liver disease: continental Europe. In: Hall P, ed. Alcoholic liver disease: pathobiology, epidemiology, and clinical aspects. New York, John Wiley & Sons, 1985, p 130
161. Lesener HR, et al. Treatment of alcoholic hepatitis with encephalopathy: comparison of prednisolone with caloric supplements. Gastroenterology 74:169, 1978
162. Lieber CS, et al. Fatty liver, hyperlipemia and hyperuricemia produced by prolonged alcohol consumption despite adequate dietary intake. Trans Assoc Am Physicians 76:289, 1963
163. Lindenbaum J, Leiber CS. Alcohol-induced malabsorption of vitamin B_{12} in man. Nature 224:806, 1969
164. Losowsky MS, Walter BE. Liver disease and malabsorption. Gastroenterology 56:598, 1969
165. Ludwig J, Viggiano TR, McGill DB, et al. Nonalcoholic steatohepatitis: Mayo clinic experiences with hitherto unnamed disease. Mayo Clin Proc 55:434–438, 1980
166. Lundy J, Raaf JH, Deakins S, Wanebo HJ, Jacobs DA, Tsung-dao L, Jacobowitz D, Spear C, Oettgen HF. The acute and chronic effects of alcohol on the human immune system. Surg Gynecol Obstet 141:212–219, 1975
167. MacSween, RNM. Pathology of viral hepatitis and its sequelae. Clin Gastroenterol 9:23–25, 1980
168. Maddrey WC, et al. Corticosteroid therapy of alcoholic hepatitis. Gastroenterology 75:193, 1978
169. Mallory FB. Cirrhosis of the liver: five different types of lesions from which it may arise. Bull Johns Hopkins Hosp 22:69, 1911
170. Marjanen L. Intracellular localization of aldehyde dehydrogenase in rat liver. J Biochem 127:633, 1972
171. Marshall JB, et al. Clinical and biochemical course of alcoholic liver disease following sudden discontinuation of alcoholic consumption. Alcoholism 7:312, 1983
172. Marubbio AT, et al. Hepatic lesions of central pericellular fibrosis in morbid obesity and after jejunoileal bypass. Am J Clin Pathol 66:684, 1976
173. McClain CJ, Cohen DA, Dinarello CA, Cannon JG, Shedofsky SI, Kaplan AM. Serum interleukin-1 (IL-1) activity in alcoholic hepatitis. Life Sci 39:1479–1485, 1986
174. McClain CJ, Cohen DA. Increased tumor necrosis factor production by monocytes in alcoholic hepatitis. Hepatology 9:349–351, 1989
175. Melendez M, et al. Distribution of HLA histocompatibility antigens: ABO blood groups, and Rh antigens in alcoholic liver disease. Gut 20:288, 1979
176. Mendenhall CL. Anabolic steroid therapy as an adjunct to diet in alcoholic hepatic steatosis. Am J Dig Dis 13:738, 1968
177. Mendenhall C, Goldberg S. Risk factors and therapy in alcoholic hepatitis. Gastroenterology 72:1100, 1977
178. Mendenhall CL, Veterans Administration Cooperative Study Group on Alcoholic Hepatitis. Alcoholic hepatitis. Clin Gastroenterol 10:417, 1981
179. Mendenhall CL, et al: Altered proline uptake by mouse liver cells after chronic exposure to ethanol and its metabolites. Gut 25:138, 1984
180. Mendenhall CL, et al. Protein-calorie malnutrition associated with alcoholic hepatitis: Veterans Administration Cooperative Study Group on Alcoholic Hepatitis. Am J Med 76:211, 1984
181. Mendenhall CL, et al. Acute and long-term survival in patients treated with oxandrolone and prednisolone. N Engl J Med 311:1464, 1984
182. Mendenhall CL, et al. Veterans Administration Cooperative Study on Alcoholic Hepatitis. III. Changes in protein-calorie malnutrition associated with 30 days of hospitalization with and without enteral nutritional therapy. JPEN 9:590, 1985
183. Mendenhall CL. The Veterans Administration Cooperative Study on Alcoholic Hepatitis: clinical and therapeutic aspects of alcoholic liver disease. In: Seitz HK, Kommerell B, eds. Alcohol related diseases in gastroenterology. Berlin, Springer-Verlag, 1985, p 304
184. Mendenhall CL, et al. Veterans Administration Cooperative Study on Alcoholic Hepatitis. II. Prognostic significance of protein-calorie malnutrition. Am J Clin Nutr 43:213–218, 1986
185. Mendenhall CL, Roselle GA, Lybecker LA. Hepatitis B vaccination: response of alcoholics with and without liver injury. Dig Dis Sci 33:263–269, 1988
186. Mendenhall CL, Gartside PS, Roselle GA, et al. Veterans Administration Cooperative Study on Alcoholic Hepatitis. V. Longevity among ethnic groups. Alcohol Alcohol 24:11–19, 1989
187. Mendenhall CL, Seeff L, Diehl AM, et al. Hepatitis B and C serologic markers: relationship to alcoholic hepatitis and cirrhosis. Proceedings of the 7th Triennial Congress, Houston, Texas, April 4–8, 1990
188. Mezey E. Intestinal function in chronic alcoholism. Ann NY Acad Sci 252:215, 1975
189. Mezey E, Potter JJ. Changes in exocrine pancreatic function produced by altered dietary protein intake in drinking alcoholics. Johns Hopkins Medical Journal 318:7, 1976
190. Mezey E, et al. Pancreatic function and intestinal absorption in chronic alcoholism. Gastroenterology 59:657, 1970
191. Mezey E, et al. Hepatic fibrogenesis in alcoholism. In: Khanna JM, Israel Y, Kalant H, eds. Alcoholic liver pathology. Toronto, Addiction Research Foundation of Ontario, 1975, p 145
192. Mezey E, et al. Hepatic collagen proline hydroxylase activity in alcoholic liver disease. Clin Chim Acta 68:313, 1976
193. Mihas AA, Bull DM, Davidson CS. Cell-mediated immunity

to liver in patients with alcoholic hepatitis. Lancet 1:951–953, 1975

194. Mills PR, Pennington TH, Kay P, MacSween RNM, Watkinson G. Hepatitis Bs antibody in alcoholic cirrhosis. J Clin Pathol 32:778–782, 1979

195. Mills PR, Follett EAC, Urquhart GED, Clements G, Watkinson G, MacSween RNM. Evidence for previous hepatitis B virus infection in alcoholic cirrhosis. Br Med J 282:437–438, 1981

196. Monroe S, et al. Mallory bodies in a case of primary biliary cirrhosis: an ultrastructural and morphological study. Am J Clin Pathol 59:254, 1973

197. Morbidity and Mortality Weekly Report. Surveillance and assessment of alcohol-related mortality: United States, 1980. MMWR 34(12):161–163, 1985

198. Morgan MY, Ross MGR, Ng. CM, Adams DM, Thomas HC, Sherlock S. HLA-B8 immunoglobins and antibody responses in alcohol related liver diseases. J Clin Pathol 33:488–492, 1980

199. Mutchnik MG, Golstein AL. In vitro thymosin effect on T lymphocytes in alcoholic liver disease. Clin Immunopathol 12:271–280, 1979

200. Mting D. Die Wirkung einer Langzeitbehandlung mit einer anabolen Substanz (Nandrolondecanoat) auf Protein-synthese und -abbau sowie Ausscheidungs- und Entgiftungsfunktion der Leber bei chronischen Leberkrankheiten und Diabetes mellitus. Klin Wochenschr 42:843, 1964

201. Nasrallah SM, Galambos JT. Aminoacid therapy of alcoholic hepatitis. Lancet 2:1276, 1980

202. Nasrallah SM, et al. Hepatic morphology in obesity. Dig Dis Sci 26:325, 1981

203. Nayak NC, et al. Indian childhood cirrhosis: the nature and significance of cytoplasmic hyalin of hepatocytes. Arch Pathol 88:631, 1969

204. Nazim M, Stamp G, Hodgson HJF. Non-alcoholic steatohepatitis associated with small intestinal diverticulosis and bacterial outgrowth. Hepatogastroenterol 36:349–351, 1989

205. Nelson S, Bagby G, Summer WR. Alcohol suppresses lipopolysaccharide-induced tumor necrosis factor activity in serum and lung. Life Sci 44:673–676, 1989

206. Nelson S, Bagby G, Summer W. Alcohol suppresses tumor necrosis factor and lung host defenses. (Abstract) Alcohol Clin Exp Res 13:330, 1989

207. Nicolaescu T, Bittman E, Stoiculescu P, Udrescu E, Bordeianu A, Bordea M, Gheorghe N, Mogos I, Vacariu A. Treatment of hepatic cirrhosis with colchicine. Med Interne 35:67–73, 1983

208. Ning M, et al. Reduction of glutamic pyruvic transaminase in pyridoxine deficiency in liver disease. Proc Soc Exp Biol Med 121:27, 1966

209. Nissenbaum M, Chedid A, Mendenhall CL, Gartside P, et al. Prognostic significance of cholestatic alcoholic hepatitis. Dig Dis Sci 35:891–896, 1990

210. Nolan JP. Alcohol as a factor in the illness of university services patients. Am J Med Sci 249:135–142, 1965

211. Ohnishi K, Okuda K. Epidemiology of alcoholic liver disease: Japan. In: Hall P, ed. Alcoholic liver disease: pathobiology, epidemiology, and clinical aspects. New York, John Wiley & Sons, 1985, p 167

212. Olmsted JB, Borisy GG. Microtubules. Annu Rev Biochem 42:507, 1973

213. Omata M, Afroudakis A, Kiew CT, Ashcavai M, Peters RL. Comparison of serum hepatitis B surface antigen and serum anticore with tissue HBsAg and hepatitis B core antigen (HBcAg). Gastroenterology 75:1003–1009, 1978

214. Orlhom M, Aldershvile J, Tage-Jensen U, et al. Prevalence of hepatitis B virus infection among alcoholic patients with liver disease. J Clin Pathol 34:1378–1380, 1981

215. Orrego H, et al. Effect of propylthiouracil in treatment of alcoholic liver disease. (Abstract) Gastroenterology 73:A39, 1977

216. Orrego H, et al. Effect of short term therapy with propylthiouracil in patients with alcoholic liver disease. Gastroenterology 76:105, 1979

217. Orrego H, et al. Assessment of prognostic factors in alcoholic liver disease Toward a global quantitative expression of severity. Hepatology 3:896, 1983

218. Orrego H, Blake JE, Blendis LM, Compton KV, Israel Y. Long-term treatment of alcoholic liver disease with propylthiouracil. N Engl J Med 317:1421–1427, 1987

219. Osborn M, et al. Visualization of a system of filaments 7–10 nm thick in cultured cells of an epithelioid line (PtK2) by immunofluorescence microscopy. Proc Natl Acad Sci USA 74:2490, 1977

220. Osler W. The principles and practice of medicine. Edinburgh, Young J. Pentland, 1892, p 444

221. Par A, Hollos I, Bajtai G, et al: Serological studies of hepatitis viruses for their etiologic role in chronic liver disease. Acta Med Acad Sci Hung 37:1–15, 1980

222. Paronetto F, Lieber CS. Cytotoxicity of lymphocytes in experimental alcoholic liver injury in the baboon. Proc Soc Exp Biol Med 153:495, 1976

223. Patek AJ, Post J. Treatment of cirrhosis of the liver by a nutritious diet and supplements rich in vitamin B complex. J Clin Invest 20:481, 1941

224. Patek AJ, et al. Dietary treatment of cirrhosis of the liver: results in 124 patients observed during a 10 year period. JAMA 138:543, 1948

225. Patrick RS. Alcoholism as a stimulus to hepatic fibrogenesis. J Alcohol 8:13, 1973

226. Pessayre D, et al. Perihexilen maleate-induced cirrhosis. Gastroenterology 76:170, 1979

227. Peters RL. Pathology of hepatocellular carcinoma. In: Okuda K, Peters RL, eds. Hepatocellular carcinoma. New York, John Wiley & Sons, 1976, p 107

228. Peters RL, et al. Post–jejunoileal bypass hepatic disease. Am J Clin Pathol 63:318, 1975

229. Petersen P. Alcoholic hyalin, microfilaments and microtubules in alcoholic hepatitis. Acta Pathol Microbiol Scand [A] 85:384, 1977

230. Pettigrew NM, et al. Evidence for a role of hepatitis B virus in chronic alcoholic liver disease. Lancet 2:724, 1972

231. Pfeifer U, Klinge O. Intracisternal hyalin in hepatocytes of human liver biopsies. Virchow Arch [B] 16:141, 1974

232. Phillips GB. Acute hepatic insufficiency of the chronic alcoholic: revisited. Am J Med 75:1, 1983

233. Phillips GB, Davidson CS. Acute hepatic insufficiency of the chronic alcoholic. Arch Intern Med 94:585, 1954

234. Phillips GB, et al. Comparative effects of a purified and an adequate diet on the course of fatty cirrhosis in the alcoholic. J Clin Invest 31:351, 1952

235. Peura DA, Stomeyer FW, Johnson LF. Liver injury with alcoholic hyaline after intestinal resection. Gastroenterology 79:128–130, 1980

236. Pierugues R, Blanc P, Barneon C, Bories P, Michel H. Short-term therapy with propylthiouracil (PTU) for alcoholic hepatitis (AH): a clinical, biochemical and histological randomized trial about 25 patients. (Abstract) Gastroenterology 96:(Pt 2)A644, 1989

237. Pirola RC, Lieber CS. Hypothesis: energy wasting in alcoholism and drug abuse. Possible role of hepatic microsomal enzymes. Am J Clin Nutr 29:90, 1976

238. Popper H. Comments: Wilson's disease. Birth Defects 4:103, 1968

239. Popper H. Pathogenesis of alcoholic cirrhosis. In: Fisher MM, Rankin JG, eds. Alcohol and the liver. New York, Plenum Press, 1976, p 289

240. Popper H, Szanto PB. Fatty liver with hepatic failure in alcoholics. J Mount Sinai Hospital 24:1121, 1957

241. Popper H, et al. Florid cirrhosis: a review of 35 cases. Am J Clin Pathol 25:889, 1955

242. Porter HR, et al. Corticosteroid therapy in severe alcoholic

Diseases of the Liver, Seventh Edition, edited by
Leon Schiff and Eugene R. Schiff. J.B. Lippincott Company, Philadelphia © 1993.

32

Cirrhosis

Harold O. Conn
Colin E. Atterbury

Dark monarch,
giver of syrups and of poisons,
regulator of salts,
from you I hope for justice:
I love life: Do not betray me! Work on!
Do not arrest my song.
—Pablo Neruda
Ode to the Liver
Translation by Oriana J. Kalant

In his classic monograph, which has withstood the challenges of one and a half centuries, Laënnec described the pathologic picture of cirrhosis and some of its clinical features and, in a footnote, proposed the name *cirrhosis* for the disorder.[286] *Cirrhosis* comes from the Greek word *kirrhos,* which means orange or tawny. This first definitive description by Laënnec is a concise and lucid example of medical writing:

The liver, reduced to a third of its ordinary size, was, so to say, hidden in the region it occupied; its external surface, lightly mamated and wrinkled, showed a greyish yellow tint: indented, it seemed entirely composed of a multitude of small grains, round or ovoid in form, the size of which varied from that of a millet seed to that of a hemp seed. These grains, easy to separate one from the other, showed between them no place in which one could still distinguish any remnant of liver tissue itself: their color was fawn or a yellowish russet, bordering on greenish; their tissue, rather moist, opaque, was flabby to the touch rather than soft, and on pressing the grains between the fingers, one could not mash but a small portion: the rest gave to the touch the sensation of a piece of soft leather.*

This early description is an inspiring starting point from which to begin a discussion of cirrhosis. English-speaking chauvinists will take pleasure, however, in noting that 25 years earlier, a good gross description and an understanding of its relation to alcohol could be found in Mathew Baillie's[25] textbook of pathology, the first in English.

Definition and History

Much more has been written about the definition of cirrhosis than is known. Much of the confusion and controversy about

its definition is based on the almost uncontrollable compulsion of the definers of cirrhosis to include various aspects of pathogenesis, which is even less well understood than the definition.

Cirrhosis can best be defined in terms of what is pathoanatomically certain. Cirrhosis is a chronic disease of the liver in which *diffuse destruction and regeneration of hepatic parenchymal cells* have occurred and in which a *diffuse increase in connective tissue* has resulted in *disorganization of the lobular and vascular architecture.* The altered vascular abnormalities of cirrhosis are at least as important as any of these other components. In fact, from a clinical point of view, the resultant portal hypertension causes serious and lethal complications. Although some observers have argued about whether the scar tissue represents de novo formation of connective tissue or whether collapse and condensation of preexisting structural tissue are responsible, all agree that the amount of connective tissue or scar is increased. Some authors think that cirrhosis is a progressive disease and that it should be defined as a chronic, *progressive* disorder. Clearly, cirrhosis, in its mature state, must have progressed, but whether it has progressed or will progress in the absence of continued injury is not clear. In all patients with cirrhosis, regardless of the presence, absence, or nature of individual clinical manifestations, the triad of parenchymal necrosis, regeneration, and scarring, which was first emphasized by Rössle,[474] is present. All other clinical, laboratory, or pathologic manifestations of cirrhosis are inconstant and represent either pathogenetic or consequential features that may be found at specific stages of the disease or in specific types of cirrhosis. Infiltration of the portal zones with leukocytes, mononuclear cells, or plasmacytes, for example, may represent inflammation associated with an initial injury, a response to continued necrosis, or part of the reparative process. Similarly, hemosiderin deposition in patients with genetically determined hemochromatosis may represent an antecedent, pathogenetic feature of the development of the cirrhosis,[435] or it may represent the subsequent deposition of iron in the cirrhotic liver, as is common in alcoholic cirrhosis.[620] No one clinical, laboratory, or pathologic feature of cirrhosis is seen in every patient.

CLASSIFICATION

The classification of cirrhosis is slightly less obscure, although controversy exists about the overlapping of certain types. The major complication is the frequent lack of correlation between the etiologic and pathologic types of cirrhosis. Alcoholic cirrhosis, for example, supposedly is characterized

---

*"This type of growth belongs to the group of those which are confused under the name of scirrhus. I believe we ought to designate it with the name of *cirrhosis,* because of its color. Its development in the liver is one of the most common causes of ascites and has the pecularity that as the cirrhosis develops, the tissue of the liver is absorbed, and its ends often, as in the subject, to disappearing entirely."

875

by uniform, micronodular formation and fine, almost ubiquitous strands of connective tissue. Large, irregularly sized nodules and broad, dense bands of scar, characteristic of postnecrotic cirrhosis, may appear in later stages. Both lesions often coexist in the same liver, so-called mixed cirrhosis.[23,479] Conversely, micronodules may occur in posthepatitic cirrhosis. In fact, expert pathologists frequently have disagreed in differentiating alcoholic from postnecrotic and posthepatitic cirrhosis in the blind histologic classification of cirrhosis.[172,184] The observation that pathologists disagreed more frequently on surgical biopsies than on percutaneous needle samples[172] has led to the facetious suggestion that the more tissue available, the more the pathologists have to disagree about. This conclusion is unfair, since these studies demonstrate not that the pathologists are deficient but rather that the histologic criteria are neither specific nor mutually exclusive. Histologically, the lesions, although usually characteristic, are not specific for any one type of cirrhosis. Typical lesions of each of the major types of cirrhosis may be seen to coexist in the same liver.[170,479] Furthermore, sometimes the gross appearance of the liver is more reliable than a small histologic sample obtained by needle biopsy. Postnecrotic cirrhosis, with its coarse nodules of variable size, is characteristic and quite different from alcoholic cirrhosis with its fine, uniform nodularity and may be distinguished with the naked eye from the posthepatitic type.[170,542]

The large number of classifications proposed testifies to the inadequacy of our knowledge about cirrhosis. These numerous classifications represent a corollary of the sarcastic "first law of pharmacology," which states that the number of forms of therapy for a specific disease is inversely proportional to their therapeutic efficacy. The profusion of classifications has led inevitably to the proposal that there is but a single type of cirrhosis that has many clinical and histologic variations. Neither this concept of lumping nor the opposite approach to classification of dividing and subdividing solves the problem.

The classification proposed here (Table 32-1) is based on the one recommended at the Fifth Pan-American Congress[460] and modified by the working group of the World Health Organization in 1978,[15] the International Association for the Study of the Liver,[300] and by us. This classification categorizes cirrhosis according to morphologic, histologic, and etiologic criteria. The arbitrary functional classification of the earlier system has been discarded.

The morphologic classification simply characterizes the gross appearance of the liver (see Table 32-1). The morphologic diagnosis as made at surgery, laparoscopy, or autopsy usually is more reliable than the histologic diagnosis.[15]

The usefulness of this morphologic classification is that it allows patterns to be studied epidemiologically and to be correlated with etiologic agents.[15]

Micronodular Cirrhosis

Micronodular cirrhosis is characterized by the uniformity of the size of the nodules, virtually all of which are less than 3 mm in diameter (Fig. 32-1). These micronodules, which are about one lobule in size, lack normal lobular organization and are surrounded by fibrous tissue (Fig. 32-2). These lobules seldom contain terminal hepatic (central) veins or portal tracts except in cardiac cirrhosis, in which they are characteristically present. Micronodular cirrhosis is seen in chronic alcoholism, biliary obstruction, hemochromatosis, venous

TABLE 32-1   *Classification of Cirrhosis*

Morphologic	Autoimmune
Micronodular	Syphilis
Macronodular	Drugs and toxins
Mixed	α_1-Antitrypsin deficiency
	Cystic fibrosis
Histologic	Galactosemia
Portal	Glycogen storage disease
Postnecrotic	Hereditary tyrosinemia
Posthepatitic	Hereditary fructose
Biliary obstruction	intolerance
Primary	Other metabolic
Secondary	Hereditary hemorrhagic
Venous outflow obstruction	telangiectasia
	Hypervitaminosis A
Etiologic	Sarcoidosis
Alcohol	Copper
Viral hepatitis	Small bowel bypass
Biliary obstruction	Indian childhood cirrhosis
Primary	Idiopathic or cryptogenic
Secondary	Unproven
Venous outflow obstruction	Malnutrition
Hemochromatosis	Mycotoxins
Hepatolenticular	Schistosomiasis
degeneration	
(Wilson's disease)	

outflow obstruction, small bowel bypass, and Indian childhood fibrosis.

Macronodular Cirrhosis

Macronodular cirrhosis (Figs. 32-3 and 32-4) is characterized by variation in nodular size, but most nodules are greater than 3 mm in diameter and may measure several centimeters across. They contain both portal triads and efferent veins, but their orientation to each other varies. There are two subtypes of macronodular cirrhosis. In one, the liver is coarsely scarred and the large nodules are surrounded by broad fibrous septa (see Fig. 32-4B). In this postnecrotic type of cirrhosis, numerous portal triads may be clumped together, presumably the consequence of the collapse of large areas of necrotic parenchyma.

In the other, the so-called posthepatitic type, macronodules are separated by slender fibrous strands that connect individual portal areas to one another (Fig. 32-5). Sometimes this pattern has been called incomplete septal cirrhosis. Efferent veins are located eccentrically within these large lobules. Incomplete septal cirrhosis is more easily diagnosed on surgical wedge than needle biopsies in which the pathologic features may be inconspicuous. This type of cirrhosis is thought to occur after a single episode of necrosis rather than after repetitive necrosis and the collapse of postnecrotic cirrhosis. There often are histologic similarities between incomplete septal cirrhosis and idiopathic portal hypertension, nodular regenerative hyperplasia, and partial nodular transformation.[500] In these disorders, an ischemic cause has been postulated related to obliterative portal venopathy with nonuniformity of portal blood to the parenchyma.[587]

Macronodular cirrhosis is sometimes a later stage of micronodular cirrhosis. When serial biopsies were examined, up to 90% of the specimens that were originally classified as micronodular were found 10 years later to be macronodular.

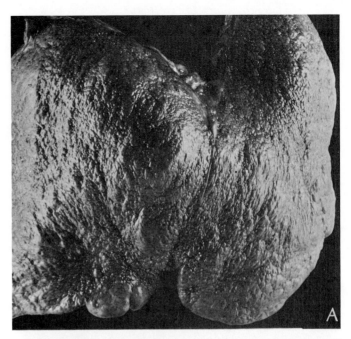
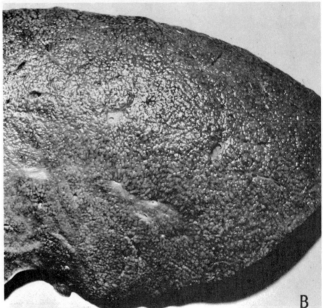

FIGURE 32-1 Micronodular cirrhosis. (**A**) Grossly the liver is large, pale, and uniformly finely nodular. (**B**) Sectioned surface of the cirrhotic liver shows the fine nodularity and regular disposition of the delicate fibrous tissue.

The mean time required for the conversion of macronodular cirrhosis from micronodular cirrhosis was around 2 years.[143]

Mixed Cirrhosis

The term *mixed cirrhosis* is used when both macrolobules and microlobules are present with equal frequency.

DIFFERENTIATION

The histologic classification of cirrhosis confirms the morphologic diagnosis and subdivides it into histologically discrete and sometimes etiologically precise categories. The postnecrotic and posthepatitic types are readily evident (see Figs.

32-4 and 32-5). Characteristic histologic findings permit the differentiation of primary and secondary biliary cirrhosis and establish the cause of venous obstruction, hemochromatosis, and α_1-antitrypsin deficiency. Histologic findings such as copper deposition or ground-glass cells may suggest Wilson's disease or chronic hepatitis B virus (HBV) infection, respectively.

The etiologic diagnosis includes established causative associations with cirrhosis. Often, however, neither the precise nature of the association nor its pathogenetic mechanism is completely understood. Also included in this classification are several suspected but unproven types of cirrhosis and several cirrhoses of unknown origin. This etiologic classification is designed to grow as new causes of cirrhosis are established.

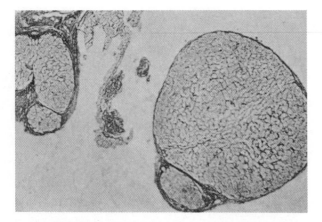

FIGURE 32-2　Micronodular cirrhosis with characteristic fragmentation of a needle biopsy specimen. Micronodules are surrounded by fibrosis (reticulin stain, × 50). (Anthony PP, et al. The morphology of cirrhosis: recommendations for definition, nomenclature, and classification by a working group sponsored by the World Health Organization. J Clin Pathol 31:395, 1978)

Pathology

The pathologic classification of cirrhosis is, in many ways, the most satisfactory and definitive type of cataloguing. It represents a static, descriptive evaluation, often at the end stage of the disease. It permits gross and microscopic descriptions and categorization into several classic types of cirrhosis. It also provides an almost infinite variety of findings, which often encourage the subclassification of less clearcut categories, as well as clues about the pathogenesis.

The simplest, least controversial pathologic classification, as suggested in Table 32-1, is followed here.

PORTAL CIRRHOSIS

The liver in portal cirrhosis (also termed alcoholic, nutritional, or micronodular cirrhosis) usually is enlarged, ranging from less than 1000 to 4000 g. The small, shrunken, hard, nodular liver, so classically described in the earlier literature,[252,449] is seen much less commonly now. In our experience, alcoholic cirrhotic livers at autopsy are usually moderately enlarged (1500 to 2000 g) and occasionally massive. Sometimes small livers are seen, most frequently in patients with advanced cirrhosis of long duration, often with severe degrees of portal hypertension. Large cirrhotic livers are most frequently found in patients with alcoholic cirrhosis with excessive fatty infiltration and active alcoholic hepatitis. These patients may die relatively early in the course of their cirrhosis of acute hepatic parenchymal failure or infection, rather than of the chronic consequences of progressive cirrhosis.

Grossly, the liver usually is golden yellow, but the color varies greatly. Cirrhotic livers may be pale yellow when they are large and filled with fat. They may be tan, brown, or reddish, depending on the degree of fatty infiltration, congestion, iron deposition, necrosis, and arterial oxygen saturation, respectively, and they may be gray or green, depending on the amount of scarring and the degree and duration of jaundice.

The surface commonly is pebbled by fine, uniform nodulations that range from 1 to 5 mm in diameter separated by a delicate reticulum of scar tissue. Traditionally, this type of cirrhosis has been known as hobnail cirrhosis, but hobnails, which are short, large-headed nails for studding shoe soles, are not known to present-day physicians. It is more appropriate nowadays to say that the liver surface resembles tanned pigskin (see Fig. 32-1). The cut surface also shows the uniform granular pattern. Sometimes in portal cirrhosis, the liver shows both granularity and nodularity; rarely, the liver is largely nodular. The nodules usually range from 5 to 12 mm in diameter, but nodules as large as 50 mm in diameter,

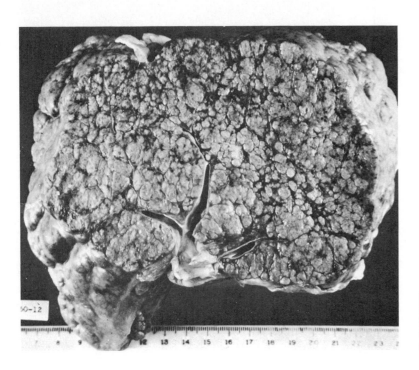

FIGURE 32-3　Macronodular cirrhosis. Grossly, the liver is coarsely nodular and shows marked variation in the pattern and character of nodulation. Broad bands of connective tissue distort the parenchyma into irregular nodules.

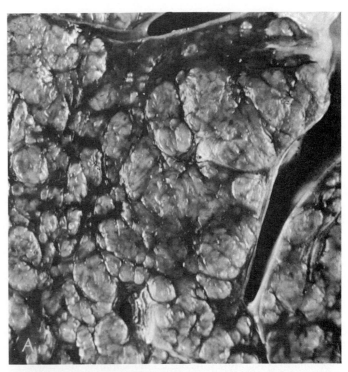

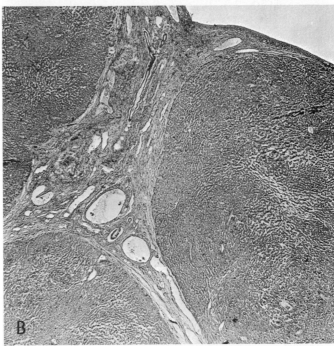

FIGURE 32-4 Macronodular cirrhosis. (**A**) Closeup of cross section emphasizes the variable size of the large regenerative nodules and the irregular nature of the scarring. (**B**) Photomicrograph shows characteristic broad septal scars. The large parenchymal nodules show no pseudolobulation but contain multiple distorted lobules, many portal areas, and asymmetrically located central veins.

separated by broad, depressed scars, which resemble those of postnecrotic cirrhosis, may characterize all or part of the liver. In general, the nodules of alcoholic cirrhosis are small and uniform in size and readily distinguishable from the large and variable nodularity of postnecrotic cirrhosis.

Microscopically, scar tissue distorts the normal architecture (Fig. 32-6; see also Fig. 32-2). Portal zones are interconnected by bands of connective tissue that divide and subdivide the normal lobular structure into islands of parenchymal cells. In some areas, stellate bands of connective tissue isolate plates of cells and even individual cells. The typical nodules are less than one lobule in size, and many lobules are segmented into much smaller pseudolobules. Some nodules are larger and formed by numbers of lobules. The strands of connective tissue usually are fine, 100 to 200 μm thick, and rarely broader than 500 μm. Bands of connective tissue may connect portal areas to one another and often to central areas. The connective tissue appears to originate from the portal areas and to advance toward the center of the lobules from the peripheral areas. In early cases of alcoholic cirrhosis, the

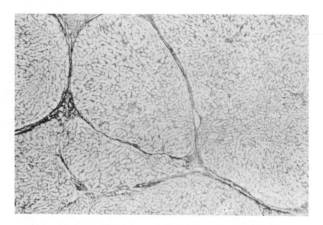

FIGURE 32-5 Macronodular, posthepatitic cirrhosis. Slender, incomplete strands of fibrosis separate the macronodules. (reticulin stain, × 24). (Anthony PP, et al. The morphology of cirrhosis: recommendations for definition, nomenclature, and classification by a working group sponsored by the World Health Organization. J Clin Pathol 31:395, 1978)

scar often can be seen to be predominantly central and to involve the portal areas secondarily. In advanced cases, the scar appears predominantly portal, and it may be impossible to appreciate the morphogenetic development of the scar tissue. Sometimes scar may replace whole areas of parenchyma, as in postnecrotic cirrhosis, and may appear as broad areas of scar in which are enmeshed arteries, veins, bile ducts, proliferating ductules, occasional individual parenchymal cells or clumps of cells, macrophages, and inflammatory cells. At times, it is a more delicate network of connective tissue that appears to be invading the lobules with fibrils of connective tissue that surround individual cells. Central veins may be eccentrically located or difficult to identify. Careful microscopic examination of many sites from the same liver often show typical portal cirrhosis in some areas and in other areas the characteristic postnecrotic pattern.[170,479] Interlobar bile ducts are unaffected, but proliferation of pseudoductules is typical.

Collagenization of the space of Disse has been shown to correlate closely with clinical decompensation and functional abnormalities.[398] This space is a lymphatic bed devoid of a basement membrane that permits maximal exposure of the hepatocytes to the circulation. The deposition of collagen in the space of Disse may be a critical pathologic lesion with functional and perhaps prognostic implications.

Hepatic parenchymal cells may appear normal, but the cytoplasm often shows altered tinctorial characteristics, sometimes staining paler and sometimes denser than normal cells. In alcoholic cirrhosis, the cytoplasm may appear to be homogeneous or particulate, and sometimes hyaline clumping, which usually is eosinophilic but may be amphophilic or even basophilic, is prominent. Such alcohol hyalin, or *Mallory bodies*,[336] which are found in both the central portion of the lobule and in proximity to the portal scars, are considered indices of alcoholic hepatitis rather than of cirrhosis per se. They are so often present in active decompensated alcoholic cirrhosis as to represent a characteristic part of the histologic picture. Popper and Schaffner[432] stress the centrilobular localization of this hyaline material in alcoholic hepatitis, but in our experience, alcoholic hyalin commonly occurs in the peripheral portions of the lobule.

Mallory bodies have been seen in the absence of cirrhosis and indeed in the absence of alcoholic liver disease. They have been described in primary biliary cirrhosis, in Wilson's disease and other diseases with prolonged cholestasis, in nonalcoholic nutritional liver disease, in hamartomas, and, occasionally, in various other types of liver disease.[162,176,418]

Mallory bodies have also been seen in recipients of various drugs, including perhexiline maleate, amiodarone, nifedipine, diethylstilbestrol, and long-term glucocorticoid therapy.[24,231,235,311]

Recent investigations have begun to clear up some of the mystery about alcohol hyalin, the homogeneous cytoplasmic bodies first described by Mallory[336] in 1911 and known since as Mallory bodies (Fig. 32-7). Leevy and associates[300] suggested that this hyaline material is immunologically important in the pathogenesis of alcoholic liver disease and that cell-mediated injury may contribute to the progression of alcoholic liver disease. Alcohol, acetaldehyde, and alcohol hyalin all stimulate lymphocyte transformation and cell-mediated hyperreactivity and cytotoxicity to autologous liver tissue.[32,244,531,616] The presence of an alcoholic hyalin antigen and an antibody to it have been demonstrated in patients with alcoholic hepatitis.[246] Although this antibody is to Mallory bodies alone, it contains other types of antibody that bind to other structures as well.[161]

Denk and colleagues[121,120] have produced Mallory bodies

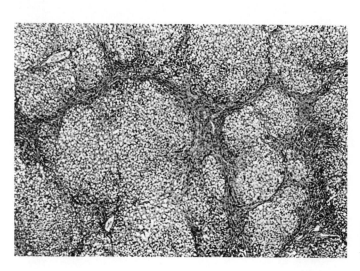

FIGURE 32-6 Alcoholic cirrhosis. Microscopically, the liver reveals fine fibrosis, micronodulation, and pseudolobule formation. Intracellular fat vacuolization is prominent.

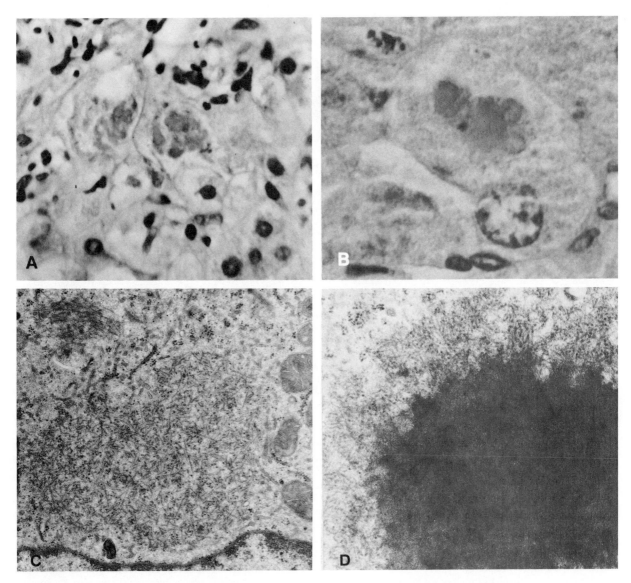

FIGURE 32-7   Mallory bodies (MBs). (**A**) Light micrograph of a human MB (× 440). (**B**) Light micrograph of a murine MB induced by griseofulvin (× 980). (**C**) Electron micrograph of a portion of a hepatocyte showing in the upper left corner aggregates of filaments in parallel arrangements characteristic of type I MBs and below it juxtanuclear clumps of moderately electron-dense, intertwining filaments characteristic of type II MBs (× 23,700). (**D**) Electron micrograph of an electron-dense, amorphous type III MB. Type II filaments surround and appear to merge with the clump (× 36,400). (These micrographs were made available by Dr. Z. Wessely. Wessely Z. Light and electron microscopy of hepatocellular changes in griseofulvin-fed mice: particular reference to Mallory bodies. Ann Clin Lab Sci 9:24, 1979)

in mice by the chronic administration of griseofulvin, an agent that has antimicrotubular and cell-activating properties and that can induce porphyria and cholestasis. Mallory bodies appear in all animals treated for 4 months with griseofulvin and disappear within 1 month after stopping griseofulvin. Mallory bodies do not appear if colchicine, another antimicrotubular agent, is administered. If griseofulvin or colchicine is given to a mouse in whom Mallory bodies have previously been induced by griseofulvin, Mallory bodies promptly reappear after 2 or 3 days.[119] These murine Mallory bodies, which appear to be identical to human Mallory bodies by ultrastructural, immunologic, and pharmacologic studies, seem to consist of intermediate-size filaments (see Fig. 32-7).

Mallory bodies have also been induced in hepatocytes after long-term feeding with dieldrin.[352] Both griseofulvin and dieldrin are carcinogens, and Mallory bodies are found in hepatocellular carcinomas induced by these agents.[162] The common denominator in Mallory body formation, whether it be induced by alcohol injury, various liver disorders, drugs, or neoplasia, appears to be cellular injury followed by proliferation of hepatocytes.[162]

Franke and coworkers[160] examined isolated purified Mallory bodies and identified them as containing prekeratin-like polypeptides assembled into unbranched, randomly oriented fimbriate rods 14 to 20 nm thick.

These filaments differ from other intermediate filaments. On polyacrylamide gel electrophoresis, they separate into six

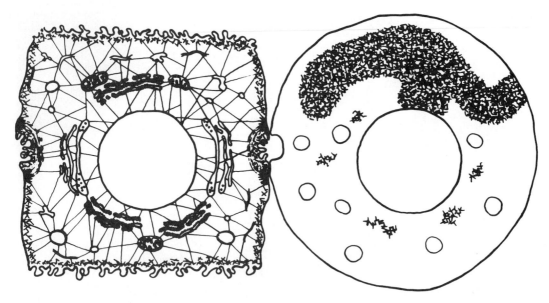

FIGURE 32-8 Artist's conception of the normal intermediate filament cytoskeleton in a hepatocyte (*left*) compared with a hepatocyte that has undergone Mallory body transformation (*right*). The normal hepatocyte has microvilli, microfilaments in the ectoplasm, and intermediate filaments that form a guy-like framework holding organelles and the nucleus in place and maintaining the polygonal shape of the cell. In contrast, the Mallory body–containing hepatocyte, attached at desmosomal connections, has lost both microfilaments and intermediate filaments, resulting in a change in shape of the hepatocyte to form a sphere (balloon degeneration). (Courtesy of Dr. S.W. French; modified from French SW. Nature, pathogenesis, and significance of the Mallory body. Semin Liver Dis 1:217, 1981)

polypeptide bands, which appear to have molecular weights between 45,000 and 66,000. Antibody to prekeratin reacts immunofluorescently with Mallory bodies from griseofulvin-treated rats and from alcohol-abused human livers. Antibodies to actin or tubulin do not react with Mallory bodies. Antisera against isolated human or murine Mallory bodies bind with the Mallory bodies in liver sections from either species.[164,515] Franke and coworkers[160] concluded that Mallory bodies are composed of hollow, intermediate-size tonofilaments that contain prekeratin.

The source of the Mallory body appears to be the hepatocyte cytoskeleton, which has intermediate filaments located throughout the cytoplasm, especially at cell borders, attached to mitochondria, the nucleus, and other organelles, and connecting to centrioles.[161,162] It is known that keratin synthesis can be altered when the environment of the cell is changed, such as by drugs or carcinogens, and it is possible that Mallory body formation results from alterations in keratin polypeptide composition rather than from toxic degeneration.[162,291] The result, whatever the mechanism, is the loss of the functions of the cytoskeleton. As shown in Figure 32-8, loss of intermediate filaments throughout the cytoplasm is accompanied by the massing of these filaments to form Mallory bodies.[161,162] Consequently, cells become ballooned and lose microvilli, the nuclei are displaced, and organization of organelles is lost. Because cells that contain Mallory bodies are prone to lysis owing to breaks in the plasma membranes, survival of the cell may be jeopardized.[161,419]

Another histologic trademark of alcoholic liver disease is the giant mitochondrion[62] (Fig. 32-9). These spherical, hyaline, eosinophilic, cytoplasmic inclusions, which resemble erythrocytes, are clearly distinguishable from Mallory bodies. They vary in size from 2 to 10 μm and have been demon-strated on electron microscopy to be megamitochondria. They occur more frequently than alcohol hyalin but are not nearly so ominous.[75]

There often is variation in cellular and nuclear size, altering dramatically the uniformity of the normal parenchymal structure (Fig. 32-10). These regenerative changes typically are accompanied by binucleate cells and increased mitotic activity. Regeneration appears to occur piecemeal in alcoholic cirrhosis compared with the large regenerating nodules characteristic of postnecrotic cirrhosis.

Necrosis is characteristically seen in the peripheral areas near the fibrous strands. When the lobular architecture is sufficiently preserved, necrosis may be prominent around the terminal hepatic (central) veins but may also be ubiquitous, although it may often be difficult to precisely identify normal landmarks in the distorted cirrhotic architecture. It is our impression that ballooning of hepatic parenchymal cells is more apt to occur near the central portion of lobules, whereas a more coagulative necrosis of cytoplasm, characterized by Mallory alcohol hyalin, tends to be located along the peripheral fibrous strands. Fibrosis tends to appear in the centrilobular areas and commonly is pericellular, as shown in Fig. 32-11. This pattern, however, is variable.

Areas of necrosis frequently contain polymorphonuclear leukocytes, which may surround or appear within necrotic or prenecrotic cells, and prominent Kupffer cells engorged with pigment. Portal areas may contain large numbers of inflammatory cells, which typically are predominantly lymphocytic and histiocytic but sometimes contain large numbers of polymorphonuclear leukocytes, eosinophils, and, occasionally, plasma cells. The inflammatory reaction that accompanies alcohol-induced hepatic damage is unpredictable. There is little relation between the type or extent of hepatocellular ne-

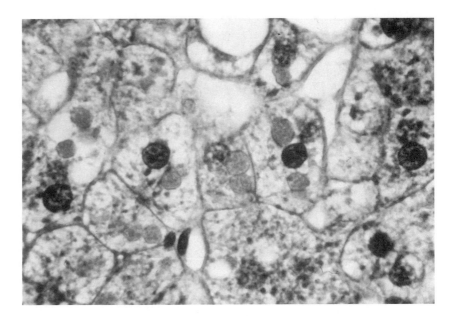

FIGURE 32-9 Giant mitochondria are shown within relatively normal-appearing hepatocytes in a patient with early, minimally active alcoholic cirrhosis. These eosinophilic, hyaline mitochondria are only slightly smaller than the hepatocyte nuclei (Masson stain, × 589).

crosis and the character, degree, or duration of inflammation.

Fatty infiltration, which is a common accompaniment of alcoholic cirrhosis but not an obligatory part of the cirrhotic picture, tends to be centrally located. When intense, fatty infiltration may involve almost every cell (Fig. 32-12). Hemosiderin, which commonly is deposited in the hepatic parenchymal cells of patients with cirrhosis, is found earliest and most intensely in the periportal areas.

POSTNECROTIC CIRRHOSIS

The liver in postnecrotic cirrhosis (also termed posthepatitic cirrhosis, healed acute yellow atrophy, or coarsely nodular cirrhosis) is characterized grossly by a misshapen, often shrunken liver (see Fig. 32-3). Broad bands of dense connective tissue divide the liver into nodules of varying size, which range from a few millimeters to 5 cm in diameter. Whole lobes may be replaced by dense, shrunken scar. The scar is grayish to greenish brown; the nodules may be tan, brown, or greenish. The scarring often is eccentric and random (see Fig. 32-4).

Microscopically, the primary feature is scarring. Coarse, irregular scars are typical, but fine strands are also present. The overall architecture is distorted by displaced but recognizable portal areas and central veins. The areas of scar tissue contain abnormal collections of portal tracts that typify the lesion and reflect the collapse and condensation of the hepatic stroma. It is widely believed that the juxtaposition of three or more portal triads abnormally placed within a single strand of scar is a hallmark of this lesion.[542] In long-standing postnecrotic cirrhosis, the scarred portal features may no longer be recognized.

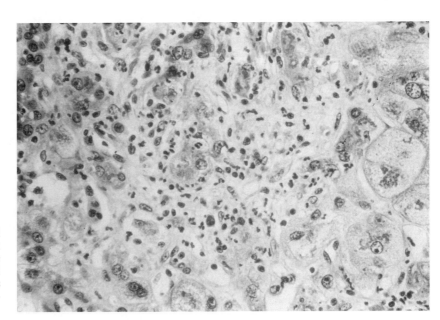

FIGURE 32-10 Variation in hepatocyte and nuclear size is shown in this photomicrograph of a portal tract of a patient with acute alcoholic hepatitis. Some of the hepatocytes are ballooned and contain Mallory bodies. Some hepatocytes are small and binucleate. A neutrophilic infiltration is seen (Masson stain, × 230).

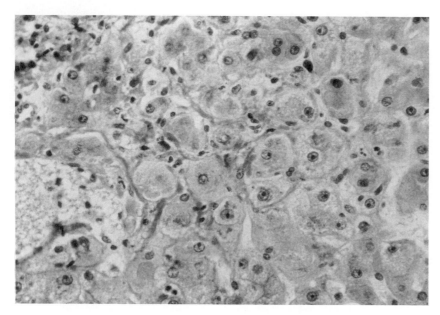

FIGURE 32-11 Centrilobular, delicate, arachnoid, pericellular fibrosis in a patient in the late healing stage of alcoholic hepatitis. Mallory hyaline is present in many of the hepatocytes, some of which are undergoing degeneration (Masson stain, × 230).

Large, regenerating nodules are the predominant parenchymal finding. Lymphocytic infiltration is typical, but plasma cells and polymorphonuclear leukocytes may be present, and often many eosinophils are seen. In the active phase, parenchymal necrosis—often piecemeal—may be present, but fatty infiltration is atypical and alcohol hyalin is seldom, if ever, present. Active necrosis reflects the changes associated with viral hepatitis, the most common cause of this type of cirrhosis. Eosinophilic, Councilman-like bodies often accompany active necrosis (Fig. 32-13).

Some authors consider posthepatitic cirrhosis (see Fig. 32-5) to be a discrete third type of cirrhosis. It appears to be intermediate between portal and postnecrotic cirrhosis in both gross and microscopic appearance, and its pathogenesis is similar to that seen in postnecrotic cirrhosis.

BILIARY CIRRHOSIS

The liver in biliary cirrhosis characteristically is dark green, firm, and granular or nodular. The deep green color is more typical of secondary than of primary biliary cirrhosis.[126] Grossly, it appears to be a green portal cirrhosis, but broad scars may predominate as in postnecrotic cirrhosis, with small or moderate-size nodules, 1 mm to 10 mm in diameter. Microscopically, the cirrhosis shows broadened portal tracts that are linked with one another. In biliary cirrhosis secondary to prolonged obstructive jaundice, the major difference is the apparent *increase* in the number of interlobar bile ducts and the absence of ductular degeneration. The characteristic finding of primary biliary cirrhosis is *reduction* in the number of interlobular bile ducts and inflammation

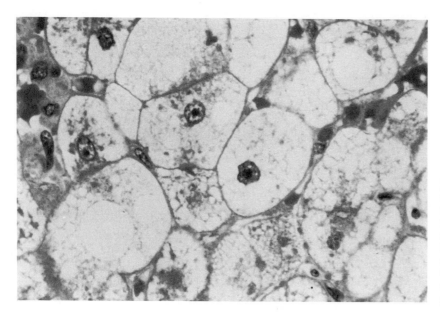

FIGURE 32-12 Microvesicular fatty deposition, also known as alcoholic foamy degeneration, is shown in this high-magnification photomicrograph from the liver of a patient with alcoholic fatty liver. The cells are characterized by the accumulation of tiny fat vesicles, which surround centrally located, shrunken nuclei. Occasional macrovesicular fat droplets are present (H&E, × 660). (Courtesy of Dr. M.H. Sjogren)

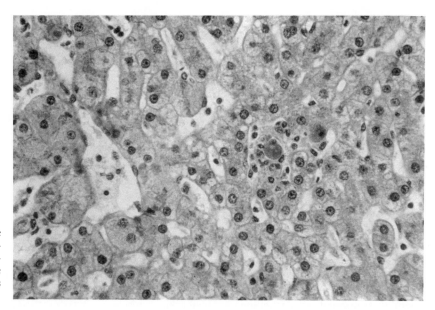

FIGURE 32-13 Two acidophilic bodies are shown in a small centrilobular focus of hepatocellular necrosis in a patient with chronic persistent non-A, non-B viral hepatitis. Also seen are swollen Kupffer cells and a few lymphocytes (Masson stain, × 230).

and degeneration of those that survive. The portal areas are heavily infiltrated with lymphocytes, plasma cells, and neutrophilic and eosinophilic leukocytes. Bile stasis is severe in both types, but bile lakes are typical of high-grade obstructive jaundice and are uncommon in primary biliary cirrhosis.

CARDIAC CIRRHOSIS

Cardiac cirrhosis is a rare lesion that develops only after prolonged, severe, right-sided congestive heart failure. For practical purposes, it develops only in patients with constrictive pericarditis or tricuspid insufficiency.[367] Unremittent, chronic congestion of the liver results in central cellular atrophy and necrosis. Congestion of sinusoids and dilatation of central veins are characteristic. Condensation of collapsed reticulum and new fiber formation combine to form fibrosis, which may connect the central areas of adjacent lobules. Sparing of the portal areas results in a reversal of the usual portal cirrhotic pattern (ie, central-to-central scarring with virtual sparing of the portal triads rather than portal-to-portal scarring with relatively normal central areas). As the disease progresses, central-to-portal and even portal-to-portal scars develop and regenerative nodules form, which may obliterate the early, characteristic central cirrhotic pattern. The central

predominance of the scar usually permits recognition. Grossly, the liver shows a finely nodular appearance with some residual nutmeg pattern of chronic passive congestion, the underlying lesion.

PATHOGENESIS OF THE PATHOLOGIC PATTERN

Morphogenetically, the development of the fibrosis is complex and not clearly understood. When large areas of parenchymal cells have undergone necrosis, as may occur in severe viral hepatitis, these empty necrotic areas collapse and undergo collagenization (Figs. 32-14 and 32-15).

The passive septa thus formed represent merely the condensation of the collapsed reticular supporting framework of the hepatic parenchyma and its metamorphosis into scar tissue. This pattern is characteristic of bridging hepatic necrosis of viral hepatitis with the linkage of adjacent portal or central areas of collapsed, necrotic stromal elements, as described by Klatskin and Boyer.[55,269] A similar pattern, occurring over a much longer period of time, develops in alcoholic liver injury (Fig. 32-16). This injury initially is centrilobular, but the process may extend in bridge-like manner to the portal tracts. Massive necrosis of whole lobules may also occur in alcoholic hepatitis and may thus cause broad areas of collapse

FIGURE 32-14 Diagrammatic relation between focal necrosis and the absence of scarring in acute hepatitis. Necrosis in acute viral hepatitis of average severity involves individual cells diffusely throughout the lobule. It may be predominantly central or diffuse, but it is contained within individual lobules, as indicated by the stippling on the left. The basic lobular architecture of the liver is unimpaired, and healing takes place by regeneration. No scar tissue is formed. After recovery, the liver is morphologically and histologically normal (*right*).

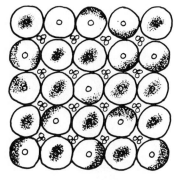

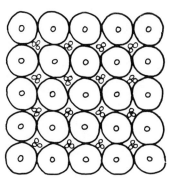

Viral hepatitis   Normal liver

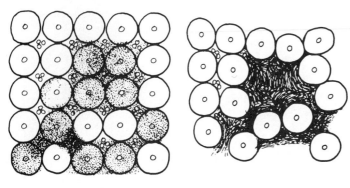

Submassive
hepatic necrosis   Postnecrotic cirrhosis

FIGURE 32-15 Diagrammatic relation between submassive (bridging) hepatic necrosis and subsequent scarring. In submassive hepatic necrosis, large areas of necrosis (*stippling*) involve whole lobules or groups of contiguous lobules or extend between the central areas of adjacent lobules or from central to portal areas. These bridges of necrosis disrupt the basic lobular structure of the liver. Wherever such large areas of necrosis develop, the empty stroma collapses and fibrous tissue formation is stimulated. As shown on the right, these areas of collapse may result in dense scar containing the condensed portal structures or in finer, more linear scars between adjacent lobules, giving rise to the patterns of postnecrotic and posthepatitic cirrhosis.

that account for the postnecrotic pattern sometimes seen in alcoholic cirrhosis.[479] In addition, active fibrogenesis is stimulated by alcoholic injury and inflammation of parenchymal, ductular, sinusoidal, and reticuloendothelial cells. This fibroplasia gives rise to active septa that radiate to the parenchyma primarily from the portal areas. These active septa, in contrast to passive septa, which give rise to static scar, represent a critical part in the progression of cirrhosis.

Simultaneously, hepatic parenchymal necrosis stimulates regeneration. Potent stimuli for hepatic parenchymal hyperplasia, which occur at the same time, further distort the random, fibrous patterns. The complex interactions of the fibrogenic and regenerative stimuli, in relation to the altered vascular pattern, the inconstant and variable inflammatory response, and the impaired functional capacity of the liver, in the face of continued alcoholic injury, result in the infinitely varied pathologic patterns seen in alcoholic cirrhosis.

Etiology and Pathogenesis

The precise etiology of cirrhosis is not known. Although some of the settings in which cirrhosis develops are obvious, the mechanisms by which these situations or agents are translated to the clinicopathologic picture of cirrhosis are unclear. Circumstantially, it appears clear that cirrhosis is associated with excessive alcohol consumption, viral hepatitis, drug-induced hepatic injury, prolonged extrahepatic biliary obstruction, the late stages of some parasitic diseases, and some genetically transmitted metabolic disorders such as hemo-

chromatosis and Wilson's disease (see Table 32-1). Despite the circumstantial indictment of malnutrition and the ritual use of the adjective *nutritional* to identify the most common type of cirrhosis, the development of cirrhosis as a consequence of pure dietary deficiency has not been established.

Studies in laboratory animals, although productive of great volumes of data, have not provided until relatively recently a reliable animal model with which to study the problem. Investigations have suggested that cirrhosis may be induced in dogs[77] by the long-term administration of alcohol and intermittent feeding, conditions not unlike those associated with alcoholic cirrhosis in humans. Similar disorders have been produced by carbon tetrachloride in rats, dimethylnitrosamine in rats and dogs,[309] and bile duct ligation in rats and dogs.[310]

The demonstration by Rubin and Lieber[478] of the production of alcoholic cirrhosis in baboons is a landmark in liver disease. These investigators showed for the first time that cirrhosis, much like human alcoholic cirrhosis, can be reproducibly caused by the administration of alcohol in laboratory animals. The authors solved the problem of the animals' natural dislike for excessive alcohol by offering them a liquid formula that provided normal amounts of high-quality protein, carbohydrate, fat, vitamins, minerals, and water. It contained ethyl alcohol, which constituted 50% of the total calories. The baboons had little choice and took the diet in amounts that maintained normal body weight. They came to like the diet and averaged from 4.5 to 8.3 g/kg of alcohol daily. This dose, which is about the equivalent of 1 to 2 qt of whiskey per day for an average-size man, caused intoxica-

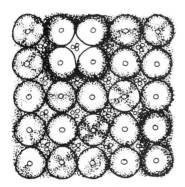
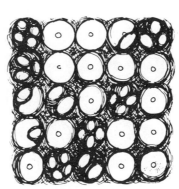

Alcoholic necrosis   Portal cirrhosis

FIGURE 32-16 Diagrammatic relation between alcoholic necrosis and portal cirrhosis. The distribution of necrosis in alcoholic hepatitis is predominantly central, but peripheral necrosis is common (*stippling on left*). The necrosis may be piecemeal, involving individual cells, or may bridge central-to-central zones or central-to-portal areas. The insidious development of scar tissue involves the centrilobular and portal areas and causes central sclerosis, portal cirrhosis, and, eventually, micronodular cirrhosis in which the lobules are subdivided into abnormal nodules and pseudolobules (*right*).

tion and perhaps alcohol addiction. In several instances, withdrawal symptoms, much like delirium tremens, were observed when alcohol was discontinued.

This diet induced fatty infiltration followed by hepatocellular necrosis, which was predominantly centrilobular in distribution, characteristic Mallory bodies, fibrosis, and, finally, cirrhosis. Histologically, the progression of hepatic pathology was similar to that of human alcoholic cirrhosis. The necrosis was predominantly central and the scarring initially was central and spread to involve the portal areas. Even the ultrastructural changes were similar to those seen in human alcoholic hepatitis. The most significant aspect of these studies is that the lesions that progressed to cirrhosis were induced *despite a normal diet*. Control animals who received a diet that contained carbohydrates with the same number of calories as contained in the alcohol remained normal. Although a primary role for malnutrition now seems untenable, the importance of secondary malnutrition is being reaffirmed.[314] It is recognized that alcohol may impair nutrient digestion, absorption, or activation.[315] Selective nutrient depletion, such as vitamin A deficiency, which is associated with hepatic lysosomal lesions, may be produced by alcohol.[306]

Several subtle differences exist between the cirrhosis produced in the baboons and that in humans. First, the disease developed in some baboons after less than 1 year of alcohol administration, a much shorter time than in humans. Second, the disease developed in more than half the laboratory animals compared with only a small percentage of human alcoholic patients. Both these differences may be consequences of greater and more constant alcohol ingestion than the human condition permits in most instances. Finally, the early development of a centrilobular cirrhosis with fibrosis connecting the central portions of lobules and sparing the portal areas is characteristic of the reverse lobulation of cardiac cirrhosis. This pattern, in our experience, is unusual in alcoholic cirrhosis. It may occur early in the course of the disease, however, before the cirrhosis is evident clinically. These exciting findings with follow-up studies should help to answer many questions about the pathogenesis of alcoholic cirrhosis.

Differences among species and the inability to control an infinite number of variables limit extrapolation of such preliminary animal data to humans. Until cirrhosis can be reproducibly induced by a single factor, presumably alcohol, in a number of species of laboratory animals and can be unequivocally shown to be responsible for human cirrhosis, the etiology must remain unproved. Multiple factors, acting individually or in concert, may be responsible for cirrhosis, and multiple factors individually or collectively may satisfy such postulates. It is probable in fact that there are many causes of cirrhosis, each of which may act differently. In the hope of deriving some general mechanism, let us consider individually those factors that, like cigarette smoking in lung cancer, are guilty by association.

ALCOHOL

Alcoholism has been present throughout recorded history, but the relation between excessive alcohol ingestion and cirrhosis was not recognized for several millennia. The association between alcohol and cirrhosis, which had apparently been recognized by Vesalius and was well known in the 17th century, is almost entirely circumstantial. It is based on the age-old observation that many heavy drinkers develop cirrhosis. This concept is supported primarily by repeated observations of a high prevalence of cirrhosis in alcoholic subjects and a low prevalence in moderate drinkers and nondrinkers. Jolliffe and Jellinek[241] collected statistics from the literature that, although uncontrolled, appear to show that cirrhosis occurs seven times more frequently in alcoholic subjects than in nondrinkers. In addition, epidemiologic data show a close correlation between fatalities from cirrhosis and the per capita consumption of alcohol[241,270] (Fig. 32-17). Furthermore, unintentional social and political experiments, such as the institution and repeal of Prohibition in the United States (Fig. 32-18) and the abrupt but transient decrease in wine consumption during the German occupation of France from 1940 to 1945,[298] provide epidemiologic evidence compatible with an etiologic association between alcohol consumption and cirrhosis. The Prohibition picture is particularly impressive, since the deprivation of alcohol was not accompanied by food deprivation, which occurred during the German occupation and that usually coexists in patients who develop alcoholic cirrhosis. Such data, however, are national, not individual, and might well reflect agents other than alcohol.

Snapper,[524] for example, rejected the alcohol hypothesis. He stated that in his opinion, the national alcohol consumption levels do *not* correlate well with the incidence of cirrhosis and implied that nutritional and other toxic factors are responsible. He argued persuasively that because cirrhosis takes 15 or more years to develop, the sharp changes in incidence observed during the U.S. Prohibition and the German occupation of France occurred too promptly to be related to alcohol consumption. His concept does not take into account the effect of cumulative alcohol-induced damage (ie, the importance of the duration of excessive alcohol consumption in the development of cirrhosis). One might thus see less cirrhosis immediately after the long-term development of the lesion has been interrupted by the withdrawal of the offending agent or a prompt rise in incidence after the resumption of alcohol in patients in whom the development of cirrhosis was transiently delayed during the obligatory abstinence.

Few investigators go so far as to reject outright the relation between excess alcohol ingestion and cirrhosis. There is, however, ongoing concern about accounting for the observation that only some heavy drinkers seem predisposed to the development of cirrhosis. Explanations have arisen from two not necessarily mutually exclusive hypotheses. The first argues that the development of cirrhosis is largely a function of alcohol consumed and the length of time over which it is ingested. The second hypothesis is that alcohol is only permissive and creates the setting for an additional factor to induce cirrhosis.[14]

The studies of Lelbach[303] have most persuasively related the development of liver damage to the degree and duration of alcohol abuse in the individual patient. In studies of alcohol addicts of more than 15 years' duration, he found severe liver damage in 75% of those with a daily alcohol consumption in excess of 160 g (about 200 mL of ethanol or 1 pt of whiskey) compared with 17% of those who consumed less than this amount.[303] The time factor was equally important. The prevalence of severe liver damage after 15 years of excessive alcohol consumption was eight times greater than after only 5 years of heavy drinking. These data support our own clinical impression that 1 pt of whiskey per day for 15 years is the critical threshold. We refer to pint-years in a man-

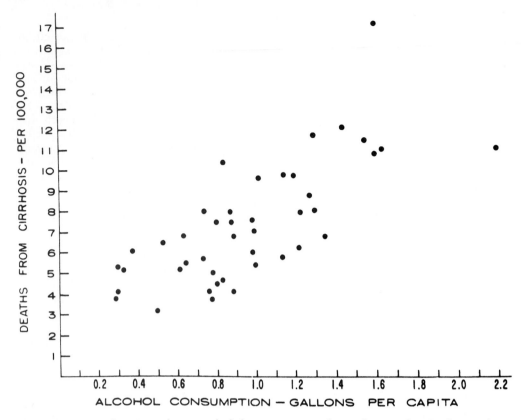

FIGURE 32-17 Association between alcohol consumption and mortality rate from cirrhosis. These data show a close, positive correlation between national alcohol consumption and the incidence of death from cirrhosis. (Klatskin G. Alcohol and its relation to liver damage. Gastroenterology 41:443, 1961. © 1961, American Gastroenterological Society)

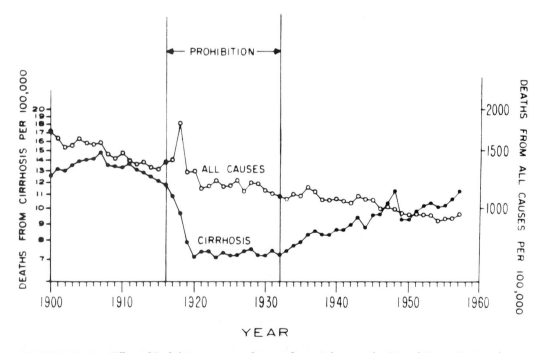

FIGURE 32-18 Effect of Prohibition on mortality rate from cirrhosis in the United States. During the period from 1900 to 1960, the overall mortality rate progressively decreased. The mortality rate from cirrhosis fell precipitously after the enactment of the 18th Amendment to the Constitution in 1916. The decreased rate was sustained until 1932, when Prohibition was repealed, after which the mortality rate from cirrhosis progressively climbed. (Klatskin G. Alcohol and its relation to liver damage. Gastroenterology 41:443, 1961. © 1961, American Gastroenterological Society)

ner analogous to the pack-years of cigarette smoking associated with the development of lung cancer. Thus, 15 pint-years, which frequently culminate in alcoholic cirrhosis, may serve as a rough index to gauge the degree of alcohol-induced liver injury and to predict the possibility of developing cirrhosis.[94] The prevalence of cirrhosis after 30 pint-years, accumulated at the rate of 1 pt/d for 30 years or 1 qt/d for 15 years, would probably be lower than in patients who consumed 2 qt/d for 7½ years. It would be fascinating but pure fantasy to attempt to validate the linearity of this relation prospectively in humans and to determine whether dose or duration predominates. There is evidence that women may be more susceptible than men.[639] For men, the level of alcohol intake at which the development of cirrhosis starts is about 60 g/d.[194,386] In women, the threshold for increased likelihood to develop cirrhosis may be as low as 20 g/d.[194,492]

It has recently been suggested that the explanation for higher toxicity of alcohol in women is that the gastric oxidation of ethanol is decreased in women.[166] This decrease was found to correlate with reduced gastric mucosal alcohol dehydrogenase. Thus, decreased first-pass metabolism of alcohol in women results in greater bioavailability of alcohol and, thereby, greater toxicity. In alcoholic men, gastric alcohol dehydrogenase activity and first-pass metabolism were about half those found in nonalcoholic men. In alcoholic women, gastric alcohol dehydrogenase activity was even lower and the first-pass metabolism of alcohol was virtually absent. No difference was noted between men and women after intravenous alcohol administration.[361,386] These observations require confirmation. Furthermore, the more rapid clearance of alcohol by women than by men when it is administered intravenously must be reconciled with decreased gastric metabolism. Is acetaldehyde dehydrogenase also decreased in women?

It is fascinating that only a small percentage of heavy drinkers develop cirrhosis. Is resistance to the ravages of alcohol absolute or relative? Does every liver have its critical pint-year requirement? It is probable that these questions can never be accurately answered.

On the other hand, no deleterious effects were observed when alcohol was administered in the hospital setting to patients recovering from alcoholic fatty liver.[547,583] In larger amounts, however, it prevented the clearing of fat from the alcoholic fatty liver.[357] These findings again imply the existence of other cofactors that may act together with alcohol.

Orrego and colleagues[399] have argued that consumption of alcohol above a threshold level is a necessary but not a sufficient condition for the development of cirrhosis. They do not deny that in the setting of alcohol consumption, the probability of developing cirrhosis increases linearly with time; they are impressed, however, that at whatever the dose or whatever the duration, many people do *not* develop cirrhosis. They therefore wonder whether it is not possible that liver damage is produced by a simultaneous combination of a primary effect produced by alcohol and a precipitating factor, which occurs randomly, independent of alcohol consumption.[399]

Partial support for this view is to be found in a prospective study from Copenhagen.[530] These investigators found that neither the duration of alcohol abuse nor the average daily consumption was related to the subsequent incidence of cirrhosis. Noteworthy is that their findings confirmed observations from Lelbach and others that above a 50 g/d threshold,

the risk of developing alcoholic cirrhosis is about 15%. They wonder whether the effect of alcohol may be permissive rather than dose-related.[529] The Copenhagen group has listed such candidate factors as genetically determined traits, nutritional impairment, and even consumption of pork.[163,529]

HBV has been suggested from time to time as being such a factor. Several studies have found that in alcoholic cirrhosis, there is either an increased prevalence of antibodies to hepatitis B surface antigen (HB_sAg),[218,359] evidence of cellular immunity to HB_sAg,[421] or an increased susceptibility of HB_sAg carriers to hepatic damage from alcohol.[581] These associations are intriguing but unproved.

An increased prevalence of antibody to hepatitis C virus (HCV) and a correlation with increased severity of alcoholic hepatitis were noted in early reports.[408] Subsequently, these phenomena were determined to represent false-positive results related to the lack of specificity of the first-generation anti-HCV test in some of these patients.[342,350] A relation exists between a positive anti-HCV test and elevated serum γ-globulin concentrations.[51,342,350]

A possible role for interactions with the histocompatibility antigens and other genetic factors is discussed later in this chapter.

From time to time, the concept is raised that it is not alcohol per se but some other factor in the alcoholic beverage that is responsible for cirrhosis. It seems clear that alcohol-associated cirrhosis in the United States occurs predominantly in whiskey drinkers; in France, Italy, Chile, and the German wine districts of Baden-Würtemberg and Rheinland-Pfalz, in wine drinkers; and in Australia and the vineyard-free parts of Germany, in beer drinkers. Alcohol is the only factor common to these diverse beverages. This concept is supported by epidemiologic studies in Canada, where cirrhosis appears to be associated with the alcoholic beverage that provides alcohol at the lowest unit cost. Such observations have not altered the well-established convictions, unsubstantiated by hard data, that cirrhosis is associated with "rotgut" whiskey, not with "good stuff"; that in northeastern France, cirrhosis is associated with the consumption of red wine but not with white; and that in Spain, cirrhosis is associated with port wine but not with sherry. It is fair to assume that Portuguese authorities have opposite opinions about the relative hepatotoxicity of sherry and port. Most data suggest it is the volume of alcohol consumed, rather than the type of beverage, that leads to cirrhosis. The ready availability of alcohol of all types in the American melting pot and the development of cirrhosis from the beverage of one's choice attest to one of the basic freedoms of American democracy.

Although it has been shown conclusively that alcohol, even in relatively small, socially acceptable, noninebriating quantities, induces fatty infiltration of the liver in humans,[319] there is no evidence that this lesion progresses to cirrhosis. In fact, fatty infiltration, which is almost invariably present after any alcohol ingestion, is rapidly reversible. Because only a small fraction—only 10% to 15%—of people who drink alcohol to excess develop cirrhosis,[241,270,530] it seems clear that fatty infiltration per se is not an obligatory precirrhotic lesion. It certainly suggests that other factors, including genetic susceptibility, which is discussed subsequently, may act as cofactors with alcohol.

Although fatty liver itself does not appear to be precirrhotic, evidence exists that there are lesions that can be present even at the fatty liver stage that may indeed presage the development of cirrhosis. Investigators from the Bronx Veterans Administration Hospital have offered evidence that perivenular fibrosis (thickening of the terminal hepatic vein) is a precursor lesion to cirrhosis.[377,578,610] Other investigators have not been able to confirm the significance of thickening around the terminal hepatic vein.[52,379] One group of these investigators found instead that lobular fibrosis and sinusoidal fibrosis are markers for progressive fibrosis and development of cirrhosis.[379] Lieber[314] has suggested that perivenular fibrosis and sinusoidal fibrosis may represent two aspects of a similar lesion surrounding vascular structures of different sizes (ie, venules and sinusoids).

It is not yet certain whether alcoholic hepatitis, which is characterized histologically by active hepatic parenchymal necrosis, the presence of characteristic Mallory hyaline cytoplasmic inclusions, and inflammation[168,207,208] and which often is accompanied by fatty infiltration, can be induced in humans by alcohol *alone* or whether other cofactors are necessary. It seems clear, however, that alcoholic hepatitis is a precirrhotic lesion.[214] Galambos[168] followed 61 such patients for a mean of 3 years and found that cirrhosis developed in 38%; even among the minority who stopped drinking, cirrhosis developed in 18%. Sorensen and his group from Copenhagen[530] found in their prospective study that the risk of subsequent development of cirrhosis was increased ninefold in patients with alcoholic hepatitis. The critical difference between fatty liver and alcoholic hepatitis is that alcoholic hepatitis embodies hepatic necrosis, the sine qua non of the experimental production of cirrhosis by any agent, and alcoholic fat deposition does not. This concept was expressed by Moon[364] in 1934, and 50 additional years of research have not increased our understanding. He wrote:

> Alcohol, even in large amounts and long continued, had caused only parenchymatous degeneration and fatty changes. These have not resulted in necrosis nor in permanent hepatic changes. However, the probability that alcohol acts as a contributing or predisposing factor *has* received experimental support. Alcohol has been found to accentuate the injurious effects of bacteria, phosphorus, chloroform, and of carbon tetrachloride, upon the livers of animals. It is probable that alcohol may similarly accentuate the effects of injurious agents upon the human liver.

This is not to say that our knowledge has not advanced since Moon. Extensive studies have been carried out on the pathways of alcohol metabolism and on associated metabolic disturbances in an attempt to define the toxicity of ethanol. This research has identified toxic effects related to the generation of NADH by oxidation of ethanol by way of the alcohol dehydrogenase (ADH) pathway, the interaction of alcohol with liver microsomes, the generation of acetaldehyde, the effects of ethanol on liver membranes, and the effects of an imbalance between oxygen delivery and the liver cells' requirements. These findings have been reviewed by Lieber,[313–318] and the role of each is discussed below.

Three pathways for ethanol metabolism exist in the hepatocyte—the ADH pathway of the cytosol, the microsomal ethanol oxidizing system (MEOS) in the endoplasmic reticulum, and the catalase pathway in peroxisomes. The major pathway is by way of ADH. In the process of oxidizing alcohol to acetaldehyde, the ADH pathway, which requires nicotinamide-adenine dinucleotide (NAD), generates an excess of reducing equivalents as free NADH.[314] The resulting altered redox state has multiple metabolic consequences, including hyperlipemia and changes in amino acid and protein metabolism. These changes may lead to cell injury and stimulation of collagen formation.

The interaction of ethanol with liver microsomes was first suggested by the morphologic observation that ethanol feeding resulted in proliferation of smooth endoplasmic reticulum (SER). Subsequently, the SER was found to be the site of the MEOS. The activity of this system depends on cytochrome P-450. The MEOS pathway of alcohol metabolism has particular importance in chronic ethanol ingestion and is a major mechanism for acceleration of ethanol metabolism at high ethanol concentrations. An ethanol-specific form of cytochrome P-450, designated as P450IIE1, is induced by chronic alcohol ingestion.[381,392] Other microsomal cytochrome P-450 isozymes can also contribute to ethanol oxidation.[317] The interaction of drugs and environmental compounds with increased cytochrome P-450 content in hepatocytes may result in increased toxicity of these compounds to liver cells. Such increased susceptibility to their toxic effects has been demonstrated for acetaminophen, phenylbutazone, halothane, cocaine, and carbon tetrachloride.[317]

The ADH and MEOS pathways, as well as the catalase pathway, generate acetaldehyde as a metabolic product. Acetaldehyde has several toxic effects: it covalently binds to protein, it may impair protein secretion, and it causes lipid peroxidation. Cell injury may result. For example, covalent binding to protein may directly injure hepatocytes or it may form acetaldehyde–protein adducts, which may have an associated immune response.[290,316–318]

Alcohol's effect on cell membranes includes changes in both their physical state and their lipid composition. Membrane function and cell integrity may, therefore, be compromised.

Alcoholic patients show a greater increase in oxygen consumption after alcohol ingestion than do nonalcoholic patients. This has been seen as energy wastage. It is postulated that this increased oxygen demand, owing either to an enhanced role of the MEOS or to relative uncoupling of reoxidation of NADH, may aggravate alcohol hepatotoxicity.

Because biochemical evidence of hepatic injury often continues despite cessation of alcohol intake, a potential role for altered humoral and cellular immunity in the pathogenesis of alcoholic liver disease has been proposed.[329,410,531,615,616] Possible humoral mechanisms have included antibodies to Mallory bodies, antibodies to antigens on hepatocyte membranes that have been altered by alcohol or its metabolites, and the triggering of liver injury by immune complexes.[233,329] The pathogenetic role of these mechanisms remains unestablished.

The evidence for the role of altered cellular immunity in the pathogenesis of alcoholic liver disease is circumstantial. It includes changes in lymphocyte population and function, changes in the response of lymphocytes to mitogens, and occurrence of abnormal tests of delayed hypersensitivity.[233]

In alcoholic hepatitis and cirrhosis, there is a reduction in peripheral blood T lymphocytes coupled with an increased number of T lymphocytes in the liver. These changes are reversible when alcohol is withdrawn and the patient improves clinically. Cytotoxicity for liver cells by peripheral blood lymphocytes has been described in other studies.[82,244]

Sera from patients with alcoholic liver disease have been found to inhibit lymphocyte transformation in vitro when phytohemagglutinin, pokeweed mitogen, and concanavalin A were used.[329]

Suppression of delayed cutaneous hypersensitivity has been shown in acute alcoholic hepatitis.[526] In vitro studies using lymphocyte transformation studies and migration inhibition indices have found lymphocyte sensitization to alcohol and acetaldehyde in alcoholic hepatitis but not cirrhosis. Patients with alcoholic hepatitis as well as alcoholic cirrhosis have shown lymphocyte sensitization to Mallory's bodies in some studies.[329,616] Whether these immunologic alterations play a role in initiating alcoholic injury or are epiphenomena is yet to be elucidated.

Fibrosis that forms nodules and distorts parenchymal architecture is one definition of cirrhosis. The mechanism by which alcohol causes fibrosis is uncertain. It may be a primary event related to toxic or immune processes or both, as in alcoholic hepatitis, or it may be an event secondary to previous acute liver injury related to host susceptibility. Whatever explanation is accepted must explain why all heavy drinkers do not develop alcoholic cirrhosis.

Fibrosis begins in the perivenular area in alcohol-induced disease[377,578] and then advances into the rest of zone 3 in a spider web or lattice manner. It then extends into the perisinusoidal area throughout the lobules, obliterating the space of Disse. Central-central and central-portal fibrous bridges develop.

Cells known to produce collagen include hepatocytes, sinusoidal endothelial cells, lipocytes, and hepatic myofibroblasts, of which the nonparenchymal cells are the major source.[358] Fibrosis is initiated by uncertain mechanisms, perhaps an effect of acetaldehyde or of hepatic inflammation, by releasing cytokines or Kupffer cell–derived factors that stimulate fibrogenesis.[334] Reactive oxygen metabolites formed during the oxidation of ethanol have also been implicated.[334]

Alcohol-Like Liver Disease in the Nonalcoholic. The spectrum of injury usually associated with alcoholic liver disease, including cirrhosis, has been documented in minimal or nondrinkers. The severity of the liver disease is milder and the frequency of complications less than in those who drink moderately or heavily. Nonetheless, one third of the patients in the nondrinking group have cirrhosis compared with two thirds of control patients whose liver disease is related to alcohol. Only 10% have clinically evident portal hypertension.[124]

Most patients with this syndrome are middle-aged women who have active medical problems such as diabetes, heart disease, hypertension, dysmenorrhea, and hypothyroidism. Consequently, the use of antihypertensive or cardiac medications, thyroid hormones, and estrogen frequently is reported in these patients. The drugs diltiazem, nifedipine, amiodarone, and diethylstilbestrol can independently produce a histologic resemblance to alcoholic hepatitis.[24,38,231,311] Although the outcome in alcohol-like liver disease is less often fatal than in alcoholic liver disease, portal hypertension and impaired hepatocellular function can be fatal.[124,434]

MALNUTRITION

Malnutrition has long been claimed to be a cause of cirrhosis or at least a major factor in its development. The evidence to support this concept is of two types. First, the production of cirrhosis in laboratory animals fed nutritionally deficient diets, especially protein-, choline-, and vitamin-deficient diets, favors this concept. Hepatic lesions that resemble cirrhosis, both postnecrotic[216] and portal in type,[217] can be produced in rats and other laboratory animals by protein- and vitamin-deficient diets.[209] It is not established that these lesions represent true cirrhosis. Although histologically compatible, they are, unlike cirrhosis in humans, apparently reversible lesions that do not exhibit the vascular consequences commonly seen in human cirrhosis. It must always be kept in mind that data derived from animal experiments, although useful in suggesting and testing hypotheses and in indicating new directions for investigation, can only be extrapolated to humans at considerable risk.

Second, the beneficial response of malnutrition–alcohol-induced lesions to high-protein diets and diet supplements supports the nutritional pathogenesis.[413] In virtually all such instances, however, excessive alcohol ingestion had coexisted with malnutrition during the development of the lesion, and diet therapy in the hospital was almost invariably accompanied by abstinence from alcohol.

A causal relation between malnutrition and human cirrhosis has not been established. The hepatic lesion closest to cirrhosis induced by protein malnutrition is kwashiorkor. This disease, which was first described by Williams[600] in Africa, has also been reported, predominantly in infants and young children, in India, Indonesia, Central America, Jamaica, and many other impoverished areas. Although it is a generalized disease characterized by retarded physical and mental growth, edema, ascites, and hypoalbuminemia, its hepatic characteristic is a large, fatty liver. There is no cirrhosis.[102,588] Ramalingaswami[443] reported that diffuse fibrosis and rarely cirrhosis may occasionally be found in children suffering from prolonged kwashiorkor. The disease is rapidly reversed by the administration of protein.[61] After recovery, the liver is normal, although in some cases, a fine fibrosis may be found. This lesion appears to be similar to the lesions induced in laboratory animals by dietary deficiencies. In adults, evidence for a malnutrition-induced lesion equivalent to kwashiorkor is scant.[510] The only indication of cirrhosis induced by malnutrition has been presented by Snapper,[523] who observed epidemic cirrhosis associated with malnutrition in Peking during the Japanese occupation. Other disorders may be responsible for or predispose to the development of cirrhosis. The prevalence of hepatitis is increased in many of the malnourished areas of the world, and underlying posthepatitic cirrhosis may account for some of the cirrhosis attributed to malnutrition. Aflatoxin, too, may play an unrecognized role in many of these areas.[457] A disorder indistinguishable from Indian childhood cirrhosis had been reported after chronic ingestion of food contaminated with aflatoxin B₁ derived from *Aspergillus flavus*.[12] Similarly, the presence of schistosomiasis and other parasitic infestations of the liver in some of the tropical areas where malnutrition occurs may complicate the problem. Certainly, malnutrition could accelerate or exacerbate such underlying lesions.

The recognition that ileojejunal bypass operations for the treatment of obesity may induce progressive fatty infiltration of the liver and even cirrhosis[129] appears to challenge the concept that malnutrition does not cause cirrhosis in humans. Such small bowel exclusion operations induce metabolically complex situations that alter absorption, enterohepatic circulation, and bile acid metabolism. Any of these abnormalities or other unrecognized consequences of these operations might conceivably induce liver damage and cirrhosis in a manner independent of malnutrition per se. Total starvation, which is in effect a protein-deficient diet, causes no significant hepatic dysfunction and in fact is associated with the disappearance of the fatty infiltration of obesity.[129]

The best conclusion is that malnutrition is undoubtedly associated with the pathogenesis of some types of cirrhosis and that famine, under certain complex, poorly studied, poorly understood situations, may cause cirrhosis in humans.

VIRAL HEPATITIS

Hepatitis A is generally held not to cause either chronic liver disease or cirrhosis.[305] Perhaps this is because hepatitis A virus (HAV) infection is cytopathic rather than immunogenic. There is less compelling evidence that HAV infection, in contrast to HBV and non-A, non-B infection, requires a contribution from the host's immune system to cause hepatocellular injury.[177] Mediation of injury by an immunopathologic process has been postulated, however.[305] At least one case of a chronic course for hepatitis A has been reported.[348]

The progression of *hepatitis B* from acute to chronic occurs in about 10% of patients, but only about 3% develop potentially progressive disease.[86] Among patients with chronic active hepatitis, the progression to cirrhosis over 2 to 5 years has been reported to be as high as 70% in retrospective studies.[117] Prospective studies have suggested that 15% to 20% of patients will develop cirrhosis by the end of 5 years.[142,312] Cirrhosis is more likely to occur in older patients, in patients who have bridging necrosis, and in patients who have persistent HBV deoxyribonucleic acid (DNA) in serum. This latter group may develop cirrhosis even if the histologic lesion is not severe.[142] There is no evidence that corticosteroid therapy alters the natural history of the histologic lesion. When chronic hepatitis B is histologically persistent (ie, limited to the portal tracts) rather than active hepatitis (ie, periportal hepatitis or confluent necrosis or both), cirrhosis is not a common consequence.[73] When hepatitis B progresses to cirrhosis, the 5-year survival is 55%; hepatic failure or the complications of cirrhosis are the most frequent cause of death.[594]

Hepatitis C not only has the propensity to become chronic, but most reported series have documented the development of cirrhosis, the prevalence of which is about 10% when biopsies are first performed.[44,108,276-278,441,483] Cirrhosis has been reported as early as 4 months to 1 year after onset of hepatitis C,[125] but a larger number of cases appear to be found between the 2nd and 4th years.[451] When these patients are observed for longer periods, the prevalence of cirrhosis appears to be 20% to 25%, but it has been as high as 50% in disease of at least 7 years' duration.[10,113,175] Until recently, when tests for specific antibody were developed, estimates of the sequelae of hepatitis C, formerly non-A, non-B hepatitis, were rather imprecise. Sixty to 80% of what was once called non-A, non-B hepatitis is found to be positive for anti-HCV.[285]

In some cases, the acute hepatitis has been symptomatic, cirrhosis has developed early, and death has occurred from hepatic failure,[125] but the more usual occurrence appears to be the slow development of cirrhosis in a clinically inapparent manner.[108] Even when cirrhosis develops insidiously, some patients may subsequently develop encephalopathy, ascites, and variceal hemorrhage.[236] These latter patients have been predominantly elderly and have received a large number of transfusions. Most patients who progress to cirrhosis

have in fact acquired their preceding hepatitis by parenteral means (transfusions, intravenous drug use, or needle stick).

The number of patients who have been followed for long periods is not large, but available data suggest that when HBV and hepatitis D virus (delta) infections are acquired simultaneously (ie, coinfection), the illness seldom progresses to chronicity.[456,519] This outcome is not the case when patients chronically infected with HBV develop delta superinfection. In such a setting, chronicity is likely to be the most frequent outcome. This conclusion is suggested by the observation that the prevalence of delta infection is three to five times higher in carriers with chronic hepatitis than in asymptomatic carriers.[466,467] It is further suggested by the finding that 90% of patients with delta infection in a Venezuelan epidemic among HBV carriers developed chronic hepatitis as opposed to only 10% of those with HBV infection alone.[466] There is some evidence that chronicity is more likely in patients with inactive infections (presence of anti-HB$_e$ in serum) than in patients who have active infection (presence of HB$_e$Ag in serum) who become superinfected.[466] In one large Italian series of patients who were chronic carriers of HB$_s$Ag and had superimposed delta infection established by intrahepatic expression of delta antigen, cirrhosis was present at initial biopsy in 23% and developed in an additional 41% over a period of observation of 2 to 6 years.[467] One third of the patients who presented with cirrhosis and one fifth of those who developed cirrhosis died during the period of observation.[467] Nearly 60% of British HB$_s$Ag carriers who were delta antibody–positive had cirrhosis as opposed to only 20% who had surface antigen alone.[595] Even when carriers of HB$_s$Ag with delta antibody are asymptomatic, 40% may have cirrhosis.[16]

Hepatitis E, the source of waterborne, enterically transmitted epidemics of hepatitis worldwide, does not become chronic and does not lead to cirrhosis.[182]

The low prevalence of cirrhosis after hepatitis of all viral etiologies, relative to the large number of patients with presumed posthepatitic cirrhosis, poses a fascinating epidemiologic paradox. The demonstration that bridging necrosis and postnecrotic cirrhosis may follow anicteric hepatitis has raised the question of whether clinically mild, inapparent hepatitis may have a worse prognosis in terms of the development of cirrhosis[269] than overt hepatitis with jaundice. Complicating the whole problem is subjective observer variability in the diagnosis of the presence[527] and type of cirrhosis[172,184] and the fact that the type of cirrhosis may differ in different portions of the liver.[170,479]

OBSTRUCTION OF THE EXTRAHEPATIC BILIARY TRACT

Any process that obstructs the biliary tree, including gallstones, neoplasms, benign strictures, extrinsic compression of any cause, or congenital or acquired atresia of the bile ducts, may in sufficient time result in secondary biliary cirrhosis. It is not, however, an invariable consequence of prolonged biliary obstruction. Less than 10% of patients with chronic biliary tract obstruction develop biliary cirrhosis.[179] Because the process takes from 3 months to more than a year to develop, it occurs more commonly with benign than with malignant causes of obstruction, since the latter may kill the patient before cirrhosis can develop. It is found more frequently with total than with partial obstruction, and this difference may explain the paradoxically less frequent occurrence of biliary cirrhosis in patients with ascending cholangitis, which is usually associated with incomplete obstruction.[126] Unilateral cirrhosis has been reported in a patient with left hepatic duct atresia.[185]

It is not clear how biliary cirrhosis develops. Review of the consequences of obstruction of the extrahepatic biliary tree may shed some light on the problem. Acute biliary tract obstruction causes the prompt appearance of hepatomegaly and dilated intrahepatic bile ducts. At first, the bile is dark, but it quickly becomes colorless, so-called white bile, which results from the suppressed secretion of bilirubin by increased intraductular pressure. Microscopically, bile duct regeneration occurs. The bile ductules, which are tortuous and distended, are lined by high cuboidal epithelium. Focal necrosis in the central areas occurs early in the process and is followed by peripheral necrosis. Periportal necrosis is more widespread and characterized by bile lakes, which appear as bile-stained areas of parenchymal necrosis presumably caused by the escape of bile from the interlobular bile ducts. Bile lakes are characteristic of high-grade mechanical obstruction of the biliary tree and are never seen in nonobstructive, intrahepatic cholestasis. If infected, the bile may become purulent and the portal areas may show acute polymorphonuclear infiltration. If cholangitis develops or an abscess forms, necrosis of the periportal areas may predominate.

Although the pathogenesis of secondary biliary cirrhosis is not fully understood, it is consistent with the pathogenetic patterns in other types of cirrhosis. The presence of periportal necrosis and inflammation may stimulate the development of portal scar. The concentric, onionskin layering of scar tissue around the portal areas is compatible with this pathogenesis. It is not known whether infection is necessary to cause biliary cirrhosis. In humans, infected biliary obstruction is less likely to be associated with biliary cirrhosis than is noninfected obstruction. Furthermore, experimental biliary cirrhosis can be produced in laboratory animals with sterile biliary tract obstruction, that is, in the absence of infection.

Histologically, it may be difficult to differentiate established secondary biliary cirrhosis from cirrhosis of other types, although the fibrous linkage from portal-to-portal areas tends to create a more regular pseudolobular pattern than the portal-to-central microlobularity of alcoholic cirrhosis or the macronodular appearance of postnecrotic cirrhosis. As the disease progresses, the pattern of necrosis to fibrosis proceeds and some portal-to-central scars develop. A dense cirrhosis may develop with unremittent biliary obstruction. Sometimes intense regenerative activity occurs, which further distorts the pattern and makes it indistinguishable from other types of cirrhosis.[126] This type of cirrhosis is not functionally benign; about half the patients develop ascites, varices, and other evidence of portal hypertension,[501] although these complications occur only with long-standing obstructive disease in which much of the parenchymal tissue has been converted into regenerative nodules.[126]

In summary, the triad of necrosis, fibrosis, and regeneration in prolonged obstructive jaundice creates a pathologically characteristic form of portal cirrhosis, which in later stages may no longer be differentiable from advanced cirrhosis of other types.

PRIMARY BILIARY CIRRHOSIS

Primary biliary cirrhosis is discussed in Chapter 16.

HEART FAILURE AND OUTFLOW OBSTRUCTION

Cardiac cirrhosis is an uncommon consequence of chronic heart failure. It is seen most frequently in patients with long-standing cardiac decompensation, especially those with tricuspid insufficiency or constrictive pericarditis. The disease is not overt clinically, and the diagnosis of cardiac cirrhosis may be difficult to make. It is seldom associated with deep jaundice or evidence of poor hepatic function, such as severe hypoalbuminemia or prolongation of prothrombin time, or manifestations of portal hypertension, such as bleeding esophageal varices or portal-systemic encephalopathy.

The liver in heart failure is enlarged, purplish, and rounded. It seldom is irregular or overtly nodular. On cut surface, the veins are prominent and dilated. The characteristic "nutmeg" liver of alternating red and yellow areas represents the reddish centrilobular areas of congestion and the normal yellowish portions of the lobule.[585]

Microscopically, the liver shows distended central veins and engorgement of the sinusoids entering them. The radiating plates of liver cells are atrophic in the central areas. The rows of hepatocytes are smaller than in the periportal areas. When severe, there may be hemorrhage into the central areas and centrilobular focal necrosis may be present. Lipofuscin pigment may be prominent in the central hepatocytes. The portal areas are relatively unaffected.

The pathogenesis of cardiac cirrhosis is compatible with the pathophysiology of heart failure and the histologic abnormalities noted above. In heart failure, reduced cardiac output results in decreased perfusion pressure of the blood entering the liver. The oxygen content of blood is greatest in the periportal areas (area 1 of Rappaport) and falls progressively as it approaches the central portion of the lobules (Rappaport's area 3), which is metabolically the most susceptible portion of the lobule.[447] The metabolic susceptibility of the central portion of the lobule is shown by the peculiarly rapid postmortem autolysis of this area in patients with chronic congestive failure.[429] Similarly, the syndrome of massive elevations of serum transaminase levels in patients after a bout of hypotension is another clinical manifestation of this anatomically localized susceptibility.[265] Presumably, the hypoxic centrilobular hepatic cells become more so during a period of shock after myocardial infarction, pulmonary embolism, or transient arrhythmia. All the injured cells simultaneously lose their enzymes into the serum, with a resultant sharp spike in transaminase activity that may reach levels of 5,000, 10,000, or even 20,000 units. This sequence of events often is fatal, but if the hypotension is transient or promptly corrected, the enormous elevation in transaminase levels may be unaccompanied by other gross distortions of liver function and the patient may survive.

In addition, the increased central venous pressure of heart failure is transmitted backward into the hepatic veins where congestion opposes the entry of portal and arterial blood to the central portion of the lobules. The localized centrilobular hypoxia results at first in sinusoidal congestion and atrophy of the hepatic cords with loss of cells and later in hemorrhage and necrosis. Loss of cells results in the collapse and condensation of the reticulum. Active necrosis stimulates collagen production, and collagenization of the collapsed reticulum and of the central veins may give rise to phlebosclerosis. It has been found in electron microscopic studies that atrophy of cells, rather than active necrosis, is the stimulus for fibrous tissue formation.[486] Finally, regenerative activity develops.

The pattern of cardiac cirrhosis fits this pathogenesis perfectly. The scar is initially centrilobular, and as it spreads into the lobule, the scars connect central areas to one another. In the presence of relatively unaffected portal areas, one sees the reverse lobulation of cardiac cirrhosis.[509] The portal areas appear to be centrally located and are surrounded by a ring of fibrous tissue bands that pass from central vein to central vein. The cirrhosis in this classic stage is characteristic and specific for cardiac cirrhosis, but later, as bile duct regeneration and portal fibrosis develop and as parenchymal regeneration takes place, the cirrhosis may lose its specific pattern.

Thus, cardiac cirrhosis is a centrizonal cirrhosis that results in loss of cells from the central portion of the liver as a consequence of centrilobular hypoxia. Central deposition of scar produces a specific type of cirrhosis that closely reflects its pathogenesis.

A lesion indistinguishable from cardiac cirrhosis may be seen in patients with chronic hepatic venous obstruction (Budd-Chiari syndrome). The pathogenesis is similar to that seen in cardiac cirrhosis, except that the initial centrilobular congestion and hepatocellular atrophy are consequences of stasis per se. Because cardiac output in this situation is normal or elevated, the Budd-Chiari syndrome may give rise to *stasis* cirrhosis.

Similarly, in venoocclusive disease, a type of Budd-Chiari syndrome induced by ingesting *Senecio* or *Crotolaria* alkaloids, a centrilobular cirrhosis may develop.[57]

It was inevitable that eventually a case of hepatocellular carcinoma complicating cardiac cirrhosis would be described.[219] A large series will no doubt be a long time in coming.

HEMOCHROMATOSIS

The pathogenesis of the cirrhosis of hemochromatosis is discussed in the section devoted exclusively to this subject (see Chap. 26).

HEPATOLENTICULAR DEGENERATION (WILSON'S DISEASE)

The pathogenesis of the cirrhosis of Wilson's disease is discussed in the section devoted exclusively to this subject (see Chap. 25).

AUTOIMMUNE DISORDERS

The pathogenesis of cirrhosis arising from chronic hepatitis and altered immunity is discussed in Chapter 24. Biliary cirrhosis has been reported as a consequence of graft-versus-host disease after bone marrow transplantation.[274,540]

SYPHILIS

Cirrhosis is a rare occurrence in syphilis, seen only when syphilis is congenital. It is a fine intralobular cirrhosis with proliferation of connective tissue that surrounds small groups of cells or individual hepatocytes.[201,461]

In 10% of acquired secondary syphilis, there is hepatitis with or without granulomas.[144,299] Treatment resolves the hepatitis but may not prevent the accumulation of collagen in the walls of the sinusoids and the spaces of Disse, but cirrhosis does not develop.[144,243]

Tertiary syphilis has erroneously been thought in the past to result in cirrhosis. It is characterized by widespread gummas that heal with fibrosis. As the fibrosis contracts, deep clefts may be produced in the liver that produce a pseudolobation of the liver called *hepar lobatum*. These deep scars may divide the liver into masses of irregular size but do not produce true cirrhosis.[201,549] Previous reports of the occurrence of cirrhosis with syphilis often were based on the finding of cirrhosis in syphilitic patients who had other epidemiologic associations or on series lacking appropriate control groups.[251,579] A historical review with likely resolution of the controversy about syphilitic cirrhosis has been published by Davies.[112]

INTRINSIC DRUG-INDUCED HEPATOTOXICITY

Carbon Tetrachloride

The solvent carbon tetrachloride represents the prototype of intrinsic hepatotoxicity. Intrinsic hepatotoxins are toxic to the livers of all species after a short, predictable latent period. The minimal toxic dose is relatively reproducible, and the severity of hepatic injury, which is characteristic for the individual compound, is roughly proportional to dosage. No signs of hypersensitivity, such as fever, rash, or eosinophilia, accompany the liver injury. Carbon tetrachloride induces diffuse fatty degeneration and centrilobular necrosis. Although often fatal, the hepatic lesion is not usually the cause of death. Usually, renal tubular injury is the lethal lesion, but sometimes the pancreatic and pulmonary lesions and other indirect consequences are fatal. Hepatic necrosis usually is not massive, and if the patient recovers, cirrhosis is rare.

The mechanism of action of carbon tetrachloride may explain this paradox. Carbon tetrachloride induces its hepatic lesion promptly, within a matter of hours after digestion. Carbon tetrachloride per se, however, is not the toxic material. Drug-metabolizing enzymes remove one chlorine atom from the molecule, forming trichloromethane, which is extremely toxic to the hepatic endoplasmic reticulum and microsomal drug-metabolizing enzyme systems.[452,453] Lipoperoxidative destruction of these susceptible organelles prevents or diminishes further activation of carbon tetrachloride and, thus, further hepatic damage. Most patients who recover regain full hepatic function, and there are no pathologic sequelae. Occasionally hepatic necrosis is massive. Several cases of bridging hepatic necrosis after carbon tetrachloride ingestion that have gone on to develop postnecrotic cirrhosis have been reported.[271] There are rare reports that recurrent or chronic exposure to carbon tetrachloride can cause cirrhosis.[427]

The terrible reputation of carbon tetrachloride, which is well deserved, has greatly restricted its commercial use. Consequently, this substance is not clinically important as a hepatotoxin or as a cause of cirrhosis but is of significance because of its well-studied mechanism of action.

Dimethylnitrosamine

Like carbon tetrachloride, dimethylnitrosamine, an anticorrosive agent, can induce cirrhosis and hepatocellular neoplasms in laboratory animals[28,330] and, apparently, postnecrotic cirrhosis in humans.[165] An immune mechanism may play a role in the pathogenesis of the fibrosis.[237]

Methotrexate

Methotrexate is a widely used antimetabolite directed against folates, which are essential for DNA synthesis and cell division. It is used in combination chemotherapy for leukemia and diverse cancers, for suppression of graft-versus-host disease after bone marrow transplantation, and as a therapeutic agent for severe psoriasis that is unresponsive to topical therapy.[240]

Its potential for hepatotoxicity has been evident for nearly 30 years. Histologic changes attributed to methotrexate include steatosis, ballooning degeneration and necrosis of hepatocytes, fibrosis, and cirrhosis. The pathologic lesion is one of portal cirrhosis, which is in no way unique. Methotrexate is thought to be an intrinsic hepatotoxin; however, the inability to consistently reproduce hepatic injury in laboratory animals leaves this classification uncertain.[619]

The extensive use of methotrexate in psoriatic patients has suggested that several factors increase the propensity to liver damage. These include increased alcohol intake, obesity, diabetes mellitus, daily dosage schedules (as opposed to weekly), preexisting liver disease, treatment with arsenic, impaired renal function, and high cumulative dose, although agreement has not been uniform about the latter.[17,387,592,612]

Studies in patients with psoriasis treated with methotrexate for 2 or more years that have performed pretreatment and posttreatment biopsies have suggested a prevalence of fibrosis and cirrhosis between 4% and 25%.[17]

A classification for liver biopsy findings in patients receiving methotrexate that was developed for monitoring therapy in patients with psoriasis is shown in Table 32-2.[471] The Psoriasis Task Force of the National Program of Dermatology recommends that liver biopsy be performed, when feasible, before starting methotrexate therapy and that patients be excluded from methotrexate therapy if there is significant preexisting liver disease. If methotrexate therapy is initiated, a repeat biopsy should be considered after a total dose of 1 g. Liver scans are of minimal value in identifying patients with methotrexate liver disease, and liver function tests identify only a few cases of methotrexate toxicity.[471] The cirrhosis often is clinically silent, although portal hypertension may occur.[83]

Methotrexate may be continued if liver biopsy changes are no more severe than grade II, but repeat biopsies should be obtained after each additional 1 to 1.5 g. Patients with grade IIIB or grade IV changes should not receive further methotrexate. Patients with grade IIIA changes may continue to receive methotrexate, but a repeat biopsy should be obtained after 6 months.[471]

Although many reports have attributed chronic liver disease to methotrexate therapy, some objective studies find that methotrexate is not to blame.[248,288] In patients who were to receive methotrexate for rheumatoid arthritis, histologic changes of chronic liver disease often were present *before* the drug was begun. Indeed, methotrexate is being used to treat patients with primary sclerosing cholangitis.[248] Some investigators have concluded that hepatotoxic substances other than methotrexate, such as alcohol, vitamin A, and arsenic, were more likely causes of the hepatic lesions.[249,611] One of these authors had previously reported methotrexate to be hepatotoxic.[612]

On the other hand, three cases from one institution are reported in which methotrexate-induced cirrhosis resulting from higher than recommended total doses of the drug in psoriasis required liver transplantation.[180] If methotrexate is withdrawn before liver disease is advanced, progression is unlikely and improvement may occur.[382]

The pathogenesis of methotrexate hepatotoxicity is unknown. It has been suggested that it may represent a toxic effect of its therapeutic mechanism of action. The major activity of methotrexate is its binding to dehydrofolic reductase, thus preventing the conversion of folic acid to its active form, folinic acid. This metabolic block may in turn slow the synthesis of nucleic acids and some amino acids.

IDIOSYNCRATIC DRUG-INDUCED HEPATOTOXICITY

Idiosyncratic hepatotoxicity, typified by α-methyldopa or halothane hepatitis, occurs rarely after a variable but prolonged latent period. Its severity is not dosage-related. It occurs in only a single species—humans—and is associated with various immunologic phenomena such as evidence of allergy, eosinophilia, and, often, abnormal immunologic reactions. Readministration of the offending drug commonly is followed by the prompt recurrence of hepatotoxicity.

It is striking that idiosyncratic hepatotoxins rarely cause cirrhosis, despite the fact that they often cause fatal hepatitis. Patients who survive massive or submassive hepatic necrosis may conceivably develop postnecrotic cirrhosis in a manner analogous to submassive necrosis in viral hepatitis. Several cases of α-methyldopa–associated cirrhosis have been reported.[507] It can be predicted with confidence that any of the drugs like α-methyldopa or oxyphenisatin that can cause chronic active hepatitis will occasionally cause cirrhosis.

MISCELLANEOUS

α_1-Antitrypsin Deficiency

The descriptive name for α_1-antitrypsin (AAT) identifies it with the α_1-globulins and correctly credits it with protection of cells against injury from trypsin and other proteases released from bacteria or dying cells. Its deficiency in serum was originally recognized as a cause of inherited liver disease in children and of an inherited predisposition to emphysema in adults.[171,506] Cirrhosis in AAT is now known also to occur in adults.

AAT deficiency results from amino acid substitution in the polypeptide core, which leads to secondary changes in the carbohydrate side chains. These changes may impede re-

TABLE 32-2 *Classification of Liver Biopsy Changes During Methotrexate Therapy*

Grade I	Normal; fatty infiltration, mild; nuclear variability, mild; portal inflammation, mild
Grade II	Fatty infiltration, moderate to severe; nuclear variability, moderate to severe; portal tract expansion, portal tract inflammation, and lobular necrosis, moderate to severe
Grade III	
IIIA	Fibrosis, mild; fibrotic septa extending into the lobules by connective tissue or reticulin stain
IIIB	Fibrosis, moderate to severe
Grade IV	Cirrhosis

(Roenigk HH Jr. Methotrexate in psoriasis: revised guidelines. J Am Acad Dermatol 19:1451, 1988)

lease from the endoplasmic reticulum of the hepatocyte. There appear to be more than 30 different inherited alleles (see Chap. 24).

The pathogenesis of cirrhosis and liver injury is unknown, but it is hypothesized that the uninhibited action of proteases, perhaps from Kupffer cells, prevents control of liver damage once the process is initiated.[370]

Of children with homozygous AAT deficiency, 25% develop cirrhosis and portal hypertension and die of complications before age 10; another 25% die of the same process by age 20; a further 25% have liver fibrosis and minimal liver dysfunction and live to adulthood, perhaps with later progression. The final 25% show no childhood evidence of progressive illness, but their fate late in adulthood is uncertain.[370]

In a series of 246 adults with homozygous (ZZ in the proteinase inhibitor or Pi classification) AAT deficiency, 59% had chronic obstructive lung disease and 12% had cirrhosis of the liver. In homozygous AAT patients over age 50, the prevalence of cirrhosis was 19%.[289] An increased prevalence of steatosis and fibrosis was also reported but not quantified.[289] As many as two thirds of patients with liver disease are reported also to have lung disease.[371,566]

There has been interest in the possibility of increased prevalence of liver disease in adults with heterozygous AAT deficiency. A convincing study based on serum analysis and liver biopsy of 1055 adults whose average age was 60 confirms an increased prevalence of at least the MZ phenotype in patients with non-B chronic active hepatitis and in cryptogenic cirrhosis.[223]

In children, liver disease related to AAT deficiency occurs only in those who are Pi ZZ homozygous.[6]

The presentation of adults with AAT-associated liver disease typically is that of hepatosplenomegaly or the overt manifestations of portal hypertension, such as variceal bleeding or ascites. An increased incidence of hepatocellular carcinoma is claimed by some to occur in AAT deficiency,[140,289] but this conclusion is not universally accepted.[191,505] If there is an increase in hepatocellular carcinoma, underlying cirrhosis may be as likely as the antitrypsin deficiency to be the inciting factor.

The diagnosis of AAT deficiency can be suggested by seeing eosinophilic globules on hematoxylin–eosin stains in liver biopsy specimens. These lesions tend to be multiple, spheroidal, hyaline, acidophilic bodies of variable size in the cytoplasm of hepatocytes near the periphery of the lobule. The demonstration that these globules are positive with periodic acid–Schiff (PAS) stain and are diastase-resistant increases the likelihood of AAT deficiency. These stains, however, are not pathognomonic.[439] For example, in alcoholic cirrhosis, PAS-positive, diastase-resistant globules occurred in nearly one third of the patients in a series in which AAT deficiency had been excluded by phenotyping.[409]

The diagnosis of AAT deficiency is also suggested by the absence or diminution of the α_1-globulin band on the serum electrophoresis pattern. Serum electrophoresis detects only severely deficient patients. When AAT deficiency is homozygous, its serum concentration is only 10% to 15% of normal. Ishak and colleagues[230] have demonstrated increased copper pigment in the peripheral pseudolobular hepatocytes, the cells in which AAT bodies are most commonly found. The significance of the copper accumulation is not known.

Functional assays of trypsin-inhibitory capacity or quan-

tification of serum AAT concentration by immunologic techniques increase the precision of the diagnosis, but even these are not always adequate for diagnosing heterozygotes in periods of hormonal or medical stress.[505] Because AAT is an acute-phase reactant, concentrations obtained during such periods may be misleading. The gold standard for diagnosis is protease inhibitor phenotyping.

The only successful therapy for severe hepatic injury from AAT deficiency is liver transplantation.

Cystic Fibrosis of the Pancreas

Cystic fibrosis has long been known to pediatricians but has had to be reckoned with only in recent years by physicians who treat adult patients. The increasing life spans of patients with cystic fibrosis into adulthood have resulted from improved nutritional management, improved use of pulmonary therapy, and the development of new antibiotics. The prevalence of hepatobiliary complications of cystic fibrosis has increased in parallel to survival.

Cystic fibrosis is the most common of the potentially lethal genetic disorders, occurring in 1 in 2000 live births. It affects the mucous secretory exocrine glands and electrolyte secretion in the eccrine sweat and parotid glands. Liver disease is thought to result from excessive intrahepatic bile duct secretion of mucus.

The pathognomonic lesion of cystic fibrosis, identifiable in 25% of patients living longer than 1 year, is characterized by bile duct proliferation, bile ducts that contain eosinophilic plugs, an inflammatory infiltrate, and fibrosis. The lesion is present in some areas but absent in others. As patients live longer, the fibrosis extends to adjacent portal areas and secondary biliary cirrhosis develops.[130]

The relation between mucous plugging and the development of cirrhosis is not solid. In fact, with age, the prevalence of focal and diffuse cirrhosis increases, whereas the presence of mucous plugging decreases.[477]

The prevalence of multilobular cirrhosis is about 10% in patients over age 25.[499] Conventional liver function tests are notoriously inadequate for the diagnosis of cirrhosis in cystic fibrosis. Portal hypertension frequently accompanies cirrhosis and may, in some instances, be the initial manifestation.[468,477]

The diagnosis of cystic fibrosis should be suspected in young adults with cirrhosis of inapparent cause and can be confirmed by measuring elevated concentrations of sodium and chloride in sweat obtained by pilocarpine iontophoresis.

Galactosemia

The congenital absence of galactose-1-phosphate-uridyl transferase is a rare disorder responsible for galactosemia. It is transmitted as an autosomal recessive trait. Hepatomegaly and jaundice usually are seen in the first week of life. Progression of the disease may result in fibrosis or cirrhosis as early as 3 to 6 months of age, perhaps as a result of the accumulation of metabolites that are toxic to hepatocytes. The liver shows severe hepatic fatty infiltration. Although necrosis is not overt, regeneration is active, and a macronodular cirrhosis may develop. The presence of multinucleated syncytial cells and the development of ductular structures in the periportal areas probably represent nonspecific, infantile responses to liver injury, rather than specific responses or clues to the nature of the lesion. The cirrhosis may be associated with ascites and other evidence of portal hypertension.[520]

Death may occur in the first year if galactose intake is not significantly curtailed.[229] Galactosemia may also result from deficiency of galactokinase, but this form of the disorder does not lead to progressive liver disease.

Glycogen Storage Disease

Most enzymatic defects that cause hepatic glycogenesis are located in the sequence of enzymes that degrade glycogen to glucose-6-phosphate. As a result of these deficiencies, glycogen accumulates in various tissues, including the liver, kidneys, intestines, heart, and skeletal and cardiac muscle. These enzymatic differences result in similar clinical presentations, most of which include fasting-induced hypoglycemia.[196]

Hepatic failure and cirrhosis invariably develop in those patients with branching enzyme deficiency (Cori type IV), in which the cirrhosis leads to death in early childhood. A variant without apparent progressive liver disease has been described.[197] In debrancher enzyme deficiency (Cori type III), fibrosis may slowly progress to cirrhosis, but it is not inevitable. Other glycogenoses with predominant hepatic manifestations, but in which cirrhosis is not expected, are types I (von Gierke) and VI. Hepatic adenomas and hepatocellular carcinoma have complicated type I disease. Adenomas have also been reported with type III glycogen storage disease.[7]

The diagnosis of glycogen storage disease is confirmed by measuring enzyme activities in liver biopsy specimens. Therapy is usually dietary, but in several forms of glycogenosis, including types I, III, and VI, portacaval anastomosis has resulted in metabolic improvement. This change may be on account of delivery of nutrients to peripheral tissues and correction of hypoinsulinemia.[7,539] Liver transplantation has been successful in several patients; amylopectin deposition in the liver is reversed, as is, more surprisingly, neuromuscular and cardiac morbidity.[502]

Hereditary Tyrosinemia

Hereditary tyrosinemia (tyrosinemia I, tyrosinosis) is an autosomal recessive defect of fumaryl acetoacetate hydrolase and maleylacetoacetate hydrolase. Hereditary tyrosinemia occurs in acute and chronic forms. The acute form usually leads to death from hepatic failure by 1 year of age. The chronic form is associated with death in the first decade. Cirrhosis may be found in both forms but is more frequent in the chronic type.[187] There is rapid morphologic change from micronodular to macronodular cirrhosis.[118] The disorder is characterized by increased α-fetoprotein in serum and aminoaciduria. One third of patients with the chronic form have had associated hepatocellular carcinoma.[589] Therapy has included diets low in tyrosine, phenylalanine, and methionine and liver transplantation, which is advised before age 2 to precede the development of cancer.[118,337]

Hereditary Fructose Intolerance

Hereditary fructose intolerance is an autosomal recessive, inherited deficiency of fructose-1-phosphate aldolase. The syndrome does not become manifest until breast or cow's milk is supplanted by fructose-containing foods. Death may occur in infancy, but some patients survive until childhood or early adulthood. In the more chronic form of the disease, cirrhosis may occur, but lesser degrees of fibrosis are more common.[389]

Other Metabolic Cirrhoses of Infancy and Early Childhood

Cirrhosis has been reported in Niemann-Pick disease, Gaucher's disease, mucopolysaccharidosis, a variant of sphingomyelin lipidosis, cystinosis, Wolman's disease, cerebrohepatorenal (Zellweger) syndrome, and neonatal adrenoleukodystrophy.[7,207,606] Cirrhosis has also been reported in adult Niemann-Pick disease.[556]

Hereditary Hemorrhagic Telangiectasia

Cirrhosis, often of the coarse, nodular type, may be part of hereditary hemorrhagic telangiectasia.[122,343] In this disorder, the scar tissue appears to contain large numbers of thin-walled telangiectases.[614] The pathogenesis is obscure.

Hypervitaminosis A

Cirrhosis from hypervitaminosis A usually is the result of excessive ingestion of commercial vitamin A–containing preparations that are available without prescription in 25,000- and 50,000-unit doses. Vitamin A doses leading to hepatotoxicity range from 25,000 units to more than 1 million units per day, which is far in excess of the recommended vitamin A daily intake of 5000 units.[177a,189] Cirrhosis typically is preceded by clinical signs and symptoms of toxicity that include hepatomegaly, hair loss, dermatologic changes, pruritus, and, sometimes, symptoms of increased intracranial pressure, such as headache, nausea, and vomiting.[189,484]

Vitamin A accumulates in Ito cells (lipocytes). Because perisinusoidal fibrosis is most evident near areas of increased Ito cell concentration, it has been suggested that such accumulation stimulates fibrogenesis. Ito cells may be fibroblast precursors.[484] Ultrastructural changes in the sinusoidal barrier morphologically similar to peliosis hepatis are also seen.[613]

The diagnosis can be suggested by history and the finding of increased serum vitamin A levels. However, plasma concentration of vitamin A and retinol-binding protein can be misleading.[489] The principal histologic finding is fat-storing (Ito) cell hyperplasia and hypertrophy.[177a] Confirmation is by increased vitamin A–like fluorescence on fluorescent microscopy or demonstration of increased vitamin A levels in liver tissue.

Sarcoidosis

Occasional cases of cirrhosis are confirmed in patients with chronic sarcoidosis and often are manifested by portal hypertension.[333] However, portal hypertension may occur in hepatic sarcoidosis without cirrhosis.[560,571] Other diseases, such as primary biliary cirrhosis, may mimic sarcoidosis or may coexist with it.[141,254,511]

Copper

Copper-induced cirrhosis is an occasional occupational hazard of the wine industry.[424] Long-term inhalation of "Bordeaux mixture," a traditional fungicide spray made up of complex copper salts, may give rise to vineyard workers' liver. This disease is characterized histologically by hyperplasia and hypertrophy of Kupffer cells, proliferation of sinusoidal lining cells, fibrosis, and, occasionally, micronodular cirrhosis and angiosarcoma. These lesions are similar to those attributed to arsenic, Thorotrast (colloidal thorium dioxide), and vinyl chloride. In Bordelaisian vineyard workers, it is safe to say that alcohol may be a potential cotoxin. Drinking water contaminated by copper produces a clinical and histologic picture similar to that of Indian childhood cirrhosis.[373,593]

Small Bowel Bypass for Obesity

Primary jejunoileal and jejunocolic anastomoses have been introduced as therapy for massive intractable obesity. An unwelcome accompaniment of successful weight loss has been the appearance of liver disease that ranges from fatty infiltration to severe central sclerosis, which may resemble alcoholic hepatitis, and micronodular cirrhosis that sometimes results in death from hepatic failure.[129,365,418] Studies involving baseline biopsies and follow-up biopsies after 3 or more years suggest that as many as one third of patients have new or progressive fibrosis, sclerosis, or central inflammation on biopsy, including those with no symptomatic or biochemical evidence of liver dysfunction.[221] Ten percent of patients in this series developed cirrhosis, including one asymptomatic patient with normal liver function tests.[221] A similar incidence of cirrhosis has been reported in other series for the initial years after bypass.[222,283,344] When cirrhosis develops, suggestive changes are usually seen in the first year after bypass but may not evolve until late in the postoperative period.[222] There is not uniform agreement on whether advancing age and degree of weight loss predispose to cirrhosis.[202,222,283] The only histologic marker before surgery that indicates a propensity to the development of cirrhosis is pericentral fibrosis.[202,345,380]

Although the pathogenesis of this problem remains a mystery, a number of imaginative hypotheses have been suggested. Among these are simple malnutrition, deficiency of essential amino acids[525] or of vitamin E,[431] a dietary imbalance in the ratio of carbohydrate to protein,[525] the absorbance of toxic peptides resulting from the maldigestion of enormous volumes of ingested food,[525] and the hepatotoxicity of lithocholic acid.[68] The last abnormality has been hypothesized to result from the impaired enterohepatic circulation of bile acids by virtue of which unabsorbed chenodeoxycholic acid is converted to lithocholic acid, a hepatotoxic substance.[525] A role in pathogenesis has been suggested for the excluded intestinal limb. Bacterial overgrowth may result in the release of endotoxin or endogenous ethanol or in changes in immune competence.[394] These intriguing explanations are hypothetical but may eventually shed some light on the pathogenesis of cirrhosis.

A prospective study of 100 consecutive gastric bypass operations for morbid obesity confirms that fatty infiltration, inflammation and necrosis resembling alcoholic hepatitis, and fibrosis are frequently found in obese patients before operation. Six percent of these patients, however, had preoperative cirrhosis that was moderate or severe.[268] It is, therefore, possible that morbid obesity itself may be a precirrhotic lesion, but cirrhosis of other causes could occur in such patients. Certainly, other disorders in which there is histologic resemblance to alcoholic hepatitis may progress to cirrhosis.[124] Cirrhosis has not been reported in other such series, however.[564] Skepticism is, therefore, still in order in accepting obesity alone as a cause of cirrhosis.

Indian Childhood Cirrhosis

Indian childhood cirrhosis is found predominantly in India and Southeast Asia. Similar cases have been reported from the Western hemisphere, including the United States.[3a,302] This disorder occurs in children between 6 months and 4 years of age. It is characterized by severe hepatocellular degeneration with Mallory bodies. Deposits of copper may also be demonstrated. Liver cell damage is accompanied by a mixed inflammatory cell infiltrate and pronounced fibrosis, which isolates individual or small groups of hepatocytes. Micronodules may be seen, but regenerative nodules are not well developed. Clinically, the disease may range from a continuing hepatitis to symptoms of decompensated cirrhosis. The cause has not been established and may be multifactorial. Alternatively, toxicity from copper-containing cooking vessels may be a cause.[4] A disorder clinically and histologically similar has been described in Europe related to contamination from corroded copper water pipes.[373,593] The disease shows familial occurrence, but there is no clear evidence that it is inherited. The disease usually is fatal. Penicillamine is not useful in advanced disease, but survival is increased when it is begun before ascites or jaundice develops.[553,554] Liver transplantation should be considered in advanced cases.

Idiopathic or Cryptogenic Cirrhosis

When morphologic cirrhosis is found and its cause cannot be surmised from historical information, histologic findings, or laboratory data, either alone or in combination, the cirrhosis is said to be idiopathic or cryptogenic. Over the years, the number of cases so labeled has fallen as markers have been found for various types of viral hepatitis and immunologic disorders and as sophistication has increased in making the diagnosis of metabolic disorders.

In urban North America, about 75% of patients with cirrhosis are thought to have alcoholic cirrhosis. Cirrhosis follows viral hepatitis or other identifiable causes in another 15%, whereas 10% of cases are cryptogenic or idiopathic. In Great Britain, cryptogenic cirrhosis accounts for nearly one third of all cases.[548]

The natural tendency is for the physician to assume that the individual patient with cryptogenic cirrhosis has underestimated or remembered incorrectly his or her alcohol intake. Although this may be true in some instances, occasionally the cirrhosis is macronodular and shows none of the histologic earmarks of alcoholic cirrhosis. Whether these patients represent posthepatitic cirrhosis after inapparent hepatitis, an environmental type of cirrhosis, a national constitutional susceptibility to cirrhosis, some completely different cause, or erroneous diagnosis is not known. The recognition of alcohol-like liver disease, which may progress to cirrhosis, in nonalcoholic patients increases the etiologic possibilities.[124,434] Chances are high that the availability of anti-HCV and the ability to detect HBV markers in hepatocytes when the markers are absent from serum will further reduce the number of cases of cirrhosis with uncertain cause.[415]

On the other hand, the clinical and biochemical presentation of cryptogenic cirrhosis is, in at least one study, different from that in patients with cirrhosis of viral or alcoholic origin. Cryptogenic cirrhosis has a greater predominance of women than does alcoholic or viral cirrhosis, is diagnosed at a more advanced age, has less marked peripheral stigmata (jaundice, spiders, palmar erythema), and has less severe abnormalities of liver function.[546]

In the final analysis, the pathogenesis of cirrhosis of any type is unknown. In some forms of cirrhosis, such as postnecrotic or cardiac cirrhosis, the precirrhotic hepatic lesion and the subsequent pathologic pattern suggest an apparent pathogenetic mechanism. Whether or not this hypothesis is correct is another matter.

GENETIC PREDISPOSITION TO CIRRHOSIS

Although there is little proof of the presence of genetic susceptibility in the development of cirrhosis, a number of circumstantial factors repeatedly raise this question. The first is the well-established observation that not all abusers of alcohol develop cirrhosis. The great majority do not. On the other hand, we have encountered alcoholic cirrhosis in eight pairs of brothers at our hospital. This prevalence seems higher than would be anticipated randomly. In addition, increased genetic susceptibility appears to be a reasonable assumption in other situations. Occasional families are described in the literature in which several members have been found to have cirrhosis in the absence of viral infections, alcohol use, or metabolic defects.[11] Recently, a familial form of incomplete septal cirrhosis was described.[289] In another family, several members were found to have the HLA haplotypes A24, B18, DRW 4X7.[11,331]

In addition to the possible association with HLA antigens in familial cirrhosis, there is a strong association between idiopathic hemochromatosis and A3 and a lesser association with B7 and B14.[34] Chronic active hepatitis has been associated with B8, CW3, or DR3.

There are less well established associations with geographic differences between alcoholic cirrhosis and the HLA antigens A1, A9, A28, B8, B13, B15, and B40.[328,329,363,493] On the other hand, HLA-B13 and B40 have also been found to be negative predictors of cirrhosis.[127] An absence of A28 has been reported as well.[329] When Eddleston and Davis[135] combined the results of seven published series, they found the frequencies of AW32, B8, B13, B27, and B37 to be higher in patients with alcoholic cirrhosis than in controls. In continental Europe, patients with B35 have an increased incidence of alcoholic cirrhosis and a more rapid progression.[339] On the other hand, in Scotland and northeastern England, no HLA-A or B locus genetic susceptibility to alcohol injury has been found.[360] These data fail to give a cohesive account of the role of HLA antigens in cirrhosis. On the other hand, a recent study has identified a gene that may influence the development of alcoholism.[50] A subsequent study has failed to confirm a genetic association with alcoholism.[174] In addition, a gene controlling type I collagen has been found to be more frequent in alcoholic patients with cirrhosis than in patients without cirrhosis.[590] These studies require confirmation.

Second, it is said that some ethnic, national, or racial groups are either predisposed to, or resistant to, the development of cirrhosis. Native Americans and the Irish are said to develop cirrhosis especially frequently, but African Americans are thought to be relatively resistant, and alcoholic cirrhosis is said to occur only rarely in Jews. Again, good data are not available to support these statements. Even more bothersome is that such data may reflect alcohol consumption rather than predisposition to alcoholic cirrhosis.

Third, an association between alcoholic cirrhosis and color blindness has been suggested,[107] but some investigators have concluded that this association is an acquired rather than a genetically determined defect.[150]

Fourth, there are several correlations of physical findings

with cirrhosis that may suggest a genetic association. Loss of chest hair, for example, has long been considered an acquired sign in male patients with cirrhosis. Some investigators have shown that chest hair is not lost but rather has never been present in patients destined to develop cirrhosis.[555] Our own observations strongly support the latter concept.[193] This point needs controlled clarification in groups of patients with various types of cirrhosis.

The situation, then and now, was well summarized by Snapper[522]:

> When many decades ago we warned the "diener" of the Department of Pathology in Vienna about the dangers of his alcoholic libations—after all, he even drank the alcohol in which the specimens had been fixed—he opened his shirt, beat his hairy chest and assured us in Viennese vernacular that hairy individuals never develop cirrhosis. Such an absolute pronouncement should probably be taken with a few grains of salt; nevertheless, it should not be disregarded completely.

Fifth, Patek and colleagues[412,414] have shown that not all rats of the same strain develop diet-induced cirrhosis and that resistance to this disease is genetically transmissible. Finally, it has recently been observed that in patients with alcoholic cirrhosis who have an increased incidence of diabetes,[106,375] the presence of a positive history of diabetes in the immediate family is far more frequent than expected.[98] This preliminary observation requires confirmation.

In summary, these diverse clues suggest that a number of genetically determined, pathogenic factors may be operative. Certainly, precedents for familial, ethnic, racial, and national susceptibility to specific diseases are well established. Assuming that a genetic predisposition exists, it is not known whether genetically predisposed people are destined to develop cirrhosis de novo or whether they are merely more susceptible to any or all of the cirrhogenic stimuli discussed above. Even more to the point, it is not known whether any of these genetic factors is of clinical significance.

Clinical Presentation

According to Feinstein's mathematical classification,[145] a disease can present in one of three ways. If one defines the universe of cirrhosis to include all patients with cirrhosis, the largest fraction or set, perhaps 60%, consists of patients who seek treatment for symptoms or signs of cirrhosis (ie, *complainant* presentation) (Fig. 32-19). In a second set, which may account for 20%, the physician discovers cirrhosis coincidentally during evaluation of some other unrelated disease, that is, lanthanic or *noncomplainant* presentation. Lanthanic is derived from the Greek word meaning to escape attention. The patients in the third set are those in whom the diagnosis of cirrhosis is established at autopsy. These three sets are overlapping (ie, the three groups are not mutually exclusive). Some patients in whom cirrhosis is found at autopsy have had the diagnosis of cirrhosis established clinically after a complainant presentation (eg, bleeding varices) or after a lanthanic presentation (eg, hepatomegaly noted during routine physical examination), but some have not been recognized clinically. In our experience, clinically undetected cirrhosis is found at autopsy in about 30%. Others have found clinically unrecognized cirrhosis to occur in 40% of patients with cirrhosis.[204] Finally, there is a fourth set that

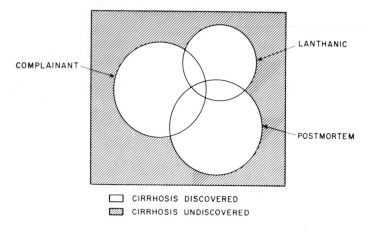

COMPLAINANT

LANTHANIC

POSTMORTEM

☐ CIRRHOSIS DISCOVERED
▨ CIRRHOSIS UNDISCOVERED

FIGURE 32-19   Modes of clinical presentation of cirrhosis. The Venn diagram shows three intersecting modes of presentation. The *complainant* set comprises patients who see physicians because of symptoms of cirrhosis. The *lanthanic* or noncomplainant set contains patients in whom cirrhosis is discovered accidentally during investigation of other, noncirrhotic disease. The *postmortem* set comprises patients whose cirrhosis was unrecognized during life and is first discovered at autopsy. A fourth group, the *unrecognized* set, is composed of patients in whom cirrhosis is never discovered.

does not overlap the other sets in whom cirrhosis remains undiscovered (ie, cirrhosis is never recognized, neither during life nor after death).

The magnitude of the fourth group is, by definition, unknown, since the factors that determine its size are unknown and speculative. Perhaps the less comprehensive medical care of the lowest socioeconomic class, which includes indigent, alcoholic individuals, the homeless, might permit a disproportionately large number of patients with silent cirrhosis to escape detection. On the other hand, one of the paradoxes of American medicine is that the lowest socioeconomic group, which often is treated in large, urban, academic hospitals, may receive better medical care than some socioeconomically higher groups.

Clinically overt, decompensated cirrhosis, in our experience, presents in three general ways. In patients in the first group, evidence of *hepatic parenchymal dysfunction* may predominate. This pattern typically is seen in relatively young patients—40 to 45 years of age—who drink excessive amounts of whiskey and, often, other alcoholic beverages as well. These patients enter the hospital acutely ill with acute alcoholic hepatitis. Most have deep jaundice, impaired coagulation, and hypoalbuminemia. If these patients survive, they tend to resume heavy drinking immediately and to return to the hospital repeatedly until they die. They appear deliberately intent on destroying themselves by their purposeful, unremitting drinking.

The second group presents with signs of *portal hypertension* (ie, vascular decompensation). In general, they are older patients, averaging about 55 to 60 years, who are more moderate drinkers. Many have drunk large quantities of wine for many years but are ethnic alcoholics rather than abusing alcoholics in the usual sense. They commonly present with ascites, esophageal varices, or portal-systemic encephalopathy and show little or no hepatic parenchymal damage.

The third group exhibits both *parenchymal damage* and *portal hypertension* and has the worst prognosis. Many are patients from the first group who have survived long enough to develop the more slowly maturing, vascular features of cirrhosis. At our institution, many patients with the vascular decompensation syndrome are of Italian ancestry. They immigrated to the New Haven area early in the 20th century and made and consumed large quantities of red wine for many years. These patients are now seldom seen. Most patients with hepatic parenchymal decompensation are of Middle European ancestry, come from the heavily industrial area

around Bridgeport, and give a history of excessive consumption of whiskey, vodka, and beer.

Although these patterns are general and not mutually exclusive, they do have important therapeutic implications. The first group, if they survive the initial admission, might well benefit from intensive psychological care, since the progress of their liver disease may be reversible if their drinking can be controlled. The second group may benefit from some of the advances made in the treatment of complications of portal hypertension—many are acceptable operative risks. Because the third group has the worst prognosis, therapy must be directed toward immediate survival rather than more long-range goals.

Clinical Features

Cirrhosis is characterized by a large number of specific findings. All may be present in some patients, and any or all may be absent in others. Most of these signs can best be discussed in a review of systems, each of which exhibits abnormalities that are specific for cirrhosis or involved in its differential diagnosis. Some are constitutional factors, which are considered next.

CONSTITUTIONAL FACTORS

General Deterioration

The most common feature of cirrhosis is deterioration of health. This failure to thrive syndrome is typified by anorexia, weight loss, weakness, and ease of fatigability. The anorexia may be masked in alcoholic cirrhosis by heavy drinking, and indeed, so may the weight loss. The metabolism of alcohol, after all, supplies 7 calories per gram. One pint of whiskey per day, therefore, provides about 1500 calories. An equivalent amount of alcohol consumed as beer furnishes even more calories. With a small amount of food, an alcoholic patient may thus maintain his or her weight for a long period. The accumulation of edema or ascitic fluid may counterbalance the loss of tissue weight and may mask weight loss, producing an absolute gain in weight. Muscle wasting may be evident peripherally despite the expansion in girth. When taking a nutritional history, it is essential for the physician to persevere and ask specifically about each meal of the past few days and the amount of each component of each meal. Similarly, one may not properly estimate the amount of alcohol consumed unless one establishes the patient's overall estimate by obtaining an hour-by-hour, glass-by-glass history and confirming it by learning the frequency and volume of alcohol purchases, the amount of money spent on alcoholic beverages, or, in the case of home wine-makers, the amount of grapes they purchase. In obtaining either a dietary or a drinking history, it is wise to speak with members of the family, bartenders, or acquaintances. Friends, however, may compound the felony. The least reliable historical data in clinical medicine are obtained in trying to determine the type and volume of alcoholic beverage consumed. Misdiagnoses of posthepatitic cirrhosis and metastatic cancer of the liver fill the records of physicians who take casual social histories. On the other hand, physicians tend to browbeat patients into exaggerating their alcohol intake and then apply a correction factor that raises the alcohol intake to the preconceived level. Nonalcoholic liver disease is not infrequently attributed to alcoholism on the basis of inaccurate histories.

Anorexia may be accompanied by abdominal unrest, nausea, vomiting, and diarrhea. Weakness and fatigue on mild exertion may be advanced despite the patient's failure to recognize them.

Jaundice

Jaundice is both a localized hepatic and a constitutional sign. It colors the skin and darkens the urine and often is the first evidence of ill health the patient or family recognizes. Jaundice ultimately results from the inability of the liver to metabolize bilirubin. The serum bilirubin normally is a reliable guide to the degree of hepatic damage. The liver's capacity to remove bilirubin may be overwhelmed by the increased bilirubin load in hemolysis. In both hepatitis and cirrhosis, hepatic parenchymal necrosis may occur in the absence of jaundice. The presence of jaundice does not necessarily correlate well with the histologic picture. In cirrhosis, hepatic parenchymal damage is a common cause of jaundice, hemolysis is common, biliary obstruction may develop in association with gallstones or pancreatitis, and other causes of jaundice may also occur. This differential diagnosis is maximally challenging.

Fever

Fever frequently is present in decompensated cirrhosis.[444,563] Whenever it occurs, one is faced with another difficult differential diagnosis. Is the fever due to an unrecognized, self-limited disease or an unrecognized bacterial infection that may be fatal if untreated, or is it a constitutional sign of decompensated cirrhosis? The fever of cirrhosis usually is low-grade and continuous, but it may reach levels of 102° to 103°F, often when alcoholic hepatitis is present. It may persist for weeks and thus qualify as a bona fide fever of unknown origin. Fever is common in alcoholic cirrhosis but much less so in nonalcoholic forms of cirrhosis. Chills seldom accompany the fever. The syndrome of necrotic fever in cirrhosis is characterized by deep jaundice, elevated serum transaminase and alkaline phosphatase levels, and leukocytosis. The serum glutamic-oxaloacetic transaminase levels are almost invariably higher than serum glutamic-pyruvic transaminase activity in alcohol-induced liver disease, reflecting a higher concentration of serum glutamic-oxaloacetic transaminase in the hepatocytes.[85] Liver biopsy, which is an important procedure in the work-up of fevers of unknown origin, is likely to show alcoholic hepatitis with active necro-

sis. The consequences of an erroneous diagnosis are too dire to risk, and an extensive search for an occult bacterial infection is mandatory. This requires examination and culture of all available body fluids; if nothing is found, a diagnostic trial of broad-spectrum antibiotics may be indicated.

It has been postulated that the fever is due to products of hepatic necrosis, to the bypassing of the liver by enteric bacterial pyrogens, and to the failure of the liver to inactivate pyrogenic steroids such as etiocholanolone. It does not respond to antibiotic therapy and may disappear only when the liver disease begins to improve.

On the other side of the coin, patients with cirrhosis may exhibit *hypothermia*, especially in the terminal stages but not infrequently with bacterial peritonitis, gram-negative bacteremia, portal-systemic encephalopathy (PSE), or the hepatorenal syndrome, all of which these patients are prone to develop.

SYSTEMIC FACTORS

No system of the body is spared in the syndrome of cirrhosis.

Alimentary System

Parotid Enlargement. Hypertrophy of the parotid gland is a frequent finding in cirrhosis,[53,534,608] occurring in about half of patients with alcoholic cirrhosis,[133] but it frequently is overlooked. It may appear early, before any signs of cirrhosis per se. The parotidomegaly is painless and reversible and may decrease rapidly in size as hepatic decompensation wanes. The gland is soft, nontender, and not fixed to the skin. It typically produces a trapezoid or lantern-jawed appearance to the face and distorts the position of the ears in which the lobes project at right angles to the face[60] (Fig. 32-20). Stenson's duct is patent. Sialographically, the duct system is normal or may show disappearance of the terminal branches, the so-called leafless tree appearance. In the older literature, the parotids tend to be hypersecretory, and the amylase activity of the saliva is about twice normal. The hypersecretory state is supported by the histologic picture, which shows hyperplasia of the parotid parenchyma, hypertrophy of the individual cells and acini, and increased xymogen granulation of the parenchymal cells.[535] A more recent study found both basal and stimulated parotid salivary flow rates to be lower in patients with cirrhosis than in controls.[133] Reductions in concentration in electrolytes, protein, and amylase were also found. The principal histologic findings were edema around the ducts and the acini as well as fatty infiltration with some fibrosis in the interstromal areas.

One cause of the parotid enlargement may, therefore, be edema and fatty infiltration. It typically occurs with malnutrition of various types, but in careful studies in repatriated prisoners of war, parotid enlargement was found to appear not during starvation but after refeeding. Malignant and other types of parotidomegaly should be excluded.

Varices. The gastrointestinal tract bears much of the brunt of cirrhosis, aside from abnormalities of the liver itself. Varices of the gastrointestinal tract develop as a consequence of the portal hypertension at the two ends of the intestinal tract—esophageal varices at the upper end and rectal varices at the other end.

Esophageal varices are, in terms of hospitalization and ultimate mortality, the single most life-threatening complica-

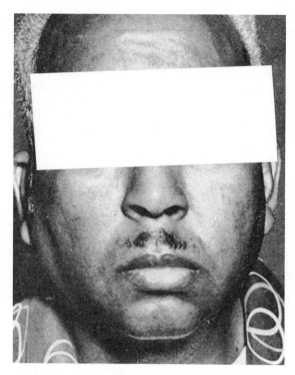

FIGURE 32-20   Bilateral parotid enlargement. (Brick IB. Parotid enlargement in cirrhosis of the liver. Ann Intern Med 49:438, 1958)

tion of cirrhosis. Admission for the management of hemorrhage from varices occupies an enormous amount of time and effort and complex techniques, as attested to by the massive bodies of literature that have accumulated regarding the diagnosis and treatment of variceal hemorrhage.[351] Despite the great amount of effort and research devoted to bleeding from varices, it continues to be the most lethal complication of cirrhosis.

Varices may be seen throughout the length of the esophagus and in the gastric fundus but bleed predominantly from the distal esophagus. In this location, they lie mainly in the lamina propria, whereas those of the stomach and the proximal esophagus lie predominantly in the submucosa. Their superficial location close to the lumen of the esophagus may, therefore, predispose them to rupture.[533]

Esophageal varices do not always imply cirrhosis. They may be seen in presinusoidal portal hypertension, such as schistosomiasis, splenic vein thrombosis, or portal arteriovenous fistulas.[116] Varices may also be seen in the absence of portal hypertension. "Downhill varices," which occur predominantly in the proximal esophagus, may result from obstruction of the superior vena cava, azygos vein, or inferior thyroid veins. Hemorrhage from these varices is rare, but it may occur.[153] Finally, there are rare reports of idiopathic varices in the absence of either portal hypertension or obstruction. Sometimes this finding is a congenital anomaly.[116,565]

Rectal varices, which develop as part of the inferior mesenteric venous collateral system and should be distinguished from hemorrhoids, may produce serious hemorrhage in patients with cirrhosis. The prevalence of rectal varices ranges from 19% in patients with cirrhosis but without portal hypertension to 59% in those who have bled from esophageal varices.[225] Hemorrhage from rectal varices, which is much less frequent and life-threatening than esophageal bleeding, may be persistent and require the perverse use of rectal tamponade using a balloon tube analogous to the Sengstaken-Blakemore tube of esophageal fame, sclerotherapy,[464] or, in refractory cases, portacaval shunt.

Sometimes a caput medusae, which results from a spontaneous portal-systemic shunt, can be seen in the periumbilical area on physical examination. Portal hypertension may lead to dilatation of the venous channels that connect the umbilical vein to the superficial epigastric veins of the anterior abdominal wall. When a hum or murmur can be heard around the umbilicus, the term Cruveilhier-Baumgarten syndrome is used.[70]

Varices of more intermediate portions of the gastrointestinal tract are less well known. Duodenal varices, which have recently been found more frequently as a result of widespread use of duodenoscopy and newer imaging techniques, will probably be shown to cause bleeding more frequently than has been recognized previously.[552] Other venous collateral vessels, including mesenteric and gallbladder varices, occasionally cause serious or even fatal bleeding in patients with cirrhosis. Such lesions can be demonstrated in vivo by angiography, laparoscopy, surgery, computed tomography (CT), and magnetic resonance imaging (MRI).

Gallstones.   The prevalence of gallstones is increased in cirrhosis of both alcoholic and nonalcoholic origin.[54,383] They occur in about 30% of patients with cirrhosis. In men, the prevalence is greater in advanced than in mild cirrhosis.[157] Cholelithiasis is not, however, a direct complication of cirrhosis. Rather, it appears to be the complication of a complication; hypersplenism causes hemolysis. The increased resulting bilirubin appears to exceed its solubility in bile. There may also be a reduction in a solubilizing component, since bile acid concentrations have been found to be decreased in the bile of patients with cirrhosis.[13,567] The resulting calcium bilirubinate stones often are amorphous and brittle.[567] This finding may explain the observation that they cause obstruction less frequently than cholesterol stones. There appears to be a lower incidence of acute cholecystitis and choledocholithiasis in patients with cirrhosis. Jaundice in cirrhosis more often reflects hepatocellular injury and seldom indicates biliary tract obstruction.[132]

Although recent investigations have suggested that cholesterol gallstones are the consequence of abnormal liver function (ie, the imbalance in bile of the normal components that maintain cholesterol in solution), cholesterol gallstones are not increased in cirrhosis. The relative absence of cholesterol gallstones in cirrhosis, despite decreased bile acid pool size,[582] presumably occurs because decreased cholesterol synthesis maintains the normal cholesterol–bile acid ratio. Conceivably, the normal solubility system of bilirubin in bile may be altered in patients with cirrhosis, predisposing them to the development of gallstones, but it seems more likely that increased red cell turnover is the critical problem.

Gallbladder Volume.   Gallbladder volume, determined echographically, is significantly greater in patients with cirrhosis (46 ± 33 mL) than in patients without cirrhosis with chronic liver disease (25 ± 14 mL) or normal control subjects (21 ± 10 mL).[151] The numbers of patients in the three groups are 90, 41, and 39, respectively. The explanation for this observation is not known. It is postulated that this phenomenon results either from decreased absorption of water and electrolytes from the gallbladders of cirrhotic patients or from diminished neural or hormonal control of gallbladder emptying. It represents another unidentified star in the constellation of cirrhosis.

Peptic Ulcer. The prevalence of peptic ulcer is increased in patients with cirrhosis.[267,528] Peptic ulcers occur in 4% to 7% of patients admitted to Department of Veterans Affairs hospitals and in 10% to 15% of patients with cirrhosis. In other studies, the prevalence of peptic ulcer is 5% to 20%, but an increased prevalence over control subjects is not always found.[65,154,178,190] Gastric acid secretion is not increased in patients with cirrhosis.[327] In laboratory animals, there is a sharp increase in gastric acid secretion after portacaval anastomosis.[211] In humans, a similar increment in gastric acid secretion has not been found.[598] More recent prospective studies of the association of portacaval shunts with peptic ulcer, using appropriate control groups, have shown that the prevalence of ulcers is no greater after shunt than in unshunted patients with equally advanced cirrhosis.[423] Although portal-systemic shunting, whether iatrogenic or spontaneous, appears important in the pathogenesis of peptic ulcer, the exact mechanism is not known.

Gastroesophageal Reflux. A controversial secondary manifestation in patients with cirrhosis who have ascites, gastroesophageal reflux, like the heartburn of pregnancy, may result from increased abdominal pressure. In pregnancy, the growing fetus is the problem; in cirrhosis, it appears to be ascites. Regurgitation of gastric contents into the esophagus seldom, if ever, is seen in patients with cirrhosis without hiatus hernia in the absence of ascites. In fact, gastroesophageal reflux, which may be present in patients with cirrhosis with tense ascites, has been reported to disappear after diuresis.[516] Manometric observations show that the lower esophageal sphincter is competent in cirrhosis and that gastroesophageal reflux is uncommon.[134]

Gastritis. Gastritis, another common concomitant of alcoholic cirrhosis, is most evident when it is the cause of upper gastrointestinal tract hemorrhage. The diagnosis of gastritis, however, usually is not made when the patient with cirrhosis has only vague epigastric distress or vomiting. Gastritis results from the effects of both portal hypertension and alcohol ingestion. Clinical evidence of increased hemorrhage from gastritis in portal hypertension is suggestive but not definitive.[295] A review of the frequency of bleeding from gastritis in patients with and without portal hypertension who were endoscoped for upper gastrointestinal tract bleeding based on five published series reveals that 38% of those with and without portal hypertension bleed from gastritis.[455] This comparison of percentages does not take into account the higher overall incidence of gastrointestinal tract bleeding in patients with portal hypertension.

The physiologic basis for bleeding from gastritis in portal hypertension may be the high prevalence of morphologic alterations in the microcirculation of the stomach in patients with cirrhosis, especially in those with esophageal varices. These alterations include arteriovenous anastomoses and dilatation of capillaries, precapillaries, and veins.[210] These

changes lead to low vascular resistance and high flow, which may play a permissive role in gastric bleeding.

Alcohol is an irritating, mildly corrosive substance. When taken as a concentrated solution, such as undiluted whiskey, and in the absence of protein or other adsorbent substances, it may at first induce self-protective emesis, later inflammation, and, eventually, erosions that may bleed. A role for alcohol has been supported by studies in laboratory animals that show alcohol potentiates mucosal abnormalities that occur in portal hypertension.[487]

Pitcher[426] suggested that in patients with cirrhosis who bleed in the hospital, varices are the most likely site, whereas in those who are admitted bleeding, erosive gastritis is the best bet.

Portal Hypertensive (Congestive) Gastropathy. A recently described entity, portal hypertensive gastropathy accounts for a number of cases of hemorrhage in patients with portal hypertension.[36,347] Although older literature did not recognize the difference, it is endoscopically and histologically distinguishable from gastritis.[110,347] It is present in 5% to 50% of patients who present with hematemesis.[36] Grossly, the endoscopist sees pink speckling, superficial reddening, or a mosaic pattern. Cherry-red spots are seen in severe gastropathy.[123] Biopsies demonstrate vascular ectasia and chronic inflammation. Ischemia and stress initiate bleeding in a congested and perhaps hypoxic gastric circulation.[488] Portal hypertension occurs more frequently in patients whose varices are treated with sclerotherapy.[110] Histomorphologic examination of tissue from endoscopic biopsies is not a reliable means of differentiating portal hypertensive gastric lesions from those unrelated to portal hypertension.[104,362]

Hemorrhage from portal hypertensive gastropathy was reduced by propranolol in a small study.[224] Similar anecdotal observations were made in studies of the prevention of hemorrhage from esophageal varices by propranolol[101,297] and by portacaval anastomosis.[481] Because both propranolol and portacaval shunts reduce the risk of hemorrhage in portal hypertension by reducing portal pressure,[199] it seems that reduction of portal pressure suppresses the risk of hemorrhage from both esophagogastric varices and congestive gastropathy.

Diarrhea. Along with vomiting, diarrhea is almost the sine qua non of the alcoholic cirrhotic syndrome. The cause is not known; a number of flimsy explanations have been offered. Pellagra, a niacin deficiency syndrome, has diarrhea as one of its prominent symptoms. It has been suggested that a forme fruste of pellagra, exhibiting only its intestinal component, may be responsible. It has also been suggested that alcohol itself or other substances in alcoholic beverages can cause diarrhea. Actually, alcohol infused chronically into the human jejunum and ileum in appropriate concentrations diminishes considerably the absorption of water and sodium by the small intestine.[353] The excess amount of saline solution in the intestinal lumen may induce a saline diuresis. Folate-deficient diets can also cause sodium and water malabsorption[205] and exaggerate the defect induced by alcohol. Because both chronic alcohol ingestion and folate deficiency, which occur together clinically, cause malabsorption of glucose, amino acids, and other substances in addition to sodium and water, a severe, chronic, unresponsive, self-perpetuating diarrhea may result.

Hypomagnesemia, which is common in both chronic alcoholism and malnutrition, has been associated with diarrhea that may be eliminated by correction of the magnesium deficit.[609] Whatever the explanation, these symptoms often complicate the management of cirrhosis.

Pancreatitis.   About one third of patients dying from alcoholic liver disease have histologic evidence of pancreatitis, predominantly chronic pancreatitis.[459] There is no increase of pancreatitis in patients with cirrhosis compared with those who have severe alcoholic hepatitis, suggesting that alcohol ingestion and not cirrhosis is the cause of the pancreatitis.

Colonic Disease.   In a series of more than 400 patients with cirrhosis undergoing colonoscopy, 8% had polyps, 20% had nonspecific edema, 10% had inflammatory changes, 25% hemorrhoids, and 4% rectal varices. Only 42% had normal findings. Unfortunately, there was no control group. When patients were stratified into parenchymal disease (viral and nonviral) and cholestatic liver disease, edema was more common in the parenchymal group and inflammatory changes were more common in the cholestatic group, reflecting the 25% prevalence of inflammatory bowel disease in the cholestatic group.[440]

Neurologic System

Portal-Systemic Encephalopathy.   PSE, the major neurologic manifestation of cirrhosis, is largely a consequence of portal-systemic shunting and, thus, may be considered a secondary complication. In patients with portacaval anastomosis, it represents a tertiary phenomenon. PSE, which is discussed in detail elsewhere, is not considered further here.

Asterixis.   The flapping tremor is the peripheral manifestation of a central nervous system metabolic abnormality. Although characteristic of PSE, it is not specific for PSE.[88] It is seen in the encephalopathy of various other metabolic disorders, including carbon dioxide narcosis, uremia, hypoglycemia, and barbiturate intoxication. The term *liver flap* is, consequently, a misnomer. Asterixis is usually accompanied by nonspecific slowing of the electroencephalogram, which also characterizes these other types of encephalopathy.

Asterixis, first described by Adams and Foley,[2] may be the consequence of metabolic suppression of the reticular activating system, which is extremely sensitive to various metabolic depressants. Suppression of the ascending reticular system is associated with depression of consciousness and arousal responses and is characterized by electroencephalographic slowing. Suppression of the descending reticular system, which is important in the maintenance of posture, muscle tone, and reflexes, may result in asterixis, rigidity, and abnormal pyramidal reflexes. Several observations provide insight into the nature of asterixis. Electromyographically, asterixis is associated with an electrical hiatus of both the active and the opposing musculature.[3,292,569] It is bilaterally asynchronous and is not temporally associated with any specific electroencephalographic abnormality. We have observed unilateral asterixis in one patient as part of the prodrome of a contralateral cerebrovascular thrombosis and in another patient long after a stroke on the hemiparetic side. Such observations indicate that asterixis is centrally determined and involves the pyramidal tracts. Intermittent asterixis was observed in a patient with Cheyne-Stokes respirations. The asterixis was most marked during hyperventilation and least evident during apnea. Assuming a latent period for the delivery of hypoxemic blood to the brain, asterixis appeared at about the same time as the nadir of intracellular oxygen content. Asterixis represents, therefore, a relatively acute and rapidly reversible phenomenon. Often associated with hyperammonemia, it can be elicited in patients with cirrhosis by the administration of ammonium salts. An electromyographically similar pattern can be produced in rabbits by the infusion of ammonium salts.

Neuropathy.   Peripheral neuropathies may be seen in alcoholic liver disease primarily related to the consumption of alcohol. Peripheral neuropathy is found in 45% of patients with alcoholic liver disease and in 22% of nonalcoholic patients with cirrhosis. In addition, autonomic neuropathy occurs in both alcoholic and nonalcoholic cirrhosis. About 45% of patients in both groups have evidence of parasympathetic damage and about 10% have sympathetic dysfunction. Two thirds of patients with peripheral neuropathy also have autonomic neuropathy.[562]

Evidence of peripheral neuropathy is also seen in nonalcoholic chronic liver disease.[275] It is not related to the severity of liver dysfunction but does appear to occur more frequently in those with previous hepatic encephalopathy and in those with other evidence of portal hypertension and portal systemic shunting, such as the presence of esophageal varices. The nerves show evidence of slowed impulse transmission and histologic abnormalities.[250,275]

Long-Tract Neurologic Signs.   These *exaggerated deep tendon reflexes*, the *Babinski sign*, and related eponymic signs occur unpredictably. Sometimes one may observe rigidity of the peripheral musculature and, rarely, the syndrome of hepatolenticular degeneration. In Wilson's disease, this neurologic syndrome is an inherited copper-associated metabolic defect, but a similar syndrome may be an acquired, noncuprogenic consequence of chronic PSE. *Portal-systemic myelopathy*, which in its severest form presents as transverse myelitis, may occur in patients with severe recurrent PSE. This demyelinating lesion, first described by Zieve and colleagues,[618] is shown in Figure 32-21. It is most frequently seen in patients with portal-systemic anastomoses.[105,293]

Some neurologic findings that typically are associated with alcoholic cirrhosis, such as *Wernicke's syndrome* and *peripheral neuritis*, are not consequences of cirrhosis but merely other diseases associated with excessive alcohol consumption, dietary inadequacies, or both.

Hematologic System

Impaired Coagulation.   Impaired coagulation is the major hematologic manifestation of cirrhosis. All the coagulation factors except factor VIII, which also originates in extrahepatic sites, are synthesized principally in the liver.[258,602] The decreased activity of any or all of these factors slows the coagulation process and, in conjunction with thrombocytopenia and various potential bleeding sites, poses a lethal threat to decompensated patients with cirrhosis. Plasma fibrinolysins, which are commonly increased in cirrhosis, may contribute to the bleeding tendency. Synthesis of inhibitors of coagulation are also reduced.[258] Dysfibrinoge-

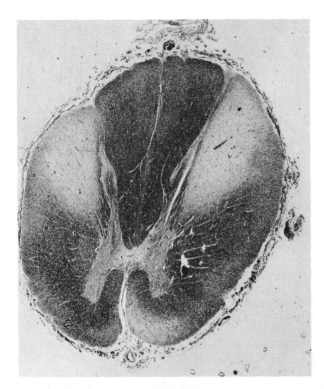

FIGURE 32-21 Pyramidal tract demyelination. Cross section of the dorsal region of the spinal cord of a cirrhotic patient with recurrent encephalopathy and spastic paraplegia. Demyelination of the pyramidal tracts is evident (luxol-fast H&E). (Courtesy of Dr. L. Zieve)

nemia from synthesis of abnormal proteins that contain an increase in sialic acid may be present in 50% to 75% of patients with chronic liver disease.[159]

Impaired coagulation is more likely to occur when hepatic parenchymal dysfunction, as in acute alcoholic hepatitis, coexists with cirrhosis. Patients who have severe histologic cirrhosis and significant manifestations of portal hypertension but who do not have parenchymal dysfunction may have normal coagulation. Even in patients with "acceptable" prothrombin times and platelet counts for the performance of invasive procedures, prolonged bleeding time (beyond 10 seconds) may be present.[48]

Disseminated Intravascular Coagulopathy. Disseminated intravascular coagulopathy may occur in decompensated cirrhosis but is not frequently an overt manifestation.[258] It is common in patients who have had peritoneovenous shunts.

Anemia, Thrombocytopenia, and Leukopenia. These hematologic disorders are among the most frequent and important of cirrhosis. *Microcytic hypochromic anemia* caused by gastrointestinal blood loss is the most common type of anemia. *Macrocytic anemia* may be seen as a consequence of folic acid deficiency and may be associated with leukopenia or thrombocytopenia. *Hemolytic anemia* occurs frequently. Sometimes active splenic hemolysis can be demonstrated, but increased erythrocyte synthesis compensates and no anemia may be detectable. Other indices of hemolysis,

such as reticulocytosis, hyperbilirubinemia, and increased serum levels of lactic dehydrogenase, may suggest that active hemolysis is occurring. The anemia typically is minimal in degree, but rarely, it may be severe enough to require blood transfusions. This form of anemia, which is almost always accompanied by splenomegaly, represents a form of hypersplenism. It is often associated with leukopenia or thrombocytopenia. Any of the formed elements may be suppressed individually or in combination. Splenectomy may promptly correct these cytopenias.

Rarely, severe hemolytic anemia may be precipitated by portacaval shunt, necessitating splenectomy in some instances. Low-grade hemolysis frequently follows portacaval shunts, but it is not clear in these instances whether the hemolysis is hypersplenic or whether it represents an intravascular consequence of portacaval vascular turbulence at the site of anastomosis, as may occur in patients with cardiac valvular prostheses or acquired valvular deformities, the so-called Waring blender syndrome.

It has been reported in a controlled investigation of hypersplenism in association with portacaval anastomosis that preexistent anemia, leukopenia, thrombocytopenia, or any combination of these features of hypersplenism disappeared as frequently in shunted patients as they did in randomly selected, unshunted patients with cirrhosis and portal hypertension.[374] Furthermore, it was found that new hypersplenism developed as frequently in the unoperated control patients as it did in those who had portacaval anastomosis. Improvements in hypersplenism often are amazingly rapid and transient. Within minutes of constructing a portacaval shunt, Schreiber and colleagues[497] reported increments in the formed elements that peaked within 2 days.

Not only may platelets be decreased in number because of splenic sequestration, but they may be reduced by platelet-associated immunoglobulin G in chronic active hepatitis and primary biliary cirrhosis[33,258] or by platelet antibodies in alcoholic cirrhosis.[31] In stable patients with cirrhosis, increased production often compensates for decreased survival related to these mechanisms.[541]

Platelets may be dysfunctional even when nearly normal in numbers. Patients with cirrhosis have a defective aggregation.[258] An intrinsic platelet abnormality related to a storage pool defect has been implicated.[287]

Zieve's Syndrome. This complex disorder is characterized by fatty infiltration of the liver, hyperlipemia, and hemolytic anemia.[617] Patients may present with abdominal pain and fever. The red blood cells may show features of an acquired pyruvate kinase deficiency.[355] Although liver damage is implicit in this disorder, cirrhosis is not necessarily present. Zieve's syndrome often is difficult to differentiate from alcohol-induced pancreatitis.

Several rare cases of *spur cell anemia* have been reported in alcoholic cirrhosis.[513] Spur cells or acanthocytes result from the accumulation of free cholesterol in red blood cell membranes and remodeling of abnormally shaped cells by the spleen. Spur-like projections are formed. This disorder is associated with hemolytic anemia and hypercholesterolemia. This phenomenon may be a variant of Zieve's syndrome.

Bone Marrow Abnormalities. Folic acid deficiency is associated with a megaloblastic marrow. In patients with blood-loss anemia, a hyperplastic, iron-depleted marrow is found. In chronic hepatocellular failure, a hyperplastic marrow is often characteristic, reflecting anemia and the need for increased erythrogenesis.

Some studies suggest that in patients with cirrhosis, humoral inhibitors of hematopoietic progenitors play a role in the development of anemia and granulocytopenia.[391]

As might be expected in patients with hyperglobulinemia, bone marrow plasmacytosis is often present. Occasionally, it is so pronounced that myelomatosis is suspected. Rarely, multiple myeloma occurs in patients with underlying cirrhosis.[137] Whether this phenomenon represents coincidence or plasmacytotic stimulus gone awry is not known. In generalized iron storage disease, excessive bone marrow hemosiderin usually accompanies the accumulation of iron in the rest of the body.

Hemosiderosis.   Hemosiderosis is another mysterious hematologic facet of cirrhosis. Modest deposition of hemosiderin occurs in the livers of 25% to 50% of patients with alcoholic cirrhosis.[89,620] Occasionally, however, massive amounts of iron are distributed throughout the body and are associated with the classic clinical signs of hemochromatosis. Indeed, a background of excessive alcohol intake so often coexists in hemosiderotic patients as to appear to be a cofactor in the pathogenesis of hemochromatosis. Accelerated hemosiderin deposition may occur after the construction of a portacaval shunt. More than 30 patients have been reported in whom disseminated iron deposition followed the construction of shunts. The full-blown syndrome of hemochromatosis has developed within 2 years after portacaval anastomosis in patients who were previously free of hepatic hemosiderin. This phenomenon has recently been shown to be significantly more common in patients with portacaval anastomosis than in randomly selected unshunted patients with cirrhosis of similar severity.[89] The pathogenesis of this association is unclear, although pancreatitis and hypersplenism, two causes of increased iron deposition, frequently are found in these hemosiderotic patients. Although portal-systemic shunting per se is related to the iron deposition, it cannot be the only factor.

Polycythemia.   Polycythemia is a paradoxical abnormality that sometimes is the clue to occult hepatocellular carcinoma.[245]

Pulmonary System

Pulmonary Oxygen Desaturation.   The pulmonary manifestations of cirrhosis may include dyspnea on review of systems, cyanosis and clubbing on physical examination, and oxygen desaturation demonstrated in the laboratory.

Dyspnea is not a frequent complaint in patients with cirrhosis except when severe ascites is present. Hyperventilation occurs frequently. Frank cyanosis is seldom seen, but clubbing of the fingers can be found in many patients with cirrhosis if carefully looked for. Cyanosis is always associated with clubbing, but the reverse is not necessarily the case[536]; even though oxygen desaturation always accompanies clubbing, there is no correlation with the degree of desaturation.

These findings of desaturation are attributed to reduced arterial oxygen concentration. Decreased arterial oxygen partial pressures have been observed in about half of decompensated patients with cirrhosis, and Po_2 levels in the range of 60 to 70 mmHg are not unusual.[354,470]

Multiple pathophysiologic processes may contribute to decreased oxygen saturation. These factors are discussed below.

RIGHT-TO-LEFT SHUNTS. Arteriovenous anastomoses have been observed within the lung (usually in the lower lobes) and on the pleural surfaces at autopsy. They resemble the spider angiomas seen on the skin.[46,485] Sometimes the existence of such shunts can be demonstrated ante mortem when intravenous, radiolabeled, macroaggregated albumin, normally trapped in the capillary network, is seen by scan to pass quickly through the lungs and be taken up by organs with high blood flow, such as the brain, kidneys, and spleen.[26,260] In addition to these microcirculatory shunts, there is evidence that some patients with cirrhosis have right-to-left shunts that involve larger vessels. Periesophageal veins in cirrhosis usually anastomose freely with mediastinal, pleuropericardial, and azygos veins. In some patients with cirrhosis, there is further anastomosis of the mediastinal venous plexus with bronchial veins and, occasionally, even pulmonary veins.[66,601] In some instances, these portopulmonary anastomoses have been large enough to permit emboli to pass from a thrombosed portal vein with resulting pulmonary embolization.[338] For significant right-to-left shunting to occur, these anatomic anastomoses must be accompanied by a pressure elevation in the portal vein branches that exceeds pulmonary venous pressure. Significant oxygen desaturation almost always occurs in the setting of esophageal varices.

On conventional chest films, intrapulmonary shunting may lead to the appearance of basilar infiltrates.[537]

In perhaps 5% of patients with cirrhosis, intrapulmonary shunting is associated with debilitating *orthodeoxia*, that is, arterial deoxygenation accentuated in the upright position and reversed in recumbency, and *platypnea*, dyspnea induced in the upright position and relieved by lying flat.[259,280,469] It is presumed that increased hypoxia in the upright position is explained by the fact that vascular shunts occur predominantly at the lung bases. Their use increases when the upright position is assumed, leading to redistribution of blood to these areas.[280]

ALTERED VENTILATION-PERFUSION RELATIONS. In patients with cardiopulmonary disease, the most frequent cause of systemic arterial hypoxemia is uneven alveolar ventilation in relation to alveolar blood flow.[87] Such mismatches of gas and blood would, therefore, not be surprising as a contributory factor to cirrhotic hypoxemia. Nonuniform ventilation may result from elevated diaphragms in patients with ascites or from cirrhotic pleural effusions, which occur in 5% to 10% of patients with cirrhosis. These same processes may also impede flow in smaller pulmonary vessels. Because altered ventilation-perfusion relations are also described in patients with cirrhosis without ascites,[470] other factors must participate in the imbalance. Premature airway closure has been described in cirrhosis with consequent gas trapping in lower lung zones and an associated low ventilation-perfusion ratio.[167,482] This may result from mechanical compression of small airways by bronchial blood vessels that have become engorged because of the azygos hypertension that accompanies portal hypertension.[482] An additional mechanism for gas and blood mismatching in cirrhosis is inappropriate pulmonary microvascular vasodilation, which has been supported by anatomic studies from patients with cirrhosis at autopsy.[111,376]

ALVEOLAR HYPOVENTILATION. General alveolar hypoventilation is a theoretic cause of arterial hypoxemia but is unlikely in most cases of cirrhosis because hyperventilation, accompanied by a mild respiratory alkalosis, commonly is seen.[212,213] It is postulated by some that hyperammonemia is the stimulus for hyperventilation, but there is a poor correlation between the ammonia content of arterial blood and the minute ventilation.[212,213]

REDUCED PULMONARY DIFFUSING CAPACITY. Reduction in pulmonary diffusing capacity may play a role in the desaturation seen in some patients. Most patients in whom diffusing capacity has been measured have had normal values,[446] but appreciable abnormalities have been found in up to 20% of patients with cirrhosis.[186,280] Diffusion defects should not be taken to imply interstitial disease. There may be instead an alveolar–capillary oxygen disequilibrium, to use the term preferred by proponents. This is anatomically associated with ten-fold increases in the diameter of thin-walled vessels in the lower lobes. It is postulated that layering of erythrocytes occurs so that only erythrocytes immediately adjacent to the capillary membrane equilibrate with alveolar gas. The problem is exacerbated when there is rapid transit, as occurs in the high cardiac output state that accompanies some forms of cirrhosis.[115,607]

SHIFTS IN OXYHEMOGLOBIN DISSOCIATION CURVE. Increased 2,3-diphosphoglycerate is reported in erythrocytes in patients with cirrhosis.[18] It increases with severity of liver disease and may be higher than in hypoxic chronic obstructive pulmonary disease.[378] These changes have been used to explain the decreased oxygen affinity of hemoglobin in patients with cirrhosis. This decreased oxygen affinity results from a shift of the oxyhemoglobin dissociation curve to the right, which may contribute to the hypoxemia in cirrhosis.[67,264,621]

HEPATOPULMONARY SYNDROME. Increasing experience with liver transplantation has led to the introduction of the term *hepatopulmonary syndrome* to describe severe, potentially reversible hypoxemia that accompanies liver disease. Pulmonologists implicate intrapulmonary vascular dilatation in particular. This phenomenon may result from circulating vasodilators or from lack of inhibition of certain vasoconstrictors.[281,282] Ventilation-perfusion relations may normalize after liver transplantation.[139]

Autoimmune Changes in the Lung. In primary biliary cirrhosis, patients may have obstructive lung disease secondary to an autoimmune process as well as interstitial lung disease, pulmonary nodules, and multiple granulomas.[584] Impairment of pulmonary function is seen predominantly in patients whose primary biliary cirrhosis is symptomatic.[570]

Primary Pulmonary Hypertension. Pulmonary hypertension without demonstrable pulmonary or cardiac disease is not a common manifestation of cirrhosis. An unselected series of 17,901 autopsies revealed a prevalence of primary pulmonary hypertension of 0.13% and 0.73% ($P < .001$) in patients with cirrhosis.[349] A prospective study has been reported from one institution in 507 patients with portal hypertension but without known pulmonary hypertension. When cardiac catheterization was performed, 2% had primary pulmonary hypertension.[200] More than half were clinically asymptomatic; the remainder had exertional dyspnea that had not aroused clinical suspicion. These numbers suggest that although infrequent, primary pulmonary hypertension occurs at least 6 times and perhaps as much as 20 times more frequently in cirrhosis than in the general population.

In most cases in which primary portal hypertension is diagnosed clinically in patients with cirrhosis, esophageal varices are present. Some reports emphasize the development of pulmonary hypertension after surgical portacaval shunts.[45,294,349]

Portal hypertension may be long-standing before pulmonary hypertension develops, but it may also be diagnosed concurrently with cirrhosis. It is thought that subclinical portal hypertension precedes the onset of symptomatic pulmonary hypertension by months or years. Quantitative histologic studies suggest that severe hepatic injury often is associated with subclinical pulmonary hypertension that might become clinically manifest with long-term patient survival.[346]

The symptom most frequently associated with pulmonary hypertension is exertional dyspnea, but syncope, precordial pain, and hemoptysis have been reported.[294]

Accentuation of the pulmonic second sound, a murmur in the second or third intercostal space or along the left lower sternal border, cardiac enlargement, prominent main pulmonary arteries, and right ventricular hypertrophy are common.[294]

The cause of pulmonary hypertension that accompanies cirrhosis is not yet established. Pathogenetic theories include the passing of emboli[503] or of humoral vasoconstrictors from the portal to the pulmonary circulation,[294,346] autoimmune mechanisms,[366] and effects of long-standing elevations in cardiac output and blood volume.[294]

Hepatic Hydrothorax. Fluid that accumulates in the pleural cavity in patients with cirrhosis is referred to as hepatic hydrothorax or cirrhotic pleural effusion. Although only 3% to 4% of all pleural effusions can be attributed to cirrhosis, the prevalence of hydrothorax in patients with cirrhosis may approach 10% in patients with ascites.[238] Most are located on the right, but they may occur on both sides or, occasionally, only on the left. Transudation from increased thoracic duct lymphatic flow was once invoked as its cause. Current evidence suggests direct passage of ascitic fluid from the abdomen through defects in the diaphragm into the pleural space.[308] Negative intrathoracic pressure also contributes to the peritoneal–pleural transfer of fluid. Ruptured blebs of pleuroperitoneum have been identified at autopsy.[322] These blebs apparently may also rupture from coughing or straining. Hepatic hydrothorax has been identified in patients without detectable ascites.[480,517] In such cases, it is assumed that the negative intrathoracic pressure favors the transport of the ascitic fluid into the pleural space at a rate equivalent to its production in the abdomen.

Hepatic hydrothorax cannot always be distinguished from pleural effusions of other cause. It is not unusual for total protein, albumin, cholesterol, and total lipids to be higher in pleural than in peritoneal fluid, perhaps because water can be more rapidly absorbed by pleural vessels.[324] Because the dissimilarity of characteristics of ascitic and pleural fluids may raise questions about the cause of the pleural effusions, the presence of a communication between the two cavities should be sought by the intraperitoneal injection of tracer amounts of technetium-99m (^{99m}Tc) sulfur colloid.

Although hepatic hydrothorax usually is an incidental finding, on some occasions, it may cause respiratory embarrassment. The primary treatment of hepatic hydrothorax is the elimination of the ascites. If the pleural effusion causes respiratory distress, thoracentesis may be necessary. An accompanying paracentesis to reduce intraabdominal pressure may decrease the pressure differential on the two sides of the diaphragm, which occurs when thoracentesis is performed alone. As the ascites is controlled, the diaphragmatic defect may heal. When repeated episodes of respiratory embarrassment occur as the result of recurrent pleural effusions, obliteration of the pleural space by instillation of nitrogen mustard, talc, or other sclerotic agents into the chest cavity may be necessary. When hydrothorax accompanied by ascites persists, a peritoneovenous shunt may be required.[220,308]

Cardiac System

Pericardial Effusion. Fluid retention leading to peripheral edema, ascites, and pleural effusion is a well-known consequence of decompensated cirrhosis. Pericardial effusion has recently been reported in a small study of patients with ascites. By echocardiographic methods, 60% of patients with ascites had pericardial effusion, which usually resolved as the ascites disappeared.[504]

Hemodynamic Changes. Between 30% and 60% of all patients with cirrhosis develop a circulatory hyperdynamic state characterized by an increase in cardiac output and a reduction in peripheral resistance. These changes are present at rest and increase with exercise. The clinical correlates of this hyperkinetic state are bounding pulses, warm hands, and capillary pulsations.

Numerous factors contribute to these circulatory changes. The increase in cardiac output can be accentuated by concurrent anemia, expansion of blood volume, and an extensive collateral circulation. Increased blood flow to the extremities and the splanchnic organs through low-resistance arterial beds also plays a role. On the other hand, ascites, which increases intraabdominal pressure and decreases venous return, may decrease cardiac output, as may diuretic therapy, recent hemorrhage, and underlying myocardial disease.[58]

The reasons for decreased peripheral resistance are not well explained. Both increased excretion and impaired hepatic inactivation of vasodilatory factors, such as glucagon or prostaglandins, have been suggested.[39,63] When arteriolar vasodilatation is present, aortic impedance is lessened and stroke output can increase without a change in myocardial contractility or ventricular preload.[446]

Despite increased cardiac output in many patients with cirrhosis, systemic blood pressure often is slightly decreased because of the accompanying low systemic resistance.[58] Hypertension is not commonly seen in patients with alcoholic cirrhosis, even though in patients without cirrhosis, alcohol has a documented pressor effect,[433] and the incidence of hypertension is increased in alcoholic patients.[272]

In alcoholic cirrhosis, alcohol may have hemodynamic consequences. Alcohol is known to be cardiotoxic. It might be expected that alcoholic cirrhosis would be accompanied by cardiomyopathy. It usually is claimed, however, that such patients tend to develop either liver disease or cardiomyopathy but not both.[458] One recent review found no evidence of either cirrhosis or alcoholic hepatitis in its series of patients with alcoholic cardiomyopathy.[301] Careful investigation reveals that even though overt cardiomyopathy is infrequent in alcoholic cirrhosis, some patients have altered left ventricular

function and are at risk of clinical decompensation in the presence of volume or pressure overload.[5]

Digoxin-Like Substances. Digoxin is detectable by radioimmunoassay in 50% to 60% of patients with cirrhosis not taking the drug because of the presence of digoxin-like substances in serum. Patients with cirrhosis who are placed on digoxin have higher digoxin levels measured than do controls who receive equivalent doses.[384]

Lymphatic System

Dumont and Mulholland[131] and the Wittes[604] showed abnormalities of the lymphatic system in cirrhosis and suggested its importance. It has long been known that in patients with portal hypertension, hepatic hilar lymphatics are distended and, when transected, discharge large volumes of lymph. These investigators have shown that in patients with cirrhosis with portal hypertension, especially those with ascites, the thoracic duct is greatly enlarged and lymph flow through the thoracic duct is enormously increased, often 10 to 15 times greater than normal. They postulated that in portal hypertension, lymph flow may decompress the hepatic and splanchnic beds. When this lymphatic flow into the peritoneal cavity surpasses the maximal capacity of the peritoneum to absorb it, ascites results. Elevated protein concentration is seen in patients with hepatic venous outflow obstruction, low protein levels occur in extrahepatic portal venous obstruction, and intermediate levels are found when both types of venous hypertension coexist.[603]

It has been suggested that the size of the communication between the thoracic duct and the subclavian vein is critical in determining the occurrence and severity of ascites. Thoracic duct drainage either externally or by anastomosis into a systemic or pulmonary vein may promptly decrease ascitic volume and portal pressure.

Indeed, peritoneovenous shunts, which have proved effective in the management of intractable ascites, may be viewed as accessory, man-made thoracic ducts.

Dermatologic System

Jaundice. Many stigmata of cirrhosis are visible in the skin. Most obvious is the bilirubin staining of elastic tissue, which gives the skin its yellow color in jaundice. Depending on the type of pigment, the color may characteristically reflect the type of jaundice, as typified by the greenish biliverdin discoloration of long-standing obstructive jaundice. Because bilirubin pigments are transported bound to albumin, localized areas of edema may be differentially more jaundiced or less jaundiced than nonedematous areas. In patients with unilateral edema caused by heart failure, which characteristically induces a low-protein edema fluid, contralateral jaundice may be observed.[402] When the edema fluid is relatively high in albumin, as in extravasated ascites, jaundice may be localized to the area of edema.[91] Similarly, hives, which are local inflammatory exudates high in protein concentration, often appear to be more jaundiced than the surrounding skin.

Spider Angiomas. Spider angiomas probably represent cutaneous manifestations of endocrine imbalances in cirrhosis. Virtually all that is known about arterial spider nevi (spider nevi) is discussed in Bean's[37] classic monograph. Histologically, spider angiomas resemble the short, corkscrew, endometrial arteries that develop and slough rapidly during the menstrual cycle. Similar spiders have been recognized on the pleural and pulmonary surfaces.[46] Other forms of telangiectasia, such as the "paper-money" facial skin have been described but are not specific for cirrhosis. It is reported that the incidence of spider angiomas and varices are similar in cirrhosis. The frequency of variceal bleeding is 50%, according to one study, when there are greater than 20 spider angiomas present. Spider angiomas greater than 15 mm in diameter are associated with an 80% frequency of bleeding.[158]

Palmar Erythema. Palmar erythema (liver palms), which characteristically involves the thenar and hypothenar eminences, the distal pads of the fingers, and often the circumungual areas on the dorsum of the fingers, usually sparing the central portion of the palm, represents an extensive collection of arteriovenous anastomoses.[514] These findings are not specific for cirrhosis because they appear in rheumatoid arthritis (rheumatoid palms) and pregnancy (palms of pregnancy). They occur with greater frequency in alcoholic cirrhosis than in cirrhosis of other causes.

Nail Changes. Nail changes of various sorts have been described in cirrhosis. Best known are Muehrcke's[372] lines. The transverse pale bands, also seen in nephrotic syndrome, were initially said to be associated with hypoalbuminemia, but whether they represent a period of increased disease activity or other factors is open to speculation. Terry[561] described white nails in cirrhosis. Red lunulae, resulting from increased arteriolar blood flow, are described in cirrhosis but are also seen in many other systemic disorders. Their presence is of no particular clinical value.[599]

Dupuytren's Contracture. Contractions of palmar fascia, which may be unilateral or bilateral, occur more commonly in patients with alcoholic cirrhosis and with chronic alcohol abuse (Fig. 32-22) than in nonalcoholic patients. The cause of this contracture of the palmar fascia is not known. The contractures correlate with the amount of alcohol consumed and not with the severity of the liver disease. Increasing age and previous hand injuries also correlate with the prevalence of Dupuytren's contractures.[19]

Chest Hair. Chest hair is commonly absent or markedly decreased in cirrhosis. Its absence is not, as is so often stated, a loss of preexisting chest hair. When asked, "When did you lose the hair from your chest?" patients with cirrhosis almost invariably answer, "I never had any!" We have been able to document this statement in many men with cirrhosis by comparing photographs taken many years earlier, before development of the cirrhosis. Seldom have we encountered a patient who has lost his pectoral hair during or after the development of cirrhosis. The chest hair pattern, like gynecomastia, is of limited diagnostic value in women. Blacks, native Americans, and Asians normally have scant chest hair, and its absence in cirrhosis is neither surprising nor meaningful. Other areas of hair distribution in the male do change, however. The pubic hair pattern typically becomes inverted and resembles the feminine pattern, the so-called female escutcheon. Axillary hair may become scant in both men and women.

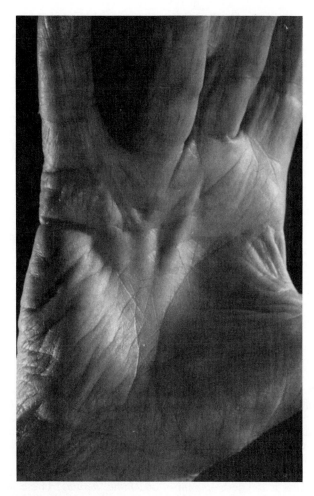

FIGURE 32-22 Dupuytren's contracture. Flexor tendons of third, fourth, and fifth digits are hypertrophied and incorporated into the thickened palmar fascia.

Vascular System

Vascular phenomena cause many of the major consequences of cirrhosis. Esophageal varices are the most dangerous of the portal-systemic collaterals by virtue of their tendency to rupture, but this venous collateral system also gives rise to some of the major metabolic derangements of cirrhosis. The pathogenesis and treatment of these manifestations are discussed elsewhere.

Portal-Systemic Encephalopathy. PSE is largely a consequence of the passage of enteric, toxic substances from the gastrointestinal tract directly into the systemic circulation instead of first passing through the liver, where these substances normally are removed. Shunting of enteric bacteria through portal-systemic collaterals instead of removal of the organisms by the hepatic reticuloendothelial system results in bacteremia. Physiologic substances that arise in the splanchnic bed, such as insulin and glucagon, may also bypass the liver with major metabolic consequences. It has been suggested that the post-portacaval shunt–hepatic failure syndrome is due to the shunting away from the liver of some hepatotrophic substances, such as insulin and glucagon.[538]

Arteriovenous communications are responsible for several abnormalities in cirrhosis. Palmar erythema, as described above,[514] represents a collection of local arteriovenous fistulas. Large numbers of such communications may exist in the lung and contribute to the severe right-to-left shunting commonly seen in cirrhosis. The functional abnormalities seen in the renal lesion of cirrhosis, the so-called hepatorenal syndrome, appear to be related to shunting of arterial blood from the cortex of the kidney to the vessels of the medulla. Arteriovenous fistulas typically occur with great profusion in the gastrointestinal tract. The purpose of these communications and the mechanism of their control are not clear.

Musculoskeletal System

Muscle Abnormalities.   Even the motor system may be involved. *Alcoholic myositis*, a complication of excessive alcohol intake rather than of cirrhosis per se, is characterized by pain and tenderness of the skeletal muscles accompanied by hyperkalemia, myoglobinuria, and elevated serum levels of glutamic oxaloacetic transaminase, creatine phosphokinase, and lactic dehydrogenase.[416] As cirrhosis advances, there is progressive reduction in lean body mass because of a high rate of muscle catabolism, which has been attributed to hyperglucagonemia.[340]

An interesting musculoskeletal manifestation of cirrhosis is seen secondary to massive ascites. In ascites, as in pregnancy, the accumulation of intraabdominal weight must be counterbalanced by increased lordosis of the spine. This posture, which in pregnant women is called the pride of pregnancy, can be called, for poetic purposes, the lordosis of cirrhosis (Fig. 32-23).

Another type of secondary musculoskeletal abnormality of ascites is the development of *abdominal hernias*. These include inguinal, ventral, umbilical, and hiatal, all of which are much more common in patients with ascites than in those without. In addition, *diastasis recti* is virtually universal in patients with ascites.

The *umbilical hernias* are potentially the most dangerous. A knuckle of bowel can become incarcerated and require surgical correction. In patients with ascites, surgical morbidity and mortality are increased and there is a high incidence of hernia recurrence. Retrospective studies suggest that these risks may be significantly reduced when herniorrhaphy is preceded by placement of a peritoneovenous shunt.[307] In some series, repair of umbilical hernias in patients with cirrhosis frequently has been followed by hemorrhage from esophageal varices presumably caused by the elevation in variceal pressure resulting from the ligation of abdominal wall portal-systemic collateral vessels.[29] Not all studies have confirmed this claim.[417]

In patients with tense ascites, the umbilical hernias may rupture, giving rise to the so-called Flood syndrome, which is eponymic rather than descriptive.[155] In most cases, the spontaneous perforation is heralded by ulceration of the skin overlying the hernia. Once perforation is established, operative management usually is indicated.[304] In addition to repair of the fascial defect, placement of a peritoneovenous shunt may be prudent to prevent reaccumulation of ascites during the immediate postoperative period.[388]

Hiatal hernias, which permit gastroesophageal reflux and may induce esophagitis, may predispose to or precipitate hemorrhage from esophageal varices.

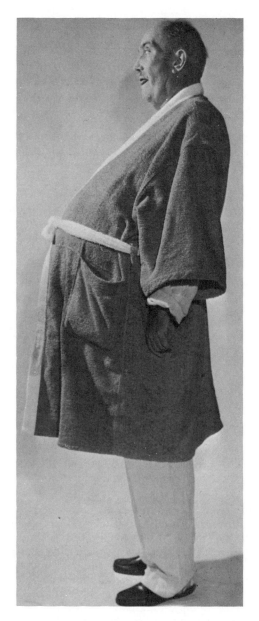

FIGURE 32-23   Lordosis of cirrhosis.

Skeletal Abnormalities

HYPERTROPHIC OSTEOARTHROPATHY.   The classic triad of periostitis, clubbing, and synovitis, a common complication of bronchogenic carcinoma, is an occasional complication of cirrhosis. This bizarre finding, more common in biliary than in alcoholic cirrhosis, is characterized by pain and tenderness along the distal long bones of the forearms and legs. Virtually all these patients exhibit clubbing of the fingers, and some of them show gynecomastia. Radiographically, there is a thin, opaque line of new bone, which is separated from the underlying, denser cortex by a narrow radiolucent band along the distal end of the diaphysis of the long bones.[138] Serum calcium and phosphorus levels are normal. Alkaline phosphatase activity is almost invariably elevated, but it is not known whether the elevation is related to the underlying liver disease or to increased osteoblastic activity.

Relative bone and liver isoenzyme levels have not been reported. It has been suggested that stimuli to periosteal growth may escape pulmonary inactivation by way of right-to-left systemic shunts. Similarly, portal-systemic shunts have been proposed to explain the failure of the liver to inactivate such substances. No such substances have been identified, however. Hypertrophic osteoarthropathy does not seem directly related to the presence or degree of hypoxemia, right-to-left shunting, or portal-systemic shunting, since only rarely do patients with these disorders develop this syndrome. It is not associated with increased growth hormone concentrations or estrogen excretion. What causes it and why it is seen much more commonly in primary biliary cirrhosis than in other types of cirrhosis are questions to be answered. The condition has been reversed by liver transplantation.

HEPATIC OSTEODYSTROPHY. Hepatic osteodystrophy has been described in cirrhosis. The results of a study of 52 patients with alcoholic cirrhosis show that osteoporosis, but not osteomalacia, characterizes these patients.[242] The mechanism is not known, but both impaired osteoblastic activity and enhanced bone resorption are likely to be present.[381a] Bone changes in primary biliary cirrhosis are discussed in Chapter 16.

Endocrine System

Many endocrine abnormalities occur, most of them presumably as consequences of the failure of the liver to conjugate or otherwise metabolize hormones. These problems may arise from hepatic parenchymal cell injury, portal-systemic shunting, or both. Sometimes, in alcoholic cirrhosis, it is difficult to differentiate the changes induced by chronic alcoholism from those caused by the liver disease itself. Most of these abnormalities are subtle changes, such as secondary hypersomatotropism and hyperinsulinemia without overt physical signs. Others are evident functionally, for example, as hyponatremia in inappropriately increased antidiuretic hormone and as hyperglycemia in diabetes. Some, such as gynecomastia, may be visible or palpable signs; others, such as testicular or prostatic atrophy, may be invisible, impalpable phenomena.

The sexual signs of cirrhosis in men are manifested by feminization and hypogonadism. The increase in femaleness and the decrease in maleness are separate syndromes.

Feminization. Feminization, which can occur in the absence of hypogonadism, is the acquisition of estrogen-induced characteristics. It occurs in both alcoholic and nonalcoholic cirrhosis but is more common in the former. Feminization is manifested by spider angiomas, palmar erythema, changes in body hair patterns, and, perhaps, gynecomastia. An iconoclastic recent study has suggested that palpable gynecomastia is not really increased in cirrhosis.[72] The study suggests that patients with alcohol-related cirrhosis and nonhepatic disorders exhibit gynecomastia in almost equal percentages. The authors suggest that the belief that palpable gynecomastia is more frequent in subjects with cirrhosis is rooted in more vigorous searches in patients with cirrhosis. We have always subscribed to the conventional wisdom and believe that our clinical experience supports it, but without hard data, we must be silent and hope that someone will pick up the gauntlet and challenge this small study.

Estradiol levels in men with cirrhosis are either normal or only slightly increased. Plasma estrone levels are moderately increased.[577] Rather than resulting from significant increases in plasma estrogens, feminization is thought to result from the increased conversion of weakly androgenic steroids to estrogens in peripheral tissues (skin, adipose tissue, muscle, bone), where they have a local effect. Chronic alcoholism may result in adrenal overproduction of such androgens. In nonalcoholic cirrhosis, feminization occurs only when cirrhosis is sufficiently advanced to result in portal-systemic shunting.[577] Such shunting allows steroidal estrogen precursors to escape the enterohepatic circulation and undergo peripheral conversion. This peripheral estrogen effect is possible without altering systemic plasma estrogen levels.[573]

Sometimes gynecomastia in cirrhosis (Fig. 32-24) has causes other than those outlined above. It may not appear during hepatic decompensation but as the patient improves, a phenomenon similar to refeeding gynecomastia, which was observed in starved prisoners after they were liberated from World War II prison camps. Widespread clinical use of spironolactone, an aglycone, may, like digitalis, induce gynecomastia.[27]

Hypogonadism. Hypogonadism in alcoholic cirrhosis is now thought to be a direct effect of alcohol and is not a manifestation of liver disease itself.[576] In nonalcoholic liver disease, it is seen with increased frequency only in hemochromatosis. Because increased iron is sometimes seen in the hypothalamus, pituitary, and testes in patients with homochomatosis, it appears to be tissue injury rather than underlying liver disease that leads to hypogonadism. Hypogonadism is manifested by testicular atrophy (Fig. 32-25), high prevalence of infertility, changes in secondary sexual characteristics, loss of libido, and impotence. Even though testicular atrophy on physical examination occurs less frequently than textbooks imply, the testes, even when not discernibly atrophic, may have a reduced number of germ cells, be oligospermic, or have many bizarre or inactive germ cells.[573] In 50% of men who are alcohol abusers, plasma testosterone levels are decreased.[574] Sex hormone–binding globulin levels are increased.[577] In addition to these indicators of gonadal

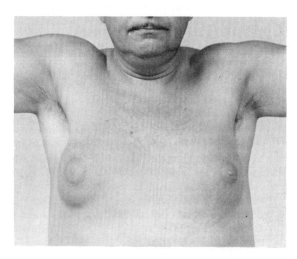

FIGURE 32-24 Gynecomastia. The patient, who had alcoholic cirrhosis and persistent ascites, had required prolonged spironolactone therapy. Gynecomastia persisted for a year after the diuretic had been stopped.

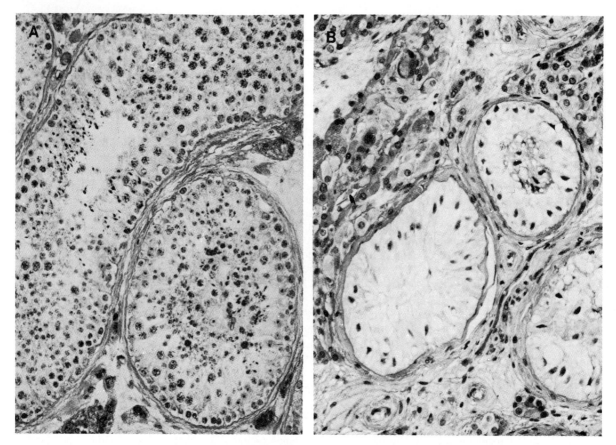

FIGURE 32-25 Testicular atrophy. (**A**) Testicular histologic specimen of normal man demonstrating active spermatogenesis in normal-size seminiferous tubules with delicate basement membranes and minimal peritubular fibrosis. Leydig cells are scarce, being widely separated by seminiferous tubules (× 250). (**B**) Testicular histologic specimen of a patient with alcoholic cirrhosis demonstrates germ cell aplasia, marked seminiferous tubular atrophy with prominent peritubular fibrosis, and condensation of Leydig cells around the seminiferous tubules (× 250). (Courtesy of Dr. D.H. Van Thiel)

failure, there is evidence of hypothalamic and pituitary dysfunction. Although plasma gonadotropins (follicle-stimulating hormone and luteinizing hormone) are not actually decreased in concentration in alcoholic liver disease, they are inappropriately low for the degree of gonadal failure.[574] This phenomenon indicates that there may be a hypothalamic defect, since in usual circumstances, a reduction in a sex steroid level would leave hypothalamic sex steroid receptors unoccupied and hypothalamic release of gonadotropin-releasing hormone (GnRH), which governs release of gonadotropin from the pituitary, would be enhanced.[573] Evidence for pituitary dysfunction also comes from diminished responses in most alcoholic men to a provocative stimulus with GnRH.[575] There are, therefore, defects in all components of the hypothalamic-pituitary-gonadal axis. In cirrhosis not of alcoholic etiology, the few studies that have been done suggest that even when there is comparably severe liver disease, nonalcoholic cirrhosis, except hemochromatosis, is not characterized by reduced testosterone or altered sperm concentration or volume.[573,576]

Impotence. Although it is a common complaint in cirrhosis, impotence seldom is the initial complaint, since more pressing symptoms usually dominate the picture. Unless this information is specifically sought by the physician,

most patients do not volunteer it. Almost invariably, decreased sexual drive precedes the impotence, but poor performance is not appreciated because of the defect in desire. The symptom often is recognized only in retrospect as sexual performance improves. Sexual capacity may return spontaneously after hepatic recompensation, and the previously deficient activity occasionally becomes excessive. The pathogenesis of impotence is not well understood, and its therapy is unsatisfactory.

It has been demonstrated that the administration of testosterone enanthate to patients with cirrhosis can increase plasma testosterone levels and normalize the male-female hormonal imbalance.[273] The authors did not mention the clinical response in these patients. We and others have used injections of testosterone enanthate in sesame oil usually with little improvement but occasionally with resounding success.

Gonadal Failure in Women. Women with alcoholic cirrhosis may show severe gonadal failure manifested by oligomenorrhea, loss of secondary sex characteristics such as breast and pelvic fat accumulation, and infertility. Women still in the reproductive years have a marked decrease in developing follicles and few or no corpora lutea.[573] Plasma levels of estradiol and progesterone are reduced.[577] Amenorrhea may also occur in decompensated cirrhosis of other causes;

normal menses may return with recovery. Pregnancies have been carried to successful conclusion in patients with cirrhosis and even in those with portacaval anastomosis.[498]

Secondary Hyperaldosteronism. Increased secretion of aldosterone is the last in a series of steps initiated by increased intrahepatic sinusoidal pressure and a key consequence of advanced cirrhosis. It is thought to be mediated by a decrease in effective plasma volume on the juxtaglomerular apparatus of the kidney, which stimulates the renin–angiotensin I–angiotensin II–aldosterone sequence. The factors that influence water balance, electrolyte concentration, and urine formation are discussed more fully in the chapter on ascites and the hepatorenal syndrome.

Diabetes. Deranged carbohydrate metabolism varies from hyperglycemia or mild glucose intolerance in one third to three fourths of patients with cirrhosis to overt diabetes in about 15%.[518] The prevalence of diabetes in patients with cirrhosis is increased.[106,375] Although diabetes is not a problem clinically, it is surprisingly common, occurring two to three times as frequently in patients with alcoholic cirrhosis as in patients without cirrhosis, thus the term *cirrhotic diabetes.* Epidemiologically, this type of diabetes is clearly secondary to the cirrhosis.[98] It usually occurs after the cirrhosis is well developed and often is found incidentally during evaluation of decompensated cirrhosis. It usually is manifested by hyperglycemia, mild glycosuria, glucose intolerance, hyperinsulinemia, and peripheral insulin resistance.[99,420,544] There seldom is evidence of the vascular lesions of diabetes mellitus, and patients are resistant to diabetic ketoacidosis. It usually can be treated with diet; occasionally it requires oral agents but seldom insulin. When a patient with cirrhosis requires insulin, the diabetes probably represents true diabetes mellitus of nonhepatogenous origin.

The pathogenesis of this metabolic disorder is not clear. It is characterized by insulin resistance, as in patients with obesity. It differs from the diabetes of obesity, which is characterized by hypoglucagonemia, by the presence of greatly increased plasma glucagon secretion.[512] It does not appear to be related to pancreatitis, hemosiderosis, hypokalemia, or hyperadrenocorticism.

The accompanying hyperinsulinemia and insulin resistance are thought to result mainly from decreased degradation of insulin by the liver,[341] although increased secretion has been demonstrated.[239] Current data suggest that the decreased degradation is primarily a result of a decrease in hepatic parenchymal function[518,544] rather than an effect of portal-systemic shunting, although the latter may contribute. Portal-systemic shunting appears to play a greater role in the hyperglucagonemia by means of pancreatic stimulation by some as yet unidentified factor.

Insulin resistance in patients with cirrhosis may be contributed to by hormonal and nonhormonal antagonists, such as hypersomatotropism, hyperglucagonemia, and increased plasma levels of free fatty acids. Defects in target tissues for insulin action have been postulated.[395] Decreased binding of insulin to adipocytes and a postreceptor defect may play major roles in the pathogenesis of insulin resistance in cirrhosis.[49,559] It is likely that there is a combined receptor-postreceptor defect.[71] The postreceptor lesion may be defective glucose storage in skeletal muscle.[373a]

The diabetes of cirrhosis typically occurs in patients with inherited susceptibility to diabetes, and this suggests that these diabetogenic influences may precipitate diabetes in patients with a genetic predisposition.

Parathyroid Hormone. Elevated parathyroid hormone levels have been observed in cirrhosis, especially primary biliary cirrhosis.[156] They have been attributed to hypovitaminosis D and secondary hyperparathyroidism. In cirrhosis other than primary biliary cirrhosis, human parathyroid hormone levels are elevated. Higher levels of parathyroid hormone correlate with higher degrees of impairment of liver function. Impaired extraction of hormone by the liver, rather than secondary hyperparathyroidism, has been suggested, but the mechanism has not been demonstrated.[266]

Orloff[397] has described a series of patients who, 3 to 9 months after portacaval shunts for variceal hemorrhage, developed a solitary parathyroid adenoma and primary hyperparathyroidism. Weakness and bone pain were presenting symptoms. Clinicians should take care not to mistake this syndrome for hepatic osteodystrophy.

Thyroid Hormones. The major thyroid hormone carrier proteins are synthesized in the liver, where thyroid hormone is also metabolized. Most triiodothyronine (T_3) is converted from thyroxine (T_4) in the liver. Patients with severe cirrhosis have low levels of T_3 but remain euthyroid.[232] Sometimes a low T_4 level is associated with a low T_3 level, usually in end-stage liver disease.[550] Although total T_3 or total T_4 is low, free T_4 is normal or high and free T_3 is normal or low. Reverse T_3, 3,3′,5′-triiodo-L-thyronine, usually is elevated.

Metabolic System

Potassium Deficiency. Hypokalemia is almost ubiquitous in alcoholic cirrhosis and common in nonalcoholic cirrhosis. Vomiting and diarrhea, which frequently are present in decompensated cirrhosis, may cause the loss of large amounts of potassium. In addition, secondary hyperaldosteronism favors the loss of potassium and interferes with intrinsic and extrinsic attempts to correct the deficit. Finally, physicians may contribute a large iatrogenic component to the potassium deficit by the use of diuretic agents, the most potent of which are strongly kaliuretic substances. The inability of the renal tubules to conserve potassium as effectively as they do sodium contributes to this developing defect. Indeed, as metabolic alkalosis appears, the tubules may paradoxically and inappropriately secrete large amounts of potassium in the face of severe kaliopenia. The metabolic alkalosis and increased intracellular-extracellular pH gradient, which develops as intracellular potassium ions are exchanged for extracellular hydrogen ions, induces potentially comagenic shifts in ammonia and amines.

Hyponatremia. Hyponatremia occurs in nearly half of hospitalized patients with cirrhosis.[406] Both dilutional and natriopenic hyponatremia occur. Increased antidiuretic hormonal activity has long been recognized, although its source, nature, and pathogenesis have never been adequately elucidated.[442] This type of dilutional hyponatremia can be effectively treated by restricting water intake. The other type of hyponatremia, which is more complex and more serious, seldom is seen in untreated patients with cirrhosis who have not been on salt-restricted diets or diuretic therapy. In this situation, the hyponatremia results from sodium loss in excess of water and often is complicated by fluid retention. This combination creates the difficult dilemma of hyponatremia with edema and ascites. Water restriction in this situation often results in progressive azotemia, and the use of diuretic drugs may exacerbate the hyponatremia. Sometimes it is difficult to tell whether fluid restriction, diuresis, or both are required. In most instances, hyponatremia represents total body hypotonicity with expansion of the intracellular fluid volume and constriction of the extracellular volume with its attendant consequences—oliguria, azotemia, and hypotension. This syndrome may respond dramatically to the administration of hypertonic saline solution to correct the extracellular sodium concentration by shifting water into the extracellular fluid,[596] which results in correction of the hyponatremia and, sometimes, diuresis. Hyponatremic encephalopathy and central pontine myelinosis are complications of hyponatremia.[406]

Hypoalbuminemia.   Hypoalbuminemia is an almost invariable finding in cirrhosis, especially alcoholic cirrhosis. It is widely held that decreased hepatic synthetic capacity for albumin is responsible. Meticulous studies, however, have indicated that although albumin synthesis sometimes is decreased, it often is normal or even increased.[475] The albumin synthetic rate does not correlate well with the serum albumin concentration. Suppression of albumin production is closely correlated with elevated SGOT levels, decreased concentration of cholesterol esters, and prolonged prothrombin time, all indications of active hepatocellular dysfunction. Many other factors contribute to the decrease in albumin concentration.[476] Alcohol specifically inhibits albumin synthesis, and this inhibition can be reversed experimentally by tryptophan. Albumin synthesis may also be affected by the nutritional state, by changes in colloid osmotic pressure, by intrahepatic pressure relations, and by altered metabolism of adrenal, testicular, ovarian, and thyroid hormones. The problem is extremely complex, since the albumin degradation rate is decreased in patients with hypoalbuminemia.[543]

Decreased serum albumin levels contribute greatly to the formation of edema and ascites and the compensatory increase in serum globulins. In addition, decreased binding of the many substances that are bound to albumin, such as bilirubin, calcium, and many drugs, results in abnormal plasma-tissue ratios and various metabolic derangements.

Oncologic Associations

Oropharyngeal Cancer.   Alcoholic cirrhosis frequently is complicated by the development of cancer of the mouth and pharynx.[255,257] Cancer of the floor of the mouth, uvula, and soft palate have also been associated independently with both alcohol consumption and smoking.[256] Because alcoholism is related to alcoholic cirrhosis by definition and to smoking by social mores, it is difficult to be certain whether oral cancer is associated with cirrhosis, alcoholism, smoking, or a combination of these factors. The association of oral cancer with alcoholism holds for the consumption of all types of alcoholic beverages—beer, wine, and whiskey—but for tobacco usage, it holds only for cigarette smoking, not for cigar or pipe smoking.

Whenever such a positive association exists, one must wonder whether Berkson's[43] bias may have been responsible for an artifactual relation. Berkson's hypothesis suggests that any two diseases will occur more commonly together in hos-

pitalized patients than their individual incidences would predict and that this comorbidity depends on the individual rates of admission to hospital for the two diseases.

As Mainland[335] has pointed out, any two lethal diseases will occur less commonly together at autopsy than would be expected on the basis of their individual incidences. The finding that oral cancer occurs *more* commonly in patients with cirrhosis than in patients without cirrhosis at autopsy, despite the statistical expectation that it should occur less frequently in cirrhosis, supports the validity of the relation.

Alcohol-Associated Neoplasia.   In alcoholic cirrhosis, there is an independent association of alcohol with cancer and an increased incidence of cancer of the esophagus, pancreas, cardia of the stomach, colon, and liver.[320] Mechanisms possibly include induction of microsomal enzymes that activate procarcinogens and impairment of DNA repair.

Cancer Metastatic to the Liver.   Several reports of a decreased incidence of hepatic metastases from nonhepatic cancers in patients with cirrhosis[321,462] have been published. They may represent examples of the Berkson-Mainland postmortem principle.[335] On the other hand, one would expect that the portal-systemic venous collaterals of cirrhosis would decrease the frequency of hepatic metastases from cancers originating in the splanchnic organs, which are disseminated by portal venous flow. Similarly, one might expect that intrahepatic arteriovenous anastomoses, which are common in cirrhosis, may reduce metastases that originate in other areas of the body and are spread by arterial dissemination. Some carefully controlled investigations have failed to confirm the negative association between hepatic metastases and cirrhosis.[188] Indeed, one study suggests that hepatic metastases from gastrointestinal tumors occurred *more* often in patients with cirrhosis than in patients without cirrhosis. On the other hand, nongastrointestinal tumors spread to the livers of patients with cirrhosis less frequently than to those of patients without cirrhosis. It is worrisome, however, that in alcoholic cirrhosis, the disproportionately frequent oropharyngeal cancers, which seldom metastasize to the liver, might falsely account for this relation.

Hepatocellular Cancer.   Hepatocellular carcinoma, which occurs with increased frequency in patients with most types of cirrhosis, is discussed in detail in Chapter 31. It is seen, in ascending order of occurrence, in alcoholic cirrhosis, posthepatitic cirrhosis, especially that associated with HBV, and hemochromatosis. Although persistence of the virus intracellularly may allow abnormal oncogenic aberrations of the genetic code to develop, the increased incidence of hepatocellular carcinoma in cirrhosis appears teleologically to represent excessive regenerative activity gone awry.

Diagnostic Procedures

Various techniques are used in the diagnosis of cirrhosis and its complications. Some deal with the evaluation of the liver itself—its size, shape, and composition. Some are biochemical, such as the so-called liver function tests, which are surprisingly useful in the differential diagnosis of liver disease,[100] and some are truly tests of liver function, which are valuable in assessing various hepatic functional capacities, such as the galactose elimination capacity or the aminopyrine transformation test. Many of them deal with the diagnosis of the complications of cirrhosis, such as esophageal varices, portal hypertension, and ascites.

LIVER BIOPSY

Percutaneous Liver Biopsy

The procedure of choice for proving the diagnosis of liver disease, percutaneous liver biopsy is safe, simple, inexpensive, and readily acceptable to the patient. The Menghini needle,[356] which is the most widely used, has compiled an impressive safety record.[325] In generalized liver diseases such as micronodular cirrhosis, it is a reliable, reproducible technique[35] that provides adequate tissue for diagnostic studies. It may be somewhat less precise in patients with macronodular cirrhosis, in whom individual samples of tissue may not necessarily be representative. Like all other procedures that require subjective evaluation, subject to histologic interpretation are error.[172,184] It is useful in establishing the type and severity of cirrhosis and, within the limits of the clinical-histologic relations, in estimating prognosis and response to therapy. It is effective in determining the cause of space-occupying lesions on liver scan, which are common in cirrhosis, by using radionuclide scan,[90] or ultrasound-guided biopsies.[561a]

Transcostal liver biopsy can be performed in cooperative patients with normal or nearly normal tests of coagulation. Sometimes prolonged prothrombin time or thrombocytopenia increases the risk of percutaneous liver biopsy. One must here weigh the potential gains against the increased risks.[20]

Coagulopathy is a contraindication to this procedure. Indeed, postbiopsy bleeding is the most common and most lethal serious complication of needle biopsy of the liver.

Liver biopsy can be performed with a variety of biopsy needles, the most widely used of which are the Menghini needle[356] and the TruCut disposable needle. A recent study[350a] reported that the rate of hemorrhage after biopsy at a single medical center was appreciably higher with the TruCut needle. Other factors than the needle itself may have been responsible,[94a] however, such as the type of patients studied and the exact technique of performing the biopsy. The presence of hepatic neoplasm appears to be the single most important risk factor.[94a,350a,350b]

Liver biopsies can be performed in children with the Menghini needle with higher, albeit acceptable, morbidity and mortality than is seen in adults.[85a]

A recent report of about 200 patients with sufficiently severe coagulopathy to contraindicate conventional needle biopsy demonstrated that transjugular biopsy could be performed safely and effectively.[104a,346a]

Transjugular Biopsy

Transjugular liver biopsy, first performed in 1964[127a] and brought to wider clinical attention by Rösch and associates in 1973,[473] is performed during hepatic vein catheterization using a long flexible biopsy needle that is advanced through the wall of the hepatic vein into the parenchyma of the liver. It can be successfully performed in 80% to 97% of cases.[346a] A core ranging from 0.3 to 2 cm is usually obtained. The procedure is a failure because of the inability to enter the hepatic

vein or to obtain a tissue core. Complications have been reported in up to 20% of cases. Major complications include perforation of the hepatic capsule with intraperitoneal hemorrhage and cardiac arrhythmia.[104a] Death has occurred in 0.1% to 0.5% (ie 1 per 200 to 1000 attempts), a figure that is somewhat higher than that observed with percutaneous biopsy with either the Menghini or the TruCut needle. A study based on 1000 tissue specimens found that enough tissue was available for evaluation of architecture in two thirds of cirrhotic livers and for almost all nonfibrotic or noncirrhotic livers.[296]

LAPAROSCOPIC BIOPSY

Another option is to perform laparoscopy. Laparoscopy has not, however, been shown to be superior to percutaneous liver biopsy in the diagnosis of cirrhosis.[403]

A series of 1000 consecutive patients who underwent both laparoscopic and liver biopsy confirmed that the frequency of diagnosis of cirrhosis was similar by both techniques (78.4% versus 78.8%) but found that the combination of the two procedures increased the diagnostic yield to 97.7% by decreasing the percentage of false negatives.[396] Advocates suggest that in addition, laparoscopy can visualize intraabdominal signs of portal hypertension and identify splenomegaly, thus increasing the information available to clinicians.

ULTRASONOGRAPHY

Ultrasonography is one of the major technologic breakthroughs in the diagnosis of hepatobiliary disease. It is as noninvasive a technique as can be envisioned. A major value is in differentiating biliary obstruction from nonobstructive, parenchymal jaundice, a differential diagnosis that may involve cirrhosis and alcoholic hepatitis. In assessment of the cirrhotic liver per se, its value is limited. Textural differences and increased attenuation may provide diagnostic insight as shown in the gray-scale ultrasonograms from Taylor's fine atlas on the subject[557] (Fig. 32-26). Attenuation of sound, however, is primarily due to concomitant fatty liver and not accurate in identifying other types of liver disease.[227,558] Liver volume can also be determined by ultrasonic scanning.[448]

Ultrasonography can determine the ratio of transverse caudate to right lobe width, a value of which below 1.3 is said to be characteristic of cirrhosis. The sensitivity of this measurement is higher in postnecrotic than in alcohol-related cirrhosis.[192] Further investigations are needed.

On occasion, an enlarged, tortuous portal vein can indicate the presence of portal hypertension (see Fig. 32-26C). In addition, ultrasonography has been used to determine the patency of portacaval anastomoses, demonstrate postshunt dilatation of the inferior vena cava, and demonstrate collateral pathways.[42,247]

COMPUTED TOMOGRAPHY

Although CT evaluation of the liver can show liver size, shape, and density more precisely and in more familiar anatomic projections than ultrasonography, its value in the diagnosis of cirrhosis is limited by its expense and relatively high radiation dosage.

The CT findings of cirrhosis are not diagnostic. Similar CT findings are observed in lymphomatous and granuloma-

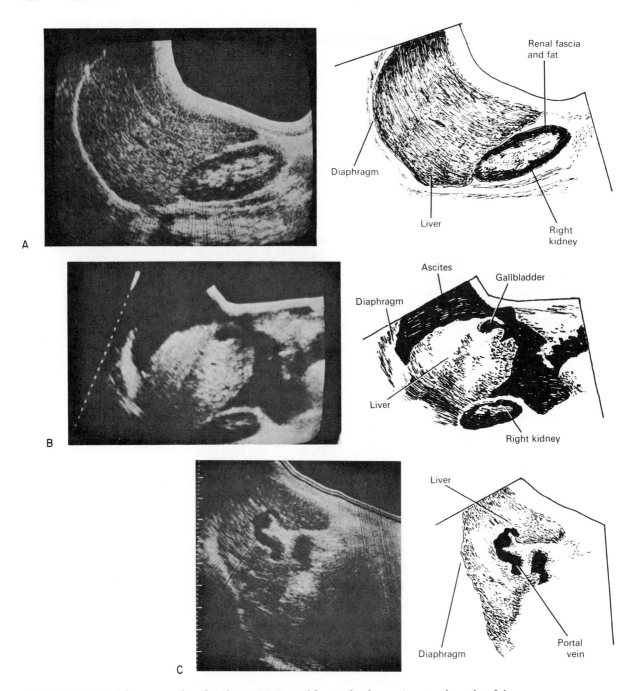

FIGURE 32-26   Ultrasonography of cirrhosis. (**A**) Normal longitudinal scan 4 cm to the right of the midline demonstrates the consistency of the liver. In this position, the liver is limited above by the right hemidiaphragm, anteriorly by the abdominal wall, and posteriorly by the right kidney, from which it is separated by the perirenal fat and fascia. These appear as a single, highly reflective interface. (**B**) Parasagittal ultrasonogram through the right lobe of the liver and right kidney shows the liver to be surrounded by ascites both on its anterior aspect and between the visceral surface of the liver and right kidney (Morison's pouch). On the anterior surface of the liver, the lumen of the gallbladder is barely seen. The liver itself displays a highly abnormal consistency with dense white echoes and inadequate penetration to the deep surface, suggesting that there is both an increase in the echoes from the liver and increased attenuation within the liver. These findings are diagnostic of diffuse intrahepatic fibrosis and consistent with cirrhosis. (**C**) A paramedian scan through the liver substance 2 cm to the right of the midline shows a diffusely abnormal liver consistency with high-level echoes. A large, highly tortuous portal vein is visible, which strongly suggests portal hypertension. (Taylor KJW. Atlas of gray scale ultrasonography. New York, Churchill Livingstone, 1978)

tous infiltrations as well as in alcoholic hepatitis.[422] It has been suggested that a ratio of the transverse widths of the caudate to right lobe greater than 0.65 on CT scanning or ultrasonography may be as accurate as the histologic diagnosis in cirrhosis. These observations require further confirmation. This phenomenon is based on shrinkage of the right lobe, which is postulated to be a consequence of more fibrous tissue in the right lobe than in the caudate lobe, and hypertrophy of the caudate lobe. Normal livers have a ratio less than 0.55.[206]

CT may be of use in confirming the cause of cirrhosis when hemochromatosis is suspected. In the absence of contrast injection, increments in the average CT density to 75 to 132 Hounsfield units are seen in patients with hemochromatosis, whereas the normal CT density of the liver is 54 to 68 Hounsfield units.[152]

Ultrasonography rather than CT usually is preferred when verification of the clinical impression of ascites is needed or when only small amounts of ascitic fluid are present. CT, however, has the additional capability of localizing the fluid collection to peritoneal, retroperitoneal, and extraperitoneal compartments. Furthermore, it is claimed that benign transudative ascites has a CT density close to urine or water, whereas malignant ascites has higher than normal CT density.[152]

In most clinical situations, the greater expense of CT probably does not justify its use in place of ultrasonography.[605]

MAGNETIC RESONANCE IMAGING

Early claims for MRI suggest that it is more sensitive than both ultrasonography and radionuclide scanning and comparable to CT scanning in the diagnosis of cirrhosis.[128,521] MRI seems to be effective in visualizing high-flow vascular structures such as portacaval anastomoses. MRI technology has not yet been applied to sufficiently large numbers of patients with cirrhosis to determine its usefulness. In one study, performed before liver biopsy, neither ultrasonography, MRI, radionuclide scanning, nor CT scanning alone or in combination could accurately make or exclude the diagnosis of parenchymal disease.[81]

RADIOISOTOPIC SCANS

Liver scans provide a simple and safe assessment of liver size, shape, and, to some degree, function. [99m]Tc sulfur colloid, which is taken up by the reticuloendothelial tissue, shows liver size and homogeneity, spleen size, and reticuloendothelial activity (Fig. 32-27). The cirrhotic liver, by virtue of its irregular parenchymal pattern and uneven distribution of blood flow, typically shows a heterogeneous appearance. A significant correlation has been observed between the span of the liver determined by percussion-palpation and by radionuclide scan.[74] Because the liver is a three-dimensional organ that assumes an infinite variety of shapes,[369] it often is impossible to accurately estimate liver size. Liver volume and weight, the most valid indices, can be calculated easily from the anterior and right lateral scans,[472] but computed, ultrasonic, and radiotomographic examinations are more precise.

Some estimate of hepatic blood flow and portal-systemic shunting can be made from the relative decrease in hepatic uptake and the increase in splenic and vertebral uptake.[69] Bircher and colleagues[47] found that liver volume does not

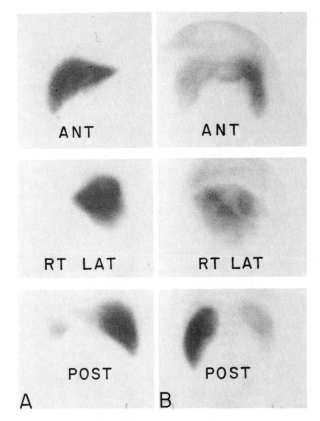

FIGURE 32-27 Technetium-99m sulfur colloid scans of the liver. (**A**) A normal scan is shown on the left. Homogeneous uptake is shown on the anterior (*upper*), right lateral (*middle*), and posterior (*lower*) projections. The liver is of normal size and shape. A small spleen, which is not seen in the anterior view, is visible on the posterior scan. No uptake by the vertebrae is seen. (**B**) An abnormal scan in a cirrhotic patient is shown on the right. Decreased and heterogeneous hepatic uptake is seen in the anterior and lateral projections. An enlarged spleen with greater uptake than the liver is seen. The clear area to the right and above the liver is caused by ascites. In the posterior scan, increased vertebral uptake is visualized.

correlate well with functional capacity but does show a close correlation with hepatic blood flow and oxygen consumption. It must be kept in mind that liver volume in disease states may not be a reliable measure of hepatic parenchymal volume. The hepatic parenchymal tissue may represent a relatively small and widely variable fraction of the total liver weight.[326]

ENDOSCOPY

The diagnosis of esophageal varices can best be made by endoscopy. Endoscopic diagnosis of esophageal varices, however, is not free of the uncertainties of observer variability.[97] This technique has the advantage of visualizing the varices themselves rather than their shadows, as is done radiologically. When the patient is bleeding, endoscopic examination can establish unequivocally the site of hemorrhage.[404] During the last quarter of the 20th century, the concept of specific endoscopic markers of impending variceal hemorrhage appeared. Although it had long been assumed that large esophageal varices were more likely to bleed than small ones, it was not until 1972 that Dagradi[109] presented data to establish this belief. Even more important, he pointed out that large (greater than 5 mm in diameter), blue-gray varices with *cherry-red spots* (Fig. 32-28) indicated a high risk of bleeding from varices. Indeed, he noted that all the patients with alcoholic cirrhosis who bled had these lesions and that their appearance de novo heralded increased risk. Groups of patients with and without these lesions were neither identified nor followed prospectively so that the degree of risk could be established.

In 1982, Paquet[407] described erosions of the surface of varices that he referred to as *black points*, which he thought represented "varices on varices," as did Dagradi about his cherry-red spots.[109] As part of a controlled trial of prophylactic endoscopic sclerotherapy, Paquet found that almost 90% of the patients with these lesions bled from varices during a 3-year period of prospective evaluation. In that study, patients with "large varices and black points or greatly prolonged prothrombin times" were studied.[407] The inclusion of patients with the latter abnormality diminished the precision of these observations.

In 1980, Beppu and colleagues[40,41] presented a complex system for predicting the risks of hemorrhage from varices. They described *cherry-red spots* that apparently were identical to those of Dagradi and to the black points of Paquet; *hemocystic spots*, which were large cherry-red spots; and *red wales*, which were linear cherry-red spots (Fig. 32-29). (Wale is a textile term for linear ridges that are characteristic of corduroy or gabardine cloth.) All these lesions were considered to be varices on varices, and we have assumed that they represent thin-walled blisters indicative of weak spots in the variceal wall. The red wale marking was thought to carry the worst prognosis of these red signs. In their classification, Beppu and

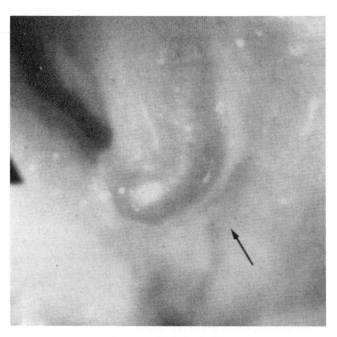

FIGURE 32-29   Red wale. This curvilinear elevation on the surface of a varix is like a cherry-red spot, a thin-walled dilatation of a varix, although the presence of these linear lesions implies a greater risk of bleeding than the round, cherry-red spots. The explanation for their linear shape and greater propensity to rupture is not known. They tend to be pale red. (Courtesy of Dr. K. Beppu)

colleagues took into account the color of the varices (blue was a more ominous prognostic sign than white), the pattern of the varices (tortuous varices were more dangerous than straight varices), and the size of the varices (the larger the varices, the more likely they would bleed). On the basis of a complicated scoring system involving all these parameters, they believed that they could predict the percentage of patients who would bleed from 0% to 100%. The North Italian Endoscopy Club for the Study and Treatment of Esophageal Varices tested these criteria in a prospective study of patients with cirrhosis who had esophageal varices and who had not previously bled from their varices.[385] They found that the risks of bleeding were much lower in Italian patients than had been predicted by the Japanese investigators, and they created a new scoring system.[234]

These important observations have initiated a rational, objective method for predicting the prognosis of varices based on the endoscopic evaluation of esophageal varices. These preliminary findings should serve as the basis for large, prospective investigations of these and other markers, perhaps in conjunction with portal pressure measurements and clinical features, to establish for different types of portal hypertension a practical system for predicting the relative risks of variceal hemorrhage.

BARIUM CONTRAST ESOPHAGOGRAPHY

Barium contrast esophagography is the time-honored method of demonstrating esophageal varices. It is safe, simple, and readily available. When the varices are large, the esophagogram shows the classic pattern (Fig. 32-30). Postprandial examination for esophageal varices appears to be more accurate

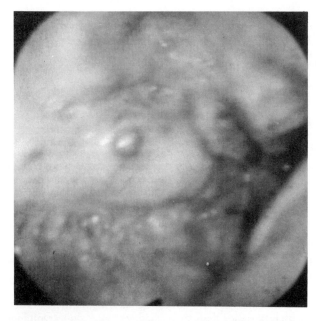

FIGURE 32-28   Cherry-red (hemocystic) spot. The elevated papule projecting from the esophageal varix in the center of this photograph is a large cherry-red spot. It represents a thin-walled variceal blister on the surface of the varix. Such lesions appear to be potential sites of rupture. In color prints, these lesions appear as dark red or purple lesions. (Courtesy of Dr. K. Beppu)

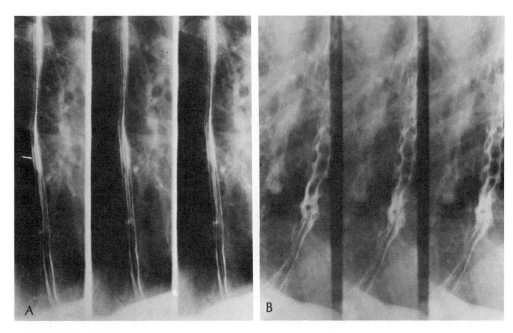

FIGURE 32-30 Esophageal varices by barium swallow. (**A**) A normal esophagogram shows delicate, parallel mucosal folds. (**B**) Large esophageal varices are seen in profile and en face on multiple films.

than the traditional fasting study, since splanchnic blood flow is increased after meals and varices are maximally distended at that time. Because observer variability can affect the diagnosis of varices appreciably,[95,96] several observers should interpret the films independently to establish a consensus diagnosis.

When the radiologic and endoscopic techniques for the diagnosis of esophageal varices were compared blindly, esophageal varices were found by each technique in about 50% of patients with cirrhosis.[95–97] The two methods agreed with each other in 70% to 75% of patients.[95,97] The disagreements were evenly distributed in a positive-negative sense and appeared to be the consequence of observer error rather than of intrinsic advantages of one method over the other.

ANGIOGRAPHY

Visualization of the portal venous system, which had previously been done by splenoportography, is accomplished during the venous phase of arteriography. Arteriography may be helpful in determining the site of upper gastrointestinal tract hemorrhage. It can demonstrate leakage of contrast material from arterial or capillary lesions such as peptic ulcer or erosive gastritis. It seldom establishes bleeding from varices. Percutaneous transhepatic portography allows direct access to the portal venous system and definitive visualization of the portal vein and its collaterals.[597] It is a more difficult and dangerous procedure than celiac or superior mesenteric arteriography. Umbilical vein catheterization has also been used to visualize the portal venous system,[580] but it requires surgical dissection of the umbilical vein, which often is unsuccessful. Celiac arteriography is not performed for the diagnosis of cirrhosis, but when performed for other reasons, the findings can support that diagnosis. It usually shows tortuosity of the intrahepatic arteries, resulting in a virtually pathognomonic corkscrew appearance.[393]

The measurement of portal pressure can best be accomplished by hepatic vein catheterization. The correlation between the wedged hepatic venous pressure and the free portal venous pressure is almost perfect in alcoholic cirrhosis[56] (Fig. 32-31). This technique, which has been greatly simplified by the introduction of a balloon catheter, permits rapid serial measurements of wedged and free hepatic venous pressure[198] and calculation of the hepatic-portal venous pressure gradient, the most critical measurement in portal hypertension.

When hepatic arteries are visualized, cirrhosis can be suggested by the tortuous, corkscrew pattern formed by arterial branches. Sometimes arteriography can differentiate hepatomas, which occur with increased frequency in cirrhosis, from regenerating nodules.[572]

SPLENOPORTOGRAPHY

For some years, splenoportography had been the standard method of measuring portal (intrasplenic) pressure and opacifying the portal venous system. It seldom is used today because the technique does not allow for simultaneous determination of the ambient intraabdominal venous pressure (ie, a baseline level) and is associated with a small but definite risk of intrasplenic hemorrhage. When successful, the technique gives good visualization of the portal system. It is particularly useful for establishing the presence or absence of patency in the portal or splenic veins when thrombosis is suspected.[23] Splenoportography is also useful in assessing the presinusoidal portal hypertension of schistosomiasis and other disorders and the presinusoidal component of nonalcoholic cirrhosis.[428]

TRANSHEPATIC PORTOGRAPHY

Because the wedged hepatic vein technique for measuring portal pressure is completely valid only in alcoholic cirrho-

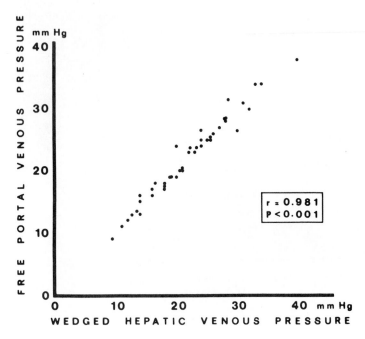

FIGURE 32-31 Relation between free portal venous pressure and wedged hepatic venous pressure. The correlation between these measurements in 43 patients with compensated alcoholic cirrhosis is almost perfect. (Viallet A, et al. Comparison of free portal venous pressure and wedged hepatic venous pressure in patients with cirrhosis of the liver. Gastroenterology 59:372, 1970)

sis, nonalcoholic cirrhosis, in which this technique underestimates portal pressure, necessitates a more direct measurement[56,428] (see Chap. 33). Visualization of the portal vein, its intrahepatic branches, the splenic vein, and collateral vessels and measurement of pressure within the portal venous system are possible by direct injection of contrast medium into the portal vein through a fine needle passed transhepatically. By redirecting the thin needle into a hepatic vein branch, a baseline pressure also can be measured for determining the portal-hepatic venous pressure gradient.[56] Contrast injections into a hepatic vein branch can be useful in confirming Budd-Chiari syndrome, in which attempts at catheterization of hepatic veins often are unsuccessful.[454]

PARACENTESIS

Abdominal paracentesis is the standard procedure for examining ascitic fluid. It is simple when the volume of ascitic fluid is large. Fluid can be removed from the midline with the patient in the sitting position or from the flank with the patient supine or in the left lateral decubitus position. When the amount of ascitic fluid is small, paracentesis may be more difficult. In this situation, the patient can be placed on hands and knees and the abdomen aspirated from below. This abdomen-dependent position has the advantage of puddling the fluid in the most dependent portion of the abdomen and floating loops of bowel away from the penetrating needle.

The usefulness of the differential analysis of ascitic fluid is suggested by Table 32-3.

Complications

Almost all the complications of cirrhosis are the complications of portal hypertension. They include hemorrhage from esophageal varices, ascites, spontaneous bacterial peritonitis, the hepatorenal syndrome, portal-systemic encephalopathy,

the hepatopulmonary syndrome and hypersplenism. Each of these subjects is discussed elsewhere in this book.

Treatment

Cirrhosis of some etiolgies has specific therapy. Examples include iron depletion in hemochromatosis, penicillamine in Wilson's disease, and corticosteroids in autoimmune chronic active hepatitis with cirrhosis. These are discussed in separate chapters. In other forms of cirrhosis, the treatment usually is the management of the principal complications—ascites, encephalopathy, and variceal hemorrhage, also discussed elsewhere.

The interventions that constitute the therapeutic armamentarium for alcoholic cirrhosis are limited. The treatment begins with convincing the patient to abstain from further alcohol consumption. In many studies, abstinence appears to improve survival,[411,436,463,491] but in others, an improved survival is not apparent.[9,405,532]

Colchicine reduces collagen synthesis by preventing polymerization of microtubules, a process necessary for collagen secretion.[59] In a double-blind, placebo-controlled trial, patients with cirrhosis of both alcoholic and nonalcoholic etiologies who received oral colchicine had improved survival and histologic improvement on liver biopsy.[261-263] These results are not universally accepted, but the physician who believes that doing something is better than doing nothing may take heart in knowing that the results appear beneficial and, perhaps even more reassuring, that the incidence of adverse effects has been low.

Patients with cirrhosis of many etiologies have been effectively treated by liver transplantation.[332] Patients with alcohol-induced cirrhosis have also been successfully transplanted, and the results are not dissimilar to the results with other kinds of liver disease. In the Pittsburgh series, the survival rate was 71%.[284] As with all other transplant candidates, patients with alcoholic cirrhosis need to be screened for sig-

TABLE 32-3 *Differential Analysis of Ascitic Fluid*

Type of Ascites	Appearance	Protein (g/dL) Mean	Protein (g/dL) Range	Leukocytes* PMN	Leukocytes* MN	Leukocytes* Total†	Cytology	Peritoneal Biopsy	Culture	pH	Amylase	Other
Cirrhotic	Clear	1.8	0.6–6.0	75	225	300 ± 400	0	NS	0	7.45	Normal	Occasionally turbid; rarely bloody
Cardiac	Clear	2.2	1.5–5.5	50	200	250 ± 200	0	NS	0	7.40	Normal	Liver biopsy diagnostic
Neoplastic	Clear or bloody	2.2	0.6–6.0	340	360	700 ± 300	+ (30%)	+ (50%)	0	7.35	Normal	Occasionally chylous
Bacterial peritonitis	Cloudy	1.0	0.6–2.2	2200	300	2500 ± 2500	0	NS	+	7.25	Normal	Positive culture
Pancreatic	Clear or bloody	3.2	1.0–5.0	900	1000	1900 ± 800	0	NS	0	7.38	Elevated (80%)	Occasionally chylous
Tuberculous	Clear	3.4	1.5–7.0	125	875	1000 ± 600	0	+ (65%)	+ (65%)	7.30	Normal	Occasionally chylous
Nephrotic	Clear	0.9	0.3–1.8	45	175	220 ± 200	0	0	0	7.38	Normal	
Postdialysis	Clear	1.3	1.0–3.0	50	200	250 ± 200	0	0	0	7.40	Normal	

PMN, polymorphonuclear leukocytes; MN, mononuclear cells; NS, nonspecific; 0, negative; +, positive.
*Mean per μL.
†Mean ± SD.

nificant injury of other organs. The ethics of transplanting or not transplanting livers in alcoholics has been discussed by several authors.[22,84,368,494]

Prognosis

Danish investigators reviewed the main causes of death among 532 patients with cirrhosis of various etiologies who were followed for up to 16 years. They found no difference in the distribution of causes of death based on the presence or absence of alcoholism. Fifty-seven percent died of liver-related causes. Of the total number of deaths, 24% were from hepatic failure, 14% gastrointestinal bleeding, 13% hepatic failure with gastrointestinal bleeding, 4% primary liver cancer, and 2% other liver-related causes. Of the non–liver-related causes, cardiovascular diseases, extrahepatic cancers, and infections were the leading causes of death. When ascites was present, a liver-related cause was found in 94%.[495] It is difficult to make meaningful statements about the prognosis of cirrhosis unless its cause, epidemiologic setting, clinical and laboratory manifestations, and histology are known and unless the findings can be put into perspective by comparison with an appropriate control group.[21] Few studies provide all this information. Published series suggest that the 5-year survival may be as high as 90% in alcoholic cirrhosis in the absence of ascites, jaundice, hematemesis, or continued drinking, and as low as 0% in patients with alcoholic cirrhosis who present with encephalopathy.[491]

Surprisingly, the survival is reported to be higher for alcoholic cirrhosis than for nonalcoholic cirrhosis in some studies,[203,491,545] but others have found the opposite to be true.[173] On the other hand, abstinence appears to improve survival[411,425,436,463,491] or has no apparent effect.[9,405,532] The effects of several factors, such as alcohol consumption or abstinence and the presence or absence of esophageal varices, are shown in Figure 32-32.

There is evidence from published papers that survival is also influenced by the patient's sex (although both males and females have had better survival in individual series),[168,169,173] race (higher mortality for blacks, especially women),[169] and social class (worse for blue-collar workers)[169] and by the therapy ordered (adrenocortical steroids worsen the prognosis in men without ascites but improve it in women with ascites).[103]

Clinical findings such as jaundice, ascites, varices, encephalopathy, spider angiomas, and bacteremia have been associated with worse prognosis.[9,80,169,173,181,195,405,449,491,545]

Assessment by peritoneoscopy, according to its advocates, allows determination of the presence or absence of regenerative nodules, size of the right hepatic lobe, formation of small lymphatic vessels, and size of the spleen, all of which are said to have prognostic significance.[551] Demanding equal time, other interventionists have found that large varices at endoscopy and high hepatic vein wedge pressure gradients also provide significant information about likely death.[30,183] The noninvasive procedure of injection of ^{99m}Tc sulfur colloid allows determination of reticuloendothelial cell phagocytic activity, predicts bacterial infection rate, and has prognostic value in cirrhosis.[465]

Laboratory findings such as serum bilirubin, hemoglobin, alkaline phosphatase, creatinine, and albumin concentrations or prothrombin time show the prognosis to be worse the more abnormal the value.[80,181,400,437,496,508]

One transplantation center has found indocyanine green half-life and monoethylglycinexylidide formation from lidocaine to provide accurate assessment of short-term prognosis.[390]

Histologic findings that suggest coexisting alcoholic hepatitis, such as necrosis, inflammation, Mallory's bodies, and eosinophilic parenchymal infiltrates, are each associated with worse prognosis.[76,400,401,496] Perversely, in one such study, the presence of cirrhosis per se did not influence the mortality risk.[400]

Child and Turcotte[78] devised a simple set of clinical and

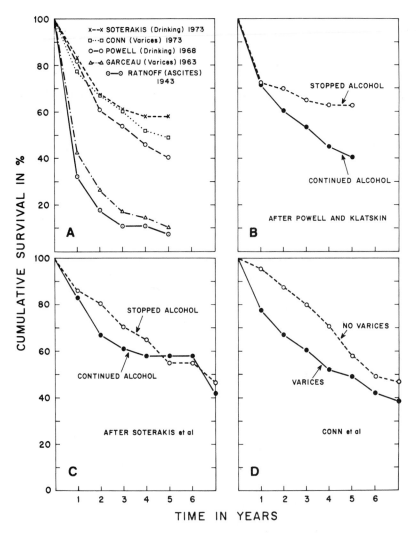

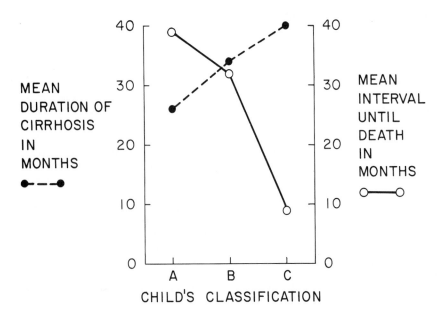

FIGURE 32-32   Effects of various factors on survival in alcoholic cirrhosis. (**A**) Comparison of cumulative survival curves of two groups of cirrhotic patients 20 years apart showing poor survival.[172,449] and three recent groups showing relative good prognosis.[436,532] The reasons for the differences are not known. (**B**) Powell and Klatskin[436] found continued alcoholic consumption associated with poor prognosis. (**C**) Soterakis and associates[532] found no difference between those patients who abstained and those who continued to drink. (**D**) We found that the prognosis of cirrhotic patients without varices was better than those with varices. The slopes were parallel, however, and suggest that the two groups represented different degrees of advancement of the cirrhotic process.

FIGURE 32-33   The association of Child-Turcotte classification and survival. Child's classification is shown on the abscissa and time in months on the ordinates. On the left ordinate, the mean interval between the clinical onset of cirrhosis and the time of classification is plotted (*closed circles, dashed line*). The duration of cirrhosis increases as the severity of cirrhosis progesses, that is, it takes longer to become Child's class C than it does B. On the right ordinate, the interval between classification and death is plotted (*open circles, solid line*). Survival is shortest for class C patients (mean, 8 months), longest for class A patients (mean, 39 months), and intermediate for class B patients (mean, 32 months).

laboratory features to help select patients with cirrhosis for portal-systemic shunt surgery. Several studies have shown that Child's criteria have prognostic value in cirrhosis and are among the best of such indicators.[8,228,490] These criteria grade patients on the basis of (1) serum bilirubin and (2) albumin concentrations, (3) severity of ascites and (4) encephalopathy, and (5) the state of nutrition, each on a 3-point scale. Although Child's classification appears to be a simple system, it is complex but surprisingly useful. We have found in systematic, prospective, unpublished studies that it is not only a useful predictor of survival in general (Fig. 32-33) but also a reliable index of the occurrence of each of the complications of portal hypertension. Because several modifications of Child's criteria are in use[438] and each scheme can be calculated in a number of ways, one must be critical in interpreting and comparing results.[93]

Other studies have assessed prognosis by combining several features. A ratio of serum bilirubin to γ-glutamyl transpeptidase was a better prognostic index than either value separately in alcoholic cirrhosis.[437] Increasingly, studies present complex computer-derived formulas that use multiple variables and variations of Cox model analysis.[64,80,181,400,496,568,586] Perhaps this approach holds promise for the future, but for the moment it is likely to remind clinicians of Aristotle's warning to bring no more precision to a topic than the subject allows.

References

1. Acalovschi M, et al. Prevalence of gallstones in liver cirrhosis: a sonographic survey. Am J Gastroenterol 23:954, 1988
2. Adams RD, Foley JM. The neurological changes in the more common types of severe liver disease. Trans Am Neurol Assoc 74:217, 1949
3. Adams RD, Foley JM. The disorder of movement in the more common varieties of liver disease. Electroencephalogr Clin Neurophysiol 5(Suppl 3):51, 1953
3a. Adamson M, et al. Indian childhood in an American child. Gastroentereology 102:1771, 1992
4. Adelson VW. Indian childhood cirrhosis as a result of copper hepatotoxicity—in all likelihood. J Pediatr Gastroenterol Nutr 6:491, 1987
5. Ahmed SS, et al. Cardiac function in alcoholics with cirrhosis: absence of overt cardiomyopathy: myth or fact? J Am Coll Cardiol 3:696, 1984
6. Alagille D. Alpha-1-antitrypsin deficiency. Hepatology 4:11S, 1984
7. Alagille D, Odievre M. Liver and biliary tract diseases in children. New York, John Wiley & Sons, 1979
8. Albers I, et al. Superiority of the Child-Pugh classification to quantitative liver function tests for assessing prognosis of liver cirrhosis. Scand J Gastroenterol 24:269, 1989
9. Alexander JF, et al. Natural history of alcoholic hepatitis. Am J Gastroenterol 56:515, 1971
10. Alter HJ. The hepatitis C virus and its relationship to the clinical spectrum of NANB hepatitis. J Gastroenterol Hepatol 5:(Suppl 1):78, 1990
11. Altman AR, et al. Idiopathic familial cirrhosis and steatosis in adults. Gastroenterology 7:1211, 1979
12. Amla I, et al. Cirrhosis in children from peanut meal contaminated by aflatoxin. Am J Clin Nutr 24:609, 1971
13. Angelin B, et al. Biliary lipid composition in patients with portal cirrhosis of the liver. Scand J Gastroenterol 15:849, 1980
14. Anonymous. Who gets alcoholic cirrhosis? Lancet 2:263, 1984
15. Anthony PP, et al. The morphology of cirrhosis: recommendations for definition, nomenclature, and classification by a working group sponsored by the World Health Organization. J Clin Pathol 31:395, 1978
16. Arico S, et al. Clinical significance of antibody to the hepatitis delta virus in symptomless HB$_s$Ag carriers. Lancet 2:356, 1985
17. Ashton RE, et al. Complications in methotrexate treatment of psoriasis with particular reference to liver fibrosis. J Invest Dermatol 79:229, 1982
18. Astrup J, Rorth M. Oxygen affinity of hemoglobin and red cell 2,3-diphosphoglycerate in hepatic cirrhosis. Scand J Clin Lab Invest 31:311, 1973
19. Attali P, et al. Dupuytren's contractures, alcohol consumption, and chronic liver disease. Arch Intern Med 147:1065, 1987
20. Atterbury CE. When not to do a liver biopsy. J Clin Gastroenterol 4:465, 1982
21. Atterbury CE. Prognosis in cirrhosis: disbelieving Cassandra. J Clin Gastroenterol 5:359, 1983
22. Atterbury CE. The alcoholic in the lifeboat: should drinkers be candidates for liver transplantation? J Clin Gastroenterol 8:1, 1986
23. Atterbury CE, Groszmann RJ. Portal venous pressure measurement and its clinical significance. In: Beker S, ed. Diagnostic procedures in the evaluation of hepatic disease. New York, Alan R Liss, 1983, p 567
24. Babany G, et al. Alcohol-like liver lesions induced by nifedipine. J Hepatol 9:252, 1989
25. Baillie M. The morbid anatomy of some of the most important parts of the human body. Albany, Barker & Southwick for Thomas, Spencer, 1795
26. Banks ER, et al. Radionuclide demonstration of intrapulmonary shunting in cirrhosis. Am J Radiol 140:967, 1983
27. Bannayan GA, Hajdu SI. Gynecomastia: clinicopathologic study of 351 cases. Am J Clin Pathol 57:431, 1972
28. Barnes JM, Magee PN. Some toxic properties of dimethylnitrosamine. Br J Ind Med 11:167, 1954
28a. Barnett JL, et al. A familial form of incomplete septal cirrhosis. Gastroenterology 102:674, 1992
29. Baron HC. Umbilical hernia secondary to cirrhosis of the liver: complications of surgical correction. N Engl J Med 263:824, 1960
30. Barrett G, et al. Hepatic venous pressure gradient as a predictor of survival in patients with cirrhosis. (Abstract) Hepatology 12:850, 1990
31. Barrison IG, et al. Platelet associated immunoglobulins in chronic liver disease. Br J Haematol 48:347, 1981
32. Barry RE, McGivan JD. Acetaldehyde alone may initiate hepatocellular damage in acute alcoholic liver disease. Gut 26:1065, 1985
33. Bassendine MF, et al. Platelet associated immunoglobulins in primary biliary cirrhosis: a cause of thrombocytopenia? Gut 26:1074, 1985
34. Bassett ML, et al. Genetic hemochromatosis. Semin Liver Dis 4:217, 1984
35. Baunsgaard P, et al. The variation of pathological changes in the liver evaluated by double biopsies. Acta Pathol Microbiol 87:51, 1979
36. Baxter JN, Dobbs BR. Portal hypertensive gastropathy. J Gastroenterol Hepatol 3:635, 1988
37. Bean WB. The cutaneous arterial spider. Medicine (Baltimore) 24:243, 1945
38. Beaugrand M, et al. Tous les inhibiteurs calciques peuvent-ils entrainer des lesions d'hepatite alcoolique? Gastroenterol Clin Biol 1:76, 1987
39. Benoit JN, et al. Role of humoral factors in the intestinal hyperemia associated with chronic portal hypertension. Am J Physiol 247:G486, 1984
40. Beppu K, et al. Prediction of variceal hemorrhage by esophageal endoscopy. Gastrointest Endosc 27:213, 1981

41. Beppu K, Japanese Research Society for Portal Hypertension. The general rules for recording endoscopic findings on oesophageal varices. Jpn J Surg 10:84, 1980

42. Berger LA, et al. The ultrasonic demonstration of portacaval shunts. Br J Surg 66:166, 1979

43. Berkson J. Limitations of the application of fourfold table analysis to hospital data. Biometric Bull 2:47, 1946

44. Berman M, et al. The chronic sequelae of non A non B hepatitis. Ann Intern Med 91:1, 1979

45. Bernthal AC, et al. Primary pulmonary hypertension after portacaval shunt. J Clin Gastroenterol 5:353, 1983

46. Berthelot P, et al. Arterial changes in the lungs in cirrhosis of the liver—lung spider nevi. N Engl J Med 274:291, 1966

47. Bircher J, et al. The significance of liver volume in patients with cirrhosis. In: Presis R, Paumgartner G, eds. The liver: quantitative aspects of structure and function. Basel, S Karger, 1973, p 87

48. Blake JC, et al. Bleeding time in patients with hepatic cirrhosis. Br Med J 301:12, 1990

49. Blei AT, et al. Insulin resistance and insulin receptors in hepatic cirrhosis. Gastroenterology 83:1191, 1982

50. Blum K, et al. Allelic association of human dopamine D2 receptor gene in alcoholism. JAMA 263:2055, 1990

51. Bode JC, et al. High incidence of antibodies to hepatitis C virus in alcoholic cirrhosis: fact or fiction? Alcohol Alcohol 26:111, 1991

52. Boitnott JK, Maddrey WC. Alcoholic liver disease. I. Interrelationships among histologic features and the histologic effects of prednisolone therapy. Hepatology 1:599, 1981

53. Bonnin H, et al. Enlarged parotid glands in alcoholic cirrhosis. Pressé Med 62:1449, 1954

54. Bouchier IAD. Postmortem study of the frequency of gallstones in patients with cirrhosis of the liver. Gut 10:705, 1969

55. Boyer JL, Klatskin G. Pattern of necrosis in acute viral hepatitis: prognostic value of bridging (subacute hepatic necrosis). N Engl J Med 283:1063, 1970

56. Boyer TD, et al. Direct transhepatic measurement of portal vein pressure using a thin needle: comparison with wedged hepatic vein pressure. Gastroenterology 72:584, 1977

57. Bras G, et al. Cirrhosis of the liver in Jamaica. J Pathol Bacteriol 82:503, 1961

58. Bredfeldt JE, Groszmann RJ. Hemodynamic aspects of portal hypertension: the effect of increased intraabdominal pressure. In: Epstein M, ed. The kidney in liver disease, ed 2. New York, Elsevier, 1983, p 281

59. Brenner DA, Alcorn JM. Therapy for hepatic fibrosis. Semin Liver Dis 10:75, 1990

60. Brick IB. Parotid enlargement in cirrhosis of the liver. Ann Intern Med 49:438, 1958

61. Brock JF, Hansen JDL. The aetiology of kwashiorkor. Leech 37:35, 1958

62. Bruguera M, et al. Giant mitochondria in hepatocytes: a diagnostic hint for alcoholic liver disease. Gastroenterology 73:1383, 1977

63. Bruix J, et al. Effects of prostaglandin inhibition on systemic and hepatic hemodynamics in patients with cirrhosis of the liver. Gastroenterology 88:430, 1985

64. Buligescu L, et al. Study of the prognosis factors in liver cirrhosis. Med Interne 25:157, 1987

65. Burra P, et al. Peptic ulcer and liver cirrhosis. Minerva Med 81:119, 1990

66. Calabresi P, Abelman WH. Portacaval and portopulmonary anastomosis in Laënnec's cirrhosis and heart failure. J Clin Invest 36:1257, 1957

67. Caldwell PRB, et al. Oxyhemoglobin dissociation curve in liver disease. J Appl Physiol 20:316, 1965

68. Carey JB Jr, et al. The metabolism of bile acids with special reference to liver injury. Medicine (Baltimore) 45:461, 1966

69. Castell DO, Johnson RB. ^{198}Au liver scan: an index of portalsystemic collateral circulation in chronic liver disease. N Engl J Med 275:188, 1966

70. Caturelli E, et al. Cruveilhier-Baumgarten syndrome without esophageal varices. J Clin Gastroenterol 11:357, 1989

71. Cavallo-Perin P, et al. On the mechanism of insulin resistance in human liver cirrhosis: evidence of a combined receptor and postreceptor defect. J Clin Invest 75:1659, 1985

72. Cavanaugh J, et al. Gynecomastia and cirrhosis of the liver. Arch Intern Med 150:563, 1990

73. Chadwick RG, et al. Chronic persistent hepatitis: hepatitis B virus markers and histological follow-up. Gut 20:372, 1979

74. Chalmers TC, et al. Clinical estimation of liver and spleen size. In: Presis R, Paumgartner G, eds. The liver: quantitative aspects of structure and function. Basel, S Karger, 1973, p 76

75. Chedid A, et al. Significance of megamitochondria in alcoholic liver disease. Gastroenterology 90:1858, 1986

76. Chedid A, et al. Prognostic factors in alcoholic liver disease. VA Cooperative Study Group. Am J Gastroenterol 86:210, 1991

77. Chey WY, et al. Effects of chronic administration of ethanol on the liver of dogs. Gastroenterology 65:533, 1973

78. Child CG III, Turcotte JG. Surgery and portal hypertension. *In* Child CG III, ed. The liver and portal hypertension. Philadelphia, WB Saunders, 1964, p 50

79. Child CG, et al. Pancreatico-duodenectomy with resection of the portal vein in the Macaca mulatta monkey and in man. Surg Gynecol Obstet 94:31, 1952

80. Christensen E, et al. Prognosis after the first episode of gastrointestinal bleeding or coma in cirrhosis: survival and prognostic factors. Scand J Gastroenterol 24:999, 1989

81. Clinical NMR Group. Magnetic resonance imaging of parenchymal liver disease: a comparison with ultrasound, radionuclide scintigraphy and x-ray computed tomography. Clin Radiol 38:495, 1987

82. Cochrane AMG, et al. Lymphocyte cytotoxicity for isolated hepatocytes in alcoholic liver disease. Gastroenterology 72:918, 1977

83. Coe RO, Bull FE. Cirrhosis and methotrexate treatment of psoriasis. JAMA 206:1515, 1968

84. Cohen C, et al. Alcoholics and liver transplantation. JAMA 265:1299, 1991

85. Cohen JA, Kaplan MM. The SGOT-SGPT ratio: an indicator of alcoholic liver disease. Dig Dis Sci 24:835, 1979

85a. Cohen MB, et al. Complications of percutaneous liver biopsy in children. Gastroenterology 102:528, 1992

86. Cohen S, Soloway RD, eds. Chronic active liver disease. New York, Churchill Livingstone, 1982

87. Comroe JH. Physiology of respiration, ed 2. Chicago, Year Book Medical Publishers, 1974

88. Conn HO. Asterixis in nonhepatic disorders. Am J Med 29:647, 1960

89. Conn HO. Portacaval anastomosis and hepatic hemosiderin deposition: a prospective, controlled investigation. Gastroenterology 62:61, 1972

90. Conn HO. Rational use of liver biopsy in diagnosis of hepatic cancer. Gastroenterology 62:142, 1972

91. Conn HO. Unilateral edema and jaundice following portacaval anastomosis. Ann Intern Med 76:459, 1972

92. Conn HO. Post liver biopsy hematoma and related phenomena. Gastroenterology 67:375, 1974

93. Conn HO. A peek at the Child-Turcotte classification. Hepatology 6:673, 1981

94. Conn HO. Alcohol content of various beverages: all booze is created equal. Hepatology 12:1252, 1990

94a. Conn HO. Liver biopsy: increased risks in patients with cancer. Hepatology 14:206, 1991

95. Conn HO, et al. A comparison of radiologic and esophagoscopic diagnosis of esophageal varices. N Engl J Med 265:160, 1961

96. Conn HO, et al. Balloon tamponade in the radiological diagnosis of esophageal varices. Gastroenterology 50:29, 1966

97. Conn HO, et al. Fiberoptic and conventional esophagoscopy

in the diagnosis of esophageal varices: a comparison of techniques and observers. Gastroenterology 52:810, 1967

98. Conn HO, et al. Cirrhosis and diabetes. I. Increased incidence of diabetes in patients with Laënnec's cirrhosis. Am J Dig Dis 14:837, 1969

99. Conn HO, et al. Cirrhosis and diabetes. II. Association of impaired glucose tolerance with portal-systemic shunting in Laënnec's cirrhosis. Am J Dig Dis 16:227, 1971

100. Conn HO, et al. The naked physician: the blind interpretation of liver function tests in the differential diagnosis of jaundice. In: Preisig R, Bircher J, eds. The liver: quantitative aspects of structure and function. Aulendorf, Editio Cantor, 1979, p 386

101. Conn HO, et al. Propranolol in the prevention of the first hemorrhage from esophageal varices. Hepatology 13:902, 1991

102. Cook GC, Hutt MS. The liver after kwashiorkor. Br Med J [Clin Res] 3:454, 1967

103. Copenhagen Study Group for Liver Diseases. Sex, ascites, and alcoholism in survival of patients with cirrhosis: effect of prednisone. N Engl J Med 291:271, 1974

104. Corbishley CM, et al. Use of endoscopic biopsy for diagnosing congestive gastropathy. J Clin Pathol 41:1187, 1988

104a. Corr P, et al. Transjugular biopsy: a review of 200 biopsies. Clin Radiol 45:238, 1992

105. Cosnett JE, et al. Shunt myelopathy: a report of 2 cases. S Afr Med J 62:215, 1982

106. Creutzfeldt W. Klinische beziehungen zwischen diabetes mellitus und leber. Acta Hepatosplenol 6:156, 1959

107. Cruz-Coke R. Colour-blindness and cirrhosis of the liver. Lancet 1:1131, 1965

108. Czaja AJ, Davis GL. Hepatitis non A non B. Mayo Clin Proc 57:639, 1982

109. Dagradi AE. The natural history of esophageal varices in patients with alcoholic liver cirrhosis. An endoscopic and clinical study. Am J Gastroenterol 57:520, 1972

110. D'Amico G, et al. Natural history of congestive gastropathy in cirrhosis. Gastroenterology 99:1158, 1990

111. Daoud FS, et al. Failure of hypoxic vasoconstriction in patients with liver cirrhosis. J Clin Invest 51:1076, 1972

112. Davies PJ. Hepatic syphilis: an historical review. J Gastroenterol Hepatol 3:287, 1988

113. Davis GL. Recombinant α-interferon treatment of non-A, non-B hepatitis: review of studies and recommendations for treatment. J Hepatol 11:S72, 1990

114. Davis GL, et al. Treatment of chronic hepatitis C with recombinant interferon alpha. N Engl J Med 321:1501, 1989

115. Davis HH, et al. Alveolar-capillary oxygen disequilibrium in hepatic cirrhosis. Chest 73:507, 1978

116. Dawson JL. Oesophageal varices: curiosities. Br Med J [Clin Res] 286:826, 1983

117. Degroote J, et al. Long-term follow-up of chronic active hepatitis of moderate severity. Gut 19:510, 1978

118. Dehner LD, et al. Hereditary tyrosinemia type I (chronic form): pathologic findings in the liver. Hum Pathol 20:149, 1989

119. Denk H, Eckerstorfer R. Colchicine-induced Mallory body formation in the mouse. Lab Invest 36:563, 1977

120. Denk H, et al. Hepatocellular hyalin (Mallory bodies) in long term griseofulvin-treated mice: a new experimental model for the study of hyalin formation. Lab Invest 32:773, 1975

121. Denk H, et al. Experimental induction of hepatocellular hyalin (Mallory bodies) in mice by griseofulvin treatment. I. Light microscopic observations. Lab Invest 35:377, 1976

122. Deviere J, et al. Hepatic telangiectasia and cirrhosis. J Clin Gastroenterol 10:111, 1988

123. DeWeert TM, et al. Congestive gastropathy and other upper endoscopic findings in 81 consecutive patients undergoing orthotopic liver transplantation. Am J Gastroenterol 85:573, 1990

124. Diehl AM, et al. Alcohollike liver disease in nonalcoholics. Gastroenterology 95:1056, 1988

125. Dienstag JL. Non A non B hepatitis. I. Recognition, epidemiology, and clinical features. Gastroenterology 85:439, 1983

126. Doehlert CA Jr, et al. Obstructive biliary cirrhosis and alcoholic cirrhosis: comparison of clinical and pathologic features. Am J Clin Pathol 25:902, 1955

127. Doffoel M, et al. Relationship between 34 HLA-A, HLA-B, and HLA-DR antigens in alcoholic cirrhosis. Hepatology 6:457, 1986

127a. Dotter CT. Catheter biopsy: experimental techniques for transvenous biopsy. Radiology 82:312, 1964

128. Doyle FH, et al. Nuclear magnetic resonance imaging of the liver: initial experience. AJR 138:193, 1982

129. Drenick EJ, et al. Effect of hepatic morphology of treatment of obesity by fasting, reducing diets and small-bowel bypass. N Engl J Med 282:829, 1970

130. d'Sant'Agnese PA, Talamo C. Cystic fibrosis of the pancreas. N Engl J Med 277:1287, 1967

131. Dumont AE, Mulholland JH. Flow rate and composition of thoracic duct lymph in patients with cirrhosis. N Engl J Med 263:471, 1960

132. Dunnington G, et al. Natural history of cholelithiasis in patients with alcoholic cirrhosis. Ann Surg 205:226, 1987

133. Dutta SK, et al. Functional and structural changes in parotid glands of alcoholic cirrhosis. Gastroenterology 96:510, 1989

134. Eckardt VF, Grace ND. Gastroesophageal reflux and bleeding esophageal varices. Gastroenterology 76:39, 1978

135. Eddleston ALWF, Davis M. Histocompatibility antigens in alcoholic liver disease. Br Med Bull 38:13, 1982

136. Edington GM. Other viral and infectious diseases. In: Macsween RNM, et al. Pathology of the liver. Edinburgh, Churchill Livingstone, 1979, p 202

137. Eliakim M, et al. Gammopathy in liver disease. In: Popper H, Schaffner F, eds. Progress in liver diseases, vol 4. New York, Grune & Stratton, 1972, p 403

138. Epstein O, et al. Hypertrophic hepatic osteoarthropathy. Am J Med 67:88, 1979

139. Erickson LS, et al. Normalization of ventilation/perfusion relationships after liver transplantation in patients with decompensated cirrhosis: evidence for a hepatopulmonary syndrome. Hepatology 12:1350, 1990

140. Eriksson S, Hagerstrand I. Cirrhosis and malignant hepatoma in an alpha-l-antitrypsin deficiency. Acta Med Scand 195:451, 1974

141. Fagan EA, et al. Multi-organ granulomas and mitochondrial antibodies. N Engl J Med 308:572, 1983

142. Fattovich G, et al. Natural history and prognostic factors for chronic hepatitis B. Gut 32:294, 1991

143. Fauerholdt L, et al. Conversion of micronodular cirrhosis into macronodular cirrhosis. Hepatology 3:928, 1983

144. Feher J, et al. Early syphilitic hepatitis. Lancet 2:896, 1975

145. Feinstein AR. Clinical judgment. Baltimore, Williams & Wilkins, 1967

146. Ferenci P, et al. Serum levels of gamma aminobutyric acid-like activity in patients with acute and chronic hepatocellular diseases. Lancet 1:811, 1983

147. Fessel JM, Conn HO. An analysis of the causes and prevention of hepatic coma. Gastroenterology 62:191, 1972

148. Fessel JM, Conn HO. Lactulose in the treatment of acute hepatic encephalopathy. Am J Med Sci 266:103, 1973

149. Fiaccadori F. La peritonite bacterienne spontanee du cirrhotique. Med Chir Dig 12:167, 1983

150. Fialkow PJ, et al. Cirrhosis and classical genetic color blindness. N Engl J Med 275:584, 1966

151. Finet L, et al. Increased fasting gallbladder volume: a new ultrasound sign of cirrhosis? Gastroenterol Clin Biol 15:676, 1991

152. Fisher MR, Gore RM. Computed tomography in the evaluation of cirrhosis and portal hypertension. J Clin Radiol 7:173, 1985

153. Fleig SW, et al. Upper gastrointestinal hemorrhage from downhill esophageal varices. Dig Dis 27:23, 1982

154. Fleig WE, et al. Is there a hepatogenic ulcer? Prospective study of the incidence of peptic ulcer in portal hypertension. Z Gastroenterol 25(Suppl 3):47, 1987
155. Flood FB. Spontaneous perforation of the umbilicus in Laënnec's cirrhosis with massive ascites. N Engl J Med 264:72, 1961
156. Fonesca V, et al. Hyperparathyroidism and low serum osteocalcin despite vitamin D replacement in primary biliary cirrhosis. J Clin Endocrinol Metab 64:873, 1987
157. Fornari F, et al. Cirrhosis of the liver: a risk factor for the development of cholelithiasis in males. Dig Dis Sci 35:1403, 1990
158. Foutch PG, et al. Cutaneous vascular spiders in cirrhotic patients: correlation with hemorrhage from esophageal varices. Am J Gastroenterol 83:723, 1988
159. Francis JL, Armstrong DJ. Acquired dysfibrogenemia in liver disease. J Clin Pathol 35:667, 1982
160. Franke WW, et al. Ultrastructural, biochemical, and immunologic characterization of Mallory bodies in livers of griseofulvin-treated mice. Lab Invest 40:207, 1979
161. French SW. Nature, pathogenesis, and significance of the Mallory body. Semin Liver Dis 1:217, 1981
162. French SW. Present understanding of the development of Mallory bodies. Arch Pathol Lab Med 107:445, 1983
163. French SW, Nanji AA. Relationship between pork consumption and cirrhosis. Lancet 1:685, 1985
164. French SW, et al. Thick microfilaments (intermediate filaments) and chronic alcohol ingestion. In: Popper H, et al, eds. Membrane alterations as basis of liver injury. Lancaster, England, St. Leonhard's House, MTP Press, 1977, p 311
165. Freund HA. Clinical manifestations and studies in parenchymatous hepatitis. Ann Intern Med 10:1144, 1937
166. Frezza M, et al. High blood alcohol levels in women: the role of decreased gastric alcohol dehydrogenase. N Engl J Med 322:95, 1990
167. Furukawa T, et al. Arterial hypoxemia in patients with hepatic cirrhosis. Am J Med Sci 287:10, 1984
168. Galambos JT. Natural history of alcoholic hepatitis. III. Histological changes. Gastroenterology 63:1026, 1972
169. Galambos JT. Cirrhosis. Philadelphia, WB Saunders 1979, p 357
170. Gall EA. Posthepatitic, postnecrotic and nutritional cirrhosis: a pathological analysis. Am J Pathol 36:241, 1960
171. Gans H, et al. Antiprotease deficiency and familial infantile liver cirrhosis. Surg Gynecol Obstet 129:289, 1969
172. Garceau AJ, et al. The natural history of cirrhosis. I. Survival with esophageal varices. N Engl J Med 268:469, 1963
173. Garceau AJ, et al. The natural history of cirrhosis. II. The influence of alcohol and prior hepatitis on pathology and prognosis. N Engl J Med 271:1173, 1964
174. Gelernter J, et al. No association between an allele at the D2 dopamine receptor gene (DRD2) and alcoholism. JAMA 266:1801, 1991
175. Genesca J, et al. Blood borne non-A, non-B hepatitis: hepatitis C. Semin Liver Dis 11:147, 1991
176. Gerber MA, et al. Hepatocellular hyaline in cholestasis and cirrhosis: its diagnostic significance. Gastroenterology 64:89, 1973
177. Gerety RJ, ed. Hepatitis A. Orlando, Academic Press, 1984
177a. Geubel AP, et al. Liver damage caused by therapeutic vitamin A administration. Gastroenterology 100:1701, 1991
178. Giacobbe A, et al. Peptic ulcer in liver cirrhosis. Minerva Dietol Gastroenterol 36:223, 1990
179. Gibson WR, Robertson HE. So-called biliary cirrhosis. Arch Pathol 28:37, 1939
180. Gilbert SC, et al. Methotrexate-induced cirrhosis requiring liver transplantation in patients with psoriasis. Arch Intern Med 150:889, 1990
181. Gines P, et al. Compensated cirrhosis: natural history and prognostic factors. Hepatology 7:122, 1987

182. Gitnick G. Hepatitis 1990. Scand J Gastroenterol 25(Suppl 175):113, 1990
183. Gluud C, et al. Prognostic indicators in alcoholic cirrhotic men. Hepatology 8:222, 1988
184. Goldblatt H. Report of pathologists on cirrhosis study. Transactions 6th Conference on Liver Injury. New York, Josiah Macy, Jr Foundation, 1947, p 9
185. Goldenberg DA, et al. Unilateral cirrhosis. Dig Dis Sci 26:843, 1981
186. Golding PL, et al. Multisystem involvement in chronic liver disease: studies on the incidence and pathogenesis. Am J Med 55:772, 1973
187. Goldsmith LA. Tyrosinemia and related disorders. In: Stanbury JB, et al, eds. The metabolic basis of inherited disease, ed 5. New York, McGraw-Hill, 1983, p 287
188. Goldstein MJ, et al. Hepatic metastases and portal cirrhosis. Am J Med Sci 252:26, 1966
189. Goodman DS. Vitamin A and retinoids in health and disease. N Engl J Med 310:1023, 1985
190. Gottardello L, et al. Ulcer and hepatic cirrhosis. Minerva Med 82:81, 1991
191. Govindarajans S, et al. Alpha-1-antitrypsin phenotypes in hepatocellular carcinoma. Hepatology 1:628, 1981
192. Goyal AK, et al. Ultrasonic diagnosis of cirrhosis: reference to quantitative measurements of hepatic dimensions. Gastrointest Radiol 15:32, 1990
193. Grace WJ, et al. Chest hair and cirrhosis of the liver. Am J Dig Dis 7:913, 1962
194. Grant BF, et al. Epidemiology of alcoholic liver disease. Semin Liver Dis 8:12, 1988
195. Graudal N, et al. The prognostic significance of bacteremia in hepatic cirrhosis. Liver 7:138, 1987
196. Greene HL. Glycogen storage disease. Semin Liver Dis 2:291, 1982
197. Greene HL, et al. A new variant of type IV glycogenosis. Hepatology 8:302, 1988
198. Groszmann RJ, et al. Wedged and free hepatic venous pressure measured with a balloon catheter. Gastroenterology 76:253, 1979
199. Groszmann RJ, et al. Hemodynamic events in a prospective randomized trial of propranolol vs placebo in the prevention of the first variceal hemorrhage. Gastroenterology 99:1401, 1990
200. Hadengue A, et al. Pulmonary hypertension complicating portal hypertension: prevalence and relation to splanchnic hemodynamics. Gastroenterology 100:520, 1991
201. Hahn RD. Syphilis of the liver. Am J Syphilis 27:529, 1943
202. Haines NW, et al. Prognostic indicators of hepatic injury following jejunoileal bypass for refractory obesity: a prospective study. Hepatology 1:161, 1981
203. Hallén J, Kroak H. Follow-up studies on unselected ten year material of 360 patients with liver cirrhosis in one community. Acta Med Scand 173:479, 1963
204. Hällen J, Norden J. Liver cirrhosis unsuspected during life: a series of 79 cases. J Chronic Dis 17:951, 1964
205. Halstead CH, et al. Intestinal malabsorption in folate-deficient alcoholics. Gastroenterology 64:526, 1973
206. Harbin WP, et al. Diagnosis of cirrhosis based on regional changes in hepatic morphology. Radiology 135:273, 1980
207. Hardwick DF, Dimmick JE. Metabolic cirrhoses of infancy and early childhood. In: Rosenberg HS, Bolande RP, eds. Perspectives in pediatric pathology, vol 3. Chicago, Year Book Publications, 1976, p 103
208. Harinasuta U, Zimmerman HJ. Alcoholic steatonecrosis. I. Relationship between severity of hepatic disease and presence of Mallory bodies in liver. Gastroenterology 60:1036, 1971
209. Hartroft WS. Experimental reproduction of human hepatic disease. In: Popper H, Schaffner F, eds. Progress in liver disease, vol 1. New York, Grune & Stratton, 1961, p 68
210. Hashizume M, et al. Morphology of gastric microcirculation in cirrhosis. Hepatology 3:1008, 1983

211. Hein MF, et al. The effect of portacaval shunting on gastric secretion in cirrhotic dogs. Gastroenterology 44:637, 1963

212. Heinemann HO. Respiration and circulation in patients with portal cirrhosis of the liver. Circulation 22:154, 1960

213. Heinemann HO, et al. Hyperventilation and arterial hypoxemia in cirrhosis of the liver. Am J Med 28:239, 1960

214. Helman R, et al. Alcoholic hepatitis: natural history and evaluation of prednisolone therapy. Ann Intern Med 74:311, 1971

215. Helwig FC, Schutz CB. A liver kidney syndrome: clinical, pathological and experimental studies. Surg Gynecol Obstet 55:570, 1932

216. Himsworth HP, Glynn LE. Massive hepatic necrosis and diffuse hepatic fibrosis (acute yellow atrophy and portal cirrhosis): their production by means of diet. Clin Sci 5:93, 1944

217. Himsworth HP, Glynn LE. Toxipathic and trophopathic hepatitis. Lancet 1:457, 1944

218. Hislop WS, et al. Serological markers of hepatitis B in patients with alcoholic liver disease: a multi-centre survey. J Clin Pathol 34:1017, 1981

219. Ho SS, et al. Hepatocellular carcinoma with cardiac cirrhosis. Med J Aust 152:553, 1990

220. Hobbs CL, et al. Peritoneovenous shunt for hydrothorax associated with ascites. Arch Surg 117:1233, 1982

221. Hocking HP, et al. Late hepatic histology after jejunoileal bypass for morbid obesity: relation of abnormalities on biopsy and clinical course. Am J Surg 141:159, 1981

222. Hocking HP, et al. Jejunoileal bypass for morbid obesity: late follow-up in 100 cases. N Engl J Med 30:995, 1983

223. Hodges R Jr, et al. Heterozygous MZ alpha-1-antitrypsin deficiency in adults with chronic active hepatitis and cryptogenic cirrhosis. N Engl J Med 304:557, 1981

224. Hosking SW, et al. The role of propranolol in congestive gastropathy of portal hypertension. Hepatology 7:437, 1987

225. Hosking SW, et al. Anorectal varices, hemorrhoids, and portal hypertension. Lancet 1:349, 1989

226. Huaux JP, et al. Hypertrophic osteoarthropathy related to end stage cholestatic cirrhosis: reversal after liver transplantation. Ann Rheum Dis 46:342, 1987

227. Igidbashian VN, et al. Hepatic ultrasound. Semin Liver Dis 9:16, 1989

228. Infante-Rivard C, et al. Clinical and statistical validity of conventional prognostic factors in predicting short term survival among cirrhotics. Hepatology 7:660, 1987

229. Ishak KG, Sharp HL. Metabolic errors and liver disease. In: MacSween R, et al, eds. Pathology of the liver. Edinburgh, Churchill Livingstone, 1979, p 28

230. Ishak KG, et al. Cirrhosis of the liver associated with alpha-1-antitrypsin deficiency. Arch Pathol 94:445, 1972

231. Ishak KG, et al. Alcoholic liver disease: pathologic, pathogenetic and clinical aspects. Alcohol Clin Exp Res 15:45, 1991

232. Israel Y, et al. Thyroid hormones in alcoholic liver disease. Gastroenterology 76:116, 1979

233. Israel Y, et al. Immune response to alcohol metabolites: pathogenic and diagnostic implications. Semin Liver Dis 8:81, 1988

234. Italian Liver Cirrhosis Project. Reliability of endoscopy in the assessment of variceal features. J Hepatol 4:93, 1987

235. Itoh S, et al. Nonalcoholic fatty liver with alcoholic hyaline after long-term glucocorticoid therapy. Acta Hepatogastroenterol 24:415, 1977

236. Jeffers LJ, et al. Post transfusion non B hepatitis resulting in cirrhosis of the liver. Hepatology 1:521, 1981

237. Jezequel AM. Dimethylnitrosamine-induced cirrhosis: evidence for an immunological mechanism. J Hepatol 8:42, 1989

238. Johnson RF, Loo RV. Hepatic hydrothorax: studies to determine the source of the fluid and report of thirteen cases. Ann Intern Med 61:385, 1964

239. Johnston DG, et al. Hyperinsulinism of hepatic cirrhosis: diminished degradation or hypersecretion? Lancet 1:10, 1977

240. Jolivet J, et al. The pharmacologic and clinical use of methotrexate. N Engl J Med 309:1094, 1983

241. Jolliffe N, Jellinek EM. Vitamin deficiencies and liver cirrhosis in alcoholism. VII. Cirrhosis of the liver. Q J Stud Alcohol 2:544, 1941

242. Jorge-Hernandez JA, et al. Bone changes in alcoholic liver cirrhosis: a histomorphometrical analysis of 52 cases. Dig Dis Sci 33:1089, 1988

243. Jozsa L, et al. Hepatitis syphilitica: a clinico-pathological study of 25 cases. Acta Hepato-Gastroenterol 2:344, 1977

244. Kakumu S, Leevy CM. Lymphocyte cytotoxicity in alcoholic hepatitis. Gastroenterology 72:594, 1977

245. Kan YW, et al. Further observations on polycythemia in hepatocellular carcinoma. Blood 18:592, 1961

246. Kanagasundaram N, et al. Alcoholic hyalin antigen (AHAg) and antibody (AHAb) in alcoholic hepatitis. Gastroenterology 73:1368, 1977

247. Kane RA, Katz SG. The spectrum of sonographic findings in portal hypertension: a subject review and new observations. Radiology 142:453, 1982

248. Kaplan MM. Methotrexate treatment of chronic cholestatic liver disease: friend or foe? Q J Med 72:757, 1989

249. Kaplan MM. Methotrexate hepatotoxicity and the premature reporting of Mark Twain's death: both greatly exaggerated. Hepatology 12:784, 1990

250. Kardel T, et al. Hepatic neuropathy: a clinical and electrophysiologic study. Acta Neurol Scand 50:513, 1974

251. Karmi G, et al. The association of syphilis with hepatic cirrhosis: a report of six cases and review of literature. Postgrad Med J 45:675, 1969

252. Karsner HT. Morphology and pathogenesis of hepatic cirrhosis. Am J Clin Pathol 13:569, 1943

253. Kaunitz JD, Lindenbaum J. The bioavailability of folic acid added to wine. Ann Intern Med 87:542, 1977

254. Keeffe EB. Sarcoidosis and primary biliary cirrhosis: literature review and illustrative case. Am J Med 83:977, 1987

255. Keller AZ. The epidemiology of lip, oral and pharyngeal cancers and the association with selected systemic diseases. Am J Public Health 53:1214, 1963

256. Keller AZ. Cirrhosis of the liver, alcoholism and heavy smoking associated with cancer of the mouth and pharynx. Cancer 20:1015, 1967

257. Keller AZ, Terris M. The association of alcohol and tobacco with cancer of the mouth and pharynx. Am J Public Health 55:1578, 1965

258. Kelly DA, Summerfield JA. Hemostasis in liver disease. Semin Liver Dis 7:182, 1987

259. Kennedy TC, Knudson RJ. Exercise aggravated hypoxemia and orthodeoxia in cirrhosis. Chest 72:305, 1977

260. Keren G, et al. Pulmonary arterio-venous fistula in hepatic cirrhosis. Arch Dis Child 58:302, 1983

261. Kershenobich D, et al. Treatment of cirrhosis with colchicine: a double-blind randomized trial. Gastroenterology 77:532, 1979

262. Kershenobich D, et al. Treatment of liver cirrhosis with colchicine: a double blind randomized trial from 1973 to 1983. (Abstract) Hepatology 4:1061, 1984

263. Kershenobich, et al. Colchicine in the treatment of cirrhosis of the liver. N Engl J Med 318:1709, 1988

264. Keys A, Snell AM. Respiratory properties of the arterial blood in normal man and in patients with disease of the liver: position of the oxygen dissociation curve. J Clin Invest 17:59, 1938

265. Killip T III, Payne MA. High serum transaminase activity in heart disease, circulatory failure and hepatic necrosis. Circulation 21:646, 1960

266. Kirch W, et al. Parathyroid hormone and cirrhosis of the liver. J Clin Endocrinol Metab 71:1561, 1990

267. Kirk AP, et al. Peptic ulceration in patients with chronic liver disease. Dig Dis 25:756, 1980

268. Klain J, et al. Liver histology abnormalities in the morbidly obese. Hepatology 10:873, 1989

269. Klatskin G. Subacute hepatic necrosis and postnecrotic cirrhosis due to anicteric infections with the hepatitis virus. Am J Med 25:333, 1958

270. Klatskin G. Alcohol and its relation to liver damage. Gastroenterology 41:443, 1961

271. Klatskin G. Toxic and drug-induced hepatitis. In: Schiff L, ed. Diseases of the liver. Philadelphia, JB Lippincott, 1969, p 517

272. Klatsky AL, et al. Alcohol consumption and blood pressure. N Engl J Med 296:1194, 1977

273. Kley HK, et al. Effect of testosterone application on hormone concentrations of androgens and estrogens in male patients with cirrhosis of the liver. Gastroenterology 76:235, 1979

274. Knapp AB, et al. Cirrhosis as a consequence of graft-versus-host disease. Gastroenterology 92:513, 1987

275. Knill-Jones RP, et al. Peripheral neuropathy in chronic liver disease: clinical, electrodiagnostic, and nerve biopsy findings. J Neurol Neurosurg Psychiatry 35:22, 1972

276. Knodell RG, et al. Development of chronic liver disease after acute non A non B post-transfusion hepatitis. Gastroenterology 72:902, 1977

277. Koretz RL. The long-term course of non A, non B post-transfusion hepatitis. Dig Dis Sci 79:893, 1980

278. Koretz RL, et al. Non A non B post transfusion hepatitis. Disaster after decades? Hepatology 2:687, 1982

279. Kountouras J, et al. Prolonged bile duct obstruction: a new experimental model for cirrhosis in the rat. Br J Exp Pathol 65:305, 1984

280. Krowka MJ, Cortese DA. Pulmonary aspects of chronic liver disease and liver transplantation. Mayo Clin Proc 60:407, 1985

281. Krowka MJ, Cortese DA. Pulmonary aspects of chronic liver disease and liver transplantation. Clin Chest Med 10:593, 1989

282. Krowka MJ, Cortese DA. Hepatopulmonary syndrome: an evolving perspective in the era of liver transplantation. Hepatology 11:138, 1990

283. Kroyer JM, Talbert W. Morphologic liver changes in intestinal bypass patients. Am J Surg 139:855, 1980

284. Kumar S, et al. Orthotopic liver transplantation for alcoholic liver disease. Hepatology 11:159, 1990

285. Kuo G, et al. An assay for circulating antibodies to a major etiologic virus of human non-A, non-B hepatitis. Science 244:362, 1989

286. Laënnec RTH. Traité de l'auscultation mediate. Paris, Chaude, 1826, p 196

287. Laffi G, et al. Evidence for a storage pool defect in platelets from cirrhosis with defective aggregation. Gastroenterology 103:641, 1992

288. Lanse SB, et al. Low incidence of hepatotoxicity associated with long-term, low-dose methotrexate in treatment of refractory psoriasis, psoriatic arthritis, and rheumatoid arthritis: an acceptable risk benefit ratio. Dig Dis Sci 30:104, 1985

289. Larsson C. Natural history and life expectancy in severe alpha anti-trypsin, Pi Z. Acta Med Scand 204:345, 1978

290. Lauterburg BH, Bilzer M. Mechanisms of acetaldehyde hepatotoxicity. J Hepatol 7:384, 1988

291. Lazarides E. Intermediate filaments: a chemically heterogeneous, developmentally regulated class of proteins. Annu Rev Biochem 51:219, 1982

292. Leavitt S, Tyler HR. Studies in asterixis. Arch Neurol 10:360, 1964

293. Lebovics E, et al. Portal-systemic myelopathy after portacaval shunt surgery. Arch Intern Med 145:1921, 1985

294. Lebrec D, et al. Pulmonary hypertension complicating portal hypertension. Am Rev Respir Dis 120:849, 1979

295. Lebrec D, et al. Propranolol for prevention of recurrent gastrointestinal bleeding in patients with cirrhosis. N Engl J Med 305:1371, 1981

296. Lebrec D, et al. Transvenous liver biopsy: an experience based on 1000 hepatic tissue samplings with this procedure. Gastroenterology 83:330, 1982

297. Lebrec D, et al. A randomized controlled study of propranolol for prevention of recurrent gastrointestinal bleeding in patients with cirrhosis: a final report. Hepatology 4:355, 1984

298. Ledermann S. In: Alcohol, Alcoolisme, Alcoholisation. Institut national d'etudes demographiques, Travaux et Documents, Cahier No. 14. Paris, Presses Universitaires de France, 1964

299. Lee RV, et al. Liver disease associated with secondary syphilis. N Engl J Med 284:1423, 1971

300. Leevy CM, et al. Disease of the liver and biliary tract: standardization of nomenclature, diagnostic criteria, and diagnostic methodology. Fogarty International Center Proceedings, No. 22, DHEW Publication No. (NIH) 76–225. Washington DC, US Government Printing Office, 1976

301. Lefkowitch JH, Fenoglio JJ Jr. Liver disease in alcoholic cardiomyopathy: evidence against cirrhosis. Hum Pathol 14:457, 1983

302. Lefkowitch JH, et al. Hepatic copper overload and featuring Indian childhood cirrhosis in an American sibship. N Engl J Med 307:271, 1982

303. Lelbach WK. Organic pathology related to volume and pattern of alcohol use. In: Gibbons RJ, et al, eds. Research advances in alcohol and drug problems, vol 1. New York, John Wiley & Sons, 1974

304. Lemmer JH, et al. Management of spontaneous umbilical hernia disruption in the cirrhotic patient. Ann Surg 198:30, 1983

305. Lemon SM. Type A viral hepatitis: new developments in an old disease. N Engl J Med 313:1059, 1985

306. Leo MA, et al. Effect of hepatic vitamin A depletion on the liver in men and rats. Gastroenterology 84:562, 1983

307. Leonetti JP, et al. Umbilical herniorraphy in cirrhotic patients. Arch Surg 119:442, 1984

308. LeVeen HH, et al. Management of ascites with hydrothorax. Am J Surg 148:210, 1984

309. Levy M. Sodium retention and ascites formation in dogs with experimental portal cirrhosis. Am J Physiol 233:F572, 1977

310. Levy M, Wexler MJ. Renal sodium retention ascites formation in dogs with experimental cirrhosis but without portal hypertension or increased splanchnic vascular capacity. J Lab Clin Med 91:520, 1978

311. Lewis JH, et al. Histopathologic analysis of suspected amiodarone hepatotoxicity. Hum Pathol 21:59, 1990

312. Liaw YF, et al. The development of cirrhosis in patients with chronic type B hepatitis: a prospective study. Hepatology 8:493, 1988

313. Lieber CS. Medical disorders of alcoholism: pathogenesis and treatment. New York, WB Saunders, 1982

314. Lieber CS. Alcohol and the liver. 1984 update. Hepatology 4:1243, 1984

315. Lieber CS. Alcohol-nutrition interaction: 1984 update. Alcohol 1:151, 1984

316. Lieber CS. Biochemical and molecular basis of alcohol-induced injury to liver and other tissues. N Engl J Med 319:1639, 1988

317. Lieber CS. Interaction of alcohol with other drugs and nutrients. Drugs 40(Suppl 3):23, 1990

318. Lieber CS. Mechanism of ethanol induced hepatic injury. Pharmacol Ther 46:1, 1990

319. Lieber CS, Rubin E. Alcoholic fatty liver. N Engl J Med 280:705, 1969

320. Lieber CS, et al. Alcohol and cancer. Hepatology 6:1005, 1986

321. Lieber MM. The rare occurrence of metastatic carcinoma in the cirrhotic liver. Am J Med Sci 233:145, 1957

322. Lieberman FL, Peters RL. Cirrhotic hydrothorax: further evidence that an acquired diaphragmatic defect is at fault. Arch Intern Med 125:14, 1970

Diseases of the Liver, Seventh Edition, edited by
Leon Schiff and Eugene R. Schiff. J.B. Lippincott Company, Philadelphia © 1993.

33

Portal Hypertension

Paul Genecin

Roberto J. Groszmann

Portal hypertension is the hemodynamic abnormality most frequently associated with serious liver disease, although it also is recognized less commonly in a variety of extrahepatic diseases. Many of the most lethal complications of liver disease are related directly to the presence of portal hypertension, including ascites, portosystemic encephalopathy, and hemorrhage from gastroesophageal varices. This chapter focuses on the pathogenesis of portal hypertension and the diseases that cause it. In addition, variceal hemorrhage and the assessment and medical management of portal hypertension are discussed in detail. The reader is referred to separate chapters that examine the other clinical consequences of this important syndrome. In addition, some of the diseases mentioned in this chapter are discussed in greater detail elsewhere. For anatomy of the portal venous system, see Chapter 1.

DEFINITION OF PORTAL HYPERTENSION

Portal hypertension is defined as a portal vein pressure in excess of the normal 5 to 10 mmHg. Direct measurement of portal pressure is difficult and portal pressure usually is estimated indirectly, as discussed later in greater detail.

Pathogenesis: Resistance and Flow

It is the aim of this section on pathophysiology to provide an overview of the circulatory derangements observed in portal hypertension. An understanding of this pathophysiology gives us a framework for understanding existing pharmacologic therapies for portal hypertension and for devising rational investigational strategies.

Ohm's law states that changes in pressure $(P_1 - P_2)$ along a blood vessel are a function of the interplay between blood flow (Q) and vascular resistance (R):

$$P_1 - P_2 = Q \times R \qquad (1)$$

The pathophysiology of portal hypertension is best approached by analyzing these components separately, although mathematical formulas necessarily oversimplify the complex and dynamic interactions that exist in biologic systems.

RESISTANCE

Resistance to the flow of blood in vessels can be expressed by Pouseuille's law:

$$R = \frac{8nL}{\pi r^4} \qquad (2)$$

where:
n = coefficient of viscosity; L = length of the vessel; and r = its radius

Under physiologic conditions, resistance is mainly a function of changes in r, which have a dramatic influence because these are taken to the fourth power. In contrast, L and n basically are constant because neither the length of a vessel nor the viscosity of blood vary greatly under usual circumstances.

The liver is the main site of resistance to portal blood flow. The normal liver may be conceptualized as a huge and distensible vascular network with very low resistance. The liver itself has no active role in regulating portal inflow; this function is provided by resistance vessels at the splanchnic arteriolar level. Hence, the liver is a passive recipient of fluctuating amounts of blood flow that it accommodates by capillary recruitment when flow increases, as in postprandial hyperemia. A normal liver can encompass a wide range of portal blood flow with minimal effect on pressure in the portal system.[141,340]

Early studies of the hepatic vascular system in portal hypertensive states contributed greatly to our understanding of resistance in the pathophysiology of portal hypertension. In McIndoe's 1928 study of corrosion casts of the vascular system in cirrhotic livers, changes in the portohepatic system are vividly described:

One of the most superficially obvious changes is the marked diminution in the total hepatic vascular bed. . . . The main trunks are attenuated and irregularly stenosed, having lost that appearance of robust strength so notable in the normal vessels. Their larger branches are given off at unusually abrupt angles and occasionally show irregular deviation to one side or the other as though pushed or pulled by an invisible force. It is among the finer branches, however, that the more profound alterations are to be seen. The tiny portal veins are distorted beyond belief, twisted and curled on themselves, and finally broken up into a network of stunted venules from which irregularly scattered terminals arise. . . . In the tree of the hepatic vein, the same change is found. . . . It is usually difficult to detect any normal central veins whatever, especially if the cirrhosis is far advanced.[256]

These gross morphologic aberrations in the portal and hepatic venous systems gave rise to the conception of portal hypertension as a vascular obliterative process in which fibrous tissue and regenerative nodules were responsible for increased resistance to the flow of blood.[10,190]

In the past 30 years, our understanding of the role of vascular resistance in the pathogenesis of portal hypertension has become considerably more detailed. Resistance to portal blood flow can be localized anywhere in the venous system, including prehepatic (such as the portal or splenic vein), intrahepatic (presinusoidal, sinusoidal, or postsinusoidal) and posthepatic. Attempts to categorize portal hypertensive syndromes according to classification systems of this type have been clinically useful.[145] Even in the normal liver, however, localization of resistance sites is incompletely understood. Experimental evidence points to various loci, including small portal veins,[382,452] hepatic sinusoids, and terminal hepatic venules.[145,382] This controversy is compounded by uncertainty about whether experimental findings in animal models such as the cat[222] can be extrapolated to humans. Moreover, in most cases, the sites of increased resistance are heterogeneous. Hence, classification of clinical syndromes according to these schemes is convenient but should be approached with caution since neat distinctions tend to dissolve with scrutiny of specific clinical entities.

The site of increased resistance to the flow of blood is defined easily in prehepatic portal hypertensive states such as splenic or portal vein obstruction. Likewise, in the uncommon syndrome of inferior vena cava web or in congestive heart failure, the posthepatic locus of obstruction is defined readily. The situation is far more complex in intrahepatic forms of portal hypertension. In these diseases, there are few pure presinusoidal, sinusoidal, or postsinusoidal lesions. For example, alcoholic liver disease is a heterogeneous collection of disorders with postsinusoidal and sinusoidal areas of obstruction to blood flow. Likewise, hepatic schistosomiasis often is defined as a presinusoidal disease, with granulomas developing in portal areas in response to the presence of parasite eggs.[17] In end-stage schistosomiasis, however, there also may be an elevation in the wedged hepatic venous pressure, reflecting an increase in resistance in the sinusoids, and correlated histologically with collagen deposition in the space of Disse and sinusoidal narrowing.[324]

Alcoholic liver disease has been a fruitful area for the generation of hypotheses about mechanisms of obstruction to the flow of blood in chronic liver disease. As stated previously, investigators initially viewed compression of portal and hepatic venules by fibrosis and regenerative nodules as the mechanism of increased intrahepatic resistance. However, several observations have added complexity to this early point of view. Portal hypertension is well described in noncirrhotic alcoholic liver disease, in the absence of significant fibrosis or regenerative nodules.[107,296] Terminal hepatic vein fibrosis or sclerosis is a histologic lesion characteristic of alcoholic liver injury that is present in noncirrhotic portal hypertensive syndromes including alcoholic hepatitis and steatosis.[108,343] Studies in baboons[237] and humans[135] have correlated development of hepatic vein sclerosis with the presence of portal hypertension. The role of terminal hepatic vein sclerosis in the pathogenesis of portal hypertension is controversial, however. Studies have demonstrated correlation[258] and lack of correlation[295] between pressure and degree of perivenular or terminal hepatic vein fibrosis.

Deposition of collagen in the space of Disse and capillarization of hepatic sinusoids are other characteristic ethanol-related lesions. Electron microscopic examination of biopsy specimens reveals an increase in the amount of collagen in the perisinusoidal space, which normally contains little or no collagen. This may progress to formation of a basement

membrane in the space of Disse, resulting not only in impairment of exchange of nutrients and oxygen between hepatocyte and sinusoid but also in physical encroachment on the sinusoid because of widening of the space of Disse, with consequent increase in sinusoidal vascular resistance.[296,318,367] Capillarization is a term introduced by Schaffner and Popper[367] to describe the dramatic change in the hepatic microcirculation in which the sinusoids evolve from highly permeable capillaries to impermeable membranes that become barriers to the transfer of important metabolic and nutrient products necessary for normal liver function. Capillarization of the sinusoids may also increase vascular resistance by impairing lymphatic drainage and causing widening of the space of Disse due to edema.

Deposition of collagen in the space of Disse has been correlated with the development of portal hypertension in a study by Orrego and colleagues.[295] Seventy alcoholic patients, including 39 without cirrhosis (30 with either normal histology or steatosis and 9 with hepatitis) underwent biopsy with quantitation of collagen in the space of Disse by electron microscopy and measurement of intrahepatic pressure using a Chiba needle. Significant correlation between degree of collagenization of the sinusoids and intrahepatic pressure was demonstrated. These findings are striking in their applicability to the subgroups of patients with noncirrhotic alcoholic liver disease. Even in the absence of fibrosis, regenerative nodules, and alcoholic hyaline, portal hypertension was correlated with a decrease in the diameter of the hepatic sinusoid due to expansion of the space of Disse by collagen. Although the validity of measurement of intrahepatic pressure as a reflection of portal pressure has been questioned,[111] these findings are provocative and have received support in a rat model of cirrhosis induced by carbon tetrachloride and phenobarbital.[334]

Defenestration of the sinusoids results in impaired nutrient and oxygen exchange between sinusoid and hepatocyte.[175,367,431] This barrier to exchange is probably a significant determinant of hepatic dysfunction in cirrhosis. Sinusoidal fenestrations have been found to be susceptible to modulation with drugs in cirrhotic models.[402,469] Research in this field may be another avenue for defining the mechanism of increased vascular resistance in the diseased liver.[146]

The clinical observation that portal hypertension in alcoholic liver disease may improve rapidly with abstinence[342] has prompted investigators to consider factors that are more dynamic than the relatively fixed anatomic lesions discussed above. Orrego and Blendis and colleagues have attempted to correlate the size or surface area of hepatocytes with pressure.[34,295,437] They postulate that hepatocyte enlargement causes encroachment on the sinusoids and thereby increases intrahepatic resistance to the flow of blood. Substances other than alcohol that also increase hepatocyte size have been correlated previously with rises in portal pressure.[88,233] These investigators estimated surface area of hepatocytes by dividing the area of photographs of biopsy specimens by the number of hepatocyte nuclei. In addition, pressure measurements (parenchymal, portal, or wedged hepatic venous) were obtained and found to correlate with hepatocyte surface area in alcoholic but not in nonalcoholic liver disease. Critics of these studies have objected to the methods of estimating cell size and portal pressure.[215,295] Nevertheless, further studies of the role of hepatocyte size in governing sinusoidal diameter and intrahepatic resistance are warranted.

Other hepatic lesions have been postulated to increase vascular resistance at the level of the hepatic sinusoid, including hepatocyte hyperplasia in biliary obstruction.[158]

Intrahepatic resistance also may be modulated by factors that are even more dynamic than flux in the size or number of hepatocytes. As in other vascular beds, sympathetic tone may contribute to portal pressure by a receptor-mediated mechanism.[467] Under normal conditions, sinusoidal perfusion is locally modulated by vascular endothelial cells that relax under the influence of the β_2-adrenergic agonist isoproterenol.[254,325] In the isolated perfused cirrhotic rat liver, isoproterenol decreases perfusion resistance.[249] Moreover, clonidine, which inhibits sympathetic nervous activity, also decreases perfusion pressure in this model, suggesting at least some component of local action on intrahepatic resistance.[249,350] Other vasodilators at high doses have similar effects.[249]

Contractile myofibroblasts have a role in the regulation of perfusion resistance in the isolated perfused liver model.[26] These cells are intermediate in structure between smooth muscle cells and fibroblasts. They proliferate around sinusoids and terminal hepatic venules in cirrhotic livers, and their density may correlate with vascular resistance.[351] Contractile myofibroblasts are thought to arise from Ito cells and also are thought to be the predominant source of collagen synthesis in ethanol-induced liver disease.[262]

Hence, increased resistance to the flow of portal blood is a phenomenon with numerous potential mechanisms and sites of localization. Some may be fixed and others susceptible to modulation by drugs. The study of reversible causes of increased intrahepatic resistance may someday yield new therapeutic agents for lowering portal pressure.

HYPERDYNAMIC FLOW

If blood flow in the portal system were fixed in the face of increased resistance, Ohm's law (equation 1) would mandate an increase in portal pressure. This is the basis for the backward flow theory of portal hypertension, which postulates that the driving force for elevation of portal pressure is increased portal vascular resistance.[465] This theory predicts a congested or hypodynamic circulatory state and seems to gain experimental support from studies in which hypoperfusion of the liver was reported.[266] According to the backward flow theory, the development of portosystemic collaterals would be insufficient to decompress the obstruction to flow created by the abnormally high portal vascular resistance, partly because of elevated portosystemic collateral resistance.[21,213]

In reality, although liver perfusion with portal blood is decreased in portal hypertension, blood flow entering the portal system actually is greatly increased by an increment made up of blood that bypasses the liver in portosystemic shunts, and which is not accounted for in studies that have reported decreased portal flow. There is a marked increase in splanchnic blood flow, with much of this flow shunted around the liver through portosystemic collaterals.[340,445] This hyperkinetic splanchnic circulation has a role in elevating portal pressure and is a factor in the maintenance of portal hypertension, even in the presence of an enormous collateral vascular bed. The development of the collateral circulation and the hyperdynamic splanchnic and systemic circulatory state have received widespread attention in recent years. The most widely studied experimental model is the rat with portal vein stenosis. Portal hypertension develops in this animal model with portosystemic shunting and a hyperdynamic circulatory state that mimic that seen in humans with portal hypertensive liver disease.[22,27,444]

The hyperdynamic circulation is observed in humans[87,203,273,356] and laboratory animals with portal hypertension.[22,232,388,444,445] This circulatory state is characterized by decreased arteriolar resistance, resulting in peripheral vasodilatation in many regional vascular beds, including the splanchnic,[22,27] renal,[444,445] and skeletal muscle circulations.[203,205] Vasodilatation is accompanied by increased cardiac index and regional blood flows.[444] Hyperkinetic blood flow is present in the splanchnic as well as systemic circulations,[87,133] with flow to the intestines, stomach, spleen, and pancreas increased by about 50% above control values.[43,232,444,445] The hyperdynamic circulation manifests in patients as warm, well perfused extremities, bounding pulses, and rapid heart rate, as well a high cardiac index and expanded blood volume.[208,273]

Recognition of the hyperdynamic circulation has led to the forward flow theory,[87,208,444] which postulates that the enormous increase in portal venous inflow cited earlier causes elevation of portal pressure, independent of resistance abnormalities in either the hepatic or portosystemic collateral vascular systems. There is consensus that elevated resistance and hyperdynamic flow contribute to portal hypertension (Fig. 33-1).[21,87,387,388,444,470]

There are several reasons for the intense research interest in the hyperdynamic circulation. The first is its role in the pathogenesis of portal hypertension. The second is that serious consequences of liver disease, including variceal hemorrhage, portosystemic encephalopathy, and ascites may be tied intimately to the presence of these hemodynamic aberrations. Last, nearly all clinically available drugs that reduce portal pressure act by ameliorating the hyperdynamic circulatory state.

The pathogenesis of the hyperdynamic circulation is slowly coming into focus. Several lines of evidence support the existence of one or more circulating vasodilators.[20,205] Such a substance might be rapidly metabolized and highly extracted by the normal liver, but it is present in increased levels in the circulation in liver disease due to portosystemic shunting or hepatocellular dysfunction. Cross-perfusion studies involving isolated hindlimb[205] and ileum[20] preparations of normal rats with blood from portal hypertensive animals resulted in a decrease in arteriolar resistance. However, this was not observed in a parabiotic model involving normal and portal hypertensive rat pairs despite documentation of extensive cross-circulation.[386]

Various vasodilators have been proposed as mediators of the hyperdynamic circulation. In particular, glucagon has been found in increased levels in animals and humans with portal hypertension,[381] and experimental data have been reported in support of a significant role for this peptide, which could mediate up to 40% of the increase in splanchnic blood flow.[20,23] Pharmacologic studies in cirrhotic patients also support a role for glucagon in mediating splanchnic vasodilatation and an increase in portal pressure.[389]

Studies of other substances, among them bile acids[39,131] and prostaglandins,[63,161,393] also have been published, without clearly identifying any single vasodilator with a predominant role in mediating the hyperdynamic circulation in portal hypertension. Recent studies[231a,384a] suggest that the

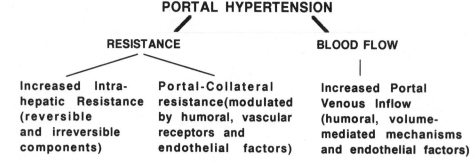

PORTAL HYPERTENSION

RESISTANCE   BLOOD FLOW

Increased Intra-   Portal-Collateral   Increased Portal
hepatic Resistance   resistance(modulated   Venous Inflow
(reversible   by humoral, vascular   (humoral, volume-
and irreversible   receptors and   mediated mechanisms
components)   endothelial factors)   and endothelial factors)

FIGURE 33-1 Factors involved in the maintenance of portal hypertension.

endothelium-derived relaxing factors such as nitric oxide may be an important component of the vasodilatory mechanism observed in portal hypertension.

Vasodilatation also may be mediated by an alteration in vascular responsiveness to pressors. A variety of studies have documented a decrease in reactivity of resistance vessels to several vasoconstrictors, including norepinephrine,[193] angiotensin,[345] and vasopressin.[345] The mechanism of decreased vascular reactivity to pressors may be down-regulation of receptors in response to increased circulating levels of vasoconstrictors such as norepinephrine and angiotensin. Circulating vasodilators and endothelial factors also may act as functional antagonists at effector sites.[201,345,384b]

Vasodilatation is central to the development of the hyperdynamic circulation, but it may not be the only condition necessary for the development of this hemodynamic syndrome. In fact, in normal humans and experimental animals, many vasodilators, while reducing peripheral resistance, cause an increase in vascular capacitance with relative vascular underfilling. This results in a decrease, or more frequently, no change in systemic blood flow.[137,299,405] Expansion of plasma volume, which has long been observed in portal hypertensive liver disease,[246,273] may be the other key factor. Studies in rats with portal vein stenosis point to a role for plasma volume expansion in the development of the hyperdynamic circulation.[132] Chronic dietary sodium restriction hinders the expansion of the plasma volume, and in turn, blunts the expression of the hyperdynamic syndrome. Marked reductions in systemic and splanchnic blood flow are observed with resulting reduction in portal pressure, underscoring the importance of hyperdynamic splanchnic blood flow in maintaining portal hypertension in this experimental model. Moreover, a reduction in plasma volume by introduction of dietary sodium restriction at the height of the hyperdynamic circulation demonstrates that systemic and splanchnic hyperemia, together with portal pressure elevation, are partially reversible. Further study of the interaction of sodium metabolism, plasma volume, and vasodilatation in the evolution of the hyperdynamic circulation are in progress, and these studies undoubtedly will be extrapolated to the clinical setting (see Fig. 33-1).

Clinical Hemodynamic Assessment

PORTAL PRESSURE

With increasing interest in therapeutic modalities for variceal hemorrhage, measurement of portal vein pressure (PVP) has much more than academic interest. Techniques for measur-

ing PVP are divided into two categories: direct and indirect. The most commonly used procedure is the indirect measurement of the hepatic vein pressure gradient (HVPG). Most of this discussion is devoted to this technique.

INDIRECT TECHNIQUES FOR MEASUREMENT OF PORTAL PRESSURE

The gradient (HVPG) between the wedged hepatic vein pressure (WHVP) and free hepatic vein pressure (FHVP) is measured by catheterization of the hepatic vein, usually with a balloon-tipped catheter[121,145,150] (Fig. 33-2). This technique is indirect because HVPG actually is a measure of pressure in the hepatic sinusoids and not the portal vein, as discussed later. A fluid-filled catheter is introduced into an antecubital or femoral vein and advanced under fluoroscopic guidance into a hepatic vein. Here it is wedged until it completely occludes a hepatic vein branch and forms a continuous column of fluid between the catheter and the blood in the vein, the sinusoid, and the portal vein. The WHVP works by the same principle as the wedged pulmonary artery pressure, which is obtained by balloon catheterization of the pulmonary artery, and which is used as an index of left atrial pressure.[121] The rate of successful hepatic vein catheterization is greater than 95%, and the procedure has been shown to be extremely safe.[50,150]

In normal liver, the sinusoidal network dissipates some of the pressure from the wedged catheter. In this situation, the static column of blood formed by the occluding balloon results in a pressure reading slightly lower than actual portal pressure (Fig. 33-3). In presinusoidal causes of portal hypertension, the catheter is not in continuity with the area of increased resistance. Therefore, the recorded pressure is that of the normal sinusoids and not of the area of increased pressure.[145] This is true to a variable degree in nonalcoholic cirrhosis (particularly in macronodular cirrhosis), because of increased presinusoidal resistance.[53,315] In these cases, HVPG underestimates PVP. In alcoholic cirrhosis, connections between sinusoids are decreased because of attenuation of the vascular bed. HVPG is virtually equal to PVP because there is little dissipation of pressure in the wedged sinusoids.[53,315,433] In pure postsinusoidal portal hypertension, the HVPG should correlate well with PVP. There are limited hemodynamic data in clinical syndromes of this type, however.

A clarification of the effect of intraabdominal pressure on PVP is important in understanding the concept of the HVPG. The pressure obtained by this method is actually the gradient between WHVP and FHVP. The FHVP is an internal reference point or zero point, which enables the investigator to subtract the variations in intraabdominal pressure

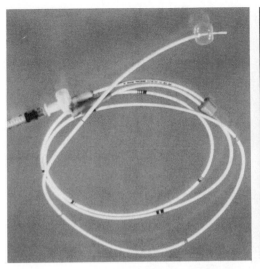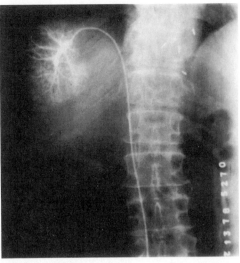

FIGURE 33-2 The left panel depicts the balloon catheter commonly used for hepatic vein pressure measurements. Free hepatic vein pressure measurements are obtained with the balloon in the collapsed state. When inflated, the balloon catheter occludes the hepatic vein and yields a wedged hepatic vein pressure. The right panel shows an inflated (wedged) balloon catheter in place in the hepatic vein with contrast material demonstrating a sinusoidal pattern. When the balloon is correctly wedged, it does not permit reflux of contrast material and demonstrates opacification of a large portion of the liver. (Modified from Groszmann RJ, Glickman M, Blei AT, et al. Wedged and free hepatic venous pressure measured with a balloon catheter. Gastroenterology 76:253, 1979)

that may cause elevation of WHVP not directly related to increases in vascular resistance or flow. The presence of ascites, for example, increases intraabdominal pressure, which is readily transmitted to the thin-walled intraabdominal venous system. In general, the inferior vena cava pressure is identical to the intraabdominal pressure, and is the internal reference point for interpreting hemodynamic measurements in the abdominal venous system. As intraabdominal pressure increases, the pressure in the inferior vena cava also rises and the PVP likewise. The gradient between PVP and intraabdominal pressure, as reflected in the HVPG, however, remains unchanged.

Another relevant point in understanding the HVPG is that the intravariceal pressure is not affected by an increase in intraabdominal pressure. This is because esophageal varices are extraabdominal and downstream from the portal circulation. The presence of ascites increases intraabdominal pressure and equally affects WHVP and FHVP but does not affect the pressure in the esophageal varix.

The major limitation of the HVPG is its inaccuracy in portal hypertensive states in which the site of increased resistance is not sinusoidal or postsinusoidal. Its advantages are simplicity and safety.[50] It enables the investigator to obtain both wedged and free pressures with the same catheter. It also can be combined with measurement of hepatic blood flow using clearance methods (discussed later). The technique is ideally suited to pharmacologic studies in which serial measurements are required. The catheter can be left safely in place for hours and the balloon tip inflated and deflated as needed.

Percutaneous Splenic Pulp Pressure

Percutaneous splenic pulp pressure measurement is the other major indirect method of estimating portal pressure.[302] It is most commonly obtained in combination with splenoportog-

raphy during assessment of splenic and portal vein thrombosis. Splenic pulp pressure is elevated in all forms of portal hypertension because of the position of the spleen at the origin of the portal system, as illustrated in Figure 33-4. Therefore, splenic pulp pressure measurements are sensitive for detecting portal hypertension but are not specific with regard to etiology. As a method of estimating portal pressure, it is attempted infrequently because of bleeding risk (1% to 2%), although this may be minimized by recent technical innovations.[61] Moreover, it does not provide an internal reference pressure, which is necessary to interpret meaningfully the splenic pulp pressure. Finally, this technique is not useful for studies in which serial measurements are needed.

DIRECT TECHNIQUES FOR MEASURING PORTAL PRESSURE

Operative Portal Vein Pressure Measurement

This technique requires direct access to the portal vascular tree during laparotomy and therefore is not useful for estimating portal pressure under usual conditions. It has obvious disadvantages in situations where serial measurements are needed. Moreover, direct portal pressure measurement is not interpretable without also obtaining a baseline intraabdominal venous pressure.

Transhepatic Portal Vein Pressure Measurement

This technique uses a thin needle or Chiba needle to cannulate an intrahepatic branch of the portal vein.[53] A catheter also can be threaded by this means into the main portal vein.[371,435] Related in methodology to transhepatic cholangiography, transhepatic portal vein catheterization usually is

Text continued on p. 942

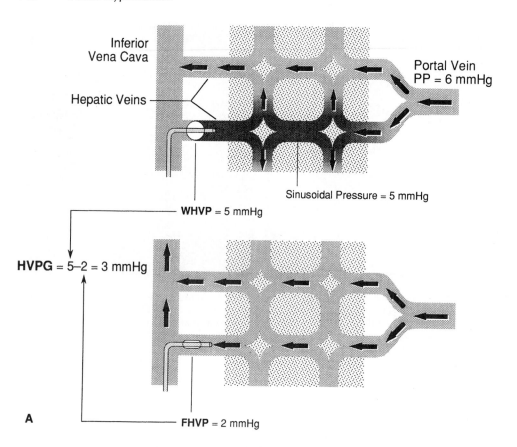

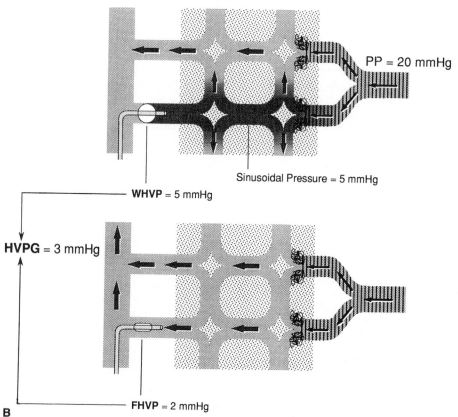

FIGURE 33-3 Illustration of the principles involved in measuring hepatic vein pressures (pressure levels are provided as examples). Stripes indicate hypertensive area; dark areas indicate stasis. (**A**) The normal liver. Due to normal dissipation of pressure through the sinusoids when the hepatic vein is occluded (*top*), the measured pressure in the hepatic vein is slightly lower than the normal portal venous pressure. This difference usually is insignificant. (**B**) Presinusoidal portal hypertension wedged hepatic venous pressure (WHVP) and hepatic vein pressure gradient (HVPG) are normal in presinusoidal portal hypertension because the intersinusoidal communications are normal and permit decompression of the static column of blood formed by the occluding balloon (*top*). The site of obstruction is depicted with twisted lines.

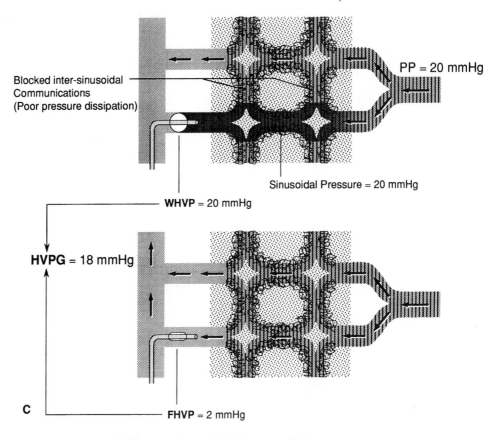

Blocked inter-sinusoidal
Communications
(Poor pressure dissipation)

PP = 20 mmHg

Sinusoidal Pressure = 20 mmHg

WHVP = 20 mmHg

HVPG = 18 mmHg

C

FHVP = 2 mmHg

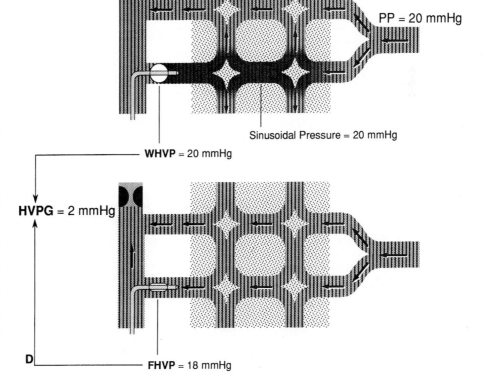

PP = 20 mmHg

Sinusoidal Pressure = 20 mmHg

WHVP = 20 mmHg

HVPG = 2 mmHg

D

FHVP = 18 mmHg

(**C**) Portal hypertension due to alcoholic cirrhosis. The portal venous pressure and the WHVP are elevated equally in sinusoidal portal hypertension; effective decompression of the static column of blood created by the occluding balloon (*top*) cannot occur at the sinusoidal level due to disruption of the normal intersinusoidal architecture. In this situation, wedged hepatic venous pressure gives an excellent approximation of actual portal pressure. (**D**) Posthepatic portal hypertension. WHVP is elevated but HVPG is normal in syndromes such as right-sided cardiac failure. The normal HVPG reflects the normal liver architecture present in these syndromes unless permanent liver injury supervenes.

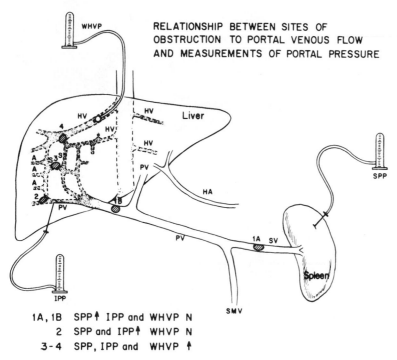

RELATIONSHIP BETWEEN SITES OF
OBSTRUCTION TO PORTAL VENOUS FLOW
AND MEASUREMENTS OF PORTAL PRESSURE

1A, 1B   SPP↑ IPP and WHVP N
2   SPP and IPP↑ WHVP N
3-4   SPP, IPP and WHVP ↑

FIGURE 33-4 This figure illustrates the relation between anatomic site of obstruction to the flow of portal blood and the pressure measurements obtained by various techniques. 1A, splenic vein obstruction; 1B, portal vein obstruction; 2, intrahepatic presinusoidal obstruction; SPP, splenic pulp pressure; IPP, intrahepatic portal pressure; WHVP, wedged hepatic vein pressure; N, normal; ↑, increase; S, sinusoids; A, intersinusoidal anastomosis. (Groszmann RJ, Atterbury CE. The pathophysiology of portal hypertension: a basis for classification. Semin Liver Dis 2:177, 1982)

simple in portal hypertensive states due to dilatation of the portal venous branches. Separate measurement of an internal reference venous pressure is necessary. The procedure is performed most safely with a thin needle under ultrasonic guidance.[270] It can be adapted for prolonged catheterization, portal venography, and angiographic embolization of collaterals in the setting of variceal hemorrhage.[371,435] Boyer and colleagues[53] found that transhepatic portal vein pressure measurement and HVPG compare favorably. There is excellent correlation of pressures using these two methods in alcoholic liver disease. Portal pressure has been found to be higher using the transhepatic method in states in which presinusoidal portal hypertension or portal vein thrombosis are present.[53,330]

Umbilical Vein Catheterization

This is a cumbersome and somewhat risky technique that is rarely used.[191]

Intrahepatic Parenchymal Pressure Measurement

This technique is similar to splenic pulp pressure measurement. Its value for estimating portal pressure is questionable and routine use is not recommended.[111]

ENDOSCOPIC MEASUREMENT OF VARICEAL PRESSURE

Although portal hypertension is a necessary condition for variceal hemorrhage, PVP has been shown to correlate poorly with risk of bleeding above the threshold HVPG gradient of 12 mmHg.[127,228] A major impetus for measuring pressure in the varix itself is to define better the relationship of this pressure to PVP and to variceal hemorrhage. Two methods are available for endoscopic measurement of variceal pressure. The first, direct variceal puncture, was first studied in the 1950s and has been used in the setting of endoscopic variceal

sclerotherapy.[301,401] Because of the risk of precipitating hemorrhage by puncturing the varix with a needle, this method should be used only in conjunction with sclerotherapy.

Pressure-sensitive gauges that can measure variceal pressure without puncturing the varix have been developed.[42,272,314,346] Polio and colleagues[314] have evaluated a pressure-sensitive capsule perfused by an air compressor using artificial varices of varying wall thickness and radius. They also studied canine mesenteric veins, demonstrating good correlation of pressures with intravariceal pressure. Some overestimation of pressure was noted in vessels with small radii at higher pressures. Bosch and colleagues[42] also demonstrated good correlation of pressures obtained in cirrhotic patients by direct puncture and by their endoscopic pressure-sensitive gauge.

The Barcelona group[346] has published a study of 70 cirrhotic patients, 47 with a history of variceal bleeding, and 23 with varices but no history of hemorrhage. These patients had variceal pressure measurement using a pressure-sensitive gauge as well as HVPG measurement. Whereas these groups had similar HVPG (20.1 ± 5.1 mmHg versus 20.4 ± 7.6 mmHg), there was a highly significant difference in variceal pressure between groups. In the group in which variceal hemorrhage had occurred, variceal pressure was 15.7 ± 2.8 mmHg versus 12.1 ± 2.6 mmHg in the group with no history of bleeding. More than 60% of bleeders but only 22% of nonbleeders were found to have variceal pressures in excess of 15 mmHg. Although the hemodynamic data in this study were not gathered during the acute hemorrhage, the findings lend support to the concept that high variceal pressure increases the risk of variceal hemorrhage.

Widespread clinical application of variceal pressure measurement is hindered by a number of problems with existing techniques. Artifact in measurement is created by esophageal contractions. The patient must be cooperative, but the effects of sedation on pressure measurements are unknown. An experienced endoscopist and an unbiased technician for obtaining pressures are necessary.

Enthusiasm for these exciting innovations must be tempered by a recognition that there is a much greater worldwide experience with the use of HVPG in clinical studies and in the bedside evaluation of the portal hypertensive patient. Until simpler, less operator-dependent techniques are developed and validated, the HVPG still should be considered the gold standard for pressure measurements in the portal system in alcoholic liver disease. In nonalcoholic liver diseases, although this measurement may underestimate portal pressure, it is still reproducible and would serve to evaluate the results of pharmacologic therapy.

Evaluation of the Splanchnic, Hepatic, and Collateral Circulation

The hemodynamic derangements that characterize portal hypertension include alterations in splanchnic and hepatic blood flow, as well as development of portosystemic collateral blood flow, which is responsible for many of the clinical features of portal hypertensive liver disease. In addition to measurement of pressure in the portal system and in esophageal varices, other important modalities exist for assessment of the splanchnic, hepatic, and collateral circulations.

UPPER GASTROINTESTINAL ENDOSCOPY

Endoscopy is necessary in any patient suspected of having portal hypertension. Not all patients with portal hypertension have varices, and risk of variceal hemorrhage does not exist in these patients. The presence of other complications of portal hypertension, such as encephalopathy and ascites, does not reliably predict presence of varices because patients with portal hypertension may develop portosystemic collaterals that are predominantly caudad.

Endoscopy also enables some stratification of patients according to risk of hemorrhage. Grading the size of varices on a scale ranging from I to IV may be useful in guiding a decision on prophylaxis against hemorrhage. Risk of bleeding increases with size of varices,[49,127,228] although this has not been a universal finding.[24] Interobserver variability in the endoscopic diagnosis and grading of varices must be considered not only in the clinical setting but also in the interpretation and comparison of published studies.[19]

Other endoscopic features of esophageal varices, including cherry-red spots, red wale markings, hemocystic spots, and blue varices could be predictive of variceal rupture.[24,286,311] Cherry red spots and red wale markings have been shown to result from dilated intraepithelial channels and dilated subepithelial superficial veins above the varix.[164] The endoscopic presence of these signs has been associated with a high transmural variceal pressure in one study.[198]

The stomach in portal hypertensive patients may reveal the presence of varices, although these may be difficult to identify because of their similar appearance to gastric folds. Other lesions, including gastritis and peptic ulceration, also are encountered frequently in cirrhotic patients, particularly alcoholics. Portal (congestive) gastropathy is an important entity that is observed in portal hypertensive patients, and is discussed in the section devoted to clinical consequences of portal hypertension.

DIAGNOSTIC IMAGING OF THE SPLANCHNIC, HEPATIC, AND COLLATERAL VASCULAR TREE IN PORTAL HYPERTENSION

The diagnostic imaging of the liver is taken up in greater detail in Chapter 9. Mention is made here only of techniques with particular bearing on the clinical assessment of portal hypertension.

Barium Studies

Although studies have demonstrated close correlation between barium esophagram using spasmolytics and endoscopy in the diagnosis of esophageal varices,[450] endoscopy has largely replaced barium studies for this purpose. Gastric varices, which may be difficult to diagnose endoscopically, also are seen occasionally in barium radiographs as polypoid filling defects in the fundus of the stomach. These may be encountered even when liver disease is not under consideration. In these cases, splenic vein thrombosis may be the cause, often because of pancreatic disease such as pancreatitis, neoplasm, or trauma. An obvious disadvantage of barium compared with endoscopy is that it is not useful for diagnosing the source of acute bleeding.

Angiography

Angiographic access to the portal vascular tree may be gained by any of the routes discussed in sections devoted to the methods of measuring portal pressure. These include umbilical vein catheterization, splenoportography, and the direct transhepatic approach.[244,394,436] In addition, visualization of the portal vein and collateral system can be accomplished by venous phase angiography after selective injection of the mesenteric artery and splenic artery. An alternative that requires a smaller dose of intravascular contrast material is digital subtraction angiography.[115] These techniques yield valuable data about the anatomy of the portocollateral system, patency of vessels, and the presence of aneurysms, fistulas, and intrahepatic vascular lesions. Many of these data also may be obtained noninvasively with ultrasonography. Hence, angiographic studies are reserved mainly for preoperative assessment and in studies in which pressure measurements are needed.

Ultrasound

Ultrasonography is the method of choice for assessment of the portal system in the patient in whom portal hypertension is suspected. This noninvasive test is extremely accurate in distinguishing the patent from the thrombosed portal vein, which is vital information in any portal hypertensive patient. Portal vein collaterals also can be identified around the azygos system, stomach, spleen, retroperitoneum, and left renal vein. Other useful findings include a congested and enlarged spleen, which is suggestive of portal hypertension, although other causes of splenomegaly also must be considered.

The caliber of the portal vein, as measured by ultrasound, also is helpful. Portal vein diameter in excess of 15 mm is very suggestive of portal hypertension, although the presence of a normal-caliber portal vein does not rule out this condition.[38] A normal portal vein increases in caliber after eating (postprandial hyperemia), and absence of this phenomenon may be a clue to the presence of portal hypertension.[356] Inability to visualize the portal vein by ultrasonography is suggestive of portal vein thrombosis. Cavernous transformation of the portal vein and echogenic thrombus within the portal vein lumen also are diagnostic of this condition.[429,457]

The reader is referred to the section on echo-Doppler flowmetry for further applications of ultrasound technology in portal hypertension.

Computed Tomography and Magnetic Resonance Imaging

These techniques have so far had less importance than ultrasonography in the assessment of the portal venous system. Although these scans may be less influenced by operator subjectivity or inexperience, they are not preferred to ultrasound. The latter technique is not limited in the scanning axis and can therefore visualize vessels from many different angles. In this way, details such as thrombus are less likely to be missed. Computed tomography (CT) should not be relied on to diagnose the presence of esophageal varices.[12] Magnetic resonance imaging (MRI) provides excellent vascular anatomic detail and is useful in the diagnosis of portal vein thrombosis and patency of surgical shunts. Its role in measurement of blood flow is mentioned later.

Scintiphotosplenoportography

After splenic injection of a radionuclide, the movement of radioactivity through the portal system can be followed for the purpose of determining patency of vessels or portacaval shunts. The presence of large shunts, however, can lead to nonvisualization of vessels and give the erroneous impression that the portal vessels are obstructed.[188]

HEPATIC BLOOD FLOW

About 25% of the cardiac output perfuses the liver under normal circumstances. A third of this flow is contributed by the hepatic artery and the remainder by the portal vein.[55,422] Portal blood flow comprises venous blood draining the stomach, intestines, pancreas, spleen, and omentum. In the hepatic sinusoids, hepatic arterial, and portal venous blood mix freely. Total hepatic blood flow is about 1860 mL/min in young healthy men and 1550 mL/min in women, as estimated by plasma clearance of indocyanine green.[473] Physiologic conditions alter hepatic blood flow. For example, splanchnic and portal blood flow increase after eating but decrease with sleep.[297,477]

Portal Vein Flow

The portal system is thought to be a passive vascular bed. Whereas decreased flow in the hepatic artery leads to a compensatory reduction in vascular resistance, decreased portal flow leads to a reduction in the cross-sectional area of the portal vasculature and a corresponding increase in portal venous resistance. Conversely, increased flow, by inducing passive dilatation of the vessel, leads to a passive decrease in portal vein resistance.[163] Moreover, there is no portal venous hyperemia in response to decreased hepatic arterial flow.[139,223] This contrasts with the behavior of the hepatic artery in response to decreased portal flow, as discussed later.

Factors that govern portal venous flow are predominantly those that control the supply of blood to the splanchnic organs. For example, feeding dramatically enhances hepatic blood flow as a result of increased splanchnic, and therefore portal, hyperemia.[170]

Resistance to the flow of portal blood in the normal liver generally is agreed to be minimal at the precapillary and si-

nusoidal level. Resistance sphincters in the region of the hepatic vein in the cat have been suggested[222] and demonstrated in the dog.[54] The existence of such sphincters in humans is speculative (unpublished data suggest that they do not exist).

Regulation of Hepatic Arterial Flow

Arterial flow to the liver is not determined by oxygen demand.[220] Under normal conditions, the liver extracts less than 50% of the supplied oxygen.[274] Under conditions of increased oxygen demand, the liver augments its oxygen extraction rather than increasing arterial flow. In chronic alcohol-fed rats, oxygen requirement by the liver increases dramatically (45%) without increased hepatic arterial flow.[62]

Autoregulation of Hepatic Arterial Flow

Flow in the hepatic artery is autoregulated.[163] This means that over at least part of the physiologic range of pressures, resistance rises with increased pressure, and pressure reduction results in decreased vascular resistance to maintain a constant flow of blood. This phenomenon has been demonstrated in several studies.[163]

Interaction Between Hepatic Arterial and Portal Venous Blood Flow

It has been known for many years that a reduction in portal flow results in an increase in hepatic arterial flow.[140,163] After portocaval anastomosis, the prognosis for recovery appears to correlate with the increase in arterial flow that follows diversion of portal blood flow.[64] The capacity of the hepatic artery to increase its flow in response to decreased portal flow ranges from 22% to 100%.[147,163] Although total hepatic blood flow is not restored to normal by hepatic arterial hyperemia, this phenomenon nevertheless has physiologic importance: it tends to increase total hepatic blood flow in situations of hemodynamic compromise such as hemorrhage.[139]

The mechanism determining the relationship between hepatic arterial and portal venous flow is undefined. A so-called hepatic arterial buffer response has been postulated, based on experiments performed in cats.[223,224] According to this hypothesis, hepatic arterial vasodilatation is mediated by an accumulation of adenosine in the space of Mall under conditions of decreased portal flow. A specific site of adenosine secretion has not been identified and it is still unknown whether adenosine is secreted constantly or is regulated by local factors such as oxygen deficit, local metabolites or endogenous vasodilators. The hypothesis is supported by several findings, however: (1) adenosine is a potent hepatic arterial vasodilator, (2) infusion of adenosine into the portal vein causes hepatic arterial vasodilatation, (3) dipyridamole, an inhibitor of uptake of adenosine, potentiates vasodilatation, and (4) adenosine blockers attenuate the buffer response.[223]

Hepatic Blood Volume

Blood makes up 25% to 30% of the volume of the liver, and hepatic blood comprises 10% to 15% of the total blood volume.[220] Hence, the liver has a major capacitance function. As hepatic venous pressure increases, sinusoidal pressure passively increases. The volume of blood contained in the liver may increase by up to 4 mL/100 g of liver for each mmHg increase in hepatic venous pressure. Hepatic blood volume may expand passively to as much as 60 mL/100 g of liver in congestive heart failure.[162] The role of the liver as a blood reservoir has been suggested by studies using animal models of hemorrhage and sympathetic nerve stimulation.[77,78,221] The applicability of these studies to humans is unknown.

MEASUREMENT OF HEPATIC BLOOD FLOW

Clearance Techniques

These techniques require injection of dyes or radiolabeled particles that are avidly extracted by the liver. If a substance is totally extracted by the liver in one pass, its clearance is equal to total hepatic blood flow; however, no substance actually possesses this property. Therefore, hepatic vein catheterization also is necessary to measure hepatic blood flow accurately. This is particularly true in the setting of clinical liver disease, where extraction of the indicator frequently is diminished.[143] Commonly used substances include dyes such as indocyanine green and bromosulphthalein, or radiolabeled bile acids. These compounds are avidly cleared by hepatocytes. Alternative substances, such as ^{32}P-colloidal chromic phosphate and heat-denatured ^{131}I-labeled albumin, are extracted by the hepatic reticuloendothelial system.

There are two methods, based on the same clearance principle, that have been used to measure hepatic blood flow, the constant infusion[56] and single-injection method.[439] In general, there is satisfactory agreement between the continuous infusion and single-injection methods.[72,439] Although the single-injection method is slightly less reliable than the constant infusion method, it has the advantage of speed (which permits repetition), and it also may provide a better estimate of extraction ratio in the presence of liver disease because dye saturation is less probable. Both clearance methods are somewhat invasive and inaccurate in the presence of severe liver disease. Extrarenal sorbitol clearance has been recently reported to be a safe, noninvasive, and reliable means of measuring parenchymal liver plasma flow in patients with normal or diseased livers.[477]

Indicator Dilution Technique

This method is invasive, requiring catheterization of the hepatic artery, or the portal vein, superior mesenteric artery, or splenic artery (any one of these vessels is sufficient if the splanchnic circulation is normal), as well as the hepatic vein. Its advantage over clearance techniques is the fact that the indicator dilution technique does not depend on liver function.[337] A known dose of an indicator is injected into one of the afferent vessels mentioned above. Hepatic blood flow is proportional to the amount of hepatic blood that has diluted the indicator, as measured in the efferent (hepatic venous) blood.[55] Commonly used indicators include ^{131}I-labeled human serum albumin and ^{51}Cr-labeled red blood cells.

In portal hypertensive liver disease, portosystemic shunting allows a certain percentage of the injected indicator to bypass the liver and escape detection in the hepatic venous blood. Therefore, Groszmann and colleagues[152] have devised a modification of the indicator dilution method that permits measurement of the amount of blood shunted around the liver through portosystemic collaterals. The indicator concentration is measured in the hepatic vein after selective injection of the splenic, superior mesenteric, and hepatic arterial circulations. Using this method, the amount of blood shunted in each regional bed can be measured.

Oral–Intravenous Pharmacokinetics

Clearance of drugs by the liver depends on blood flow (rate of delivery) and intrinsic ability of the liver to metabolize the drug in question.[204] Substances such as propranolol, indocyanine green, and lidocaine are rapidly extracted by the liver and their clearance is determined by hepatic blood flow. In contrast, poorly extracted compounds such as antipyrine and warfarin undergo blood flow-independent hepatic clearance. Their rate of disappearance from the circulation depends on the metabolic activity of hepatic enzymes.[204] Hepatic blood flow can be measured by administering simultaneous oral and intravenous doses of a drug (one of the doses radiolabeled) that is highly extracted and completely metabolized by the liver, as well as completely absorbable by the gastrointestinal tract. DL-Propranolol has been used for this purpose, with ^{3}H-labeled propranolol administered intravenously and the unlabeled drug given orally.[204]

Inert Gas Washout

Inert gases such as krypton-85 and xenon-133 establish an immediate equilibrium between tissues and blood according to a specific partition coefficient. Gas may be administered by intraparenchymal, intrasplenic, or portal vein injection.[159,218,377] Less invasive methods such as inhalation[369] and intraluminal gastrointestinal tract administration also have been reported. This technique also has been adapted to estimate portosystemic shunting. After the establishment of equilibrium between liver and blood, the rate of washout of the inert gas is measured using an external counting device. The rate of washout is proportional to flow of blood to the liver. Although accurate and reproducible, there are several disadvantages to inert gas washout for measurement of hepatic blood flow. First, in hepatic steatosis and other conditions that affect the composition of the liver, the coefficient of partition differs from that of a normal liver. This coefficient also must be adjusted for hematocrit. Second, the inert gas washout technique measures only blood flow that perfuses the sinusoids and underestimates total flow in the presence of hepatic arteriovenous or portohepatic venous shunts.

Echo-Doppler and Related Methods

All of the methods of measuring hepatic blood flow discussed so far are cumbersome and invasive. They are likely to be replaced in the near future by echo-Doppler flowmetry and related techniques. Echo-Doppler flowmetry is inexpensive, noninvasive, and capable of efficiently obtaining serial measurements.[356] Sonographic techniques are well accepted in clinical practice in cerebrovascular and peripheral vascular disease.

Initial echo-Doppler studies involving the abdominal circulation were uncontrolled, and were greeted with skepticism in the scientific literature regarding their reliability and their methodology, which may be limited by subjectivity and bias.[65] A study in normal volunteers and cirrhotic patients underscores the contention that there is a high degree of interobserver variability and intraobserver variability for a given parameter over time.[357] The technical pitfalls and limitations of the method also have been demonstrated.[306] Echo-Doppler flowmetry, however, has been subjected to scrutiny in clinical protocols involving normal controls as well as patients with portal hypertensive liver disease.[356] From these studies, a better understanding of the value as well as limitations of this methodology is emerging.

Based on the Doppler effect, echo-Doppler flowmetry actually measures the movement of red blood cells rather than blood flow per se. It measures the direction and velocity of red blood cell flow. B-mode ultrasound can be used to measure cross-sectional area of a blood vessel and volume of flow can be estimated by multiplying velocity by area. The superior mesenteric artery provides 75% of the blood flow entering the portal system and may be used as a representation of portal flow.

Mathematical elaboration of the velocity wave form in echo-Doppler flowmetry of arteries yields another useful hemodynamic parameter, the pulsatility index (PI):

$$PI = \frac{\text{peak-to-peak velocity}}{\text{mean velocity}} \qquad (3)$$

This ratio has been related to the resistance in the vascular bed under examination.[321] Its clinical usefulness has been validated in controlled studies comparing the superior mesenteric artery PI of alcoholic cirrhotic patients with that of healthy controls.[356]

Color-Doppler is another ultrasound technique for studying blood flow that has been applied to the splanchnic circulation.[16] This method uses B-mode imaging of the blood vessel as well as two-dimensional flow signals, which are converted into colors. This technique permits determination of the presence of blood flow and can distinguish flow direction as well the difference between laminar and turbulent flow.

Magnetic Resonance Imaging

Magnetic resonance imaging has been used to provide details of human vascular anatomy. For example, MRI can accurately diagnose portal vein thrombosis and surgical shunt patency. Portal blood flow measurements using direct bolus imaging have been shown to agree closely with measurements obtained with Doppler ultrasound under a variety of physiologic conditions.[347] This technique may be free of certain limitations of the ultrasound technique such as nonvisualization of the portal vein due to obesity or the presence of intestinal gas. The role of MRI in measurement of portal blood flow is likely to evolve rapidly.

ESTIMATION OF AZYGOS BLOOD FLOW

The gastroesophageal collaterals, including esophageal varices, drain for the most part into the azygos vein.[44,46,49,71,434] Measurement of azygos blood flow, therefore, provides an index of blood flow through this collateral system. Its main limitation is that it cannot distinguish flow in varices from that in periesophageal veins. Bosch and Groszmann[44] have developed a method of measuring azygos blood flow that uses continuous thermal dilution. The azygos vein is easily catheterized, often in the course of other hemodynamic investigations. Blood flow measurement is performed using the continuous thermal dilution method, a well accepted method of measuring flow in single vessels.[122,122a] Azygos flow is calculated by the equation:

$$\text{azygos blood flow} = \frac{Q_i \times 1.08\ T_b - T_i - 1}{T_b - T_m} \qquad (4)$$

where:

Q_i = the rate of infusion of indicator (5% dextrose); 1.08 = the constant representing the ratio of density and specific heat of 5% dextrose and blood; T_b = the baseline azygos blood temperature (all temperatures degrees centigrade); T_i = the baseline temperature of the indicator and blood during infusion, sensed by an external thermistor[44,49,122a]

Measurement of azygos blood flow is easily adapted for serial measurements. Moreover, it is well tolerated and reproducible. Correlation of increased azygos blood flow with presence of portal hypertension and, in fact, with degree of portal pressure elevation, have been demonstrated.[44,49] The size and pressure of esophageal varices, which correlate with risk of hemorrhage, have been shown to parallel azygos blood flow.[42,49] Moreover, shunt surgery,[44,49] balloon tamponade,[49] variceal sclerotherapy, and pharmacologic therapies[40,44,49] such as vasopressin, somatostatin, and β-blockers,[48,73] have all resulted in significant drops in azygos blood flow.

Data indicate that in at least 15% of patients, variceal blood flow drains in other veins such as the cervical veins and not in the azygos vein. In these patients, measurement of azygos blood flow may not reflect flow in the superior collateral bed.[196]

VARICEAL BLOOD FLOW

Transesophageal real-time two-dimensional Doppler echography has also been adapted to the measurement of blood flow in gastroesophageal varices, azygos vein, intercostal veins, and thoracic aorta. This technique may be a valuable tool in assessing the hemodynamic effects of various pharmacologic compounds on the ascending collateral system in portal hypertension.[406]

Classification of Portal Hypertensive States

For a discussion of the pitfalls of attempting to classify clinical syndromes in portal hypertension according to the site of presumed resistance to the flow of portal venous blood, the reader is referred to the earlier section dealing with resistance in the pathogenesis of portal hypertension. Nevertheless, such a classification is helpful in organizing a miscellaneous group of disorders according to a system that has some anatomic basis. Accordingly, this system can be conceptualized hemodynamically by considering the relationship between portal pressure and wedged hepatic venous pressure. The main categories are prehepatic, intrahepatic (classified according to the predominant anatomic site of resistance relative to the hepatic sinusoid), and posthepatic portal hypertension syndromes.

PREHEPATIC PORTAL HYPERTENSIVE SYNDROMES

Splanchnic Arteriovenous Fistula

Arteriovenous fistulas in the spleen and splanchnic vascular bed may manifest with portal hypertension, ascites, and varices. Other features include an abdominal bruit, often in the right upper quadrant, as well as abdominal pain. Arteriovenous fistulas may be congenital as in hereditary hemorrhagic telangiectasia or they may be the consequence of trauma, rupture of splenic or hepatic arterial aneurysms, or hepatocellular carcinoma.[316,448] The initial hemodynamic consequence of arteriovenous fistula may be increased portal blood flow. There is evidence to suggest that secondary hepatoportal sclerosis, with fibrosis of portal radicles, and thickening and sclerosis of the portal veins, may develop in response to arterial flow into the portal system.[104,260] In a canine model of splanchnic arteriovenous fistula, the portal vein is arterialized by anastomosis to the hepatic artery, leading to muscularis hypertrophy and venular thickening.[383,384,481] Hence, these prehepatic forms of portal hypertension may elicit an intrahepatic presinusoidal increase in resistance. Ligation or selective embolization of these fistulas does not necessarily reverse portal hypertension,[104] and portosystemic shunt surgery may also be required.

Splenic Vein Thrombosis

Occlusion of the extrahepatic portal system may occur at the level of the splenic or portal vein. Symptoms of portal hypertension, particularly variceal hemorrhage, in the presence of normal liver function, histology, and HVPG should lead to suspicion of these disorders.[358] Splenic vein thrombosis is particularly important to diagnose because it is readily treatable with splenectomy.

Pancreatic disease is a common cause of isolated splenic thrombosis because of the position of the splenic vein posterior to the pancreas. Acute and chronic pancreatitis, pancreatic carcinoma, pseudocyst, trauma, and other causes have been reported.[219,390,408] Diagnosis is best made by venous phase angiography, although ultrasound, contrast CT, and splenoportography all may be used.

In splenic vein thrombosis, gastric varices may be present in the absence of esophageal varices because the left coronary vein is still in continuity with the patent portal vein. This condition may be referred to as left-sided, or sinistral, portal hypertension. The course of collateral blood flow may be through short gastric veins to the gastric submucosal plexus, leading to isolated gastric varices that anastomose with the portal vein through the coronary vein. Alternatively, gastric veins may connect with esophageal submucosal veins, leading to gastroesophageal varices that shunt blood into the portal system or vena cava. Finally, blood may cross the gastroepiploic system through omental varices into the portal system. In one series of 51 patients, 49% had isolated gastric varices, 43% had gastroesophageal varices, and only 8% had esophageal varices alone.[271] Cytopenias and splenomegaly are not reliably present.[326,390]

Portal Vein Thrombosis

In portal vein thrombosis, the lumen of the portal vein may be replaced by several collateral vessels, giving rise to so-called cavernous transformation of the portal vein.[378] This disease, which is encountered in the pediatric population, may have its origin in umbilical vein infection in some cases.[419] Nearly a quarter of nonpediatric cases of portal vein thrombosis are associated with cirrhotic liver disease, although overall, the incidence of portal vein thrombosis in cirrhosis is less than 1%,[293] and overdiagnosis of this condition may be the result of failure to opacify the portal system with contrast material because of retrograde flow. Myriad other causes are reported, including coagulopathic conditions (eg, deficiency of protein C,[294,425] inflammatory bowel disease, myeloproliferative syndromes,[424] collagen vascular disease,[310] paroxysmal nocturnal hemoglobinuria, and retroperitoneal fibrosis). Hepatocellular carcinoma is an important consideration in portal vein thrombosis, particularly in the patient with known cirrhotic liver disease. Compression or invasion of the portal vein by hepatocellular or pancreatic carcinoma also are encountered. Portal vein thrombosis may result from trauma (including postoperative), pancreatitis and other pancreatic diseases, abdominal sepsis, and as a complication of endoscopic variceal sclerotherapy.[6,225] In addition,

pregnancy and oral contraceptives have been associated with portal vein thrombosis.[75]

The incidence of portal vein thrombosis is difficult to determine. In one series of 602 patients presenting with portal hypertension, 47 (7.8%) had portal vein thrombosis with normal livers.[18] All manifested with variceal hemorrhage. In 29 of the 47 patients, the etiology could not be identified.

The most serious symptom of portal vein thrombosis is variceal hemorrhage, which frequently is recurrent and well tolerated in children. Liver function and histology are normal. Splenomegaly and cytopenias are not reliably present, and are seen more commonly in children. For obscure reasons, ascites may be encountered in some patients, raising questions about the necessity for sinusoidal hypertension in the pathogenesis of ascites.[259,458] Likewise, encephalopathy may be encountered but not frequently.[259] Stigmata of chronic liver disease, such as vascular spiders and palmar erythema, are absent.

The systemic and splanchnic hemodynamic profile of portal vein obstruction has been described.[226] As expected, the HVPG is normal. Hepatic blood flow is decreased compared with both cirrhotic and normal controls, whereas the elevated cardiac index and low systemic vascular resistance characteristic of the hyperdynamic systemic circulatory state in cirrhotic patients, also are seen in the patients with portal vein thrombosis, all of whom also have large portosystemic collaterals.

The diagnosis of portal vein thrombosis is made readily with venous phase angiography. Reports suggest that MRI soon will become the first-line diagnostic method, because it is at least as accurate as contrast CT, and may be more accurate than ultrasound.[235,479] Splenoportography rarely is necessary today in diagnosing portal vein thrombosis. Treatment is surgical when possible; the reader is referred to Chapter 34 for further discussion. Alternative therapy is available in the form of endoscopic sclerotherapy for patients who are unable or unwilling to undergo some form of surgical treatment.[18,86,399,403]

Splenomegaly as a Cause of Portal Hypertension

Most patients with splenomegaly unrelated to liver disease do not develop portal hypertension. There are many reports, however, of portal hypertension with complications including ascites and variceal hemorrhage in miscellaneous diseases including leukemia, lymphoma, polycythemia vera, myelophthisis with myeloid metaplasia, Gaucher's disease, and others.[7,33,242,290,348,407] In some instances, splenectomy may normalize portal pressure; in these cases, portal hypertension is due, in part, to hyperdynamic portal venous inflow from the enlarged spleen.[239,242,407] HVPG would be predicted to be normal in portal hypertension due to splenomegaly, but it is not always so.[7,348] In most cases, however, as in hematologic diseases that commonly infiltrate the liver, this is due to increased vascular resistance secondary to presinusoidal or intrahepatic infiltration (in this latter category the HVPG is increased).[373]

POSTHEPATIC PORTAL HYPERTENSION SYNDROMES

Inferior Vena Cava Obstruction

Posthepatic obstruction can take place in the inferior vena cava (IVC) or at the level of the heart in any disease that raises right-sided cardiac pressure. Causes of mechanical IVC obstruction include venous thrombosis, tumor, cysts, abscesses, and membranous obstruction by a web. There is overlap in clinical presentation between these extrahepatic syndromes, Budd-Chiari syndrome (resulting from hepatic vein thrombosis), and nonthrombotic occlusion of small hepatic veins (venoocclusive disease). Because the hepatic circulation has no valves, obstruction at any point distal to the sinusoids results in sinusoidal hypertension and retrograde flow in the portal vein and collaterals. The histologic picture of posthepatic obstruction is sinusoidal congestion with areas of centrilobular infarction.

The lesion of membranous obstruction of the IVC is a fibrous web found above the hepatic veins, although the hepatic veins themselves also may be involved. The disease is encountered most commonly in young adults in the Far East and Africa, although cases have been described elsewhere.[167,195,391,474] Membranous obstruction of the IVC usually is a subacute disease, with a many years of symptoms, in contrast to thrombotic occlusion of the IVC or hepatic veins (Budd-Chiari syndrome), which often is clinically more dramatic. The disease may be complicated by hepatocellular carcinoma.[474]

Clinical features of IVC obstruction include congestive hepatomegaly, which may be painful when acute, ascites, and gastroesophageal varices with hemorrhage. IVC obstruction frequently can be distinguished from other causes of portal hypertension by the presence of vena cava collaterals. Vena cava collaterals may be distinguished by their presence on the back, where portal vein collaterals are not encountered. We have encountered the case of a patient with Laennec's cirrhosis complicated by refractory ascites. A dramatic venous collateral pattern later developed on the pa-

tient's back, and was shown angiographically to result from compression of the IVC by the hypertrophic liver (Fig. 33-5). Another typical feature of IVC obstruction is venous stasis with lower extremity edema.

The diagnosis is made angiographically by demonstrating a web or other filling defect in the IVC below the level of the diaphragm with a collateral venous pattern. The hepatic veins, approached through the right heart, are usually patent, particularly on the right, and pressure studies disclose a high WHVP but a normal HVPG resulting from high IVC pressure.[171] Patients with IVC web may have correction of their hemodynamic abnormality by excision.

Cardiac Disease

When pressure rises in the right chambers of the heart from constrictive pericarditis, valvular disease such as mitral stenosis with tricuspid insufficiency, or cardiomyopathy of any cause, the pressure is transmitted through a valveless venous system from IVC to hepatic veins to hepatic sinusoids and into the portal system. The consequence is a picture similar to that of hepatic vein occlusion, IVC web, or any syndrome of obstruction to hepatic venous outflow. Indeed, the liver in right-sided heart failure has the same histologic features as in the latter entities. The patient with this syndrome may have symptoms of intractable ascites and hepatocellular dysfunction, which are difficult to distinguish from other causes of portal hypertension.

The hemodynamic abnormalities in the portal system in congestive heart failure have been described using pulsed Doppler flowmetry.[174] Portal flow is directly influenced by the hemodynamic events in the right heart in severe congestive heart failure. Increased pulsatility in the portal vein is ob-

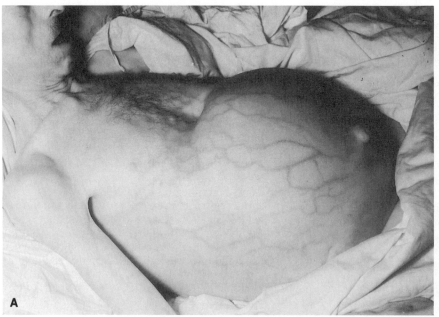
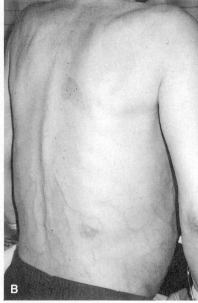

FIGURE 33-5 (A) Typical pattern of abdominal wall collaterals observed in portal hypertensive liver disease. (B) Collateral pattern of inferior vena cava obstruction, with dilated veins on the back. This pattern is not encountered in portal hypertension in the absence of inferior vena cava obstruction. (A from Reynolds T. Portal hypertension. In: Schiff L, Schiff E, eds. Diseases of the liver, ed 5. Philadelphia, JB Lippincott, 1982, p 393)

served in severe failure, corresponding to increased resistance to portal blood flow in the presence of increased right-sided cardiac pressures. Pulsatility is shown to decrease with treatment of congestive failure in some cases. Portal blood flow also varies markedly with the phase of the cardiac cycle. Anterograde flow peaks during ventricular diastole but decreases in velocity during systole and in some cases reverses direction.

INTRAHEPATIC CAUSES OF PORTAL HYPERTENSION

Intrahepatic causes of portal hypertension have been classified according to the anatomic zone of obstruction to portal blood flow within the liver. Hence, these syndromes are divided into presinusoidal, sinusoidal, and postsinusoidal categories. In reality, many of these diseases cause liver lesions that overlap zones, particularly in advanced cases.

Presinusoidal portal hypertension results from obstruction in the small intrahepatic portal veins. Review of Chapter 5 will remind the reader that the portal vein is one component of the portal triad, which also consists of branches of the hepatic artery and bile duct. Injury to the portal vein at the level of the portal triad may be the consequence of lesions in the artery, bile duct, or triad as a whole.

Schistosomiasis

Hepatic schistosomiasis is a leading cause of portal hypertension worldwide. Early in the course of hepatic schistosomiasis, portal hypertension is the consequence of a granulomatous reaction resulting from deposition of parasite eggs in the portal venules. The inflammatory response leads to fibrosis and obliteration of portal venules, with manifestations of portal hypertension in the absence of significant hepatocellular injury. As the disease progresses, fibrosis extends into the sinusoid. Hence, early schistosomiasis results in a normal HVPG, whereas advanced disease may result in an increased HVPG. This may be the consequence of inflammation and fibrosis spilling over into the sinusoids, or it may result from compensatory increase in hepatic arterial flow in response to decreased hepatic portal venous flow.[3,17,95,298,323,324] This important disease is taken up in much greater detail in Chapter 47.

Sarcoidosis

Chapter 57 is devoted to granulomatous diseases of the liver, of which sarcoidosis is foremost. Although the liver may be involved histologically in most cases of sarcoidosis, clinical liver dysfunction is rare. Likewise, portal hypertension is an unusual, although well recognized, manifestation of hepatic sarcoidosis.[247,264,427] Sarcoid granulomas frequently localize in the portal areas of liver lobule, resulting in injury to portal veins. Early disease is predominantly presinusoidal, with normal sinusoidal pressure, whereas advanced disease leads to fibrosis and cirrhosis, with sinusoidal as well as presinusoidal obstruction to portal blood flow.

Myeloproliferative Diseases

The syndrome of portal hypertension with myeloproliferative diseases that cause splenomegaly has been mentioned previously. Myeloproliferative diseases, including systemic mastocytosis,[154] leukemias, lymphomas, and myelosclerosis also may cause presinusoidal (and probably also sinusoidal) por-

tal hypertension due to direct infiltration by malignant cells.[100,373]

Malignant Disease in the Liver

Portal hypertension is well described as a complication of hepatocellular carcinoma, independent of the propensity of this cancer to arise in cirrhosis and in other portal hypertensive liver diseases.[277] Portal hypertension may arise as a consequence of hepatic artery–portal vein fistula, compression of the portal trunk by tumor, invasion of the portal vein, and portal vein thrombosis. Portal venous hemodynamics in hepatoma are studied increasingly with Doppler flowmetry in lieu of celiac–mesenteric angiography.[289]

Transudative ascites and gastroesophageal varices may result from portal hypertension in primary and metastatic carcinoma in the liver.[176,353] This may be the consequence of embolization of the portal venules, compression of the intrahepatic portal tree by tumor that replaces hepatic parenchyma, or by extension of tumor into the portal system. Hepatic vein and IVC obstruction due to malignancy also are recognized. The subject of cancer in the liver is considered further in Chapter 44.

Nodular Regenerative Hyperplasia

Hepatic histologic lesions that fall in the spectrum of nodular regenerative hyperplasia (NRH) are referred to by a variety of labels, including micronodular transformation, diffuse and focal nodular hyperplasia, and partial nodular transformation. These have been the subject of a study and attempt at reclassification.[453] The subject is reviewed in detail in Chapter 5. Manifestations of portal hypertension probably are not as frequent as review of the collected literature would suggest, and in a series of 64 cases, only 1 patient had varices (compared with 73 of 135 in the literature), and 4.7% had ascites (compared with 26% in the literature).[453]

NRH is not a single disease but a nonspecific reaction to a variety of injuries. It is characterized by nodular transformation of the hepatic parenchyma without fibrous tissue between nodules. The cause of NRH seems to be heterogeneity of blood supply. Whereas acini with inadequate blood supply atrophy, other acini with greater blood flow either hypertrophy or stand out in contrast to atrophic acini as spherical nodules. This process may be the result of diseases that decrease the flow of blood in portal venules. Thrombosis of these vessels has been described in association with NRH in polycythemia vera and other hematologic disorders.[454] Compromised arterial flow to the liver acinus has been associated with NRH in rheumatoid arteritis; secondary injury to portal venules in this condition may be severe enough to result in portal hypertension.[344,379] Injury to arteries may be the consequence of immune complexes in Felty's syndrome and polyarteritis nodosa.[35,276] The lesion also has been described in toxic liver injury from vinyl chloride,[317] and in the toxic oil syndrome.[397] Numerous other conditions in which regional hepatic blood flow may be affected have been described in association with NRH, including collagen vascular diseases, malignancies of many kinds, congestive heart failure, diabetes, atherosclerosis, and old age.[453] This lesion also has been observed in the early stages of primary biliary cirrhosis (PBC), in which inflammation of bile ducts leads to obliteration of small portal veins and portal hypertension in some cases even before cirrhosis is present.[275]

NRH may cause portal hypertension with normal or increased HVPG, reflecting variable involvement of the sinusoids in this lesion. A presinusoidal element probably always is present.[349,454] The pathogenesis of portal hypertension in NRH is probably obliterative venopathy, as stated previously. The presence of nodules, which may press on the portal system, also has been postulated to play a role, although nodularity is present in most cases without clinical evidence for portal hypertension.[453]

Primary Biliary Cirrhosis

Primary biliary cirrhosis is discussed in greater depth in Chapter 16. In a prospective study of 265 patients enrolled without gastroesophageal varices and followed for a median of 5.6 years, varices eventually developed in 31%, with half of these patients eventually experiencing hemorrhage.[136] In an earlier series, 4% of patients presented initially with portal hypertension.[380] The pathogenesis of portal hypertension early in PBC may be injury to portal venules due to their proximity to inflamed bile ducts. This may lead to portal hypertension in the absence of fully developed cirrhosis.[275] With progression of disease, obstruction to the flow of portal blood is not only at the presinusoidal level but also in the sinusoids because of the development of cirrhosis.[192] In PBC and other causes of advanced nonalcoholic (macronodular) cirrhosis, the pathologic lesion is heterogeneous. Areas of normal architecture with intersinusoidal collaterals are interspersed with cirrhotic nodules. This may explain the presence of both presinusoidal and sinusoidal hypertension, with a gradient between portal vein pressure and HVPG.[315] This is in contrast to alcoholic cirrhosis, in which the pathologic abnormality is uniform, with loss of intersinusoidal communications between nodules of equal size, resulting in a HVPG that approximates actual portal pressure.

Chronic Active Hepatitis

As stated previously, the HVPG underestimates portal pressure in diseases in which obstruction to the flow of portal blood is presinusoidal, and in which connections between sinusoids are preserved. In pure presinusoidal disease, HVPG may be normal. In chronic active hepatitis of any cause, the early lesion is localized predominantly in the portal triad. With progression of chronic active hepatitis to involve the liver lobule, there is an increase in the HVPG that reflects morphologic changes. The roles of hepatocyte size, cell volume density, volume density of sinusoids, Disse's space, and Disse's space collagen in the evolution of the portal hypertension in chronic hepatitis have been studied.[430] In particular, hepatocyte size and Disse's space collagen increase with severity of disease and seem to correlate with increases in HVPG. Hence, the evolution of portal hypertension in precirrhotic chronic hepatitis is probably multifactorial.[430]

Idiopathic Portal Hypertension

Idiopathic portal hypertension is known by numerous names, including Banti's syndrome (after Guido Banti, whose descriptions date to the 1880s),[13] noncirrhotic portal fibrosis,[361] and hepatoportal sclerosis. The syndrome is recognized predominantly in Japan[291] and India.[361] In India, up to 30% of portal hypertensive patients have this disease,[364] with a predominance of men with a mean age of 25 to 35 years.[361] In contrast, Japanese patients are likely to be 10 to 20 years older and female.[291,292]

Idiopathic portal hypertension is characterized by gastroesophageal variceal hemorrhage in a young patient with prominent splenomegaly. Ascites, encephalopathy, jaundice, and other signs of liver failure are not common but are encountered in end-stage disease. Hypersplenism with anemia and thrombocytopenia is frequent. Variceal hemorrhage that complicates this disease generally is well tolerated and is not associated with the dismal prognosis of variceal bleeding in cirrhotic patients, possibly because idiopathic portal hypertension usually is encountered in young patients with good hepatic function and without comorbid disease.[52,364,410] Moreover, with treatment of varices by sclerotherapy or portocaval anastomosis, rates of rebleeding and death are extremely low.[287]

There is no satisfactory explanation of the etiology of idiopathic portal hypertension. Exposure to toxins such as arsenic[101] and others[52,359] have been postulated, without confirmation. Likewise, hypotheses that this disease results from chronic bacterial infection,[52,359] malarial infection,[374] immunologic derangements,[283] or genetic predisposition[363,409] remain to be substantiated.

The main clinical entity from which idiopathic portal hypertension must be distinguished is extrahepatic portal vein obstruction. Nevertheless, these two diseases may be part of the same spectrum, since the main lesion in idiopathic portal hypertension has been described as "obliterative portal venulopathy of the liver,"[282] with patchy segmental subendothelial thickening of intrahepatic portal veins, thrombus formation with variable obliteration or recanalization, and scarring and fibrosis of the portal tracts. Fibrosis is prominent in the extrahepatic portal vein and its intrahepatic branches. Although grossly the liver surface may appear nodular,[284] the liver is not cirrhotic. Other features are widening and fibrosis of the space of Disse, as well as capillarization of the sinusoids.[359]

The hemodynamic profile of idiopathic portal hypertension has been described, with differences noted between patients in Japan and India. All patients have increased splenic and portal pressure,[52,359,365] whereas Japanese patients are reported also to have elevated HVPG.[292] In contrast, Indian patients may have either normal or raised HVPG.[359,365] There is no clear explanation of this difference. Splanchnic hemodynamic studies from Japan, in which portal and hepatic vein catheterization as well as Doppler flowmetry were used, demonstrate dramatic increases in splenic and mesenteric arterial flow, as well as portal vascular resistance compared with controls (patients with chronic persistent hepatitis who lacked portal hypertension).[288] These findings support the hypothesis that hyperdynamic splanchnic blood flow as well as increased intrahepatic portal resistance play roles in the pathogenesis of portal hypertension in this disease.

The patient with idiopathic portal hypertension must be distinguished by liver biopsy from the well compensated cirrhotic patient. Extrahepatic portal vein obstruction must be excluded. Splenoportography has been the most common means of imaging the portal vein in India, although celiac angiography and ultrasonography also may be used. Finally, the diagnosis of tropical splenomegaly syndrome must be considered. This disease is encountered in areas where malaria is prevalent, and is due to deranged immunologic response to chronic malaria infection.[168] It is dominated by splenomegaly without prominent portal hypertension.

Wilson's Disease

The lesion causing portal hypertension in Wilson's Disease has been thought to be presinusoidal.[411] As in many diseases, however, a mixed profile of presinusoidal portal hypertension with elevation of the HPVG also has been described.[53]

Vinyl Chloride, Arsenic, Vitamin A, Mercaptopurine, Azathiaprine and Thioguanine, and Others

A variety of drugs and toxins have been associated with the development of portal hypertensive liver disease in the absence of cirrhosis. Among these, arsenic is a well known cause of portal hypertension. Probably due to vascular injury, a wide spectrum of arsenic-related lesions is recognized. The best described is a portal venular injury,[101] but angiosarcoma,[110] perisinusoidal fibrosis,[96] peliosis hepatitis in association with angiosarcoma,[110] and venoocclusive disease with centrilobular sinusoidal dilatation and perisinusoidal fibrosis[216] also have been observed. Although the mechanism of vascular lesions is speculative, it may be similar to that of 6-mercaptopurine and 6-thioguanine, which are antimetabolites that interfere with the synthesis of DNA.[234]

Noncirrhotic portal fibrosis is seen with various toxic injuries, with angiographic findings, including cutoff of portal vein radicles in the absence of portal vein thrombosis, similar to the radiographic findings described in Indian patients with idiopathic portal hypertension. Fibrosis may be minimal by light microscopy but perisinusoidal fibrosis is observed by electron microscopy. Nodular regenerative hyperplasia also is recognized, in keeping with the hypothesis that this lesion is a response to obliterative portal venopathy.[376] Etiologic agents in addition to arsenic include vinyl chloride,[418,438] vitamin A,[354] mercaptopurine, azathiaprine,[278] busulfan, chlorambucil, and others.[376] Manifestations of this syndrome are hepatosplenomegaly, ascites, gastroesophageal hemorrhage, and jaundice.

Other Causes of Intrahepatic Portal Vein Obstruction

Numerous other causes of obstruction to the flow of portal blood at the presinusoidal level have been reported. Many of these are discussed in separate chapters but are worthy of brief mention here. Congenital hepatic fibrosis is a well described form of noncirrhotic portal hypertension that results from fibrosis in the portal triads and leads to gastroesophageal varices and splenomegaly in children. Cystic fibrosis also is a condition of childhood and is discussed in Chapter 44. Ascites, splenomegaly with hypersplenism, and bleeding gastroesophageal varices have been reported in less than 5% of patients with cystic fibrosis in several series.[370,392,404] The cause of portal hypertension in this disease is biliary cirrhosis.

Acute and Fulminant Viral Hepatitis.   Portal hypertension with all its complications has been described in severe acute and fulminant hepatitis of various causes. A significant correlation has been demonstrated between HVPG and severity of hepatitis, as indicated by encephalopathy, serum bilirubin elevation, albumin concentration, and coagulopathy. Histologically, portal hypertension seems to correlate with degree of collapse of sinusoids with reduction in intrahepatic vascular space due to hepatic necrosis.[426] Other factors, such as inflammatory infiltration of the liver and ballooning of hepatocytes, probably also are at play.

Hepatic Cirrhosis.   Cirrhotic liver disease is discussed in depth in Chapter 32. The hemodynamic abnormalities present in cirrhosis are covered in this chapter in the section pertaining to the pathogenesis of portal hypertension.

Peliosis Hepatitis.   Peliosis is a rare histologic lesion characterized by blood-filled cavities without zonal preference within the liver lobule, varying from less than 1 mm to centimeters in diameter. This condition rarely is dominated clinically by portal hypertension, although in one series of 12 patients, 7 had symptoms of portal hypertension or elevation of HVPG (HVPG was not obtained in the remaining patients).[476] The disease is associated with azathioprine toxicity in transplant recipients and is encountered in various other diseases, including tuberculosis, Hodgkin's disease, anabolic steroid use, systemic light-chain disease,[476] and acquired immunodeficiency syndrome.[309] In acquired immunodeficiency syndrome, peliosis has been demonstrated to share similarities with bacillary angiomatosis and to be caused by infection with *Rochalimaea henselae*, which also may be a cause of fevers and bacteremia in these patients.[393a] Cases in which massive hepatomegaly, ascites, and anemia due to blood sequestration in the peliotic liver exist, have been described, and the clinical features have resolved with appropriate antimicrobial therapy.[127a]

Peliosis is postulated to result from injury to the sinusoidal barrier, resulting in dilatation of the sinusoidal lumen or enlargement of the space of Disse.[476] These sinusoidal abnormalities as well as obstruction to the flow of portal blood due to the compressive effect of blood-filled cavities both may contribute to portal hypertension in peliosis hepatitis.

Alcoholic Hepatitis.   The complex subject of hepatotoxicity due to ethanol is covered in detail in a separate chapter. Mention also is made of portal hypertension in cirrhotic and noncirrhotic liver injury due to alcohol in the section of Chapter 32 on pathogenesis of portal hypertension.

Budd-Chiari Syndrome.   Although Budd-Chiari syndrome is named to honor Budd (1846) and Chiari (1899), the syndrome of hepatic vein thrombosis was described originally by Lambroan in 1842. The disease usually is the result of systemic coagulopathic conditions that predispose to venous thrombosis, including myeloproliferative states, paroxysmal nocturnal hemoglobinuria, malignancy, pregnancy, oral contraceptive use, and protein C deficiency. As a consequence of hepatic vein occlusion, the liver becomes congested with dilated sinusoids and areas of central necrosis, which progress to fibrosis in chronic cases. Ascites is a major manifestation of Budd-Chiari syndrome because of elevated sinusoidal pressure. In Budd-Chiari syndrome, the hepatic artery becomes the main source of hepatic blood flow, whereas the direction of flow in the portal system becomes hepatofugal. The clinical consequences are hepatomegaly, which is painful when acute, ascites, and gastroesophageal varices with hemorrhage. The syndrome may be observed in association with IVC obstruction, with the additional findings of peripheral edema and the characteristic pattern of dilated collaterals on the back. The pathogenesis, manifestations, diagnosis, and management of this important and treatable cause of portal hypertension are discussed at length in Chapter 40.

Membranous obstruction of the hepatic veins gives rise to a clinical syndrome with hemodynamic similarities to Budd-Chiari syndrome. The disease is encountered principally in the the Far East and South Africa. Further discussion may be found in the section of this chapter devoted to IVC obstruction.

Venoocclusive Disease. Noncirrhotic portal hypertensive disease due to occlusion of small hepatic veins is venoocclusive disease. The disease often manifests acutely with jaundice, congestive (frequently painful) hepatomegaly, ascites, and gastroesophageal varices. Venoocclusive disease is recognized as a toxic injury. The most notorious cause is so-called bush tea disease, which is encountered in Jamaica and results from ingestion of pyrrolizidine alkaloids of *Senecio* and *Crotalaria* plants.[60] The syndrome also is recognized in cancer patients and organ transplant recipients because of exposure to cytotoxic drugs,[25,142,255,327] and after radiation to the liver.[332] Further discussion of injury to the hepatic vascular system may be found in the section Chapter 27 dealing with drug toxicity as a cause of portal hypertension, as well as in the chapter devoted to drug-induced liver injury.

Clinical Assessment

In any patient suspected of having portal hypertension, the clinician should include an inventory of physical signs of liver disease, of which the best recognized are jaundice, spider angiomas, palmar erythema, testicular atrophy, gynecomastia, and clues to the presence of portosystemic encephalopathy such as altered mental status, asterixis, and fetor hepaticus. Splenomegaly is a helpful clue that is present in most patients with portal hypertension. The spleen is best palpated with the patient lying on the right side and inhaling deeply while the examiner applies light pressure to the left upper quadrant. Spleen size, however, correlates poorly with portal venous pressure.[464] Moreover, splenomegaly may be present in many disease states in the absence of portal hypertension. Portal hypertensive patients may have findings suggestive of a hyperdynamic circulatory state, including bounding pulses, warm, well perfused extremities, and arterial hypotension.

Ascites is a complication of great importance in portal hypertensive liver disease. The presence of ascites supports a diagnosis of portal hypertension if conditions such as malignancy, congestive heart failure, and peritoneal inflammatory disease are excluded. The subject of ascites, including its pathogenetic relationship to portal hypertension, complications, and management are taken up in detail in Chapter 35.

The presence of dilated abdominal veins supports a diagnosis of portal hypertension. Umbilical vein–epigastric vein shunts result in dilated collaterals on the anterior abdominal wall, whereas portal vein–parietal peritoneal shunts may result in a venous pattern on the flanks. These collaterals are best visualized with infrared photography if the diagnosis is in question, although frequently the finding is obvious (see Fig. 33-5). The caput medusae represents tortuous collateral veins around the umbilicus and can be a dramatic finding.

The Cruveilhier-Baumgarten murmur is a bruit that is appreciated by auscultation with the stethoscope in the epigastrium between the umbilicus and the sternum. This murmur results from a large collateral connection between the portal system and the umbilical vein remnant in the falciform ligament. Its intensity and pitch may vary, leading to different descriptions of the murmur in the same patient. Increases in intraabdominal pressure (as with the Valsalva maneuver) may

cause the Cruveilhier-Baumgarten murmur to become louder, and it can be diminished by pressing on the skin above the umbilicus. A palpable thrill may be detectable in patients with a loud murmur.

Dilated abdominal collaterals must be distinguished from the collaterals that arise in response to obstruction in the IVC. The latter syndrome causes prominent flank veins and dilated veins on the back. A collateral venous pattern on the back never is encountered in portal hypertension alone. Rarely a patient with cirrhosis may present with IVC obstruction and dilated veins on the back due to compression of the IVC by large regenerative nodules. The distinction is best made angiographically.

The laboratory approach to the patient with liver disease is the subject of Chapter 4; there are no laboratory tests diagnostic of portal hypertension. Thrombocytopenia, leukopenia, and anemia frequently are encountered in patients with hypersplenism, but their presence is not sensitive or specific with respect to etiology. The cytopenias that result from hypersplenism rarely are a cause of clinical complications in themselves.

Clinical Consequences

The clinical consequences of portal hypertension are myriad. Some are the subject of this chapter, including the evolution of portosystemic collaterals, plasma volume expansion, the hyperdynamic circulation, varices and congestive gastropathy, and splenomegaly. Ascites, portosystemic encephalopathy, and renal failure are tied intimately to the hemodynamic derangements of portal hypertension, but these are the topics of separate chapters.

ESOPHAGEAL VARICES

Esophageal varices are part of the system of spontaneous portosystemic collaterals that develop in portal hypertensive states to provide conduits for the flow around the liver. In humans, portosystemic shunting of blood occurs between the short gastric and coronary veins and the esophageal, azygous, and intercostal veins; the superior and the middle and inferior hemorrhoidal veins; the paraumbilical plexus and the venous system of the abdominal organs that are juxtaposed with the retroperitoneum and abdominal wall; and the left renal vein and splanchnic, adrenal, and spermatic veins. Dilatation of preexisting embryonic channels is thought to be the main mechanism of evolution of these collaterals.[160]

The anatomy of esophageal varices has been studied with vascular casts.[197] Intraepithelial channels in the lower esophagus drain blood shunted from the portal system into a superficial venous plexus, which in turn communicates with adventitial veins through a plexus of large deep intrinsic veins through perforating vessels that traverse the muscular layers. The deep intrinsic veins dilate to become varices, localized to the lamina propria in the distal esophagus, where they are poorly buttressed by surrounding connective tissue.[285,398] Of all the portosystemic collaterals, these are clinically the most important because of their propensity to bleed (Fig. 33-6).

A threshold portal pressure has been shown to exist in humans, below which esophageal varices are not encountered.[127] Elevation above this pressure (a HVPG of 11 to 12 mmHg), however, is not a sufficient condition for causing

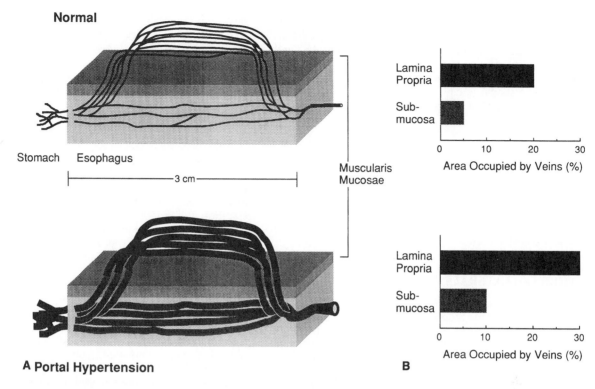

FIGURE 33-6 In portal hypertension, both the size and number of veins increase in the plexus of veins that normally is located in the distal esophagus, 2 to 3 cm above the lower esophageal sphincter. (**A**) Comparison of normal distal esophageal angioarchitecture with the portal hypertensive state in which vessels in the lamina propria dilate disproportionately. (**B**) The relative area occupied by veins in the lamina propria of the distal esophagus is greater in portal hypertension compared with normal. These findings explain, in part, the propensity of varices in the distal esophagus to develop and bleed. (Modified from Spence RAJ. The venous anatomy of the lower esophagus in normal subjects and patients with varices: an image analysis study. Br J Surg 71:739, 1984; and Noda T. Angioarchitectural study of esophageal varices with special reference to variceal rupture. Virchows Arch [A] 404:381, 1984)

varices to develop, since many patients with HVPG in excess of 12 mmHg do not have varices.

Other factors besides portal pressure therefore are involved in the development of esophageal varices. One important factor may be blood flow through the gastroesophageal collaterals. Azygos blood flow is an index of gastroesophageal collateral blood flow that has been demonstrated to increase exponentially with increasing portal pressure.[44,49] Higher azygos blood flows are encountered in patients with larger compared with smaller esophageal varices.[49] The fact that patients with high azygos vein blood flow do not necessarily have varices, however, indicates that high collateral flow also is not a sufficient condition for the development of varices.[49] Other factors may be direction of collateral blood flow; varices and variceal hemorrhage are correlated with the presence of cephalad collaterals.[180] In addition, pressure in the lower esophageal sphincter has been postulated to play a role.[5,37,263,243,398]

GASTRIC VARICES

Isolated gastric varices in the absence of esophageal varices are rare, with a reported incidence of 8% to 12% in patients with varices in two large series.[362,456] Gastroesophageal varices, in contrast, were present in many patients (123 of 230 patients) in one series.[456] A combination of endoscopy and splenoportovenography may be necessary to verify the presence of gastric varices, which may be difficult to diagnose. This may account for the variability in incidence reported in the literature. Recently, endoscopic sonography has been shown to be useful in identifying gastric varices.

Most gastric varices are supplied by the short or posterior gastric veins, and are present in the fundus or lesser curvature of the stomach.[252] Large gastric varices are infrequent, and in their presence, esophageal varices are less likely to be found.[456] Hemodynamic studies in patients with large gastric varices have demonstrated a lower portal pressure, large gastrorenal shunts, less risk of hemorrhage, but somewhat greater likelihood of portosystemic encephalopathy.[456]

PORTAL HYPERTENSIVE GASTROPATHY

Portal hypertensive gastropathy is a lesion that is recognized with increasing frequency. This topic has been the subject of several studies and reviews.[99,149,253] In one series, 65 of 127 patients with portal hypertension of various etiologies had endoscopically diagnosed congestive gastropathy, of whom 28 had severe or persistent lesions.[253] In another series of 81 nonalcoholic cirrhotic patients, 28% had gastric mucosal abnormalities consistent with congestive gastropathy.[102] The appearance of the gastric mucosa is beefy red (focal or diffuse), with small intramucosal hemorrhages and a white reticular pattern surrounding hyperemic areas (mosaic pattern).

Cherry red spots also are observed. In this condition, the mucosal and submucosal vascular architecture is altered by dilated veins, ectatic capillaries, thickening of arterioles, and submucosal arteriovenous communications. Bleeding from congestive gastropathy may be diffuse and severe[253]; propranolol has been shown to have a beneficial effect in acute and long-term control of bleeding in this syndrome.[308]

PULMONARY HYPERTENSION

Pulmonary hypertension is a rare complication of all types of portal hypertension, occurring in 1% to 2% of patients in a large prospective study.[156] Most patients are asymptomatic. The syndrome is independent of severity of liver dysfunction and degree of portal pressure elevation. Dyspnea is the most frequent manifestation.

OTHER COLLATERALS

Gastroesophageal collaterals have the greatest clinical importance because of their propensity to bleed. In addition, significant anorectal varices may develop through connections between the portal system and the middle and superior hemorrhoidal veins. In one prospective series, anorectal varices were found in 44% of 100 patients with cirrhosis and in 59% of those who had bled from esophageal varices. These collaterals are thought to be distinct from hemorrhoids.[173]

The umbilical vein remnant may dilate and serve as a conduit for blood from the left portal into the systemic circulation through the epigastric veins of the abdominal wall. The characteristic physical finding of dilated paraumbilical veins is known as the caput medusae. Collaterals also may develop between the portal system and the posterior abdominal wall and through the liver capsule and diaphragm. In addition, large spontaneous anastomoses between the portal system and the left renal vein may evolve; these may be large enough to simulate a surgical shunt.[217]

LYMPHATIC FLOW

In addition to portosystemic collaterals, there is increased lymphatic flow in portal hypertension. This probably arises in intrahepatic portal hypertension from increased lymph formation due to congestion in the sinusoids. The normal lymphatic flow in the direction of the hilum of the liver is increased, with enlargement of hilar lymphatics demonstrated in autopsy specimens.[8] Increased lymphatic flow contributes to the formation of ascites.

Variceal Hemorrhage

Just as varices are not encountered in patients with HVPG of less than 11 to 12 mmHg, likewise variceal hemorrhage in patients (mainly with alcoholic cirrhosis) seldom if ever occurs at portal pressures below this level.[49,127,434] Many patients with varices and HVPG greatly in excess of 12 mmHg never experience variceal bleeding, however. It seems obvious that higher portal pressure should predispose to bleeding (or rebleeding) of esophageal varices, and this has been borne out in some,[187,267,328,434,441] but not all studies.[228,394,442] Indirect support for this relationship is provided by observations that

expansion of blood volume increases portal pressure and can precipitate hemorrhage.[51] Moreover, patients with higher posthemorrhage portal pressures have a greater risk of rebleeding.[441] Thus, although there is not a linear increase in incidence of bleeding with increases in portal pressure above the threshold, the degree of elevation in portal pressure has been described as having a permissive effect on the risk of hemorrhage from esophageal varices.[313]

There have been conflicting reports about the relationship of portal pressure to size of esophageal varices, as determined endoscopically.[98,127,228,434,442,468] Methodologic problems have been observed in the studies in which a direct relationship has been reported,[313] and, in general, there does not appear to be a clear correlation between degree of portal pressure elevation and size of varices. There is a general relationship between variceal size and risk of bleeding: the larger the varix, the higher the risk of rupture.[127,187,228,442] This correlation, however, is far from exact, and a significant percentage of patients bleed from small varices.[49,228,434]

The pressure in varices has been correlated with portal pressure in endoscopic studies using pressure-sensitive capsules and direct puncture techniques, as discussed previously. Pressure in the portal vein, and presumably in the varix, is probably in a constant state of flux, depending on various physiologic conditions such as phase of the respiratory cycle, coughing, Valsalva, and meal ingestion. The gradient between portal vein and esophageal luminal pressure is affected by these dynamic conditions, although the degree to which these fluctuations are reflected in variceal pressure remains to be determined.[331] Likewise, a direct correlation between variceal pressure and risk of hemorrhage remains to be defined.

The concept of variceal wall tension has been introduced to account for several variables that play a role in the pathogenesis of variceal hemorrhage.[144,313] Based on Frank's modification of LaPlace's law:

$$\text{variceal wall tension (T)} = (TP_1 - TP_2)(r \times w^{-1}) \quad (5)$$

where:

$TP_1 - TP_2$ (transmural pressure) = the difference between intraluminal varix pressure and esophageal luminal pressure (for practical purposes, this gradient can be thought of as portal pressure); r = the radius of the varix; w = the wall thickness of the varix

Tension (T) of the varix therefore is a property of the vessel wall that can be thought of as an inwardly directed force that opposes an expanding force proportional to transmural pressure and vessel radius and inversely proportional to wall thickness.

As the varix distends, variceal wall tension, or the resistance to further distension, increases. At high levels of distention, the elastic limit of the vessel wall is approached and small increments of increase in TP or vessel radius are associated with large changes in wall tension, as illustrated in Figure 33-7. When the elastic limit of the varix is reached, further distention cannot be counteracted by further increase in wall tension.[70,79] At this point, variceal rupture occurs. In blood vessels, an increase in pressure results in an increase in radius and a corresponding decrease in wall thickness. Hence, in vessels that are poorly supported by connective tissue, such as varices in the lamina propria of the distal esophagus, changes in pressure would be expected to have a greater impact on vessel radius and accelerate the approach of the

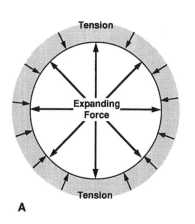

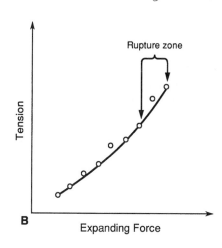

FIGURE 33-7 (A) Illustration of the concept of variceal wall tension, which is an inwardly directed force that opposes an outwardly directed or expanding force. At the point at which the expanding force exceeds the capacity of the vessel to increase its wall tension, rupture of the vessel occurs. (B) This concept is illustrated from data derived from studies in artificial varices constructed from latex tubes. (Modified from Polio J, Groszmann RJ. Hemodynamic factors involved in the development and rupture of esophageal varices: a pathophysiologic approach to treatment. Semin Liver Dis 6:318, 1986)

varix to its elastic limit. The concept that wall tension in distensible blood vessels increases out of proportion to increases in TP (due to expanding radius and wall thinning), has been demonstrated experimentally.[116] The interplay of vessel size, wall thickness, and transmural pressure has been studied in an experimental system using latex tubes, further clarifying these concepts.[313]

Local conditions in the distal esophagus, particularly esophagitis due to gastroesophageal reflux, also have been postulated to play a role in variceal rupture.[238] Although early autopsy studies seemed to bear out this hypothesis,[83] more recent studies based on histologic examination of esophageal specimens obtained at the time of surgical transection procedures have not confirmed the presence of significant inflammatory changes in the mucosa overlying esophageal varices.[400] Moreover, there is no statistical difference in esophageal motility or pH measurements in patients with varices and in control subjects.[106] In agreement with these observations, a placebo-controlled, double-blind study of cimetidine in prophylaxis of variceal hemorrhage revealed no efficacy.[245] The consensus of opinion now favors the view that variceal rupture is not correlated with the presence of acid–peptic esophageal disease.

A number of clinical criteria have been found useful in predicting variceal hemorrhage. The Northern Italian Endoscopic Club has proposed a prognostic index that stratifies patients with cirrhosis according to 1-year probability of bleeding. Based on a prospective study of 321 patients (of whom 26.5% bled), multiple regression analysis disclosed a relationship between risk of bleeding and severity of liver disease (modified Child class), size of varices, and the presence of so-called red wale markings on the varices.[286] The latter are longitudinal dilated venules that resemble whip marks.[286,311] Other numerical grading systems based on size of varices and other endoscopic features also have been reported.[395] These endoscopic signs of impending variceal rupture can be correlated with thinning of the variceal wall. Size of varices and wall thickness are clinical manifestations of two of the major variables in the variceal wall tension formula.

Once variceal rupture occurs, the factors that govern the severity of the bleed include the size of the hole in the varix, the TP (or for practical purposes, the pressure in the varix), and the viscosity of blood. This can be expressed as follows:

$$\text{severity of bleed} \propto (\text{TP}_1 - \text{TP}_2) \times \frac{\text{area of variceal rent}}{\text{blood viscosity}} \quad (6)$$

At higher pressures and in the presence of a larger tear in the varix wall, hemorrhage is more severe. Factors influencing TP, which relate to portal pressure, have been mentioned previously. Factors determining the size of the rent are not well defined. Blood viscosity, however, which is inversely related to the hematocrit,[116] is worth dwelling on here because events during variceal hemorrhage, some of them iatrogenic, may have significant influence on the severity of the bleed. Anemia resulting from blood loss, reexpansion of blood volume with intravenous fluids, and the dilutional effect of high circulating levels of antidiuretic hormone all reduce hematocrit, decrease blood viscosity, and may exacerbate hemorrhage. Moreover, volume overexpansion may adversely affect portal pressure.[51,240] Studies in hemorrhaged portal vein stenosed rats suggest that volume expansion sufficient to normalize systemic blood pressure results in an increase in portal pressure to levels even greater than baseline.[211] Although these data cannot be extrapolated directly to humans, they do suggest a need for study of the hemodynamic effects of volume reexpansion in the clinical setting of variceal hemorrhage.

PROGNOSIS AFTER VARICEAL HEMORRHAGE

In the presence of varices, a patient with cirrhosis has a 25% to 33% risk of hemorrhage. After the initial hemorrhage, the risk of rebleeding is great (up to 70%) and is highly dependent on the severity of underlying liver disease. This risk is especially great during the first few weeks after the index hemorrhage. Subsequently, risk decreases progressively until it reaches levels close to those (20% to 30%) observed in patients who have never bled. Likewise, the initial variceal hemorrhage is associated with high mortality; patients with severe liver disease (Child's grade C) have about 50% 2-week survival and only about 10% survive 1 year. The outlook is somewhat better for less ill patients, but even Child's grade A patients have only about 50% 5-year survival. These data derive from studies involving mainly alcoholic cirrhotics.[312]

MANAGEMENT

Hemorrhage from esophageal varices is likely to be a clinically dramatic event, with hematemesis, melena, or hematochezia. Hemodynamic indications of hemorrhage such as orthostatic hypotension and tachycardia are frequent. Insidious bleeding from varices is encountered less frequently and is a diagnosis of exclusion. A patient with severe liver disease also may present in coma; alteration in mental status in a patient with signs of liver disease therefore should prompt the clinician to consider the possibility of bleeding.

Identification of the bleeding source is of critical importance and should be considered as soon as steps are being taken to stabilize the patient hemodynamically. A nasogastric tube should be passed immediately. Failure to obtain fresh blood or coffee grounds from the stomach does not rule out an upper tract source of bleeding. If blood is aspirated from the stomach, however, a search for a lower tract source is obviated. Hematemesis is a clear indicator of upper tract hemorrhage. Hematochezia frequently is encountered with massive variceal bleeding and should not be assumed to originate from a lower tract source.

Endoscopy should be undertaken as soon as the patient can tolerate it. The diagnosis of variceal hemorrhage is likely in a patient known to have varices, but other sources of bleeding such as gastropathy, peptic ulceration, and Mallory-Weiss tears also are encountered. A barium esophagram may be helpful in the diagnosis of large varices but has no role in evaluation of a patient with bleeding.

The treatment of the hemorrhagic complications of portal hypertension can be broadly divided into management of the acute episode, and the prevention of the initial bleeding episode (primary prophylaxis) and subsequent episodes (secondary prophylaxis; Fig. 33-8). Approaches to the management of acute hemorrhage are discussed in the next section.

NONPHARMACOLOGIC TREATMENT OF ACUTE VARICEAL HEMORRHAGE

Endoscopic Sclerotherapy

At the time of endoscopic diagnosis of esophageal variceal hemorrhage, emergency endoscopic sclerotherapy (ES) should be undertaken. The technical aspects of this procedure are discussed in Chapter 11. In numerous studies, the procedure has been shown to control acute hemorrhage in about 90% of cases, and permits a more leisurely decision regarding long-term therapy.[241,414,461] Even in cases in which acute bleeding has ceased, ES may be undertaken at the time of initial endoscopy for prevention of immediate and long-term rebleeding. After immediate control of hemorrhage, many clinicians continue with ES with repeated injections on a weekly basis until varices are obliterated, followed by periodic surveillance and repetition if necessary. The data

supporting efficacy of ES for control of rebleeding and survival are summarized in following sections.

An initial report of endoscopic ligation for acute and chronic treatment of bleeding esophageal varices has been published in the form of a randomized trial in which this technique is compared with endoscopic sclerotherapy.[404a] The findings suggest that ligation of varices may be somewhat more effective and safer than sclerotherapy, which was associated with esophageal strictures and infections such as pneumonia. In addition, the mortality rate was lower in patients treated with endoscopic ligation than in sclerotherapy control patients. More controlled trials are needed before firm recommendations can be made about this promising new technique. Worldwide experience with sclerotherapy is vastly greater, as discussed later.

For the 5% to 10% of patients in whom hemostasis cannot be achieved, surgical options exist, including portosystemic shunting, devascularization and transection procedures, and orthotopic liver transplantation. These are discussed elsewhere, with the exception of transjugular intrahepatic portosystemic shunts (TIPSs), which are discussed later. At this time, we consider ES to be the most practical and effective form of treatment of the acute hemorrhagic episode. As the reader will appreciate from the discussion of prophylaxis against variceal bleeding and rebleeding, however, the recommendations for long-term treatment depend on the clinical situation.

Balloon Tamponade

Several devices for control of variceal hemorrhage by tamponade are available. The Senkstaken-Blakemore tube is a triple-lumen tube with gastric and esophageal balloons as well as a tube for aspiration of the stomach. The Minnesota tube has a larger gastric balloon and a lumen for aspiration of the esophagus. The Linton-Nachlas tube, which is used for gastric variceal hemorrhage, has a large gastric balloon and lumens for suctioning the contents of the stomach and esophagus. Success rates for acute control of variceal hemorrhage with balloon tamponade are reported in the 80% to 100% range.[117,155,417]

In two randomized trials of balloon tamponade versus vasopressin (or derivative)–nitroglycerin, tamponade was equivalent to[117] or superior to[417] pharmacologic treatment in acute control of bleeding. In a study comparing tamponade with ES, ES was superior both with respect to immediate control of hemorrhage (100% of 23 patients at 24 hours versus 80%

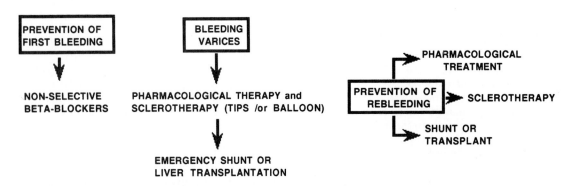

FIGURE 33-8 Schematic depiction of the treatment modalities for portal hypertension and variceal bleeding as discussed in the text.

of 20 patients in the tamponade group) and prevention of relapse at 7 days.[268]

Balloon tamponade should not be continued past 24 hours and has no role in long-term control of bleeding.[268] Moreover, the risks of tamponade are well known.[84] These consist mainly of aspiration pneumonia and esophageal rupture. Complications were reported in 15% of 186 patients treated with tamponade in one series, and nearly half of these were fatal.[155] Its use should be restricted to situations in which sclerotherapy is ineffective in controlling bleeding, and continued only until the patient is stable enough to undergo surgery. In many centers, the use of pharmacologic agents to control hemorrhage precedes a trial of balloon tamponade. This choice hinges partly on the experience of the specific center.

Percutaneous Transhepatic Embolization of Gastroesophageal Varices

This procedure involves catheterization of the gastric collaterals that supply blood to varices through the transhepatic route mentioned in the sections on transhepatic measurement of portal pressure and angiographic imaging of the portal system. A variety of sclerosing agents have been infused with varying degrees of success in controlling acute bleeding but with poor (about 50%) rates of long-term control.[236,244,371]

The procedure is less effective than ES for variceal hemorrhage and much less effective than the other medical and surgical options discussed elsewhere for prophylaxis against rebleeding. Transhepatic embolization therefore is reserved for the unusual situation in which a bleeding patient is not a surgical candidate and all other nonsurgical modalities have failed.

Transjugular Intrahepatic Portosystemic Shunting

Transjugular intrahepatic portosystemic shunting is an angiographic technique for cannulation of the portal vein by the transjugular route, followed by the introduction of an expandable stent to construct an intrahepatic shunt between the portal circulation and the hepatic vein. This innovative technique is hemodynamically similar to a side-to-side portocaval shunt. A number of small uncontrolled series have been published in which TIPS provided control of variceal hemorrhage after more-conventional means had failed.[347a,478] Preliminary results are also promising for improvement of ascites. Reported complications (eg, occlusion, stent migration, and encephalopathy) are few. Data are insufficient, however, to make conclusions about the safety and efficacy of TIPS in comparison with any of the conventional modalities for controlling acute variceal hemorrhage.

TIPS should be reserved for situations in which all conventional means of controlling acute hemorrhage have failed. It should be considered when a surgical shunt is believed to pose excessive risk (or is refused), and possibly as a substitute for surgical shunt to stabilize a refractory variceal bleeder before orthotopic liver transplantation.[347a,347b] It is hoped that TIPS will soon be compared with sclerotherapy or banding in the acute management of variceal hemorrhage in prospective, randomized, controlled trials.

Surgical Treatment

This important topic is taken up in a separate chapter. The reader is referred to Figure 33-8 for our view of the approach to the treatment and prevention of variceal bleeding, taking into consideration all available modalities, including shunting procedures and orthotopic liver transplantation.

PHARMACOTHERAPY OF ACUTE VARICEAL HEMORRHAGE

There are two major categories of drugs used for treatment of portal hypertension: vasoconstrictors and vasodilators. Vasoconstrictors reduce portal blood flow and portal pressure by their action on the splanchnic vascular system. In contrast, vasodilators ideally act by reducing intrahepatic vascular resistance (and therefore portal pressure) without decreasing peripheral or portal–collateral resistance. Only the vasoconstrictors vasopressin and somatostatin (and the vasodilator nitroglycerin in conjunction with vasopressin) are used in the treatment of acute hemorrhage. Miscellaneous other agents also undergoing study reduce pressure or blood flow in the gastroesophageal variceal system by mechanisms other than vasoconstriction or vasodilation. Drugs used (or potentially useful) for the chronic treatment of portal hypertension are discussed later in the section devoted to long-term treatment of portal hypertension.

Vasoconstrictors

The mechanism of action of these drugs in the treatment of portal hypertension is splanchnic vasoconstriction, which results in a reduction in portal venous inflow and portal pressure. Consequently, these drugs decrease blood flow in the gastroesophageal collateral system. The splanchnic arterial vasoconstrictors in clinical use are vasopressin, triglycylvasopressin (tGLVP, also known as glypressin and terlipressin), somatostatin, and β-adrenergic blockers.

Vasopressin and Triglycyl-Vasopressin. Vasopressin is an endogenous nonapeptide that causes splanchnic vasoconstriction when infused into humans and experimental animals,[32,372] resulting in reductions in portal venous inflow, portal pressure, and flow in gastroesophageal collaterals. The decrease in HVPG has been shown to correlate well with a decrease in intravariceal pressure.[41] Two forms of the drug, lysine 8-vasopressin and arginine 8-vasopressin, differ by one amino acid. Pitressin, the drug that was used most commonly in the United States, is a mixture of these two forms. Synthetic arginine vasopressin is available as well. The vasopressin molecule interacts with two receptors, the V_1 receptor, which is found in vascular smooth muscle, and the V_2 receptor, which is localized to renal collecting tubule epithelial cells. The binding of vasopressin to the V_1 receptor results in activation of phospholipase C. This enzyme cleaves phosphatidylinositol biphosphate, yielding diacylglycerol and inositol triphosphate. The latter compound causes release of calcium from the endoplasmic reticulum, whereas diacylglycerol activates protein kinase C.[76] Increase in free cytosolic calcium and activation of protein kinase C result in vascular smooth muscle contraction.

Although vasopressin has a relatively greater vasoconstrictive effect on splanchnic resistance vessels,[31,368] the drug is not highly selective. While decreasing splanchnic, renal, and cutaneous blood flow, vasopressin increases flow to skeletal muscle.[368] Furthermore, the reduction in the portosystemic pressure gradient during vasopressin infusion reduces flow through collaterals, as demonstrated by azygos blood flow thermodilution measurements.[49] Compression of the submucosal varices by increasing lower esophageal sphincter pressure also has been postulated to occur with vasopressin therapy.[19]

Vasopressin toxicity manifests with systemic vasoconstriction, reduction of cardiac output due to increased cardiac afterload, bradycardia, and direct impairment of cardiac contractility.[480] Therefore, this drug should not be used in patients with suspected alcoholic cardiomyopathy or coronary disease. Severe arrhythmias, myocardial infarction, respiratory failure, cerebrovascular accidents, bowel necrosis, and local tissue necrosis have been reported.[85,91,105,114] Hyponatremia due to antidiuresis also has been reported.[209] In addition, vasopressin therapy may complicate hemorrhage by releasing plasminogen activator,[105] although the clinical significance of this may be obscured by its tendency to increase factor VIII release,[80] as well as by the variability in coagulation profile in a patient with liver disease who is hemorrhaging and receiving blood products. The incidence of vasopressin toxicity is not reduced by direct infusion into the superior mesenteric artery compared with peripheral infusion,[85] partly because the liver is not the main site of vasopressin metabolism.

Vasopressin has long been considered the first-line treatment of acute variceal hemorrhage, although its toxicity and overall failure to control half of bleeding episodes, as well as questions about whether it actually reduces transfusion requirements, make it far from ideal. There also is evidence to suggest relative hyposensitivity of the splanchnic vascular bed to the therapeutic effects of vasopressin during active bleeding, compared with hemodynamically stable controls.[210,421] Of three placebo-controlled North American trials of vasopressin, only one[114] was double-blind.[91,248] Other trials comparing intraarterial with intravenous infusion also have been reported.[85,186] Results from these trials are not strikingly consistent, with control of variceal hemorrhage (using differing dosages and definitions of therapeutic success) varying from 29%[114] to 71%.[91]

tGLVP (also known as glypressin or terlipressin) is a prodrug of vasopressin. This compound has received some attention because it does not require constant infusion and may have fewer adverse cardiac effects compared with vasopressin.[120,447,451] Because of its slow mechanism of release, bolus intravenous injections of tGLVP are possible. Since blood levels are low, the drug has been postulated to cause less cardiotoxicity. Bolus injections of tGLVP in dogs, however, decrease cardiac output and increase mean arterial pressure to the same degree as a continuous intravenous infusion of vasopressin.[32] Although tGLVP has been reported to be superior to vasopressin in several reports,[32,117,451] the experimental designs and the low numbers of patients in these trials do not suggest an advantage over continuous intravenous vasopressin.

Vasopressin–Nitroglycerin. The addition of the potent venous dilator nitroglycerin to vasopressin results in reduction of portal pressure while limiting the vasoconstrictor toxicity of vasopressin.[153] Although initial studies reported in 1986 demonstrated reduction in frequency of toxic side effects with the addition of sublingual[475] or intravenous[134,460] nitroglycerin to vasopressin, a decrease in requirement for blood transfusions was not observed in comparison with vasopressin alone. A subsequent study using vasopressin plus transdermal nitroglycerin has demonstrated both a decrease

in transfusion requirement and reduction in need for balloon tamponade or portocaval anastomosis to control acute bleeding.[45]

Although vasopressin is not an ideal treatment for variceal hemorrhage, the recommendation is to use the drug in combination with nitroglycerin as an initial measure to provide time for more definitive treatment. The starting intravenous vasopressin infusion rate should be 0.4 IU/min, with upward titration to a maximum rate of 1 IU/min. Vasopressin does not need to be tapered but may be discontinued abruptly without acutely increasing portal pressure.[329] Nitroglycerin should be simultaneously infused intravenously or administered sublingually or transdermally in a dose that maintains systolic arterial pressure at about 100 mmHg.

Somatostatin

Somatostatin is an endogenous peptide that reduces splanchnic blood flow in animals[183] and humans.[449] Originally isolated from the hypothalamus, it also has been found in gut epithelial cells, pancreatic islets, and elsewhere.[36,336] Two major somatostatin molecules have been sequenced—S-14 and S-48. The carboxyl terminal of the 14–amino acid sequence is responsible for the bioactivity of somatostatin. Endogenous somatostatin undergoes hepatic metabolism with a half-life of 1 to 3 minutes in normals and 1.2 to 4.8 minutes in cirrhotics.[269] Octreotide, a synthetic analogue, has a longer half-life and is more potent than the native hormone.[269] The molecular basis of somatostatin's activity is not clearly defined. It has been shown to reduce the production of cyclic adenosine monophosphate in gastric parietal cells and other cell types.[305] Other actions may not be dependent on cAMP. For example, it also alters cytomembrane potassium permeability, resulting in modulation of calcium-mediated intracellular activation.[336]

Somatostatin is used to treat gastroesophageal bleeding because of its ability to decrease splanchnic as well as azygos blood flow.[46] Somatostatin infusion over 60 minutes at a rate of 10 μg/min has been shown to decrease splanchnic blood flow by 30% in healthy adults with a return to baseline within 10 minutes after stopping the infusion.[449] Somatostatin has been postulated to decrease splanchnic blood flow by blocking the release of vasoactive peptides such as glucagon, vasoactive intestinal peptide, calcitonin gene-related peptide, and substance P.[385] These vasodilatory peptides may be present in portal hypertensive states due to hypersecretion, portosystemic shunting, or decreased hepatocellular clearance.

In contrast to vasopressin, the clinical effects of somatostatin appear to be confined to the splanchnic vascular system, without the systemic toxicity observed with vasopressin.[47,347c] In a randomized trial of somatostatin versus vasopressin, efficacy in controlling hemorrhage was about equal (53% and 58%, respectively).[209] In this and other studies, favorable results and a lower incidence of toxicity were reported with somatostatin.[184] An additional study of somatostatin versus vasopressin demonstrated a slight advantage for somatostatin in control of acute bleeding with less toxicity but somewhat greater incidence of early rebleeding and no advantage with respect to survival.[355]

The first placebo-controlled, double-blind trial of somatostatin in controlling variceal hemorrhage was published in 1989, with the unexpected finding that the drug lacked efficacy compared with placebo.[423] This may have been the result of a greater than expected rate of hemorrhage control in the placebo group (83% in 30 hours). A subsequent randomized, double-blind, placebo-controlled trial of somatostatin infusion over 5 days in 120 subjects has documented successful control of bleeding in 59% of treated subjects compared with 36% of the placebo group. Decreases in transfusion requirement and need for balloon tamponade also were demonstrated.[69] The role for somatostatin in control of acute variceal hemorrhage is not yet defined. Results of large randomized trials comparing somatostatin with vasopressin–nitroglycerin (which is much less expensive) are needed to clarify this issue.

Long-Term Treatment of Portal Hypertension

The discussion of long-term treatment of portal hypertension is divided into primary prophylaxis of variceal hemorrhage (primary prophylaxis) and prophylaxis against variceal hemorrhage. The three modalities in common use are drug therapy (mainly β-blockade), ES, and shunt surgery. The reader is referred to the appropriate chapters for further details concerning ES and surgery. Discussion here focuses on the merits of ES and portal decompressive surgery compared with drug therapy. First, we discuss pharmacologic agents that are available (or may potentially become available in the future) for chronic treatment or portal hypertension.

PHARMACOLOGIC AGENTS

β-Adrenergic Blockers

Propranolol and other nonselective β-adrenergic antagonists are the best-studied drugs available for chronic therapy of portal hypertension. Propranolol reduces portal pressure acutely and chronically in portal hypertensive patients.[229] This effect appears to be independent of type of portal hypertension, since patients with prehepatic portal hypertension also respond clinically.[59,194] Likewise, patients with various types of cirrhosis, including alcoholic, postnecrotic, and cryptogenic cirrhosis experience reduction in portal pressure with β-adrenergic blockade.[202] There are several reports of other nonselective β-adrenergic blockers in treating portal hypertension, with results similar to those reported in studies of propranolol. These agents include nadolol, mepindolol, and sotalol.[57,130]

The mechanism of the portal hypotensive effect of propranolol is a reduction in splanchnic or portal venous inflow. This is the result of a dual effect of nonselective β-blockade on cardiac output (mediated by β_1-adrenergic blockade) and splanchnic vasoconstriction (mediated by β_2-adrenergic blockade, resulting in unopposed α-adrenergic vasoconstriction).[212,320] Although β_1- and β_2-adrenergic blockers also lower portal pressure, the magnitude of the effect has been demonstrated in portal hypertensive rats to be less than that of nonspecific β-adrenergic antagonists.[212] Selective β_1-adrenergic blockade in patients is likewise less efficacious than nonselective β-blockade.[261,459]

Most clinical series have reported a rate of nonresponse ranging from 0% to 50%. In one study, after a 40-mg oral dose of propranolol, 60% of patients experienced reduction in HVPG, but only 30% had decreases of more than 20%, and even with higher doses, 20% or more do not respond.[125] Blood levels, heart rate reduction, severity of liver failure, and a variety of other hemodynamic, clinical, and laboratory parameters have all been shown to correlate poorly with β-blocker-induced decrease in HVPG.[58,125,185] Whereas portal pressure response to β-blockade is unpredictable, a consistent decrease in azygos blood flow has been observed.[48,73]

Although discussions of drug therapy of portal hypertension tend to focus on variceal hemorrhage, there also are data to support a role for propranolol in treatment of congestive gastropathy.[172,308] Moreover, the addition of isosorbide-5-mononitrate to propranolol may enhance the portal pressure reduction seen with β-adrenergic blockade.[124]

Propranolol therapy appears to be quite safe. Impotence and fatigue are reported.[440] Renal function does not seem to be affected.[15] Hepatic encephalopathy may rarely be attributed to β-blockers in patients with severe liver disease.[15] In patients without severe hepatocellular dysfunction or history of encephalopathy, however, propranolol does not alter cerebral blood flow, arterial ammonia, or neuropsychological functions.[74] Although cases of bleeding after cessation of propranolol therapy are reported, so-called rebound bleeding is not sufficiently well documented to justify avoiding its use.[227] The presence of bradycardia, chronic bronchospastic lung disease, insulin-dependent diabetes, and peripheral vascular disease should be considered contraindications to therapy with β-adrenergic blockers.

Propranolol is a first-line therapy for long-term treatment of portal hypertension. The drug should be dosed at 10 to 20 mg twice a day and titrated on a weekly basis up to a maximum of 160 mg twice a day. If available, patients who are started on propranolol should have baseline HVPG measurements. A reduction in the HVPG to levels below 12 mmHg has been demonstrated to protect against variceal bleeding and increase survival.[90,148] In view of the relative safety of the drug, however, it should not be withheld in situations where pressure measurements are unavailable. In this situation, the dose should be increased to achieve the maximal effect without inducing toxic side effects (severe bradycardia or arterial hypotension).

Vasodilators

Organic nitrates, α_2-agonists, calcium channel blockers, and 5-hydroxytryptamine antagonists are vasodilators that reduce portal pressure by decreasing intrahepatic vascular resistance or by dilating portosystemic collaterals. In vivo, however, many if not all vasodilators paradoxically induce reflex splanchnic arterial vasoconstriction in response to systemic vasodilation and venous pooling (Fig. 33-9). They therefore reduce portal pressure also by decreasing portal venous inflow. The ideal vasodilator would have relatively high selectivity for receptors in the hepatic vascular bed. Contractile myofibroblasts that line the hepatic sinusoids and fibrous septa in cirrhosis have been postulated to contribute to the increased resistance to portal blood flow in portal hypertension.[26,382] Investigators have used the isolated perfused cirrhotic rat liver to study the action of various vasodilators on receptors in the intrahepatic portal circulation.[11,26]

Organic Nitrates

Administration of short-acting (nitroglycerin) or long-acting (isosorbide dinitrate, 5-isosobide mononitrate) organic nitrates results in intracellular formation of nitric oxide and 5-nitrosothiol, leading to stimulation of guanylate cyclase and generation of cyclic guanosine monophosphate. The consequence is venodilation, which results from a decrease in calcium concentration in vascular smooth muscle cells due to decreased permeability to extracellular calcium and inhibi-

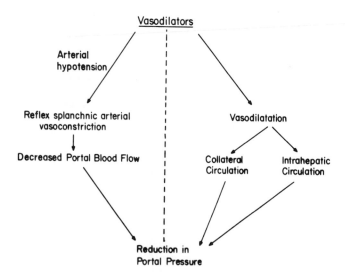

FIGURE 33-9 Illustration of the portal pressure–lowering effect of vasodilators. The mechanism of the portal flow–reducing effect of vasodilators is triggered by arterial hypotension and venous pooling.

tion of release of intracellular calcium from the sarcoplasmic reticulum.[109]

Sublingual and oral isosorbide-5-mononitrate have been shown to decrease portal pressure in cirrhotic patients.[119,169] Studies in portal hypertensive rats have provided insights into possible mechanisms. In rats, nitroglycerin reduces mean arterial pressure and induces venous pooling, thus activating low-pressure baroreceptors; in this way, it triggers splanchnic arterial vasoconstriction with consequent reduction in portal venous inflow and portal pressure.[214] The effect of nitrates on portal venous inflow appears to be dose dependent.[30] At low doses of isosorbide dinitrate, arterial pressure decreases by 10%, with reduction in portal venous inflow. At high nitrate doses, however, splanchnic arterial vasodilation is observed and the portal venous inflow is unaffected. Nevertheless, portal pressure decreases, probably by reducing portocollateral and intrahepatic resistance.

Several studies demonstrate a decrease in HVPG with organic nitrate therapy in cirrhosis.[29,165,257] Although alterations in systemic arterial blood pressure appear to correlate poorly with reduction in HVPG,[214] a correlation has been observed between the fall in the cardiac index, the increase in the systemic vascular resistance, and reduction in HVPG.[165] The effect of nitrates on the collateral circulation, as estimated by azygos blood flow, is variable. Increases and decreases in azygos blood flow have been observed,[126,280] suggesting that nitrates lower portal pressure by reducing portal venous inflow in some cases and by reducing portocollateral resistance in others.[28] This variability may be a result of dose differences, variability in the hepatic extraction, or the development of nitrate tolerance.[109] Another action of organic nitrates may be relaxation of myofibroblasts in the fibrous septa and in sinusoidal areas of the liver.

To summarize, nitrates have a clearly defined role in the clinical management of portal hypertension when used in combination with vasopressin to control gastroesophageal hemorrhage. Data suggest that the propranolol–nitroglycerin combination is worthy of further long-term clinical stud-

ies.[123] Likewise, the role of nitrates as single agents for treatment or portal hypertension needs to be better defined.

Clonidine
Clinical use of clonidine as a treatment for portal hypertension is premature because there are as yet no randomized, controlled trials evaluating this drug. Promising preliminary data have been reported in cirrhotic patients.[265,466] The drug has been observed to normalize peripheral norepinephrine levels,[1] to normalize cardiac output,[1] and to reduce HVPG without decreasing hepatic blood flow in humans.[265] Because clonidine exerts only a small effect on intrahepatic resistance in the isolated perfused cirrhotic rat liver, it is doubtful that its main mechanism of action is at this level.[249] Studies in cirrhotic rats suggest that the main effect of α_2-adrenergic blockade is to increase splanchnic arteriolar resistance, thereby decreasing portal venous inflow.[350] This study raises the question whether the clinical effect of clonidine therefore is not at the level of intrahepatic resistance but instead is mediated by a decrease in portal flow induced by reflex splanchnic vasoconstriction.

Calcium Channel Blockers
Despite encouraging animal studies using verapamil,[249,333] there are no satisfactory studies demonstrating efficacy in humans. Two studies in humans with cirrhosis suggest that there is little if any clinical role for this class of drugs in the treatment of portal hypertension.[279]

5-Hydroxytryptamine Receptor Antagonists
Studies of 5-hydroxytryptamine (5-HT; serotonin) blockers were prompted by the observation that this compound may be important in increasing portal vascular resistance. In fact, in portal hypertensive rats, Cummings and colleagues[97] demonstrated a greatly increased sensitivity to 5-HT in isolated mesenteric venous strips, which can be blocked with a 5-HT type 2 ($5-HT_2$) blocking agent, ketanserin, with resulting reduction in portal pressure. Clinical studies with ketanserin corroborated a portal pressure–lowering effect, but the drug is not in use because of undesirable complications in cirrhotic patients.[157,446]

ICI 169, 369 and ritanserin are $5-HT_2$ receptor antagonists with a greater binding affinity for 5-HT receptors than ketanserin.[97] Clinical studies using these compounds are eagerly anticipated, based on animal studies that suggest that they may be devoid of systemic hemodynamic toxicity, and may reduce portal vascular resistance without decreasing hepatic blood flow.[189,251] Mastai and colleagues[251] have postulated that the mechanism of portal pressure reduction in ritanserin therapy is an alteration in intrahepatic or portocollateral resistance.

Molsidomine
Molsidomine is a venodilator with antianginal properties similar to nitrates. Unlike with nitrates, however, tachyphylaxis has not been observed with molsidomine and it has minimal effects on arterial pressure. The acute effects of this agent in portal hypertensive alcoholic patients have been reported.[443] HVPG was reduced by about 15% with simultaneous decreases in hepatic blood flow, mean arterial pressure, and cardiac output. The role of molsidomine in the long-term treatment of portal hypertension is yet unexplored.

Constrictors of the Lower Esophageal Sphincter

Drugs of this class, including intravenous pentagastrin, domperidone, and metaclopramide, by constricting the lower esophageal sphincter, may decrease intravariceal pressure by impairing blood flow toward the variceal vessels. Preliminary reports suggest that further study of these agents is warranted.[199,243,250,263]

RESULTS OF CLINICAL TRIALS OF β-ADRENERGIC BLOCKADE, ENDOSCOPIC SCLEROTHERAPY, AND PORTAL DECOMPRESSIVE SURGERY IN PRIMARY PROPHYLAXIS AGAINST VARICEAL HEMORRHAGE

Despite the tremendous mortality (about 50%) associated with variceal hemorrhage,[66,138] only about 30% of patients experience bleeding over a period of 27 months after the presence of varices is diagnosed.[9,93] Therefore, identification of patients at risk for hemorrhage is a high priority, and excellent studies documenting endoscopic criteria that predict likelihood of bleeding have been published.[286] Because of the poor prognosis for patients with variceal hemorrhage, considerable attention has been focused on primary prophylaxis. Several conclusions can be drawn from review of studies in this field. First, the use of surgical shunts for prophylaxis against first variceal hemorrhage rightly has been abandoned despite significant reduction in the frequency of bleeding. This is because of a great excess in relative risk of mortality in all major studies.[92,93,182,338] Likewise, the use of prophylactic ES is not supported by existing data.

Despite numerous studies, there is marked heterogeneity of outcome of prophylactic ES trials, both with respect to bleeding and mortality.[4,113,118,200,303,311,319,360,366,420,452,471,472] Interpretation of these reports is confounded by a high degree of variability in risk of bleeding in the control groups, as demonstrated in a recent detailed metaanalysis that included many of these studies.[300]

Data concerning β-adrenergic blockade for primary prophylaxis in patients with large varices has been published in six full reports.[4,90,177,179,231,307] All demonstrate a reduction of bleeding rate in the treated groups, which reaches statistical significance in four studies.[4,90,177,307] It remains uncertain whether β-blockade favorably affects mortality, but this may be difficult to prove for statistical reasons.[300] Further studies also are needed to evaluate whether an increase in mortality may exist in certain subgroups.[179] Nevertheless, β-blockade is easy, inexpensive, and relatively free of adverse side effects in most patients. Therefore, this therapy should be used in patients with large varices who are thought to be at high risk for hemorrhage, provided that specific clinical contraindications (such as heart failure or obstructive lung disease) are not present. Insufficient data are available to make clear recommendations about prophylaxis in patients without large varices. Likewise, extrapolation of these data to patients with nonalcoholic liver disease must be made with caution since most of the patients studied have been alcoholic.

As previously stated, there have been no recognized clinical, laboratory, or hemodynamic parameters that can to used to predict a therapeutic response to β-blockade. This problem has been addressed in a recent cooperative study from New Haven, Boston, and Barcelona,[90] which provides evidence that reduction in HVPG to less than 12 mmHg is a useful index of treatment efficacy. Reduction of HVPG to this level was demonstrated to protect against variceal hemorrhage and to increase survival. Therefore, the use of hepatic venous pressure measurements is highly recommended, with the goal of reduction of HVPG to less than 12 mmHg. Other clinical parameters, such as reduction in heart rate, should not be viewed as adequate substitutes for HVPG in centers where this test is available.

RESULTS OF CLINICAL TRIALS OF β-ADRENERGIC BLOCKADE, ENDOSCOPIC SCLEROTHERAPY, AND PORTAL DECOMPRESSIVE SURGERY IN PROPHYLAXIS AGAINST RECURRENT VARICEAL HEMORRHAGE (THERAPEUTIC TRIALS)

β-Blockade Versus Placebo

Compared with placebo, relative risk of recurrent variceal hemorrhage decreased significantly in patients receiving β-blockers in all reported randomized trials.[68,82,89,128,129,230,322,375,440] The effect on mortality was somewhat more heterogeneous, with a nonsignificant reduction only in relative risk of death, when the results of seven of the studies are pooled in a metaanalysis.[68,82,128,129,230,300,322,440]

Endoscopic Sclerotherapy Versus Placebo

Endoscopic sclerotherapy was compared with placebo in eight randomized clinical therapeutic trials.[14,67,94,206,304,396,412,462] The rebleeding risk was significantly reduced in all but one trial.[412] Moreover, although the therapeutic response was heterogeneous, careful metaanalysis of the available data has revealed this variability to be in the magnitude rather than in the direction of the clinical response.[300] A significant reduction in pooled relative risk of death also is noted with ES. This risk reduction is not observed with either β-blockade or surgery.[178,300]

Portocaval Shunt Surgery Versus Placebo

Portocaval shunt was compared with placebo in four studies,[181,339,341,352] and found to be highly efficacious in preventing rebleeding in all studies. Despite increased portosystemic encephalopathy after shunt surgery, this well described complication was not more commonly encountered in the treated groups compared with the control groups because of the high risk of developing portosystemic encephalopathy after variceal hemorrhage. Although three of the four trials reported a decrease in mortality after portocaval anastomosis, pooled relative risk of death is not significantly decreased when the four trials are combined in a metaanalysis.[300]

Endoscopic Sclerotherapy Versus Shunt Surgery

There are several published studies comparing shunt surgery with ES.[81,166,207,347,400a,415,455] Compared with ES, shunt surgery was superior for reducing risk of rebleeding in all studies in which these data were reported. Neither form of treatment prevailed with respect to relative risk of death from rebleeding. In two studies,[166,455] however, patients who rebled after ES were shunted with good outcomes. In the remaining studies, 11% to 31% of patients originally randomized to ES also eventually underwent surgery for recurrent hemorrhage.

β-Adrenergic Blockade
Versus Endoscopic Sclerotherapy

Metaanalysis of the five available studies[2,103,112,416,463] reveals little difference between these modalities with respect to rebleeding and risk of death.[300]

Several conclusions can be drawn from the foregoing discussion. First, of the three modalities, only ES has been shown to decrease not only the risk of rebleeding but also the risk of death after initial variceal hemorrhage. In addition to the controlled trials mentioned, numerous long-term studies provide support for the view that ES should be the first-line treatment for acute bleeding as well as part of a program of prophylaxis against rebleeding. In the event of uncontrollable esophageal variceal hemorrhage or refractory bleeding from gastric varices, the patient may then undergo a shunt procedure or orthotopic liver transplantation; devascularization and esophageal transection procedures also are options in some cases.[241,413] Finally, it is fair to state that therapeutic trials comparing any modality with placebo no longer are justifiable, based on the available studies that demonstrate that any therapy decreases rebleeding rate compared with placebo (and sclerotherapy, at least, also decreases mortality).

Despite these points, clear guidelines have not yet been established for prophylaxis against rebleeding from esophageal varices. Although the ES data would suggest that this is the treatment of choice, it is more invasive and cumbersome than drug therapy. Moreover, no treatment surpasses shunt surgery for efficacy in prevention of rebleeding, although there are problems with this intervention that need to be solved before it can be considered a first-line therapy. Further large studies comparing these forms of treatment are needed before firm conclusions can be made. It is especially crucial further to investigate pharmacologic therapy because this probably will be the most practical and best-accepted form of treatment. Major areas for further investigation will focus on optimizing drug dosage, defining clinical indices of efficacy, and exploring new classes and combinations of drugs for treatment of portal hypertension.

RECOMMENDATIONS

We recommend the following approach to the patient with portal hypertension and gastroesophageal varices (see Fig. 33-8). For the patient with large varices who has never bled, the first choice is long-term treatment with nonselective β-adrenergic blockade. Since bleeding risk in patients with small varices appears to be low, the clinician can follow such patients without intervention. Further studies may provide data supporting pharmacologic therapy in patients with small varices.

The initial variceal hemorrhage is treated best with ES at the time of the diagnostic endoscopy. Pharmacologic therapy may be useful if these diagnostic and therapeutic interventions cannot be performed immediately, or to stabilize the patient until they can be performed. Balloon tamponade always can be used as an alternative option pending definitive treatment if ES and pharmacologic therapy fail. TIPS may also become an option in this setting.[478] However, before a role can be defined for TIPS in long-term prevention of rebleeding, it must be studied in controlled prospective trials in large numbers of patients. The use of TIPS for this indication is currently not recommended outside the context of such trials. If hemorrhage cannot be controlled, we recommend surgical intervention, which also may include orthotopic liver transplantation for patients with poor hepatic reserve.

In patients in whom the acute bleeding is controlled without surgery, transplantation still should be considered if hepatic reserve is poor, since this class of patients otherwise has a poor prognosis for rebleeding and death. In the remainder of patients, the clinician is faced with the choice of long-term ES, β-adrenergic blockade, or surgical decompression. The needs of the individual patient as well as the resources of the medical center dictate the preferable form of treatment.

References

1. Albillos A, Banares R, Barrios C, et al. Chronic oral clonidine administration in patients with alcoholic cirrhosis: hemodynamic and liver function effects. Gastroenterology 102:248, 1992
2. Alexandrino P, Martins Alves M, Correia JP. Propranolol or endoscopic sclerotherapy in the prevention of recurrence of variceal bleeding: a prospective, randomized controlled trial. J Hepatol 7:175, 1988
3. Andrade Z. Hepatic schistosomiasis: morphologic aspects. In: Popper H, Schaffner F, eds. Progress in liver diseases, vol 2. New York, Grune & Stratton, 1965, p 228
4. Andreani T, Poupon RE, Balkau BJ, et al. Preventive therapy of first gastrointestinal bleeding in patients with cirrhosis: results of a controlled trial comparing propranolol, endoscopic sclerotherapy and placebo. Hepatology 12:1413, 1990
5. Aronsen KF, Bjorkman L, Lindstrom K, et al. The mechanism of lysine-vasopressin in bleeding esophageal varices. Acta Chir Scand 145:231, 1979
6. Ashida H, Kotoura Y, Nishioka A, et al. Portal and mesenteric venous thrombosis as a complication of endoscopic sclerotherapy. Am J Gastroenterol 84:306, 1989
7. Aufses AH. Bleeding varices associated with haematologic disorders. Arch Surg 80:655, 1960
8. Baggenstoss AH, Cain JC. The hepatic hilar lymphatics of man: their relation to ascites. N Engl J Med 256:531, 1957
9. Baker LA, Smith C, Lieberman G. The natural history of esophageal varices: a study of 115 cirrhotic patients in whom varices were diagnosed prior to bleeding. Am J Med 26:228, 1959
10. Baldus WP, Hoffbauer FW. Vascular changes in the cirrhotic liver as studied by injection technic. Am J Dig Dis 8:689, 1963
11. Ballet F, Chretien Y, Rey C, et al. Differential response of normal and cirrhotic liver to vasoactive agents: a study in the isolated perfused liver. J Pharmacol Exp Ther 244:283, 1988
12. Balthazar EJ, Naidich DP, Megibow AJ, et al. CT evaluation of esophageal varices. AJR 148:131, 1987
13. Banti G. Splenomegalie mit Leberzirrhose: Beitrage zur pathologischen. Anat Allgemeinen Pathol 24:21, 1889
14. Barsoum MS, Bolous FI, El-Rooby AA, et al. Tamponade and injection sclerotherapy in the management of bleeding oesophageal varices. Br J Surg 69:76, 1982
15. Bataille C, Bercoff E, Pariente EA, et al. Effects of propranolol on renal blood flow and renal function in patients with cirrhosis. Gastroenterology 86:129, 1984
16. Becker CD, Cooperberg PL. Sonography of the hepatic vascular system. AJR 150:999, 1988
17. Beker S, Valencia-Parparcen J. Portal hypertension syndrome: a comparative analysis of bilharzial fibrosis and hepatic cirrhosis. Am J Dig Dis 13:1047, 1968
18. Belli L, Romani F, Riolo F, et al. Thrombosis of portal vein in absence of hepatic disease. Surg Gynecol Obstet 169:46, 1989
19. Bendtsen F, Skovgaard LT, Sorensen TIA, et al. Agreement among multiple observers on endoscopic diagnosis of esophageal varices before bleeding. Hepatology 11:341, 1990
20. Benoit JN, Barrowman JA, Harper SL, et al. Role of humoral

factors in the intestinal hyperemia associated with chronic portal hypertension. Am J Physiol 247:G486, 1984

21. Benoit JN, Womack WA, Hernandez L, et al. "Forward" and "backward" flow mechanisms of portal hypertension: relative contributions in the rat model of portal vein stenosis. Gastroenterology 89:1092, 1985

22. Benoit JN, Womack WA, Korthuis RJ, et al. Chronic portal hypertension: effects on gastrointestinal blood flow distribution. Am J Physiol 250:G535, 1986

23. Benoit JN, Zimmermann H, Premeu AJ, et al. Role of glucagon in splanchnic hyperemia of chronic portal hypertension. Am J Physiol 251:G674, 1986

24. Beppu K, Inokuchi K, Koyanagi N, et al. Prediction of variceal hemorrhage by esophageal endoscopy. Gastrointest Endosc 27:213, 1981

25. Berk P, Popper H, Kreuger G, et al. Diagnosis and management of the Budd-Chiari syndrome. Am J Surg 160:128, 1990

26. Bhathal PS, Grossman HJ. Reduction of the increased portal vascular resistance of the isolated perfused cirrhotic rat liver by vasodilators. J Hepatol 1:325, 1985

27. Blancet L, Lebrec D. Changes in splanchnic blood flow in portal hypertensive rats. Eur J Clin Invest 12:327, 1982

28. Blei AT, Ganger D, Fung HL, et al. Organic nitrates in portal hypertension. Eur Heart J 9:205, 1988

29. Blei AT, Garcia-Tsao G, Groszmann RJ, et al. Hemodynamic evaluation of isosorbide dinitrate in alcoholic cirrhosis: pharmacokinetic–hemodynamic interactions. Gastroenterology 93:576, 1987

30. Blei AT, Gottstein J. Isosorbide dinitrate in experimental portal hypertension: a study of factors that modulate the hemodynamic response. Hepatology 6:107, 1986

31. Blei AT, Groszmann RJ. Vasopressin and vasoconstrictors. In: Shepherd AP, Granger DN, eds. The physiology of the intestinal circulation. New York, Raven Press, 1984, p 377

32. Blei AT, Groszmann GJ, Gusberg R, et al. Comparison of vasopressin and triglycyl-lycine vasopressin on splanchnic and systemic hemodynamics in dogs. Dig Dis Sci 25:688, 1980

33. Blendis L, Banks D, Romboer C, et al. Spleen blood flow and splanchnic haemodynamics in blood dyscrasias and other splenomegalies. Clin Sci 38:73, 1970

34. Blendis LM, Orrego H, Crossley IR, et al. The role of hepatocyte enlargement and hepatic pressure in cirrhotic and non-cirrhotic alcoholic liver disease. Hepatology 2:539, 1982

35. Blendis LM, Parkinson MC, Shilkin KB, et al. Nodular regenerative hyperplasia of the liver in Felty's syndrome. Q J Med 43:25, 1974

36. Bloom SR, Polak JM. Somatostatin. Br Med J 295:288, 1987

37. Boesky S, Pedersen SA. The effect of vasopressin on resting gastroesophageal sphincter pressure in man. Scand J Gastroenterol 9:587, 1974

38. Bolondi L, Gandolfi L, Arienti V, et al. Ultrasonography in the diagnosis of portal hypertension: diminished response of portal vessels to respiration. Radiology 142:167, 1982

39. Bomzon A, Finberg JPM, Tovbin D, et al. Bile salts, hypotension and obstructive jaundice. Clin Sci 67:177, 1984

40. Bosch J. Effect of pharmacological agents on portal hypertension: a haemodynamic appraisal. Clin Gastroenterol 14:169, 1985

41. Bosch J, Bordas JM, Mastai R, et al. Effects of vasopressin on the intravariceal pressure in patients with cirrhosis: comparison with the effects on portal pressure. Hepatology 8:861, 1988

42. Bosch J, Bordas JM, Rigau J, et al. Non-invasive measurement of the pressure of esophageal varices using an endoscopic gauge: comparison with measurements by variceal puncture in patients undergoing endoscopic sclerotherapy. Hepatology 6:667, 1986

43. Bosch J, Enriquez R, Groszmann RJ. Chronic bile duct ligation in the dog: hemodynamic characterization of a portal hypertensive model. Hepatology 3:1002, 1983

44. Bosch J, Groszmann RJ. Measurement of azygos venous blood flow by a continuous thermodilution technique: an index of blood flow through gastroesophageal collaterals in cirrhosis. Hepatology 4:424, 1984

45. Bosch J, Groszmann RJ, Garcia-Pagan JC, et al. Association of transdermal nitroglycerin to vasopressin infusion in the treatment of variceal hemorrhage: a placebo-controlled clinical trial. Hepatology 10:962, 1989

46. Bosch J, Kravetz D, Mastai R, et al. Azygos venous blood flow in cirrhosis: effects of balloon tamponade, vasopressin, somatostatin and propranolol. Hepatology 3:855, 1983

47. Bosch J, Kravetz D, Rodes J. Effects of somatostatin on hepatic and systemic hemodynamics in patients with cirrhosis of the liver: comparison with vasopressin. Gastroenterology 80:518, 1981

48. Bosch J, Mastai R, Kravetz D, et al. Effects of propranolol on azygos venous blood flow and hepatic and systemic hemodynamics in cirrhosis. Hepatology 4:1200, 1984

49. Bosch J, Mastai R, Kravetz D, et al. Measurement of azygous venous blood flow in the evaluation of portal hypertension in patients with cirrhosis: clinical and hemodynamic correlation in 100 patients. J Hepatol 1:125, 1985

50. Bosch J, Mastai R, Kravetz D, et al. Hemodynamic evaluation of patients with portal hypertension. Semin Liver Dis 6:309, 1986

51. Boyer JL, Chatterjee C, Iber FL, et al. Effect of plasma-volume expansion on portal hypertension. N Engl J Med 275:750, 1966

52. Boyer JL, Sengupta KP, Biswas SK, et al. Idiopathic portal hypertension: comparison with the portal hypertension of cirrhosis and extrahepatic portal vein obstruction. Ann Intern Med 66:41, 1967

53. Boyer TD, Triger DR, Horisawa M, et al. Direct transhepatic measurement of portal vein pressure using a thin needle: comparison with wedged hepatic vein pressure. Gastroenterology 72:584, 1977

54. Bradley SE. The hepatic circulation. In: Hamilton WF, Dow P, eds. Handbook of physiology. Washington, DC, American Physiological Society, 1963, p 1387

55. Bradley SE. Variations in hepatic blood flow in man during health and disease. N Engl J Med 240:456, 1949

56. Bradley SJ, Ingelfinger FJ, Bradley GP, et al. The estimation of hepatic blood flow in man. J Clin Invest 24:890, 1945

57. Braillon A, Cales P, Lebrec D. Comparison of short-term effects of mepindolol and propranolol on splanchnic and systemic haemodynamics in patients with cirrhosis. Int J Clin Pharmacol Res 5:223, 1985

58. Braillon A, Cales P, Valla D, et al. Influence of the degree of liver failure on systemic and splanchnic hemodynamics and on response to propranolol in patients with cirrhosis. Gut 27:1204, 1986

59. Braillon A, Moreau R, Hadengue A, et al. Hyperkinetic circulatory syndrome in patients with presinusoidal portal hypertension: effect of propranolol. J Hepatol 9:312, 1989

60. Bras G, Jelliffe D, Stuart, K. Veno-occlusive disease of liver with nonportal type of cirrhosis, occurring in Jamaica. Arch Pathol 57:285, 1954

61. Brazzini A, Hunter DW, Darcy MD, et al. Safe splenoportography. Radiology 162:607, 1987

62. Bredfeldt JE, Riley EM, Groszmann RJ. Compensatory mechanism in response to an elevated hepatic oxygen consumption in chronic ethanol-fed rats. Am J Physiol 248:G507, 1985

63. Bruix J, Bosch J, Kravetz D, et al. Effects of prostaglandin inhibition on systemic and hepatic hemodynamics in patients with cirrhosis of the liver. Gastroenterology 88:430, 1985

64. Burchnell AR, Morena AH, Panke WF, et al. Hepatic artery flow improvement after portacaval shunt: a single hemodynamic correlate. Ann Surg 184;289, 1978

65. Burns P, Taylor K, Blei AT. Doppler flowmetry and portal hypertension. Gastroenterology 92:824, 1987

66. Burroughs AK, D'Heygere F, McIntyre N. Pitfalls in studies

of prophylactic therapy for variceal bleeding in cirrhotics. Hepatology 6:1407, 1986

67. Burroughs AK, D'Heygere F, Phillips A, et al. Prospective randomized trial of chronic sclerotherapy for prevention of variceal rebleeding, with use of the same protocol to treat rebleeding in all patients: single interim analysis. J Hepatol 3:S25A, 1986

68. Burroughs AK, Jenkins WJ, Sherlock S, et al. Controlled trial of propranolol for the prevention of recurrent variceal hemorrhage in patients with cirrhosis. N Engl J Med 309:1539, 1983

69. Burroughs AK, McCormick PA, Hughes MD, et al. Randomized, double-blind, placebo-controlled trial of somatostatin for variceal bleeding: emergency control and prevention of early variceal rebleeding. Gastroenterology 99:1388, 1990

70. Burton AC, ed. Physical principles of circulatory phenomena: the physical equilibrium of the heart and blood vessels. In: Handbook of physiology: circulation. Bethesda, MD, 1962, p 85

71. Butler H. The veins of the esophagus. Thorax 6:267, 1951

72. Caesar J, Shaldon S, Chiandussi L, et al. The use of indocyanine green in the measurement of hepatic blood flow and as a test of hepatic function. Clin Sci 21:43, 1961

73. Cales P, Braillon J, Jiron M, et al. Superior portosystemic collateral circulation estimated by azygos blood flow in patients with cirrhosis. J Hepatol 1:37, 1985

74. Cales P, Pierre-Nicolas M, Guell A, et al. Propranolol does not alter cerebral blood flow and functions in cirrhotic patients without previous hepatic encephalopathy. Hepatology 9:439, 1989

75. Capron JP, LeMay JL, Muir JR, et al. Portal vein thrombosis and fatal pulmonary thromboembolism associated with oral contraceptive treatment. J Clin Gastroenterol 3:295, 1981

76. Caramelo C, Okada K, Tsai, P, et al. Interaction of arginine vasopressin and angiotensin II on Ca^{2+} mobilization and contraction in rat cultured vascular smooth muscle cells. Kidney Int 38:47, 1990

77. Carneiro JJ, Donal DE. Change in liver blood flow and blood content in dogs during direct and reflex alteration of hepatic sympathetic nerve activity. Circ Res 40:150, 1975

78. Carneiro JJ, Donal DE. Blood reservoir function of dog spleen, liver and intestine. Am J Physiol 232:H67, 1977

79. Caro CG, Pedley TJ, Schroter RC, Seed WA, eds. The mechanics of the circulation. Oxford, Oxford University Press, 1978, p 86

80. Cash JD, Gader AMA, DaCosta J. The release of plasminogen activator and factor VIII to lysine vasopressin, arginine vasopressin, 1-desamino-8-d-arginine vasopressin, angiotensin and oxytocin in man. Br J Haematol 27:363, 1974

81. Cello JP, Grendell JH, Crass RA, et al. Endoscopic sclerotherapy versus portacaval shunt in patients with severe cirrhosis and acute variceal hemorrhage: long-term follow-up. N Engl J Med 316:11, 1987

82. Cerbelaud P, Lavignolle A, Perrin D, et al. Propranolol et prévention des récidives de rupture de varice oesophagienne du cirrhotique. Gastroenterol Clin Biol 18:A10, 1986

83. Chiles NH, Baggenstoss AN, Butt HR, et al. Esophageal varices: comparative incidence of ulceration and spontaneous rupture as a cause of fatal hemorrhage. Gastroenterology 25:565, 1953

84. Chojkier M, Conn HO. Esophageal tamponade in the treatment of bleeding varices. Dig Dis Sci 25:267, 1980

85. Chojkier M, Groszmann RJ, Atterbury CE, et al. A controlled comparison of continuous intra-arterial and intravenous infusions of vasopressin in hemorrhage from esophageal varices. Gastroenterology 77:540, 1979

86. Cohen D, Mansour A. Extrahepatic portal hypertension: long-term results. Prog Pediatr Surg 10:129, 1977

87. Cohn JN, Khatri IM, Groszmann RJ, et al. Hepatic blood flow in alcoholic liver disease measured by an indicator dilution technique. Am J Med 53:704, 1972

88. Colman JC, Britton RS, Orrego H, et al. Relation between osmotically induced hepatocyte enlargement and portal hypertension. Am J Physiol 245:G382, 1983

89. Colombo M, de Franchis F, Tommasini M, et al. Beta-blockade prevents recurrent gastrointestinal bleeding in well-compensated patients with alcoholic cirrhosis: a multicenter randomized controlled trial. Hepatology 9:433, 1989

90. Conn HO, Grace ND, Bosch J, et al. Propranolol in the prevention of the first hemorrhage from esophagogastric varices: a multicenter, randomized clinical trial. Hepatology 13:902, 1991

91. Conn HO, Ramsby GR, Storer EH, et al. Intra-arterial vasopressin in the treatment of upper gastrointestinal hemorrhage: a prospective controlled trial. Gastroenterology 68:211, 1975

92. Conn HO, Lindenmuth WW, May CJ, et al. Prophylactic portacaval anastomosis in cirrhotic patients with esophageal varices. N Engl J Med 272:1255, 1965

93. Conn HO, Lindenmuth WW, May, CJ, et al. Prophylactic portacaval anastomosis. Medicine 51:27, 1972

94. The Copenhagen Esophageal Varices Sclerotherapy Project. Sclerotherapy after first variceal hemorrhage in cirrhosis: a randomized multicenter trial. N Engl J Med 311:1594, 1984

95. Coutinho A. Hemodynamic studies of portal hypertension in schistosomiasis. Am J Med 44:547, 1968

96. Cowlishaw JL, Pollard EJ, Cowe, AE, et al. Liver disease associated with chronic arsenic ingestion. Aust NZ J Med 9:310, 1979

97. Cummings SA, Groszmann RJ, Kaumann A. Hypersensitivity of mesenteric veins to 5-hydroxytryptamine and ketanserin induced reduction of portal pressure in portal hypertensive rats. Br J Pharmacol 89:501, 1986

98. Dagradi AE. Esophageal varices, splenic pulp pressure and "directional" flow patterns in alcoholic liver cirrhosis. Am J Gastroenterol 59:15, 1973

99. D'Amico G, Montalbano L, Pagliaro L, et al. Natural history of congestive gastropathy in cirrhosis. Gastroenterology 99:1558, 1990

100. Datta DV, Grover SL, Saini VK, et al. Portal hypertension in chronic leukaemia. Br J Haematol 31:279, 1975

101. Datta DV, Mitra SK, Chuttani PN, et al. Chronic oral arsenic intoxication as a possible etiological factor in idiopathic portal hypertension (non-cirrhotic portal fibrosis) in India. Gut 20:378, 1979

102. DeWeert TM, Gostout CJ, Wiesner RH. Congestive gastropathy and other upper endoscopic findings in 81 consecutive patients undergoing orthotopic liver transplantation. Am J Gastroenterol 85:573, 1990

103. Dollet JM, Champigneulle B, Patris A, et al. Sclerotherapie endoscopique contre propranolol après hemorrhage par rupture de varices oesophagiennes chez le cirrhotique: resultats a 4 ans d-une étude randomizée. Gastroenterol Clin Biol 12:234, 1988

104. Donovan AJ, Reynolds TB, Mikkelsen W, et al. Systemic-portal arteriovenous fistulas: pathologic and hemodynamic observations in two patients. Surgery 66:474, 1969

105. Douglas JG, Forrest JAH, Prowse CV, et al. Effects of lysine-vasopressin and glypressin on the fibrinolytic system in cirrhosis. Gut 20:565, 1979

106. Eckardt VF, Grace ND. Gastroesophageal reflux and bleeding esophageal varices. Gastroenterology 76:39, 1979

107. Edmondson H, Peters R, Reynolds T, et al. Sclerosing hyaline necrosis of the liver in the chronic alcoholic. Ann Intern Med 59:646, 1963

108. Edmondson HA, Peters RL, Frankel HH, et al. The early stage of liver injury in the alcoholic. Medicine 46:119, 1967

109. Elkayam U. Tolerance to organic nitrates: evidence, mechanisms, clinical relevance, and strategies for prevention. Ann Intern Med 114:667, 1991

110. Falk H, Herbert JT, Edmonds L, et al. Review of four cases

of childhood hepatic angiosarcoma: elevated environmental arsenic exposure in one case. Cancer 47:382, 1981

111. Fenyves D, Pomier-Layrargues G, Willems B, Cole J. Intrahepatic pressure measurement: not an accurate reflection of portal vein pressure. Hepatology 8:211, 1988

112. Fleig WE, Stange EF, Schonborn W, et al. Propranolol (P) versus endoscopic sclerotherapy (EVS) for the prevention of recurrent hemorrhage in cirrhosis: final analysis of a randomization clinical trial. J Hepatol 7(Suppl):S32, 1988

113. Fleig WE, Stange EF, Wordehoff D, et al. A randomized trial comparing prophylactic (PS) and therapeutic sclerotherapy in cirrhotic patients with large oesophageal varices and no previous hemorrhage. J Hepatol 7(Suppl):S128, 1988

114. Fogel MR, Knauer CM, Andres LL, et al. Continues intravenous vasopressin in active upper gastrointestinal bleeding. Ann Intern Med 96:565, 1982

115. Foley WD, Stewart ET, Milbrath JR, et al. Digital subtraction angiography of the portal venous system. AJR 140:495, 1983

116. Folkow B, Neil E, eds. Circulation. London, Oxford University Press, 1971, p 14

117. Fort E, Sautereau D, Silvain C, et al. A randomized trial of terlipressin plus nitroglycerin vs. balloon tamponade in the control of acute variceal hemorrhage. Hepatology 11:678, 1990

118. Franchis R, the North Italian Endoscopic Clubs. Prophylactic sclerotherapy (ST) in high risk cirrhotics selected by endoscopic criteria: interim report of a multicenter randomized controlled trial. J Hepatol 7(Suppl):S23, 1988

119. Freeman JG, Barton JR, Record CO. Effect of isosorbide dinitrate, verapamil and labetalol on portal pressure in cirrhosis. Br Med J 1985;291:561,

120. Freeman JG, Lishman AJ, Cobden I, Record CO. Terlipressin (glypressin) versus vasopressin in the early treatment of esophageal varices. Lancet 2:66, 1982

121. Friedman EW, Weiner RS. Estimation of hepatic sinusoid pressure by means of venous catheters and estimation of portal pressure by hepatic vein catheterization. Am J Physiol 165:527, 1951

122. Fronek AW. Measurement of flow in single blood vessels including cardiac output by local thermodilution. Circ Res 8:175, 1960

122a. Ganz W, Swan HJC. Measurement of blood flow by the thermodilution technique. In: Bloomfield DA, ed. Dye curves: the theory and practice of indicator dilution. Baltimore, University Park Press, 1974, p 245

123. Garcia-Pagan JC, Feu F, Bosch J, et al. Propranolol compared with propranolol plus isosorbide-5-mononitrate for portal hypertension in cirrhosis. Ann Intern Med 114:869, 1991

124. Garcia-Pagan JC, Navasa M, Bosch J, et al. Enhancement of portal pressure reduction by the association of isosorbide-5-mononitrate to propranolol administration in patients with cirrhosis. Hepatology 11:230, 1990

125. Garcia-Tsao G, Grace ND, Groszmann RJ, et al. Short term effects of propranolol on portal venous pressure. Hepatology 6:101, 1986

126. Garcia-Tsao G, Groszmann RJ. Portal hemodynamics during nitroglycerin administration in cirrhotic patients. Hepatology 7:805, 1987

127. Garcia-Tsao G, Groszmann RJ, Fisher RL, et al. Portal pressure, presence of gastroesophageal varices and variceal bleeding. Hepatology 5:419, 1985

127a. Garcia-Tsao G, Panzini L, Yoselevitz M, et al. Bacillary peliosis hepatis as a cause of acute anemia in a patient with the acquired immunodeficiency syndrome. Gastroenterology 102:1065, 1992

128. Garden OJ, Mills PR, Birnie GG, et al. Propranolol in the prevention of recurrent variceal hemorrhage in cirrhotic patients. Gastroenterology 98:185, 1990

129. Gatta A, Merkel C, Sacerdoti D, et al. Nadolol for prevention of variceal rebleeding in cirrhosis: a controlled clinical trial. Digestion 37:22, 1987

130. Gatta A, Sacerdoti D, Merkel C, et al. Effects of nadolol treatment on renal and hepatic hemodynamics and function in cirrhotic patients with portal hypertension. Am Heart J 108:1167, 1984

131. Genecin P, Polio J, Colombato LA, et al. Bile acids do not mediate the hyperdynamic circulation in portal hypertensive rats. Am J Physiol 259:G21, 1990

132. Genecin P, Polio J, Groszmann RJ. Na restriction blunts expansion of plasma volume and ameliorates hyperdynamic circulation in portal hypertension. Am J Physiol 259:G498, 1990

133. Giltin N, Grahame GR, Kreel L, et al. Splenic blood flow and resistance in patients with cirrhosis before and after portacaval anastomosis. Gastroenterology 59:208, 1970

134. Gimson AE, Westaby D, Hegarty J, et al. A randomized trial of vasopressin and vasopressin plus nitroglycerin in the control of acute variceal hemorrhage. Hepatology 6:410, 1986

135. Goodman ZD, Ishak KG. Occlusive venous lesions in alcoholic liver disease: a study of 200 cases. Gastroenterology 83:786, 1982

136. Gores GJ, Wiesner RH, Dickson ER, et al. Prospective evaluation of esophageal varices in primary biliary cirrhosis: development, natural history, and influence on survival. Gastroenterology 96:1552, 1989

137. Graham RM, Pettinger WA. Drug therapy: prazosin. N Engl J Med 300:232, 1979

138. Graham DY, Smith JL. The course of patients after variceal hemorrhage. Gastroenterology 80:800, 1981

139. Greenway CV, Lawson AE, Stark RD. The effect of hemorrhage on hepatic artery and portal vein flows in the anesthetized cat. J Physiol (Lond) 193:375, 1967

140. Greenway CV, Oshiro G. Intrahepatic distribution of portal and hepatic arterial blood flows in anesthetized cats and dogs and the effects of portal occlusion, raised venous pressure and histamine. J Physiol (Lond) 227:473, 1972

141. Greenway CV, Stark RD. Hepatic vascular bed. Physiol Rev 51:23, 1971

142. Griner P, Elbadani A, Packman C. Veno-occlusive disease of the liver after chemotherapy of acute leukemia. Ann Intern Med 85:578, 1976

143. Groszmann RJ. The measurement of liver blood flow using clearance techniques. Hepatology 3:1039, 1983

144. Groszmann RJ. Reassessing portal venous pressure measurements. Gastroenterology 80:1611, 1984

145. Groszmann RJ, Atterbury CE. The pathophysiology of portal hypertension: a basis for classification. Semin Liver Dis 2:177, 1982

146. Groszmann RJ, Blei A, Atterbury CE. Portal hypertension. In: Arias IM, Popper H, Jakoby WB, Schachter DA, Shafritz DA, eds. The liver: biology and pathobiology, ed 2. New York, Raven Press, 1988, p 1147

147. Groszmann RJ, Blei AT, Kniaz JL, et al. Portal pressure reduction induced by partial mechanical obstruction of the superior mesenteric artery in the anesthetized dog. Gastroenterology 75:187, 1978

148. Groszmann RJ, Bosch J, Grace ND, et al. Hemodynamic events in a prospective randomized trial of propranolol versus placebo in the prevention of a first variceal hemorrhage. Gastroenterology 99:1401, 1991

149. Groszmann RJ, Colombato LA. Gastric vascular changes in portal hypertension. Hepatology 8:1708, 1988

150. Groszmann RJ, Glickman M, Blei AT, et al. Wedged and free hepatic venous pressure measured with a balloon catheter. Gastroenterology 76:253, 1979

152. Groszmann RJ, Kotelanski B, Cohn JN. Circulation of portosystemic shunting from the splenic and mesenteric beds in alcoholic liver disease Am J Med 53:715, 1972

153. Groszmann RJ, Kravetz D, Bosch J, et al. Nitroglycerin improves the hemodynamic response to vasopressin in portal hypertension. Hepatology 2:757, 1982

154. Grundfest A, Cooperman AM, Ferguson R, et al. Portal hy-

pertension associated with systemic mastocytosis and spleno-megaly. Gastroenterology 78:370, 1980

155. Haddock G, Garden OJ, McKee RF, et al. Esophageal tam-ponade in the management of acute variceal hemorrhage. Dig Dis Sci 24:913, 1989

156. Hadengue A, Lebrec D, Benhamou J-P. Pulmonary arterial hypertension in patients with portal hypertension. In: Okuda K, Benhamou J-P, eds. Portal hypertension: clinical and phys-iological aspects. Tokyo, Springer-Verlag, 1991, p 401

157. Hadengue A, Lee SS, Moreau R, et al. Beneficial hemody-namic effects of ketanserin in patients with cirrhosis: possible role of serotonergic mechanisms in portal hypertension. Hep-atology 7:644, 1987

158. Hadjis NS, Blumgart LH. Role of liver atrophy, hepatic resec-tion and hepatocyte hyperplasia in the development of portal hypertension in biliary disease. Gut 28:1022, 1987

159. Hall C, Bergan A, Henriksen, JE. Washout of intraparenchy-mally injected xenon 133 as a parameter of liver blood flow in the dog. Scand J Clin Invest 35:635, 1975

160. Halvorsen JF, Myking AO. The porto-systemic collateral pat-tern in the rat: an angiographic and anatomic study after par-tial occlusion of the portal vein. Eur Surg Res 6:183, 1974

161. Hamilton G, Phing RCF, Hulton RA, et al. The relationship between prostacyclin activity and pressures in the portal vein. Hepatology 2:236, 1982

162. Hanson KM. Liver. In: Johnson PC, ed. Peripheral circula-tion. New York, John Wiley & Sons, 1978, p 285

163. Hanson KM, Johnson PC. Local control of hepatic arterial and portal venous flow in the dog. Am J Physiol 211:712, 1966

164. Hashizume M, Kitano S, Sugimachi K, et al. Three-dimen-sional view of the vascular structure of the lower esophagus in clinical portal hypertension. Hepatology 8:1482, 1988

165. Hayes PC, Westaby D, Williams R. Effect and mechanism of action of isosorbide-5-mononitrate. Gut 29:752, 1988

166. Henderson JM, Kutner MH, Millikan WJ Jr, et al. Endo-scopic variceal sclerosis compared with distal splenorenal shunt to prevent recurrent variceal bleeding in cirrhosis: a pro-spective, randomized trial. Ann Intern Med 112:262, 1990

167. Hirooka M, Kimura C. Membranous obstruction of the he-patic portion of the inferior vena cava. Arch Surg 100:656, 1970

168. Hoffman SL, Piessens WF, Ratiwayanti S, et al. Reduction of suppressor T lymphocytes in the tropical splenomegaly syn-drome. N Engl J Med 310:337, 1984

169. Hollemans R, Naije R, Nols P, et al. Treatment of portal hy-pertension with isosorbide dinitrate alone and in combination with vasopressin. Crit Care Med 11:536, 1983

170. Hopkinson BR, Schener WG. The electromagnetic measure-ment of liver blood flow and cardiac output in conscious dogs during feeding and exercise. Surgery 63:970, 1968

171. Horisawa M, Yokoyama T, Juttner H, et al. Incomplete mem-branous obstruction of the inferior vena cava. Arch Surg 111:599, 1976

172. Hosking SW, Kennedy HJ, Seddon I, et al. The role of pro-pranolol in congestive gastropathy of portal hypertension. Hepatology 7:437, 1987

173. Hosking SW, Smart HL, Johnson AG, et al. Anorectal var-ices, haemorrhoids, and portal hypertension. Lancet 1:349, 1989

174. Hosoki T, Arisawa J, Marukawa T, et al. Portal blood flow in congestive heart failure: pulsed duplex sonographic findings. Radiology 174:733, 1990

175. Huet PM, Goresky CA, Villeneuve JP, et al. Assessment of liver microcirculation in human cirrhosis. J Clin Invest 70:1234, 1982

176. Hyun BH, Singer EP, Sharrett RH. Esophageal varices and metastatic carcinoma of the liver: a report of three cases and review of the literature. Arch Pathol 77:292, 1976

177. Ideo, G, Bellati G, Fesce E, et al. Nadolol can prevent the

178. Infante-Rivard C, Esnaola S, Villeneuve JP. Role of endo-scopic variceal sclerotherapy in the long-term management of variceal bleeding: a meta-analysis. Gastroenterology 96:1087, 1989

179. The Italian Multicenter Project for Propranolol in Prevention of Bleeding. Propranolol for prophylaxis of bleeding in cir-rhotic patients with large varices: a multicenter, randomized clinical trial. Hepatology 8:1, 1988

180. Jackson FC. Directional flow patterns in portal hypertension. Arch Surg 87:307, 1963

181. Jackson FC, Perrin EB, Felix RW, et al. A clinical investi-gation of the portacaval shunt: survival analysis of the thera-peutic operation. Ann Surg 174:672, 1971

182. Jackson FC, Perrin EB, Smith AG, et al. A clinical investi-gation of the portacaval shunt. II. Survival of the prophylactic operation. Am J Surg 115:22, 1968

183. Jaspan J, Polonsky J, Lewis M, et al. Reduction of portal vein blood flow by somatostatin. Diabetes 28:888, 1979

184. Jenkins SA, Baxter JN, Corbett WA, et al. A prospective ran-domized controlled clinical trial comparing somatostatin and vasopressin in controlling acute variceal hemorrhage. Br Med J 290:275, 1985

185. Jiron MI, Delhotal B, Lebrec D. Relationship between dose, blood level and haemodynamic response in patients with cir-rhosis receiving propranolol. Eur J Clin Pharmacol 28:353, 1985

186. Johnson WE, Widrich WC, Ansell JE, et al. Control of bleeding varices by vasopressin: a prospective randomized study. Ann Surg 186:369, 1977

187. Joly JG, Marleau D, Legare A, et al. Bleeding from esopha-geal varices in cirrhosis of the liver. Can Med Assoc J 104:576, 1971

188. Kashiwagi T, Kamada T, Abe H. Dynamic studies of the por-tal hemodynamics by scintiphotosplenoportography: stream-line flow in the human portal vein. Gastroenterology 69:1292, 1975

189. Kaumann AJ, Morgan JS, Groszmann RJ. ICI 169, 369 se-lectively blocks 5-hydroxytryptamine-2 receptors and lowers portal pressure in portal hypertensive rats. Gastroenterology 95:1601, 1988

190. Kelty RH, Baggenstoss AH, Butt HR. The relation of the re-generated liver nodule to the vascular bed in cirrhosis. Gas-troenterology 15:285, 1950

191. Kessler R, Tice D, Zimmon D. Value, complications and limitations of umbilical vein catheterization. Surg Gynecol Obstet 136:526, 1973

192. Kew M, Varma R, Dos Santos H, et al. Portal hypertension in primary biliary cirrhosis. Gut 12:830, 1971

193. Kiel JW, Pitts V, Benoit JN, et al. Reduced vascular sensitivity to norepinephrine in portal hypertensive rats. Am J Physiol 248:G192, 1985

194. Kiire CF. Controlled trial of propranolol to prevent recurrent variceal bleeding in patients with non-cirrhotic portal fibrosis. Br Med J 298:1363, 1989

195. Kimur, C, Matsuda S, Koie H, et al. Membranous obstruc-tion of the hepatic portion of the inferior vena cava: clinical study of nine cases. Surgery 72:551, 1972

196. Kimura T, Moriyasu F, Kawasaki T. Relationship between esophageal varices and azygos vein evaluated by cineportog-raphy. Hepatology 13:858, 1991

197. Kitano S, Terblanche J, Kahn D, et al. Venous anatomy of the lower oesophagus in portal hypertension: practical impli-cations. Br J Surg 73:525, 1986

198. Kleber G, Sauerbruch T, Fischer G, et al. Pressure of intra-oesophageal varices assessed by fine needle puncture: its rela-tion to endoscopic signs and severity of liver disease in patients with cirrhosis. Gut 30:228, 1989

199. Kleber G, Sauerbruch T, Gottfried F, et al. Reduction of

transmural oesophageal variceal pressure by metoclopramide. J Hepatol 12:362, 1991

200. Koch H, Henning H, Grimm H, et al. Prophylactic sclerosing of esophageal varices: results of a prospective controlled study. Endoscopy 18:40, 1986

201. Kock NG, Tibblin S, Schenk WG. Modification by glucagon of the splanchnic vascular responses to activation of the sympathicoadrenal system. J Surg Res 11:12, 1971

202. Kong CW, Lay CS, Tsai YT, et al. Hemodynamic effect of propranolol on portal hypertension in patients with HBs-Ag positive cirrhosis. Dig Dis Sci 31:1303, 1986

203. Kontos HH, Shapiro W, Mauck HP, et al. General and regional circulatory alterations in cirrhosis of the liver. Am J Med 37:526, 1964

204. Kornhauser DM, Wood AJJ, Vestal RE, et al. Biological determinants of propranolol disposition in man. Clin Pharmacol Ther 23:165, 1978

205. Korthuis RJ, Benoit JN, Kvietys PR, et al. Humoral factors may mediate increased rat hindquarter blood flow in portal hypertension. Am J Physiol 249:H827, 1985

206. Korula J, Balart LA, Radvan G, et al. A prospective randomized controlled trial of chronic esophageal variceal sclerotherapy. Hepatology 5:584, 1985

207. Korula J, Yellin A, Yamada S, et al. A prospective randomized controlled comparison of chronic endoscopic variceal sclerotherapy and portal-systemic shunt for variceal hemorrhage in Child's class A cirrhotics. Gastroenterology 92:1745, 1987

208. Kowalski HJ, Adelmann WH. The cardiac output at rest and in Laennec's cirrhosis. J Clin Invest 32:1025, 1953

209. Kravetz D, Bosch J, Teres J, et al. A controlled comparison of continuous somatostatin and vasopressin infusions in the treatment of acute variceal hemorrhage. Hepatology 4:442, 1984

210. Kravetz D, Cummings SA, Groszmann RJ. Hyposensitivity to vasopressin in a hemorrhage-transfused rat model of portal hypertension. Gastroenterology 93:170, 1987

211. Kravetz D, Sikuler E, Groszmann RJ. Splanchnic and systemic hemodynamics in portal hypertensive rats during hemorrhage and blood volume restitution. Gastroenterology 90:1232, 1986

212. Kroeger R, Groszman RJ. The effect of selective blockade of B2-adrenergic receptors on portal and systemic hemodynamics in a portal hypertensive model. Gastroenterology 88:896, 1985

213. Kroeger RJ, Groszmann RJ. Increased portal venous resistance hinders portal pressure reduction during the administration of β-adrenergic blocking agents in a portal hypertensive model. Hepatology 5:97, 1985

214. Kroeger RJ, Groszmann RJ. The effect of the combination of nitroglycerin and propranolol on splanchnic and systemic hemodynamics in a portal hypertensive rat model. Hepatology 5:425, 1985

215. Krogsgaard K, Gluud C, Henriksen JH, et al. Correlation between liver morphology and portal pressure in alcoholic liver disease. Hepatology 4:699, 1984

216. Labadie H, Stoessel P, Callard P, et al. Hepatic venoocclusive disease and presinusoidal fibrosis secondary to arsenic poisoning. Gastroenterology 99:1140, 1990

217. Lam KC, et al. Spontaneous portosystemic shunt: relationship to spontaneous encephalopathy and gastrointestinal hemorrhage. Dig Dis Sci 26:346, 1981

218. Lam PIJ, Mathic RT, Harper AM, et al. A simple technique of measuring liver blood flow: intrasplenic injection of xenon 133. Acta Chir Scand 145:95, 1979

219. Lankisch PG. The spleen in inflammatory pancreatic disease. Gastroenterology 98:509, 1990

220. Lautt WW. Hepatic vasculature: a conceptual review. Gastroenterology 73:1163, 1977

221. Lautt WW. Hepatic nerves: a review of their functions and effects. Can J Physiol Pharmacol 58:105, 1980

222. Lautt WW, Greenway CV, Legare DJ, et al. Localization of intrahepatic portal vascular resistance. Am J Physiol 251:G375, 1986

223. Lautt WW, Legare DJ, MS. Adenosine as putative regulator of hepatic arterial flow (the buffer response). Am J Physiol 248:H331, 1985

224. Lautt WW, Legare DJ, Ezzat WR. Quantitation of the hepatic arterial buffer response to graded changes in portal blood flow. Gastroenterology 98:1024, 1990

225. Leach SD, Meier GH, Gusberg RJ. Endoscopic sclerotherapy: a risk factor for splanchnic venous thrombosis. J Vasc Surg 10:9, 1989

226. Lebrec D, Bataille C, Bercoff E, et al. Hemodynamic changes in patients with portal venous obstruction. Hepatology 3:550, 1983

227. Lebrec D, Bernuau J, Rueff B, et al. Gastrointestinal bleeding after abrupt cessation of propranolol administration in cirrhosis. N Engl J Med 307:560, 1982

228. Lebrec D, DeFleury P, Rueff B, et al. Portal hypertension, size of esophageal varices, and risk of gastrointestinal bleeding in alcoholic cirrhosis. Gastroenterology 79:1139, 1980

229. Lebrec D, Hillon P, Munoz C, et al. The effect of propranolol on portal hypertension in patients with cirrhosis: a hemodynamic study. Hepatology 2:523, 1982

230. Lebrec D, Poynard T, Berneau J, et al. A randomized controlled study of propranolol for prevention of recurrent gastrointestinal bleeding in patients with cirrhosis: a final report. Hepatology 4:355, 1984

231. Lebrec D, Poynard T, Capron JP, et al. Nadolol for prophylaxis of gastrointestinal bleeding in patients with cirrhosis: a randomized study. J Hepatol 7:118, 1988

231a. Lee FY, Groszmann RJ. Nw-nitro-L-arginine corrects the systemic vascular hyporesponsiveness to methoxamine in portal hypertension. Hepatology 16:1043, 1992

232. Lee SS, Girod C, Broullon A, et al. Hemodynamic characterization of chronic bile duct-ligated rats: effect of pentobarbital sodium. Am J Physiol 251:G176, 1986

233. Leevy CM, ten Hove W, Opper A. et al. Influence of ethanol and microsomal drugs on hepatic hemodynamics. Ann NY Acad Sci 170:315, 1970

234. Leonard A, Lauwerys RR. Carcinogenicity, teratogenicity and mutagenicity of arsenic. Mutat Res 75:49, 1980

235. Levy HM, Newhouse, JH. MR imaging of portal vein thrombosis. AJR 151:283, 1988

236. L'Hermine C, Chastenet P, Delemazure O, et al. Percutaneous transhepatic embolization of gastroesophageal varices: results in 400 patients. AJR 152:755, 1989

237. Lieber CS, Zimmon DS, Kessler RE, et al. Portal hypertension in experimental alcoholic liver injury. Clin Res 24:478, 1976

238. Liebowitz HR. Pathogenesis of esophageal varix rupture. JAMA 175:874, 1961

239. Lindor K, Rakela J, Perrault J, et al. Noncirrhotic portal hypertension due to lymphoma: reversal following splenectomy. Dig Dis Sci 32:1056, 1987

240. Losowsky MS, Atkenson M. Intravenous albumin in the treatment of diuretic-resistant ascites in portal cirrhosis. Lancet 2:386, 1961

241. Low DE, Kozarek RA, Ball TJ, et al. Endoscopic variceal sclerotherapy as primary treatment for bleeding esophageal varices. J Clin Gastroenterol 11:253, 1989

242. Lukie B, Card R. Portal hypertension complicating myelofibrosis: reversal following splenectomy. Can Med Assoc J 117:771, 1977

243. Lunderquist A, Alwmark A, Gullstrand P, et al. Pharmacologic influence of esophageal varices: a preliminary report. Cardiovasc Intervent Radiol 6:65, 1983

244. Lunderquist A, Vang J. Transhepatic catheterization and obliteration of the coronary vein in patients with portal hypertension. N Engl J Med 291:646, 1974

245. MacDougall BRD, Williams R. A controlled clinical trial of cimetidine in the recurrence of variceal hemorrhage: implications about the pathogenesis of hemorrhage. Hepatology 3:69, 1983

246. Maddrey WC, Boyer JL, Sen NN. Plasma volume expansion in portal hypertension. Johns Hopkins Med J 125:171, 1969

247. Maddrey W, Johns C, Boitnott J, et al. Sarcoidosis and chronic hepatic disease: a clinical and pathologic study of 20 patients. Medicine 49:375, 1970

248. Mallory A, Schaefer JW, Cohen JR, et al. Selective intra-arterial vasopressin infusion for upper gastrointestinal tract hemorrhage. Arch Surg 115:30, 1980

249. Marteau P, Ballet F, Chazouillères O, et al. Effect of vasodilators on hepatic microcirculation in cirrhosis: a study in the isolated perfused rat liver. Hepatology 9:820, 1989

250. Mastai R, Grande L, Bosch J, et al. Effects of metoclopramide and domperidone on azygous venous blood flow in patients with cirrhosis and portal hypertension. Hepatology 6:1244, 1986

251. Mastai R, Rochelau B, Huet PM. Serotonin blockade in conscious, unrestrained cirrhotic dogs with portal hypertension. Hepatology 9:265, 1989

252. Mathur SK, Dalvi AN, Someshwar V, et al. Endoscopic and radiological appraisal of gastric varices. Br J Surg 77:432, 1990

253. McCormack TT, Sims J, Eyre-Brook I, et al. Gastric lesions in portal hypertension: inflammatory gastritis or congestive gastropathy? Gut 26:1226, 1985

254. McCoskey RS. A dynamic and static study of the hepatic arterioles and hepatic sphincters. Am J Anat 119:455, 1966

255. McDonald GB, Sharma P, Matthews D, et al. Veno-occlusive disease of the liver after bone marrow transplantation: diagnosis, incidence and predisposing factors. Hepatology 4:123, 1984

256. McIndoe AH. Vascular lesions of portal cirrhosis. Arch Pathol 5:23, 1928

257. Merkel C, Gianfranco F, Renzo Z, et al. Effects of isosorbide dinitrate on portal hypertension in alcoholic cirrhosis. J Hepatol 4:174, 1987

258. Mikakawa H, Lida S, Leo MA, et al. Pathogenesis of precirrhotic portal hypertension in alcohol-fed baboons. Gastroenterology 88:143, 1985

259. Mikkelsen WP. Extrahepatic portal hypertension in children. Am J Surg 111:333, 1966

260. Mikkelsen WP, et al. Extra- and intrahepatic portal hypertension without cirrhosis (hepatoportal sclerosis). Ann Surg 162:602, 1965

261. Mills PR, Rae AP, Farah DA, et al. Comparison of three adrenoreceptor blocking agents in patients with cirrhosis and portal hypertension. Gut 25:73, 1984

262. Minato Y, Hasumura Y, Takeuchi J. The role of fat-storing cells in Disse space fibrogenesis in alcoholic liver disease. Hepatology 3:559, 1983

263. Miskowiak J. How the lower oesophageal sphincter affects submucosal oesophageal varices. Lancet 1:1284, 1978

264. Mistilis S, Green J, Schiff L. Hepatic sarcoidosis with portal hypertension. Am J Med 36:470, 1964

265. Moreau B, Lee SS, Hadenque A, et al. Hemodynamic effects of a clonidine-induced decrease in sympathetic tone in patients with cirrhosis. Hepatology 7:149, 1987

266. Moreno AH, Burchell AR, Rousselot LM, Panke WF, Slafsky F, Burke JH. Portal blood flow in cirrhosis of the liver. J Clin Invest 46:436, 1967

267. Moreno AH, Rousselot LM, Panke WF. Studies on portal hypertension. Surg Clin North Am 38:421, 1958

268. Moreto M, Zaballa M, Bernal A, et al. A randomized trial of tamponade or sclerotherapy as immediate treatment for bleeding esophageal varices. Surg Gynecol Obstet 167:331, 1988

269. Morgan JS, Groszmann RJ. Somatostatin in portal hypertension. Dig Dis Sci 34:40S, 1989

270. Moriyasu F, Nishida O, Ban N, et al. Measurement of vascular resistance in patients with portal hypertension. Gastroenterology 90:710, 1986

271. Moosa AR, Sadd MA, Isolated splenic vein thrombosis. World J Surg 9:384, 1985

272. Mosimann R. Non-aggressive assessment of portal hypertension using endoscopic measurement of variceal pressure: preliminary report. Am J Surg 143:212, 1982

273. Murray JF, Dawson AM. Sherlock S. Circulatory changes in chronic liver disease. Am J Med 24:358, 1958

274. Myers JD. The hepatic blood flow and splanchnic oxygen consumption in man: their estimation from urea production or bromsulphthalein excretion during catheterization of the hepatic veins. J Clin Invest 26:1130, 1947

275. Nakanuma Y, Ohta G. Nodular hyperplasia of the liver in primary biliary cirrhosis of early histological stages. Am J Gastroenterol 82:8, 1987

276. Nakanuma Y, Ohta G, Sasaki K. Nodular regenerative hyperplasia of the liver associated with polyarteritis nodosa. Arch Pathol Lab Med 108:133, 1984

277. Nakashima T. Vascular changes and hemodynamics in hepatocellular carcinoma. In: Okuda K, Peters J, eds. Hepatocellular carcinoma. New York, John Wiley & Sons, 1976, p 169

278. Nataf C, Feldmann G, Lebrec D, et al. Idiopathic portal hypertension (perisinusoidal fibrosis) after renal transplantation. Gut 20:531, 1979

279. Navasa M, Bosch J, Reichen J, et al. Effects of verapamil on hepatic and systemic hemodynamics and liver function in patients with cirrhosis and portal hypertension. Hepatology 8:850, 1988

280. Navasa M, Chesta J, Bosch J, et al. Reduction of portal pressure by isosorbide-5-mononitrate in patients with cirrhosis. Gastroenterology 96:110, 1989

281. Nayak NC. Pathology of non-cirrhotic portal fibrosis in India. In Okuda K, Omata M, eds. Idiopathic portal hypertension. Tokyo, University of Tokyo Press, 1983, p 37

282. Nayak NC, Ramalingaswami B. Obliterative venopathy of the liver. Arch Pathol 87:359, 1969

283. Nayyar AD, Sharma BK, Sarin SK, et al. Characterization of peripheral blood lymphocytes in patients with non-cirrhotic portal fibrosis: a comparison with cirrhosis and healthy controls. Proceedings of the 28th Annual Conference of the Indian Society of Gastroenterology. Bhopal, 1987, p B3

284. Nayak NC. Pathology of non-cirrhotic portal fibrosis in India. In Okuda K, Omata M, eds. Idiopathic portal hypertension. Tokyo, University of Tokyo Press, 1983, p 37

285. Noda T. Angioarchitectural study of esophageal varices with special reference to variceal rupture. Virchows Arch [A] 404:381, 1984

286. The North Italian Endoscopic Club for the Study and Treatment of Esophageal Varices. Prediction of the first variceal hemorrhage in patients with cirrhosis of the liver and esophageal varices: a prospective multicenter study. N Engl J Med 319:983, 1988

287. Nundy S, Tandon BN. The proximal lieno-renal shunt in the management of varices. In: Okuda D, Omata M, eds. Idiopathic portal hypertension. Tokyo, University of Tokyo Press, 1983, p 535

288. Ohnishi K, Sato S, Nomura F, et al. Splanchnic hemodynamics in idiopathic portal hypertension: comparison with chronic persistent hepatitis. Am J Gastroenterol 84:403, 1989

289. Ohnishi K, Sato S, Tsunoda S, et al. Portal venous hemodynamics in hepatocellular carcinoma: effects of hepatic artery embolization. Gastroenterology 93:591, 1987

290. Oishi N, Swisher S, Stormont J, et al. Portal hypertension in myeloid metaplasia. Arch Surg 81:80, 1960

291. Okuda K. Idiopathic portal hypertension. In: Thomas HC, Jones EA, eds. Recent advances in hepatology. Edinburgh, Churchill Livingstone, 1986, p 93

292. Okuda K, Kono K, Ohnishi I, et al. Clinical study of eighty-six cases of idiopathic portal hypertension and comparison with cirrhosis with splenomegaly. Gastroenterology 86:600, 1984

293. Okuda K, Ohnishi K, Kimura K, et al. Incidence of portal vein thrombosis in liver cirrhosis. An angiographic study in 708 patients. Gastroenterology 89:279, 1985

294. Orozco H, Guraieb E, Takahashi T, et al. Deficiency of protein C in patients with portal vein thrombosis. Hepatology 8:1110, 1988

295. Orrego H, Blendis LM, Crossley IR, et al. Correlation of intrahepatic pressure with collagen in the Disse space and hepatomegaly in humans and in the rat. Gastroenterology 80:546, 1981

296. Orrego H, Medline A, Blendis LM, et al. Collagenization of the Disse space in alcoholic liver disease. Gut 20:673, 1979

297. Orrego J, Mena I, Baraona E, et al. Modifications in hepatic blood flow and portal pressure produced by different diets. Am J Dig Dis 10:239, 1965

298. Paes-Alves C, Alves A, Abreu W, et al. Hepatic artery hypertrophy and sinusoidal hypertension in advanced schistosomiasis. Gastroenterology 72:126, 1977

299. Pagani MS, Vatner SF, Braunwald E. Hemodynamic effects of intravenous nitroprusside in the conscious dog. Circulation 57:144, 1978

300. Pagliaro L, Burroughs AK, Sorensen TIA, et al. Therapeutic controversies and randomised controlled trials (RCTs): prevention of bleeding and rebleeding in cirrhosis. Gastroenterol Int 2:71, 1989

301. Palmer E. Determination of venous pressure within esophageal varices. JAMA 146:570, 1951

302. Panke WF, Bradley EG, Moreno AH, et al. Techniques, hazards and usefulness of percutaneous splenic portography. JAMA 169;1032, 1959

303. Paquet HJ. Prophylactic endoscopic sclerosing treatment of the esophageal wall in varices: a prospective controlled randomized trial. Endoscopy 14:4, 1982

304. Paquet KJ, Feussner H. Endoscopic sclerosis and esophageal balloon tamponade in acute hemorrhage from esophagogastric varices: a prospective controlled randomized trial. Hepatology 5:580, 1985

305. Park J, Chiba T, Yamada T. Mechanisms for direct inhibition of canine gastric parietal cells by somatostatin. J Biol Chem 262:14190, 1987

306. Parvey HR, Eisenberg RL, Giyanani V, et al. Duplex sonography of the portal venous system: pitfalls and limitations. AJR 152:765, 1989

307. Pascal JP, Cales P, Multicentre Study Group. Propranolol in the prevention of first upper gastrointestinal tract hemorrhage in patients with cirrhosis of the liver and esophageal varices. N Engl J Med 317:856, 1987

308. Perez-Ayuso RM, Pique JM, Bosch J, et al. Propranolol in prevention of recurrent bleeding from severe portal hypertensive gastropathy in cirrhosis. Lancet 337:1431, 1991

309. Perkocha LA, Geaghan SM, Yen B. Clinical and pathological features of bacillary peliosis hepatitis in association with human immunodeficiency virus infection. N Engl J Med 323:1581, 1990

310. Pertuiset E, Tribout B, Wechsler B, et al. Systemic lupus erythematosus presenting with portal venous thrombosis. Am J Med 86:501, 1989

311. Piai G, Cipolletta L, Claar, et al. Prophylactic sclerotherapy of high-risk esophageal varices: results of a multicentric prospective controlled trial. Hepatology 8:1495, 1988

312. Pinto HC, Abrantes A, Esteves AV, et al. Long-term prognosis of patients with cirrhosis of the liver and upper gastrointestinal bleeding. Am J Gastroenterol 84:1239, 1989

313. Polio J, Groszmann RJ. Hemodynamic factors involved in the development and rupture of esophageal varices: a pathophysiologic approach to treatment. Semin Liver Dis 6:318, 1986

314. Polio J, Hanson J, Sikuler E, et al. A critical assessment of a pressure sensitive capsule for endoscopic measurement of variceal pressure. Gastroenterology 92:1109, 1987

315. Pomier-Layrargues G, Kusielewicz D, Willems B, et al. Presinusoidal portal hypertension in non-alcoholic cirrhosis. Hepatology 5:415, 1985

316. Ponsky J, Hoffman M, Rhodes R. Arteriovenous fistula and portal hypertension secondary to islet-cell tumor of the pancreas. Surgery 85:408, 1979

317. Popper H, Maltoni C, Sellikoff IJ. Vinyl chloride-induced hepatic lesions in man and rodents: a comparison. Liver 1:7, 1981

318. Popper H, Paronetto F, Schaffner F, et al. Studies on hepatic fibrosis. Lab Invest 10:265, 1961

319. Potzi R, Bauer P, Reichel W, et al. Prophylactic endoscopic sclerotherapy of oesophageal varices in liver cirrhosis: a multicentre prospective controlled trial in Vienna. Gut 30:873, 1989

320. Price HL, Cooperman LH, Warden JC. Control of the splanchnic circulation in man: role of beta-adrenergic receptors. Circ Res 1 21:333, 1967

321. Qamar MI, Read AE, Skidmore R, et al. Pulsatility index of superior mesenteric artery blood velocity waveforms. Ultrasound Med Biol 12:773, 1986

322. Queuniet AM, Czernichow P, Lerebours E, et al. Etude contrôlée du propranolol dans la prévention des récidives hémorragiques chez les patients cirrhotiques. Gastroenterol Clin Biol 11:41, 1987

323. Raia S, Mies S, Macedo AL, Portal hypertension in schistosomiasis. Clin Gastroenterol 14:57, 1985

324. Ramos OL, Saad F, Leser WP. Portal hemodynamics and liver cell function in hepatic schistosomiasis. Gastroenterology 47:241, 1964

325. Rappaport AM. Hepatic blood flow: morphologic aspects and physiologic regulation. In: Devitt NB, ed. Liver and biliary tract. Physiology I. International review of physiology, vol 21. Baltimore, University Park Press, 1980

326. Ravenna P. Splenoportal venous obstruction without splenomegaly. Arch Intern Med 72:786, 1943

327. Read AE, Wiesner RH, LaBreque DR, et al. Hepatic veno-occlusive disease associated with renal transplantation and azathioprine therapy. Ann Intern Med 104:651, 1986

328. Ready JB, Robertson AD, Goff JS, et al. Assessment of the risk of bleeding from esophageal varices by continuous monitoring of portal pressure. Gastroenterology 100:1403, 1991

329. Ready JB, Robertson AD, Rector WG. Effects of vasopressin on portal pressure during hemorrhage from esophageal varices. Gastroenterology 100:1411, 1991

330. Rector WG, Redeker AG. Direct transhepatic assessment of hepatic vein pressure and direction of flow using a thin needle in patients with cirrhosis and Budd-Chiari syndrome: an effective alternative to hepatic vein catheterization. Gastroenterology 86:1395, 1984

331. Reding P, Urbain D, Grivegnee A, et al. Portal venous esophageal luminal pressure gradient in cirrhosis. Hepatology 6:98, 1986

332. Reed G, Cox A. The human liver after radiation injury: a form of veno-occlusive disease. Am J Pathol 48:597, 1966

333. Reichen J. Verapamil favorably influences hepatic microvascular exchange and function in rats with cirrhosis of the liver. J Clin Invest 78:448, 1986

334. Reichen J, Egger B, Ohara N, et al. Determinants of hepatic functions in liver cirrhosis in the rat: a multivariate analysis. J Clin Invest 82:2069, 1988

336. Reichlin S. Somatostatin (second of two parts). N Engl J Med 309:1556, 1983

337. Reichma S, Davis WD, Storaash JP, et al. Measurement of hepatic blood flow by indicator dilution techniques. J Clin Invest 37:1848, 1958

338. Resnick RH, Chalmers TC, Ishiara A, et al. A controlled

study of prophylactic portacaval shunts: a final report. Ann Intern Med 70:675, 1969

339. Resnick RH, Iber FL, Ishiara A, et al. A controlled study of the therapeutic portacaval shunt. Gastroenterology 67:843, 1974

340. Reynolds T. Portal hypertension. In: Schiff L, Schiff E, eds. Diseases of the liver, ed 5. Philadelphia, JB Lippincott, 1982, p 393

341. Reynolds TB, Donavan AJ, Mikkelsen WP, et al. Results of a 12 year randomized trial of portacaval shunt in patients with alcoholic liver disease and bleeding varices. Gastroenterology 80:1005, 1981

342. Reynolds TB, Geller H, Kuzma O, et al. Spontaneous decrease in portal pressure with clinical improvement in cirrhosis. N Engl J Med 263:734, 1960

343. Reynolds TB, Hidmura R, Michell H, et al. Portal hypertension without cirrhosis in alcoholic liver disease. Ann Intern Med 70:497, 1969

344. Reynolds WJ, Wanless IR. Nodular regenerative hyperplasia of the liver in a patient with rheumatoid vasculitis: a morphometric study suggesting a role for hepatic arteritis in the pathogenesis. J Rheumatol 11:838, 1984

345. Richardson PDI, Withrington PG. The inhibition of glucagon of the vasoconstrictor actions of noradrenaline, angiotensin and vasopressin on the hepatic arterial vascular bed. Br J Pharmacol 57:93, 1976

346. Rigau J, Bosch J, Bordas JM, et al. Endoscopic measurement of variceal pressure in cirrhosis: correlation with portal pressure and variceal hemorrhage. Gastroenterology 96:873, 1989

347. Rikkers LF, Burnett DA, Valentine GD, et al. Shunt surgery versus endoscopic sclerotherapy for long-term treatment of variceal bleeding: early results of a randomized trial. Ann Surg 206:261, 1987

347a. Ring EJ, Lake JR, Roberts JP, et al. Using transjugular intrahepatic shunts to control variceal bleeding before liver transplantation. Ann Intern Med 116:304, 1992

347b. Roberts JP, Ring E, Lake JR, et al. Intrahepatic portocaval shunt for variceal hemorrhage prior to liver transplantation. Transplantation 52:160, 1991

347c. Rodriguez-Perez F, Groszman RJ. Pharmacologic treatment of portal hypertension. Gastrointesterol Clin North Am 21:1, 1992

348. Rosenbaum DL, et al. Hemodynamic studies of the portal circulation in myeloid metaplasia. Am J Med 41:360, 1966

349. Rougier P, Degott C, Rueff B, et al. Nodular regenerative hyperplasia of the liver: report of six cases and review of the literature. Gastroenterology 75:169, 1978

350. Roulot D, Braillon A, Gaudin C, et al. Mechanisms of a clonidine-induced decrease in portal pressure in normal and cirrhotic conscious rats. Hepatology 10:477, 1989

351. Rudolph R, McClure WJ, Woodward M. Contractile fibroblasts in chronic alcoholic cirrhosis. Gastroenterology 76:704, 1979

352. Rueff B, Prandi D, Degos F, et al. A controlled study of therapeutic portacaval shunt in alcoholic cirrhosis. Lancet 2:655, 1976

353. Ruprecht AL, Kinney TD. Esophageal varices caused by metastasis of carcinoma to the liver. Am J Dig Dis 1:145, 1956

354. Russell RM, Boyer JL, Bagheri SA, et al. Hepatic injury from chronic hypervitaminosis A resulting in portal hypertension and ascites. N Engl J Med 291:435, 1974

355. Saari A, Klvilaakso E, Inberg M, et al. Comparison of somatostatin and vasopressin in bleeding esophageal varices. Am J Gastroenterol 85:804, 1990

356. Sabbá C, Ferraioli G, Genecin P, et al. Evaluation of postprandial hyperemia in superior mesenteric artery and portal vein in healthy and cirrhotic humans in an operator-blind echo-Doppler study. Hepatology 13:714, 1991

357. Sabbá C, Weltin GG, Cicchetti DV, et al. Observer variability in echo-Doppler measurements of portal flow in cirrhotic patients and normal volunteers. Gastroenterology 98:1603, 1990

358. Salem AA, Warren WD, Tyras DH. Splenic vein thrombosis: a diagnosable and curable form of portal hypertension. Surgery 74:961, 1973

359. Sama SK, Bhargawa S, Gopi N, et al. Non-cirrhotic portal fibrosis. Am J Med 51:160, 1971

360. Santangelo WC, Dueno MI, Estes BL, et al. Prophylactic sclerotherapy of large esophageal varices. N Engl J Med 318:814, 1988

361. Sarin SK. Non-cirrhotic portal fibrosis. Gut 30:406, 1989

362. Sarin SK, Kumar A. Gastric varices: profile, classification, and management. Am J Gastroenterol 84:1244, 1989

363. Sarin SK, Malhotra V, Mehra NK, et al. Familial aggregation of non-cirrhotic portal fibrosis; a study of four families. Am J Gastroenterol 82:1130, 1987

364. Sarin SK, Sachdev G, Nanda R. Follow-up of patients after variceal eradication: a comparison of patients with cirrhosis, non-cirrhotic portal fibrosis and extrahepatic obstruction. Ann Surg 201:78, 1986

365. Sarin SK, Sethi KK, Nanda R. Measurement and correlation of wedged hepatic, intrahepatic, intrasplenic and intravariceal pressures in patients with cirrhosis of liver and non-cirrhotic portal fibrosis. Gut 28:260, 1987

366. Sauerbruch T, Wotzka R, Kopcke W, et al. Prophylactic sclerotherapy before the first episode of variceal hemorrhage in patients with cirrhosis. N Engl J Med 319:8, 1988

367. Schaffner F, Popper H. Capillarization of the hepatic sinusoids in man. Gastroenterology 44:239, 1963

368. Schmid PG, Abboud FM, Wendling MG, et al. Regional vascular effects of vasopressin: plasma levels and circulatory responses. Am J Physiol 227:998, 1974

369. Schmitz-Feuerhake I, Huchzermeyer H, Reblin T. Determination of the specific blood flow of the liver by inhalation of radioactive rare gases. Acta Hepatol Gastroenterol (Stuttgart) 22:150, 1975

370. Schuster S, Schwachmann H, Toyawa W, et al. The management of portal hypertension in cystic fibrosis. J Pediatr Surg 12:201, 1977

371. Scott J, et al. Percutaneous transhepatic obliteration of gastroesophageal varices. Lancet 2:53, 1976

372. Shaldon S, Dolle W, Guevara L, et al. Effect of pitressin on the splanchnic circulation in man. Circulation 24:797, 1961

373. Shaldon S, Sherlock S. Portal hypertension in the myeloproliferative syndrome and the reticuloses. Am J Med 32:758, 1962

374. Sharma BK, Malhotra P, Sarin SK, et al. Malarial antibody studies in patients with non-cirrhotic portal fibrosis. Proceedings of the 28th Annual Conference of Indian Society of Gastroenterology. Bhopal, 1987, p B5

375. Sheen IS, Chen TY, Liaw YF. Randomized controlled study of propranolol for prevention of recurrent esophageal bleeding in patients with cirrhosis. Liver 9:1, 1989

376. Shepherd P, Harrison DJ. Idiopathic portal hypertension associated with cytotoxic drugs. J Clin Pathol 43:206, 1990

377. Sheriff SB, Smart RC, Taylor I. Clinical study of liver blood flow in man measured by 133 xenon clearance after portal vein injection. Gut 18:1027, 1977

378. Sherlock S. Extrahepatic portal venous hypertension in adults. Clin Gastroenterol 14:1, 1985

379. Sherlock S, Feldman CA, Moran B, et al. Partial nodular transformation of the liver with portal hypertension. Am J Med 40:195, 1966

380. Sherlock S, Scheuer PJ. The presentation and diagnosis of 100 patients with primary biliary cirrhosis. N Engl J Med 289:674, 1973

381. Sherwin R, Joshi P, Hendley R, et al. Hyperglucagonemia in Laennec's cirrhosis. N Engl J Med 290:239, 1974

382. Shibayama Y, Nakata K. Localization of increased hepatic vascular resistance in liver cirrhosis. Hepatology 5:643, 1985

383. Shilling J, McKee F. Late follow-up on experimental hepatic-portal arteriovenous fistula. Surg Forum 5:392, 1954

384. Siderys H, Judd D, Herendeen T. The experimental produc-

tion of elevated portal pressure by increasing portal vein flow. Surg Gynecol Obstet 120:514, 1965

384a. Sieber C, Groszmann RJ. In vitro hyporeactivity to methoxamine in mesenteric vessels of portal hypertensive rats: reversal by nitric oxide blockade. Am J Physiol 262:996, 1992

384b. Sieber C, Groszmann RJ. Nitric oxide mediates the in vitro hyporeactivity to vasopressors in mesenteric vessels of portal hypertensive rats. Gastroenterology 103:235, 1992

385. Sieber C, Mosca G, Groszmann RJ. Effect of natural somatostatin (SRIF-14) and its analogue SMS 201–995 (SMS) on splanchnic vascular resistance. Gastroenterology 100:A250, 1991

386. Sikuler E, Groszmann RJ. Hemodynamic studies in a parabiotic model of portal hypertension. Experientia 41:1323, 1985

387. Sikuler E, Groszmann RJ. Interaction of flow and resistance in maintenance of portal hypertension in a rat model. Am J Physiol 250:G205, 1986

388. Sikuler E, Kravetz D, Groszmann RJ. Evolution of portal hypertension and mechanisms involved in its maintenance in a rat model. Am J Physiol 248:G618, 1985

389. Silva G, Navasa M, Bosch J, et al. Hemodynamic effects of glucagon in portal hypertension. Hepatology 11:668, 1990

390. Simpson WG, Schwartz RW, Strodel WE. Splenic vein thrombosis. South Med J 83:417, 1990

391. Simson IW. Membranous obstruction of the inferior vena cava and hepatocellular carcinoma in South Africa. Gastroenterology 82:171, 1982

392. Sinaasappel M. Hepatobiliary pathology in patients with cystic fibrosis. Acta Paediatr Scand [Suppl] 363:45, 1989

393. Sitzmann JV, Bulkley GB, Mitchell MC, et al. Role of prostacyclin in the splanchnic hyperemia contributing to portal hypertension. Ann Surg 209:322, 1989

393a. Slater LN, Welch DF, Min KW. *Rochalimaea henselae* causes bacillary angiomatosis and peliosis hepatis. Arch Intern Med 152:602, 1992

394. Smith-Laing G, Camilo ME, Dick R, Sherlock S. Percutaneous transhepatic portography in the assessment of portal hypertension: clinical correlations and comparison of radiographic techniques. Gastroenterology 78:197, 1980

395. Snady H, Feinman L. Prediction of variceal hemorrhage: a prospective study. Am J Gastroenterol 83:519, 1988

396. Soderlund C, Ihre T. Endoscopic sclerotherapy versus conservative management of bleeding oesophageal varices. Acta Chir Scand 151:449, 1985

397. Solis-Herruzo JA, Vidal JV, Colina F, et al. Nodular regenerative hyperplasia of the liver associated with the toxic oil syndrome. Hepatology 6:687, 1986

398. Spence RAJ. The venous anatomy of the lower esophagus in normal subjects and patients with varices: an image analysis study. Br J Surg 71:739, 1984

399. Spence RA, Johnston GW, Odling-Smee GW, et al. Bleeding esophageal varices with long term follow up. Arch Dis Child 59:336, 1984

400. Spence RAJ, Sloan JM, Johnston GW. Histologic factors of the esophageal transection ring as clues to the pathogenesis of bleeding varices. Surg Gynecol Obstet 159:253, 1984

400a. Spina GP, et al. Distal splenorenal shunt vs endoscopic sclerotherapy in the prevention of variceal rebleeding: first stage of a randomized controlled trial. Ann Surg 211:178, 1990

401. Staritz M, Poralla T, Meyer zum Buschenfelde KH. Intravascular oesophageal pressure (IOVP) assessed by endoscopic fine needle puncture under basal conditions, Valsalva's manoeuvre and after glyceryltrinitrate application. Gut 26:525, 1985

402. Steffan AM, Gendrault JL, Kirn A. Increase in the number of fenestrae in mouse endothelial liver cells by altering the cytoskeleton with cytochalasin B. Hepatology 7:1230, 1987

403. Stellen GP, Litty JR. Esophageal endosclerosis in children. Surgery 98:970, 1985

404. Stern R, Stevens D, Boat T, et al. Symptomatic hepatic diseases in cystic fibrosis: incidence, course, and outcome of portal systemic shunting. Gastroenterology 70:645, 1976

404a. Stiegman GV, Goff JS, Michaletz-Onody PA, et al. Endoscopic sclerotherapy as compared with endoscopic ligation for bleeding esophageal varices. N Engl J Med 326:1527, 1992

405. Styles M, Coleman AJ, Leary WP. Some hemodynamic effects of sodium nitroprusside. Anesthesiology 38:173, 1973

406. Sukigara M, Shimoji K, Ohata M, et al. Effects of propranolol and nitroglycerin on cephalad collateral venous flow in patients with cirrhosis: evaluation using transesophageal real-time two-dimensional Doppler echography. Am J Gastroenterol 83:1248, 1988

407. Sullivan A, Rheinlander H, Weintraub L. Esophageal varices in agnogenic myeloid metaplasia: disappearance after splenectomy. Gastroenterology 66:429, 1974

408. Sutton JP, Yarborough D, Richards D. Isolated splenic vein thrombosis. Arch Surg 100:623, 1970

409. Taneja V, Mehra NK, Sarin SK. HLA studies in non-cirrhotic portal fibrosis. Tissue Antigen 30:184, 1987

410. Tandon BN, Nundy S, Nayak NC. Non-cirrhotic portal hypertension in Northern India: clinical features and liver function tests. In: Okuda K, Omata M, eds. Idiopathic portal hypertension. Tokyo, University of Tokyo Press, 1983, p 377

411. Taylor W. Wilson's disease, portal hypertension and intrahepatic vascular obstruction. N Engl J Med 260:1160, 1959

412. Terblanche J, Bornman PC, Kahn D, et al. Failure of repeated injection sclerotherapy to improve long term survival after oesophageal variceal bleeding: a five-year prospective controlled clinical trial. Lancet 2:1328, 1983

413. Terblanche J, Kahn D, Bornman PC. Long-term injection sclerotherapy treatment for esophageal varices: a 10-year prospective evaluation. Ann Surg 210:725, 1989

414. Terblanche J, Krige JE, Bornman PC. Endoscopic sclerotherapy. Surg Clin North Am 70:341, 1990

415. Teres J, Bordas JM, Rodes J. Sclerotherapy versus distal splenorenal shunt in the elective treatment of variceal hemorrhage: a randomized controlled trial. Hepatology 7:430, 1987

416. Teres J, Bosch J, Bordas JM, et al. Endoscopic sclerotherapy (ES) versus propranolol (PR) in the elective treatment of variceal bleeding: preliminary results of a randomized controlled clinical trial. J Hepatol 5(Suppl):408:S210, 1987

417. Teres J, Planas R, Panes J, et al. Vasopressin/nitroglycerin infusion vs. esophageal tamponade in the treatment of acute variceal bleeding: a randomized controlled trial. Hepatology 11:964, 1990

418. Thomas LB, Popper H, Berk PD, et al. Vinyl chloride induced liver disease: from idiopathic portal hypertension (Banti's syndrome) to angiosarcomas. N Engl J Med 292:17, 1975

419. Thompson EN, Sherlock S. The aetiology of portal vein thrombosis with particular reference to the role of infection and exchange transfusion. Q J Med 33:465, 1964

420. Triger DR, Johnson AG. Prophylactic sclerotherapy of oesophageal varices: a preliminary report. Gut 3A:102, 1985

421. Tsai Y, Lee F, Lin H, et al. Hyposensitivity to vasopressin in patients with hepatitis B-related cirrhosis during acute variceal hemorrhage. Hepatology 13:407, 1991

422. Tystrup N, Winkler K, Mellemgaard K, et al. Determination of arterial blood flow and oxygen supply in man by clamping the hepatic artery during surgery. J Clin Invest 41:447, 1962

423. Valenzuela JE, Schubert T, Fogel MR, et al. A multicentre, randomized, double-blind trial of somatostatin in the management of acute hemorrhage from esophageal varices. Hepatology 10:958, 1989

424. Valla D, Casadevall N, Huisse MG, et al. Etiology of portal vein thrombosis in adults: a prospective evaluation of primary myeloproliferative disorders. Gastroenterology 94:1063, 1988

425. Valla D, Denninger MH, Delvigne JM, et al. Portal vein thrombosis with ruptured oesophageal varices as presenting manifestation of hereditary protein C deficiency. Gut 29:856, 1988

426. Valla D, Flejou JF, Lebrec D, et al. Portal hypertension and ascites in acute hepatitis: clinical, hemodynamic and histological correlations. Hepatology 10:482, 1989

427. Valla D, Pessegueiro-Miranda H, Degott C, et al. Hepatic sarcoidosis with portal hypertension. A report of seven cases. Q J Med 63:531, 1987

428. Vallance P, Moncada S. Hyperdynamic circulation in cirrhosis: a role for nitric oxide? Lancet 1:776, 1991

429. Van Gasbeke D, Avni EF, Delcour C, et al. Sonographic features of portal vein thrombosis. AJR 144:749, 1985

430. Van Leeuwen, Howe SC, Scheuer PJ, et al. Portal hypertension in chronic hepatitis: relationship to morphological changes. Gut 31:339, 1990

431. Varin F, Huet PM. Hepatic microcirculation in the perfused cirrhotic rat liver. J Clin Invest 76:1904, 1985

432. The Veterans Affairs Cooperative Variceal Sclerotherapy Group. Prophylactic sclerotherapy for esophageal varices in men with alcoholic liver disease: a randomized, single-blind, multicenter clinical trial. N Engl J Med 324:1779, 1991

433. Viallet A, Joly JG, Marleau D, et al. Comparison of free portal venous pressure and wedged hepatic venous pressure in patients with cirrhosis of the liver. Gastroenterology 59:372, 1970

434. Viallet A, Marleau, Huet M, et al. Hemodynamic evaluation of patients with intrahepatic portal hypertension: relationship between bleeding varices and the portohepatic gradient. Gastroenterology 69:1297, 1975

435. Viamonte M, et al. Transhepatic obliteration of gastroesophageal varices: results in acute and nonacute bleeders. AJR 129:237, 1977

436. Viamonte M Jr, LePage J, Lunderquist A, et al. Selective catheterization of the portal vein and its tributaries: preliminary report. Radiology 114: 456, 1975

437. Vidins EI, Britton RS, Medline A, et al. Sinusoidal caliber in alcoholic and nonalcoholic liver disease: diagnostic and pathogenic implications. Hepatology 5:408, 1985

438. Villeneuve JP, Huet PM, Joly JG, et al. Idiopathic portal hypertension. Am J Med 61:459, 1976

439. Villeneuve JP, Huot R, Marleau D, et al. The estimation of hepatic blood flow with indocyanine green: comparison between continuous infusion and single injection methods. Am J Gastroenterol 77:233, 1982

440. Villeneuve JP, Pomier-Layrargues G, Infante-Rivard C, et al. Propranolol for the prevention of recurrent variceal hemorrhage: a controlled trial. Hepatology 6:1239, 1986

441. Vinel JP, Cassigneul J, Levade M, et al. Assessment of short term prognosis after variceal bleeding in patients with alcoholic cirrhosis by early measurement of portohepatic gradient. Hepatology 6:116, 1986

442. Vinel JP, Cassigneul J, Louis A, et al. Clinical and prognostic significance of portohepatic gradient in patients with cirrhosis. Surg Gynecol Obstet 155:347, 1982

443. Vinel JP, Monnin JL, Combis JM, et al. Hemodynamic evaluation of molsidomine: a vasodilator with antianginal properties in patients with alcoholic cirrhosis. Hepatology 11:239, 1990

444. Vorobioff J, Bredfeldt JE, Groszmann RJ. Hyperdynamic circulation in portal-hypertensive rat model: a primary factor for maintenance of chronic portal hypertension. Am J Physiol 244:G52, 1983

445. Vorobioff J, Bredfeldt JE, Groszmann RJ. Increased blood flow through the portal system in cirrhotic rats. Gastroenterology 87:1120, 1984

446. Vorobioff J, Garcia-Tsao G, Groszmann RJ, et al. Long term hemodynamic effects of ketanserin, a 5-hydroxytryptamine blocker, in portal hypertensive patients. Hepatology 9:88, 1989

447. Vosnik J, Jedlicka K, Mulder JL, Cort JH. Action of the triglycyl hormonogen of vasopressin (glypressin) in patients with liver cirrhosis and bleeding esophageal varices. Gastroenterology 72:605, 1977

448. Waes LV, Demeulanaere L, Damme W, et al. Hepaticoportal fistula and portal hypertension. Dig Dis Sci 24:565, 1979

449. Wahren J, Felig P. Influence of somatostatin on carbohydrate disposal and absorption in diabetes mellitus. Lancet 2:1213, 1976

450. Waldram R, Nunnerley H, Davis M, et al. Detection and grading of oesophageal varices by fibre-optic endoscopy and barium swallow with and without Buscopan. Clin Radiol 28:137, 1977

451. Walker S, Stiehl A, Raedsch R, Kommerell B. Terlipressin in bleeding esophageal varices: a placebo-controlled, double-blind study. Hepatology 6:112, 1986

452. Wanless IR. Pathophysiology of non-cirrhotic portal hypertension: a pathologist's perspective. In: Boyer JL, Bianchi L, eds. Liver cirrhosis. Lancaster, England, Falk Foundation MTP Press, 1987, p 293

453. Wanless IR. Micronodular transformation (nodular regenerative hyperplasia) of the liver: a report of 64 cases among 2,500 autopsies and a new classification of benign hepatocellular nodules. Hepatology 11:787, 1990

454. Wanless IR, Godwin TA, Allen F, et al. Nodular regenerative hyperplasia of the liver in hematologic disorders: a possible response to obliterative venopathy. Medicine 59:367, 1980

455. Warren WD, Henderson JM, Millikan WJ, et al. Distal splenorenal shunt vs. endoscopic sclerotherapy for long-term management of variceal bleeding. Ann Surg 203:454, 1986

456. Watanabe K, Kimura K, Matsutani S, et al. Portal hemodynamics in patients with gastric varices: a study in 230 patients with esophageal and/or gastric varices using portal vein catheterization. Gastroenterology 95:434, 1988

457. Webb LJ, Berger LA, Sherlock S. Grey-scale ultrasonography of portal vein. Lancet 2:675, 1977

458. Webb LJ, Sherlock S. The aetiology, presentation and natural history of extra-hepatic portal venous obstruction. Q J Med 48:627, 1979

459. Westaby D, Bihari DJ, Gimson AES, et al. Selective and non-selective beta receptor blockade in the reduction of portal pressure in patients with cirrhosis and portal hypertension. Gut 25:121, 1984

460. Westaby D, Gimson A, Hayes PC, et al. Haemodynamic response to intravenous vasopressin and nitroglycerin in portal hypertension. Gut 29:372, 1988

461. Westaby D, Hayes PC, Gimson AE, et al. Controlled clinical trial of injection sclerotherapy for active variceal bleeding. Hepatology 9:274, 1989

462. Westaby D, MacDougall BR, Williams F. Improved survival following injection sclerotherapy for esophageal varices: final analysis of a controlled trial. Hepatology 5:827, 1985

463. Westaby D, Polson RJ, Gimson AE, et al. A controlled trial of oral propranolol compared with injection sclerotherapy for the long-term management of variceal bleeding. Hepatology 11:353, 1990

464. Westaby S, Wilkinson SP, Warren R, et al. Spleen size and portal hypertension. Digestion 17:63, 1978

465. Whipple AO. The problem of portal hypertension in relation to hepatosplenopathies. Ann Surg 122:449, 1945

466. Willett IR, Esler M, Jennings G, et al. Sympathetic tone modulates portal venous pressure in alcoholic cirrhosis. Lancet 2:939, 1986

467. Willett IR, Jennings G, Esler M, et al. Sympathetic tone modulates portal venous pressure in alcoholic cirrhosis. Lancet 2:939, 1986

468. Willoughby EO, David D, Smith D, et al The significance of small esophageal varices in portal cirrhosis. Gastroenterology 47:375, 1964

469. Wisse E, DeZanger RB, Charels K, et al. The liver sieve: considerations concerning the structure and function of endothelial fenestrae, the sinusoidal wall and the space of Disse. Hepatology 5:683, 1985

470. Witte CL, Witte MH, Bair G, et al. Experimental study of

hyperdynamic vs stagnant mesenteric blood flow in portal hypertension. Ann Surg 179:304, 1974

471. Witzel L, Wolbergs E, Merki H. Prophylactic endoscopic sclerotherapy of oesophageal varices: a prospective controlled trial. Lancet 1:773, 1985

472. Workehoff D, Spech HJ. Prophylaktische Osophagusvarizen-sklerosieriung. Dtsch Med Wochenschr 112:947, 1987

473. Wynne HA, Cope LH, Mutch E, et al. The effect of age upon liver volume and apparent liver blood flow in healthy man. Hepatology 9:297, 1989

474. Yamamot S, Yokoyama T, Takeshige K, et al. Budd-Chiari syndrome with obstruction of the inferior vena cava. Gastroenterology 54:1070, 1968

475. Yang-Te T, Chii-Shyan L, Kwok-Hung L, et al. Controlled trial of vasopressin plus nitroglycerin vs. vasopressin alone in the treatment of bleeding esophageal varices. Hepatology 6:406, 1986

476. Zafrani E, Cazier A, Baudelot A, et al. Ultrastructural lesions of the liver in human peliosis. Am J Physiol 114:349, 1984

477. Zeeh J, Lange H, Bosch J, et al. Steady-state extrarenal sorbitol clearance as a measure of hepatic plasma flow. Gastroenterology 95:749, 1988

478. Zemel G, Katzen BT, Becker GJ, et al. Percutaneous transjugular portosystemic shunt. JAMA 266:390, 1991

479. Zirinsky K, Markisz JA, Rubenstein WA. MR imaging of portal venous thrombosis: correlation with CT and sonography. AJR 150:283, 1988

480. Zito RA, Diez A, Groszmann RJ. Comparative effects of nitroglycerin and nitroprusside on vasopressin-induced cardiac dysfunction in the dog. J Cardiovasc Pharmacol 5:586, 1983

481. Zuidema G, Gaisford W, Abel M, et al. Segmental portal arterialization of canine liver. Surgery 53:689, 1975

Diseases of the Liver, Seventh Edition, edited by Leon Schiff and Eugene R. Schiff. J.B. Lippincott Company, Philadelphia © 1993.

34

Surgical Management of Portal Hypertension

J. Michael Henderson

History

Enthusiasm for surgical methods to manage the complications of portal hypertension has waxed and waned for over a century. Controversy has existed since Nicolai Eck, with no supportive data, declared in 1877 that portal diversion to the general circulation could be safely applied in humans.[29] Pavlov, the physiologist, systematically demonstrated the consequences of total portal diversion, and advised caution in considering this as a treatment for portal hypertension in humans.[40] Sporadic reports of portosystemic shunts, such as Vidal's "forced" shunt in 1903,[136] reinforced Pavlov's data showing protein intolerance, encephalopathy, sepsis, and death. Alternative approaches such as omentopexy were advocated by Drummond and Morrison[28] and Talma[125] and might be considered the forerunners of partial portosystemic shunts.

Surgical intervention for portal hypertension from 1900 to 1940 largely was limited to splenectomy, omentopexy, and devascularization procedures.[25] Shunt surgery was reintroduced in 1945 by Whipple and the Columbia group[152] because of a recognition that (1) variceal bleeding was not controlled by splenectomy and devascularization; (2) new methods of venous anastomosis promised improved shunt patency; (3) observation in advanced cirrhosis indicated spontaneous reduction or loss of portal flow[83,84]; and (4) studies with careful dietary protein manipulation in animals with portal diversion showed that encephalopathy could be controlled.[153] The initial outstanding clinical results of this group are testimony to their skill and attention to detail. Variceal bleeding could be controlled: enthusiasm for decompressive surgical shunt was high. Within a decade, however, came the realization that there was a cost to control of bleeding in an accelerated liver failure and encephalopathy. This era of doubt led to prospective, randomized, controlled studies in the 1960s and 1970s to define the place of total portosystemic shunts. First, prophylactic portacaval shunts,[16,63,101] made before the first bleed, and then therapeutic shunts,[64,102,103,109] made after the initial bleed, showed no improvement in survival. The mode of death could be changed from bleeding to hepatic failure.

The 1970s and 1980s have seen a plethora of new methods for treatment of the complications of portal hypertension. Selective variceal decompression was introduced independently by Warren and colleagues in the United States,[143] and by Inokuchi in Japan[57] in the late 1960s. The recognition that bleeding was best controlled by a shunt, but that the cirrhotic liver needs continued portal perfusion, characterized this concept. Sclerotherapy, initially used by Craford and Frenckner in 1939,[19] was reintroduced by Johnston and Rogers,[67] Terblanche and colleagues,[127] and Paquet and Oberhammer[96] in the 1970s. This method has the appeal of wide applicability and relative simplicity. Pharmacologic reduction of portal hypertension by Lebrec and colleagues[78] in the 1980s appeared finally to be taking the need for surgery out of treatment options.

The 1990s, however, are witnessing a swing back toward surgical therapy for portal hypertension in appropriately selected patients. This has been precipitated by two events. First, it has been recognized that endoscopic sclerotherapy and pharmacologic reduction of portal pressure do not provide adequate control of variceal bleeding for all patients.[94,151] Second, liver transplantation has come of age through the 1980s, making it a viable clinical treatment option.[121] Surgical enthusiasm is rekindled[115] with the mandate to define which patients with portal hypertension require surgical procedures for control of variceal bleeding, and which procedure they require.

Anatomy

The liver has a dual blood supply through the hepatic artery and portal vein. The arterial anatomy is highly variable, but most commonly the celiac axis carries the arterial supply to the liver through a single hepatic artery.[21] A replaced or accessory right artery arises from the superior mesenteric artery in 20% of subjects, and an accessory left artery from the left gastric artery occurs in 20% of patients.

The portal vein and sinusoids develop from the vitelline veins, which drain the foregut, midgut, and hindgut.[21] The major tributaries to the portal vein are the splenic, superior mesenteric, and inferior mesenteric veins, which unite behind the neck of the pancreas to form the portal vein.[26] Further venous inflow from the foregut comes through the left gastric (coronary), gastroepiploic, and pancreatic veins. The portal vein itself is 10 to 15 mm in diameter and 5 to 8 cm long. It extends upward behind the pancreas and then in the posterior fold of the free edge of the gastrohepatic ligament to the liver hilus. Anterior to it lie the bile duct and the hepatic arteries. The portal vein bifurcates into right and left branches, with the right directly entering liver substance and dividing early, whereas the left portal vein has a longer extrahepatic course as it passes to base of the falciform ligament. The umbilical vein entered the left vein in fetal life, and may reopen in portal hypertension.

Portal venous and hepatic arterial blood mix to enter the functional unit of the liver lobule. Having traversed the sinusoids of these lobules, blood is drained by the hepatic venules, to lobular, segmental, and the main right, middle, and left hepatic veins.

The sites of natural collateral communication between the portal and systemic circulations, which may open significantly in portal hypertension, are (1) at the gastroesophageal and anorectal junctions, (2) at sites of fetal obliteration such as in the umbilical vein, and (3) in the retroperitoneum, particularly where the gastrointestinal tract has a visceral surface directly in contact with a parietal surface.

The venous anatomy of the distal esophagus and proximal stomach has been reevaluated in the past decade with corrosion casts,[72,118] ultrasound,[82] and angiographic methods.[135] These studies have shown the patterns of normal and portal hypertensive venous anatomy. Submucosal and paraesophageal veins intercommunicate with perforating vessels, which are most prominent at the gastroesophageal junction.

Pathophysiology

Normal portal pressure is 5 to 10 mmHg, with portal flow in the range 1 to 1.5 L/min. The volume of portal flow is set by events in the feeding tributaries, but despite significant fluctuations in flow, portal pressure remains remarkably constant. Total liver blood flow is regulated by intrinsic and extrinsic mechanisms.[77] Intrinsic regulation of total flow is maintained through a hepatic arterial buffer response to changes in portal flow. Extrinsic regulation is maintained through neural and humoral influences.

Portal hypertension is present when portal pressure exceeds 12 mmHg. Direct and indirect methods for measurement of portal pressure are discussed elsewhere. The major changes associated with this rise in portal pressure that are common to all etiologies of portal hypertension are reduction in portal flow to the liver and the development of portosystemic collaterals. The most clinically significant of the collateral pathways are gastroesophageal varices, because of their propensity to bleed. The other main pathophysiologic determinant of outcome is the presence or absence of liver disease. Most portal hypertension occurs secondary to cirrhosis, and the associated hepatocellular damage adversely affects survival. Portal hypertension due to portal vein thrombosis or hepatosplenic schistosomiasis is associated with normal hepatocellular function, and thus has a better prognosis than cirrhosis. Decisions of appropriate surgical therapy in the management of portal hypertension should be based on definition of its etiology and severity.

Evaluation Methods

The surgeon is asked to evaluate the patient with portal hypertension for surgical treatment of variceal bleeding, ascites, or for liver transplantation. By this stage in his or her disease, the patient usually has been fully evaluated by a hepatologist and has a clear definition of disease etiology and status. Specific points of emphasis that the surgeon should attend to are emphasized.

Clinical Assessment

A careful history clarifies the nature of bleeding, its frequency, and transfusion requirement. The occurrence and severity of ascites is determined from the history and diuretic requirement, with emphasis on whether it occurs at the time

of an acute event or is present at all times. More difficult to assess is the rate of progression of the liver disease. Complaints such as general malaise, anorexia, weight loss, muscle weakness, and abdominal pain are nonspecific signs and symptoms. In patients with known cirrhosis, a key question to assess the severity of disease is, can they can still perform their daily activities or is their life-style impaired by their disease? Physical examination should look for spider angiomas, liver palms, ascites, jaundice, muscle wasting, and assess hepatosplenomegaly, ascites, and hepatic encephalopathy.

Laboratory Testing

Hematologic evaluation measures a full blood profile with hemoglobin, hematocrit, white blood count, and platelets. Coagulation defects are common in liver disease, and are screened for with prothrombin time and partial thromboplastin time. In-depth analysis of coagulation by measurement of fibrinogen and the individual coagulation factors gives a measure of hepatic synthetic capacity.

Biochemical measurements of conventional liver tests may be entirely normal or grossly disturbed in patients with portal hypertension. Bilirubin, and serum glutamic oxaloacetic and pyruvic transaminases are indicators of acute hepatocyte injury. Alkaline phosphatase and serum γ-glutamyl transferase may be indicative of biliary obstruction or bile duct damage. Decreased serum albumin may indicate impaired synthesis by the liver and suggests advanced disease.

Child's classification[13] brings together a combination of clinical and laboratory findings, which have been shown to be of prognostic significance for patients undergoing shunt surgery. The combination of ascites and encephalopathy, with measurement of bilirubin, albumin, and prothrombin time has been used to standardize disease stage (Table 34-1).

Finally, the specific serologic markers for underlying hepatitis, primary biliary cirrhosis, and autoimmune disease complete the laboratory evaluation.

Liver Biopsy

Before surgical therapy can be considered, most patients with portal hypertension require liver biopsy. Percutaneous needle biopsy confirms the diagnosis and assesses disease activity. The surgeon's interest in the biopsy are (1) identification of cirrhosis, (2) classification of a morphologic etiology and stage of the cirrhosis, and (3) identification of the degree of activity of the parenchymal disease with necrosis and inflammation.

Endoscopy

Upper gastrointestinal endoscopy is performed primarily in patients with portal hypertension to assess varices.

TABLE 34-1   *Child-Pugh Classification**

	1 Point	*2 Points*	*3 Points*
Bilirubin (mg/dL)	<2	2–3	>3
Albumin (g/dL)	>3.5	2.8–3.5	< 2.8
Prothrombin (↑ s)	1–3	4–6	>6
Ascites	None	Slight	Moderate
Encephalopathy	None	1–2	3–4

*Grades: A, 5–6 points; B, 7–9 points; C, 10–15 points.

In the patient who is bleeding actively, or has just stopped bleeding, it is important to identify the bleeding site and exclude other sources of bleeding such as peptic ulcer disease. In the patient undergoing an elective endoscopy, varices should be graded for size, tortuosity, and bleeding risk factors. The latter have been defined by the Japanese[5] and Italian groups,[61] with red risk signs, varices on varices, and size the most important prognostic signs.

Radiology

The radiologic methods for assessing portal hypertension are ultrasound combined with Doppler study of the vessels, computed tomography (CT) scanning, and angiography.[9,88,89] Ultrasound assesses hepatic morphology, and visualizes the portal and hepatic veins. When ultrasound is combined with Doppler study, flow is visualized in the portal and hepatic veins, and in the vena cava. CT visualizes the liver parenchyma for morphologic assessment, and may define fatty change or focal abnormalities such as hepatocellular carcinoma. Dynamic CT enhances the parenchyma to improve imaging, and visualizes the main vessels and collateral varices.

Liver angiography is used in portal hypertension, to measure venous pressure, and to visualize arterial and venous anatomy. The main methods are (1) arterial injection of the celiac or splenic and superior mesenteric arteries followed through to the venous phase, (2) splenoportography, (3) venous catheterization of hepatic veins with pressure measurements, and (4) direct transhepatic portography. There are clinical situations in which each of these methods may be indicated. These techniques have been discussed elsewhere in more detail but bear emphasis in this chapter because of their importance in surgical decision making.

Quantitative Hepatic Function Assessment

The final outcome of most management methods for the treatment of complications of portal hypertension ultimately depends on hepatic reserve. Standard liver function tests do not assess hepatocellular reserve. A patient with advanced cirrhosis may have entirely normal standard biochemical test results if his or her disease is stable at the time of assessment. The liver's synthetic capacity must be severely reduced to decrease serum albumin and increase prothrombin time. Measurements of rate processes for the metabolism or production of substances by the liver offer a means of assessing hepatocyte reserve.[7] Tests that have been used are the galactose elimination capacity,[132] low-dose galactose clearance,[45] antipyrine clearance,[3] caffeine clearance,[100] monoethylglycinexylidide production,[90] and urea synthesis rates.[108] Although these have not had widespread acceptance, the increasing application of liver transplantation to patients with portal hypertension puts a burden on defining which patients are reaching end-stage liver disease.

A summary of the surgical evaluation of patients with portal hypertension follows:

ASSESS BLEEDING RISK
• Endoscopy
• Angiography

ASSESS LIVER FAILURE RISK
• Clinical
• Biochemical or hematologic
• Liver biopsy
• Quantitative tests

This should address the risk of variceal bleeding and the severity of the underlying liver disease. A primary question to be answered at this evaluation is whether the patient requires liver transplantation at this time or is likely to in the near future. Second, if the patient is not a candidate for transplantation or does not require transplantation, what are reasonable therapy options based on his or her risk for bleeding and liver failure?

Surgical Methods

This section presents the available surgical options for management of the complications of portal hypertension, outline the anticipated outcomes, and address the indications for the use of each procedure. Each therapy may be required in different stages of management, or in different patient populations as outlined in subsequent sections of this chapter. An institution managing patients with portal hypertension should have all these therapies available, or have an appropriate referral route for them.

SCLEROTHERAPY

Endoscopic variceal sclerosis was introduced by the ear, nose, and throat surgeons in the 1930s using the rigid esophagoscope.[19] The ability to visualize and directly inject varices, followed by compression with the rigid scope, obtained some success. The introduction of total portosystemic shunts in the 1940s, however, temporarily obscured the need for this approach. Dissatisfaction with total portosystemic shunts in the 1970s led to the reintroduction of sclerotherapy, again by surgeons, using rigid esophagoscopes. The 1980s saw the application of sclerotherapy using flexible endoscopy and, by the end of that decade, some definition of its role in overall patient management.[44]

Initial trepidation at injecting a large, high-pressure varix at the end of a flexible endoscope soon was replaced with enthusiasm when it became apparent that acute bleeding could be stopped, that varices could be obliterated, and that this method offered a widely applicable form of therapy. From a technical standpoint, sclerotherapy uses a flexible endoscope with either intravariceal or paravariceal injection under differing circumstances[146]; it is equally efficacious with a variety of different sclerosing agents[71]; finally, variceal obliteration can be achieved more rapidly with weekly sclerotherapy sessions rather than sessions every other week.[147] Complications are relatively minor, including retrosternal burning, mild dysphagia, mucosal ulceration, microperforation, and esophageal stricture.[113,117] More significant complications such as true perforation, deep ulceration, and systemic embolization of sclerosant have been reported.[24,114]

Sclerotherapy works by direct variceal ablation and fibrous scarring of the mucosa. This does not alter the portal hemodynamics. There is no change in portal perfusion patterns, and no adverse affect on the liver itself as a direct result of the treatment. The risk of major venous thrombosis of the portal superior mesenteric or splenic veins does not appear to be high; although there have been case reports suggesting this, these have not documented the status of the veins before injection.[55,131] In a series of patients followed with presclerotherapy and postsclerotherapy angiography over 2 to 5 years, no instances of major vessel thrombosis could be documented.[69] The same population showed no change in quantitative liver function over this time.

The results of sclerotherapy have been extensively reported. In acute variceal bleeding, endoscopic sclerotherapy controls acute bleeding in 90% of patients.[4,95,150] In prevention of recurrent bleeding, randomized studies show that sclerotherapy lessens the risk of bleeding compared with no therapy,[18,74,128,148] is equivalent to propranolol in control of bleeding,[1,33] but is not as efficacious as shunt surgery.[107,120,129,144] Sclerotherapy does not improve survival compared with any of the other therapies. The overall rebleeding rate through sclerotherapy at 3- to 5-year follow-up is about 50%, but half of these cases are controlled by repeated injection. The data suggest that there are two patterns of rebleeding[53]: early rebleeding in the first few months is associated with failure to obliterate large varices, whereas late rebleeding at 2 to 4 years usually is due to gastric variceal rebleeding or portal gastropathy.

Sclerotherapy is an appropriate initial therapy in management of variceal bleeding. Acute bleeding is controlled, and the initial course of sclerotherapy gives time fully to evaluate the patient, to determine whether he or she is likely to rebleed, and to select an appropriate surgical rescue therapy should there be rebleeding or progressive hepatic failure.[37]

DECOMPRESSIVE SHUNT SURGERY

Decompressive shunts for portal hypertension fall into three groups: (1) total portosystemic shunts decompress all portal hypertension, (2) partial portosystemic shunts reduce portal hypertension to about 12 mmHg, and (3) selective shunts decompress the varices but maintain portal hypertension. This section briefly describes the major shunts in each of these groups, outlines their physiologic goals, and summarizes current experience.

Total Portosystemic Shunts

Pathophysiologically, there are two distinctly different methods for total portosystemic shunt. Both reduce portal venous pressure from about 30 mmHg to 8 to 10 mmHg, and deprive the liver of all portal venous flow. Figure 34-1 illustrates the classic end-to-side portacaval shunt, or the Eck fistula. This technically easy shunt isolates 6 to 8 cm of the portal vein from its bifurcation proximally, and turns the splanchnic end posterior for end-to-side anastomosis to the infrahepatic inferior vena cava. The hepatic end of the portal vein is ligated at its bifurcation. Thus, the intestinal, splenic, and gastroesophageal segments of the portal venous bed are decompressed, but the liver itself maintains a high sinusoidal pressure. This shunt controls variceal bleeding but does not alter or improve ascites.

The second group of total portosystemic shunts are the side-to-side shunts, some of which are illustrated in Figure 34-2. These interposition shunts,[27] or their variations with direct side-to-side portacaval, cavomesenteric,[14] mesoatrial,[12] or central splenorenal shunt,[79] not only decompress the splanchnic bed but also decompress the obstructed liver sinusoids. In contrast to the Eck fistula, the portal vein is left intact and serves as an outflow track from the sinusoids. Study of these types of shunt have shown clearly that if they are large enough to decompress portal hypertension, they are not associated with any continuing prograde portal flow.[35,123] In those that use prosthetic material as an interposition graft, there is a risk of thrombosis.[116] The two advantages of side-to-side shunts over the end-to-side portacaval shunt are that they control ascites and they decompress the obstructed sinusoids of acute Budd-Chiari syndrome.

Technical details of these operations are beyond the scope of this text, but some general points should be made. The portal vein, superior mesenteric vein, and infrahepatic vena cava are relatively robust vessels, allowing for safe anastomosis. The procedures are relatively easy to perform by iso-

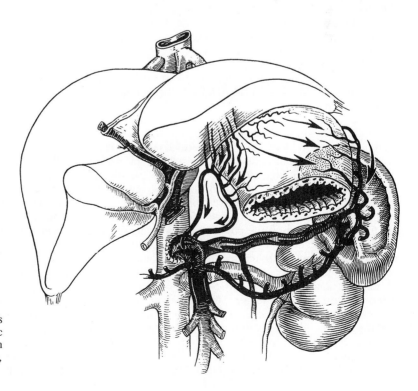

FIGURE 34-1 End-to-side portacaval shunt (Eck's fistula). Portal hypertension is reduced, but the hepatic sinusoids remain obstructed. (Henderson JM, Warren WD. Portal hypertension. Curr Probl Surg 25:173, 1988)

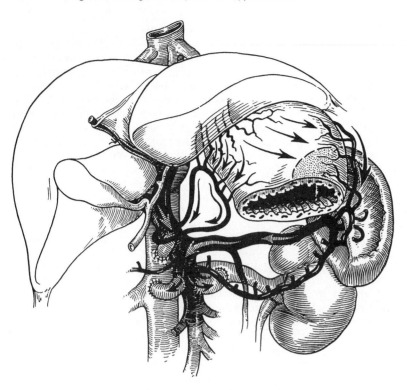

FIGURE 34-2 Interposition, or side-to-side, total portosystemic shunts. Both portal hypertension and the high sinusoidal pressure are relieved by these operations. (Henderson JM, Warren WD. Portal hypertension. Curr Probl Surg 25:174, 1988)

lating an adequate length of vessel before anastomosis. Patency and flow in the shunt should be confirmed either by intraoperative flow and pressure measurement or with angiography within the first week after surgery. In the era of transplantation, shunts in the hepatic hilus should be avoided in patients who may become transplantation candidates.

The results of total portosystemic shunts have been well defined. Bleeding control is excellent in over 90% of patients. This advantage has been more than offset, however, by the high rate of hepatic failure and encephalopathy. Randomized trials of prophylaxis[16,63,101] of the initial bleed and therapy[64,102,103,109] to prevent rebleeding have shown parallel results. Operative mortality is of the order 8% to 15%. Five-year survival is about 35% to 50% with 10-year survival of 20% to 25%. The unanswered question with total portosystemic shunts is, which patients will tolerate them? If this 20% to 25% subset of patients for whom adequate hepatic function is maintained on hepatic arterial flow alone could be identified, total shunts would offer an excellent management method for variceal bleeding in those selected patients. Portal diversion is not tolerated by all patients, however, and in those with incapacitating encephalopathy or progressive hepatic failure, restoration of portal flow can reverse the changes of encephalopathy and liver failure.[41,97]

The indications for total portosystemic shunts in the 1990s are limited. The end-to-side portacaval shunt rarely should be performed. Side-to-side total portosystemic shunts are indicated for patients with massive continued bleeding that cannot be controlled by endoscopic sclerotherapy. Control of bleeding is rapid, and liver failure can be addressed if and when it occurs. If the patient is a potential liver transplantation candidate, the choice should be a mesocaval shunt so that the hepatic hilus is not disturbed.[8,20] The total abolition of portal hypertension makes a side-to-side shunt the operation of choice for ectopic variceal bleeding. Finally, side-to-side total portosystemic shunts are indicated for the man-

agement of acute Budd-Chiari syndrome in which there is ongoing hepatocyte necrosis from congestion.

Partial Portosystemic Shunts

Partial portosystemic shunts aim to reduce portal hypertension to 12 mmHg. Although the concept of being able to reduce portal hypertension sufficiently to control variceal bleeding without depriving the liver of all prograde portal flow seems untenable, careful hemodynamic data have documented that this can be achieved. This critical portal pressure is 12 mmHg, which is the same pressure documented in pharmacologic studies as the cutoff point below which variceal bleeding is not seen.[39]

Partial portosystemic shunts are interposition shunts with a limited-size graft Figure 34-3. Sarfeh and colleagues[112] systematically have reduced the size of portacaval H-grafts and documented that with an 8-mm graft, portal pressure falls to 12 mmHg, and that prograde portal flow is maintained in 80% of patients. This shunt is combined with variceal inflow ligation, primarily of the left gastric vein, and incorporates the concept of controlled collateralization. Data from these studies suggest that further collateral formation may not occur when portal pressure is reduced to 12 mmHg.

The technical aspects of this operation have been well defined by its originators. Adequate exposure of the portal vein and inferior vena cava is critical. The anastomosis should be longer than the diameter of the graft and made with an everting suture. Early postoperative documentation of patency and flow should be made in the first week. An initial thrombosis rate of about 20% is anticipated for these small grafts, but, when identified, thrombosis can be opened with direct infusion of urokinase.

Results of partial portosystemic shunt in limited series have shown good control of bleeding.[6,66,110] Maintenance of portal flow has resulted in a lower incidence of encephalopathy and liver failure than seen with total shunts. Prospective

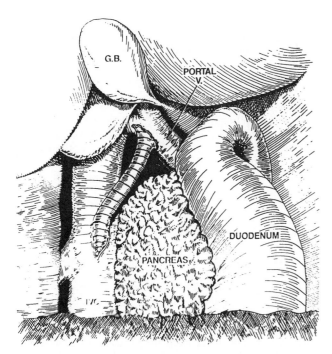

FIGURE 34-3 Partial portosystemic shunt is achieved by a small-bore (8-mm) portacaval interposition graft. (Sarfeh IJ, Rypins EB, Mason GR. A systematic appraisal of portacaval H-graft diameters: clinical and hemodynamic perspectives. Ann Surg 204:358, 1986)

randomized studies comparing total and partial decompression are underway, and should provide documentation as to whether partial shunts offer a significant advantage.

Limited-size interposition mesocaval shunts apply the same concept, and have been advocated.[94] There are insuf-ficient data to show whether the hemodynamic advantages of the interposition portacaval small-bore shunts are achieved similarly with the mesocaval equivalent.

Selective Variceal Decompression

The pathophysiologic concept behind selective variceal decompression is to provide a low-pressure decompressive shunt for gastroesophageal varices, while at the same time maintaining portal hypertension to maintain portal venous flow to the liver. This concept was born of the observations that shunts provided the best control for variceal bleeding, and that portal perfusion was essential to maintain hepatic function in the cirrhotic liver. The two operative methods have been distal splenorenal shunt (DSRS)[143] and coronary caval shunt.[58]

DSRS is illustrated in Figure 34-4. It divides the splenic vein at its juncture with the superior mesenteric vein, isolates the vein from the posterior surface of the pancreas, and turns it down to an anastomosis with the left renal vein.[140] The second component of this procedure is to isolate the low-pressure gastrosplenic drainage segment from the high-pressure splanchnic-to-portal axis. This is achieved by interruption of the coronary vein both at its junction with the portal vein and above the pancreas, interruption of the colonic vessels, which pass from the transverse mesocolon to the inferior ramus on the splenic vein, and interruption of the gastroepiploic arcade along the greater curve of the stomach. The technical difficulty of DSRS has been overemphasized, and this operation can be performed by surgeons proficient in management of portal hypertension. The essential steps are as follows: make an adequate exposure of the pancreas through the lesser sac, with the added component of taking down the splenic flexure of the colon from the inferior pole of the spleen. Next, mobilize the whole of the pancreas from the superior mesenteric vein to the splenic hilus, then dissect

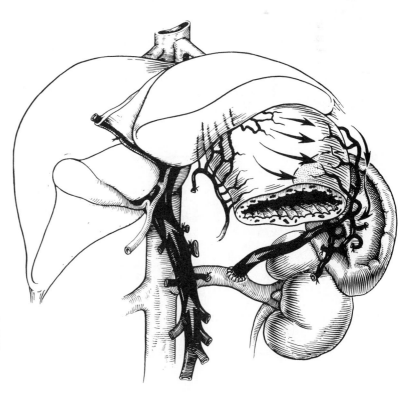

FIGURE 34-4 Distal splenorenal shunt selectively decompresses gastroesophageal varices through the spleen, while at the same time portal hypertension is sustained to keep prograde portal flow to the liver. (Henderson JM, Warren WD. Portal hypertension. Curr Probl Surg 25:177, 1988)

the splenic vein out of the pancreas, commencing at the superior mesenteric end, dissecting the posterior surface before the anterior surface. Sufficient length of vein must be isolated to come down easily to the left renal vein without kinking. The anastomosis should be carefully aligned and made without tension. A meticulous separation of the communications between the portal and splenic venous systems improves maintenance of long-term portal perfusion.

The widespread application of DSRS in many countries around the world is testimony to its success.[51,59,65,76,80,86,91,98,111] The results of DSRS indicate that bleeding control is as good as with total portosystemic shunt.[49,106] In most series, over 90% of patients have satisfactory bleeding control, with the time of highest risk for rebleeding being in the first month to 6 weeks. In this time interval, the short gastric veins and the renal vein accommodate the increased flow from the varices.[104] Long-term patency of DSRS has been excellent because of the high-flow, vein-to-vein end anastomosis, with late thrombosis being unusual. Maintenance of portal perfusion is achieved in 90% of patients with nonalcoholic cirrhosis at late follow-up.[46,48,141] With standard DSRS, however, although 90% of patients with alcoholic cirrhosis maintain portal flow initially, 50% lose portal perfusion in the first 6 to 12 months.[48] Failure to maintain portal flow in the alcoholic population is associated with significantly poorer survival (Fig. 34-5).[47,141,156] Prospective, randomized trials comparing DSRS with total shunts have been conducted in populations with 83% having alcoholic cirrhosis.[17,32,42,75,85,99] The failure to show any significant advantage to DSRS may be associated with the choice of this patient population. Definition of large pancreatic siphoning collaterals from the high-pressure portal vein to the low-pressure shunt identified this pathway as the

culprit in loss of portal perfusion.[48] This led to the operative modification of entire splenopancreatic disconnection, which was associated with improved maintenance of portal flow in 84% of patients with alcoholic cirrhosis.[50] This improved maintenance of portal perfusion was associated with improved survival.

Randomized studies also have compared DSRS with endoscopic sclerotherapy.[107,120,129,144] The four trials that have been conducted all show significantly improved control of bleeding with the shunt. In three of the studies, there was no significant difference in survival between the two randomized groups. In the fourth study,[53] there was significant survival advantage at all time points for the patients randomized to sclerotherapy (Fig. 34-6). This sclerotherapy group, however, is in reality a combined sclerotherapy–surgical salvage group. Of the patients randomized to sclerotherapy, 58% had rebleeding, and 35% required surgical rescue for uncontrolled rebleeding. In this trial, the advantage of initial sclerotherapy and subsequent surgical rescue was seen only in patients with alcoholic cirrhosis. In patients with nonalcoholic disease, the significantly better control of bleeding suggests initial DSRS for patients who are good surgical risks.

The indications for DSRS for variceal bleeding are (1) patients with nonalcoholic liver disease who are good surgical risks, and (2) patients with alcoholic cirrhosis who fail sclerotherapy. DSRS also fulfills an important criteria in the transplantation era by avoiding dissection in the hepatic hilus.

Intrahepatic Shunts

The creation of a direct intrahepatic fistula from the portal vein to a hepatic vein or intrahepatic vena cava is an appealing way of relieving portal hypertension. Advances in radiologic techniques and improvement in expandable stents have led to renewed interest.[15,92,105,122] Pathophysiologically, this is a total portosystemic shunt, with the aim of creating an anastomosis between a main portal vein and the systemic circulation.

An intrahepatic shunt is made by access through the internal jugular vein, with direct puncture through the hepatic substance from a hepatic vein to the portal vein to identify the path for the shunt. The artificial track so created is then balloon-dilated and an expandable metal stent placed. In theory, the stent may be sized in a manner similar to that already described for partial portal decompression. The technical capability has been demonstrated in both animals and patients, and is particularly appealing for patients with variceal bleeding who are likely to need transplantation in the near future. The ability to control bleeding and relieve portal hypertension before transplantation should improve their general condition.[122]

Results are too preliminary to make any generalizations about the applicability of this method. The preliminary results from a group with a high level of expertise are encouraging,[122] but further data must be accumulated before widespread use is advocated.

DEVASCULARIZATION PROCEDURES

Devascularization procedures as management of variceal bleeding recognize the importance of maintaining portal perfusion to maximize hepatic function in cirrhosis. In contrast to shunt procedures, which emphasize the importance of decompression to control variceal bleeding, this surgical

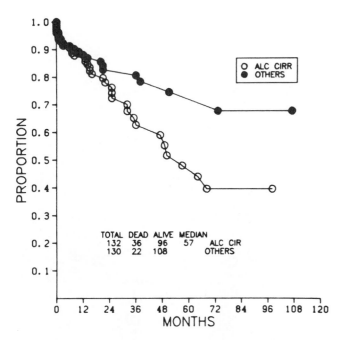

FIGURE 34-5 Survival of alcoholic (O) and nonalcoholic (●) patients after distal splenorenal shunt. There was significantly improved survival in patients with nonalcoholic disease. (Warren WD, et al. Ten years of portal hypertensive surgery at Emory. Ann Surg 195:532, 1982)

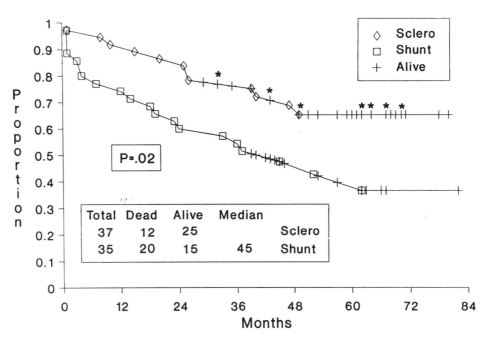

FIGURE 34-6 Survival curves for patients randomized to distal splenorenal shunt (□) or sclerotherapy (◇). There is a significantly improved survival (*P* < .02) to the sclerotherapy group at all time points, but 38% of this group required surgical rescue in the 5 years of study follow-up. Asterisks indicate those who crossed over and are still alive. (Henderson JM, Kutner MH, Millikan WJ, et al. Endoscopic variceal sclerosis compared with distal splenorenal shunt to prevent recurrent variceal bleeding in cirrhosis: a prospective randomized trial. Ann Intern Med 112:265, 1990)

Total	Dead	Alive	Median	
37	12	25		Sclero
35	20	15	45	Shunt

P=.02

approach is prepared to accept a higher risk of rebleeding so as better to maintain hepatic function. The components to devascularization procedures are splenectomy, gastric and esophageal devascularization, and esophageal transection (Fig. 34-7).

The techniques of devascularization vary enormously in their extent, with the risk of rebleeding correlating with the extent of the devascularization. The most extensive devascularizations combine thoracotomy and laparotomy to en-sure adequate devascularization. Sugiura and colleagues[124] and Idezuki and coworkers[56] devascularize from the pylorus to the inferior pulmonary veins, and have a rebleeding rate of less than 5%. Devascularization limited to a laparotomy at best isolates 8 cm of the esophagus and leaves intact some of the perforating veins to the submucosal varices. Adequate ligations of the other inflow tracts, which are predominately the left gastric system and short gastric veins, are essential components to this procedure. Lesser devascularization,

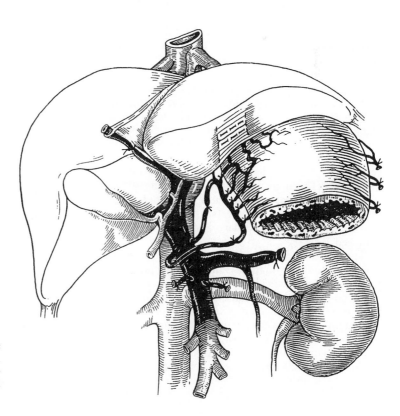

FIGURE 34-7 Devascularization procedures have the component parts of splenectomy, gastric and esophageal devascularization, and esophageal transaction. (Henderson JM, Warren WD. Portal hypertension. Curr Probl Surg 25:183, 1988)

leaving the spleen in situ, has been advocated but is associated with increased risk of rebleeding. Simple esophageal transection with a staple gun anastomosis without further attempt at devascularization appears to be an inadequate operative approach.[11,130]

The anticipated outcomes from devascularization procedures vary significantly in different patient populations. The exceedingly favorable outcome achieved in Japan, with an 80% long-term survival, indicates a patient population with stable liver disease. This population can undergo the extensive devascularization procedures with relatively low operative morbidity and mortality.[12] In contrast, series from Europe[119] and the United States,[23,70] with patients with more advanced and unstable liver disease, have been associated with higher operative and long-term mortalities. It is probable that the performance of these extensive procedures in higher-risk patients has led to lesser degrees of devascularization, and hence to higher rebleeding rates.

The indications for devascularization procedures are governed by patient populations. These procedures should be used in patient populations in whom they have been shown to be effective. In the United States, patients with nonalcoholic cirrhosis who have no vessels suitable for selective shunt procedures may be managed by devascularization. The picture is even less clear in patients with alcoholic cirrhosis, in whom control of the variceal bleeding probably is of primary importance, and can be achieved better with a shunt procedure.

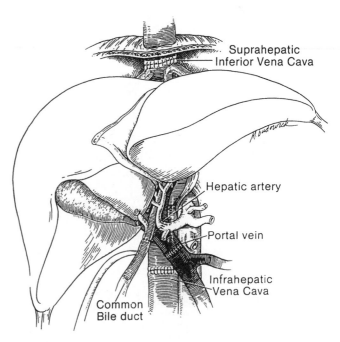

FIGURE 34-8   Orthotopic liver transplant replaces the cirrhotic liver and both removes portal hypertension and restores hepatic function. (Henderson JM, Warren WD. Portal hypertension. Curr Probl Surg 25:185, 1988)

LIVER TRANSPLANTATION

Should all patients with complications of portal hypertension who require surgery be managed by liver transplantation? Appealing as this concept may be, it is both impractical and unnecessary.

Liver transplantation, by removal of the diseased cirrhotic liver and replacement with a new liver, relieves both the portal hypertension and restores normal hepatic function (Fig. 34-8). This ideal is offset, however, by the significant operative and perioperative risks, by the risk of long-term immunosuppression, by the limitation of donor organs, and by the fact that not all such patients are suitable candidates for transplantation. Nevertheless, the question of current or future candidacy for transplantation always should be asked in patients with portal hypertension being considered for surgery.[6,8,20,81,115,155] Management decisions are influenced by the answer. The indication for liver transplantation remains end-stage liver disease, and an enthusiasm for transplantation in the patient with complications of portal hypertension who has not reached end-stage liver disease should be discouraged.

The decision on the need for transplantation should be based on careful evaluation. This has three phases. The initial decision is medical necessity for liver transplantation, which combines clinical status, standard laboratory tests, and more specialized tests such as serologic markers, biopsy, and quantitative tests to determine whether the liver disease can be managed in any lesser way. Once it is determined that there is medical necessity, the evaluation should focus on medical contraindications. Careful assessment of other organ systems may provide absolute or relative contraindications such as malignancy, sepsis, and cardiac, pulmonary, or renal

dysfunction. The final phase of evaluation is psychosocial suitability, which should receive careful consideration.

In the context of this chapter, the anticipated outcome after transplantation is good for appropriately selected patients. Variceal bleeding is controlled by relief of portal hypertension, and hepatic function is restored to normal provided the graft functions well. Increasing evidence points to the risk of recurrent hepatitis in patients requiring transplantation for end-stage cirrhosis secondary to viral hepatitis. This creates uncertainty as to its role in such patients. Current survival figures show a 75% to 80% survival rate after 1 year and a 70% survival rate at 2 years after liver transplantation.[62] In large series that included a significant number of patients with variceal bleeding, the outcome in this latter group was equivalent to that of the transplantation population as a whole.[6,62,155] The necessity to comply with a lifelong medical regimen to avoid rejection must be emphasized in preoperative evaluation and selection. The risks of immunosuppression, both from infection and in the development of tumors, are real, and need to be understood by the patient. Despite these risks, however, liver transplantation has dramatically altered the outlook and survival for patients with end-stage liver disease and the complications of portal hypertension. It undoubtedly is part of the overall armamentarium for the management of such patients.

MANAGEMENT ALGORITHMS FOR VARICEAL BLEEDING

Prophylaxis

The appropriate prophylactic therapy to reduce the risk of the first variceal bleed is pharmacologic reduction of portal pressure.[36] Many randomized studies have documented a lower incidence of initial bleed in patients treated with a nonselective β-blocker.[43] Survival advantage has been documented in some but not all of these studies.[10] Identification of varices in patients with cirrhosis who have not bled entails a 30% risk of bleeding in the next 2 years. β-Blockers reduce this risk to less than 20%.

Endoscopic sclerotherapy is not advocated as therapy to prevent the first bleed,[126] based on randomized studies. There are favorable[93,154] and unfavorable[134] studies, but overall there is no significant advantage with prophylactic sclerotherapy. In large part, this is because of the relatively low risk for initial variceal bleed, with only one in three patients at risk, dictating the need for prophylactic therapy with a low morbidity. New studies focusing on identification of patients at higher risk for initial variceal bleed may reopen the question of the role of sclerotherapy in this setting.[22]

Prophylactic surgery to prevent the initial variceal bleed is not indicated. Studies in the 1960s compared prophylactic portacaval shunts with standard medical management and showed an increased morbidity and mortality in the surgically treated groups, which outweighed the risk of bleeding.[16,63,101] A multicenter study of portal nondecompressive surgery conducted in Japan has reopened this question, however.[60] In a randomized study in which surgical therapy was either extensive devascularization or selective shunt, both significantly lower bleeding and significantly improved survival were documented at late follow-up in the surgery group. Is this type of surgical procedure that much superior to total portosystemic shunt? This question remains unanswered, and most would agree that the group at greatest risk for that initial variceal bleed are those with poorest hepatic function, indicating that prophylactic surgery is not a rational approach.

Acute Variceal Bleeding

The primary treatment for patients with acute variceal bleeding should be endoscopic variceal sclerotherapy. Figure 34-9 provides a treatment algorithm for the management of acute variceal bleeding.

The patient with known or suspected portal hypertension who presents with upper gastrointestinal bleeding initially should be resuscitated, as for any patient with hypovolemic hemorrhagic shock. If the patient has ascites or is undergoing diuretic therapy, resuscitation should differ in that sodium should be restricted. Blood loss requires blood replacement, and intravascular volume should be repleted with fresh frozen plasma or 5% albumin. Minimizing infusion of lactated Ringer's solution or normal saline pays benefits over the next week. If ongoing massive bleeding occurs, the patient should be given pitressin, 20 IU in 200 mL of 5% dextrose infused over 20 minutes for a bolus effect. Early endoscopy should be undertaken either in the emergency room or as soon as the patient is transferred to the intensive care unit. This endoscopy is both diagnostic and therapeutic. The site of bleeding should be localized by visualization either of active bleeding or of a platelet plug on a varix. It is equally important to exclude other sources of bleeding. If an active bleeding varix is identified, or a platelet plug visualized, injection sclerotherapy of that varix should be undertaken immediately. If no bleeding source is identified, and other causes of upper gastrointestinal bleeding are excluded, the esophageal varices should be sclerosed. Acute variceal bleeding is controlled after this regimen in 90% of patients. The patient should then pass on to a phase of full evaluation and decisions on management to prevent recurrent bleeding, as discussed later.

In the 5% to 10% of patients in whom acute bleeding cannot be controlled by endoscopic sclerotherapy, further measures may be required. It is in this small minority of patients that balloon tamponade is required to control the bleeding temporarily. Placement of a balloon tube should be viewed as an opportunity to stabilize the patient and prepare him or her for an alternative treatment modality. The aim should be to deflate the balloon within 12 to 24 hours for either further sclerotherapy or for surgical intervention. In the phase of tamponade, the patient should have arteriography, be fully stabilized from a hemodynamic point of view, and have optimal coagulation.

The surgical role for management of acute variceal bleeding is minimal. Only the patient whose bleeding cannot be controlled by the above methods should be considered for emergency surgery. In a patient with continued massive bleeding in this setting, a total portosystemic shunt with a large (14- to 18-mm) mesocaval or portacaval H-graft shunt relieves the portal hypertension and almost always stop the bleeding.

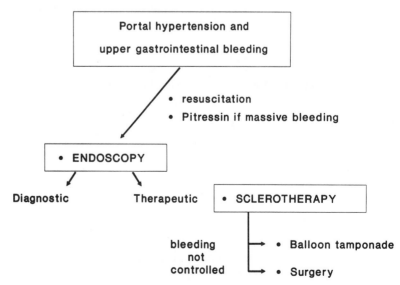

FIGURE 34-9 Algorithm for management of acute variceal bleeding.

Prevention of Recurrent Variceal Bleeding

The high risk of further bleeding dictates the need for definitive therapy to reduce that risk.[38] All treatment modalities may be required in management of different patients to prevent recurrent variceal bleeding. These treatments include pharmacologic reduction of portal pressure, endoscopic sclerotherapy of varices, decompressive shunt procedures, devascularization operations, and liver transplantation. A treatment algorithm for the management of these patients is given in Figure 34-10.

The most important step in management of patients to prevent recurrent variceal bleeding is a full evaluation. The two important decision steps are determining what the risks are for continued or recurrent bleeding, and what the risks are for hepatic failure. This evaluation should be completed within a week after stabilization of acute variceal bleeding. In the patient with good hepatic function, the emphasis of management should be on prevention of recurrent bleeding. In the patient with poor liver function, treatment focuses on improving this, or consideration for transplantation.

The patient with nonalcoholic disease who has good hepatic function should be managed with DSRS. Alternatively, the nonalcoholic patient who is a good surgical risk may be managed with endoscopic sclerotherapy with or without a β-blocker. Data indicate that there is a 30% to 50% chance of rebleeding with such a management regimen but that half of those rebleeding episodes can be controlled with further sclerotherapy. This decision should take into account other factors such as geographic location and local available expertise.

In the patient with alcoholic cirrhosis and good hepatic function, data suggest that sclerotherapy should be the initial line of management. The data are not clear on whether this should be combined with a β-blocker,[149] and ongoing studies should clarify this. The risk of rebleeding with this regimen remains 30% to 50%, but surgical management, usually with DSRS, should be reserved for those who fail sclerotherapy.[37] Appropriate management of the underlying liver disease should be integral to this management regimen. Stopping drinking and actively participating in a rehabilitation program probably are as important as the specific therapy for variceal bleeding. Ultimately, the patient's survival is going to be determined by his or her liver disease, and it is important to emphasize this phase of management.

Patients with poor hepatic function, as defined by Child's class C, or more rigorously defined with quantitative hepatic function testing, should be viewed as potential liver transplantation candidates. In patients who fulfill candidacy criteria, treatment should be liver transplantation. Many patients with poor hepatic function, however, do not fulfill these criteria because of concomitant medical disease, active alcoholism, or patient choice. The alternatives are not good. Management of the bleeding with sclerotherapy may buy time while other issues are addressed. A major question is the reversibility of the underlying liver disease.

Evaluation has been emphasized as critical in these decisions and should be an ongoing process. It is the behavior of the liver disease over time that best determines whether the patient has good or poor hepatic function. When this picture is not clear at initial assessment, endoscopic sclerotherapy offers a holding therapy that may allow this longitudinal determination to be made. For example, if variceal bleeding has been associated with acute decompensation of a reversible process in the liver, the risk for further bleeding may lessen as that acute disease is treated. Conversely, the initial bleed may precipitate a more rapid decline in an already advanced cirrhosis, and it may become apparent over the next month or two that there is no alternative but transplantation for end-stage liver disease.

EXTRAHEPATIC PORTAL VEIN THROMBOSIS

The distinguishing feature of this group of patients with variceal bleeding is that they have normal livers. In contrast to the patient with cirrhosis, bleeding is better tolerated in these patients because they do not have hepatic decompensation.[145] The other main clinical presentation of these patients is mas-

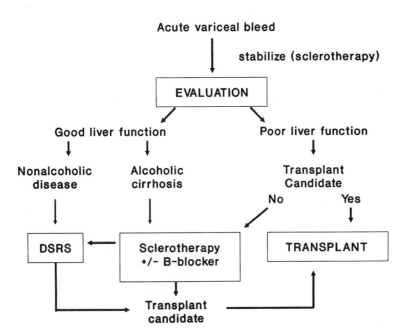

FIGURE 34-10 Algorithm for prevention of recurrent variceal bleeding.

sive splenomegaly and hypersplenism. The associated thrombocytopenia is a source of alarm for the managing physician, although it frequently causes no problem for the patient. Splenectomy in this situation is contraindicated because it removes the best treatment option for these patients should they have variceal bleeding.[30]

Pathophysiology

Extrahepatic portal vein obstruction results from either thrombosis, agenesis, or atresia of the portal vein. The high venous pressure in the gastrointestinal and splenic beds results in gastroesophageal varices with a risk of bleeding, splenomegaly, and hypersplenism. Hemodynamically, these patients maintain excellent portal perfusion of their liver through cavernous transformation of the portal vein, whereby many variceal channels collateralize back to the liver, which has sinusoids under normal pressure.

Management

Management of the acute bleeding episode in these patients should be the same as for patients with cirrhosis. Sclerotherapy usually stops the acute bleeding episode. Definitive management is more controversial. Because they tolerate bleeding episodes well, a conservative management approach has been advocated[145]; however, repeated bleeding episodes managed simply by transfusion is untenable when definitive control can be achieved. Endoscopic sclerotherapy has been applied successfully,[54,68] but does carry a risk of recurrent bleeding. Surgical management has incorporated both total and selective shunts.[2,34,138,139] Review of a collected series in 1982 showed that in the previous 20 years, traditional total shunts were associated with a 50% rebleeding rate.[34] From the same series, 68% rebled after nonshunt operations. Use of DSRS has had a more favorable outcome. In 75% of patients, the splenic vein is open for a sufficient length to allow DSRS.[142] Bleeding control has been greater than 90%, but 25% of patients have required balloon dilation in the first 6 months because of anastomotic stricture secondary to the abnormal splenic vein. Dilation at that time has resulted in excellent long-term patency. In addition, selective shunt has allowed long-term maintenance of portal perfusion of the liver in these patients through their collaterals. Splenic size falls to 30% to 50% of preoperative volume and is associated with a significant increase in platelet counts. Finally, quantitative data have shown no deterioration in hepatic function after selective shunt.[142]

The recommendation for patients with variceal bleeding secondary to portal vein thrombosis should be for a selective shunt if they have an adequate splenic vein for this procedure. This gives definitive control of bleeding and returns them to a normal life expectancy.

HEPATOSPLENIC SCHISTOSOMIASIS

Hepatosplenic schistosomiasis is a worldwide public health problem that is the most common cause of portal hypertension in some parts of the world. It may account for over 80% of portal hypertension seen in some areas of Africa, South America, and Asia.[31,98]

Pathophysiology

Portal hypertension follows infestation of the liver by schistosomal eggs. The adult worms shed their eggs into the portal vein, and they provoke a significant reaction in the terminal portal venule. The granuloma formation and portal fibrosis obstruct the intrahepatic branches of the portal vein. In the setting of pure schistosomiasis, hepatic function is well maintained; however, many of these patients have concomitant hepatitis. Massive splenomegaly also is a feature, and portal hypertension is aggravated in part by the high flow from the huge spleen.

Management

Access to medical care may be limited in many of the countries where this problem dominates. In these patients, variceal bleeding is the usual mode of death. Definitive control of variceal bleeding is therefore required. Total portosystemic shunts proved unsatisfactory because of accelerated hepatic failure. Dissatisfaction with this approach led to widespread application of splenectomy and devascularization.[98] Significant rebleeding accompanied this approach, however. Series of selective shunts have shown favorable outcome.[31,98,111] Good bleeding control has been achieved, hepatic function has been maintained, and encephalopathy has been a minor problem. Data suggest that this population is optimally managed by DSRS.

BUDD-CHIARI SYNDROME

Budd-Chiari syndrome is extensively discussed in Chapter 40. There are two surgical options—decompressive shunt for acute Budd-Chiari syndrome and liver transplantation for advanced end-stage disease.

Pathophysiology

Budd-Chiari syndrome brings together a group of diseases with the common parameter of hepatic venous outflow obstruction. In the acute setting, sinusoidal congestion and dilation lead to hepatocyte necrosis and ultimately to fibrosis. With ongoing hepatocyte necrosis, the surgeon's role is to provide sinusoidal decompression.

An alternative presentation of Budd-Chiari syndrome is the patient with repeated lesser episodes in which small areas of the liver are progressively obstructed, undergoing destruction and fibrosis with marked scarring. In this situation, the liver is markedly fibrotic and the patient has end-stage disease.

Management

In this unusual cause of portal hypertension, the surgeon plays a role in management to provide either hepatic decompression or hepatic replacement. In the acute setting, the need for sinusoidal decompression is dictated by the biopsy finding of ongoing hepatocyte necrosis.[52] Decompression is provided by a side-to-side total portosystemic shunt. The type of shunt is dictated by the status of the intrahepatic inferior vena cava.[52,73,137] If the inferior vena cava is open and there is no significant pressure gradient between the right atrium and the infrahepatic vena cava, a portacaval or mesocaval H-graft shunt provides decompression. In this situation, the portal vein acts as an outflow tract from the obstructed sinusoids, which results in lowering of sinusoidal pressure and halting of the ongoing hepatic necrosis. In the patient in whom the inferior vena cava is obstructed or thrombosed, a suprahe-

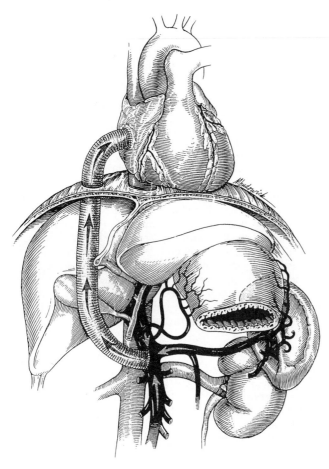

FIGURE 34-11   Mesoatrial shunt is a side-to-side total portal systemic shunt that bypasses intrahepatic inferior vena caval obstruction. (Henderson JM, Warren WD. Portal hypertension. Curr Probl Surg 25:213, 1988)

patic shunt is required. This usually is achieved with a mesoatrial shunt, which again is a side-to-side type shunt.[12] This is illustrated in Figure 34-11, which shows a long prosthetic graft taken from the superior mesenteric vein through the diaphragm to the right atrium. The goal of this therapy again is to use the portal vein as an outflow tract and provide sinusoidal decompression.

Concurrent with these surgical management methods, a full hematologic evaluation is required because a significant percentage of these patients have an underlying myeloproliferative disorder.[133] The surgeon should be particularly concerned that this condition is defined accurately and treated concurrently with surgery; otherwise, shunt thrombosis occurs.

Liver transplantation for Budd-Chiari syndrome is indicated for end-stage disease. This usually is manifest by the markedly fibrotic liver shown on biopsy, and by diminished hepatocellular reserve. Technically, this is one of the more difficult transplantation procedures because the liver has developed multiple collaterals to the diaphragm. Emphasis again should be placed on evaluation for etiologic factors in development of Budd-Chiari syndrome, because underlying myeloproliferative disorders must be treated aggressively to avoid rethrombosis.

Results

The results of decompressive shunts for acute Budd-Chiari syndrome have been satisfactory.[52,73,137] The liver disease is stabilized and the main symptom of ascites is resolved. The late (10 to 20 years) follow-up of these patients is awaited because the continued portaprival state of this liver ultimately may lead to hepatic failure.

The results of liver transplantation in Budd-Chiari syndrome have been limited, but reported small series indicate an outcome equivalent to that for other disease etiologies.

Summary

Surgical management is a component of overall management in patients with portal hypertension. Variceal bleeding is the main complication that may require surgical treatment. The choice of operation should be based on full evaluation of the risks for further bleeding and for liver failure. The main surgical treatments in use are DSRS and liver transplantation, but there are indications for use of total shunts and devascularization procedures.

References

1. Alexandrino PJ, Alves MM, Pinto-Correia J. Propranolol or endoscopic sclerotherapy in the prevention of recurrence of variceal bleeding: a prospective, randomized controlled trial. J Hepatol 7:175–185, 1988
2. Alvarez F, Bernard O, Brunelle F, et al. Portal obstruction in children: results of surgical portosystemic shunts. J Pediatr 103:703–707, 1983
3. Andreasen PG, Ranek L, Statland BE, Tygstrup N. Clearance of antipyrine: dependence on quantitative liver function. Eur J Clin Invest 4:120, 1974
4. Barsoum MS, Boulous FI, El-Robby A, et al. Tamponade and injection sclerotherapy in the management of bleeding esophageal varices. Br J Surg 69:76–78, 1982
5. Beppu K, Inokuchi K, Kayanagi N, et al. Prediction of variceal hemorrhage by esophageal endoscopy. Gastrointest Endosc 27:213–218, 1981
6. Bismuth H, Adam R, Mathur S, Sherlock D. Options for elective treatment of portal hypertension in cirrhotic patients in the transplantation era. Am J Surg 160:105–110, 1990
7. Branch RA. Drugs as indicators of hepatic function. Hepatology 2:97–105, 1982
8. Brems JJ, Hiatt JR, Klein AS, et al. Effect of prior portasystemic shunt on subsequent liver transplantation. Ann Surg 209:51–56, 1989
9. Burns P, Taylor K, Blei AT. Doppler flowmetry and portal hypertension. Gastroenterology 92:824–826, 1987
10. Burroughs AK, D'Heygere F, McIntyre N. Pitfalls in studies of prophylactic therapy for variceal bleeding in cirrhotics. Hepatology 6:1407–1413, 1986
11. Burroughs AK, Hamilton G, Phillips A, et al. A comparison of sclerotherapy with staple transection of the esophagus for the emergency control of bleeding from esophageal varices. N Engl J Med 321:857–862, 1989
12. Cameron JL, Maddrey WC. Mesoatrial shunt: a new treatment for Budd-Chiari syndrome. Ann Surg 187:402–406, 1978
13. Child CG. The liver and portal hypertension. Philadelphia, WB Saunders, 1964, p 50
14. Clatworthy HW, Wall T, Watman RN. A new type of portal to systemic venous shunt for portal hypertension. Arch Surg 71:588–596, 1955
15. Colapinto RF, Stronell RD, Gildiner M, et al. Formation of

intrahepatic portosystemic shunts using a balloon dilatation catheter: preliminary clinical experience. AJR 140:709–714, 1983

16. Conn HO, Lindenmuth WW, May CJ, et al. Prophylactic portacaval anastomosis: a tale of two studies. Medicine 51:27–40, 1972

17. Conn HO, Resnick RF, Grace ND, et al. Distal splenorenal shunt vs portalsystemic shunt: current status of a controlled trial. Hepatology 1:151–160, 1981

18. The Copenhagen Esophageal Varices Sclerotherapy Project. sclerotherapy after first variceal hemorrhage in cirrhosis: a randomized multicenter trial. N Engl J Med 311:1594–1600, 1984

19. Crafoord C, Frenckner P. New surgical treatment of varicose veins of the esophagus. Acta Otolaryngol 27:422–429, 1939

20. Crass RA, Keeffe EB, Pinson CW. Management of variceal hemorrhage in the potential liver transplant candidate. Am J Surg 157:476–478, 1989

21. Davies DV, Davies F, eds. Gray's anatomy, ed 33. London, Longmans, 1962, pp 826–829

22. de Franchis R, and the North Italian Endoscopic Club. Prediction of the first variceal hemorrhage in patients with cirrhosis of the liver and esophageal varices. N Engl J Med 319:983, 1988

23. DelGuercio LRM, Hodgson WJB, Morgan JC, et al. Splenic artery and coronary vein occlusion for bleeding esophageal varices. World J Surg 8:680–687, 1984

24. DePuey EG, Richards WO, Millikan WJ, Henderson JM. Scintigraphic detection of pulmonary embolization of esophageal variceal sclerosant. Endoscopy 20:91–94, 1988

25. Donovan AJ, Cavey PC. Early history of the portacaval shunt in humans. Surg Gynecol Obstet 147:423–428, 1978

26. Douglass BC, Baggenstoss A. Holinshead W. The anatomy of the portal vein and its tributaries. Surg Gynecol Obstet 91:562, 1950

27. Drapanas T. Interposition mesocaval shunt for treatment of portal hypertension. Ann Surg 176:435, 1972

28. Drummond D, Morison RA. A case of ascites due to liver cirrhosis cured by operation. Br Med J 2:728–729, 1896

29. Eck NV. On the question of ligature of the portal vein. Voen Med Zh 130:1, 1877

30. El-Khishen MA, Henderson JM, Millikan WJ, et al. Splenectomy is contraindicated for thrombocytopenia secondary to portal hypertension. Surg Gynecol Obstet 160:233, 1985

31. Ezzat FA, Abu-Elmagd KM, Aly IY, et al. Distal splenorenal shunt for management of variceal bleeding in patients with schistosomal hepatic fibrosis. Ann Surg 204:566–573, 1986

32. Fischer JE, Bower RH, Atamian S, et al. Comparison of distal and proximal splenorenal shunts: a randomized prospective trial. Ann Surg 194:531–544, 1981

33. Fleig WE, Stange EF, Hunecke R, et al. Prevention of recurrent bleeding in cirrhotics with recent variceal hemorrhage: prospective, randomized comparison of propranolol and sclerotherapy. Hepatology 7:355–361, 1987

34. Fonkalsrud EW, Myers NA, Robinson MJ. Management of extrahepatic portal hypertension in children. Ann Surg 180:487, 1974

35. Fulenwider JT, Nordlinger BM, Millikan WJ, et al. Portal pseudoperfusion, an angiographic illusion. Ann Surg 189:257–248, 1979

36. Grace NA. A hepatologist's view of variceal bleeding. Am J Surg 160:26–31, 1990

37. Grace ND. Prevention of recurrent variceal bleeding: is surgical rescue the answer? Ann Intern Med 112:242–244, 1990

38. Graham DY, Smith JL. The course of patients after variceal hemorrhage. Gastroenterology 80:800–809, 1981

39. Groszmann RJ, Bosch J, Grace ND, et al. Hemodynamic events in a prospective randomized trial of propranolol versus placebo in the prevention of a first variceal hemorrhage. Gastroenterology 99:1401–1407, 1990

40. Hahn M, Massen O, Nenki M, et al. De eckssche fistel zwischen der unteren hohlvene and der pfortaden und folgen fur den organismus. Arch Exp Pathol Pharmacol 32:162–210, 1893

41. Hanna SS, Smith RB III, Henderson JM, Millikan WJ, Warren WD. Reversal of hepatic encephalopathy after occlusion of total portasystemic shunts. Am J Surg 142:285–289, 1981

42. Harley HAJ, Morgan T, Redeker AG, et al. Results of a randomized trial of end-to-side portacaval shunt and distal splenorenal shunt in alcoholic liver disease and variceal bleeding. Gastroenterology 91:802–809, 1986

43. Hayes PC, Davis JM, Lewis JA, Bouchier IAD. Meta analysis of value of propranolol in prevention of variceal hemorrhage. Lancet 336:153–156, 1990

44. Health and Public Policy Committee. Endoscopic sclerotherapy for esophageal varices. Ann Intern Med 100:608, 1984

45. Henderson JM, Kutner MH, Bain RP. First-order clearance of plasma galactose: the effect of liver disease. Gastroenterology 83:1090–1096, 1982

46. Henderson JM, Warren WD. A method for measuring quantitative hepatic function and hemodynamics in cirrhosis: the changes following distal splenorenal shunt. Jpn J Surg 3:157–168, 1986

47. Henderson JM, Millikan WJ, Wright-Bacon L, Kutner MH, Warren WD. Hemodynamic differences between alcoholic and non-alcoholic cirrhotics following distal splenorenal shunt: effect on survival? Ann Surg 198:325–334, 1983

48. Henderson JM, Gong-Liang J, Galloway J, et al. Portaprival collaterals following distal splenorenal shunt: incidence, magnitude, and associated portal perfusion changes. J Hepatol 1:649–661, 1985

49. Henderson JM. Variceal bleeding: which shunt? Gastroenterology 91:1021–1023, 1986

50. Henderson JM, Warren WD, Millikan WJ, Galloway JR, Kawasaki S, Kutner MH. Distal splenorenal shunt with splenopancreatic disconnection: a four-year assessment. Ann Surg 210:332–341, 1989

51. Henderson JM, Millikan WJ, Galloway JR. The Emory perspective of distal splenorenal shunt in 1990. Am J Surg 160:54–59, 1990

52. Henderson JM, Warren WD, Millikan WJ, Galloway JR, Kawasaki S, Stahl RL, Hertzler G. Surgical options, hematologic evaluation and pathologic changes in Budd-Chiari syndrome. Am J Surg 159:41–50, 1990

53. Henderson JM, Kutner MH, Millikan WJ, et al. Endoscopic variceal sclerosis compared with distal splenorenal shunt to prevent recurrent variceal bleeding in cirrhosis: a prospective randomized trial. Ann Intern Med 112:262–269, 1990

54. Howard ER, Stringer MD, Mowat AP. Assessment of injection sclerotherapy in the management of 152 children with esophageal varices. Br J Surg 75:404–408, 1988

55. Hunter GC, Steinkirchner T, Burbige EJ, et al. Venous complications of sclerotherapy for esophageal varices. Am J Surg 156:497–501, 1988

56. Idezuki Y, Sanjo K, Bandai Y, Kawasaki S, Ohashi K. Current strategy for esophageal varices in Japan. Am J Surg 160:98–104, 1990

57. Inokuchi K. A selective portocaval shunt. Lancet 2:51, 1968

58. Inokuchi K, Kobayashi M, Ogawa Y, et al. Results of left gastric venacaval shunt for esophageal varices: analysis of one hundred clinical cases. Surgery 78:628, 1975

59. Inokuchi K, Sugimachi K. The selective shunt for variceal bleeding: a personal perspective. Am J Surg 160:48–53, 1990

60. Inokuchi K, Cooperative Study Group of Portal Hypertension in Japan. Improved survival after prophylactic portal nondecompressive surgery for esophageal varices: a randomized controlled trial. Hepatology 2:1–6, 1990.

61. The Italian Liver Cirrhosis Project. Reliability of endoscopy in the assessment of variceal features. J Hepatol 4:93–98, 1987.

62. Iwatsuki S, Starzl TE, Todo S, et al. Liver transplantation in

the treatment of bleeding esophageal varices. Surgery 104:697–705, 1988

63. Jackson FC, Perrin EB, Smith AG, et al. A clinical investigation of the portacaval shunt: 2. survival analysis of the prophylactic operation. Am J Surg 115:22–42, 1968

64. Jackson FC, Perrin EB, Felix R, et al. A clinical investigation of the portacaval shunt: analysis of the therapeutic operation. Ann Surg 174:672–701, 1971

65. Jin G. Current status of the distal splenorenal shunt in China. Am J Surg 160:93–97, 1990

66. Johansen K. Partial portal decompression for variceal hemorrhage. Am J Surg 157:479–482, 1989

67. Johnston GW, Rogers HW. A review of 15 years experience in the use of sclerotherapy in the control of acute hemorrhage from esophageal varices. Br J Surg 60:797, 1973

68. Kahn D, Terblanche J, Kitano S, Bornman P. Injection sclerotherapy in adult patients with extrahepatic portal venous obstruction. Br J Surg 74:600–602, 1987

69. Kawasaki S, Henderson JM, Riepe SP, et al. Endoscopic variceal sclerosis does not increase the risk of portal venous thrombosis. Gastroenterology 102:206, 1992

70. Keagy BA, Schwartz JA, Johnson G. Should ablative operations be used for bleeding esophageal varices? Ann Surg 203:463–469, 1986

71. Kitano S, Iso Y, Yanaga H, et al. Trial of sclerosing agents in patients with oesophageal varices. Br J Surg 75:751–753, 1988

72. Kitano S, Terblanche J, Kahn D, Bornman PC. Venous anatomy of the lower esophagus in portal hypertension: practical implications. Br J Surg 73:525–531, 1986

73. Klein AS, Cameron JL. Diagnosis and management of the Budd-Chiari Syndrome. Am J Surg 160:128–133, 1990

74. Korula J, Balart LA, Radvan G, et al. A prospective, randomized controlled trial of chronic esophageal variceal sclerotherapy. Hepatology 5:584–589, 1985

75. Langer B, Taylor BR, Mackenzie DR, et al. Further report of a prospective randomized trial comparing distal splenorenal shunt with end-to-side portacaval shunt. Gastroenterology 88:424–429, 1985

76. Langer B, Taylor BR, Greig PD. Selective or total shunts for variceal bleeding. Am J Surg 160:75–79, 1990

77. Lautt WW, Greenway CV. Conceptual view of the hepatic vascular bed. Hepatology 5:952–963, 1987

78. Lebrec D, Nouel O, Corbic M, et al. Propranolol, a medical treatment for portal hypertension? Lancet 2:180–182, 1980

79. Linton RR, Ellis DS. Emergency and definitive treatment of bleeding esophageal varices. JAMA 160:1017–1023, 1956

80. Maffei-Faccioli A, Geruuda GE, Neri D, et al. Selective variceal decompression and its role relative to other therapies. Am J Surg 160:60–66, 1990

81. Mazzaferro V, Todo S, Tzakis AG, Stieber AC, Makowka L, Starzl TE. Liver transplantation in patients with previous portasystemic shunt. Am J Surg 160:111–114, 1990

82. McCormack TT, Rose JD, Smith PM, et al. Perforating veins and blood flow in esophageal varices. Lancet 2:1442–1444, 1983

83. McIndoe AH. Vascular lesions of portal cirrhosis. Arch Pathol 5:23–40, 1928

84. McMichael J. Local vascular changes in splenic anemia. Edinburgh Medical Journal 38:1–29, 1931

85. Millikan WJ, Warren WD, Henderson JM, et al. The Emory prospective randomized trial: selective versus nonselective shunt to control variceal bleeding—ten-year follow-up. Ann Surg 201:712–722, 1985

86. Myberg JA. Selective shunts: the Johannesburg experience. Am J Surg 160:67–74, 1990

87. National Institutes of Health Consensus Development Conference Statement. Liver transplantation. Hepatology 1:107S–110S, 1983

88. Nordlinger BM, Nordlinger DF, Fulenwider JT, et al. Angiography in portal hypertension: clinical significance in surgery. Am J Surg 139:132, 1980

89. Oliver TW, Sones PJ. Hepatic angiography: portal hypertension. In: Bernardino ME, Sones PJ, eds. Hepatic radiology. New York, Macmillan, 1984, pp 243–275

90. Oellerich M, Berdelski M, Lautz HV, et al. Lidocaine metabolite formation as a measure of liver function in patients with cirrhosis. Ther Drug Monit 12:219–226, 1990

91. Orozco H, Mercado HA, Takahashi T, et al. Role of the distal splenorenal shunt in management of variceal bleeding in Latin America. Am J Surg 160:86–89, 1990

92. Palmaz JC, Garcia F, Sibbitt RR, et al. Expandable intrahepatic portacaval shunt in dogs with chronic portal hypertension. AJR 147:125–1254, 1986

93. Paquet KJ. Prophylactic endoscopic sclerosing treatment of the esophageal wall in varices: a prospective controlled trial. Endoscopy 27:213–218, 1982

94. Paquet KJ, Mercado MA, Gad HA. Surgical procedures for bleeding esophagogastric varices when sclerotherapy fails: a prospective study. Am J Surg 160:43–47, 1990

95. Paquet KJ, Feussner H. Endoscopic sclerosis and esophageal balloon tamponade in acute hemorrhage from esophagogastric varices: a prospective controlled randomized trial. Hepatology 5:580–583, 1985

96. Paquet KJ, Oberhammer E. Sclerotherapy of bleeding oesophageal varices by means of endoscopy. Endoscopy 10:7–12, 1978

97. Potts JR III, Henderson JM, Millikan WJ, Sones PJ, Warren WD. Restoration of portal venous perfusion and reversal of encephalopathy by balloon occlusion of portal systemic shunt. Gastroenterology 87:208–212, 1984

98. Raia S, Mies S, Macedo AL. Surgical treatment of portal hypertension in schistosomiasis. World J Surg 8:738–752, 1984

99. Reichle FA, Fahmy WE, Golsorkhi M. Prospective comparative clinical trial with distal splenorenal and mesocaval shunts. Am J Surg 137:13–21, 1979

100. Renner E, Wietholtz H, Hugnenin P, et al. Caffeine: a model compound for measuring liver function. Hepatology 4:38–46, 1984

101. Resnick RH, Chalmers TC, Ishihara AM, et al. A controlled study of the prophylactic portacaval shunt: a final report. Ann Intern Med 70:675–688, 1969

102. Resnick RH, Iber FL, Ishihara AM, et al. A controlled study of the therapeutic portacaval shunt. Gastroenterology 57:843–857, 1974

103. Reynolds TB, Donovan AJ, Mikkelsen WP, et al. Results of a 12-year randomized trial of portacaval shunt in patients with alcoholic liver disease and bleeding varices. Gastroenterology 80:1005–1011, 1981

104. Richards WO, Pearson TC, Henderson JM, Millikan WJ, Warren WD. Evaluation and treatment of early hemorrhage of the alimentary tract after selective shunt procedures. Surg Gynecol Obstet 164:530–536, 1987

105. Richter GM, Noeldge G, Palmaz JC, et al. Transjugular intrahepatic portacaval stent shunt: preliminary clinical results. Radiology 174:1027–1030, 1990

106. Rikkers LF. Is the distal splenorenal shunt better? Hepatology 8:1705–1707, 1988

107. Rikkers LF, Burnett DA, Volentine GD, et al. Shunt surgery versus endoscopic sclerotherapy for long-term treatment of variceal bleeding: early results of a randomized trial. Ann Surg 206:261–271, 1987

108. Rudman D, DiFulco TJ, Galambos JT, et al. Maximal rates of excretion and synthesis of urea in normal and cirrhotic subjects. J Clin Invest 52:2241–2249, 1973

109. Rueff B, Degos F, Prandi D, et al. A controlled study of the therapeutic portacaval shunt in alcoholic cirrhosis. Lancet 1:655–659, 1976

110. Rypins EB, Sarfeh IJ. Small-diameter portacaval H-graft for variceal hemorrhage. Surg Clin North Am 70:395–404, 1990

111. Salam AA, Ezzat FA, Abu-Elmagd KM. Selective shunt in schistosomiasis in Egypt. Am J Surg 160:90–92, 1990

112. Sarfeh IJ, Rypins EB, Mason GR. A systematic appraisal of

portacaval H-graft diameters: clinical and hemodynamic perspectives. Ann Surg 204:356–363, 1986

113. Sarin SK, Nanda R, Vij JC, et al. Oesophageal ulceration after sclerotherapy: a complication or an accompaniment? Endoscopy 18:44, 1986

114. Sauerbruch T. Holl J, Ruckdeschel G, et al. Bacteriaemia associated with endoscopic sclerotherapy of oesophageal varices. Endoscopy 17:170, 1985

115. Shields R. Bleeding esophageal varices and the surgeon. Br J Surg 78:513–515, 1991

116. Smith RB, Warren WD, Salam AA, et al. Dacron interposition shunts for portal hypertension: an analysis of morbidity correlates. Ann Surg 192:9–17, 1980

117. Smith PM. Variceal sclerotherapy: further progress. Gut 28:645–649, 1987

118. Spence RAJ. The venous anatomy of the lower esophagus in normal subjects and in patients with varices: an image analysis study. Br J Surg 71:739–744, 1984

119. Spence RAJ, Johnston GW. Results in 100 consecutive patients with stapled esophageal transection for varices. Surg Gynecol Obstet 160:323–329, 1985

120. Spina GP, Santambrogio R, Opocher E, et al. Distal splenorenal shunt versus endoscopic sclerotherapy in prevention of variceal rebleeding. Ann Surg 211:178–186, 1990

121. Starzl TE, Demetris AJ, Van Thiel DH. Medical progress: liver transplantation. N Engl J Med 321:1014, 1989

122. Sternbeck M, Ring E, Gordon R, et al. Intrahepatic portocaval shunt: a bridge to liver transplantation in patients with refractory variceal bleeding. Gastroenterology 100:A801, 1991

123. Stipa S, Ziparo V, Anza M, et al. A randomized controlled trial of mesenteric caval shunt with autologous jugular vein. Surg Gynecol Obstet 153:353–356, 1981

124. Sugiura M, Futagawa S. Esophageal transection with paraesophagogastric devascularizations (the Sugiura procedure) in the treatment of esophageal varices. World J Surg 8:673–682, 1984

125. Talma S. Chirurgische oeffnung neuer Seitenbahnen fur das Blut der Vena Porta. Klin Wochenschr 35:833–836, 1898

126. Terblanche J. Sclerotherapy for prophylaxis of variceal bleeding. Lancet 1:961–963, 1986

127. Terblanche J. Northover JMA, Bornmann PC, et al. A prospective controlled trial of sclerotherapy in the long-term management of patients after esophageal variceal bleeding. Surg Gynecol Obstet 148:323–333, 1979

128. Terblanche J. Bornmann PC, Kahn D, et al. Failure of repeated injection sclerotherapy to improve long-term survival after oesophageal variceal bleeding: a five year prospective controlled clinical trial. Lancet 2:1328–1332, 1983

129. Teres J, Bordas JM, Bravo D, et al. Sclerotherapy vs distal splenorenal shunt in the elective treatment of variceal hemorrhage: a randomized controlled trial. Hepatology 7:430–436, 1987

130. Teres J, Baroni R, Bordas JM, et al. Randomized trial of portacaval shunt, stapling transection and endoscopic sclerotherapy in uncontrolled variceal bleeding. J Hepatol 4:159–167, 1987

131. Thatcher BS, Sivak MW, Ferguson R, et al. Mesenteric venous thrombosis as a possible complication of endoscopic sclerotherapy: a report of two cases. Am J Gastroenterol 81:126–129, 1988

132. Tygstrup N. The galactose elimination capacity in control subjects and patients with cirrhosis of the liver. Acta Med Scand 175:281, 1964

133. Valla D, Casadevali N, Lacombe C, et al. Primary myeloproliferative disorders and hepatic vein thrombosis: a prospective study of erythroid colony formation in vitro in 20 patients with Budd-Chiari Syndrome. Ann Intern Med 103:329–334, 1985

134. The Veterans Affairs Cooperative Variceal Sclerotherapy Group. Prophylactic sclerotherapy for esophageal varices in men with alcoholic liver disease: a randomized, single blind, multicenter clinical trial. N Engl J Med 324:1779–1784, 1991

135. Vianna A, Hayes PC, Moscoso G, et al. Normal venous circulation of the gastroesophageal junction: a route to understanding varices. Gastroenterology 93:876–889, 1987

136. Vidal E. Traitment chirurgical des ascites. Presse Med 11:747, 1903

137. Vons C, Bourstyn E, Bonnet P, et al. Results of portal systemic shunts in Budd-Chiari syndrome. Ann Surg 203:366–370, 1986

138. Voorhees AB, Chaitman E, Schneider S, et al. Portal systemic encephalopathy in the non-cirrhotic patient: effect of portal systemic shunt. Arch Surg 107:659–663, 1973

139. Warren WD, Millikan WJ, Smith RB, et al. Noncirrhotic portal vein thrombosis: physiology before and after surgery. Ann Surg 192:341, 1980

140. Warren WD, Millikan WJ. Selective transplenic decompression procedure: changes in technique after 300 cases. Contemp Surg 18:11–32, 1981

141. Warren WD, Millikan WJ, Henderson JM, et al. Ten years of portal hypertensive surgery at Emory: results and new perspective. Ann Surg 195:530–542, 1982

142. Warren WD, Henderson JM, Millikan WJ, et al. Management of variceal bleeding in patients with non-cirrhotic portal vein thrombosis. Ann Surg 207:623–634, 1988

143. Warren WD, Zeppa R, Foman JS. Selective transplenic decompression of gastroesophageal varices by distal splenorenal shunt. Ann Surg 166:437, 1967

144. Warren WD, Henderson JM, Millikan WJ, et al. Distal splenorenal shunt versus endoscopic sclerotherapy for long-term management of variceal bleeding. Ann Surg 203:454–462, 1986

145. Webb LJ, Sherlock S. The etiology, presentation and natural history of extrahepatic portal venous obstruction. Q J Med 48:627–639, 1979

146. Westaby D, Macdougall BRD, Melia W, et al. A prospective randomized study of two sclerotherapy techniques for esophageal varices. Hepatology 3:681–684, 1983

147. Westaby D, Melia WM, MacDougall BRD, et al. Injection sclerotherapy for oesophageal varices: a prospective randomized trial of different treatment schedules. Gut 25:129, 1984

148. Westaby D, Macdougall BRD, Williams R. Improved survival following injection sclerotherapy for esophageal varices: final analysis of a controlled trial. Hepatology 5:827–830, 1985

149. Westaby D, Melia W, Hegarty J, et al. Use of propranolol to reduce the rebleeding rate during injection sclerotherapy prior to variceal obliteration. Hepatology 6:673, 1986

150. Westaby D, Hayes PC, Grimson AES, et al. Controlled clinical trial of injection sclerotherapy for active variceal bleeding. Hepatology 9:274–277, 1989

151. Westaby D, Williams R. Status of sclerotherapy for variceal bleeding in 1990. Am J Surg 160:32–37, 1990

152. Whipple AO. The problem of portal hypertension in relation to the hepatosplenopathies. Ann Surg 122:449, 1945

153. Whipple GH, Robscheit-Robbins FS, Hawkins WB. ECK fistula liver is subnormal in producing hemoglobin and plasma proteins on diets rich in liver and iron. J Exp Med 81:171, 1945

154. Witzel L. Wolbergs E, Merki H. Prophylactic endoscopic sclerotherapy of oesophageal varices, Lancet 1:773, 1985

155. Wood RP, Shaw BW, Rikkers LF. Liver transplantation for variceal hemorrhage. Surg Clin North Am 70:449–461, 1990

156. Zeppa R, Hensley GT, Levi JU, et al. The comparative survival of alcoholics versus non-alcoholics after distal splenorenal shunt. Ann Surg 187:510, 1978

Diseases of the Liver, Seventh Edition, edited by Leon Schiff and Eugene R. Schiff. J.B. Lippincott Company, Philadelphia © 1993.

35

Ascites

Bruce A. Runyon

The patient with ascites is a common diagnostic and therapeutic challenge to the internist and gastroenterologist. Cirrhotic ascites is associated with significant morbidity and mortality as a result, in part, of both the severe underlying liver disease and the ascites per se. Half the patients in whom cirrhosis is detected before development of decompensation (ie, before development of ascites, jaundice, encephalopathy, or gastrointestinal hemorrhage) have ascites in 10 years[38] (Fig. 35-1). Once ascites or other evidence of decompensation is present, the expected mortality rate is about 50% in just 2 years[23] (Fig. 35-2). Much information is available on pathogenesis, diagnosis, and treatment of ascites, and this information should improve survival of patients with this condition. In this chapter, much of this information is reviewed.

The word *ascites* is of Greek derivation (*askos*) and refers to a bag or sack. The word is a singular noun that signifies the condition of pathologic fluid accumulation within the abdominal cavity. The adjective *ascitic* is used in conjunction with the word *fluid* to describe the liquid per se.

Diagnosis and Differential Diagnosis

The most common setting in which ascites develops is the patient with known cirrhosis or the patient with a risk factor for development of cirrhosis (eg, alcohol abuse). As jaundice develops or the patient loses muscle mass, or deteriorates in another fashion, the abdomen swells, frequently as body weight increases. In this context, the diagnosis is readily suspected from the patient's history and is confirmed easily by the presence of shifting dullness on physical examination and by a successful abdominal paracentesis. Some patients are less cognizant of their physical appearance and weight; in this setting, when there is not a large volume of fluid, the diagnosis may be suspected first on physical examination. The presence of abdominal fullness and bulging flanks should lead to percussion of the flanks. If the amount of flank dullness is greater than usual (ie, if the percussed air–fluid level is higher than normally found on the lateral aspect of the abdomen with the patient supine), shifting of the dullness should be checked. If there is no flank dullness, there is no reason to check for shifting dullness. About 1500 mL of fluid must be present before dullness is detected.[18] If no flank dullness is present, the patient has less than a 10% chance of having large-volume ascites.[18] Fluid wave and puddle sign were found to be much less helpful in a study of physical findings in patients with small-volume ascites.[18]

A thick panniculus abdominis, gaseous distention of the bowel, and an ovarian mass can be confused with the presence of ascites. An obese abdomen may be diffusely dull to percussion, and an attempt at paracentesis (if there is significant suspicion of ascites) or abdominal ultrasound may be required to settle the question. Ultrasound can detect as little as 100 mL of fluid in the abdomen.[41] Gaseous distention should be apparent on percussion. Ovarian masses characteristically cause tympanitic flanks with central dullness.

Although parenchymal liver disease is the cause of ascites formation in most patients evaluated by internists, about 22% of patients have a cause other than liver disease (Table 35-1). About 5% of patients with ascites have two causes of ascites formation (ie, mixed ascites). Usually these patients have cirrhosis as well as one of the following: peritoneal carcinomatosis, hepatocellular carcinoma, or peritoneal tuberculosis. Because tuberculosis is curable and potentially fatal, one must not assume that a patient has *only* liver disease as the cause of ascites formation, if the clinical situation is atypical. For example, if the ascitic fluid lymphocyte count is unusually high or there is persistent unexplained fever in the setting of cirrhosis, peritoneal tuberculosis may be present. Interpretation of ascitic fluid analysis is difficult in patients with mixed ascites but crucial to appropriate diagnosis and treatment (see section on ascitic fluid analysis). Additionally, not all patients with liver disease and ascites have cirrhosis. Ascites regularly develops along with hepatic coma as a manifestation of acute liver failure in viral hepatitis. Because fulminant liver failure itself is uncommon, however, the total number of ascites patients who have acute liver failure is small. The 80% acute mortality rate in patients with ascites due to acute hepatic failure (unless liver transplantation is performed) is much worse than that observed in patients with ascites due to chronic liver disease. One percent of the large series detailed in Table 35-1 involved fulminant hepatic failure, and 1.5% occurred in the setting of acute hepatitis superimposed on cirrhosis.

Cancer is an uncommon cause (only 12%) of ascites formation as seen by the hepatologist or general internist. Unfortunately, most patients with malignancy-related ascites (except ovarian cancer and lymphoma) survive only a few weeks after onset of fluid retention.[130] If a delay in diagnosis occurs because of confusion about the diagnosis, many of these patients die during the hospitalization for which they presented with ascites. The physician's goal in treating this subgroup of ascites patients should be to make a rapid diagnosis and maximize the time that the patient can spend out of the hospital. Not all malignancy-related ascites is due to peritoneal carcinomatosis; the characteristics of the ascitic fluid and the treatments vary depending on the pathophysiology of ascites formation (eg, peritoneal carcinomatosis versus massive liver

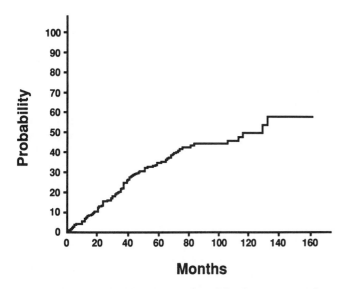

FIGURE 35-1 Cumulative probability of developing ascites after diagnosis of cirrhosis in 293 patients. (Gines P, Quintero E, Arroyo V, et al. Compensated cirrhosis: natural history and prognostic factors. Hepatology 7:125, 1987)

TABLE 35-1 *Causes of Ascites**

Cause	Patients (%)
Parenchymal liver disease	78
Cirrhosis and alcoholic hepatitis	69
Mixed ascites	5
Acute hepatitis with underlying cirrhosis	1.5
Chylous cirrhotic ascites	1.5
Fulminant hepatic failure	1
Malignancy	12
Heart failure	5
Tuberculosis	2
Pancreatic	1
Nephrogenous (dialysis ascites)	0.6
Chlamydia	0.6
Nephrotic	0.6
Surgical peritonitis in the absence of liver disease	0.6

*Based on a series of 1200 paracenteses performed in a predominantly inpatient hepatology–general internal medicine setting.

metastases versus malignant lymph node obstruction chylous ascites[130]; also see section on ascitic fluid analysis).

In 1912, heart failure was the cause of ascites in more than half the patients evaluated.[15] Apparently, improved treatment of heart failure and decreasing prevalence of heart disease have led to its decline to about 5% as a cause of ascites formation. Ascites currently is an uncommon complication of heart disease.[112] Meanwhile, liver disease has increased dramatically as a cause of ascites—from about 10% in 1912 to 78% today.

In the United States, tuberculous peritonitis is a disease of Asian and Latin American immigrants to the West coast and of poor blacks on the East coast. It is a rare disease; many internists have never made the diagnosis. Despite the fact that the series detailed in Table 35-1 was collected largely from the 1200-bed Los Angeles County Hospital (which houses many of these high-risk subgroups of patients), only about six cases of tuberculous peritonitis are diagnosed per year (Runyon BA, unpublished observations, June 1990). Half of these patients are found to have underlying cirrhosis (ie, mixed ascites). Although patients with liver disease are not unusually prone to the hepatotoxicity of antituberculous therapy, they tolerate drug toxicity less well than do patients with normal livers. Therefore, the diagnosis of mixed tuberculous and cirrhotic ascites is unusual but important. Underdiagnosis and lack of antituberculous therapy can lead to unnecessary deaths from uncontrolled tuberculosis, whereas overdiagnosis and overtreatment could lead to unnecessary deaths from the hepatotoxicity of isoniazid.

Pancreatitic ascites develops as a complication of severe acute pancreatitis or as a complication of chronic pancreatitis with pancreatic duct rupture or leakage from a pseudocyst. Patients with this form of ascites also may have underlying cirrhosis. Pancreatic ascites may be complicated by bacterial infection. This combination is frequently misdiagnosed and usually fatal.

Nephrogenous ascites is a poorly understood form of fluid overload that develops in patients undergoing hemodialysis.[70] On careful evaluation, many of these patients are found to have underlying chronic liver disease. The presence of underlying liver disease may be the reason fluid overload develops more readily in them than in dialysis patients who do not have liver disease.

In sexually active, young women with fever and neutrocytic ascites, chlamydia peritonitis should be placed near the top of the differential diagnosis. Chlamydia causes a modern-day Fitz-Hugh-Curtis syndrome.[78] This rapidly responds to doxycycline and is one of the few curable causes of ascites formation.

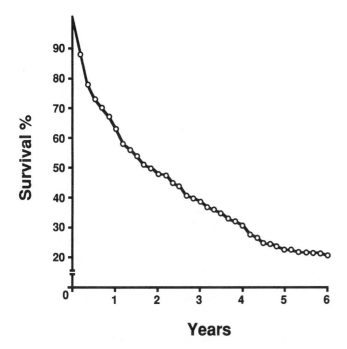

FIGURE 35-2 Survival in a series of 1155 patients with decompensated cirrhosis. (D'Amico G, Morabito A, Pagliaro L, Marubini E. Survival and prognostic indicators in compensated and decompensated cirrhosis. Dig Dis Sci 31:471, 1986)

Although nephrotic syndrome used to be a common cause of ascites formation in children, it is rare in adults, causing less than 1% in the series reported in Table 35-1.

Pathologic accumulations of fluid in the peritoneal cavity of some patients develop due to leakage from a ruptured viscus (eg, bile ascites in the setting of a ruptured gallbladder).[110] The ascitic fluid analysis can be crucial to making a preoperative diagnosis of this condition (see section on ascitic fluid analysis).

Conditions excluded from or not encountered in the series detailed in Table 35-1 include ambulatory peritoneal dialysis fluid, Budd-Chiari syndrome, myxedema ascites, ascites associated with benign ovarian disease, and ascites associated with connective tissue diseases. The iatrogenic form of ascites associated with peritoneal dialysis usually is under the management of nephrologists. Although Budd-Chiari syndrome is regularly (if not always) complicated by ascites, hepatic vein thrombosis itself is rare enough that it causes less than 1% (probably less than 0.1%) of ascites. Ascites in patients with myxedema appears to be cardiac ascites, related to the subtle heart failure that develops in these patients.[5,69] Treatment of the thyroid insufficiency cures the fluid retention. Most ascites that is caused by ovarian disease involves peritoneal carcinomatosis.[130] Meigs' syndrome (ie, ascites and pleural effusion caused by benign ovarian neoplasms) is no longer a common cause of ascites formation; I have never encountered a convincing example of Meigs' syndrome. Serositis with ascites formation may complicate systemic lupus erythematosus.[138]

Pathogenesis

ASCITES FORMATION IN LIVER DISEASE

Simplistically, ascites forms in severe chronic or acute liver disease as a result of portal hypertension, baroreceptor activation, and neurohumorally mediated abnormalities in renal perfusion, with resulting sodium retention. The clinically apparent problem is that of intravascular and extravascular volume overload. The site of spillover of fluid is the peritoneal cavity—because of the portal hypertension.

The questions that have puzzled investigators in this field are (1) what is the *initial* event? and (2) why is there neurohumoral excitation (which should be characteristic of volume depletion) in the setting of volume overload? Animals (including humans) have sophisticated and duplicative systems for detection and preservation of normal or near normal vascular perfusion pressures and intravascular osmolality. The animal's ability to sense abnormalities in intravascular *volume* status (especially volume overload), however, is limited and is linked largely to pressure receptors. This may partially explain the paradox of dramatic volume overload in the face of sympathetic nervous traffic and hormone levels that are indicative of intravascular volume depletion.

All investigators in the field of the pathogenesis of ascites formation agree that patients are intravascularly volume overloaded once they reach the stage of large-volume ascites. The controversy hinges on the initial stimulus for fluid retention. The first proposed theory (ie, the underfill theory) states that the spillover of fluid into the peritoneal cavity is primary and that because of the resulting intravascular hypovolemia, the kidneys retain sodium.[146] Based on this theory, investigators measured blood volume and, to their surprise, it was found to be uniformly high in patients with cirrhosis.[64] The over-

flow theory was proposed, in large part, to explain the hypervolemia detected in cirrhosis. According to this theory, urinary sodium retention is primary and spillover into the peritoneal cavity is a direct result of intravascular hypervolemia.[62]

During the three decades that have passed since these theories were first proposed, data have been published in support of both. Both, in fact, may be partially correct. Both theories apparently assumed that there was only one stage in the formation of ascites. Now we recognize so-called compensated and decompensated stages and that there is a spectrum of renal failure in patients with cirrhosis. Hepatorenal syndrome is the extreme end of the spectrum. The most recent theory, the peripheral arterial vasodilation hypothesis, has proposed that both the underfill and overflow theories of ascites formation are correct but that each is operative at a different stage.[143] The first abnormality that develops *en route* to fluid retention, according to this theory, is peripheral arterial vasodilation. Intravascular underfilling occurs because the compartment enlarges. This theory is based in part on observations in soldiers who were vasodilated due to arteriovenous fistulas.[28] Compression of a fistula was found to increase urinary sodium excretion acutely and dramatically despite stable indices of renal perfusion.[28] This led to the concept that effective distribution of blood rather than total blood volume was important in influencing renal behavior.[28]

The vasodilation hypothesis proposes that in the early compensated stage of cirrhosis (ie, before fluid retention occurs), the intravascular hypervolemia suppresses renin, aldosterone, vasopressin, and norepinephrine concentrations such that abnormally elevated levels of these hormones usually are not detected. Also, these patients usually have normal indices of renal function. The ability of such patients to handle a salt load or to escape from mineralocorticoid administration, however, is not entirely normal.[25] As the state of vasodilation worsens, renal function deteriorates and plasma levels of vasoconstrictor, sodium-retentive hormones increase; ascites develops (ie, decompensation occurs). Hepatorenal syndrome is the extreme end of the spectrum.

Data supporting decreased effective volume have been generated by the technique of head-out water immersion.[29] Redistributing blood volume centrally (ie, to the cardiopulmonary compartment) by immersion in warm water to the neck increases urine sodium excretion in patients with cirrhosis and ascites. The central redistribution of a stable total intravascular volume apparently increases effective volume and improves, at least temporarily, the sodium avid state.

Data supporting the overflow theory have come from studies involving careful attention to the sequence of events leading to sodium retention in a dog model of cirrhosis and ascites.[61] Urine sodium precedes ascites formation in these dogs, confirming the overflow theory.

Intrahepatic portal hypertension plays a crucial role in ascites formation. Ascites rarely develops in patients with prehepatic portal hypertension. Fluid retention develops only in patients with high sinusoidal pressure. Ascites does not develop in patients or dogs with cirrhosis but normal portal pressures due to surgical decompression.[155] A low-pressure hepatic baroreceptor has been demonstrated in dogs; increases in hepatic venous pressure instantaneously increase renal sympathetic nerve activity.[57] In turn, increased renal sympathetic activity causes urine sodium retention.[26]

The site of ascites formation also depends on the presence of portal hypertension. Theoretically, fluid could form from the surface of the liver or the gut; however, the data support the liver as the site of ascites formation. The hepatic sinusoid lacks a basement membrane and is therefore more permeable than the bowel.[42] Lymph flow is related linearly to pressure. The large hydrostatic pressure gradient present in the portal hypertensive liver leads to loss of intravascular fluid across the hepatic sinusoids into the space of Disse, and weeping of the fluid from the liver surface as extravasated lymph. Older animal experiments also confirm the liver as the source of ascites formation. If the liver of a portal hypertensive dog is moved into the chest, the dog develops a pleural effusion rather than ascites.[32] If the liver is placed in a cellophane bag in situ, fluid forms within the bag.[53]

A flurry of papers on atrial natriuretic peptide in the setting of cirrhosis has been published.[37,140] It was hoped that studying this peptide would help in understanding ascites formation and its treatment. The unresponsiveness of patients with cirrhosis and ascites to infusion of synthetic peptide, however, has dampened enthusiasm for the importance of this hormone in the pathogenesis and treatment of ascites.[140]

In summary, in the early phase of ascites formation, there is vasodilation and renal retention of sodium with eventual overflow of fluid into the peritoneal cavity from the hepatic sinusoids. After ascites is formed, underfilling assumes a more prominent role. The sequestration of intravascular fluid in the abdomen in large quantities results in decreased effective intravascular volume and triggers (1) increased nonosmotic secretion of antidiuretic hormone, (2) renin and aldosterone release, (3) further stimulation of sympathetic nervous system activity, and (4) further sodium and water retention. The cycle is self-perpetuating.

ASCITES FORMATION IN OTHER SETTINGS

The mechanism of ascites formation in patients with malignancy-related ascites depends on the location of the tumor. Peritoneal carcinomatosis appears to cause ascites formation by exudation of proteinaceous fluid by tumor cells lining the peritoneum, with entry of extracellular fluid into the peritoneal cavity for reestablishment of oncotic balance.[89] Little information is available on the cause of ascites formation in patients with massive liver metastases.[44,89,130] Presumably stenosis or occlusion of portal veins due to extrinsic compression by tumor nodules or tumor emboli leads to portal hypertension. Ascites then forms because of portal hypertension.[130] In the United States, most patients with hepatocellular carcinoma have underlying portal hypertension; fluid retention does not develop in some of these patients until the tumor becomes relatively large and replaces a significant percentage of the liver parenchyma. Alternatively, in the setting of liver cancer, tumor-induced portal vein thrombosis may contribute to the patient's portal hypertension and predispose to fluid retention. Chylous ascites due to malignancy appears to be caused by lymph node involvement by tumor and rupture of chyle-containing lymphatics.

Ascites forms in high-output and low-output heart failure. In the former condition, decreased peripheral resistance appears to initiate salt and water retention, whereas in the latter situation a diminished cardiac output is the first event.[142] Both of these initial events lead to a decreased effective arterial blood volume and subsequent activation of the vasopressin, renin–aldosterone, and sympathetic nervous systems. In turn, there is renal vasoconstriction and sodium and water retention.[142] Fluid then weeps from the congested hepatic si-

nusoids as lymph, as in cirrhotic ascites. As mentioned, myxedema ascites is cardiac ascites.[69]

As in peritoneal carcinomatosis, tuberculous peritonitis probably causes ascites formation because of exudation of proteinaceous fluid by tubercles lining the peritoneum and entry of extracellular fluid into the peritoneal cavity for reestablishment of oncotic balance. Presumably, coccidiodes (a rare form of inflammatory ascites), chlamydia peritonitis, and some cases of surgical peritonitis result in ascites formation by the same mechanism as with tuberculosis.

Ascites forms in the setting of pancreatitis or biliary leak by leakage of pancreatic juice or bile into the peritoneal cavity or by a chemical burn of the peritoneum. Extracellular fluid then enters to reestablish oncotic equilibrium. The ascitic fluid retains some of the unique characteristics of the source fluid (eg, high amylase concentration), modified to some degree by the added extracellular fluid.

After abdominal surgery, especially extensive retroperitoneal dissection as in distal splenorenal shunt or radical pelvic lymphadenectomy for testicular carcinoma, lymphatics may be transected and leak lymph for variable periods of time.[13,73] The formation of ascites in this condition is similar to that in malignant chylous ascites (ie, lymphatic leak). The presence or absence of chyle in the ascitic fluid depends on where the tear is in the lymphatic system, that is, whether it is in chyle-containing channels or not.

It is postulated that in nephrotic syndrome loss of protein in the urine leads to decreased effective arterial blood volume and activated vasopressin, renin–aldosterone, and sympathetic nervous systems, with resulting renal sodium and water retention.[142]

Patient Evaluation

HISTORY

Most ascites is due to liver disease and most liver disease in the United States is caused by alcohol. Therefore, most patients with ascites abuse alcohol. Ascites frequently develops as a part of the patient's first decompensation of alcoholic liver disease. Ascites can develop early in alcoholic liver disease in the precirrhotic stage of alcoholic hepatitis. Patients often state that the increasing abdominal girth has been noted for only a short time, but the laxity of the abdominal wall and the severity of the liver disease indicate a longer chronology. Patients with alcoholic liver disease who intermittently reduce alcohol consumption may experience wet–dry cycles in terms of fluid retention also. The cycles of ascites may be separated by years of normal sodium balance and tend to parallel alcohol consumption. In contrast, patients with nonalcoholic liver disease in whom ascites develop tend to be persistently fluid overloaded, probably due to the late stage at which ascites forms in nonalcoholic liver disease and the lack of effective therapy other than liver transplantation.

When the patient has a long history of stable cirrhosis and then has ascites, the possibility of hepatocellular carcinoma should be considered as the cause for decompensation. Patients with ascites also should be questioned about risk factors for liver disease other than alcohol (eg, intravenous drug use, homosexuality, transfusions, acupuncture, tattoos, country of origin).

Patients with ascites who have histories of cancer should be suspected of having malignancy-related ascites. Breast, colon, and pancreatic cancer are regularly complicated by ascites.[130] Patients with malignancy-related ascites frequently have abdominal pain, whereas cirrhotic ascites usually is not associated with abdominal pain unless there is superimposed bacterial peritonitis or alcoholic hepatitis.

Patients with cardiac ascites often have histories of heart failure or restrictive lung disease. Alcoholics with ascites may have alcoholic cardiomyopathy or liver disease.

Tuberculous peritonitis usually is manifested by fever and abdominal pain in a patient who has emigrated recently from an endemic area. Half the patients with tuberculous peritonitis have underlying cirrhosis as a second cause for ascites formation.

Patients who have ascites and anasarca in the setting of diabetes should be suspected of having nephrotic ascites. Ascites developing in a patient with cold intolerance, lethargy, altered bowel motility, and change in the skin should prompt measurement of thyroid function. Serositis in connective tissue diseases may be complicated by ascites.[138]

PHYSICAL EXAMINATION

The details of the physical examination in detecting ascites are discussed at the beginning of the chapter. The fluid wave has not been found to be of much value in detection of ascites.[18] The puddle sign can detect 120 mL of fluid, but feeble patients cannot cooperate in the performance of this test; patients must remain in a hands-on-knees position during the examination.

The presence of palmar erythema or large pulsatile vascular spiders is suggestive of the presence of parenchymal liver disease. The presence of pathologically large abdominal wall collateral veins suggests that portal hypertension is present. The presence of large veins on the flanks and dorsum of the patient suggests inferior vena cava blockage by a fibrous caval web or malignant obstruction. A firm nodule in the umbilicus, the Sister Mary Joseph nodule, is suggestive of peritoneal carcinomatosis—usually from a gastric primary. The neck veins of patients with ascites always should be examined for distention in pursuit of a cardiac origin of ascites. Some patients with cardiac ascites have bulging forehead veins that can be seen across the room; some have no visible jugular venous distention. When patients with liver disease have peripheral edema, it usually is in the lower extremities and spares the arms. Nephrotics and patients with cardiac failure may have leg and arm edema (eg, anasarca).

Ascites may be quantified using the following system:

1 +   Detectable only by careful examination
2 +   Easily detected but of relatively small volume
3 +   Obvious ascites but not tense
4 +   Tense ascites

This system works relatively well for patients with chronic ascites and flaccid abdominal wall muscles, but patients with acute onset ascites and good musculature, as in fulminant hepatic failure, may have a tense abdomen without a large volume of fluid.

ABDOMINAL PARACENTESIS

In the past, many physicians avoided diagnostic paracentesis in the evaluation of the patient with ascites, in part because of concern over complications of paracentesis. In view of the documented safety of this procedure and the frequency of ascitic fluid infection, however, paracentesis should be (1) performed as a routine part of the evaluation of new onset ascites, (2) should be repeated as part of the admission physical examination of patients hospitalized with ascites, and (3) should be repeated again during hospitalization if the patient shows any signs or symptoms suggestive of infection.[108]

Choice of Needle Entry Site and Needle

Many physicians have been taught to tap the flank (ie, one of the lower abdominal quadrants); however, both studies that assessed the complications of paracentesis recommended a midline site.[67,108] The midline caudad to the umbilicus is avascular unless there is an unusual collateral vein there, whereas the lower quadrants carry arteries and veins. Puncture of vessels may lead to hematoma formation.

Needles inserted in the midline should be placed *caudad* to the umbilicus. A large collateral frequently is located in the midline *cephalad* to the umbilicus in the setting of portal hypertension; this area should be avoided. The urinary bladder is in the midline, but this structure does not rise above the symphysis pubis in adults unless there are neurologic problems or significant obstruction in the neck of the bladder. Although it is reasonable for the patient to empty the bladder before paracentesis, it is not really necessary. I have entered the bladder only once in more than 1000 paracenteses; it was not problematic. Urologists intentionally sample urine routinely in patients with distended bladders by suprapubic puncture.

Surgical scars pose the most significant problems in selection of a site for needle entry of the abdominal wall. Needles inserted near abdominal wall scars may enter the bowel, which may be adherent to the serosal surface of the abdomen.[108] The needle must be placed several centimeters from the scar. A midline scar precludes midline paracentesis. If a lower quadrant is chosen as the site of paracentesis in this setting, it is necessary to avoid placing the needle near an enlarged liver or spleen and to avoid entering a subcutaneous vessel. Some physicians choose the right lower quadrant to avoid the sigmoid colon or spleen; others choose to tap the left side to avoid the cecum or liver. Neither of these recommendations is supported by data. When a midline site is inappropriate because of scar, I prefer to enter either flank at a site two fingerbreadths cephalad and two fingerbreadths medial to the anterior superior iliac spine. Whichever flank is more dull to percussion is selected as the site for needle entry. This usually requires that the patient be placed in the semirecumbent position, the lateral decubitus position, or the face-down, hands-on-knees position.[108] The hands–knees position is the most clumsy; fortunately, it is required in only 5% of taps.[108] If the patient is too weak to maintain the hands–knees position, it may be necessary to position the patient prone between two beds with the operator approaching the abdomen from below. Ultrasound guidance is required in only 3% of paracenteses—usually in the patient with multiple abdominal scars.[108]

I prefer to use standard metal 1.5-inch needles—22-gauge for diagnostic taps and 18-gauge for therapeutic taps. Spinal needles (ie, 3.5-inch needles) are needed only 6% of the time.[108] Bare steel needles are preferable to plastic-sheathed cannulas because of the risk of the sheath shearing off into the peritoneal cavity and the tendency of the plastic sheath to kink. Metal needles do not puncture bowel unless there is scar or severe gaseous bowel distention. The steel needle can be left in the abdomen during a therapeutic tap for 60 minutes without injury, unless the needle is allowed to drift subcutaneously. Larger-bore needles may speed drainage but leave larger defects if they inadvertently are allowed to enter vessels or the bowel. A multihole disposable needle is needed but is not yet available.

Technique of Diagnostic Paracentesis
The skin is disinfected with an iodine solution. The skin and subcutaneous tissue should be infiltrated with a local anesthetic. Drapes, gown, hat, and mask are optional but sterile gloves should be used when actually obtaining the fluid. The sterile paper package insert in which the gloves are enclosed can be used as a sterile field on which to place syringes, needles, etc. If sterile gloves are not used, there may be a high prevalence of skin contaminants growing from the cultures that are obtained. If fluid could be obtained easily in a few seconds in 100% of patients, sterile gloves might not be needed. It frequently is necessary to disconnect the syringe from the needle and manipulate the needle to obtain fluid, however; this cannot be accomplished in a sterile fashion without use of sterile gloves.

The manner in which the needle is inserted is important in preventing continued leakage of fluid after the needle is withdrawn. Use of a Z-tract minimizes leakage. To create a Z-tract, the operator uses one gloved hand to move the skin about 2 cm caudad in relation to the deep abdominal wall and then inserts the paracentesis needle. The skin is not released until the needle has penetrated the peritoneum and fluid begins to flow. When the needle is removed, the skin slips back into its original position and seals the needle pathway. If the needle is inserted without a Z, the fluid leaks out easily because its pathway is straight. The needle should be advanced slowly in 5-mm increments. If it is inserted in one rapid motion, vessels and bowel may be impaled by the needle. A slow insertion allows the operator to see a flash of blood if a vessel is entered; then the needle can be withdrawn before further damage is done. A slow insertion also allows the bowel to float away from the needle without needle penetration of the bowel. The syringe that is attached to the needle should not be aspirated until the there is fluid visible in the needle hub. If there is continuous suction on the needle insertion, bowel or omentum may be drawn to the end of the needle as soon as the needle enters the peritoneal cavity—giving the appearance of a dry tap. Therefore, the needle should be inserted about 5 mm, then the syringe aspirated for a few seconds while the needle is stationary, then advanced, then aspirated, and so forth until the peritoneum is entered and fluid is aspirated. A slow insertion also allows time for the elastic peritoneum to tent over and be pierced by the needle. Once fluid is flowing, the needle should be stabilized so that its position can be maintained to ensure a steady flow. It is not unusual for flow to stop as bowel or omentum are suctioned over the bevel of the needle. When flow ceases, the syringe is removed from the needle, and the needle is twisted 90 degrees and then inserted in 1- to 2-mm increments until dripping of fluid from the needle hub is achieved. The syringe is then reattached and fluid is aspirated. Occasionally, fluid cannot be aspirated but it drips nicely from the needle hub. In this situation, as in a lumbar puncture, fluid is allowed to drip into a sterile container for collection.

Indications
Abdominal paracentesis is probably the most rapid and cost-effective method of diagnosing the cause of ascites and the only method of detecting ascitic fluid infection. In view of the 10% to 27% prevalence of ascitic fluid infection at the time ascites patients are admitted to the hospital, a surveillance tap may detect unexpected infection at the time of hospitalization.[114] Not all patients with ascitic fluid infection are symptomatic; detection of infection at an early asymptomatic stage may reduce mortality.[86] Therefore, I advocate sampling ascitic fluid in all inpatients and outpatients with *new onset* ascites and in all patients admitted to the hospital with ascites (ie, a tap at the time of each hospitalization). Paracentesis should be *repeated* in outpatients and inpatients in whom signs or symptoms of infection develop. Signs, symptoms, and laboratory test abnormalities suggestive of infection include hypotension, abdominal pain or tenderness, fever, encephalopathy, renal failure, acidosis, and peripheral leukocytosis.

Contraindications
The only prospective study published regarding paracentesis complications in patients with ascites documented no deaths or infections due to the paracentesis per se.[108] Complications included 2 of 229 (0.9%) transfusion-requiring abdominal wall hematomas, and 2 of 229 (0.9%) small hematomas. Seventy-one percent of the patients who underwent paracentesis had an abnormal prothrombin time; 21% had a prothrombin time prolonged by at least 5 seconds.[108] A continuation of this study involving more than 1000 paracenteses has confirmed the safety reported in the initial smaller study and documented no more transfusion-requiring hematomas (Runyon BA, unpublished observations, June 1990).

There are few contraindications to paracentesis. Coagulopathy is a potential contraindication; however, most patients with cirrhotic ascites have coagulopathy. Coagulopathy has precluded me from performing a paracentesis only when there was clinically evident primary fibrinolysis or disseminated intravascular coagulation; these conditions occur less than once per 1000 taps. There is no cutoff of coagulation parameters beyond which paracentesis should not be performed. Even patients with severe prolongation of prothrombin time usually have a trivial ascitic fluid red blood cell (RBC) count after multiple paracenteses. Cirrhotics without clinically obvious coagulopathy do not bleed excessively from needlesticks unless a blood vessel is entered.[108]

It is the policy of some physicians to give prophylactic blood products (fresh frozen plasma or platelets) routinely before paracentesis in cirrhotics with coagulopathy. This practice is not supported by data. Transfusion-requiring hematoma develops in only 0.9% of patients who undergo paracentesis without prophylactic transfusions of plasma or platelets.[108] Therefore, about 50 to 100 units of fresh frozen plasma or platelets would have to be given to prevent transfusion of about 2 units of RBCs. Also, the risk of posttransfusion hepatitis is about 5%; over 50% of patients with cirrhosis die when superimposed hepatitis develops. A 2% to 3% risk of death from hepatitis superimposed on cirrhosis is not an acceptable alternative to a small reduction in risk of paracentesis-related hematoma.

DIFFERENTIAL DIAGNOSIS BY ASCITIC FLUID ANALYSIS

Gross Appearance of the Fluid
Most ascitic fluid is transparent and yellow-tinged. Deeply bile-stained ascitic fluid from jaundiced patients is less bile-

stained than paired serum. Fluid as dark as molasses usually indicates biliary perforation.[110] The opacity of most cloudy ascitic fluid specimens is caused by neutrophils. The presence of particulate matter, such as neutrophils, leads to a shimmering effect when a glass tube of the fluid is held in front of a bright light. Absolute neutrophil counts under 1000/μL may be nearly clear. Counts over 5000/μL are cloudy, and counts over 50,000/μL have a purulent consistency.

Ascitic fluid specimens are occasionally blood-tinged or frankly bloody. An RBC count of 10,000/μL is the threshold for a pink appearance; smaller concentrations result in clear or turbid fluid. Ascitic fluid with an RBC count greater than 20,000/μL is distinctly blood tinged. Many ascitic fluid specimens are bloody because of a traumatic tap in the setting of cirrhosis; these specimens are heterogeneously bloody and clot. In contrast, nontraumatic or remotely traumatic bloody ascitic fluid is homogenously pigmented and does not clot because it has already clotted and lysed. Some patients with portal hypertension have bloody hepatic lymph leading to bloody ascitic fluid, perhaps because of rupture of high-pressure lymphatics. Half the samples from patients with hepatocellular carcinoma that I have encountered are bloody, but only about 10% of samples from patients with peritoneal carcinomatosis have this appearance.[108] Overall, only 22% of malignancy-related samples (including primary liver cancer) are bloody.[108] Although many physicians are of the opinion that tuberculosis results in bloody ascites, less than 5% of tuberculosis samples are hemorrhagic in my experience.

There is a spectrum of milkiness in ascitic fluid, ranging from slightly cloudy, opalescent fluid, to completely opaque chylous fluid. The most opaque milky fluid has a triglyceride concentration of over 200 mg/dL, usually over 1000 mg/dL. Fluids that look like dilute skim milk usually have a concentration between 100 and 200 mg/dL. A substantial minority of cirrhotic ascitic fluid samples are not transparent but not frankly milky. In this condition, which I label *opalescent* ascitic fluid, the cloudiness of the fluid has been found to be caused by a slightly elevated triglyceride concentration—50 to 200 mg/dL.[120] The lipid usually layers out in the refrigerator over a 48- to 72-hour interval.

Pancreatic ascites may appear tea-colored, due to the effect of pancreatic enzymes on ascitic fluid RBCs. Such fluid may have to be centrifuged to spin the RBCs down and reveal the discolored supernatant. In hemorrhagic pancreatitis, the fluid may be so darkly pigmented that it appears black. Malignant melanoma also can result in black ascites.

Ascitic Fluid Tests

Some physicians order every test that they can think of when analyzing ascitic fluid. This practice can be expensive and can be more confusing than helpful, especially when unexpectedly abnormal results are encountered. The price tag on ordering all routine tests is in excess of $500. An algorithm approach to ascitic fluid analysis is more appropriate. Screening tests are performed on the initial specimen, and additional testing is performed (usually necessitating another paracentesis) based on the results of the screening tests. Most specimens consist of uncomplicated cirrhotic ascites. Usually, no further testing is needed in this setting.

Based on cost analysis, I have developed a list of routine, optional, unusual, and unhelpful tests (Table 35-2). The strategy used in this algorithm is discussed below.

TABLE 35-2   *Ascitic Fluid Laboratory Data to Be Obtained on Patients With Ascites*

Routine
Cell count
Albumin
Culture in blood culture bottles

Optional
Total protein
Glucose
Lactate dehydrogenase
Amylase
Gram stain

Unusual
Tuberculosis smear and culture
Cytology
Triglyceride
Bilirubin

Unhelpful
pH
Lactate
Cholesterol
Fibronectin

Cell Count.   The cell count is the single most helpful ascitic fluid test. If only one drop of fluid is obtained, it should be sent for cell count. Only a few microliters are required for a standard manual hemocytometer count. The fluid should be submitted in an anticoagulant tube (ie, EDTA) to prevent clotting. Because the decision to begin empiric antibiotic treatment of suspected ascitic fluid infection is based largely on the rapidly available absolute neutrophil count rather than the not so rapidly available culture, the cell count is more important than the culture in the early approach to these patients with regard to ascitic fluid infection.

The mean total white blood cell (WBC) count in uncomplicated cirrhotic ascites is reported to be 281 ± 25 cells/μL; the upper limit is said to be 500 cells/μL.[6] During diuresis in patients with cirrhosis and ascites, however, the cells exit the peritoneal cavity more slowly than the fluid and the mean ascitic fluid WBC count has been shown to increase to over 1000 cells/μL.[48] I have encountered several examples of end-of-diuresis WBC counts of over 3000/μL and one example of 7000/μL. Before a patient can be diagnosed as having a diuresis-related elevation of ascitic fluid WBC count, however, three criteria must be fulfilled: (1) a prediuresis count must be available and must be normal, (2) there must be a predominance of lymphocytes, and (3) there must be no unexplained clinical signs or symptoms (eg, fever or abdominal pain).

The mean percentage of polymorphonuclear cells (PMNs) in uncomplicated cirrhotic ascites is 27% ± 2%.[6] The upper limit absolute PMN count in uncomplicated cirrhotic ascitic fluid usually is stated to be 250/μL.[6] Fortunately, the short life expectancy (hours) of PMNs results in relative stability in the absolute PMN count during diuresis (42 to 68 cells/μL from the beginning to end, difference not significant).[48] Therefore, the 250-cell/μL cutoff pertains even at the end of diuresis.

infection and cirrhosis. If the ascitic fluid glucose is unusually low in a patient with neutrocytic ascites, measurement of a serum glucose may explain the ascitic fluid hypoglycemia and lead to potentially life-saving emergency administration of glucose intravenously. Measurement of serum bilirubin or triglyceride concentration may be of value in comparison with their ascitic fluid concentrations. Measurement of serum α-fetoprotein concentration (which is always higher in serum than in ascitic fluid) may be of value in detecting hepatocellular carcinoma as the explanation for clinical deterioration of a patient with known cirrhosis.[130]

Complications

INFECTION

Ascitic fluid infection can be classified into five categories based on culture, PMN count, and presence or absence of a surgical source of infection:

- Spontaneous ascitic fluid infection
  - SBP
  - Monomicrobial nonneutrocytic bacterascites
  - Culture-negative neutrocytic ascites
- Secondary bacterial peritonitis
  - Gut perforation
  - Nonperforation
  - Polymicrobial bacterascites

An abdominal paracentesis must be performed and ascitic fluid must be analyzed before a confident diagnosis of ascitic infection can be made. A clinical diagnosis of infected ascitic fluid without a paracentesis is not enough.

Definitions

Of the three types of spontaneous ascitic fluid infection, the prototype form is SBP. This diagnosis is made when there is a positive ascitic fluid culture (essentially always a monomicrobial infection) and there is an elevated ascitic fluid absolute PMN count (ie, at least 250 cells/μL), without an evident intraabdominal source of infection that requires surgical treatment.[52] When Harold Conn coined the phrase *spontaneous bacterial peritonitis* in 1975, his goal was to distinguish this form of infection from surgical peritonitis.[21] I agree with the importance of this distinction. Therefore, although many patients with SBP have a focus of infection (eg, urinary tract infection or pneumonia), they are labeled SBP unless the focus requires surgical intervention, as in ruptured viscus.

The criteria for a diagnosis of monomicrobial nonneutrocytic bacterascites (MNB) include a positive ascitic fluid culture for a single organism, an ascitic fluid PMN count of less than 250 cells/μL, and no evident intraabdominal source of infection that requires surgical treatment.[115] The adjective *monomicrobial* is used to distinguish this form of ascitic fluid infection from polymicrobial bacterascites (see later discussion). In the older literature, this condition was either grouped with SBP or called *asymptomatic bacterascites*.[20] Because many patients with bacterascites have symptoms, the modifier *asymptomatic* does not seem appropriate.[115] The absence of PMNs in this variant has implications for prognosis as well as for understanding the pathogenesis and natural history of ascitic fluid infection (see later discussion).

Culture-negative neutrocytic ascites (CNNA) is diagnosed when (1) the ascitic fluid culture grows no bacteria, (2) the ascitic fluid PMN count is at least 250 cells/μL, (3) no antibiotics have been given (even a single dose usually makes the culture negative), and (4) there is no other explanation for an elevated PMN count (eg, hemorrhage into ascites, peritoneal carcinomatosis, tuberculosis, or pancreatitis).[126] This variant of ascitic fluid infection seldom is diagnosed when sensitive culture methods are used.[122,136]

Secondary bacterial peritonitis is diagnosed when (1) the ascitic fluid culture is positive (usually for multiple organisms), (2) the PMN count is at least 250 cells/μL, and (3) there is an identified intraabdominal surgically treatable primary source of infection (eg, perforated gut, perinephric abscess).[1,125] The importance of distinguishing this variant from SBP is that secondary peritonitis usually is treated with antibiotics *and* surgery, whereas SBP essentially always is treated *only* with antibiotics.[1] Performing a laparotomy in the setting of SBP or treating secondary peritonitis with antibiotics and no surgical intervention usually results in the death of the patient.

Polymicrobial bacterascites is diagnosed when (1) multiple organisms are cultured from ascitic fluid and (2) the PMN count is less than 250 cells/μL.[123] This diagnosis should be suspected when (1) the paracentesis is difficult because of ileus or is traumatic, (2) stool or air are aspirated into the paracentesis syringe, and (3) multiple organisms but no PMNs are seen on Gram stain. Polymicrobial bacterascites essentially is diagnostic of inadvertent gut perforation by the paracentesis needle.

Setting

For all practical purposes, the spontaneous variants of ascitic fluid infection (ie, SBP, CNNA, and MNB) occur only in the setting of severe liver disease. Spontaneous infection of noncirrhotic ascites is rare enough to be the subject of case reports.[58,102,160] Ninety-five percent of patients with SBP have an elevated serum bilirubin and 98% have an abnormal prothrombin time.[52] Radionuclide liver–spleen scan demonstrates marked colloid redistribution, indicating shunting of portal blood away from reticuloendothelial cells. The liver disease usually is chronic, as in cirrhosis, but may be acute, as in fulminant hepatic failure, or subacute, as in alcoholic hepatitis. SBP is most common in alcoholic cirrhosis, but that is probably because alcoholic cirrhosis is the most common cause of ascites formation in the United States. All forms of cirrhosis have been reported to be complicated by spontaneous ascitic fluid infection. Ascites is a prerequisite to development of SBP; fluid almost always is clinically detectable at the time of infection. It is unlikely that SBP precedes the development of ascites. Usually, this infection develops at the time of maximum ascites volume. Although nephrotic ascites regularly was complicated by SBP in the preantibiotic era, use of diuretics and antibiotics have made SBP uncommon in this setting.

About half of SBP episodes are detected at the time of admission to the hospital; the remainder develop during hospitalization.[52] Some retrospective studies have collected data in the absence of an admission surveillance paracentesis and then reported that most cases developed during hospitalization. If admission paracenteses had been routine in these studies, more episodes probably would have been detected on admission.

Secondary bacterial peritonitis and polymicrobial bacterascites can develop in ascites of any type. The only prerequisite, in addition to the presence of ascites, for development of the former infection is the presence of a surgical source of infection (eg, ruptured viscus or perinephric abscess).[1] The latter infection occurs due to needle entry of the bowel during attempted paracentesis.[123]

Pathogenesis

In 1975, Harold Conn used the adjective *spontaneous* in describing bacterial peritonitis in the ascites patient to indicate that the infection appeared from nowhere. During the past 5 years, the pathogenesis and natural history of the spontaneous forms of ascitic fluid infection have become more clear (Fig. 35-4). The enteric nature of most organisms that cause these infections implicates the gut as their source.[52] The pneumococcus is the only frequently isolated organism that does not reside in the gut. The body of available evidence suggests that SBP, CNNA, and MNB are probably the result of colonization of susceptible ascitic fluid as a result of spontaneous bacteremia (see Fig. 35-4). Although direct transmural migration of bacteria from the gut into ascites has been postulated as a route of colonization of ascitic fluid, this has been documented in humans only after loss of gut mucosal integrity and in an animal model only after irritation of the visceral peritoneum.[105,144] If organisms could easily traverse the gut wall and directly enter the fluid, polymicrobial infections would be the rule rather than the exception, and the flora of spontaneous ascitic fluid infections would be more representative of the flora of the gut. Although *Escherichia coli* and *Klebsiella pneumoniae* are present in the gut, they are outnumbered by two to four orders of magnitude by anaerobes and enterococci. Yet anaerobes and enterococci seldom cause spontaneous ascitic fluid infection.[52]

Monomicrobial infections imply that the source of the infection also is monomicrobial, or that there is a filter mechanism or a series of filters between a polymicrobial source, such as the gut, and the ascitic fluid. Studies in rodents have demonstrated that under certain circumstances bacteria can translocate from the gut lumen across the mucosa into submucosal lymphatics and be detected in mesenteric lymph nodes.[9] Circumstances that promote translocation include bacterial overgrowth in the gut, chemotherapy-induced immunodeficiency, thermal burn, and hemorrhagic shock.[8] Translocation may explain how bacteria access the bloodstream in shock, leukemia, thermal burn, and multiple trauma.[24] Patients with cirrhosis have altered gut flora, which would promote translocation.[68] The inability of anaerobes to translocate also is of interest.[8] The presence of gram-negative bacteria-derived endotoxin in the peripheral blood of cirrhotic patients also lends credence to the likelihood of translocation in this setting.[66]

Perhaps the gut mucosa is abnormally permeable in the setting of cirrhosis, leading to promotion of translocation of bacteria from the gut to mesenteric lymph nodes and on to peripheral blood (see Fig. 35-4). Bacteremia is common in patients with severe liver disease.[43] More than 50% of patients with SBP have bacteremia documented at the time of diagnosis of peritoneal infection.[52] The flora of spontaneous bacteremia is similar to that of SBP and MNB and also is monomicrobial.[43,52]

Complement is synthesized in the liver, and cirrhotic patients with severe enough liver disease to develop ascites usually have serum complement deficiency.[134] Neutrophil dysfunction and reticuloendothelial system dysfunction also are common in cirrhosis.[91,99] These defects in host defense against infection would be expected to lead to frequent

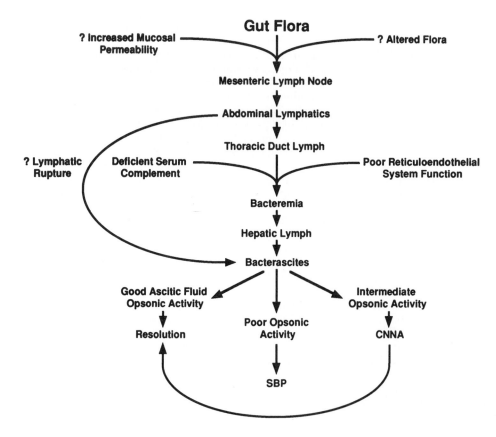

FIGURE 35-4 Pathogenesis of spontaneous ascitic fluid infection.

and prolonged bacteremia. Cirrhotic rats with ascites have been shown uniformly to develop bacteremia after intratracheal exposure to pneumococci; these rats also have more prolonged bacteremia and more fatalities compared with cirrhotic rats without ascites and compared with normal rats.[72]

Alternatively, spontaneous ascitic fluid infection could be a result of translocation of bacteria from the gut into mesenteric lymphatics with rupture of the high-pressure lymphatics and direct leakage of bacteria-laden lymph into the ascitic fluid.[27] Intraabdominal lymphatic rupture is not uncommon, as evidenced by the frequency of chylous and lipid-laden ascitic fluid in the setting of portal hypertension.[92,120] If direct lymphatic rupture is the source of ascitic fluid bacteria, bacteremia would be secondary to thoracic duct contamination with peritoneal bacteria.

In summary, there is circumstantial evidence favoring the gut as the source of most of the bacteria that cause spontaneous ascitic fluid infection. Translocation of bacteria from the gut to the mesenteric lymphatics of normal rodents is common under certain circumstances.[8,9,24] Perhaps it is more common in the setting of cirrhosis. Seeding of ascitic fluid with gut-derived bacteria could then be the result of at least two possible bacterial routes (see Fig. 35-4). Mesenteric lymphatic bacteria could (1) pass through lymph nodes, on to the thoracic duct, bloodstream and then leak across the sinusoids of the liver as ascites forms from the blood, or (2) directly leak into ascitic fluid due to intraabdominal lymphatic rupture.

Once bacteria enter the fluid in the abdomen, by whatever route, a battle ensues between the organism's virulence factors and the host's immune defenses. Several studies shed some light on the events that take place in this battle.[107,113,115,128,134] The protein concentration does not change with development of spontaneous infection.[128] Low-protein concentration ascitic fluid (eg, less than 1 g/dL) has been shown to be particularly prone to SBP.[107] The opsonic activity (endogenous antimicrobial activity) of human ascitic fluid correlates directly with the fluid's protein concentration.[134] Patients with deficient ascitic fluid opsonic activity have been shown to be predisposed to SBP.[113] Patients with detectable ascitic fluid opsonic activity are protected from SBP unless a particularly virulent organism (eg, *Salmonella* sp) is involved.[113,160]

Studies in both humans with cirrhosis and rats with experimental cirrhosis demonstrate that MNB is common.[115,135] In both humans and rats, most episodes (up to 62%) of bacterascites resolve without antibiotic treatment.[115,135] The fluid frequently becomes sterile without an evident PMN response. Apparently the host defense mechanisms are able to eradicate the invading bacteria on most occasions. Perhaps it is only when the defenses are particularly weak or the organism is particularly virulent that uncontrolled fatal infection develops. The patients with clinically apparent ascitic fluid infection may represent only the "tip of the iceberg." Bacterascites probably is much more common than SBP. Only frequent surveillance paracenteses would settle this question. Perhaps patients with cirrhotic ascites regularly have their ascitic fluid colonized by bacteria, and almost just as regularly, the colonization resolves in these patients. The entry of PMNs into the fluid probably signals failure of opsonins in combination with peritoneal macrophages to control the infection. As a rule, MNB resolves spontaneously in rats and humans, whereas SBP frequently is fatal.[115,135] In summary, MNB probably represents an early stage of ascitic fluid infection that can resolve to sterile non-neutrocytic ascites or progress to SBP.

Most episodes of CNNA are diagnosed using insensitive culture methods where there are insufficient numbers of bacteria to reach the threshold of detectability.[122,136] Blood culture bottles can detect a single organism in the cultured aliquot of fluid, whereas the conventional method of culture probably requires at least 100 organisms per milliliter[122] (Table 35-4). Even when optimal culture methods are used, however, no bacteria grow in the neutrocytic ascitic fluid of a small percentage of patients.[122] A study of rapid sequential paracenteses (before initiation of antibiotic treatment) in patients with CNNA demonstrated that in most cases the PMN count dropped spontaneously and the culture remained negative.[118] In the setting of sensitive culture technique, CNNA probably represents spontaneously resolving SBP in which the tap is performed after all bacteria have been killed by host defenses but before the PMN count has normalized.

The pathogenesis of secondary bacterial peritonitis is no mystery compared with the pathogenesis of SBP. When the gut perforates into the ascitic fluid, billions of bacteria flood in. When there is secondary peritonitis without a frank perforation (eg, a perinephric abscess or empyema of the gallbladder), bacteria cross inflamed tissue planes and enter ascites.

The pathogenesis of polymicrobial bacterascites also is apparent.[123] The paracentesis needle enters the bowel and bowel contents are released. Fortunately, this event is rare. Even when needle puncture occurs, it usually resolves without antibiotic therapy, especially in high-protein ascites.[123]

Signs and Symptoms

Although 87% of SBP patients reported in 1990 were symptomatic at the time of diagnosis of infection, the symptoms or signs of infection may be subtle or misinterpreted.[115] Minor changes in mental status that would be detected only by family members or a physician who is extremely familiar with the patient, may be the sole clinical evidence of infection. Unless such changes prompt paracentesis, the diagnosis and treatment of the ascitic fluid infection may be delayed. Delays in initiation of therapy usually result in a fatal outcome. The signs and symptoms manifested in all five variants of ascitic fluid infection are listed in Table 35-5.

It is of interest to compare these clinical parameters in patients with SBP reported in 1985 with those reported in

TABLE 35-4 *Quantitation of Ascitic Fluid Bacteria*

Colony Count (organisms/mL)	Episodes (%)
>10,000	7
1000–10,000	11
100–1000	11
10–100	7
1–10	21
<1	43
<10	64
≤1	54

(Data from Runyon BA, Canawati HN, Akriviadis EA. Optimization of ascitic fluid culture technique. Gastroenterology 95:1351, 1988)

TABLE 35-5 *Signs and Symptoms of Ascitic Fluid Infection**

	SBP	MNB	CNNA	2BP	PMB
Fever	68	57	50	33	10
Abdominal pain	49	32	72	67	10
Tender abdomen	39	32	44	50	10
Rebound	10	5	0	17	0
Decreased bowel sounds	12	2	28	83	0
Mental status	54	50	61	33	0

SBP, spontaneous bacterial peritonitis; MNB, monomicrobial nonneutrocytic bacterascites; CNNA, culture-negative neutrocytic ascites; 2BP, secondary bacterial peritonitis; PMB, polymicrobial bacterascites.
*Data presented as percentage of the total number of patients in that group.
(Data from Runyon and Hoefs,[125,126] Runyon,[115] and Runyon and colleagues[123])

TABLE 35-6 *Prevalence of the Variants of Ascitic Fluid Infection at the Time of Hospital Admission*

Subtype	Prevalence (%)
SBP	6–11
MNB	2–7
CNNA	2–7
PMB	~0.1
2BP	0–2
Total infected on admission	10–27

SBP, spontaneous bacterial peritonitis; MNB, monomicrobial nonneutrocytic bacterascites; CNNA, culture-negative neutrocytic ascites; PMB, polymicrobial bacterascites; 2BP, secondary bacterial peritonitis.
(Data from Pinzello and colleagues,[86] Hoefs and Runyon,[52] Runyon,[107,115] Akriviadis and Runyon BA,[1] Runyon and Hoefs,[126] and Runyon and associates[123])

1990.[52,115] Some symptoms are less frequently present now. For example, the prevalence of abdominal pain and tenderness appears to be less frequent in recent years. Rebound tenderness and ileus have markedly decreased from about 50% to about 10%, whereas fever and mental status change have remained relatively stable. These differences in clinical evidence of infection indicate that the infection is being diagnosed earlier in recent years. Earlier treatment may explain the lower recent mortality, as is discussed later.

Prevalence

Before the 1980s, abdominal paracentesis was not performed regularly because of fear of complications of the procedure and because the utility of ascitic fluid analysis in the differential diagnosis of ascites was not fully recognized. Now that the complication rate is known to be under 1% and the serum–ascites albumin gradient has increased the diagnostic accuracy of ascitic fluid analysis, routine paracentesis is performed at the time of admission of many ascites patients.[49,83,93,108,127,133] Routine admission paracenteses have provided data on the prevalence of ascitic fluid infection; 10% to 27% of ascites patients (whether or not they have symptoms of infection) are found to have SBP or a variant thereof on admission.[86,107] Overall, about 10% of ascites patients are infected at the time of admission; of the subgroup of patients with cirrhotic ascites, about 27% are infected. The prevalence of the subtypes of ascitic fluid infection is listed in Table 35-6. Of patients with culture-positive ascitic fluid, about two thirds have neutrocytic ascitic fluid (ie, SBP) and one third have MNB.[115] The prevalence of CNNA among series of neutrocytic ascitic fluid depends largely on culture technique.[122,126,136] Polymicrobial bacterascites is present in only about 1 per 1000 patients.[123] Secondary bacterial peritonitis occurs in only 0% to 2% of ascites patients at the time of admission to the hospital.[86] About 15% of patients whose signs and symptoms initially resemble SBP are shown to have secondary peritonitis; too often this diagnosis is made at autopsy.[1]

No studies of the frequency of SBP in outpatients have been published. SBP or a variant may be a common cause of death of cirrhotic patients who die at home.

Flora

E coli streptococci (mostly pneumococci) and *Klebsiella* sp cause most episodes of SBP and MNB (Table 35-7). CNNA is by definition culture-negative. Polymicrobial bacterascites is by definition polymicrobial. The most apparent difference between the spontaneous forms of ascitic fluid infection and the nonspontaneous forms is that the former nearly always are monomicrobial and the latter usually are polymicrobial. Although older papers report that about 6% of SBP cases were caused by anaerobes, this is probably a reflection of the presence of unrecognized secondary bacterial peritonitis cases in series of purported SBP cases.[152] The high prevalence of polymicrobial infection among episodes of anaerobic "SBP" further support the contention that these represent misdiagnosed secondary peritonitis.[152] Anaerobes cause about 1% of cases of SBP.[115,122,136] The infrequency of anaerobic SBP probably is due to the relatively high pO$_2$ of ascites and the inability of anaerobes to translocate across the gut mucosa.[8,145] The prevalence of pneumococcal SBP appears to be increasing; as of 1988, 25% of SBP cases were caused by this organism compared with an aggregate average of 8% in seven older series.[52,122] This may reflect the fragility of this organism and the improvements in culture methods. Fungi do not cause SBP. Fungal infection of ascitic fluid occurs only in the setting of disseminated systemic mycosis in the immunosuppressed patient, or in secondary peritonitis with gut release of fungi into ascitic fluid.[1,122]

One series of patients with MNB reported a predominance of gram-positive organisms,[86] whereas a larger series reported flora similar to that of SBP.[115] Gram-negative organisms do not colonize the skin, and must be interpreted as pathogens, whereas gram-positives are routine skin flora and must be considered contaminants in the absence of a PMN response. *Staphylococcus epidermidis* cannot be interpreted as a pathogen in ascitic fluid unless there is a foreign body (eg, peritoneovenous shunt) present. α-Hemolytic streptococcus also should be considered a skin contaminant, unless there is a PMN response or bacteremia with the same organism. Failure to use sterile technique when performing a paracentesis or failure to sterilize the blood culture bottle tops with iodine before inoculation increases the presence of contaminants in the cultures.

TABLE 35-7 *Flora of Ascitic Fluid Infection**

Organism	SBP	MNB	CNNA	PMB	2BP
Monomicrobial					
Escherichia coli	37	27	0	0	20
Klebsiella pneumoniae	17	11	0	0	7
Pneumococcus	12	9	0	0	0
Streptococcus viridans	9	2	0	0	0
Staphylococcus aureus	0	7	0	0	13
Miscellaneous gram-negative	10	14	0	0	7
Miscellaneous gram-positive	14	30	0	0	0
Polymicrobial	1	0	0	100	53

SBP, spontaneous bacterial peritonitis; MNB, monomicrobial nonneutrocytic bacterascites; CNNA, culture-negative neutrocytic ascites; PMB, polymicrobial bacterascites; 2BP, secondary bacterial peritonitis.
*Data reported as percentages of total in that group.
(Data from Akriviadis and Runyon,[1] Runyon,[115] Runyon and Hoefs,[126] and Runyon and colleagues[123])

Risk Factors

Patients with cirrhosis are unusually prone to bacterial infections because of multiple defects in immune defense (see section on pathogenesis). This concept is rather new and is only beginning to be widely appreciated. In a prospective study performed in Barcelona, 46% of 187 consecutive cirrhotic patients had bacterial infection (ranging from asymptomatic urinary tract infections to fatal sepsis) at the time of admission to the hospital, or contracted infection during hospitalization.[99] Thirty-five percent of 87 women with primary biliary cirrhosis contracted bacteriuria (70% *E coli*, 7% *Klebsiella* sp, 6% *Streptococcus* sp) during a 12-month period.[14]

The low-protein (opsonin-deficient) ascitic fluid risk factor was discussed earlier. The colloid redistribution of the liver–spleen scan is indicative of these patients' inability to rapidly remove particulate matter from the blood; this phenomenon would be expected to result in frequent and prolonged bacteremia.[99] Marked colloid redistribution has been demonstrated to be a risk factor for SBP and spontaneous bacteremia.[99]

Some physicians have been taught that paracentesis itself poses a significant risk of causing ascitic fluid infection. This theoretical risk was not substantiated in the only published prospective study of paracentesis complications; no instances of needle-induced ascitic fluid infection were reported.[108] In this study, SBP was statistically more likely to be diagnosed at the time of the first paracentesis compared with subsequent taps.[108] The most likely setting in which to expect iatrogenic peritonitis is when the paracentesis needle enters the bowel inadvertently during attempted paracentesis. Fortunately, this is unusual (see section on prevalence). Skin flora (eg, *Staphylococcus aureus*) would be expected to be isolated if poor paracentesis technique were the cause of many cases of SBP, yet skin flora seldom are isolated.[115,122]

Gastrointestinal hemorrhage is temporally associated with development of spontaneous bacteremia and SBP.[98,106] This has not been clearly demonstrated to be a cause-and-effect relation, but circumstantial evidence supports the possibility. Experimental animals have prolonged bacteremia when inoculated with bacteria at the time of bloodletting, suggesting an acute deterioration in reticuloendothelial system function due to hemorrhage.[3,82,97] Also, invasive procedures performed in relation to gastrointestinal bleeding (eg, endoscopy,

intravascular catheter placement) also may predispose to bacteremia.

Diagnosis

An accurate and timely diagnosis of ascitic fluid infection requires a low threshold for performing a paracentesis and a high index of suspicion for infection. Clinical deterioration in a patient with ascites always should raise the suspicion, especially if there is fever or abdominal pain. If the ascitic fluid PMN is elevated, the working diagnosis is ascitic fluid infection until proven otherwise. Although peritoneal carcinomatosis, pancreatitis, hemorrhage into ascites, pancreatitis, and tuberculosis can lead to an elevated ascitic fluid PMN count, most cases of neutrocytic ascitic fluid are due to infection. A majority of PMNs in the WBC differential lends further credence to the diagnosis of infection. An elevated absolute ascitic fluid PMN count with a predominance of neutrophils in a clinical setting compatible with infection (eg, febrile cirrhotic patient) should prompt empiric antibiotic therapy (see later discussion).

Once the presumptive diagnosis of ascitic fluid infection is made, the next consideration should be: is there a surgically treatable source of infection? Secondary peritonitis should be *considered* in any patient with neutrocytic ascites. Because of the rarity of SBP in peritoneal carcinomatosis or cardiac ascites, however, a surgical source of peritonitis should be *presumed* in these conditions until proven otherwise. Surprisingly, even with free perforation of the colon into ascitic fluid, a classic surgical abdomen does not develop.[1] Peritoneal signs require contact of inflamed visceral and parietal peritoneal surfaces. This does not happen when there is a large volume of fluid present. Therefore, clinical signs and symptoms do not separate patients with secondary peritonitis from those with SBP.[1] Gut perforation can be suspected and pursued if neutrocytic ascitic fluid analysis meets two of the following three criteria (see Fig. 35-2): total protein greater than 1 g/dL, glucose less than 50 mg/dL, and LDH greater than 225 mU/mL (or above the upper limit of normal for serum).[1,125] Except for gallbladder rupture, essentially all ascitic fluids culture multiple organisms in the setting of a perforated viscus.[1] If multiple organisms and PMNs are seen on Gram stain, the likelihood of perforation is high. Brown ascitic fluid with a bilirubin concentration greater than 6 mg/

dL (and greater than the serum level) is indicative of biliary or upper gut perforation into ascites.[110]

The initial ascitic fluid analysis is helpful in delineating which patients are likely to have a ruptured viscus (see Fig. 35-3). These patients need an emergent (within minutes) radiologic evaluation to confirm and localize the site of rupture. Older patients should have a water-soluble contrast enema first to rule out perforated colonic diverticulum; younger patients, who are more likely to have a perforated duodenal ulcer, should have a water-soluble upper gastrointestinal contrast study first.[1] If perforation is documented, emergency intervention is mandatory to maximize survival; survivors have been reported. Antibiotic therapy without surgical intervention in the treatment of a ruptured viscus is predictably unsuccessful.

Patients with *nonperforation* secondary peritonitis tend *not* to have a diagnostic *initial* ascitic fluid analysis.[1,125] Fortunately, it is less urgent to make the diagnosis of secondary peritonitis in nonperforation peritonitis compared with perforation peritonitis. Therefore, there may be time to evaluate the response of the ascitic fluid culture and PMN count to treatment. These parameters have been shown to be helpful in distinguishing secondary from spontaneous peritonitis.[1,125] The best time to perform a single repeat paracentesis to assess response is after 48 hours of treatment; by 48 hours, essentially every SBP patient who has been treated with an appropriate antibiotic has a PMN count lower than the pretreatment value and a negative culture.[1] Before 48 hours of treatment (ie, at 12 or 24 hours), the PMN count may be higher than baseline even in SBP. Also, the culture remains positive in secondary peritonitis and becomes rapidly negative in SBP (see Fig. 35-3).[1,125]

Treatment

Patients with ascitic fluid PMN counts of at least 250 cells/μL in a clinical setting compatible with ascitic fluid infection should receive empiric antibiotics.[114] Patients with hemorrhage into ascites, peritoneal carcinomatosis, pancreatic ascites, or tuberculous peritonitis may have an elevated PMN count that is not related to SBP. These patients usually do not require empiric treatment. If the situation initially is unclear, however, the physician should err on the side of overtreatment, as long as nonnephrotoxic antibiotics are used. Usually, patients with uninfected neutrocytic ascitic fluid (except those with hemorrhage) have a predominance of lymphocytes in their ascitic fluid differential; this helps distinguish them from patients with SBP, in which PMNs predominate. Patients with bloody ascites should have a corrected PMN count calculated (see section on cell count). Patients with bloody ascites do not need antibiotics unless their corrected PMN count is at least 250 cells/μL.

Patients with MNB are special cases regarding empiric antibiotic treatment. Many episodes resolve without treatment.[115] Because of the hospitalization mortality rate (22% to 43%) associated with MNB, however, treatment appears to be warranted in many patients.[86,115] By definition, the PMN count is less than 250 cells/μL in this variant of ascitic fluid infection.[115] Because of this variant, the PMN count cannot be the only parameter on which to hinge the decision about empiric therapy. Most of the patients whose MNB colonization does not resolve and progresses to SBP have signs or symptoms of infection.[115] Therefore, patients with cirrhotic ascites who have *convincing signs or symptoms of in-*fection should receive treatment regardless of the PMN count in ascitic fluid. Empiric treatment can be discontinued after only 2 to 3 days if the culture remains negative and suspicion of infection has diminished.

Patients with *asymptomatic* MNB should undergo repeat paracentesis for cell count and culture, once it is known that the initial culture is growing bacteria. If the PMN count has risen above 250/μL in the follow-up ascitic fluid analysis, treatment should be started. Patients in whom no PMN response or clinical evidence of infection has developed do not require treatment.[115] These are the patients whose own immune defenses have probably eradicated the colonization.

When initially faced with a patient who has CNNA, the physician does not know that the culture is destined to be nogrowth. Therefore, empiric treatment should be given. When the preliminary report demonstrates no growth, it is helpful to repeat the paracentesis to assess the response of the PMN count to therapy. A decline in PMN count confirms a response to treatment and probably warrants a few more days of therapy. A stable PMN count, especially if there is not a predominance of PMNs, indicates that a nonbacterial (or mycobacterial) cause of the neutrocytosis is present. Cytology and culture for tuberculosis may be appropriate. Because improper culture techniques result in negative cultures, one of the most important methods to reduce the prevalence of CNNA in a hospital that still is using the conventional method of culture is to convince the microbiology laboratory to convert to the optimal method of culture.[122,136]

The ascitic fluid Gram stain is not particularly helpful in the choice of empiric antibiotic. I have not found that the Gram stain allowed a narrowed spectrum of antibiotic coverage in even 1 patient of about 300 with SBP. Only about 10% of Gram stains demonstrate organisms in early-detected SBP.[122] The actual utility of the Gram stain is in assisting with the differential diagnosis of spontaneous versus nonspontaneous ascitic fluid infection.[1,122,125] Sheets of multiple different types of bacteria are found in gut perforation; this requires coverage of anaerobic flora in addition to coverage of aerobic and facultative anaerobic flora, as well as an emergency search for a source for the bacteria.[1] Therefore, a positive Gram stain may lead to broader spectrum coverage rather than narrower coverage. Choosing narrow-spectrum coverage (eg, penicillin) based on a misinterpreted Gram stain may lead to the patient's death from uncontrolled infection before it is known that the isolated organism is resistant to the antibiotic that is in use.

Patients with suspected ascitic fluid infection require relatively broad-spectrum therapy until the results of susceptibility testing are available. The recommendation for choice of empiric treatment has changed over the past 20 years. In 1971, the combination of a first-generation cephalosporin and kanamycin was recommended.[20] In 1978, the combination of ampicillin and gentamicin was suggested.[157] Neither of these recommendations was supported by data; no susceptibility testing or efficacy data were provided.[20,157] Now it is known that the volume of distribution of gentamicin does not correlate with total body weight or estimated dry body weight in patients with ascites, and that the glomerular filtration rate of patients with ascites is not accurately estimated by serum creatinine or even creatinine clearance.[35,80] Therefore, it is difficult to give appropriate loading or maintenance doses of gentamicin to these patients. To do so, scientifically, requires that an immediate ascitic fluid and serum level of the gentamicin be obtained after each dose, so that adequate but nontoxic levels are achieved and maintained. Even if toxic doses are avoided, nephrotoxicity develops in up to 73% of cirrhotic patients.[16,76,77]

A number of nonaminoglycoside options are available. Aztreonam is a new monobactam that has been used in SBP. Unfortunately, its gram-positive coverage is negligible, and an unacceptable 19% superinfection rate has been documented with this drug.[4] Nearly 100% of SBP flora are susceptible to chloramphenicol or most third-generation cephalosporins.[52] Unfortunately, chloramphenicol is not bactericidal for gram-negative bacteria; fatal relapses are common, just as in chloramphenicol-treated gram-negative meningitis.[19] The first- and second-generation cephalosporins cover less than 75% of the flora of SBP (Runyon BA, unpublished observations). Because organisms that are resistant to the empiric antibiotic may cause the patient's death before the susceptibility testing results are available, broad-spectrum bactericidal drugs must be used for empiric treatment. Some third-generation cephalosporins are bactericidal and have an adequate spectrum of coverage. Cefotaxime, one of the early third-generation cephalosporins, has been shown to be superior to ampicillin plus tobramycin in a controlled trial.[30] This drug covered 98% of the flora, was more efficacious, and did not result in superinfection or nephrotoxicity in this trial.[30] This drug or a similar third-generation cephalosporin probably is the treatment of choice for suspected SBP. For cefotaxime, 2-g intravenous doses are appropriate, and the dosing interval is 8 to 12 hours—8 hours for a serum creatinine less than about 3 mg/dL and 12 hours for more severe renal failure.[121] Dosing interval does not *have* to be altered in renal failure (because of the lack of toxicity of the drug), but dosing more frequently than every 12 hours in the setting of frank renal failure simply is unnecessary and more expensive than less frequent dosing. Ascitic fluid levels can exceed 300 μg/mL in the setting of renal failure and dosing every 8 hours.[121] Dosing more frequently than every 8 hours is not necessary because high ascitic fluid concentrations (greater than 20-fold the minimal inhibitory concentrations of more than 90% of the flora) of the drug are attained after one dose and are sustained during dosing every 8 hours.[121]

When susceptibility testing results are available, a more narrow spectrum drug usually can be substituted (eg, pneumococci usually are sensitive to penicillin and most *E coli* species are sensitive to ampicillin).

Most infectious disease experts treat life-threatening infections with 10 to 14 days of therapy. There are no data, however, to support this duration of treatment of spontaneous ascitic fluid infection. The ascitic fluid culture becomes sterile after one dose of cefotaxime in 86% of patients.[1] The ascitic fluid PMN count, in general, drops exponentially after treatment is started such that the PMN count after 48 hours of therapy is always less than the pretreatment value in patients with spontaneous ascitic fluid infection treated with appropriate antibiotics.[1,129] A randomized controlled trial involving 100 patients has demonstrated that 5 days of treatment is as efficacious as 10 days in the treatment of SBP and CNNA.[132]

Patients suspected of having secondary peritonitis require broader-spectrum empiric antibiotic coverage than those with SBP, in addition to an emergency evaluation to assess the need for surgical intervention (see Fig. 35-3). Cefotaxime plus metronidazole provides excellent initial empiric therapy of suspected secondary peritonitis while the radiologic work-up is underway.[1]

Surprisingly, needle perforation of the bowel (polymicrobial bacterascites) is relatively well tolerated. Peritonitis developed in only 10% (1 of 10) of patients with needle perforation of the gut into ascitic fluid; only 0.06% (1 of 1578) of paracenteses were documented to cause peritonitis in this large study.[123] The paracentesis-related peritonitis was not fatal. It appears that patients with low-protein ascitic fluid are at most risk for development of a PMN response and clinical peritonitis related to needle perforation of the gut.[123] Most of the patients with high-protein ascites (eg, greater than 1 g/dL) did not even receive antibiotics and yet did well; however, most physicians probably would feel uncomfortable withholding antibiotic treatment if needle perforation is suspected. If a decision to treat is made, anaerobic coverage should be included, such as cefotaxime and metronidazole. If a decision not to treat is made, follow-up paracentesis is helpful in following the PMN count and culture. If the number of organisms does not decrease or a PMN response occurs, antibiotic treatment should be initiated.

Prognosis

In the past, despite treatment, 48% to 95% of patients with spontaneous ascitic fluid infection died during the hospitalization in which the diagnosis was made.[20,51,86] The mean weighted mortality rate in the seven largest series as of 1985 was 78%.[52] The most recent series report the lowest mortality rate.[132,154] This is probably a reflection of earlier detection of infection in the 1990s as well as avoidance of nephrotoxic antibiotics. In the older series, about half the SBP patients died of the infection despite antibiotic treatment; now under 5% of patients die of infection if timely and appropriate antibiotics are used.[132] Because of the severity of the underlying liver disease, however, even now many patients are cured of their infection and yet die of liver or renal failure or gastrointestinal bleeding. Because spontaneous ascitic fluid infection is a marker of end-stage liver disease, it has been proposed as an indication for liver transplantation in a patient who is otherwise a candidate.[114]

In the past, a delay in diagnosis was, at least in part, responsible for the excessive mortality. If the physician waited until convincing signs and symptoms of infection developed in the patient before performing a paracentesis, the infection was likely to be advanced by the time the diagnosis is made. There have been no reported survivors of SBP when the diagnosis is made after the creatinine has risen above 4 mg/dL. To maximize survival, it is important to perform paracentesis on hospital admission so that infection can be diagnosed and treated early. In addition, paracentesis should be repeated during hospitalization if any deterioration occurs—including pain, fever, mental status change, renal failure, acidosis, peripheral leukocytosis, or gastrointestinal bleeding.

Early diagnosis and surgical intervention reduce the hospitalization mortality of secondary peritonitis into the same range as that of SBP, about 50%.[1] Without surgical intervention, the mortality rate approaches 100%.

Prevention

All series of patients with SBP report recurrences. The older series did not report a high rate, in part because few patients survived the first episode. A prospective study reported in

1988 documents a 69% recurrence rate at 1 year.[154] An ascitic fluid protein concentration of less than 1 g/dL was the best predictor of recurrence. This impressive recurrence rate has prompted studies of antibiotic prophylaxis. Norfloxacin, 400 mg/d orally, has been reported successfully to prevent recurrences of SBP with essentially no toxicity, development of bacterial resistance, or superinfection.[39]

Antibiotic prevention of SBP in the setting of low-protein ascitic fluid or gut hemorrhage also has been reported.[98,148] Norfloxacin is effective in the former situation and a triple-drug nonabsorbable combination in the latter.[98,148]

TENSE ASCITES

Some patients with ascites do not seek medical attention until their intraabdominal fluid exerts such pressure on their diaphragms that they can no longer breath comfortably. The volume of fluid required before tenseness occurs usually is about 10 L. In young patients with good muscle tone, however, a tense abdomen may develop with only a few liters of fluid. Rapid accumulation of fluid (eg, after surgery in a patient with no prior fluid retention) does not give the abdominal wall time to stretch; these patients also can have small-volume tense ascites.

Tense ascites requires urgent treatment—therapeutic paracentesis. Tense ascites can be drained without untoward hemodynamic effects.[22,45,46,95] Total paracentesis (ie, removal of all mobilizable fluid) has been demonstrated to be safe.[153] Therapeutic paracentesis of cirrhotic ascites is less problematic than the textbooks and folklore of medicine would indicate. Many physicians were taught that large-volume paracentesis leads to hemodynamic disasters. This concept, however, was based on anecdotal observations in small numbers of patients and has been disproven by carefully conducted controlled trials.[95,153]

ABDOMINAL WALL HERNIAS

Abdominal wall hernias (usually umbilical or incisional, occasionally inguinal) are common in patients with ascites. Unfortunately, there is little published information available about these hernias. In one study, 17% of cirrhotic patients with ascites were found to have umbilical hernias at the time of admission to the hospital.[7] During 4-year follow-up, 14% of these patients' hernias incarcerated, 35% developed skin ulceration, and 7% ruptured.[7] Surgical treatment should be considered electively in all patients with hernias and ascites. The hernia recurs in 73% of patients who have ascites at the time of hernia repair but in only 14% of patients who have no ascites at the time of repair.[131] Therefore, ascites should be medically removed before surgery. If skin ulceration, crusting, or black discoloration develop, surgery should be performed semiemergently. Emergent surgery should be performed for rupture or incarceration that is unresponsive to medical therapy.[59] Rupture (ie, Flood's syndrome—an eponym as well as a descriptive label), is the most feared complication of abdominal hernias. The mortality rate of this complication is 11% to 43% overall—100% if there is preoperative jaundice or if the prothrombin time is prolonged to more than 2.5 seconds.[59] If surgical repair of Flood's syndrome is delayed, fatal *S aureus* peritonitis usually develops.

PLEURAL EFFUSIONS

Pleural effusions are common in patients with cirrhotic ascites. They usually are unilateral and right sided but occasionally may be bilateral with the amount of fluid on the right being greater than that on the left. When there is a unilateral left-sided effusion, tuberculosis should be high in the differential diagnosis.[74]

When the effusion is large and obscures most of the right lung, it is referred to as hepatic hydrothorax.[63] Most carefully studied examples of hepatic hydrothorax have been shown to be due to a small defect in the right hemidiaphragm. Occasionally, a hydrothorax results in sudden shortness of breath as the abdomen decompresses. On rare occasions, ascites is undetected in the face of a large pleural effusion.[101]

The predominant symptom associated with hepatic hydrothorax is shortness of breath. Infection of this fluid occurs, usually a result of SBP and transmission of bacteria across the diaphragm.[161] Usually the fluid resembles ascites, but the total protein is higher (by 0.75 to 1 g/dL) in the pleural fluid than in ascites because the pleural fluid is subject to different pressures than those of the portal bed.[63]

Treatment of hepatic hydrothorax usually is more difficult than anticipated.[124] These large right-sided effusions tend to occur in patients who are the least compliant or most refractory. Some authors have recommended tetracycline sclerosis using a chest tube. Chest tube insertion with suction, however, has been reported to lead to serious fluid and protein depletion and death.[124] Once a chest tube is inserted, usually it becomes difficult to remove. Clamping the tube may lead to a leak of fluid around the tube's insertion site. Peritoneovenous shunt can be considered in the patient with hepatic hydrothorax and large-volume ascites, but it frequently is a morbid procedure and the shunt usually clots after a short period of time (see section on refractory ascites). Direct surgical repair of the defect can be considered, but typically these patients are poor operative candidates. Medical therapy (ie, sodium restriction and diuretics) probably is the safest and most effective form of therapy for hepatic hydrothorax.

Treatment

Ascites is not always due to liver disease (see Table 35-1). Not all patients with ascites respond to routine salt restriction and diuretics. Therefore, an accurate diagnosis of the cause of ascites formation is important so that treatment can be tailored appropriately. The SAAG is helpful in therapeutic decision making. Patients with low SAAG ascites usually do not respond to salt restriction and diuretics, whereas patients with a high SAAG usually are responsive.

NON–PORTAL HYPERTENSION–RELATED (LOW-ALBUMIN GRADIENT) ASCITES

The most common form of low-albumin gradient ascites is peritoneal carcinomatosis.[130] Peripheral edema in these patients responds to diuretics, but the ascitic fluid usually does not; edema-free patients treated with diuretics lose only intravascular volume without loss of ascites.[89] The cornerstone of treatment of peritoneal carcinomatosis is therapeutic paracentesis.[22,46] Patients with peritoneal carcinomatosis usually live only a matter of weeks; therefore, the total number of taps required to minimize symptoms is not great. Patients with ovarian malignancy are an exception to this rule. They may have a good response to surgical debulking and chemotherapy. Peritoneovenous shunts are said to be more effective and less morbid in malignant ascites than in cirrhotic ascites[47]; however, in view of the short life expectancy of these patients, a hospitalization for placement of a shunt may not be appropriate.

Tuberculous peritonitis is cured by antituberculous therapy; there is no point in using diuretics unless the patient has concomitant portal hypertension from cirrhosis. Pancreatic ascites may resolve spontaneously or may require endoscopic stenting or operative intervention. A postoperative lymphatic leak may resolve spontaneously, or may require surgical intervention or peritoneovenous shunting.[73] Chlamydial peritonitis is cured by doxycycline therapy.[78] Nephrogenous ascites (dialysis ascites) may respond to vigorous dialysis.[70]

PORTAL HYPERTENSION–RELATED (HIGH-ALBUMIN GRADIENT) ASCITES

The most common cause of portal hypertension-related ascites is cirrhosis, usually caused by alcohol abuse. One of the most important steps in treating this form of ascites is to treat the underlying liver disease by convincing the patient to stop drinking alcohol. With time and healing of the reversible component of alcoholic liver disease, the ascites may resolve or at least convert from being refractory to medical therapy to being nonrefractory to medical therapy. Patients with autoimmune chronic active hepatitis, iron storage disease, or Wilson's disease should receive specific therapy for those diseases; this may improve their overall liver function and increase ease of management of their ascites. These diseases seem to be less reversible than alcoholic liver disease, however, and by the time ascites is present, the patients may be better candidates for liver transplantation than protracted medical therapy.

Patients who are determined to have cirrhotic ascites based on history, physical examination, and ascitic fluid analysis usually require hospitalization for diagnosis and management of their liver disease as well as their fluid overload, especially if the fluid retention is of new onset. Frequently, ascites formation is only part of the overall picture of decompensation of liver disease. Although outpatient treatment of ascites patients can be successful, frequently it fails and an intensive period of inpatient education and treatment is required. Once the patient realizes that the diet and diuretics actually are effective, he or she frequently is more compliant with the regimen.

Precipitating Cause

In the initial management of the patient with ascites, it usually is of value to determine the precipitating cause of ascites formation. Frequently, ascites accumulates because of noncompliance either with the dietary sodium or diuretics, or ascites may accumulate because of the fluid resuscitation given in the treatment of variceal hemorrhage. Education about compliance may help prevent future hospitalizations for ascites. Ascites that is initiated by variceal hemorrhage may resolve after the bleeding is controlled without need for long-term diuretics.

Diet

In portal hypertension–related ascites, fluid loss and weight change are directly and predictably related to sodium balance. Dietary sodium restriction is essential; the patient and the patient's cook (who frequently is not the patient) should be educated by a dietitian in a salt-restricted diet. The more contact the dietician has with the patient and cook, the better. A severe sodium-restricted diet (eg, 500 mg/d or 22 mEq/d sodium) is feasible in an inpatient setting; however, it is an unrealistic diet for most outpatients. Most patients do not follow a diet that contains less than 2 g/d sodium. The advantage of a 500-mg/d diet while in hospital is more rapid loss of ascites because of a more negative sodium balance. On the other hand, the advantage of a less restricted, 2-g/d hospital diet is the probability that the patient will be able to follow the diet at home and the opportunity to tailor a diuretic regimen that will match the salt intake in and out of the hospital.

Fluid Restriction

Fluid restriction of all patients with ascites is inappropriate. There is no evidence that fluid restriction speeds weight loss. It is the sodium restriction that is important. Although rapidly developing hyponatremia (eg, postoperative hyponatremia in a previously healthy patient) is associated with high mortality, the chronic hyponatremia usually seen in cirrhotic ascites patients is far less morbid. Attempts to correct it rapidly can be much worse that the hyponatremia itself. The only indication for fluid restriction in the cirrhotic ascites patient is severe hyponatremia. I do not fluid-restrict ascites patients unless their serum sodium drops below 120 mEq/L. Cirrhotic patients usually do not have symptoms from hyponatremia until the sodium is below 110 mEq/L or unless the decline in sodium is rapid. To fluid-restrict everyone serves only to alienate patients, nurses, and dieticians. Indiscriminant fluid restriction may lead to hypernatremia.

Urinary Sodium Concentration

Twenty-four-hour urinary sodium measurements are useful in patients with portal hypertension–related ascites, both in assessing the need for diuretic therapy and in monitoring its progress. Completeness of collection is notoriously difficult to achieve but can be assessed by measurement of urinary creatinine. Cirrhotic men should excrete 15 to 20 mg/kg/d of creatinine and women 10 to 15 mg/kg/d. Many patients have less than 10 mEq of sodium in a 24-hour urine collection, obtained before diuretic administration. These patients cannot be managed successfully with dietary sodium restriction alone and need diuretic therapy or intermittent paracentesis. Those with less than 5 mEq/d usually need relatively high doses of diuretics and do respond to the starting regimen of 100 mg spironolactone and 40 mg furosemide orally daily. If a patient has more than 25 mEq sodium in the initial 24-hour urine and has not recently received diuretics, he or she may be undergoing a spontaneous natriuresis. Only the approximately 10% of patients who have significant spontaneous natriuresis can be considered for dietary sodium restriction alone (ie, without diuretics).[150] Although a 24-hour collection for baseline assessment of the avidity of sodium retention is optimal, a "spot" urinary sodium concentration assessment is a satisfactory substitute in many cases. Even if the patient is receiving diuretics at the time of admission, a urine collection for sodium can be helpful. Many patients have essentially no urine sodium despite diuretics, indicating the need for higher doses or alternative treatment.

If body weight is not declining satisfactorily, this may be due to inadequate natriuresis or failure properly to restrict sodium intake, or both. Monitoring 24-hour urinary sodium excretion and daily weight usually clarifies the problem. Because urinary excretion is the most important route of excretion of sodium in the absence of diarrhea or hyperthermia, dietary intake and urinary excretion should be equivalent if the weight is stable. If the weight is increasing despite urinary losses in excess of prescribed dietary intake, one can assume that the patient is eating more than his or her allotted salt.

Diuretics

Single-agent diuretic therapy, such as spironolactone or amiloride, frequently is effective in the treatment of patients with cirrhotic ascites—starting with a minimum of 100 or 10 mg/d, respectively. Amiloride is more expensive but is more rapidly effective and does not cause gynecomastia, as spironolactone occasionally does. Spironolactone is the mainstay of treatment of cirrhotic ascites. It was effective in one study in 95% of patients as a single agent compared with the 58% efficacy of furosemide alone.[84] The half-life of spironolactone in normal control patients is about 24 hours but is markedly prolonged in cirrhosis.[151,156] There is no reason to administer the drug in multiple doses per day in view of its long half-life. Single daily doses of pills are most appropriate and enhance compliance; 100-mg spironolactone pills are available. In general, spironolactone *and* furosemide are used together, starting with 100 mg/d spironolactone and 40 mg/d furosemide, then increasing both drugs simultaneously as needed. If weight loss or urine sodium is inadequate, diuretics are increased up to doses of about 400 mg/d spironolactone and about 160 mg/d furosemide. Higher doses can be given, but further increments in urine sodium are marginal. If diuresis is inadequate on high doses of two diuretics, one can add 25 to 50 mg hydrochlorothiazide or 5 mg metolazone.[71] Unfortunately, these three-drug combinations can cause a massive urine sodium loss with profound hyponatremia. Also, this triple therapy can be difficult to manage for outpatients. The ratio of spironolactone and furosemide can be adjusted to correct serum potassium problems. Combined with a sodium-restricted diet, the aldactone–furosemide regimen has been demonstrated, in a study that screened almost 4000 patients, to achieve a successful diuresis in more than 90% of cirrhotic subjects.[149]

Intravenous furosemide causes an acute reduction in glomerular filtration rate in these patients and should be avoided. If rapid weight loss is desired, therapeutic paracenteses should be performed[22,45,46,95,153] (see section on refractory ascites). For patients who have massive edema, there is no limit to the daily weight loss; once the edema has resolved, 0.5 kg/d probably is a reasonable maximum.[88] If patients manifest encephalopathy, serum sodium less than 120 mEq/L despite fluid restriction, or serum creatinine greater than 2 mg/dL, diuretics usually are stopped and then carefully reinstituted after the reason for discontinuation improves. The ratio of the doses of the diuretics is adjusted to maintain a normal serum potassium. Serious hyperkalemia despite adjustment of diuretics usually indicates intrinsic renal disease (eg, diabetic nephropathy or IgA nephropathy). Many of the patients in whom complications of diuretic treatment develop are considered failures of first-line treatment

and require second-line therapy. Prostaglandin inhibitors, such as nonsteroidal antiinflammatory drugs, should not be used in patients with ascites because they curtail diuresis, may promote renal failure, and cause gastrointestinal bleeding.[75]

Complete removal of ascites may not always be achieved[96]; however, diuresis-mediated concentration of ascitic fluid increases the fluid's opsonic activity 10-fold, and theoretically may be of value in attempting to prevent spontaneous ascitic fluid infection.[137] Maximum concentration of opsonins occurs at the end of diuresis. It is reasonable to attempt to achieve a dry abdomen in order to minimize risk of infection and to decrease risk of abdominal wall hernias and hepatic hydrothorax.

Duration of Hospitalization

Patients with ascites frequently occupy hospital beds for 30 to 60 or more days. Many days are used suboptimally because of confusion about diagnosis and treatment and because of iatrogenic problems. Although a dry abdomen is a reasonable goal to pursue in an attempt to minimize risk of ascitic fluid infection and to prevent the development of hernias and hepatic hydrothorax, it need not be a prerequisite for discharge from the hospital. The patient may finally achieve a dry abdomen as an outpatient. Several studies have chosen a dry abdomen as a study endpoint.[95,153] There is no specific reason, however, to retain patients in the hospital only for treatment of their fluid retention, if they are ready for discharge otherwise and if they are responding to their medical regimen.

Refractory Ascites

A patient with refractory ascites is defined as having fluid overload unresponsive to inpatient salt restriction and diuretic treatment. The failure may be manifested by minimal to no weight loss despite high-dose diuretics or development of complications of diuretics. Multiple studies have shown that less than 10% of cirrhotic ascites patients are refractory to standard medical therapy.[84,149,150] Second-line therapy options include portacaval shunt (of historical interest only), Paris pump (of historical interest only), peritoneovenous shunt, therapeutic paracenteses, and liver transplantation. In the 1960s, portacaval shunts were used for treatment of ascites, but operative complications, in particular portosystemic encephalopathy, led to an abandonment of this practice.[31] In Europe in the 1970s, the Paris pump was used to ultrafilter ascitic fluid and then reinfuse it intravenously.[81] Unfortunately, disseminated intravascular coagulation and other complications were common with this procedure, and this form of treatment was not popularized in the United States.

In the mid-1970s, the peritoneovenous shunt was promoted as a new physiologic treatment in the management of ascites.[60] It initially was unclear to some physicians whether this new tool should be used for initial therapy or should be reserved only for treatment of patients who were refractory to diuretics. Reports of shunt failure and fatal complications of shunt insertion rapidly sobered the enthusiasm for this treatment and have removed it from first-line therapy of cirrhotic ascites. Reported complications include recovery room pulmonary edema, variceal hemorrhage (from fluid overload), disseminated intravascular coagulation, thromboembolic phenomena including superior vena cava thrombosis, pseudocyst formation, peritoneal fibrosis, and bacterial infection.[79] Shunt failure due to thrombosis continues to be a serious problem. Most shunts clot in less than a year's time. Second-generation shunts (eg, Denver shunts) have not reduced the shunt failure rate.[33]

The study that placed peritoneovenous shunts in the third-line category of options for therapy of cirrhotic ascites was the Veterans Administration Cooperative Study.[149] Almost 4000 alcoholic cirrhotic ascites patients were screened for entry into this study. Patients who were refractory to standard medical therapy were randomized to either continued diuretic therapy plus therapeutic paracentesis or peritoneovenous shunt (including use of Denver shunts in patients who clotted LeVeen shunts). This study documented (1) no improved survival in shunted patients compared with medically treated patients, (2) excessive infections in shunted patients, (3) continued need for sodium restriction and diuretics despite a functional shunt, (4) frequent shunt failure, and (5) most importantly, *only about 10% failure of diuretic therapy*.[149] Shunted patients did have slightly shorter hospitalizations and slightly longer periods before readmission. Removal of most of the ascitic fluid during surgery before shunt insertion, use of perioperative antiplatelet therapy, replacement of ascites with saline, and administration of intraoperative intravenous furosemide have decreased the incidence of perioperative complications.[139] Even before the Veterans Administration study was published, however, most hepatologists had severely curtailed use of this device. It is difficult today to find a surgeon who has experience with and enthusiasm for these peritoneovenous shunts; peritoneovenous shunting is reserved for the small group of patients who fail both diuretic *and* paracentesis therapy (see discussion later). This does not happen often—only when patients cannot or will not return for outpatient paracentesis.

Abdominal paracentesis is one of the oldest medical procedures. From the time of Celsus, who is credited with first describing the technique in about 20 BC, until the late 1940s, therapeutic paracentesis was essentially the only available therapy for ascites. Before 1950, volumes of ascitic fluid were removed by means of large trocars in outpatient clinics in minutes without incident. In the early 1950s, diuretics became available as reports of complications of therapeutic paracentesis were published. This laborious procedure rapidly fell out of favor as a treatment option for patients with ascites. The 1980s saw renewed interest in therapeutic paracentesis, partly because of dissatisfaction with the prolonged hospitalizations required for treatment of ascites with diuretics and partly because of dissatisfaction with peritoneovenous shunts.[36,149] Also in the 1980s, scientific data on large-volume (5-liter) paracentesis were reported.[36,56,85] Patients were treated with daily taps followed by colloid infusion or single taps without intravenous colloid infusion. These patients tolerated large-volume taps well, just as the patients did in the 1940s. In fact, therapeutic paracentesis plus colloid infusion was found to lead to fewer minor asymptomatic changes in electrolytes and serum creatinine than those associated with diuretic therapy in one large randomized controlled trial.[36] No differences in morbidity or mortality could be demonstrated in this study, however.[36] Physically removing the fluid predictably was found to be faster than diuretic treatment in achieving a dry abdomen. Some physicians have concluded from this study that therapeutic paracentesis should be first-line therapy for patients with tense cirrhotic ascites, but not all physicians agree with this conclusion. In view of the ease and efficacy of diuretic therapy in over 90% of patients, ther-

apeutic paracentesis probably should be reserved for treatment of tense ascites and ascites that is refractory to diuretic therapy. Also, therapeutic paracentesis lacks the ascitic fluid opsonin-conserving advantage of diuresis; in theory, depletion of opsonins by paracentesis could predispose to spontaneous bacterial peritonitis.[119]

One practical issue in therapeutic paracentesis is that of colloid replacement. Should colloid be given? How much? Which colloid? In one study, patients were randomized to receive albumin (10 g/L of fluid removed) versus no albumin, after therapeutic paracentesis.[40] The group that received no albumin showed statistically significantly more (asymptomatic) changes in electrolytes, plasma renin, and serum creatinine than the albumin group, but it had no more clinical morbidity or mortality. The authors of this study recommend routine albumin infusion after therapeutic paracentesis; however, not all physicians agree with this recommendation. Albumin infusions markedly increase albumin degradation.[100,158] In one older study, 58% of infused albumin was accounted for by increased degradation, and a 15% increase in serum albumin led to a 39% increase in degradation.[100] Albumin is expensive—$2 to $25 a gram or *$100 to $1250 a tap*. It is difficult to justify the expense of routine albumin infusion after every therapeutic paracentesis worldwide based on the data at hand. At the University of Southern California Liver Unit, some 1000 paracenteses are performed per year; about half are therapeutic. Therapeutic paracentesis *without* colloid infusion has been routine for decades in this Unit. Postparacentesis problems related to volume depletion have not been apparent.

Another study has compared the colloid dextran 70 with albumin after large-volume paracentesis.[87] Dextran 70 (8 g/L of fluid removed) led to renin increases in more patients than did albumin (8 g/L). There were no differences in electrolyte imbalance or clinically relevant complications between groups, however.

Finally, orthotopic liver transplantation should be considered in the treatment options of a refractory ascites patient who is otherwise a transplant candidate. The 12-month survival of patients with ascites refractory to medical therapy is only 25%.[11] Transplantation has a 12-month survival three times this value.

Summary of Treatment of Cirrhotic Ascites

The mainstay of therapy of patients with cirrhotic ascites is dietary sodium restriction and diuretics. Standard medical therapy is effective in 90% of patients. Therapeutic paracentesis should be performed to treat tense ascites acutely and as second-line treatment of chronic ascites in the 10% of patients who are refractory to medical therapy. Data are insufficient to determine whether colloid replacement is necessary after therapeutic paracentesis. Use of colloid has been shown to prevent laboratory abnormalities; however, withholding colloid has not been shown to result in increased morbidity or mortality. Dextran appears to be as effective as albumin in preventing asymptomatic laboratory abnormalities after paracentesis. If a physician feels compelled to give postparacentesis colloid while awaiting more data, use of the less expensive dextran would seem appropriate. Peritoneovenous shunting is third-line therapy and should be reserved for special circumstances, such as ascites due to surgical lymphatic tear that does not respond to medical therapy, and for patients with ascites refractory to medical treatment with circumstances that preclude chronic therapeutic paracenteses. Patients with refractory ascites who are liver transplant candidates should be prioritized for transplantation.

References

1. Akriviadis EA, Runyon BA. The value of an algorithm in differentiating spontaneous from secondary bacterial peritonitis. Gastroenterology 98:127, 1990
2. Albillos A, Cuervas-Mons V, Millan I, et al. Ascitic fluid polymorphonuclear cell count and serum to ascites albumin gradient in the diagnosis of bacterial peritonitis. Gastroenterology 98:134, 1990
3. Altura BM, Hershey SG. Sequential changes in reticuloendothelial system function after acute hemorrhage. Proc Soc Exp Biol Med 139:935, 1972
4. Ariza J, Gudiol F, Dolz C, et al. Evaluation of aztreonam in the treatment of spontaneous bacterial peritonitis in patients with cirrhosis. Hepatology 6:906, 1986
5. Baker A, Kaplan M. Central congestive fibrosis of the liver in myxedema. Ann Intern Med 77:927, 1972
6. Bar-Meir S, Lerner E, Conn HO. Analysis of ascitic fluid in cirrhosis. Dig Dis Sci 24:136, 1979
7. Belghiti J, Rueff B, Fekete F. Umbilical hernia in cirrhotic patients with ascites. (Abstract) Gastroenterology 84:1363, 1983
8. Berg RD. Translocation of indigenous bacteria from the intestinal tract. In: Hentges DJ, ed. Human intestinal microflora in health and disease. New York, Academic Press, 1983, p 333
9. Berg RD, Garlington AW. Translocation of certain indigenous bacteria from the gastrointestinal tract to the mesenteric lymph nodes and other organs in a gnotobiotic mouse model. Infect Immun 23:403, 1979
10. Bobadilla M, Sifuentes J, Garcia-Tsao G. Improved method for bacteriological diagnosis of spontaneous bacterial peritonitis. J Clin Microbiol 27:2145, 1989
11. Bories P, Garcia-Compean D, Michel H, et al. The treatment of refractory ascites by the LeVeen shunt: a multi-center controlled trial (57 patients). J Hepatol 3:212, 1986
12. Boyer TD, Kahn A, Reynolds TB. Diagnostic value of ascitic fluid lactic dehydrogenase, protein, and WBC levels. Arch Intern Med 138:1103, 1978
13. Brown MW, Burk RF. Development of intractable ascites following upper abdominal surgery in patients with cirrhosis. Am J Med 80:879, 1986
14. Burroughs AK, Rosenstein IJ, Epstein O, et al. Bacteriuria and primary biliary cirrhosis. Gut 25:133, 1984
15. Cabot RC. The causes of ascites: a study of 5000 cases. Am J Med Sci 143:1, 1912
16. Cabrera J, Arroyo V, Ballesta AM, et al. Aminoglycoside nephrotoxicity in cirrhosis. Gastroenterology 82:97, 1982
17. Cardozo PL. A critical evaluation of 3000 cytologic analyses of pleural fluid, ascitic fluid, and pericardial fluid. Acta Cytol 10:455, 1966
18. Cattau EI, Benjamin SB, Knuff TE, et al. The accuracy of the physical exam in the diagnosis of suspected ascites. JAMA 247:1164, 1982
19. Cherubin CE, Marr JS, Sierra MF, et al. Listeria and gram-negative bacillary meningitis. Am J Med 71:199, 1981
20. Conn HO, Fessel JM. Spontaneous bacterial peritonitis in cirrhosis: variations on a theme. Medicine 50:161, 1971
21. Correia JP, Conn HO. Spontaneous bacterial peritonitis in cirrhosis: endemic or epidemic. Med Clin North Am 59:963, 1975:
22. Cruikshank DP, Buchsbaum HJ. Effects of rapid paracentesis. JAMA 225:1361, 1973
23. D'Amico G, Morabito A, Pagliaro L, Marubini E. Survival
and prognostic indicators in compensated and decompensated cirrhosis. Dig Dis Sci 31:468, 1986
24. Deitch EA, Winterton J, Li M, et al. The gut as a portal of entry of bacteria. Ann Surg 205:681, 1987
25. Denison EK, Lieberman FL, Reynolds TB. 9-Alpha-fluorohydrocortisone induced ascites in alcoholic liver disease. Gastroenterology 61:497, 1971
26. DiBona G, Herman PJ, Sawin LL. Neural control of renal function in edema-forming states. Am J Physiol 254:R1017, 1988
27. Dumont AE, Mulholland JH. Flow rate and composition of thoracic duct lymph in patients with cirrhosis. N Engl J Med 263:471, 1960
28. Epstein FH, Post RS, McDowell M. The effect of an arteriovenous fistula on renal hemodynamics and electrolyte excretion. J Clin Invest 32:233, 1953
29. Epstein M. Renal effects of head-out water immersion in man: implications for an understanding of volume homeostasis. Physiol Rev 58:529, 1978
30. Felisart J, Rimola A, Arroyo V, et al. Randomized comparative study of efficacy and nephrotoxicity of ampicillin plus tobramycin versus cefotaxime in cirrhotics with severe infections. Hepatology 5:457, 1985
31. Franco D, Vons C, Traynor O, et al. Should portosystemic shunt be reconsidered in the treatment of intractable ascites in cirrhosis? Arch Surg 123:987, 1988
32. Freeman S. Recent progress in the physiology and biochemistry of the liver. Med Clin North Am 37:109, 1953
33. Fulenwider JT, Galambos JD, Smith RB, et al. LeVeen vs. Denver peritoneovenous shunts for intractable ascites of cirrhosis. Arch Surg 121:351, 1986
34. Geake TMS, Spitaels JM, Moshel MG, et al. Peritoneoscopy in the diagnosis of tuberculous peritonitis. Gastrointest Endosc 27:66, 1981
35. Gill MA, Kern JW. Altered gentamicin distribution in ascitic patients. Am J Hosp Pharm 36:1704, 1979
36. Gines P, Arroyo V, Quintero E, et al. Comparison of paracentesis and diuretics in the treatment of cirrhotics with tense ascites: results of a randomized study. Gastroenterology 93:234, 1987
37. Gines P, Jimenez W, Arroyo V, et al. Atrial natriuretic factor in cirrhosis with ascites: plasma levels, cardiac release, and splanchnic extraction. Hepatology 8:636, 1988
38. Gines P, Quintero E, Arroyo V, et al. Compensated cirrhosis: natural history and prognostic factors. Hepatology 7:12, 1987
39. Gines P, Rimola A, Planas R, et al. Norfloxacin prevents spontaneous bacterial peritonitis recurrence in cirrhosis: results of a double-blind, placebo-controlled trial. Hepatology 12:716, 1990
40. Gines P, Tito L, Arroyo V, et al. Randomized comparative study of therapeutic paracentesis with and without intravenous albumin in cirrhosis. Gastroenterology 94:1493, 1988
41. Goldberg BB, Goodman GA, Clearfield HR. Evaluation of ascites by ultrasound. Radiology 96:15, 1970
42. Granger DN, Miller T, Allen R, et al. Permselectivity of cat liver blood-lymph barrier to endogenous macromolecules. Gastroenterology 77:103, 1979
43. Graudal N, Milman N, Kirkegaard E, et al. Bacteremia in cirrhosis of the liver. Liver 6:297, 1986
44. Greenway B, Johnson PJ, Williams R. Control of malignant ascites with spironolactone. Br J Surg 69:441, 1982
45. Guazzi M, Polese A, Magrini F, et al. Negative influences of ascites on the cardiac function of cirrhotic patients. Am J Med 59:165, 1975
46. Halpin TF, McCann TO. Dynamics of body fluids following rapid removal of large volumes of ascites. Am J Obstet Gynecol 110:103, 1971
47. Helzberg JH, Greenberger NJ. Peritoneovenous shunt in malignant ascites. Dig Dis Sci 30:1104, 1985
48. Hoefs JC. Increase in ascites WBC and protein concentrations

during diuresis in patients with chronic liver disease. Hepatology 1:249, 1981

49. Hoefs JC. Serum protein concentration and portal pressure determine the ascitic fluid protein concentration in patients with chronic liver disease. J Lab Clin Med 102:260, 1983

50. Hoefs JC. Globulin correction of the albumin gradient: correlation with measured serum to ascites colloid osmotic pressure gradients. Hepatology 16:396, 1992

51. Hoefs JC, Canawati HN, Sapico FL, et al. Spontaneous bacterial peritonitis. Hepatology 2:399, 1982

52. Hoefs JC, Runyon BA. Spontaneous bacterial peritonitis. Dis Month 31:1, 1985

53. Hyatt RE, Smith JR. The mechanism of ascites: a physiologic appraisal. Am J Med 16:434, 1954

54. Johnson WD. The cytological diagnosis of cancer in serous effusions. Acta Cytol 10:161, 1966

55. Kajani MA, Yoo YK, Alexander JA, et al. Serum-ascites albumin gradients in nonalcoholic liver disease. Dig Dis Sci 35:33, 1990

56. Kao HW, Rakov NE, Savage E, et al. The effect of large volume paracentesis on plasma volume: a cause of hypovolemia? Hepatology 5:403, 1985

57. Kostreva DR, Castener A, Kampine JP. Reflex effects of hepatic baroreceptors on renal and cardiac sympathetic nerve activity. Am J Physiol 238:R390, 1980

58. Kurtz RC, Bronzo RL. Does spontaneous bacterial peritonitis occur in malignant ascites? Am J Gastroenterol 77:146, 1982

59. Lemmer JH, Strodel WE, Knol JA. Management of spontaneous umbilical hernia disruption in the cirrhotic patient. Ann Surg 198:30, 1983

60. LeVeen HH, Christoudias G, Ip M, et al. Peritoneovenous shunting for ascites. Ann Surg 180:580, 1974

61. Levy M, Allotey JB. Temporal relationships between urinary salt retention and altered systemic hemodynamics in dogs with experimental cirrhosis. J Lab Clin Med 92:560, 1978

62. Lieberman FL, Denison EK, Reynolds TB. The relationship of plasma volume, portal hypertension, ascites, and renal sodium retention in cirrhosis: the overflow theory of ascites formation. Ann NY Acad Sci 70:202, 1970

63. Lieberman FL, Hidemura R, Peters RL, Reynolds TB. Pathogenesis and treatment of hydrothorax complicating cirrhosis with ascites. Ann Intern Med 64:341, 1966

64. Lieberman FL, Reynolds TB. Plasma volume in cirrhosis of the liver: its relation to portal hypertension, ascites, and renal failure. J Clin Invest 46:1297, 1967

65. Loewenstein MS, Rittgers RA, Feinerman AE, et al. CEA assay of ascites and detection of malignancy. Ann Intern Med 88:635, 1978

66. Lumsden AB, Henderson JM, Kutner MH. Endotoxin levels measured by a chromogenic assay in portal, hepatic and peripheral venous blood in patients with cirrhosis. Hepatology 8:232, 1988

67. Mallory A, Schaefer JW. Complications of diagnostic paracentesis in patients with liver disease. JAMA 239:628, 1978

68. Martini GA, Phear EA, Ruebner B, Sherlock S. The bacterial content of the small intestine in normal and cirrhotic subjects: relation to methionine toxicity. Clin Sci 16:35, 1957

69. Mauer K, Manzione NC. Usefulness of the serum-ascites albumin gradient in separating transudative from exudative ascites: another look. Dig Dis Sci 33:1208, 1988

70. Mauk PM, Schwartz JT, Lowe JE, et al. Diagnosis and course of nephrogenic ascites. Arch Intern Med 148:1577, 1988

71. McHutchison JG, Pinto PC, Reynolds TB. Hydrochlorothiazide as a third diuretic in cirrhotics with refractory ascites. (Abstract) Hepatology 10:719, 1989

71a. McHutchison JG, Runyon BA. Spontaneous bacterial peritonitis. In: Surawicz CM, Owen RL, eds. Gastrointestinal and hepatic infections. Philadelphia, WB Saunders, 1993

72. Mellencamp MA, Preheim LC. Pneumococcal pneumonia in a rat model of cirrhosis: effects of cirrhosis on pulmonary defense mechanisms against *Streptococcus pneumoniae*. J Infect Dis 163:102, 1991

73. Miedema EB, Bissada NK, Finkbeiner AE, et al. Chylous ascites complicating retroperitoneal lymphadenectomy for testis tumors: management with peritoneovenous shunting. J Urol 120:377, 1978

74. Mirouze D, Juttner HU, Reynolds TB. Left pleural effusion in patients with chronic liver disease and ascites: prospective study of 22 cases. Dig Dis Sci 26:984, 1981

75. Mirouze D, Zipser RD, Reynolds TB. Effect of inhibitors of prostaglandin synthesis on induced diuresis in cirrhosis. Hepatology 3:50, 1983

76. Moore RD, Smith CR, Lietman PS. Increased risk of renal dysfunction due to interaction of liver disease and aminoglycosides. Am J Med 80:1093, 1986

77. Moore RD, Smith CR, Lipsky JJ, et al. Risk factors for nephrotoxicity in patients treated with aminoglycosides. Ann Intern Med 100:352, 1984

78. Muller-Schoop JW, Wang SP, Munzinger J, et al. Chlamydia trachomatosis as possible cause of peritonitis and perihepatitis in young women. Br Med J 1:1022, 1978

79. Norfray JF, Henry HM, Givens JD, et al. Abdominal complications from peritoneal shunts. Gastroenterology 77:337, 1979

80. Papadakis MA, Arieff AI. Unpredictability of clinical evaluation of renal function in cirrhosis: prospective study. Am J Med 82:945, 1987

81. Parbhoo SP, Ajdukiewicz, Sherlock S. Treatment of ascites by continuous ultrafiltration and reinfusion of protein concentrate. Lancet 1:949, 1974

82. Pardy BJ, Spencer RC, Dudley HAF. Hepatic reticuloendothelial protection against bacteremia in experimental hemorrhagic shock. Surgery 81:193, 1977

83. Pare P, Talbot J, Hoefs JC. Serum-ascites albumin concentration gradient: a physiologic approach to the differential diagnosis of ascites. Gastroenterology 85:240, 1983

84. Perez-Ayuso RM, Arroyo V, Planas R, et al. Randomized comparative study of efficacy of furosemide vs. spironolactone in nonazotemic cirrhosis with ascites. Gastroenterology 84:961, 1983

85. Pinto PC, Amerian J, Reynolds TB. Large-volume paracentesis in nonedematous patients with tense ascites: its effect on intravascular volume. Hepatology 8:207, 1988

86. Pinzello G, Simonetti RG, Craxi A, et al. Spontaneous bacterial peritonitis: a prospective investigation in predominantly nonalcoholic cirrhotic patients. Hepatology 3:545, 1983

87. Planas R, Gines P, Arroyo V, et al. Dextran-70 versus albumin as plasma expanders in cirrhotic patients with tense ascites treated with total paracentesis. Gastroenterology 99:1736, 1990

88. Pockros PJ, Reynolds TB. Rapid diuresis in patients with ascites from chronic liver disease: the importance of peripheral edema. Gastroenterology 90:1827, 1986

89. Pockros PJ, Esrason KT, Nguyen C, et al. Mobilization of malignant ascites with diuretics is dependent on ascitic fluid characteristics. Gastroenterology 103:1302, 1992

90. Press OW, Press NO, Kaufman SD. Evaluation and management of chylous ascites. Ann Intern Med 96:358, 1982

91. Rajkovic IA, Williams R. Abnormalities of neutrophil phagocytosis, intracellular killing, and metabolic activity in alcoholic cirrhosis and hepatitis. Hepatology 6:252, 1986

92. Rector WG. Spontaneous chylous ascites of cirrhosis. J Clin Gastroenterol 6:369, 1984

93. Rector WG, Reynolds TB. Superiority of serum-ascites albumin difference over the ascites total protein concentration in separation of "transudative" and "exudative" ascites. Am J Med 77:83, 1984

94. Reynolds TB. Rapid presumptive diagnosis of spontaneous bacterial peritonitis. Gastroenterology 90:1294, 1986

95. Reynolds TB. Therapeutic paracentesis: have we come full circle? Gastroenterology 93:386, 1987

96. Reynolds TB, Lieberman FL, Goodman AR. Advantages of treatment of ascites without sodium restriction and without complete removal of excess fluid. Gut 19:549, 1979

97. Rhodes RS, Depalma RG. Intestinal barrier function in hemorrhagic shock. J Surg Res 14:305, 1973

98. Rimola A, Bory F, Teres J, et al. Oral, nonabsorbable antibiotics prevent infection in cirrhotics with gastrointestinal hemorrhage. Hepatology 5:463, 1985

99. Rimola A, Soto R, Bory F, et al. Reticuloendothelial system phagocytic activity in cirrhosis and its relation to bacterial infections and prognosis. Hepatology 4:53, 1984

100. Rothschild M, Oratz M, Evans C, Schreiber SS. Alterations in albumin metabolism after serum and albumin infusions. J Clin Invest 43:1874, 1964

101. Rubinstein D, McInnes IA, Dudley FJ. Hepatic hydrothorax in the absence of clinical ascites: diagnosis and management. Gastroenterology 88:188, 1985

102. Runyon BA. Spontaneous bacterial peritonitis associated with cardiac ascites. Am J Gastroenterol 79:796, 1984

103. Runyon BA. Ascitic fluid "humoral tests of malignancy." Hepatology 6:1443, 1986

104. Runyon BA. Elevated ascitic fluid fibronectin: a non-specific finding. J Hepatol 3:219, 1986

105. Runyon BA. Fatal bacterial peritonitis secondary to nonobstructive colonic dilatation (Ogilvie's syndrome) in cirrhotic ascites. J Clin Gastroenterol 8:687, 1986

106. Runyon BA. Gastrointestinal hemorrhage markedly increases the risk of development of spontaneous bacterial peritonitis. (Abstract) Gastroenterology 90:1763, 1986

107. Runyon BA. Low-protein-concentration ascitic fluid is predisposed to spontaneous bacterial peritonitis. Gastroenterology 91:1343, 1986

108. Runyon BA. Paracentesis of ascitic fluid: a safe procedure. Arch Intern Med 146:2259, 1986

109. Runyon BA. Amylase levels in ascitic fluid. J Clin Gastroenterol 9:172, 1987

110. Runyon BA. Ascitic fluid bilirubin concentration as a key to the diagnosis of choleperitoneum. J Clin Gastroenterol 9:543, 1987

111. Runyon BA. Ascitic fluid culture technique. Hepatology 8:983, 1988

112. Runyon BA. Cardiac ascites: a characterization. J Clin Gastroenterol 10:410, 1988

113. Runyon BA. Patients with deficient ascitic fluid opsonic activity are predisposed to spontaneous bacterial peritonitis. Hepatology 8:632, 1988

114. Runyon BA. Spontaneous bacterial peritonitis: an explosion of information. Hepatology 8:171, 1988

115. Runyon BA. Monomicrobial nonneutrocytic bacterascites: a variant of spontaneous bacterial peritonitis. Hepatology 12:710, 1990

116. Runyon BA, Antillon MR. Ascitic fluid pH and lactate: insensitive and nonspecific tests in detecting ascitic fluid infection. Hepatology 13:929, 1991

117. Runyon BA, Antillon MR, Akriviadis EA, McHutchison JG. Bedside inoculation of blood culture bottles with ascitic fluid is superior to delayed inoculation in the detection of spontaneous bacterial peritonitis. J Clin Microbiol 28:2811, 1990

118. Runyon BA, Antillon MR, McHutchison JG. Short term natural history of spontaneous bacterial peritonitis and culture-negative neutrocytic ascites prior to antibiotic treatment. Hepatology (submitted for publication)

119. Runyon BA, Antillon MR, Montano AA. Effect of diuresis versus therapeutic paracentesis on ascitic fluid opsonic activity and serum complement. Gastroenterology 97:158, 1989

120. Runyon BA, Akriviadis EA, Keyser AJ. The opacity of portal hypertension-related ascites correlates with the fluid's triglyceride concentration. Am J Clin Pathol 96:142, 1991

121. Runyon BA, Akriviadis EA, Sattler F, et al. Ascitic fluid and serum cefotaxime and desacetylcefotaxime levels in patients treated for bacterial peritonitis. Dig Dis Sci 36:1782, 1991

122. Runyon BA, Canawati HN, Akriviadis EA. Optimization of ascitic fluid culture technique. Gastroenterology 95:1351, 1988

123. Runyon BA, Canawati HN, Hoefs JC. Polymicrobial bacterascites: a unique entity in the spectrum of infected ascitic fluid. Arch Intern Med 146:2173, 1986

124. Runyon BA, Greenblatt M, Ming RHC. Hepatic hydrothorax is a relative contraindication to chest tube insertion. Am J Gastroenterol 81:566, 1986

125. Runyon BA, Hoefs JC. Ascitic fluid analysis in the differentiation of spontaneous bacterial peritonitis from gastrointestinal tract perforation into ascitic fluid. Hepatology 4:447, 1984

126. Runyon BA, Hoefs JC. Culture-negative neutrocytic ascites: a variant of spontaneous bacterial peritonitis. Hepatology 4:1209, 1984

127. Runyon BA, Hoefs JC. Is the concept of "exudative" ascites useful? (Letter) Hepatology 4:982, 1984

128. Runyon BA, Hoefs JC. Ascitic fluid analysis before, during, and after spontaneous bacterial peritonitis. Hepatology 5:257, 1985

129. Runyon BA, Hoefs JC. Spontaneous vs secondary bacterial peritonitis: differentiation by response of ascitic fluid neutrophil count to antimicrobial therapy. Arch Intern Med 146:1563, 1986

130. Runyon BA, Hoefs JC, Morgan TR. Ascitic fluid analysis in malignancy-related ascites. Hepatology 8:1104, 1988

131. Runyon BA, Juler GL. Natural history of umbilical hernias in patients with and without ascites. Am J Gastroenterol 80:38, 1985

132. Runyon BA, McHutchison JG, Antillon MR, et al. Short-course vs long-course antibiotic treatment of spontaneous bacterial peritonitis: a randomized controlled study of 100 patients. Gastroenterology 100:1737, 1991

133. Runyon BA, Montano AA, Akriviadis EA, et al. The serum–ascites albumin gradient is superior to the exudate–transudate concept in the differential diagnosis of ascites. Ann Intern Med 117:215, 1992

134. Runyon BA, Morrissey R, Hoefs JC, Wyle F. Opsonic activity of human ascitic fluid: a potentially important protective mechanism against spontaneous bacterial peritonitis. Hepatology 5:634, 1985

135. Runyon BA, Sugano S, Kanel G, Mellencamp M. A rodent model of cirrhosis and spontaneous bacterial peritonitis. Gastroenterology 100:489, 1991

136. Runyon BA, Umland ET, Merlin T. Inoculation of blood culture bottle with ascitic fluid: improved detection of spontaneous bacterial peritonitis. Arch Intern Med 147:73, 1987

137. Runyon BA, Van Epps DE. Diuresis of cirrhotic ascites increases its opsonic activity and may help prevent spontaneous bacterial peritonitis. Hepatology 6:396, 1986

138. Wilkins KW, Hoffman GS. Massive ascites in systemic lupus erythematosus. J Rheumatol 12:571, 1985

139. Salem HH, Dudley FJ, Merrett A, et al. Coagulopathy of peritoneovenous shunts: studies on the pathogenic role of ascitic fluid collagen and value of antiplatelet therapy. Gut 24:412, 1983

140. Salerno F, Badalamenti S, Incerti P, Capozza L, Mainardi L. Renal response to atrial natriuretic peptide in patients with advanced liver cirrhosis. Hepatology 8:21, 1988

141. Sampliner RE, Iber FL. High protein ascites in patients with uncomplicated hepatic cirrhosis. Am J Med Sci 256:257, 1974

142. Schrier RW. Pathogenesis of sodium and water retention in high-output and low-output cardiac failure, nephrotic syndrome, cirrhosis, and pregnancy. N Engl J Med 319:1065, 1988

143. Schrier RW, Arroyo V, Bernardi M, Epstein M, Henriksen JH, Rodes J. Peripheral arterial vasodilation hypothesis: a proposal for the initiation of renal sodium and water retention in cirrhosis. Hepatology 8:1151, 1988

144. Schweinberg FB, Seligman AM, Fine J. Transmural migration of intestinal bacteria: a study based on the use of radioactive Escherichia coli. N Engl J Med 242:47, 1950

145. Sheckman P, Onderdonk AB, Bartlett JG. Anaerobes in spontaneous peritonitis. Lancet 2:1223, 1977

146. Sherlock S, Shaldon S. The aetiology and management of ascites in patients with hepatic cirrhosis: a review. Gut 4:95, 1963

147. Singh MM, Bhargava AN, Jain KP. Tuberculous peritonitis. N Engl J Med 281:1091, 1969

148. Soriano G, Guarner C, Teixido M, et al. Selective intestinal decontamination prevents spontaneous bacterial peritonitis. Gastroenterology 100:477, 1991

149. Stanley MM, Ochi S, Lee KK, et al. Peritoneovenous shunting as compared with medical treatment in patients with alcoholic cirrhosis and massive ascites. N Engl J Med 321:1632, 1989

150. Strauss E, DeSa MDFG, Lacet CMC, et al. Standardization of a therapeutic approach for ascites due to chronic liver disease: a prospective study of 100 cases. Hepatology 7:409, 1987

151. Sungaila I, Bartle WR, Walker SE, et al. Spironolactone pharmacokinetics and pharmacodynamics in patients with cirrhotic ascites. Gastroenterology 102:1680, 1992

152. Targan SR, Chow AW, Guze LB. Role of anaerobic bacteria in spontaneous peritonitis of cirrhosis. Am J Med 62:397, 1977

153. Tito L, Gines P, Arroyo V, et al. Total paracentesis associated with intravenous albumin management of patients with cirrhosis and ascites. Gastroenterology 98:146, 1990

154. Tito L, Rimola A, Gines P, et al. Recurrence of spontaneous bacterial peritonitis in cirrhosis: frequency and predictive factors. Hepatology 8:27, 1988

155. Unikowsky B, Wexler MJ, Levy M. Dogs with experimental cirrhosis of the liver but without intrahepatic hypertension do not retain sodium or form ascites. J Clin Invest 72:1594, 1983

156. Varin E, Benoit F, Theoret Y, et al. Metabolism of spironolactone in control and cirrhotic subjects. Hepatology (Abstract) 10:616, 1989

157. Weinstein MP, Iannini PB, Stratton CW, et al. Spontaneous bacterial peritonitis: a review of 28 cases with emphasis on improved survival and factors influencing prognosis. Am J Med 64:592, 1978

158. Wilkinson P, Sherlock S. The effect of repeated albumin infusions in patients with cirrhosis. Lancet 2:1125, 1962

159. Wilson JAP, Suguitan EA, Cassidy WA, et al. Characteristics of ascitic fluid in the alcoholic cirrhotic. Dig Dis Sci 24:645, 1979

160. Wolfe GM, Runyon BA. Spontaneous *Salmonella* infection of high protein non-cirrhotic ascites. J Clin Gastroenterol 12:430, 1990

161. Xiol X, Castellote J, Baliellas C, et al. Spontaneous bacterial empyema in cirrhotic patients: analysis of eleven cases. Hepatology 11:365, 1990

Diseases of the Liver, Seventh Edition, edited by Leon Schiff and Eugene R. Schiff. J.B. Lippincott Company, Philadelphia © 1993.

36

Renal Complications in Liver Disease

Murray Epstein

Liver disease frequently is accompanied by a variety of alterations in renal function and electrolyte metabolism[43] (Table 36-1). These complications of liver disease are diverse and vary from those that have little clinical significance to others that constitute serious complications requiring therapeutic intervention.

Providing an overview of such a large and complex subject has made it necessary to select the information presented and to establish rather arbitrary priorities as to which areas receive more detailed discussion. In this review, emphasis is placed on abnormalities of renal sodium and water handling and on the syndromes of acute intrinsic renal failure (acute tubular necrosis [ATN]) and the hepatorenal syndrome (HRS), which often supervene in patients with severe liver disease.

Renal Sodium Handling

CLINICAL FEATURES

Patients with Laennec's cirrhosis manifest a remarkable capacity for sodium chloride retention; indeed, such patients frequently excrete urine that is virtually free of sodium.[34,43,63,67,77,83] As a result, there is excessive accumulation of extracellular fluid that eventually becomes evident as clinically detectable ascites and edema. Cirrhotic patients who are unable to excrete sodium continue to gain weight and accumulate ascites and edema as long as the dietary sodium content exceeds the maximal urinary sodium excretion. If access to sodium is not curtailed, the relentless retention of sodium may lead to the accumulation of vast amounts of ascites (on occasion up to 30 L). By contrast, weight gain and ascites formation promptly cease when sodium intake is restricted to a level below that of the maximal renal sodium excretion.

The abnormality of renal sodium handling in cirrhosis should not be regarded as a static and unalterable condition. Rather, cirrhotic patients in whom salt retention has occurred may undergo a spontaneous diuresis, followed by a return to avid salt retention.[67,83] Although a significant number of patients who are maintained on a sodium-restricted dietary program may demonstrate a spontaneous diuresis,[11] there is inadequate information about the incidence with which this

Portions of this chapter have been adapted from two earlier reviews by the author: Epstein M. Renal sodium handling in liver disease; and Epstein M. The hepatorenal syndrome. In: Epstein M, ed. The kidney and liver disease, ed 3. Baltimore, Williams & Wilkins, 1988, pp 3–30, 89–118.

occurs. Sometimes spontaneous diuresis occurs within a few days but more often within a few weeks after hospital admission. There is no reliable way of predicting which patients will demonstrate it and which will not.

Although ascites often is considered to be an indicator of decompensated hepatic disease, such is not always the case. The onset of ascites often can be related directly to an increased dietary sodium intake and is more a reflection of salt loading than of progressive alterations in hepatic function. Occasionally, a history of increased intake of salted foods in the period before the development of ascites can be elicited. The use of sodium-containing remedies such as antacids must be considered in these people.

Even when such precipitating events are ruled out, it is evident that there is a poor relation between abnormalities in renal sodium handling and the presence or absence of compensation. Although it frequently is stated that the abnormalities in renal sodium handling are restricted to the patient with frankly decompensated cirrhosis (ie, presence of clinically demonstrable ascites or edema), a review of the available data attempting to correlate renal sodium handling with a degree of compensation lends little support to this concept. It is not possible to predict the presence or magnitude of the impairment of renal sodium handling in the cirrhotic patient merely on the basis of the absence of ascites or edema.

Finally, the primary renal excretory abnormality causing fluid retention is a disturbance of sodium, rather than of water excretion. Many sodium-retaining patients with ascites and edema still are capable of excreting large volumes of dilute urine when given excessive amounts of water without sodium. When the water is ingested with sodium, however, it is not excreted.[97,126]

In contrast to the wealth of available data on renal sodium handling in cirrhosis, there is a paucity of information in *humans* on this subject in hepatic conditions other than cirrhosis.[35,40] In contradistinction to patients with Laennec's cirrhosis, in whom renal sodium retention is common, patients with primary biliary cirrhosis (PBC) do not appear to manifest this abnormality. Chaimovitz and coworkers[17] have assessed the natriuretic and diuretic response to extracellular fluid volume expansion in patients with PBC and demonstrated that the natriuretic and diuretic response exceeded that observed in both healthy normal volunteers and in edema-free patients with Laennec's cirrhosis. The authors suggested that a common mechanism may underlie both the augmented natriuretic response to volume expansion in their PBC patients and the rarity of fluid retention observed in this type of cirrhosis.

TABLE 36-1 *Renal Abnormalities in Liver Disease*

Parenchymal liver disease with secondary impairment of renal
    function
    Deranged renal sodium handling
    Impaired renal water excretion
    Impaired renal concentrating ability
    Hepatorenal syndrome
    Acute renal failure
    Glomerulopathies, associated with:
        Cirrhosis
        Acute viral hepatitis
        Chronic viral hepatitis
    Impaired renal acidification
Extrahepatic biliary obstruction with secondary impairment of
    renal function: acute renal failure

PATHOGENESIS

The pathogenetic events leading to the deranged sodium homeostasis of cirrhosis are exceedingly complex and remain the subject of continuing controversy. Rather than offer an exhaustive review of the diverse alterations in liver structure and function and the perturbations in circulatory homeostasis that may contribute to the renal sodium retention of liver disease, this discussion considers two major concepts that have received much attention.

An examination of the pathogenetic events leading to the deranged sodium homeostasis of cirrhosis is simplified by a consideration of so-called afferent events and efferent events.

A discussion of afferent events usually includes consideration of the detector element responsible for the recognition of the degree of volume alterations as well as a consideration of the extracellular fluid translocations or sequestrations into serous spaces or interstitial fluid compartments that characterize advanced liver disease. Because the afferent derangements that supervene in advanced liver disease have been reviewed in depth,[35,41] the concepts of a diminished effective volume and the overflow theory of ascites formation are reviewed here only briefly. The major emphasis is placed on the efferent events mediating sodium retention.

In considering the afferent events, it is worthwhile to consider two concepts that have been cited frequently in the pathogenesis of the abnormal sodium retention of liver disease—the role of a diminished effective volume and the overflow theory of ascites formation.

Afferent Events

Role of Diminished Effective Volume (Underfill Theory). Traditionally, it has been proposed that ascites formation in cirrhotic patients begins when a critical imbalance of Starling forces develops in the hepatic sinusoids and splanchnic capillaries (Fig. 36-1). This causes the formation of an excessive amount of lymph, exceeding the capacity of the thoracic duct to return lymph to the circulation.[6,24,130] Consequently, excess lymph accumulates in the peritoneal space as ascites, with a resultant contraction of circulating plasma volume. Thus, as ascites develops, there is a progressive redistribution of plasma volume. Although *total* plasma

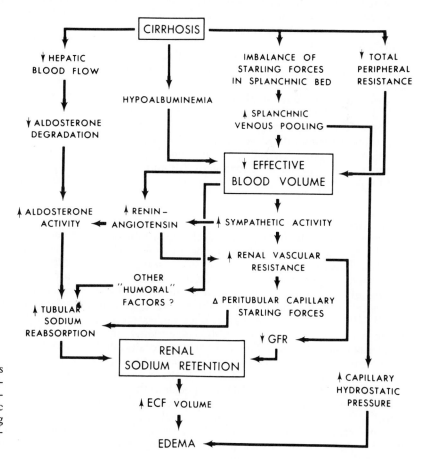

FIGURE 36-1 Schematic drawing of the factors operative in the traditional or underfill theory of sodium retention in cirrhosis. As can be seen, an imbalance of Starling forces in the hepatosplanchnic microcirculation is not the sole mechanism. Acting in concert, these factors promote a reduction in effective plasma volume.

volume may be increased in this setting, the physiologic circumstance may mimic a reduction in plasma volume (a reduced effective plasma volume). The diminished effective volume is thought to constitute an afferent signal to the renal tubule to augment salt and water reabsorption. The traditional formulations thus suggest that the renal retention of sodium is a *secondary* rather than a primary event.

The term *effective* plasma volume refers to that part of the total circulating volume that is effective in stimulating volume receptors. The concept is somewhat elusive, because the actual volume receptors remain incompletely defined. A diminished effective volume may reflect subtle alterations in systemic hemodynamic factors such as decreased filling of the arterial tree, a diminished central blood volume, or both. Because the stimulus is unknown and the afferent receptors are incompletely elucidated, alterations in effective volume must be defined in a functional manner, such as the kinetic response to volume manipulation.

Overflow Theory of Ascites Formation. During the past decade, an alternative hypothesis has been proposed. Lieberman and Reynolds and their associates[88,89] proposed the overflow theory of ascites formation. In contrast to the traditional formulation, the overflow theory suggests that the initiating or primary event is the inappropriate retention of excessive amounts of sodium by the kidneys, with a resultant expansion of plasma volume. In the setting of abnormal Starling forces (both portal venous hypertension and a reduction in plasma colloid osmotic pressure) in the portal venous bed and hepatic sinusoids, the expanded plasma volume is sequestered preferentially in the peritoneal space as ascites. Thus, according to this formulation, renal sodium retention and plasma volume expansion *precede* rather than follow the formation of ascites.

Since the promulgation of the overflow theory of ascites formation, controversy has centered on which of the two hypotheses is correct. Evidence cited in support of the overflow theory includes the demonstration that plasma volume is increased in cirrhosis with ascites, and the finding that increases in measured plasma volume have not been observed in cirrhotic patients with ascites undergoing a spontaneous diuresis also has been cited as evidence in support of the overflow hypothesis. Additional support derives from a series of elegant investigations carried out during the past decade by Levy[86,87] on dogs with experimental portal cirrhosis, investigations that demonstrate that renal sodium retention is the initial event and precedes the formation of ascites.

Although these observations collectively support the overflow theory of ascites formation, a number of clinical observations in *humans* are inconsistent with such a formulation. Thus, rapid volume expansion with exogenous solutions including saline, mannitol, and albumin frequently results in a transient improvement in renal sodium and water handling.[110,124,129] The results of many earlier studies must be considered inconclusive because of the confounding effects of the experimental designs. Studies from our laboratory during the past 25 years have circumvented many of the experimental problems of earlier studies by applying a unique investigative tool, the water immersion model, to the assessment of renal function and volume–hormonal relations.[39,58,61] Specifically, in contrast to saline administration, (1) water immersion is associated with a decrease in body weight, rather than the increase that attends saline infusion; (2) the volume stimulus of immersion is promptly reversible

after cessation of immersion, in contrast to the relatively sustained hypervolemia that follows saline administration, and thus constitutes an important attribute in minimizing any risk to the patient; and (3) the volume stimulus of immersion occurs in the absence of changes in plasma composition.[39,58,61]

Studies in 32 patients with decompensated cirrhosis demonstrated a striking normalization of renal sodium handling after water immersion. As shown in Figure 36-2, immersion resulted in marked natriuresis and kaliuresis in most of these patients. During the final hour of immersion, $U_{Na}V$ was 20-fold greater than it was during the prestudy hour. Thus, the marked antinatriuresis of cirrhosis was reversed promptly by a manipulation that merely altered the distribution of plasma volume without increasing (and often decreasing) total plasma volume. Indeed, in many instances, the natriuresis of such patients exceeded markedly the response manifested by normal subjects to the identical procedure. Taken together, these studies lend strong support to the concept that a diminished *effective* intravascular volume is a major determinant of the enhanced tubular reabsorption of sodium in patients with established cirrhosis.

Although I believe that the available evidence favors a prominent role for a diminished effective volume in mediating the avid sodium retention of many cirrhotic patients, it is important to underscore that these two formulations (ie, diminished effective volume and overflow theory) may not be mutually exclusive. Virtually all the available clinical studies of deranged sodium homeostasis were carried out at a time when decompensation was well established, with little information available about the incipient stage of sodium retention. The two ostensibly differing formulations may be reconciled by viewing the pathogenesis of abnormal sodium retention in cirrhosis as a complex clinical constellation in which differing forces participate in varying degrees as the derangement in sodium homeostasis evolves. Thus, it is conceivable that a primary defect in renal sodium handling may assume a more prominent role in the early stages of cirrhosis and a diminished effective volume may constitute the major determinant of sodium retention in many patients once the derangement is established.

Peripheral Vasodilation Theory. An additional theory has been promulgated to account for the pathogenesis of ascites formation—the peripheral vasodilation theory.[41] In some aspects, it is similar to the traditional underfill theory in that it focuses on the pivotal role of a diminished effective blood volume. The principal distinguishing feature, however, is the notion that the contracted effective volume is attributable primarily to an early increase in vascular capacitance. Thus, peripheral vasodilation is the initial determinant of intravascular underfilling, and an imbalance between the expanded capacitance and available volume constitutes a diminished effective volume. This concept brings the hypothesis into accord with some experimental observations that were not consistent with the original postulate. For example, careful balance studies in animals with experimental cirrhosis have shown clearly that sodium retention precedes ascites formation.[86]

Effectors of Renal Sodium Retention

The initial attempts to explain the abnormalities of renal sodium handling focused on the decrement in glomerular filtration rate (GFR), which occurs frequently in patients with

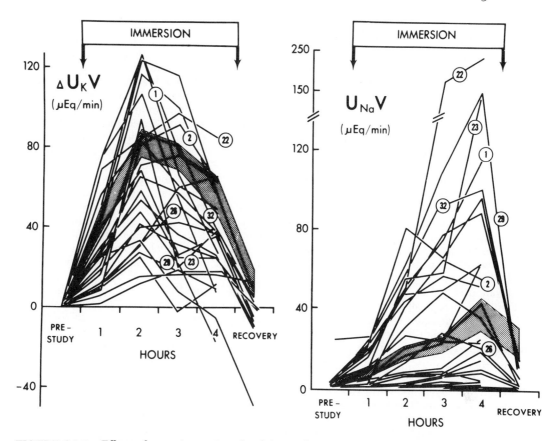

FIGURE 36-2 Effects of water immersion after 1 hour of quiet sitting (prestudy) on rate of sodium excretion ($U_{Na}V$) and potassium excretion (U_KV) in a large group of patients with alcoholic liver disease. The circled numbers represent individual patients. Data for U_KV are expressed in terms of absolute changes from prestudy hour (ΔU_KV). The shaded area represents the SEM for 14 normal control subjects undergoing an identical immersion study while ingesting an identical diet of 10 mEq sodium/100 mEq potassium per day. More than half of the cirrhotic patients manifested an appropriate or exaggerated natriuretic response. In general, the increase in $U_{Na}V$ was associated with a concomitant increase in ΔU_KV.

advanced liver disease. A number of observations indicate, however, that a decrease in GFR cannot constitute the major determinant of the abnormalities in renal sodium handling. Many observers have reported derangements in renal sodium handling despite preserved GFR. In fact, avid sodium reabsorption has been observed even in the face of supranormal GFR.[18,83]

Although the weight of evidence demonstrates that the renal sodium retention accompanying cirrhosis is attributable primarily to enhanced tubular reabsorption rather than to alterations in the filtered load of sodium, the precise nephron sites that are operative remain the subject of continuing controversy.[18,20,60,83]

The mediators of the enhanced tubular reabsorption of sodium in cirrhosis and their relative participation in the avid sodium retention have not been elucidated completely. Several mechanisms have been implicated or suggested, including hyperaldosteronism, alterations in intrarenal blood flow distribution, an increase in sympathetic nervous system activity, alterations in the endogenous release of renal prostaglandins, the possible role of a humoral natriuretic factor, and atrial natriuretic factor. These mechanisms and their interrelations are summarized schematically in Figure 36-2.

Role of Hyperaldosteronism. Cirrhosis frequently is associated with increased levels of aldosterone in the urine

as well as in peripheral plasma. The elevation of plasma aldosterone levels is attributable to both an increased adrenal secretion and decreased metabolic degradation of the hormone.[26,50,55,109] The rate of hepatic degradation is related directly to hepatic blood flow, which is markedly decreased in patients with decompensated cirrhosis.

Nevertheless, the etiologic relation between the hyperaldosteronism and the encountered sodium retention has not been fully delineated. The traditional viewpoint held that aldosterone is a *major* determinant of the sodium retention.[55] In contrast to this long-held traditional view, many lines of evidence have challenged the predominant etiologic role of elevated plasma aldosterone levels in mediating the sodium retention of cirrhosis. First, the widely held view that plasma aldosterone levels usually are elevated in advanced liver disease is probably an oversimplification.[55] Furthermore, increasing evidence demonstrates a dissociation between sodium excretion and plasma aldosterone in diverse clinical and experimental conditions,[55,109] thereby challenging the predominance of elevated plasma aldosterone levels in mediating the sodium retention of cirrhosis. Unfortunately, none of these studies attempted to assess in a kinetic manner the responses of plasma aldosterone and renal sodium excretion to acute volume manipulation. My coworkers and I investigated the role of aldosterone in mediating the abnormal renal sodium handling in cirrhosis by carrying out studies using a newly developed investigative tool, the model of head-out water immersion. Immersion studies during chronic spironolactone administration permitted a further elucidation of the relative contribution of aldosterone to the sodium retention.[59] Spironolactone administration without immersion resulted in only a modest increase in sodium excretion. In contrast, there was a marked increase in sodium excretion when immersion was carried out during chronic spironolactone administration, thereby indicating that the major contribution to the natriuresis was an enhanced distal delivery of filtrate.[59]

More compelling evidence mitigating against a predominant role for aldosterone in prompting the antinatriuresis of cirrhosis is derived from delete immersion studies kinetically assessing the relation of plasma aldosterone responsiveness to renal sodium handling.[50] Despite profound suppression of plasma aldosterone to comparable nadir levels in 16 cirrhotic patients, half of the patients manifested an absent or markedly blunted natriuretic response during immersion.[50] This demonstration of a dissociation between the suppression of circulating aldosterone and the absence of the natriuresis in these subjects lends strong support to the interpretation that aldosterone often is not the primary determinant of the impaired sodium excretion of cirrhosis.

Role of Renal Prostaglandins and Renal Sodium Handling. Evidence indicating that prostaglandins participate in mediating the sodium retention of cirrhosis should be considered. Because several studies indicate that alterations in prostaglandin release constitute a determinant of the natriuretic response to extracellular fluid volume expansion,[51] it is probable that alterations in renal prostaglandin synthesis may contribute to the derangements in renal sodium handling. Several studies have demonstrated clearly that the administration of nonsteroidal antiinflammatory drugs (NSAIDs; which act as inhibitors of prostaglandin synthetase) to patients with decompensated cirrhosis results in profound decrements of renal hemodynamics, GFR, and sodium excretion.[13,133] These provocative observations suggest a role for renal prostaglandins as determinants of the abnormal sodium retention of cirrhosis.

Because these studies have examined the effect of inhibiting endogenous production of renal prostaglandins, it was of great interest to assess an opposite experimental manipulation, namely, augmentation of endogenous prostaglandins.[51] We used water immersion to the neck, which redistributes blood volume with concomitant central hypervolemia and enhances prostaglandin E (PGE) excretion in normal subjects.[52] It was demonstrated that decompensated cirrhotic patients manifested an increase in mean PGE excretion that was three-fold greater than that observed in normal subjects studied under identical conditions.[51] This was attended by a marked natriuresis and an increase in creatinine clearance. Collectively, these observations suggest that derangements in renal PGE production contribute to the renal dysfunction of cirrhosis, including sodium retention. It is tempting to postulate that in the setting of cirrhosis of the liver, enhancement of prostaglandin synthesis is a compensatory or adaptive response to incipient renal ischemia.

It has been suggested that sulindac differs from other NSAIDs by sparing *renal* but inhibiting *systemic* prostaglandins.[16,21] This is reflected by the lack of an effect on urinary PGE_2 excretion and on other putative endpoints of renal prostaglandin synthesis such as renin release and response to furosemide, whereas inhibition of systemic prostaglandins is reflected by the decreased production of thromboxane by platelets.[14] If such findings are extrapolated to cirrhotic patients, one might anticipate that sulindac would be associated with the lowest incidence of sodium retention. Despite these impressive preliminary results, it has not been established whether sulindac is indeed renal sparing in cirrhotic patients. Indeed, Brater and associates[14] have reported that sulindac did not differ from ibuprofen in its ability to decrease urinary PGE_2 and that both decreased the pharmacodynamics of response to furosemide. Daskalopoulos and coworkers[28] compared the effects of sulindac and indomethacin on furosemide-induced augmentation of PGE_2 and on renal sodium and water handling. Although only indomethacin reduced creatinine clearance, urinary volume, sodium, and PGE_2 *before* furosemide administration, these differences were virtually abolished after furosemide administration. That is, indomethacin appeared only slightly more potent in reducing the diuresis (55% versus 38%), natriuresis (67% versus 52%), and PGE_2 release (81% versus 74%). Thus, under conditions of furosemide-enhanced prostaglandin activity, sulindac does affect renal function. To the extent that the ability to augment renal prostaglandin synthesis constitutes an important adaptive response in disorders characterized by decreased renal perfusion, the observations of Daskalopoulos and associates[28] merit attention. Additional studies are necessary to define the differences between sulindac and indomethacin in patients with cirrhosis, both under basal conditions and during maneuvers that alter (ie, augment) renal prostaglandin production.

Role of Sympathetic Nervous System Activity. An increase in sympathetic nervous system activity also contributes to the sodium retention in cirrhosis.[33] Thus, the decrease in central blood volume should favor an increase in renal sympathetic activity.[33,123] Furthermore, studies have demonstrated that an increase in sympathetic tone promotes an antinatriuresis both by altering intrarenal hemodynamics and by a direct tubular effect.[33]

Although these theoretic considerations suggest a role for the sympathetic nervous system in the sodium retention of cirrhosis, only relatively little data are available that bear directly on this possibility. Bichet and coworkers[9] have reported that patients with advanced cirrhosis manifest elevated concentrations of plasma catecholamines. These investigators proposed that the encountered catecholamine changes accounted for the impaired sodium and water handling in their patients.

Only recently have studies been initiated to assess the activity of the sympathetic nervous system in cirrhotic humans by measuring plasma catecholamine levels during basal conditions and after postural manipulations.[48,75,76,107] Ring-Larsen and colleagues[107] have determined plasma norepinephrine (NE) and epinephrine concentrations in differing vascular beds of cirrhotic patients at the time of hepatic venous catheterization. Based on differences in regional NE levels, they concluded that the elevated NE levels in patients with cirrhosis were attributable to enhanced sympathetic nervous system activity rather than decreased metabolism.

Bichet and coworkers[9] examined the potential role of increased sympathetic activity in mediating the impaired sodium and water excretion in cirrhosis. They reported that patients with advanced cirrhosis manifest elevated concentrations of plasma NE. In addition to documenting an increase in NE, they correlated plasma NE levels with the ability to excrete an acute water load in 26 patients with cirrhosis.

Although most observers agree that mean peripheral NE levels are elevated in cirrhotic patients,[50–52] it is an oversimplification to suggest that such alterations in catecholamine metabolism affect all cirrhotic patients with deranged sodium and water homeostasis. We examined the relation between plasma NE levels and renal sodium and water handling during immersion-induced central blood volume expansion.[48] Although mean NE levels were elevated for the group as a whole, more than half of the patients with decompensated cirrhosis manifested appropriate (nonelevated) NE levels. Furthermore, NE levels did not correlate with alterations in renal sodium or water excretion[48] (Figs. 36-3 and 36-4).

The available data on the role of the sympathetic nervous system in cirrhotic humans may be summarized as fragmentary and inconclusive. More direct indices of autonomic activity (such as renal venous NE levels rather than peripheral plasma levels) are required to determine whether diminished

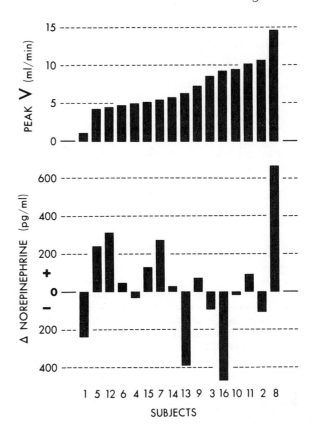

FIGURE 36-4 Relation between renal water handling (**upper panel**) and alterations in plasma norepinephrine (NE) (**lower panel**) during immersion in 16 cirrhotic patients. The numbers along the horizontal axis designate individual patients. As can be seen, the magnitude of the diuresis, as assessed by peak V, varied independently of ΔNE (nadir minus prestudy NE) during immersion ($r = .239$; NS). (Epstein M, Larios O, Johnson G. Effects of water immersion on plasma catecholamines in decompensated cirrhosis: implications for deranged sodium and water homeostasis. Miner Electrolyte Metab 11:25–34, 1985)

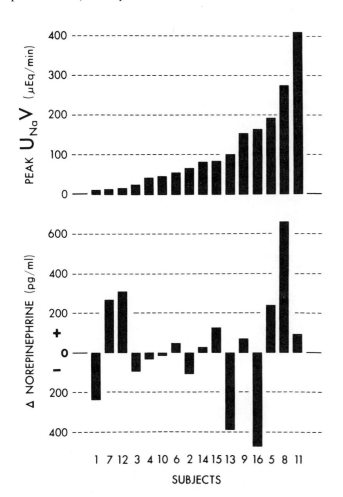

FIGURE 36-3 Relation between renal sodium excretion (**upper panel**) and alterations in plasma norepinephrine (NE) (**lower panel**) during immersion in 16 cirrhotic patients. The numbers along the horizontal axis designate individual patients. As can be seen, the magnitude of the natriuresis, as assessed by peak $U_{Na}V$, varied independently of ΔNE (nadir minus prestudy NE) during immersion ($r = .256$; NS). (Epstein M, Larios O, Johnson G. Effects of water immersion on plasma catecholamines in decompensated cirrhosis: implications for deranged sodium and water homeostasis. Miner Electrolyte Metab 11:25–34, 1985)

effective volume with a concomitant increase in sympathetic activity, both in the kidney and in other regional vascular beds, contributes to the sodium retention of cirrhosis.[66]

Role of Humoral Natriuretic Factor. Several lines of evidence have suggested the possibility that a circulating natriuretic factor constitutes a component part of the biologic control system regulating sodium excretion in humans.[15] The presence of this natriuretic factor also has been demonstrated in *normal* subjects during immersion-induced volume expansion[47] and during mineralocorticoid escape. Because this natriuretic factor is operative in uremia and because it also has been proposed to play a role in the regulation of sodium excretion in normal physiologic states, it is conceivable that deficiencies of this hormone could mediate, at least in part, the sodium retention of cirrhosis (see Fig. 36-2). Implicit in this concept is the hypothesis that sodium retention results from a failure to elaborate natriuretic hormone when extracellular fluid volume increases in response to renal sodium retention.

Several preliminary observations using bioassay systems are consistent with such a formulation.[64,93] Additional studies are needed to assess the precise role of a natriuretic factor in the pathogenesis of sodium retention in cirrhosis.

Role of Atrial Natriuretic Factor. In contrast to cardiac glycoside–like compounds, there are additional circulating natriuretic factors that can be differentiated by virtue of their failure to inhibit Na^+-K^+-ATPase. These mediators have been called atrial natriuretic factors (ANF) or atriopeptins. It has been shown that mammalian atria contain potent natriuretic and vasoactive peptides, which have been referred to as ANF and auriculin.[31,90] Several laboratories have purified, sequenced, and synthesized atrial peptides that have the natriuretic and vasoactive properties of crude atrial extract. Studies in intact animals have demonstrated that ANF decreases blood pressure and increases GFR and sodium excretion without a sustained increase in renal plasma flow. In addition, synthetic auriculin decreased renin secretory rate, plasma renin levels, and plasma aldosterone levels. Taken together, these observations suggest an important potential role for ANF in the regulation of blood pressure, renal function, and sodium–volume homeostasis.

In light of several lines of evidence suggesting that stretch receptors residing in the atria may participate in regulating volume homeostasis,[69] it is tempting to attribute a cardinal role to this peptide in modulating renal sodium handling in both normal people and in patients with edematous disorders including chronic liver disease. Specifically, the sodium retention and activation of the renin–angiotensin–aldosterone system in patients with cirrhosis may result from a failure to elaborate ANF when extracellular fluid volume increases in response to renal sodium retention.

Despite such theoretic considerations, evidence indicates that a deficiency of circulating ANF levels per se does not account for the sodium retention. Most studies have demonstrated that plasma ANF levels in cirrhotic patients with ascites are not suppressed; indeed, they tend to be elevated, exceeding those of normal subjects studied under similar conditions.[41,45,54] Studies of ANF responsiveness using stimulatory maneuvers, including water immersion and peritoneovenous shunting, disclosed that ANF is released appropriately.[45,54]

Studies encompassing infusions of ANF and maneuvers that augment ANF release, including water immersion and peritoneovenous shunting, all have disclosed that some patients manifest renal refractoriness to ANF. It is conceivable that renal vasoconstriction mediated by diverse mechanisms, including activation of the renin–angiotensin and the sympathetic nervous system, impede the ability of ANF to promote a natriuresis.[53,54]

SUMMARY

It is apparent that the renal sodium retention of advanced liver disease is a complex pathophysiologic constellation with numerous and diverse causes, each one of which may be operative to a varying degree during the course of the disease. Figure 36-5 represents an attempt to integrate these diverse findings and to summarize some of the mechanisms whereby these diverse hormonal mediators may act in concert to induce sodium retention.

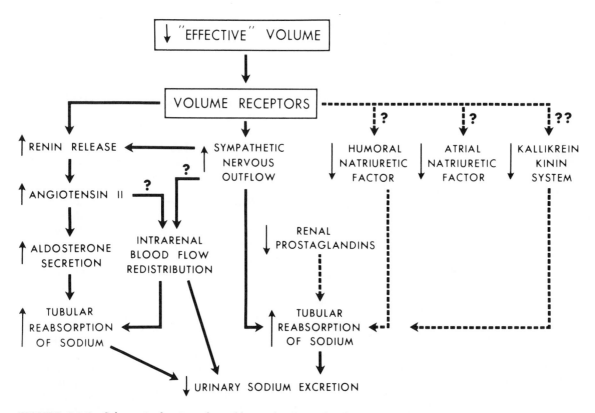

FIGURE 36-5 Schematic drawing of possible mechanisms whereby a diminished effective volume results in sodium retention. The solid arrows indicate pathways for which evidence is available. The dashed lines represent proposed pathways, the existence of which remains to be established. (Epstein M. Renal sodium handling in liver disease. In: The kidney in liver disease, ed 3. Baltimore, Williams & Wilkins, 1988, pp 3–30)

Management of Ascites and Edema

It is well established that ascites is associated with many unwanted side effects in the patient with liver disease.[23] Clearly, the marked accumulation of ascites is associated with significant discomfort. Ascites enhances the two prime precipitants of variceal bleeding—high portal pressure, which favors rupture of the varices, and gastroesophageal reflux, which may lead to erosion of the varices. Furthermore, it has been suggested that ascites is the sine qua non of spontaneous bacterial peritonitis.[25] Finally, the frequent association of ascites with the development of HRS raises the possibility that ascites may play an essential role in its pathogenesis.

Although ascites is indeed the "root of much evil," the decision to relieve ascites with diuretic agents should not be automatic. On the one hand, several studies have suggested that diuretic therapy in the cirrhotic patient may be associated with a substantial risk of adverse effects. Sherlock[116] surveyed diuretic-related complications occurring in a group of cirrhotic patients treated from 1962 to 1965 and reported an incidence of encephalopathy varying from 22% to 26% (depending on the diuretic used), hyponatremia varying from 40% to 49%, and azotemia (blood urea nitrogen greater than 40 mg/dL) ranging from 20% to 40%. The incidence of hypokalemia was marked (as high as 64%), and this complication persisted, albeit at a much lessened frequency, even when potassium-sparing diuretics such as spironolactone and amiloride were added. Although it may be argued that this 22-year-old survey may be unrepresentative and that this study was uncontrolled in nature, a subsequent report by Naranjo and coworkers[94] using a prospective drug surveillance program suggests that diuretic-induced complications in the cirrhotic patient continue to constitute formidable problems.

A RATIONAL APPROACH

The approach to the cirrhotic patient with ascites should be grounded on the realization that ascites, unless massive, may not require complete mobilization treatment per se. The initial goal of any treatment program should be an attempt to induce weight loss resulting from a spontaneous diuresis by consistent and scrupulous adherence to a well balanced diet with rigid dietary sodium restriction (250 mg/d). The sodium intake prescribed for cardiac patients (1200 to 1500 mg/d) is not sufficiently restrictive for the cirrhotic patient, who continues to gain weight on such a regimen. Although the frequency with which such dietary management successfully relieves ascites is unsettled, a sodium-restricted diet still should be prescribed to all patients, because it is impossible to predict which patients will respond.

In some symptomatic patients, however, less rigid sodium restriction may be advisable for several reasons. First, as a consequence of the anorexia, the patient eats only part of the meals offered and thus only a fraction of the daily sodium allowance. Second, in malnourished patients, nutrition clearly must have a priority over rigid sodium restriction.

When the response to dietary management is inadequate or when the imposition of rigid dietary sodium restriction is not feasible because of cost or unpalatability of the diet, the use of diuretic agents may be considered.

The rational basis of diuretic therapy lies in an understanding of the mechanisms and sites of action of the diuretic agent, coupled with an understanding of the pathophysiology of sodium retention in cirrhosis. Because the attributes and efficacy of the varying diuretic agents are reviewed in detail elsewhere,[37] only therapeutic considerations that are unique to the cirrhotic patient are considered here. When diuretics are used, the therapeutic aim is a gradual diuresis not exceeding the capacity for mobilization of ascitic fluid. Shear and associates[113] have demonstrated that ascites absorption averages about 300 to 500 mL/d during spontaneous diuresis and has as its upper limits 700 to 900 mL/d. Thus, any diuresis that exceeds 900 mL/d (in the ascitic patient without edema) is mobilized at the expense of the plasma compartment, with resultant volume contraction (Fig. 36-6).

Finally, the dangers of diuretic-associated hypokalemia should be emphasized.[100] Because total body potassium depletion frequently is associated with cirrhosis, the use of any diuretic that acts proximal to the distal potassium-secretory site may result in profound hypokalemia. Because of the frequently observed temporal relation between diuretic therapy and the development of hepatic encephalopathy, and the

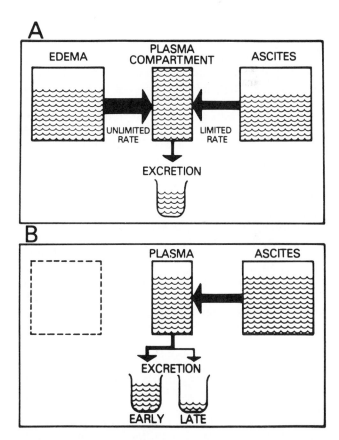

FIGURE 36-6 Schematic depiction of the mobilization and formation of fluid in extracellular fluid compartments in patients with fluid retention. The key to understanding this diagram is the realization that the rate of ascites mobilization is limited, whereas that of edema is relatively unlimited. (**A**) In the presence of ascites and edema, edema is recruited in an unlimited manner to equal the rate of diuresis. (**B**) In ascitic patients without edema, the rate of mobilization of ascitic fluid is limited (700 to 900 mL/d). Thus, any diuresis that exceeds 900 mL/d must be mobilized at the expense of the plasma compartment. (Adapted from a drawing by A. Miller, in Gabuzda GJ. Cirrhotic ascites: an etiologic approach to management. Hosp Pract 8[8]:67–74, 1973)

probability that the enhanced renal ammonia production of hypokalemia may be related to the encephalopathy,[100] great care should be exercised in monitoring and correcting potassium derangements in the cirrhotic patient receiving diuretics. The overriding consideration in diuretic therapy, however, is that its use as the sole indication of cosmetic improvement be clearly contraindicated.

CHOICE OF A DIURETIC AGENT

As discussed earlier, there is considerable sodium retention at both proximal and distal tubular sites in patients with liver disease. Although at first glance one may consider the therapeutic use of agents that act primarily by inhibiting proximal tubular reabsorption, such as carbonic anhydrase inhibitors or osmotic diuretics, they should not be prescribed. In general, despite their ability to promote proximal tubular rejection of filtrate, these agents, when administered *alone*, are only weakly natriuretic. This is attributable primarily to an enhancement of sodium reabsorption at distal tubular sites, which tends to counteract the proximal tubular effect of the drug.

If there is no compelling reason for rapidly mobilizing excessive fluid, one can initiate therapy with one of the distal potassium-sparing diuretics. Although such diuretics induce merely a modest natriuresis, this feature in a sense commends their use. With such drugs, the physician is less likely to exceed the guidelines suggested by Shear and coworkers.[113]

One can start with spironolactone, 100 mg daily. If this dosage of spironolactone does not induce a natriuresis, the dosage may be increased in stepwise fashion every 3 to 5 days to a maximum of 400 mg/d. Spironolactone's onset of action is slow, requiring 3 to 5 days for the peak effect to become manifest, so natriuresis does not occur during the initial 2 to 3 days of therapy. Such a regimen results in natriuresis in about half the patients.

Unfortunately, spironolactone is not free of side effects. It causes gynecomastia in a large fraction of cirrhotic patients who receive large doses. To circumvent this problem, it has been suggested that the other potassium-sparing diuretics, triamterene or amiloride, may constitute alternative medications for such patients. Both are nonsteroidal, natriuretic, potassium-sparing agents that both promote sodium excretion and limit potassium excretion even in the absence of mineralocorticoids. All three potassium-sparing diuretics have the potential to induce hyperkalemia (and hyperchloremic acidosis), which sometimes is of serious proportions.

If no natriuresis occurs with the maximal dosage of spironolactone, furosemide (Lasix), 40 to 80 mg/d, should be added. If no natriuresis is observed on this regimen, the physician should reassess dietary intake to ensure that the patient is not cheating. If dietary sodium intake is being restricted and if hepatic and renal function show no deterioration, one should consider increasing furosemide dosage in a stepwise fashion to a maximum of 240 mg/d.

Finally, in an attempt to minimize the complications of diuretic therapy, it has been proposed that intermittent administration is safer than continuous treatment. From the limited data available, such rest periods appear advisable. At the least, they provide adequate time to observe and detect any adverse effects and discontinue the therapy if so indicated.

DRUG–DIURETIC INTERACTIONS

For patients receiving spironolactone therapy, it would be wise to avoid the use of aspirin as an analgesic.[125] Although the interfering effect of aspirin on spironolactone-induced diuresis in cirrhotic ascitic patients has not been evaluated, observations made in normal subjects are sufficiently striking to advise that no aspirin-containing analgesics be used in patients who are undergoing spironolactone therapy. In normal subjects who were receiving exogenous mineralocorticoids, 600 mg of aspirin markedly blunted the effect of spironolactone.[125]

The detrimental effects of NSAIDs merit emphasis. NSAIDs are potent inhibitors of prostaglandin synthesis. In light of suggestions that the renal effects of loop diuretics may be attributable, at least in part, to an increased renal production of PGE_2,[19,29,118] it might be anticipated that the administration of NSAIDs may affect the natriuretic effect of loop diuretics. Studies have confirmed such suggestions.[5]

Studies in edematous patients with cirrhosis and cardiac failure have demonstrated that NSAIDs decreased the natriuretic response to furosemide.[92,132] Although NSAIDs cause a concomitant reduction of creatinine clearance, the available evidence suggests that these agents exert their effect primarily by an inhibition of the tubular action of furosemide rather than by an impairment of renal hemodynamics.[102] Regardless, the clinical importance is founded in a realization that NSAIDs often impair the natriuretic effects of *all* diuretics.

COMBINED THERAPY WITH THIAZIDE-TYPE AND LOOP DIURETIC AGENTS FOR RESISTANT SODIUM RETENTION

True resistance to conventional diuretic regimens is relatively unusual.[49] When true resistance is encountered, one proposed approach to management is the combined use of a thiazide-type diuretic with a loop diuretic. The addition of a relatively small dose of a diuretic agent that acts mainly in the cortical diluting segment of the distal nephron (eg, metolazone or thiazides) to a large but apparently ineffective dose of a potent loop diuretic agent (ie, furosemide, bumetanide, or ethacrynic acid) might not be expected to produce a massive natriuretic response. Nevertheless, a synergistic effect of such a combination has been documented in several reports, and successful fluid removal has occurred in patients with previously resistant severe sodium retention associated with diverse disorders, including hepatic cirrhosis.[49]

There is no question that diuretic combinations can constitute a highly efficacious means to relieve refractory edema. Nevertheless, despite the positive aspects of these regimens, increasing experience has resulted in disturbing observations regarding morbidity. Specifically, there is a growing awareness that the use of such combinations may be attended by a wide array of complications, including massive fluid and electrolyte losses and circulatory collapse.[96] Of particular concern in the cirrhotic patient is a major risk of profound hypokalemia that may occur with an alarming rapidity. Furthermore, such patients with a diminished effective volume are at risk of developing the HRS, ATN, and hepatic encephalopathy if an overly rapid diuresis occurs. As we explained in an editorial,[96] the potential risk may only rarely be justifiable in patients with liver disease. Rather, if there are compelling reasons for mobilizing excessive fluid (as discussed earlier), the physician should resort to the use of large-volume paracentesis or possibly the peritoneojugular shunt.

THERAPEUTIC PARACENTESIS

Because therapeutic paracentesis may induce hypovolemia, hyponatremia, renal failure, and encephalopathy, until recently its use in the treatment of refractory ascites has been limited. Previous studies have demonstrated a varied decrease in plasma volume after paracentesis. Furthermore, it has been suggested that ascites per se may have a negative influence on cardiac function. Several groups of investigators have reevaluated the effects of large-volume (4 to 25 L/d) or total paracentesis (complete mobilization of ascites in only one paracentesis session), concluding that these modalities constitute effective and relatively safe therapy for mobilizing ascites.[3] Extensive studies of Arroyo and associates have clearly established a role for large-volume paracentesis in the therapeutic armamentarium of refractory ascites. Their experience and that of others would dictate that there are relatively few side effects associated with this procedure. In addition, a number of investigators have demonstrated that less expensive plasma expanders such as dextran 70 can be successfully substituted for albumin.

There are several ongoing controlled trials comparing therapeutic paracentesis to peritoneovenous shunt in the management of patients with refractory ascites. We await their findings.

In summary, paracentesis has been shown to be highly effective in eliminating ascites with few adverse effects. The systemic and renal hemodynamic disturbances that lead to the refractoriness of ascites remain unmodified, however. Consequently, patients reaccumulate ascites rapidly, thereby requiring frequent paracentesis.

Renal Water Handling in Cirrhosis

CLINICAL FEATURES

The serum sodium level is determined by the balance of water in relation to that of sodium: too much water causes hyponatremia; too little causes hypernatremia. Hyponatremia connotes a serum sodium concentration (S_{Na}) below the lower limit of normal, that is, less than 135 mEq/L. In the cirrhotic patient, exchangeable sodium is increased. Therefore, if the patient is hyponatremic, the amount of water retained must be disproportionately greater than that of sodium. That is, there must be a specific defect in renal water excretion (ie, diluting capacity).

Impairment of renal diluting capacity occurs frequently in cirrhosis.[36,126] Hyponatremia, the expression of this impaired capacity to excrete water, is a commonly encountered clinical problem in cirrhotic patients. Indeed, hyponatremia probably represents the single most common electrolyte abnormality that confronts the physician treating patients with cirrhosis of the liver. For example, 20 of 50 (40%) patients with cirrhosis admitted to a liver unit in 1 year by Arroyo and associates[2] were found to have a serum sodium concentration below 130 mEq/L.

Although it has been suggested that this abnormality correlates with the severity of the hepatic disease, a critical review of the available data suggests that it is difficult to relate

the capacity of water diuresis with specific clinical features.[114,126] Whereas most compensated patients (ie, those without clinical evidence of ascites or edema, or both) excrete water normally, decompensated patients (those with ascites or edema, or both) manifest widely varying responses to oral water loading. Furthermore, prospective studies have indicated that the transition from compensation to decompensation, or vice versa, is not necessarily accompanied by concomitant changes in renal water handling.[126]

Aside from the increased frequency of spontaneous hyponatremia, there is an increased propensity for hyponatremia to develop in association with diuretic administration in patients with decompensated cirrhosis. Indeed, in an earlier survey of diuretic-related complications, Sherlock[116] observed that hyponatremia occurred in over 40% of cirrhotic patients treated with chlorothiazide, furosemide, or chlorothiazide plus spironolactone. Subsequent studies have confirmed the heightened susceptibility of cirrhotic patients to this complication.

The symptoms of hyponatremia associated with severe liver disease do not differ from those found in dilutional hyponatremia of other etiologies. Therein lies a diagnostic dilemma. These symptoms (difficulty in mental concentration, anorexia, headache, apathy, nausea, vomiting, and, occasionally, seizures) also can be observed in patients with hepatic coma or precoma but with normal serum sodium concentration. Thus, it often is difficult to ascertain if symptoms relate to the hyponatremia itself or to severe liver disease. In addition, one may observe an increase in serum sodium levels without significant changes in symptoms.

PATHOGENESIS

The mechanisms responsible for the impairment in renal water excretion in cirrhosis have not been elucidated completely, but several possibilities have been proposed. The two principal mechanisms are a decreased delivery of filtrate to the diluting segments of the nephron and enhanced antidiuretic hormone (ADH) activity. Additional mechanisms include a decrease in the release of endogenous renal prostaglandins and an increase in sympathetic nervous system activity.

Decreased Delivery of Filtrate to Diluting Segments of the Nephron

Theoretic considerations suggest that a decreased delivery of filtrate to the diluting segments of the nephron contribute to the impaired water excretion of cirrhotic patients. Many decompensated cirrhotic patients manifest a decrease in GFR.[35,41] Furthermore, much evidence suggests avid reabsorption of filtrate along the proximal tubule.[20,41,110] The demonstration that free water generation is improved in some cirrhotic patients after expansion with infusions of hypotonic saline or isotonic mannitol or saline and albumin[41,110,129] supports a role for increasing distal delivery of filtrate in the enhancement of water excretion.

Elevated Levels of Antidiuretic Hormone

Several lines of evidence suggest that the impairment in water excretion is attributable to increased levels of ADH, with a resultant increased back-diffusion of free water in the collecting tubule. Most of the experimental evidence supporting a role for vasopressin has been indirect, involving an assessment of the responses to the administration of agents that either alter ADH release or interfere with its peripheral actions. Thus, the ingestion of alcohol increased urine flow and decreased urine osmolality in severely decompensated cirrhotic patients with normal GFR.[122] Subsequently, the administration of demeclocycline, a tetracycline derivative that appears to antagonize the peripheral action of ADH, has been shown to enhance free water generation in patients with cirrhosis and ascites.[32]

The development of sensitive and specific radioimmunoassays for ADH has provided a more precise delineation of the frequency with which ADH levels are elevated. The available reports suggest that decompensated cirrhosis is associated with a wide spectrum of ADH levels varying from normal to elevated values.[7,62,104] The possible mechanisms for increased vasopressin levels in cirrhosis are multiple. It has been proposed that enhanced vasopressin activity may be mediated by known nonosmotic stimuli, including a decrease in peripheral resistance and arterial pressure.[8] Alternatively, abnormalities in the metabolic clearance of vasopressin may contribute to the increase in the vasopressin activity.

Alterations in Renal Prostaglandin Metabolism

Alterations in renal prostaglandins may contribute to the antidiuresis of cirrhosis by several mechanisms.[98,103] Prostaglandins have been shown to exert a number of functional effects on urinary concentrating and diluting mechanisms, and these have been reviewed in depth by Stokes[121] and by Raymond and Lifschitz.[103] The overall action of prostaglandins appears to be that of promoting free water excretion, and several mechanisms have been proposed to account for this effect. Although the role of renal prostaglandins is not yet fully established, most studies suggest that a relative diminution of renal prostaglandins may contribute to the antidiuresis of cirrhosis.[36,98,103] Such a formulation does not necessarily imply an absolute decrease in renal prostaglandins. Rather, a relative deficiency characterized by levels that may be appropriate in absolute terms but insufficient in light of the marked elevation of vasoconstrictor hormones may contribute to the pathogenesis of renal water retention.

Increase in Sympathetic Nervous System Activity

It is possible that an increase in efferent renal sympathetic nerve activity (ERSNA) also may contribute to the water retention of cirrhosis. Alterations in adrenergic nervous activity can modify renal water handling by several mechanisms.[33,123] Several studies have attempted to demonstrate a correlation between peripheral plasma NE levels and the impairment in renal water excretion,[9] demonstrating negative correlations between plasma NE and renal water excretion. Although most observers agree that mean peripheral NE levels are elevated in many cirrhotic patients, it would appear to be an oversimplification to suggest that such alterations in catecholamine metabolism affect all cirrhotic patients with deranged sodium and water homeostasis. Although an etiologic role for increased ERSNA is probable, more direct indices of autonomic activity are required to determine whether a diminished effective volume with concomitant increase in sympathetic activity, both in the kidney and in other areas, contributes to the water retention of cirrhosis.

TREATMENT

The impaired diluting ability afflicting many patients with advanced liver disease may have important implications for management. As has been emphasized, hyponatremia connotes a dilutional state secondary to an impaired capacity to excrete water. A sine qua non of this observation is that the rational basis for treating hyponatremia is fluid restriction. Regardless of the degree of dilutional impairment, appropriate fluid restriction eventually repairs this abnormality.

As a caveat, it must be emphasized that in many hospitals it is difficult to adhere to the physician's orders for fluid restriction. As examples, paramedical and nursing personnel may not consider the fluids administered with medication as part of the fluid restriction. We often are dismayed to observe pitchers of water and several containers of juice inadvertently placed at the bedside of patients thought to be severely fluid restricted. Thus, patients who ostensibly are on rigid fluid restriction may indeed be receiving 1500 or even 2000 mL/d fluid. It is not surprising that the serum sodium level of such patients does not increase or may even decrease. Because of this problem, it frequently is necessary to resort to absolute fluid restriction with levels approaching 0 to 200 mL/d for the first few days to initiate the return of the serum sodium level toward normal.

Although hyponatremia frequently is attributed to diuretic therapy, such an inference is somewhat simplistic. Although diuretics impair renal diluting ability, the diuresis that follows diuretic administration is characterized by a urine that is hypotonic relative to plasma. Therefore, hyponatremia does not ensue if concomitant water restriction is sufficient. Nevertheless, if the patient becomes severely hyponatremic while receiving diuretics, diuretic administration may have to be discontinued. This is particularly true in an outpatient setting because fluid restriction cannot be rigidly controlled.

Because many patients with advanced liver disease manifest an impairment of renal diluting ability, one may inquire when therapy should be instituted to normalize this disturbance. In light of experimental evidence suggesting that hyponatremia of even moderate degree (125 mEq/L or less) may result in irreversible neurologic deficits if allowed to persist, it seems reasonable to treat hyponatremia in all liver disease patients in whom the serum sodium level is less than 130 mEq/L.

Another major consideration sometimes not given sufficient attention is the inappropriate use of drugs that may adversely affect renal diluting capacity. Specifically, there may be numerous drugs administered to the cirrhotic patient that could impair renal diluting capacity. Examples include NSAIDs and chlorpropamide. For a more complete listing, the reader is referred to another source.[36]

The use of agents that block the hydroosmotic effect of ADH, such as demeclocycline, for the correction of hyponatremia in cirrhosis has been suggested by various investigators.[32,91] In view of the numerous reports of the appearance of renal failure in such patients treated with demeclocycline,[32,91] this drug should not be administered to cirrhotic patients.

Finally, in rare circumstances, the physician may be forced to consider the use of dialysis for the correction of severe hyponatremia in cirrhosis.[106] Such heroic measures, however, rarely are necessary, even in the most severely decompensated cirrhotic patient.

Another development that holds promise is the possible availability of vasopressin antagonists. The discovery of diuretic vasopressin analogues by Manning and Sawyer has spurred interest in designing vasopressin receptor antagonists as potential specific water diuretic (aquaretic) agents.[82,120] The mechanism of action is most probably antagonism of vasopressin at the renal epithelial receptor.

Syndromes of Acute Azotemia

ATN occurs with increased frequency in patients with hepatic and biliary disease. Although acute azotemia may often represent classic ATN, cirrhotic patients may also manifest a unique form of renal failure for which a specific cause cannot be elucidated—HRS. The following section reviews the spectrum of acute azotemic syndromes, including HRS and ATN in the setting of hepatic and biliary disease.

HEPATORENAL SYNDROME

Progressive oliguric renal failure commonly complicates the course of patients with advanced hepatic disease.[38] Although this condition has been designated by many names, including *functional renal failure* and *the renal failure of cirrhosis*, the more appealing albeit less specific term *hepatorenal syndrome* commonly has been used to describe this syndrome. For the purposes of this discussion, HRS may be defined as unexplained progressive renal failure occurring in patients with liver disease in the absence of clinical, laboratory, or anatomic evidence of other known causes of renal failure.

Clinical Features

A review of the clinical features of HRS reveals marked variability in both the clinical presentation and clinical course.[38] In the United States, HRS occurs usually in cirrhotic patients who are alcoholic, although cirrhosis is not a sine qua non for the development of HRS. HRS may complicate other liver diseases, including acute hepatitis and hepatic malignancy.[56,108,128] Renal failure may develop with great rapidity, often occurring in patients in whom normal serum creatinine levels have been documented within a few days of onset of HRS. The serum creatinine level may be a poor index of renal function in patients with chronic liver disease, often masking markedly reduced GFRs.[38] Implicit in such a formulation is the concept that HRS represents a progression in patients who already have markedly impaired renal function.

Numerous reports have emphasized the development of renal failure after events that reduce effective blood volume, including abdominal paracentesis, vigorous diuretic therapy, and gastrointestinal tract bleeding, although it can occur in the absence of an apparent precipitating event. In this context, several careful observers have noted that HRS patients seldom arrive in the hospital with preexisting renal failure. Rather, HRS seems to develop in the hospital, raising questions as to whether events in the hospital might precipitate this syndrome.[38] Virtually all HRS patients have ascites, which often is tense, and clinical stigmata of portal hypertension usually are present. The degree of jaundice is extremely variable. Although most reports suggest that HRS occurs in patients who manifest evidence of severe hepatocellular disease, HRS can occur with minimal jaundice and with little evidence of severe hepatic dysfunction.

Most patients have a modest decrease in systemic blood pressure, but significant hypotension occurs usually as a terminal event. Most patients die within 3 weeks of onset of azotemia, although occasional recoveries occur.[70] Rare patients have survived for several months with mild azotemia.

HRS patients manifest a rather characteristic urine excretory pattern, voiding urine that is practically sodium-free and retaining the capacity to concentrate urine to a modest degree.

Pathogenesis

Several lines of evidence have lent strong support to the concept that the renal failure in HRS is functional in nature. Despite the severe derangement of renal function, pathologic abnormalities are minimal and inconsistent.[38,115] Furthermore, tubular functional integrity is maintained during the renal failure, as manifested by an unimpaired sodium reabsorptive capacity and concentrating ability. Finally, more direct evidence is derived from the demonstration that kidneys transplanted from patients with HRS are capable of resuming normal function in the recipient.[84]

Despite extensive study, the precise pathogenesis of HRS remains obscure. Many studies using diverse hemodynamic techniques have documented a significant reduction in renal perfusion.[46,81,112] Because a similar reduction of renal perfusion is compatible with urine volumes exceeding 1 L in many patients with chronic renal failure,[79] it is unlikely that a reduction in mean blood flow per se is responsible for the encountered oliguria.

Our laboratory has applied the xenon-133 washout technique and selective renal arteriography to the study of HRS and has demonstrated a significant reduction in both mean renal blood flow and preferential reduction in cortical perfusion.[46] In addition, we carried out simultaneous renal arteriography to delineate further the nature of the hemodynamic abnormalities.[46] Selective renal arteriograms disclosed marked beading and tortuosity of the interlobar and proximal arcuate arteries and an absence of both distinct cortical nephrograms and vascular filling of the cortical vessels (Fig. 36-7A). Postmortem angiography carried out on the kidneys of five patients studied during life disclosed a striking normalization of the vascular abnormalities, with reversal of all the vascular abnormalities in the kidneys (see Fig. 36-7B). The peripheral vasculature filled completely, and the previously irregular vessels became smooth and regular. These findings provide additional strong evidence for the functional basis of the renal failure, operating through active renal vasoconstriction.

Although renal hypoperfusion with preferential renal cortical ischemia has been shown to underlie the renal failure of HRS, the factors responsible for sustaining the reductions in cortical perfusion and the suppression of filtration in HRS have not been elucidated. Several major possibilities have been suggested, including the renin–angiotensin system, alterations in the endogenous release of renal prostaglandins, an increase in sympathetic nervous system activity, changes in the kallikrein–kinin system, and endotoxemia. These proposed mechanisms and their interrelations are summarized schematically in Figure 36-8.

Renin–Angiotensin System. Several lines of evidence have suggested a role for the renin–angiotensin axis in sustaining the vasoconstriction in HRS.[78] Patients with de-

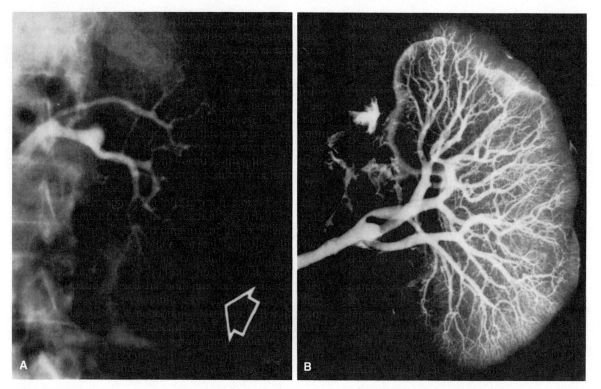

FIGURE 36-7 (A) Selective renal arteriogram performed in a patient with oliguric renal failure and cirrhosis. Note the extreme abnormality of the intrarenal vessels, including the primary branches off the main renal artery and the interlobar arteries. The arcuate and cortical arterial system is not recognizable, nor is a distinct cortical nephrogram present. The arrow indicates the edge of the kidney. (B) Postmortem angiogram on the same kidney with the intraarterial injection of micropaque in gelatin as the contrast agent. Note filling of the renal arterial system throughout the vascular bed to the periphery of the cortex. The peripheral arterial tree that did not opacify in vivo now fills completely. The vascular attenuation and tortuosity are no longer present. The vessels also were histologically normal. (Epstein M, Berk DP, Hollenberg NK, et al. Renal failure in the patient with cirrhosis: the role of active vasoconstriction. Am J Med 49:175–185, 1970)

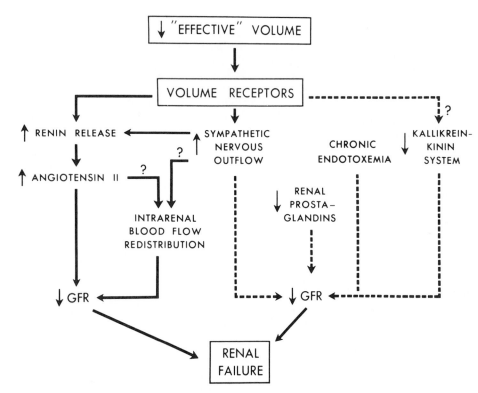

FIGURE 36-8 Schematic representation of possible mechanisms whereby a diminished effective volume might modulate a number of hormonal effectors, eventuating in renal failure. Solid arrows indicate pathways for which evidence is available; dashed arrows represent proposed pathways, the existence of which remains to be established.

Syndromes of Acute Azotemia

compensated cirrhosis with or without HRS frequently manifest marked elevations of plasma renin–angiotensin levels attributable to both decreased hepatic inactivation of renin and increased renin secretion by the kidney (Fig. 36-9).[78,111] Often, the elevation of plasma renin–angiotensin occurs despite the presumed failure of hepatic synthesis of the α_2-globulin, renin substrate. There are at least two alternative explanations for the persistence of high renin levels in cirrhosis. First, it is possible that the renal hypoperfusion is the primary event, with a resultant activation of the renin–angiotensin system. Alternatively, the activation of the renin–angiotensin system (perhaps in response to a diminished effective blood volume) may constitute the primary event. In light of compelling experimental evidence that angiotensin plays an important role in the control of the renal circulation,[79] it is tempting to speculate that enhanced angiotensin levels contribute to the renal vasoconstriction and reduction in glomerular filtration rate of renal failure in cirrhosis (see Fig. 36-9).

Renal Prostaglandins.   It is probable that renal prostaglandins participate in mediating the renal failure of cirrhosis. Initially, this possibility was assessed by examining the renal hemodynamic response to the administration of exogenous prostaglandins.[1] Unfortunately, the relevance of such studies in cirrhotic patients is tenuous, because other studies suggest that any action of prostaglandins on the kidney must be as a local tissue hormone.[44,103] Thus, any evaluation of the physiologic role of prostaglandins on renal function necessitates an experimental design in which the endogenous production of the lipids is altered. Indeed, subsequent investigations of the role of prostaglandins on renal function have focused on comparisons before and after the administration of inhibitors of prostaglandin synthetase. Such studies have demonstrated that the administration of inhibitors of prosta-

glandin synthetase (both indomethacin and ibuprofen) resulted in a lowering of plasma renin activity and plasma aldosterone levels and marked decrements in GFR.[13,133]

Thromboxanes and Renal Function in Cirrhosis.   Thromboxane levels are elevated in cirrhotic patients with renal dysfunction.[105,135] Studies conducted by Zipser and coworkers[135] suggest that the ratio of the vasodilator PGE_2 to the vasoconstrictor prostaglandin thromboxane A_2 (TxA_2)—the ratio PGE_2/TxA_2—rather than the absolute levels of PGE_2 may modulate the renal vasoconstriction of HRS. Urinary excretion of PGE_2 and thromboxane B_2 (TxB_2, the nonenzymatic metabolite of TxA_2) was measured in 14 patients with HRS. It was observed that whereas PGE_2 levels were decreased compared with those of healthy controls and patients with ATN, TxB_2 levels were markedly elevated. The authors interpreted their data to suggest that an imbalance of vasodilator and vasoconstrictor metabolites of arachidonic acid contributes to the pathogenesis of HRS. Additional studies are needed to confirm such alterations.

There has been an attempt to modify the course of HRS by administration of selective inhibitors of thromboxane synthesis.[134] Whereas *nonspecific* cyclooxygenase inhibitors, such as indomethacin and aspirin, reduce both thromboxane and prostaglandin synthesis to varying degrees in different biologic systems, *selective* inhibitors of thromboxane synthesis preserve or possibly increase the production of other metabolites of arachidonic acid, such as the potent vasodilator prostacyclin. Zipser and associates[134] administered the thromboxane synthetase inhibitor, dazoxiben, to patients with alcoholic hepatitis and progressive azotemia. Although administration of dazoxiben reduces the urinary excretion of the thromboxane metabolite TxB_2 by about half, PGE_2 and 6-keto prostaglandin $F_{1\alpha}$ ($PGF_{1\alpha}$) were essentially unaltered. Despite reduction in thromboxane excretion, there was no

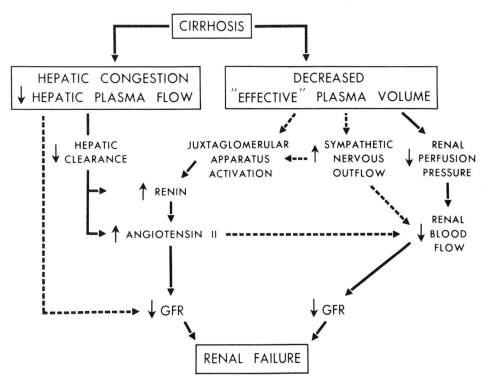

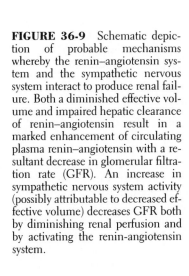

FIGURE 36-9 Schematic depiction of probable mechanisms whereby the renin–angiotensin system and the sympathetic nervous system interact to produce renal failure. Both a diminished effective volume and impaired hepatic clearance of renin–angiotensin result in a marked enhancement of circulating plasma renin–angiotensin with a resultant decrease in glomerular filtration rate (GFR). An increase in sympathetic nervous system activity (possibly attributable to decreased effective volume) decreases GFR both by diminishing renal perfusion and by activating the renin-angiotensin system.

consistent reversal of the progressive renal deterioration.[134] Unfortunately, most of the patients had far advanced disease and may not have been capable of responding to therapeutic interventions. Additional studies with selective thromboxane inhibitors in patients with widely varying degrees of acute renal insufficiency are required to establish definitively the role of TxA_2 as a major determinant of the renal vasoconstriction in HRS.

Kallikrein–Kinin System. The available evidence suggests that bradykinin and other kinins synthesized in the kidney may participate in the modulation of intrarenal blood flow and renal function. Measurements of plasma prekallikrein levels in patients with HRS disclosed undetectable levels in many such patients,[95] raising the possibility that the decrease in prekallikrein levels results in diminished kinin formation. Because bradykinin has been suggested to be a physiologic renal vasodilator, it is possible that failure of bradykinin formation may contribute to the renal cortical vasoconstriction encountered in HRS.

Endotoxins. It has been proposed that systemic endotoxemia may participate in the pathogenesis of the renal failure of cirrhosis.[12,38] The increased endotoxin levels might result from incomplete hepatic inactivation and portosystemic shunts of material of gastrointestinal origin in cirrhotic patients. Because several investigators have indeed demonstrated a high frequency of positive Limulus assays in cirrhotic patients with renal failure but not in the absence of renal failure, it is conceivable that endotoxins might contribute to the pathogenesis of the renal failure. This interesting hypothesis awaits additional study and confirmation.

Endotoxemia is appealing as a possible humoral agent, not only because it may cause renal vasoconstriction but also because it may produce vasodilatation in other circulatory beds and may be a treatable condition.[12] It has been proposed that the endotoxemia of cirrhosis induced nitric oxide synthesis in peripheral blood vessels directly, or indirectly through cytokines, and that this increased nitric oxide synthesis and release accounts for the associated hyperdynamic circulation.[127]

Although endotoxemia frequently is observed in patients with chronic liver disease, its role in contributing to the development of renal failure is unclear. Attempts to correlate the occurrence of renal failure with the presence of endotoxemia are conflicting. On the one hand, Clemente and associates[22] observed endotoxemia in 9 of 22 patients with HRS but not in any cirrhotic patients with normal GFRs. On the other hand, Gatta and colleagues[68] demonstrated that in patients with cirrhosis without overt renal failure, renal vasoconstriction did not seem to be related to endotoxemia.

Coratelli and colleagues[27] have observed two patients before and after the development of HRS and demonstrated the appearance of endotoxemia coincident with the development of HRS.

ACUTE INTRINSIC RENAL FAILURE

Although much attention has been directed to HRS, it must be emphasized that cirrhotic patients are no less vulnerable than noncirrhotic patients to the development of acute intrinsic renal failure (ATN). Indeed, a review of several published series discloses that among liver disease patients who manifested renal failure, the etiology of the renal failure was

more commonly ATN than HRS.[38] The increased frequency of ATN relates to the hypotension, bleeding dyscrasias, infection, and multiple metabolic disorders that often complicate the course of these patients.

Finally, the association between obstructive jaundice and ATN merits comment. Dawson[30] noted that of patients undergoing operation for the relief of obstructive jaundice, the incidence of ATN was many times greater than that encountered in a comparable group of nonjaundiced patients. It was further noted that the greater the degree of jaundice, the greater the risk of ATN. The demonstration that the risk of ATN is higher in the most deeply jaundiced patients prompted an investigation of the mechanisms in the Gunn rat (a species unable to conjugate bilirubin).[4] These studies suggest that circulating *conjugated* bilirubin was responsible for the increased proclivity toward development of renal failure in jaundiced animals. There is a lack of unanimity of opinion, however, regarding the uniqueness of the association of biliary tract disease and ATN.[10]

Differential Diagnosis

The abrupt onset of oliguria in a cirrhotic patient does not necessarily imply the presence of HRS. Prerenal causes are important to differentiate, particularly because they constitute reversible conditions if recognized and treated in the incipient phase. Volume contraction or cardiac pump failure may present as a pseudohepatorenal syndrome. Furthermore, as already mentioned, it is common for classic ATN to develop in patients with alcoholic cirrhosis. In many instances, the differentiation from HRS can be made readily by recognition of the precipitating event and by characteristic laboratory findings. Table 36-2 lists laboratory features helpful in differentiating the three principal causes of acute azotemia in the patient with liver disease. The most uniform finding in the urine of HRS patients is a strikingly low sodium concentration, usually less than 10 mEq/L, and occasionally as low as 2 to 5 mEq/L. Similarly, prerenal azotemia is associated with low urinary sodium concentrations. In contrast, patients with oliguric ATN frequently have urinary sodium concentrations exceeding 30 mEq/L and usually even higher. Both HRS and prerenal azotemia manifest well-maintained urinary concentrating ability characterized by a urine/plasma osmolality ratio greater than 1.0, whereas ATN patients excrete an isosmotic urine. Urine/plasma creatinine ratio is greater than 30 in both prerenal failure and HRS, whereas it is less than 20:1 in ATN. Proteinuria is absent or minimal in HRS.

In summary, the finding of a low urinary sodium concentration in the presence of oliguric ATN precludes the diagnosis of ATN. Only when prerenal failure and ATN are excluded can the diagnosis of HRS be established.

Treatment

The management of the HRS generally has been discouraging in view of the absence of any effective treatment modality. Because knowledge about the pathogenesis of HRS is inferential and incomplete, therapy must be primarily supportive. The initial step in management is not to equate decreased renal function with HRS but rather to search diligently for and treat correctable causes of azotemia such as volume contraction, cardiac decompensation, and urinary tract obstruction. The diagnosis of ATN should be considered, because cirrhotic patients with ATN may recover if supported with dialytic therapy.

TABLE 36-2 *Differential Diagnosis of Acute Azotemia in a Patient With Liver Disease: Important Differential Urinary Findings*

Urinary Finding	Prerenal Azotemia	Hepatorenal Syndrome	Acute Renal Failure
Sodium concentration (mEq/L)	<10	<10	>30
Urine/plasma creatinine ratio	>30:1	>30:1	<20:1
Osmolality	At least 100 mOsm greater than plasma osmolality	At least 100 mOsm greater than plasma osmolality	Equal to plasma osmolality
Sediment	Normal	Unremarkable	Casts, cellular debris

Once the correctable causes of renal functional impairment are excluded, the mainstay of therapy is careful restriction of sodium and fluid intake. Although a number of specific therapeutic measures have been attempted, only orthotopic liver transplantation has proved to be of practical value. Attempts at volume expansion with different exogenous expanders and exchange transfusion have resulted in only transient improvement in renal hemodynamics and function without significant improvement in the outcome.[38,80,124] Similarly, attempts at reinfusion of ascites using peritoneal fluid that has been concentrated have not provided any lasting improvement.

Dialysis has been reported to be ineffective in the management of HRS. My own experience, however, suggests that such a sweeping condemnation should be qualified. Although most of the published literature indeed suggests a dismal prognosis for patients who undergo dialysis, such reports have dealt with patients with chronic end-stage liver disease.[99] Our experience suggests that in selected patients, that is, patients with *acute* hepatic dysfunction in whom there is reason to believe that the renal failure may reverse coincident with resolution of the acute hepatic insult, dialytic therapy is indicated.[57,99]

A relatively recent development in the management of HRS is the introduction of the peritoneojugular shunt.[42,101,119] The past several years have witnessed a flurry of enthusiasm for the use of the peritoneojugular shunt (LeVeen shunt) in the management of HRS. Unfortunately, many reports have been anecdotal, with insufficient details to allow critical assessment. Even where sufficient data were available, we must conclude most putative successes occurred in patients who were not clearly documented to have HRS; rather, many patients probably had reversible azotemia secondary to a diminished effective blood volume. Furthermore, there is increasing awareness that the widespread use of the peritoneojugular shunt has been attended by a wide array of complications.[42,73]

The few well-documented cases in which the peritoneojugular shunt was successful in reversing HRS do not justify the growing and uncritical trend to resort to this modality in the treatment of virtually any cirrhotic patient with azotemia. The peritoneojugular shunt cannot yet be viewed as established therapy until its value is determined by appropriate peer-reviewed clinical trials. I would consider its use in hemodynamically stable HRS patients in whom hypovolemia has been clearly excluded. It is hoped that in the next few years several ongoing clinical trials will assist us in selecting those HRS candidates who stand to benefit most from such a procedure.

Orthotopic Liver Transplantation. Orthotopic liver transplantation (OLTX) has become the accepted treatment for end-stage liver disease.[71,74] Many of these patients present with varying degrees of concomitant renal dysfunction, including HRS. OLTX has been reported to reverse HRS acutely.[72,80a] Recently, Gonwa and colleagues[71] reviewed the extensive experience of the Baylor University transplant group and have reported a good, long-term survival with return of acceptable renal function for prolonged periods. They retrospectively reviewed the first 308 patients undergoing OLTX. The incidence of HRS was 10.5%. HRS patients manifested an increase in GFR from a baseline of 20 ± 4 mL/min to a mean of 33 ± 3 mL/min at 6 weeks, with a further increase to 46 ± 6 mL/minute at 1 year. GFR remained stable at 2 years after surgery (38 ± 6 mL/min). There was no difference in perioperative (90-day) mortality rates between HRS and non-HRS patients, despite a worse preoperative status and a rockier postoperative course. The actuarial 1- and 2-year survival rate for the HRS patients was 77%, not different from non-HRS patients. These investigators concluded that with aggressive pretransplant and posttransplant management, excellent results can be anticipated after OLTX in patients with HRS.

Newer Experimental Modalities. As noted previously, NSAIDs have been shown to induce reversible decrements in renal perfusion and renal function in patients with decompensated cirrhosis.[13,44,133] Conversely, we have shown that augmentation of renal prostaglandins induced by water immersion is associated with marked increments in creatinine clearance.[51] Fevery and associates[65] attempted to extend these observations by investigating the effects of administration of a PGE$_1$ analogue (misoprostol) on renal function in four patients with alcoholic cirrhosis and HRS. In response to misoprostol, 0.4 mg orally four times daily, and albumin infusions, urine volume increased three- to four-fold. Concomitantly, serum creatinine levels diminished. All patients had hyponatremia that normalized with misoprostol administration. Although the experience is preliminary, it raises the possibility that provision of exogenous prostaglandins may have a salutary role in the management of HRS.

Vasoconstrictor Therapy. As noted, patients with decompensated liver disease manifest a hyperdynamic circulation characterized by increased cardiac index and heart rate, as well as decreased systemic vascular resistance.[41] Indeed, the peripheral vasodilation theory postulates that peripheral vasodilation and an early increase in vascular capacitance constitute cardinal events in the pathogenesis of ascites and HRS. There has been renewed interest in the hemodynamic arrangement and attempts to improve renal function by countervailing this hyperdynamic state. Lenz and colleagues[85] investigated the effects of infusion of ornipressin on renal and circulatory function. They demonstrated that ornipressin reversed the hyperdynamic state. Concomitantly, there is improvement in renal function as assessed by a more than 70% increase in creatinine clearance and a doubling in urine flow. These preliminary observations lend support to the concept that the peripheral vasodilation of liver disease contributes importantly to the renal dysfunction. Consequently, maneuvers that counter the vasodilatation may possibly prove of benefit in improving renal function.

Summary

Renal functional abnormalities in patients with advanced liver disease constitute complex pathophysiologic constellations with numerous and diverse causes. Although our understanding of the many ways in which the liver affects renal processes is inevitably incomplete, it is apparent that the past several years have witnessed much progress in the delineation of the abnormalities of renal sodium and water handling that characterize advanced liver disease. Advances in the measurement of renal vasoactive hormones (including renal eicosanoids), which have been demonstrated to affect renal hemodynamics and renal sodium handling, are providing a basis for a more complete understanding of the mechanisms that promote sodium retention in cirrhosis. These insights provide a more rational basis for the management of the patient with liver disease who has impairment of renal sodium and water excretion.

Although there has been some progress in characterizing the pathogenesis of HRS, therapy of this disorder is largely empiric. Any future breakthroughs in the definitive treatment of HRS will be predicated on greater clarification of mechanisms and delineation of mediators. The role of hemodialysis has undergone reappraisal, and it is apparent that dialysis may be warranted as a supportive measure in some patients with reversible hepatic dysfunction. Preliminary studies suggest that the shunt may have a role in the management of selected patients with HRS.

References

1. Arieff AI, Chidsey CA. Renal function in cirrhosis and the effects of prostaglandin A₁. Am J Med 56:695, 1974
2. Arroyo V, Rodes J, Gutierrez-Lizarraga MA, et al. Prognostic value of spontaneous hyponatremia in cirrhosis with ascites. Dig Dis 21:249, 1976
3. Arroyo V, Ginés P, Planas R, et al. Paracentesis in the management of cirrhotics with ascites. In Epstein M, ed. The kidney in liver disease, ed 3. Baltimore, Williams & Wilkins, 1988, pp 578–592
4. Baum M, Stirling GA, Dawson JL. Further study into obstructive jaundice and ischaemic renal damage. Br Med J 2:229, 1969
5. Benet LZ. Pharmacokinetics/pharmacodynamics of furosemide in man: a review. J Pharmacokinet Biopharm 7:1, 1979
6. Better OS, Schrier RW. Disturbed volume homeostasis in patients with cirrhosis of the liver. Kidney Int 23:303, 1983
7. Bichet D, Szatalowicz V, Chaimovitz C, et al. Role of vaso-

8. pressin in abnormal water excretion in cirrhotic patients. Ann Intern Med 96:413, 1982
8. Bichet DG, Groves BM, Schrier RW. Mechanisms of improvement of water and sodium excretion by immersion in decompensated cirrhotic patients. Kidney Int 24:788, 1983
9. Bichet DG, VanPutten VJ, Schrier RW. Potential role of increased sympathetic activity in impaired sodium and water excretion in cirrhosis. N Engl J Med 307:1552, 1982
10. Bismuth H, Kuntziger H, Corlette MB. Cholangitis with acute renal failure. Ann Surg 181:881, 1975
11. Bosch J, Arroyo V, Rodes J, et al. Compensacion espontanea de la ascites en la cirrosis hepatica. Rev Clin Esp 133:441, 1974
12. Bourgoignie JJ, Valle GA. Endotoxin and renal dysfunction in liver disease. In: Epstein M, ed. The kidney in liver disease, ed 3. Baltimore, Williams & Wilkins, 1988, pp 486–507
13. Boyer TD, Zia P, Reynolds TB. Effect of indomethacin and prostaglandin A₁ on renal function and plasma renin activity in alcoholic liver disease. Gastroenterology 77:215, 1979
14. Brater DC, Anderson S, Baird B, et al. Effects of ibuprofen, naproxen, and sulindac on prostaglandins in men. Kidney Int 27:66, 1985
15. Buckalew VM Jr. Natriuretic hormone. In: Epstein M, ed. The kidney in liver disease, ed 3. Baltimore, Williams & Wilkins, 1988, pp 417–428
16. Bunning RD, Barth WF. Sulindac: a potentially renal-sparing nonsteroidal antiinflammatory drug. JAMA 248:1864, 1982
17. Chaimovitz C, Rochman J, Eidelman S, et al. Exaggerated natriuretic response to volume expansion in patients with primary biliary cirrhosis. Am J Med Sci 274:173, 1977
18. Chaimovitz C, Szylman P, Alroy G, et al. Mechanism of increased renal tubular sodium reabsorption in cirrhosis. Am J Med 52:198, 1972
19. Chennavasin P, Sciwell R, Brater DC. Pharmacokinetic-dynamic analysis of the indomethacin–furosemide interaction in man. J Pharmacol Exp Ther 215:77, 1980
20. Chiandusi L, Bartoli E, Arras S. Reabsorption of sodium in the proximal renal tubule in cirrhosis of the liver. Gut 19:497, 1978
21. Ciabottoni G, Cinotti GA, Pierucci A, et al. Effects of sulindac and ibuprofen in patients with chronic glomerular disease: evidence for the dependence of renal function on prostacyclin. N Engl J Med 310:279, 1984
22. Clemente C, Bosch J, Rodes J, et al. Functional renal failure and haemorrhagic gastritis associated with endotoxaemia in cirrhosis. Gut 18:556, 1977
23. Conn HO. Diuresis of ascites: fraught with or free from hazard. Gastroenterology 73:619, 1977
24. Conn HO. The rational management of ascites. In: Popper H, Schaffner F, eds. Progress in liver disease, vol 4. New York, Grune & Stratton, 1972, pp 269–288
25. Conn HO, Fessell JM. Spontaneous bacterial peritonitis in cirrhosis: variations on a theme. Medicine 50:161, 1971
26. Coppage WS Jr, Island DP, Cooner AE, et al. The metabolism of aldosterone in normal subjects and in patients with hepatic cirrhosis. J Clin Invest 41:1672, 1962
27. Coratelli P, Passavanti G, Munno I, et al. New trends in hepatorenal syndrome. Kidney Int 28:S143, 1985
28. Daskalopoulos G, Kronborg I, Katkov, et al. Sulindac and indomethacin suppress the diuretic action of furosemide in patients with cirrhosis and ascites: evidence that sulindac affects renal prostaglandins. Am J Kidney Dis 6:217, 1985
29. Data JL, Rane A, Gerkens J, et al. The influence of indomethacin on the pharmacokinetics, diuretic response and hemodynamics of furosemide in the dog. J Pharmacol Exp Ther 207:431, 1978
30. Dawson JL. The incidence of postoperative renal failure in obstructive jaundice. Br J Surg 52:663, 1965
31. De Bold AJ, Borenstein HR, Veress AT, et al. A rapid and potent natriuretic response to intravenous injection of atrial myocardial extracts in rats. Life Sci 28:89, 1981

In the sixth study,[249] a BCAA-enriched solution was compared with glucose. Both groups received lactulose. About one half of both groups of patients improved, and two thirds of both groups survived, despite the fact that nitrogen balance became positive in the BCAA group but remained negative in the control group. There seemed, therefore, to be no advantage to the BCAA therapy.

It is difficult to determine the efficacy of BCAA from these six investigations, in which different amounts of BCAA were administered in different ways for different durations in comparison with four different forms of therapy. Two of the six studies showed BCAA to be beneficial, but four did not. In one additional investigation, BCAA plus lactulose was found to be better than BCAA or lactulose alone. The differences, however, are not impressive.

BCAA also has been used in the nutritional management of patients with cirrhosis with chronic recurrent PSE. Several randomized trials have been reported. One of them by Eriksson and coworkers[72] studied a small number of patients in a randomized, double-blind, crossover study. The patients received either 30 g pure BCAA per day for 14 days orally or an equicaloric carbohydrate placebo. Similar percentages of patients improved, remained unchanged, or deteriorated under the two forms of therapy despite transient increments in plasma BCAA levels.

The second study, which was a double-blind trial by Horst and colleagues,[107] compared progressive increments in dietary protein intake (up to 70 g/d) with a BCAA-enriched, AAA-depleted mixture of essential amino acids (Hepatic Aid) in 37 stable patients with cirrhosis who were prone to develop PSE. In both groups, nitrogen balance improved from negative to strongly positive. Dietary protein induced PSE in half the patients studied. The BCAA mixture caused PSE in only one patient ($P < .01$), but this patient died. It seems clear that the BCAA diet was less comagenic than conventional dietary protein.

In a similar study, Christie and colleagues[45] compared a different solution of BCAA-enriched amino acids (Travasorb-Hepatic), a casein diet. The BCAA content of the amino acid solution was 22 g/d, compared with 9 g/d in the casein diet. In this double-blind trial, no difference in the frequency of PSE was noted, although both groups that had been in negative nitrogen balance became strongly positive.

As in the studies of BCAA in acute PSE, there are no consistent benefits reported in the randomized clinical trials. The studies, however, use different amounts of BCAA and compare them with different control diets. I believe that in patients who are intolerant to dietary protein, a trial on BCAA-enriched solutions of amino acids is indicated.

It has long been known that different sources of protein have different coma-producing potential. Meat protein is more comagenic than dairy protein, which is more so than vegetable protein. Vegetable protein, therefore, appears to be an ideal source of dietary nitrogen for patients with cirrhosis who frequently are in negative nitrogen balance. There are several theories to explain why vegetable protein does not induce encephalopathy. The concentration of methionine, which can induce PSE and fetor hepaticus,[194] is low in vegetable protein. The content of AAA is low in vegetable protein, and the content of BCAA is high. Vegetable protein, therefore, is ideal food for the correction of the plasma amino acid patterns of PSE. Several crossover studies have been performed in patients with cirrhosis and chronic PSE, and each

has shown that vegetable protein diets induce less encephalopathy than equal amounts of meat protein.[96,238,239] Improvement was accompanied by reduction in asterixis and in blood ammonia concentration, and improvement in EEG and psychometric tests. Doubling the amount of methionine by doubling the amount of vegetable protein did not make the diet more comagenic, nor did the addition of an equal amount of pure methionine to the vegetable protein diet. Furthermore, high-fiber vegetable diets reduced the glucose concentration and were especially useful in patients with cirrhosis and diabetes,[239] a disorder that is unusually common in cirrhosis. In one such study, vegetable protein was better tolerated than meat protein, but there was no improvement in the BCAA/AAA ratio.[123] Its mechanism of action remains a mystery. Vegetable protein has been shown to decrease the urea synthesis rate, urea excretion, and the blood urea nitrogen, and to increase fecal nitrogen excretion.[263] Conceivably, vegetable fiber, which contains complex, unabsorbed, undigested carbohydrates, acts like lactulose, which is metabolized by bacteria in the lower bowel with the production of acid and catharsis. Some investigators have noted no differences in the clinical or laboratory responses of patients with cirrhosis and HE given equal amounts of either animal or vegetable protein.

Another approach that should be considered is based on an observation of Thompson and associates[230] on dogs with Eck fistulas. When offered dry, standard dog chow diets, the dogs lost weight and HE developed; when given a palatable, nutritionally complete, liquid diet, the dogs gained weight, thrived, and exhibited no neurologic deterioration. The authors concluded that simply making the diet palatable was the answer. Zieve and Zieve[278] concluded that increasing the ratio of carbohydrate to protein in the diet probably was responsible. It seems simple enough to test in patients.

Another therapeutic candidate is L-dopa. Fischer and Baldessarini[83] have suggested that PSE may result from the accumulation in central nervous system neurons of abnormal, inert amines, instead of physiologically active amines, such as dopamine or norepinephrine. Like ammonia, amines may arise from the bacterial degradation of proteins in the gut, may be adversely affected by an increased extracellular–intracellular pH gradient, and may be reduced by antibiotic or lactulose therapy or by the other antiammonia measures used. L-Dopa has been used in hepatic coma with enthusiasm in uncontrolled series.[83,188] In controlled clinical trials of L-dopa in hepatic coma, the results have been unimpressive,[140,157] and L-dopa is not considered viable therapy for PSE. Bromocriptine, a pharmacologic relative of L-dopa, may have met a similar fate. Although a preliminary anecdotal report of bromocriptine was enthusiastic,[164] the one clinical trial reported so far shows no beneficial results.[236]

The use of *sodium benzoate* represents a clever biochemical strategy for bypassing the urea cycle while augmenting the renal excretion of ammonia.[242a] This approach permits the ammonia to be excreted as hippuric acid rather than as urea. Phenylacetate, which combines with glutamine to form phenylacetylglutamine, also can be used to convert ammonia into a renally excreatable substance.[12] Uribe and colleagues[242b] compared sodium benzoate syrup, 6 g/d, with lactulose syrup, 40 mL/d (ie, 27 g). They showed that most patients with PSE in both groups improved—10 of 11 (91%) with benzoate versus 7 of 10 (70%) with lactulose. Side effects were less common with the benzoate therapy.

A word of caution: in mice, sodium benzoate in very large doses appears to intensify ammonia intoxication.[181b] This dose is proportionally about 50 times greater than that given to humans by Uribe and coworkers (500 versus 10 mg/kg). This paradoxical effect of large doses of benzoate can be prevented by the prior administration of L-carnitine.[181c]

Finally, surgical removal or short-circuiting of the colon (colectomy, ileosigmoidostomy) has been done successfully. Unfortunately, the operative mortality is discouragingly high in patients with chronic recurrent PSE.[196,200] PSE in patients with surgical portal-systemic shunts may be improved by ligation[258] or embolic occlusion of the anastomosis.[235]

NONNITROGENOUS ENCEPHALOPATHY

Hepatic coma induced by nonnitrogenous substances is characterized by essentially the same clinical picture as the nitrogenous type, except that blood ammonia levels either are normal or minimally elevated. Approximately one third of cases of HE are nonnitrogenous in origin. This syndrome may be induced by any substance or metabolic disorder that itself may depress consciousness. Among the most common substances are sedatives, depressants, and analgesics. Normal doses of barbiturates, for example, may produce overdose effects due to impaired drug catabolism by the liver. In one characteristic patient with cirrhosis, we found the explanation for episodic nonnitrogenous hepatic precoma in the nurses' notes. This patient was found on several consecutive mornings difficult to rouse, confused, and with asterixis. Review of the nurses' notes revealed that the "coma" was preceded each evening by conventional doses of medication for sleep. Discontinuation of these hypnotic drugs "cured" the hepatic coma.

Similarly, normal doses of preoperative medications such as Demerol to patients with cirrhosis before esophagoscopy or equivalent procedures often will induce surprisingly severe and prolonged HE with normal blood ammonia levels. We believe that patients with portacaval shunts are especially susceptible to such effects, and particularly to the postural abnormalities associated with phenothiazines and other tranquilizing drugs. These effects can be prevented by avoiding such drugs in patients with incipient hepatic coma or by administering one quarter or one half the usual dosage to patients with cirrhosis who previously have experienced episodes of hepatic coma or who are suspected of being unduly sensitive. It is easier to add small doses than it is to remove overdoses. Similarly, small doses of analgesia after surgery in patients with cirrhosis, especially after portacaval shunts, will avoid many episodes of postoperative "hepatic" coma.

Primary treatment of such episodes consists of discontinuation of the offending drug. An antiammonia program also may be instituted, because the effects of ammonia intoxication and drug-induced coma appear to be additive or even synergistic in susceptible patients. Metabolic disorders such as hypoxemia, carbon dioxide narcosis, hypoglycemia, myxedema, or generalized infection seem to potentiate the toxic effects of ammonia or other precipitants of encephalopathy. Correction of such metabolic derangements in conjunction with the antiammonia program usually is effective.

In summary, the patient with hepatic coma should be carefully evaluated for the precipitating cause or causes. Eradication of the cause usually reverses the encephalopathy. Therapy based on pathogenetic principles should be rationally designed for the individual patient. As understanding of these disorders improves, so does therapy.

References

1. Adams RD, et al. The neurological disorder associated with liver disease. In: Metabolic and toxic diseases of the nervous system, vol 32. Baltimore, Williams & Wilkins, 1953, p 198
2. Aguglia U, et al. Nonmetabolic causes of triphasic waves: a reappraisal. Clin Electroencephalogr 21:120, 1990
3. Alagille D, et al. Long-term neuropsychological outcome in children undergoing portal-systemic shunts for portal vein obstruction without liver disease. J Pediatr Gastroenterol Nutr 5:861, 1986
4. Allen SI, Conn HO. Observations on the effect of exercise on blood ammonia concentration in man. Yale J Biol Med 33:133, 1960
5. Amendt BA, et al. Short-chain acyl-coenzyme A dehydrogenase deficiency. J Clin Invest 79:1303, 1987
6. Atterbury CE, et al. Neomycin-sorbitol and lactulose in the treatment of acute portal-systemic encephalopathy. Am J Dig Dis 23:398, 1978
7. Baertl JM, et al. Relation of acute potassium depletion to renal ammonium metabolism in patients with cirrhosis. Clin Invest 42:696, 1983
8. Baraldi M, et al. Toxins in hepatic encephalopathy: the role of the synergistic effect of ammonia, mercaptans and short chain fatty acids. Arch Toxicol [Suppl] 7:103, 1984
9. Basile AS, et al. Elevated brain concentrations of 1,4-benzodiazepines in fulminant hepatic failure. N Engl J Med 325:473, 1991
10. Basile AS, et al. The pathogenesis and treatment of hepatic encephalopathy: evidence for the involvement of benzodiazepine receptor ligands. Pharmacol Rev 43:27, 1991
11. Bass P. Cathartic properties of lactitol, lactulose and related carbohydrates. In: Conn HO, Bircher J, eds. Hepatic encephalopathy: syndromes and therapies. East Lansing, MI, Medi-Ed Press, 1993
12. Batshaw ML, et al. Treatment of inborn errors of urea synthesis: activation of alternative pathways of waste nitrogen synthesis and excretion. N Engl J Med 306:1387, 1982
13. Bauer AG, et al. Hyperprolactinemia in hepatic encephalopathy: the effect of infusion of an amino acid mixture with excess branched chain amino acids. Hepatogastroenterology 30:174, 1983
14. Berk DP, Chalmers T. Deafness complicating antibiotic therapy of hepatic encephalopathy. Ann Intern Med 73:393, 1970
15. Bernardi M, et al. Plasma norepinephrine, weak neurotransmitters, and renin activity during active tilting in liver cirrhosis: relationship with cardiovascular homeostasis and renal function. Hepatology 3:56, 1983
16. Bernthal P, et al. Cerebral CT scan abnormalities in cholestatic and hepatocellular disease and their relationship to neuropsychologic test performance. Hepatology 7:107, 1987
17. Bessman AN, Mirick GS. Blood ammonia levels following the ingestion of casein and whole blood. J Clin Invest 37:990, 1958
18. Bessman SP, Bradley JE. Uptake of ammonia by muscle: its implications in ammoniagenic coma. N Engl J Med 253:1143, 1955
19. Bickford RG, Butt HR. Hepatic coma: the electroencephalographic pattern. J Clin Invest 34:790, 1955
20. Bircher J, Ullrich D. Clinical pharmacology of nonabsorbed disaccharides. In: Conn HO, Bircher J, eds. Hepatic encephalopathy: syndromes and therapies. East Lansing, MI, Medi-Ed Press, 1993
21. Bircher J, et al. Treatment of chronic portalsystemic encephalopathy with lactulose. Lancet 1:890, 1966

22. Bircher J, et al. Erstmaligne von lactitol in der behandlung de porto-systemischen enzephalopathie. Schweiz Med Wochenschr 112:1306, 1982
23. Bird SP, et al. Effects of lactulose and lactitol on protein digestion and metabolism in conventional and germ free animal models: relevance of the results to their use in the treatment of portal-systemic encephalopathy. Gut 31:1403, 1990
24. Blom HJ, et al. The role of methanethiol in the pathogenesis of hepatic encephalopathy. Hepatology 13:445, 1991
25. Bosman DK, et al. Changes in brain metabolism during hyperammonemia and acute liver failure: results of a comparative ^{1}H-NMR spectroscopy and biochemical investigation. Hepatology 12:281, 1990
26. Bove KE, et al. The hepatic lesion in Reye's syndrome. Gastroenterology 69:685, 1975
27. Brown T, et al. Transiently reduced activity of carbamyl phosphate synthetase and ornithine transcarbamylase in liver of children with Reye's syndrome. N Engl J Med 294:861, 1976
28. Brusilow SW, Horwich AL. Urea cycle enzymes. In: Scriver CR, Beaudet AL, Sly WS, et al, eds. The metabolic basis of inherited disease. New York, McGraw-Hill, 1989, p 629
29. Bruton CJ, et al. Hereditary hyperammonemia. Brain 93:423, 1970
30. Butt HR, Mason HL. Fetor hepaticus: its clinical significance and attempts at clinical isolation. Gastroenterology 26:829, 1954
31. Butterworth RF, et al. Ammonia: key factor in the pathogenesis of hepatic encephalopathy. Neurochem Pathol 6:1, 1987
32. Butterworth RF, Pomier Layrargues G, eds. Hepatic encephalopathy: pathophysiology and treatment. Clifton, NJ, Humana Press, 1990
33. Cabrera J, et al. Aminoglycoside nephrotoxicity in cirrhosis: value of urinary β$_2$-microglobulin to discriminate functional renal failure from acute tubular damage. Gastroenterology 82:97, 1982
34. Cales P, et al. Propranolol does not alter cerebral blood flow and functions in cirrhotic patients without previous hepatic encephalopathy. Hepatology 9:439, 1989
35. Canalese J, et al. Controlled trial of dexamethasone and mannitol for the cerebral oedema of fulminant hepatic failure. Gut 23:625, 1982
36. Canzanello VJ, et al. Hyperammonemic encephalopathy during hemodialysis. Ann Intern Med 99:190, 1983
37. Capocaccia L, et al. Influence of phenylethanolamine on octopamine plasma determination in hepatic encephalopathy. Clin Chim Acta 93:371, 1979
38. Capocaccia L, et al. Hepatic encephalopathy in chronic liver failure. London, Plenum Press, 1984, p 393
39. Capocaccia L. Long-term treatment with lactitol and lactulose. In: Conn HO, Bircher J, eds. Hepatic encephalopathy: syndromes and therapies. East Lansing, MI, Medi-Ed Press, 1993
40. Carithers RL Jr, et al. Methylprednisolone therapy in patients with severe alcoholic hepatitis. Ann Intern Med 110:685, 1989
41. Cerra FB, et al. Disease-specific amino acid infusion (F080) in hepatic encephalopathy: a prospective, randomized, double-blind, controlled trial. JPEN 9:288, 1985
42. Challenger F, Walshe JM. Methyl mercaptan in relation to foetor hepaticus. Biochem J 59:372, 1955
43. Chen S, et al. Mercaptans and dimethyl sulfide in the breath of patients with cirrhosis of the liver. J Lab Clin Med 75:628, 1970
44. Chen S, et al. Volatile fatty acids in the breath of patients with cirrhosis of the liver. J Lab Clin Med 75:622, 1970
45. Christie ML, et al. Enriched branched-chain amino acid formula versus a casein-based supplement in the treatment of cirrhosis. JPEN 9:671, 1985
46. Colombo JP, et al. Liver enzymes in the Eck fistula rat: I. urea cycle enzymes and transaminases. Enzyme 14:353, 1973

47. Conn HO. Asterixis in nonhepatic disorders. Am J Med 29:647, 1960
48. Conn HO. The Trailmaking and Number Connection Tests in assessing mental state in portalsystemic encephalopathy. Am J Dig Dis 22:541, 1977
49. Conn H, et al. Hepatic encephalopathy: management with lactulose and related carbohydrates. In: Conn HO, Bircher J, eds. Hepatic encephalopathy: syndromes and therapies. East Lansing, MI, Medi-Ed Press, 1993
50. Conn HO. Assessment of the severity of hepatic encephalopathy. In: Rodes J, Arroyo V, eds. Therapy in liver diseases. Barcelona, Ediciones Doyma SA, 1991, p 277
51. Conn HO, Bircher J, eds. Hepatic encephalopathy: syndromes and therapies. East Lansing, MI, Medi-Ed Press, 1993
52. Conn HO, Lieberthal MM. The hepatic coma syndromes and lactulose. Baltimore, Williams & Wilkins, 1979, p 112
53. Conn HO, et al. A comparison of lactulose and neomycin in the treatment of portal-systemic encephalopathy: a double-blind controlled trial. Gastroenterology 72:573, 1977
54. Conn HO, et al. Cirrhosis and diabetes: II. association of impaired glucose tolerance with portal-systemic shunting in Laënnec's cirrhosis. Am J Dig Dis 16:227, 1971
55. Cooper AJL, et al. The metabolic fate of ^{13}N-labeled ammonia in rat brain. J Biol Chem 254:4982, 1979
56. Cosnett JE, et al. Shunt myelopathy: a report of 2 cases. S Afr Med J 62:215, 1982
57. Davies MG, et al. Flash visual evoked responses in the early encephalopathy of chronic liver disease. Scand J Gastroenterol 25:1205, 1990
58. DeBruijn KM, et al. Effect of dietary protein manipulations in subclinical portal-systemic encephalopathy. Gut 24:53, 1983
59. DeMagno EP, et al. Ornithine transcarbamylase deficiency: a cause of bizarre behavior in a man. N Engl J Med 315:744, 1986
60. Derr RF, Zieve L. Effect of fatty acids on the disposition of ammonia. J Pharmacol Exp Ther 197:675, 1976
61. DerSimonian R. Parenteral nutrition with branched-chain amino acids in hepatic encephalopathy: meta analysis. Hepatology 11:1083, 1990
62. Doffoel M, et al. Hyperammoniemie indulte par le propranolol chez le cirrhotique. Role du rein et influence de la gravite de la cirrhose. Gastroenterol Clin Biol 11:123, 1987
63. Doizaki WM, Zieve L. An improved method for measuring blood mercaptans. J Lab Clin Med 90:849, 1977
64. Drage JS (coordinator). The diagnosis and treatment of Reye's syndrome. NIH Consensus Development Conference Summary, Bethesda, National Library of Medicine, 4:1, 1981
65. Ede RJ, Williams R. Hepatic encephalopathy and cerebral edema. Semin Liver Dis 6:107, 1986
66. Ede RJ, et al. Controlled hyperventilation in the prevention of cerebral oedema in fulminant hepatic failure. J Hepatol 2:43, 1986
67. Egberts EH, et al. Branched chain amino acids in the treatment of latent portal-systemic encephalopathy: a double-blind placebo controlled crossover study. Gastroenterology 88:887, 1985
68. Egense J, Schwartz M. Recurrent hepatic coma following ureterosigmoidostomy. Scand J Gastroenterol 7(Suppl):149, 1970
69. Elkington SG, et al. Lactulose in the control of portal-systemic encephalopathy. N Engl J Med 281:408, 1969
70. Elsass P, et al. Encephalopathy in patients with cirrhosis of the liver: a neuropsychological study. Scand J Gastroenterol 13:241, 1978
71. Ericson G, et al. Unilateral asterixis in a dialysis patient. JAMA 240:671, 1978
72. Eriksson LS, et al. Branched-chain amino acids in the treatment of chronic hepatic encephalopathy. Gut 23:801, 1982
73. Eriksson LS, Conn HO. Branched-chain amino acids in the

management of hepatic encephalopathy: an analysis of variants. Hepatology 10:228, 1989

74. Faraj BA, et al. Evidence for central hypertyraminemia in hepatic encephalopathy. J Clin Invest 67:395, 1981

75. Farber MO, et al. The oxygen affinity of hemoglobin in hepatic encephalopathy. J Lab Clin Med 98:135, 1981

76. Ferenci P, et al. Serum levels of gamma aminobutyric acid-like activity in patients with acute and chronic hepatocellular diseases. Lancet 1:811, 1983

77. Ferenci P, et al. Successful longtime treatment of chronic hepatic encephalopathy (HE) with a benzodiazepine antagonist. Hepatology 7:1064, 1987

78. Ferenci P, et al. Overestimation of serum concentrations of γ-aminobutyric acid in patients with hepatic encephalopathy by the γ-aminobutyric acid-radioreceptor assay. Hepatology 8:69, 1988

79. Ferenci P, Jones EA. GABA and benzodiazepines in hepatic encephalopathy. In: Conn HO, Bircher J, eds. Hepatic encephalopathy: syndromes and therapies. East Lansing, MI, Medi-Ed Press, 1993

80. Fessel JM, Conn HO. An analysis of the causes and prevention of hepatic coma. Gastroenterology 62:191, 1972

81. Fiaccadori F, et al. Branched-chain enriched amino acid solutions in the treatment of hepatic encephalopathy: a controlled trial. Ital J Gastroenterol 17:5, 1985

81a. Finlayson MAJ, et al. Relationship of education to neurophysiological measures in brain-damaged and non–brain-damaged adults. J Consult Clin Psychol 45:536, 1977

82. Fisch BJ, Klass DW. The diagnostic specificity of triphasic wave patterns. Electroencephalogr Clin Neurophysiol 70:1, 1988

83. Fischer JE, Baldessarini RJ. False neurotransmitters and hepatic failure. Lancet 2:75, 1971

84. Fischer JE, Baldessarini RJ. Pathogenesis and therapy of hepatic coma. In: Popper H, Schaffner F, eds. Progress in liver diseases, vol 5. New York, Grune & Stratton, 1976, p 363

85. Fischer JE, et al. The effect of normalization of plasma amino acids on hepatic encephalopathy in man. Surgery 80:77, 1976

86. Flannery DB, et al. Current status of hyperammonemic syndromes. Hepatology 2:495, 1985

89. Gabuzda GJ, Hall PW III. Relation of potassium depletion to renal ammonium metabolism and hepatic coma. Medicine 45:481, 1966

90. Gammal SH, et al. Reversal of the behavioral and electrophysiological abnormalities of an animal model of hepatic encephalopathy by benzodiazepine receptor ligands. Hepatology 11:371, 1990

91. Gilberstadt S, et al. Psychomotor performance defects in cirrhotics without overt encephalopathy. Arch Intern Med 140:519, 1980

92. Gilchrist JM, Coleman RA. Ornithine transcarbamylase deficiency: adult onset of severe symptoms. Ann Intern Med 106:556, 1987

93. Gimson AES, et al. Late onset hepatic failure: clinical, serological and histological features. Hepatology 6:288, 1986

94. Gitlin N, et al. The diagnosis and prevalence of subclinical hepatic encephalopathy in apparently healthy, ambulant, non-shunted patients with cirrhosis. J Hepatol 3:75 1986

95. Goodman MW, et al. Mechanism of arginine protection against ammonia intoxication in the rat. Am J Physiol 247:G290, 1984

96. Greenberger NJ, et al. Effect of vegetable and animal protein diets in chronic hepatic encephalopathy. Am J Dig Dis 22:845, 1977

97. Gullino P, et al. Studies on the metabolism of amino acids and related compounds in vivo: I. toxicity of essential amino acids, individually and in mixtures, and the protective effect of L-arginine. Arch Biochem Biophys 64:319, 1956

98. Hanid MA, et al. Intracranial pressure in pigs with surgically induced acute liver failure. Gastroenterology 76:123, 1979

99. Hanid MA, et al. Clinical monitoring of intracranial pressure in fulminant hepatic failure. Gut 21:866, 1980

100. Hassall E, et al. Hepatic encephalopathy after portacaval shunt in a noncirrhotic child. J Pediatr 105:439, 1984

101. Haussinger D, et al. Liver carbonic anhydrase and urea synthesis: the effect of diuretics. Biochem Pharmacol 35:3317, 1986

102. Heird WC, et al. Hyperammonemia resulting from intravenous alimentation using a mixture of synthetic L-amino acids: a preliminary report. J Pediatr 81:162, 1972

103. Heredia D, et al. Lactitol vs. lactulose in the treatment of chronic recurrent portal-systemic encephalopathy. J Hepatol 7:106, 1988

104. Herlong HF, et al. The use of ornithine salts of branched-chain ketoacids in portal systemic encephalopathy. Ann Intern Med 93:545, 1980

105. Heubi JE, et al. Reye's syndrome: current concepts. Hepatology 7:155, 1987

106. Hirayama C, et al. A controlled clinical trial of nicotinohydroxamic acid and neomycin in advanced chronic liver disease. Digestion 25:115, 1982

107. Horst D, et al. Comparison of dietary protein with an oral, branched chain-enriched amino acid supplement in chronic portal-systemic encephalopathy: a randomized controlled trial. Hepatology 4:279, 1984

108. Hortnagl H, et al. Substance P is markedly increased in plasma of patients with hepatic coma. Lancet 1:480, 1984

109. Hourani BT, et al. Cerebrospinal fluid glutamine as a measure of hepatic encephalopathy. Arch Intern Med 127:1033, 1971

110. Hsia YE. Inherited hyperammonemic syndromes. Gastroenterology 67:347, 1974

111. Imler M, et al. Importance de l'hyperammoniemie d'origine renale dans la pathogenie des comas hepatiques declenches chez les cirrhotiques par les diuretiques generateurs d'hypokaliemie. Pathol Biol 17:5, 1969

112. Imler M, et al. Etude comparative du traitement de l'encephalopathie port-cave par le lactulose, les bacilles lactiques et les antibiotiques. Therapeutique 47:237, 1971

113. Ishak KG, et al. Alcoholic liver disease: pathologic, pathogenetic and clinical aspects. Alcoholism 15:45, 1991

114. Jenkins JG, et al. Reye's syndrome: assessment of intracranial monitoring. Br Med J 294:337, 1987

115. Joelsson B, et al. Portal-systemic encephalopathy: Influence of shunt surgery and relations to serum amino acids. Scand J Gastroenterol 21:900, 1986

116. Jones EA, et al. The neurobiology of hepatic encephalopathy. Hepatology 4:1235, 1984

117. Jones EA. Hepatic encephalopathy and GABA-ergic neurotransmission. In: Conn HO, Bircher J, eds. Hepatic encephalopathy: syndromes and therapies. East Lansing, MI, Medi-Ed Press, 1993

118. Jonung T, et al. A comparison between meat and vegan protein diet in patients with mild chronic hepatic encephalopathy. Clin Nutr 6:169, 1987

119. Kabadi UM, et al. Elevated plasma ammonia levels in hepatic cirrhosis: role of glucagon. Gastroenterology 88:750, 1985

120. Kaufman JJ. Ammoniagenic coma following ureterosigmoidostomy. J Urol 131:743, 1984

121. Kerlan RK, et al. Portal-systemic encephalopathy due to a congenital portocaval shunt. AJR 139:1013, 1982

122. Kersh ES, Rifkin H. Lactulose enemas. Ann Intern Med 78:81, 1973

123. Keshavarzian A, et al. Dietary protein supplementation from vegetable sources in the management of chronic portal systemic encephalopathy. Am J Gastroenterol 79:945, 1984

124. Kreis R, et al. Metabolic disorders of the brain in chronic hepatic encephalopathy detected with H-1 MR spectroscopy. Radiology 182:19, 1992

125. Lam KC, et al. Role of a false neurotransmitter, octopamine

in the pathogenesis of hepatic and renal encephalopathy. Scand J Gastroenterol 8:465, 1973

126. Lanthier PL, Morgan MY. Lactitol in the treatment of chronic hepatic encephalopathy: an open comparison with lactulose. Gut 26:415, 1985

127. Lauterburg BH, et al. Hepatic functional deterioration after portacaval shunt in the rat: effects on sulfobromophthalein transport maximum, indocyanine green clearance, and galactose elimination capacity. Gastroenterology 71:221, 1976

128. Leavitt S, Tyler HR. Studies in asterixis. Arch Neurol 10:360, 1964

129. Lebek G, Luginbuhl M. Effects of nonabsorbed disaccharides on human intestinal flora. In: Conn HO, Bircher J, eds. Hepatic encephalopathy: syndromes and therapies. East Lansing, MI, Medi-Ed Press, 1993

130. Lebovics E, et al. Portal-systemic myelopathy after portacaval shunt surgery. Arch Intern Med 145:1921, 1985

131. Lembeck F, et al. Elimination of substance P from the circulation of the rat and its inhibition by bacitracin. Naunyn Schmiedebergs Arch Pharmacol 305:9, 1978

132. Lerman BB, et al. Hepatic encephalopathy precipitated by fecal impaction. Arch Intern Med 139:707, 1979

133. Levy LJ, et al. The use of the visual evoked potential (VEP) in delineating a state of subclinical encephalopathy: a comparison with the number connection test (NCT). J Hepatol 5:211, 1987

134. Liehr H, et al. Lactulose: a drug with antiendotoxin effect. Hepatogastroenterology 27:1, 1980

135. Limberg B, et al. Correction of altered plasma amino acid pattern in cirrhosis of the liver by somatostatin. Gut 25:1291, 1984

136. Lischner MW, et al. Natural history of alcoholic hepatitis: I. the acute disease. Am J Dig Dis 16:481, 1971

137. Lockwood AH, et al. The dynamics of ammonia metabolism in man: effects of liver disease and hyperammonemia. J Clin Invest 63:449, 1979

138. Loguercio C et al. Psychometric tests and "latent" portal-systemic encephalopathy. Br J Clin Pract 38:407, 1984

139. Lowenstein JM. Ammonia production in muscle and other tissues: the purine nucleotide cycle. Physiol Rev 52:382, 1972

140. Lunzer M. Treatment of chronic hepatic encephalopathy with levodopa. Gut 15:555, 1974

141. MacBeth WAAG, et al. Treatment of hepatic encephalopathy by alteration of intestinal flora with *Lactobacillus acidophilus.* Lancet 1:399, 1965

142. Manning RT. A nomogram for estimation of pNH$_3$. J Lab Clin Med 63:297, 1964

143. Marchesini G, et al. Insulin and glucagon levels in liver cirrhosis: relationship with plasma amino acids imbalance of chronic hepatic encephalopathy. Dig Dis Sci 24:594, 1979

144. Marchesini G, et al. Prevalence of subclinical hepatic encephalopathy in cirrhotics and relationship to plasma amino acid imbalance. Dig Dis Sci 25:763, 1980

145. Marchesini G, et al. Long-term oral branched-chain amino acid treatment in chronic hepatic encephalopathy: a randomized double-blind casein-controlled trial. J Hepatol 11:92, 1990

146. Marshall, et al. Pentobarbital therapy for intracranial hypertension in metabolic coma: Reye's syndrome. Crit Care Med 6:1, 1978

148. Masala A, et al. Failure of nomifensine to reduce serum prolactin levels in patients with hepatic encephalopathy. J Endocrinol Invest 8:25, 1985

149. McLain CJ, et al. Hyperprolactinemia in portal-system encephalopathy. Dig Dis Sci 26:353, 1981

150. McClain CJ, et al. The effect of lactulose on psychomotor performance tests in alcoholic cirrhotics without overt hepatic encephalopathy. J Clin Gastroenterol 6:325, 1984

151. McDermott WV Jr. Diversion of urine to the intestines as a factor in ammoniagenic coma. N Engl J Med 256:460, 1957

152. McDermott WV, Adams RD. Episodic stupor associated with an Eck fistula in the human with particular reference to the metabolism of ammonia. J Clin Invest 33:1, 1954

153. McGhee A, et al. Comparison of the effects of hepatic-acid and a casein modular diet on encephalopathy, plasma amino acids and nitrogen balance in cirrhotic patients. Ann Surg 197:288, 1983

154. McWilliam RC, Stephenson JBP. Life-threatening intracranial hypertension in Reye's syndrome treated with intravenous thiopentone. Pediatrics 144:383, 1985

155. Mendenhall CL, et al. A new therapy for portal systemic encephalopathy. Am J Gastroenterol 81:540, 1986

156. Meyers S, Lieber CS. Reduction of gastric ammonia by ampicillin in normal and azotemic subjects. Gastroenterology 70:244, 1976

157. Michel H, et al. Treatment of cirrhotic hepatic encephalopathy with L-dopa: a controlled trial. Gastroenterology 70:207, 1980

158. Michel H, et al. Treatment of acute hepatic encephalopathy in cirrhotics with a branched-chain amino acids enriched versus a conventional amino acids mixture: a controlled study of 70 patients. Liver 5:282, 1985

159. Mills PR, et al. A study of zinc metabolism in alcoholic cirrhosis. Clin Sci 64:527, 1983

160. Minuk GY, et al. Elevated serum γ-aminobutyric acid levels in children with Reye's syndrome. J Pediatr Gastroenterol Nutr 4:528, 1985

161. Minuk GY. Gamma-aminobutyric acid (GABA) production by eight common bacterial pathogens. Scand J Infect Dis 18:465, 1986

162. Moore EW, et al. Distribution of ammonia across the blood-cerebrospinal fluid barrier in patients with hepatic failure. Am J Med 35:350, 1963

163. Morgan MH, et al. Clinical and electrophysiological studies of peripheral nerve function in patients with chronic liver disease. Clin Sci 57:31, 1979

164. Morgan MY, et al. Successful use of bromocriptine in the treatment of a patient with chronic portal-systemic encephalopathy. N Engl J Med 296:793, 1977

165. Morgan MH, et al. Treatment of hepatic encephalopathy with metronidazole. Gut 23:1, 1982

166. Morgan MY, Hawley KE. Lactitol vs. lactulose in the treatment of acute hepatic encephalopathy in cirrhotic patients: a double-blind, randomized trial. Hepatology 7:1278, 1987

167. Morgan MY. Lactitol for the treatment of hepatic encephalopathy. In: Conn HO, Bircher J, eds. Hepatic encephalopathy: syndromes and therapies. East Lansing, MI, Medi-Ed Press, 1993

168. Mortensen PB, et al. The degradation of amino acids, proteins, and blood to short-chain fatty acids in colon is prevented by lactulose. Gastroenterology 98:353, 1990

169. Mullen KD. Benzodiazepine compounds and hepatic encephalopathy. N Engl J Med 325:509, 1991

170. Munro HN. Insulin, plasma amino acid imbalance, and hepatic coma. Lancet 1:722, 1975

171. Munoz SJ, et al. Elevated intracranial pressure and computed tomography of the brain in fulminant hepatocellular failure. Hepatology 13:209, 1991

172. Mutchnick MG, et al. Portal-systemic encephalopathy and portal anastomosis: a prospective, controlled investigation. Gastroenterology 66:1005, 1974

173. Muto Y, Takahashi Y: Gas chromatographic determination of plasma short chain fatty acids in diseases of the liver. Journal of the Japanese Society of Internal Medicine 53:828, 1964

174. Nance FC, et al. Ammonia production in germ-free Eck fistula dogs. Surgery 70:169, 1971

175. Nance FC, et al. Role of urea in the hyperammonemia of germ-free Eck fistula dogs. Gastroenterology 66:108, 1974

176. Naparstek Y, et al. Transient cortical blindness in hepatic encephalopathy. Isr J Med Sci 15:854, 1979

177. Naylor CD, et al. Parenteral nutrition with branched-chain amino acids in hepatic encephalopathy: a meta-analysis. Gastroenterology 97:1033, 1989

178. Noda S, et al. Hip flexion-abduction to elicit asterixis in unresponsive patients. Ann Neurol 18:96, 1985

179. Norenberg MD. A light and electron microscopic study of experimental portal-systemic (ammonia) encephalopathy. Lab Invest 36:618, 1977

180. Norenberg MD. Immunohistochemistry of glutamine synthetase. In: Hertz L, Kvamme E, McGeer EG, Schousboe A, eds. Glutamine, glutamate and GABA in the central nervous system. New York, Alan R. Liss, 1983, p 95

181. Norenberg MD. The role of astrocytes in hepatic encephalopathy. Neurochem Pathol 6:13, 1987

181a. Norenberg MD. Astrocytes in hepatic encephalopathy. In: Grisolia S, et al, eds. Cirrhosis, hepatic encephalopathy, and ammonium toxicity. New York, Plenum, 1990, p 81

181b. O'Connor JE, Ribelles M, Grisolia S. Potentiation of hyperammonemia by sodium benzoate in animals: a note of caution. Eur J Pediatr 138:186, 1982

181c. O'Connor JE, Costell M, Grisolia S. The potentiation of ammonia toxicity by sodium benzoate is presented by L-carnitine. Biochem Biophys Res Commun 145:817, 1987

182. Oei LT, et al. Cerebrospinal fluid glutamine levels and EEG findings in patients with hepatic encephalopathy. Clin Neurol Neurosurg 81:59, 1979

183. Ono J, et al. Tryptophan and hepatic coma. Gastroenterology 74:196, 1974

184. Orlandi F, et al. Clinical trials of lactulose and lactitol therapy in hepatic encephalopathy. In: Conn HO, Bircher J, eds. Hepatic encephalopathy: syndromes and therapies. East Lansing, MI, Medi-Ed Press, 1993

185. Orlandi F, et al. Comparison between neomycin and lactulose in 173 patients with hepatic encephalopathy: a randomized clinical study. Dig Dis Sci 26:498, 1981

186. Orloff MJ, Peskin GW. The effect of formaldehyde on experimental ammonia intoxication. Surg Forum 10:295, 1960

187. Pappas SC, et al. Visual potentials in a rabbit model of hepatic encephalopathy: comparison of hyperammonemic encephalopathy, posital coma, and coma induced by synergistic neurotoxins. Gastroenterology 86:546, 1984

188. Parkes JD, et al. Levodopa in hepatic coma. Lancet 2:1341, 1970

189. Parsons-Smith BG, et al. The electroencephalograph in liver disease. Lancet 1:867, 1957

190. Partin JC, et al. Mitochondrial ultrastructure in Reye's syndrome: encephalopathy and fatty degeneration of the viscera. N Engl J Med 258:1339, 1971

191. Patil DH, et al. Comparative modes of action of lactitol and lactulose in the treatment of hepatic encephalopathy. Gut 28:255, 1987

192. Pedretti G, et al. Rifaximin versus neomycin on hyperammoniemia in chronic portal systemic encephalopathy of cirrhotics: a double-blind, randomized trial. Ital J Gastroenterol 23:175, 1991

193. Peter B, et al. Influence de l'alpha-ceto-glutarate de L(+) ornithine sur l'hyperammoniémie provoquée des cirrhotiques. Ann Gastroenterol Hepatol 10:179, 1974

194. Phear, et al. Methionine toxicity in liver disease and its prevention by chlortetracycline. Clin Sci 15:93, 1956

195. Phillips GB, et al. The syndrome of impending hepatic coma in patients with cirrhosis of the liver given certain nitrogenous substances. N Engl J Med 247:239, 1952

196. Picone SB Jr, et al. Abdominal colectomy for chronic encephalopathy due to portal-systemic shunt. Arch Surg 118:33, 1983

197. Raabe W. Synaptic transmission in ammonia intoxication. Neurochem Pathol 6:145, 1987

198. Reding P, et al. Oral zinc supplementation improves hepatic encephalopathy: results of a randomized controlled trial. Lancet 2:493, 1984

199. Rehnstrom SH, et al. Chronic hepatic encephalopathy: a psychometrical study. Scand J Gastroenterol 121:305, 1977

200. Resnick RH, et al. A controlled trial of colon bypass in chronic hepatic encephalopathy. Gastroenterology 54:1057, 1968

201. Reynolds TB, et al. A controlled study of the effects of L-arginine on hepatic encephalopathy. Am J Med 25:359, 1958

202. Riggio O, et al. Lactitol in prevention of recurrent episodes of hepatic encephalopathy in cirrhotic patients with portal-system shunt. Dig Dis Sci 34:823, 1989

203. Rikkers L, et al. Subclinical hepatic encephalopathy: detection, prevalence, and relationship to nitrogen metabolism. Gastroenterology 75:462, 1978

204. Rosen HM, et al. Plasma amino acid patterns in hepatic encephalopathy of differing etiology. Gastroenterology 72:483, 1977

205. Rosenberg LE, Fenton WA. Disorders of propionate and methylmalonate metabolism. In: Scriver CR, Beaudet WS, Valle D, eds. The metabolic basis of inherited disease, 6th ed. New York, McGraw-Hill, 1989, p 821

206. Rossi-Fanelli F, et al. Branched-chain amino acids vs. lactulose in the treatment of hepatic coma: a controlled study. Dig Dis Sci 27:929, 1982

207. Rothstein JD, et al. Cerebrospinal fluid content of diazepam binding inhibitor in chronic hepatic encephalopathy. Ann Neurol 26:57, 1989

208. Rowe PC, et al. Inborn errors of metabolism in children with Reye's syndrome. JAMA 260:3167, 1988

209. Samtoy B, DeBeukelaer MM: Ammonia encephalopathy secondary to urinary tract infection with *Proteus mirabilis*. Pediatrics 65:294, 1980

210. Sandford NL, Saul RE. Assessment of hepatic encephalopathy with visual evoked potentials compared with conventional methods. Hepatology 8:1094, 1988

211. Scevola D, et al. Lattitolo e neomicina: monoterapia o terapia combinata nella prevenzione e nel trattamento dell'encelfalopatia epatica? Clin Ter 129:105, 1989

212. Schafer DF, Jones EA. Hepatic encephalopathy and the γ-aminobutyric acid neurotransmitter system. Lancet 1:18, 1982

213. Schafer DF, et al. Colonic bacteria: a source of γ-aminobutyric acid in blood. Proc Soc Exp Biol Med 167:301, 1981

214. Schafer DF, et al. Visual evoked potentials in a rabbit model of hepatic encephalopathy: I. sequential changes and comparisons with drug-induced comas. Gastroenterology 86:540, 1984

215. Schafer VK, et al. Influence of an orally administered protein mixture enriched in branched chain amino acids on the chronic hepatic encephalopathy (CHE) of patients with liver cirrhosis. Z Gastroenterol 19:356, 1981

216. Schenker S, Brady CE III. Pathogenesis of hepatic encephalopathy. In: Conn HO, Bircher J, eds. Hepatic encephalopathy: syndromes and therapies. East Lansing, MI, Medi-Ed Press, 1993

217. Schomerus H, et al. Latent portasystemic encephalopathy: I. nature of cerebral functional defects and their effect on fitness to drive. Dig Dis Sci 26:622, 1981

218. Seegmiller JE, et al. The plasma ammonia and glutamine content in patients with hepatic coma. J Clin Invest 33:984, 1954

219. Short EM, et al. Evidence for X-linked dominant inheritance of ornithine transcarbamylase deficiency. N Engl J Med 288:7, 1973

220. Silberman R. Ammonia intoxication following ureterosigmoidostomy in a patient with liver disease. Lancet 2:937, 1958

221. Sinatra F, et al. Abnormalities of carbamyl phosphate synthetase and ornithine transcarbamylase in liver of patients with Reye's syndrome. Pediatr Res 9:829, 1975

222. Soeters PB. Nitrogen metabolism in the gut. In: Conn HO, Bircher J, eds. Hepatic encephalopathy: management with

lactulose and related carbohydrates. East Lansing, MI, Medi-Ed Press, 1988, p 31

223. Stabenau JR, et al. The role of pH gradient in the distribution of ammonia between blood and cerebrospinal fluid, brain and muscle. J Clin Invest 38:373, 1959

224. Stahl J. Studies of the blood ammonia in liver disease: its diagnostic, prognostic, and therapeutic significance. Ann Intern Med 58:1, 1963

225. Strauss E, et al. Treatment of hepatic encephalopathy: a randomized clinical trial comparing a branched chain enriched amino acid solution to oral neomycin. Nutr Supp Serv 6:18, 1986

226. Summerskill WHJ. Aguecheek's disease. Lancet 2:288, 1955

226a. Summerskill WHJ, et al. The neuropsychiatric syndrome associated with hepatic cirrhosis. Q J Med 25:245, 1956

227. Summerskill WHJ, et al. The management of hepatic coma in relation to protein withdrawal and certain specific measures. Am J Med 23:59, 1957

228. Tarver D, et al. Precipitation of hepatic encephalopathy by propranolol in cirrhosis. Br Med J 287:585, 1983

229. Testa R, Eftimiadi C, Sukkar GS, et al. A non absorbable rifamycin for treatment of hepatic encephalopathy. Drugs Exp Clin Res 11:387, 1985

230. Thompson JS, et al. Adequate diet prevents hepatic coma in dogs with Eck fistulas. Surg Gynecol Obstet 162:126, 1986

231. Thomson A, Visek WJ. Some effects of induction of urease immunity in patients with hepatic insufficiency. Am J Med 35:804, 1963

232. Tobe BA. The metabolism of the volatile amines: II. observations on the use of L-arginine L-glutamate in the therapy of acute hepatic encephalopathy. Can Med Assoc J 85:591, 1961

233. Tsukiyama K, et al. Electromyographic studies on the flapping tremor, especially its relationship to hyperammonemia. Folia Psychiatrica et Neurologica Japonica 15:21, 1961

234. Tuomisto J. Neuropharmacological intervention on the pituitary-hypothalamic relationship. Ann Clin Res 10:120, 1978

235. Uflacker R, Piske et al. Chronic portal-systemic encephalopathy: embolization of portal-systemic shunts. Radiology 165:721, 1987

236. Uribe M, et al. Treatment of chronic portal systemic encephalopathy with bromocriptine. Gastroenterology 76:1347, 1979

237. Uribe M, et al. Controlled study of lactose versus neomycin plus cathartics in the management of chronic portal-systemic encephalopathy. Gastroenterology 76:1300, 1979

238. Uribe M, et al. Treatment of chronic portal systemic encephalopathy with vegetable and animal protein diets: a controlled cross-over study. Dig Dis Sci 27:119, 1982

239. Uribe M, et al. Beneficial effect of vegetable protein diet supplemented with *Psyllium plantago* in patients with hepatic encephalopathy and diabetes mellitus. Gastroenterology 88:901, 1985

240. Uribe M, et al. Treatment of chronic portal-systemic encephalopathy with lactose in lactase deficient patients. Dig Dis Sci 25:924, 1980

241. Uribe M, et al. Acidifying enemas (lactitol and lactose) vs. nonacidifying enemas (tap water) to treat acute portal-systemic encephalopathy: a double-blind, randomized clinical trial. Hepatology 7:639, 1987

242. Uribe M, et al. Lactitol, a second-generation disaccharide for treatment of chronic portasystemic encephalopathy: a double-blind, crossover, randomized clinical trial. Dig Dis Sci 32:1345, 1987

242a. Uribe M. Treatments of portal-systemic encephalopathy: the old and new treatments. In: Grisolia S, ed. Cirrhosis, hepatic encephalopathy and ammonium toxicity. New York, Plenum, 1990, p 235

242b. Uribe M, et al. Hyperammonemic hepatic encephalopathy treated with sodium benzoate: final report of a double-blind evaluation. (Abstract) Hepatology 10:589, 1989

243. van Berlo CLH, et al. Is increased ammonia liberation after bleeding in the digestive tract the consequence of complete

absence of isoleucine in hemoglobin?: a study in pigs. Hepatology 10:315, 1989

244. van Der Rijt CCD, et al. Overt hepatic encephalopathy precipitated by zinc deficiency. Gastroenterology 100:1114, 1991

245. van Velthuijsen JA. Lactitol: chemical and biological properties. In: Conn HO, Bircher J, eds. Hepatic encephalopathy: syndromes and therapies. East Lansing, MI, Medi-Ed Press, 1993

246. van Vugt H, et al. Galactosamine hepatitis, endotoxemia, and lactulose. Hepatology 3:236, 1983

247. van Waes L, et al. Emergency treatment of portal-systemic encephalopathy with lactulose enemas: a controlled study. Acta Clin Belg 34:122, 1979

248. Victor M, et al. The acquired (non-Wilsonian) type of chronic hepatocerebral degeneration. Medicine 44:345, 1965

249. Vilstrup H, et al. Branched chain enriched amino acid versus glucose treatment of hepatic encephalopathy: a double-blind study of 65 patients with cirrhosis. J Hepatol 10:291, 1990

250. Vince A, et al. Effect of lactulose on ammonia production in a fecal incubation system. Gastroenterology 74:544, 1978

251. Voorhees AB, et al. Portal-system encephalopathy in the noncirrhotic patient. Arch Surg 107:659, 1973

252. Wahren J, et al. Is intravenous administration of branched chain amino acids effective in the treatment of hepatic encephalopathy?: a multicenter study. Hepatology 3:475, 1983

253. Walker S, et al. The use of ornithine salts of branched-chain acids in hyperammonemia in patients with cirrhosis of the liver: a double-blind crossover study. Digestion 24:105, 1982

254. Walker S, et al. Oral keto analogs of branched-chain amino acids in hyperammonemia in patients with cirrhosis of the liver: a double-blind crossover study. Digestion 24:105, 1982

255. Walshe JM. The effect of glutamic acid on the coma of hepatic failure. Lancet 1:1075, 1953

256. Ware AJ, et al. Cerebral edema: a major complication of massive hepatic necrosis. Gastroenterology 61:877, 1971

257. Warren KS, et al. Ammonia metabolism and hepatic coma in hepatosplenic schistosomiasis. Ann Intern Med 62:1113, 1965

258. Warren WD, et al. Ten years of portal hypertension surgery at Emory: results and new perspectives. Ann Surg 195:530, 1982

259. Weber FL Jr. The effect of lactulose on urea metabolism and nitrogen excretion in cirrhotic patients. Gastroenterology 77:518, 1979

260. Weber FL, Reiser BJ. Relationship of plasma amino acids to nitrogen balance and portal-systemic encephalopathy in alcoholic liver disease. Dig Dis Sci 27:103, 1982

261. Weber FL, Jr, Veach GI. The importance of the small intestine in gut ammonium production in the fasting dog. Gastroenterology 77:235, 1979

262. Weber FL Jr, et al. Effects of lactulose and neomycin on urea metabolism in cirrhotic subjects. Gastroenterology 82:213, 1982

263. Weber FL Jr, et al. Effects of vegetable diets on nitrogen metabolism in cirrhotic subjects. Gastroenterology 89:538, 1985

264. Webster LT Jr, Gabuzda GJ. Effect of portal blood ammonium concentration and of administering methionine to patients with hepatic cirrhosis. J Lab Clin Med 50:426, 1957

265. Wiesner RH. Does propranolol precipitate hepatic encephalopathy? J Clin Gastroenterol 8:74, 1986

266. Windus-Podehl G, et al. Encephalopathic effect of phenol in rats. J Lab Clin Med 101:586, 1983

267. Young LS, Hewitt WL. Activity of five aminoglycoside antibiotics in vitro against gram-negative bacilli and *Staphylococcus aureus*. Antimicrob Agents Chemother 4:617, 1973

268. Zaki AEO, et al. Experimental studies of blood brain barrier permeability in acute hepatic failure. Hepatology 4:359, 1984

269. Zeneroli ML, et al. Prevalence of brain atrophy in liver cirrhosis patients with chronic persistent encephalopathy. J Hepatol 4:283, 1987

270. Zeneroli ML, et al. Visual evoked potential diagnostic tool for the assessment of hepatic encephalopathy 25:291, 1984

270a. Zenerol ML, et al. Interindividual variability of the Number Connection Test. (Letter) J Hepatol 16:263, 1992
271. Zieve L, Brunner G. Encephalopathy due to mercaptans and phenols. In: McCandless DW, ed. Cerebral energy metabolism and metabolic encephalopathy. New York, Plenum Press, 1985, p 179
272. Zieve FJ, et al. Synergism between ammonia and fatty acids in the production of coma: implications for hepatic coma. J Pharmacol Exp Ther 191:10, 1974
273. Zieve L. Encephalopathy due to short- and medium-chain fatty acids. In: McCandless DW, ed. Cerebral energy metabolism and metabolic encephalopathy. New York, Plenum Press, 1985, p 163
274. Zieve L, et al. Synergism between mercaptans and ammonia or fatty acids in the production of coma: a possible role for mercaptans in the pathogenesis of hepatic coma. J Lab Clin Med 83:16, 1974
275. Zieve L, et al. Toxicity of a fatty acid and ammonia: interactions with hypoglycemia and Krebs cycle inhibition. J Lab Clin Med 101:930, 1983
276. Zieve L, et al. Brain methanethiol and ammonia concentrations in experimental hepatic coma and coma induced by injections of various combinations of these substances. J Lab Clin Med 104:655, 1984
277. Zieve L, et al. Ammonia, octanoate and mercaptan depress regeneration of normal rat liver after partial hepatectomy. Hepatology 5:28, 1985
278. Zieve L, et al. The dietary prevention of hepatic coma in Eck fistula dogs: ammonia and the carbohydrate to protein ratio. Hepatology 7:196, 1987
279. Zimmerman HJ, Ishak KG. Valproate-induced hepatic injury: analyses of 23 fatal cases. Hepatology 2:591, 1982
280. Zimmon DS. Oxyhemoglobin dissociation in patients with hepatic encephalopathy. Gastroenterology 52:647, 1967

Diseases of the Liver, Seventh Edition, edited by
Leon Schiff and Eugene R. Schiff. J.B. Lippincott Company, Philadelphia © 1993.

38

Hemostatic Disorders in Liver Disease

Justine Meehan Carr

Hemorrhagic sequelae of liver disease were recognized and described more than a century ago.[32] Bleeding complications and abnormal coagulation test results still frequently accompany liver disease. Because of the primary role of the liver in the synthesis of coagulation factors and regulating proteins, the diagnosis of acquired coagulopathies in patients with impaired liver function often poses a diagnostic dilemma both at the bedside and in the laboratory.

Normal Coagulation and the Role of the Liver

Under normal conditions, blood circulates through the vasculature without appreciable coagulation or hemorrhage.[53] When vessel injury occurs, three hemostatic responses are initiated: (1) the vessel constricts; (2) platelets adhere at the site of damage and, subsequently, aggregate; and (3) fibrin clot is formed and modified. The hemostatic response occurs in a stepwise, integrated manner. In primary hemostasis, vessels constrict and a temporary platelet plug is formed. Secondarily, the platelet plug is reinforced with a durable fibrin clot. The fibrin clot is modified and, after tissue healing, ultimately dissolved by fibrinolytic components. The failure of any part of the hemostatic response may contribute to hemorrhage. The coexistence of multiple defects in the hemostatic system may have an additive effect, resulting in a profound hemorrhagic catastrophe.

Vasoconstriction is an immediate but probably minor response to vascular injury.[269] Small arteries and veins contract so as to decrease blood flow to the area. If hemorrhage occurs in a closed compartment, such as a joint space, local pressure causes collapse of small vessels, thereby contributing to local control.[208] In the absence of local tissue tension, as in gastrointestinal bleeding or hemorrhage from a large vessel, bleeding is more difficult to control.[208]

Platelets serve two functions. First, they form a primary hemostatic plug. Second, they serve as a template for the generation of fibrin by way of the coagulation cascade. Platelet plug formation occurs in two phases—platelet adhesion, which occurs within seconds, followed by platelet aggregation, which is complete within minutes.[203] Platelet adhesion to the injured vessel requires the secretion of von Willebrand factor by endothelial cells and the availability of platelet membrane glycoprotein Ib as a receptor for von Willebrand factor.[207,235] Once adhesion occurs, platelets undergo a shape change with a coincident release of various mediators, including adenosine diphosphate (ADP), which stimulates

platelets to aggregate and form the primary platelet plug. The aggregated platelets then provide the surface on which the fibrin plug is formed. In addition, platelets serve as a source of phospholipid, in the form of platelet factor 3, required for the conversion of prothrombin to thrombin by factor Xa.[164]

The exposed subendothelial components activate the coagulation cascade, either through contact activation of the intrinsic pathway or through expression of tissue factor at the site of injury with consequent extrinsic pathway activation (Fig. 38-1). It is now recognized that the intrinsic and extrinsic pathways are not entirely independent of each other. In vitro and in vivo studies support the observation that factor VII–tissue factor also activates factor IX.[15,137,182] Through a complex sequence of reactions, clotting factor precursors are converted to their active form with the eventual generation of thrombin. Thrombin then transforms fibrinogen to fibrin, and fibrin is cross-linked by factor XIIIa to form a stable fibrin clot.

When fibrin is formed, plasminogen is bound to the clot. Tissue plasminogen activator is released from endothelial cells and then binds to the fibrin clot. On the fibrin surface, plasminogen is cleaved, plasmin is generated, and fibrin degradation ensues[53,141] (Fig. 38-2). Remodeling and eventual dissolution of the clot permit subsequent wound healing with the formation of fibrous tissue.[53] In abnormal states, such as disseminated intravascular coagulation (DIC), plasmin may also be present in the blood, where it can degrade fibrinogen and factors V, VIII, and XIII.[152]

Modulation of coagulation and fibrinolysis occurs at various sites, as listed in Figures 38-1 and 38-2.[85] Control of coagulation is achieved by several measures. The liver inactivates activated factors.[67,83] Further, natural inhibitors to various factors are present in plasma. Antithrombin III (ATIII) is a major inhibitor of thrombin as well as factors XIIa, XIa, Xa, and IXa.[14] ATIII also inhibits plasma kallikrein and plasmin.[239] The activity of ATIII is increased 1000-fold in the presence of heparin, heparan, or contact with endothelial cells, which are coated with heparan sulfate.[59]

Protein C is a second major inhibitor. This vitamin K–dependent glycoprotein is synthesized in the liver and inactivates factors Va and VIIIa.[93,230] In addition, protein C enhances fibrinolysis by inactivating plasminogen activator inhibitor type 1.[248] Protein C is activated when thrombin is bound to the endothelial cell membrane protein thromboodulin.[185] Both anticoagulant and profibrinolytic activities of protein C are accelerated in the presence of the cofactor protein S, another vitamin K–dependent protein.[64,69] Activated protein C is inactivated by α_1-antitrypsin and protein C inhibitor.[229,245]

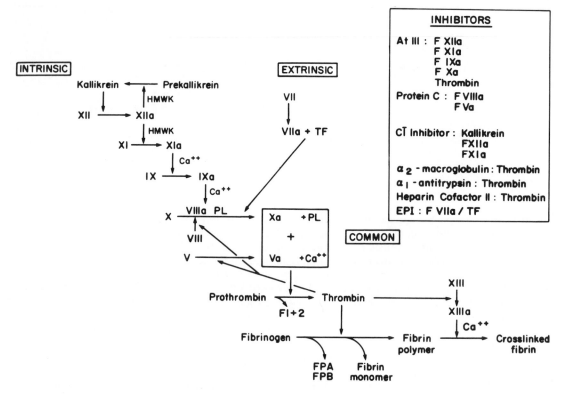

FIGURE 38-1 Overview of coagulation cascade. Factor VII and tissue factor can also activate factor IX. HMWK, high-molecular-weight kininogen; PL, phospholipid; TF, tissue factor; FPA, fibrinopeptide A; FPB, fibrinopeptide B; AT III, antithrombin III; EPI, extrinsic pathway inhibitor, also known as lipoprotein associated coagulation inhibitor. (Carr JM. Disseminated intravascular coagulation in cirrhosis. Hepatology 10:103, 1989)

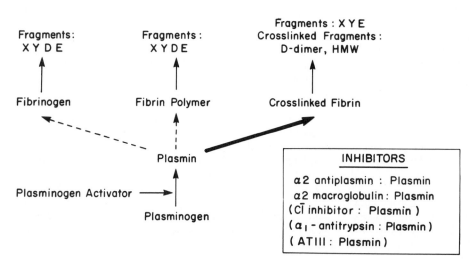

FIGURE 38-2 Fibrinolytic pathway. Plasmin is formed when plasminogen is activated. Activation may be accomplished either by tissue (or urokinase) plasminogen activator or by contact phase of coagulation (factor XIIa or kallikrein). Under physiologic conditions, tissue plasminogen activator is released from endothelial cells and binds to fibrin polymer where plasminogen is activated to form plasmin. Plasmin then digests fibrin clots (*heavy line*), yielding the unique high-molecular-weight (HMW) degradation fragments and fragment D-dimer. In the pathologic condition disseminated intravascular coagulation, excess plasmin is generated, and in addition to degrading cross-linked fibrin, it degrades fibrinogen and non–cross-linked fibrin, yielding degradation fragments X, Y, D, and E (*dashed lines*). The major inhibitor of plasmin is α_2-antiplasmin; other, minor inhibitors are indicated in parentheses. The major inhibitors of plasminogen activator are plasminogen activator inhibitor 1 and plasminogen activator inhibitor 2. (Carr JM. Disseminated intravascular coagulation in cirrhosis. Hepatology 10:103, 1989)

Heparin cofactor II, a glycoprotein synthesized by the liver, inactivates thrombin in the presence of heparin or dermatan sulfate.[121,237] Extrinsic pathway inhibitor (also called lipoprotein-associated coagulation inhibitor) inhibits coagulation initiated by the VIIa–tissue factor complex by binding to factor Xa.[31,194,211] The site of synthesis of extrinsic pathway inhibitor is still not certain.[175] The major inhibitor of plasmin is α_2-antiplasmin, which is synthesized in the liver.[209] α_2-Macroglobulin, a second-line inhibitor of plasmin[113] and thrombin,[1] is synthesized by macrophages[117] and, possibly, hepatocytes.[131] Tissue plasminogen activator is inhibited by plasminogen activator inhibitor 1, which is secreted by endothelial cells but also found in platelets.[221]

The liver plays a central role in hemostasis. In addition to its synthetic function, the liver serves as a key site for clearance of activated clotting factors and plasminogen activators.[67,83,92]

Coagulation Disorders in Liver Disease

THROMBOCYTOPENIA AND THROMBOPATHY

Both quantitative and qualitative platelet defects may occur in patients with liver disease. Thrombocytopenia often is found in patients with cirrhosis who have portal hypertension and congestive splenomegaly. In a normal person, about 30% of the total platelet mass is traversing the spleen at any one time. In stress, such as hemorrhage, these platelets are readily available for hemostasis.[7,256] In patients with portal hypertension and cirrhosis, up to 90% of the platelets may pool in the expanded cordal compartments of the spleen. Although the measurable platelet count is low (often 50,000 to 100,000/μL), the total platelet mass is normal and the platelets are available participants in hemostasis.[7] Platelet transfusion in these patients often yields no increment in platelet count because transfused platelets may also be sequestered in the spleen.[7,236]

Thrombocytopenia commonly is seen in patients with alcoholic liver disease, where several causes are possible. First, splenic pooling of platelets may occur if cirrhosis with portal hypertension is present. Second, alcohol has a direct toxic effect on platelets and lowers the platelet count after 10 days of binge drinking in an otherwise well-nourished person.[145] The mechanism is thought to be ineffective thrombopoiesis combined, in some cases, with decreased platelet survival.[227] Finally, alcoholic patients may have inadequate diets with limited folate ingestion—a problem compounded by the fact that alcohol can interfere with utilization of available folate.[226] The manner whereby alcohol interferes with folate metabolism is not well understood. Folate is critical for DNA synthesis; therefore, because of the high proliferative rate of marrow cells, folate deficiency often is manifested as a depression of platelets or of white or red cells or pancytopenia.

Mild thrombocytopenia may develop during acute hepatitis, occurring in one study in 16% of patients without hepatic failure and 52% of patients with hepatic failure.[95] The cause is multifactorial, resulting in part from congestive splenomegaly. In addition, platelet production may be impaired by viral invasion of megakaryocytes[11,172] or platelets.[216] Finally, immune-mediated platelet destruction may also occur.[125] Thrombocytopenia usually resolves with hepatic recovery. Several weeks to months after the onset of acute hepatitis, a subset of patients may develop aplastic anemia,

possibly as a result of stem cell destruction by the virus.[160,206] Aplastic anemia has also been observed among patients with severe hepatitis who undergo liver transplantation. In one study, 9 of 32 patients (28%) who received a liver transplant for non-A, non-B hepatitis developed aplastic anemia.[243] This complication was not seen in the patients who received a transplant for reasons other than non-A, non-B hepatitis.[243] In a prospective study of 19 patients with severe hepatitis-associated aplastic anemia, there was no increased representation of patients with anti–hepatitis C virus antibodies.[190]

One additional cause of thrombocytopenia in patients with liver disease and hemorrhage is dilution. Thrombocytopenia may occur in a patient with a major hemorrhage who is being transfused with red blood cells and plasma but not receiving platelets.

Various qualitative platelet defects have also been described in patients with liver disease, but these defects are not seen in all patients. In acute fulminant hepatitis, abnormal ultrastructure, increased glass bead retention, and impaired platelet aggregation to ADP have been described.[205] Platelet dysfunction has been described in a case of a patient with thrombocytosis and extrahepatic biliary obstruction from pancreatic cancer.[134] The patient's platelets did not aggregate with collagen, epinephrine, or ristocetin and ADP-induced aggregation was reduced.[134] Bleeding times in patients with acute hepatic failure may be prolonged more than would be predicted by the platelet count.[206] The qualitative platelet defects are thought to be minor contributors to the overall coagulopathy of acute hepatic failure except in cases of severe thrombocytopenia.

Many studies have also reported platelet dysfunction in chronic liver disease.[10,40,136,181,184,206,233] As in acute hepatic disease, disproportionately long bleeding times have been reported.[10,151,206] In vitro abnormalities have included decreased adhesiveness of platelets to glass beads[136] and impaired aggregation to ADP,[10,184,206,233,234] epinephrine,[184] thrombin,[233] and ristocetin.[40] In concordance with the abnormal ristocetin agglutination, decreased membrane glycoprotein I has been observed.[181] Decreased platelet factor 3 has also been described.[148] Qualitative platelet defects are not found in all patients with cirrhosis, however.[222] Indeed, some authors question whether the observed platelet dysfunction in liver disease has any clinical significance.[97]

ALTERED SYNTHESIS OF COAGULATION FACTORS: VITAMIN K DEFICIENCY

Vitamin K is necessary for factors II, VII, IX, and X as well as protein C and protein S to be biologically active.[228] After synthesis of these factors, vitamin K serves as a cofactor for a hepatic carboxylase that converts glutamic acid residues in the amino-terminal region of the proteins to γ-carboxyglutamic acid residues.[74,224] The γ-carboxyglutamic acid is the site for attachment of calcium, which is critical for the function of the factors.[29] When vitamin K is unavailable or blocked by an antagonist, the amount of γ-carboxyglutamic acid is reduced and the proteins become inert.[91,223] Although present immunologically, functional laboratory tests reveal depressed levels of these proteins.[99,115]

Vitamin K is a fat-soluble vitamin found in abundance in green, leafy vegetables.[3] Small amounts of the vitamin are also synthesized by bacteria in the large intestine.[158] The daily dietary requirement for vitamin K is between 1 and 3 μg/kg body weight.[21,89] Because vitamin K is fat-soluble, absorption from the small intestine requires the presence of bile salts.[114,218] Patients with either extrahepatic biliary tract obstruction or intrahepatic obstruction from parenchymal disease may be at risk for vitamin K deficiency. Patients with partial biliary tract obstruction treated with cholestyramine for pruritus are also at risk because cholestyramine binds bile salts and further impairs vitamin K absorption. Patients with inadequate vitamin K intake may become deficient if they receive antibiotics, thereby abolishing intestinal flora as a source of vitamin K.[4] Clinical deficiency can develop within 1 to 3 weeks.[4] Spontaneous hemorrhage may occur if the deficiency is not treated.

ALTERED SYNTHESIS OF CLOTTING FACTORS: DYSFIBRINOGENEMIA

Patients with cirrhosis, chronic active liver disease, acute hepatic failure, or hepatoma may develop dysfibrinogenemia.[86,104,106,107] In patients with obstructive jaundice, dysfibrinogenemia is uncommon.[86,142] The dysfibrinogenemia is characterized by excess sialic acid residues on the beta and gamma chains of fibrinogen.[154] These residues interfere with fibrin polymerization.[154] The fibrinogen level may be normal, but the thrombin time and often the reptilase time are prolonged.[154]

Assessment of the risk of hemorrhage in a patient with dysfibrinogenemia is difficult for several reasons. First, the question of whether this represents a hemorrhagic risk is unclear, since most patients with hereditary dysfibrinogenemias with impairment of fibrin monomer polymerization have no bleeding complications.[102] Second, dysfibrinogenemia often occurs in patients with significant impairment of hepatic function and impaired synthesis of other coagulation factors, so that the unique contribution of dysfibrinogenemia to hemorrhage cannot be assessed.[106] In one study of patients bleeding from esophageal varices, however, the patients with abnormal fibrin polymerization had a worse prognosis than those who lacked this defect.[107]

DEPRESSED SYNTHESIS OF CLOTTING FACTORS

Because most clotting factors are synthesized in the liver, depressed levels of various clotting factors often are found in hepatic failure. The type of liver disease may influence the constellation of clotting factor deficiencies.

Factor VII

Factor VII has the shortest half-life of the clotting factors (about 5 to 6 hours) and is synthesized in the liver. Prolongation of the prothrombin time, which reflects factor VII activity, may serve as a sensitive indicator of impaired synthetic function.[95] Impairment of clotting factor synthesis often is seen in acute hepatitis as well as in cirrhosis. In acute liver disease, the prothrombin time prolongation correlates with the severity of the hepatocellular damage, the likelihood of bleeding, and the overall prognosis.[70,95,165,219] In chronic liver disease, depression of factor VII reflects loss of hepatic parenchymal cells and usually correlates with severity of disease,[254] although factor V levels may correlate to a greater degree.[66,186]

Fibrinogen

Fibrinogen is synthesized predominantly in the liver. The normal plasma level is between 150 and 300 mg/dL and the

half-life is 3 to 5 days.[52] Megakaryocytes produce some fibrinogen as well, but the role of megakaryocytic fibrinogen is uncertain.[244] Fibrinogen is an acute-phase reactant, and plasma levels may increase eight-fold in the face of an inflammatory stimulus.[132] This response to inflammation is mediated by the peptide hepatocyte-stimulating factor II.[81] Fibrinogen degradation is also a stimulus to fibrinogen synthesis, increasing fibrinogen production up to 20-fold.[88] This response is initiated by fibrinogen degradation products (FDP) by way of hepatocyte-stimulating factor.[210] In acute hepatitis without hepatic failure, fibrinogen levels are high, as would be expected of an acute-phase reactant.[95,138] In acute hepatitis with hepatic failure, the levels often are low.[95,138] Failure of fibrinogen to respond as an acute-phase reactant in acute hepatitis or cirrhosis is a poor prognostic sign.[197] In addition to impaired synthesis of fibrinogen, the hypofibrinogenemia may result from extravascular losses or coexistent DIC,[192] although the presence of DIC has been difficult to establish conclusively in many cases.[17,24,35,36,225,232,247,251] In chronic stable liver disease, fibrinogen levels usually are normal or mildly increased. In advanced disease, levels fall as a result of impaired synthesis, extravascular losses, or increased catabolism.[222]

Factor VIII

Factor VIII:C (coagulant) circulates in a complex with von Willebrand factor, which is synthesized in the endothelium and megakaryocytes.[118,122,170] The site of synthesis for factor VIII:C has not been established conclusively. Evidence from organ transplantation experience in hemophilia suggests that the liver is a major site of synthesis.[143,259] Further, factor VIII antigen has been identified in human hepatocytes.[268] However, messenger RNA for factor VIII has been found in spleen and lymph nodes as well as in liver, an observation that suggests the likelihood of extrahepatic synthesis of factor VIII.[265] Patients with severe hepatic failure often have normal or elevated factor VIII:C levels, which further suggests the possibility of extrahepatic synthesis.[40,126,163,183,249] Alternatively, factor VIII:C levels may remain high because of the liver's inability to degrade the factor VIII complex.[219]

Factor V

Factor V is synthesized both in the liver and in megakaryocytes.[98,155,173,180,264] Transfusion of normal platelets into a factor V–deficient patient partially corrects the deficiency.[28] Endothelial cells may synthesize factor V as well.[43] Factor V usually is low in patients with cirrhosis, hepatoma, or chronic liver disease but normal or elevated in patients with obstructive jaundice, primary biliary cirrhosis, or metastatic tumor in the liver.[42,126,195,246] The degree of depression of the factor V level often is a prognostic indicator in chronic liver disease.[66,186,198] How often factor V deficiency contributes to hemorrhage in these patients is not clear. Patients with congenital factor V deficiency have levels that range from 0% to 10% of normal. Patients with the inherited deficiency may be asymptomatic or have bruisability and epistaxis, whereas spontaneous hemarthroses are rare.[200]

OTHER FACTORS AND INHIBITORS

Plasma concentrations of contact activation factors XII and XI, prekallikrein, and high-molecular-weight kininogen may be reduced in acute liver disease but appear to alter the clinical course very little.[138] Factor XIII may also be reduced in

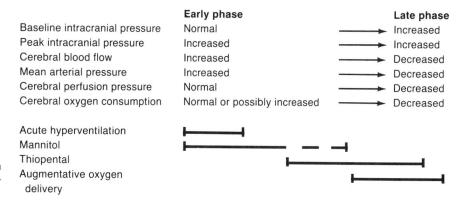

	Early phase	Late phase
Baseline intracranial pressure	Normal	→ Increased
Peak intracranial pressure	Increased	→ Increased
Cerebral blood flow	Increased	→ Decreased
Mean arterial pressure	Increased	→ Decreased
Cerebral perfusion pressure	Normal	→ Decreased
Cerebral oxygen consumption	Normal or possibly increased	→ Decreased

Acute hyperventilation
Mannitol
Thiopental
Augmentative oxygen delivery

FIGURE 39-3 Schematic representation of the characteristics and management of cerebral edema.

320 mOsm. In patients with coexisting oliguric renal failure, the administration of mannitol needs to be coupled with the removal of three times the administered volume by ultrafiltration after 15 minutes. When the cerebral perfusion pressure falls below 50 mmHg, inotropic support should be instituted and the delivery of oxygen to the brain optimized. At this stage, the patient should be supine to maximize cerebral perfusion.[18] Cerebral edema resistant to these associated measures may respond to sodium thiopental, using initial bolus doses of 185 to 500 mg (median, 250 mg) over 15 minutes, followed by infusions of 50 to 250 mg/h for up to 4 hours.[31] The limitations of this approach are hypotension, reversible by dose reduction, and possible impairment of white cell function. The prophylactic use of dexamethasone was not found to be effective in reducing cerebral edema.[14] Most patients who survive cerebral edema revert to normal neurologic function, but occasional cases with a residual deficit have been reported.[76]

RENAL FAILURE

The incidence of oliguric renal failure, defined by a urine output of less than 300 mL/24 h and serum creatinine levels less than 300 μmol/L in the presence of adequate intravascular pressures, is 75% after an acetaminophen overdose and 30% in other cases of fulminant hepatic failure.[79] Renal failure after acetaminophen overdose appears to be a consequence of direct renal toxicity and usually is established before the development of advanced encephalopathy. Patients with other causes of fulminant hepatic failure develop renal impairment when the encephalopathy is advanced, and it is usual to progress through a stage of functional renal failure (urinary sodium below 10 mmol/L, urine/plasma osmolarity ratio of more than 1.1) before demonstrating the characteristics of tubular damage. Impaired urea synthesis may result in a considerable disparity between serum urea and creatinine levels, so the latter should be used to monitor renal function in fulminant hepatic failure.

Reduced intravascular filling pressures, secondary either to hypovolemia or vasodilatation, may contribute to deteriorating renal function, and appropriate treatment is important. Infusion of dopamine, 2 to 4 μg/kg/h, may reverse or slow the deterioration in renal function by increasing renal blood flow in patients who are not anuric. The use of high-dose furosemide is not advised, and considerable care is indicated when using other potentially nephrotoxic drugs, including high doses of mannitol and aminoglycosides. Fulminant hepatic failure complicated by renal failure was once considered to have a poor prognosis,[111] but recent survival figures for such patients are as high as 50% in acetaminophen-overdose patients, and 30% in patients with viral hepatitis A and B.[79]

Renal support is usually instituted before the conventional indications for hemodialysis become established. Continuous hemofiltration systems, either arteriovenous or venovenous, are well tolerated and usually effective. They are associated with less hemodynamic instability and less potentiation of cerebral edema than conventional hemodialysis and are thus preferable in patients with advanced encephalopathy. Hemodialysis has advantages, however, in patients who require prolonged renal support after recovery from encephalopathy, a scenario that is especially common in acetaminophen-induced fulminant hepatic failure. Despite the coexisting coagulopathy, heparin is needed to protect the remaining coagulation factors, and requirements are often higher than in uncomplicated renal failure.[97] Prostacyclin and regional citration are alternatives to heparin in patients with significant clinical coagulopathy.

METABOLIC DISORDERS

Hypoglycemia is common and may precede the onset of grade 3 encephalopathy, resulting in a precipitous deterioration in mental state. In established encephalopathy, the clinical signs and symptoms of hypoglycemia are masked, and the blood glucose levels should be measured hourly and supplemental glucose administered intravenously when the level falls below 3.5 mmol/L (63 mg/dL). The hypoglycemia is a consequence of increased circulating insulin levels, impaired gluconeogenesis, and inability to mobilize glycogen stores.

Metabolic acidosis is present in 30% of patients who develop fulminant hepatic failure after an acetaminophen overdose and is associated with a particularly high mortality—more than 90% if the arterial pH is less than 7.3 on the second or subsequent days after the overdose.[77,79] This acidosis precedes the onset of encephalopathy and is independent of renal function. In contrast, a metabolic acidosis is found in 5% of patients with other causes of fulminant hepatic failure, occurring later in the disease process and also associated with a poor outcome.[77] Increased serum lactate levels have been documented in patients with metabolic acidosis,[7] possibly reflecting tissue hypoxia resulting from impaired oxygen extraction caused by microvascular shunting of blood away from actively respiring tissues. The latter may be due to changes in microvascular tone, increased capillary permeability, or fibrin and cellular aggregate microemboli.[109] Impaired tissue oxygen extraction is associated with a poor prognosis, and its management is considered in more detail later. Treatment modalities directed at the manifestations of tissue hypoxia in blood (eg, sodium bicarbonate and hemodialysis) are ineffective.

In most cases of fulminant hepatic failure, an alkalosis is more frequently encountered. It probably is a combination of respiratory and metabolic abnormalities and often is associated with hypokalemia. Hyponatremia also is seen commonly in fulminant hepatic failure and is dilutional in origin. Hypophosphatemia occurs,[23] especially in patients with normal renal function. Phosphate replenishment may be indicated to improve diaphragmatic contractility, but caution is necessary because levels rise rapidly when renal impairment develops.

CARDIOVASCULAR SYSTEM AND HEMODYNAMICS

As mentioned previously, systolic hypertension in a patient with grade 4 encephalopathy indicates a paroxysm of increased intracranial pressure. Circulatory failure is another common cause of death in fulminant hepatic failure. The initial hemodynamic abnormalities are similar to those found in septic shock and are typified by a high cardiac output with a reduction in systemic peripheral vascular resistance and diastolic blood pressure. Relative hypovolemia secondary to vasodilation results in decreased central venous, pulmonary artery, and left atrial end-diastolic pressures. Measurement of all these parameters is necessary because a disparity between right- and left-sided pressures may result in an erroneous assessment of fluid requirements. Volume replacement should be with an appropriate combination of blood (if the hemoglobin is reduced), colloid (plasma or human albumin), and crystalline (5% to 10% dextrose) solutions. Persistent hypotension in patients with adequate intravascular volumes is associated with a poor prognosis. Inotropes may be used, but unless they facilitate a therapeutic procedure (eg, orthotopic liver transplantation or hemodialysis), they rarely improve the outcome. Dopamine and dobutamine are relatively ineffective, but noradrenaline and adrenaline increase the mean arterial pressure and systemic vascular resistance.[110] Adrenaline is more likely to increase the cardiac output if this is also compromised. Neither noradrenaline nor adrenaline improves oxygen consumption in this setting,[110] and manipulations to produce a parallel improvement in oxygen delivery and consumption indices are necessary. Prostacyclin has been shown to increase oxygen extraction and consumption in fulminant hepatic failure,[7,110] while N-acetylcysteine has also been shown to improve the hemodynamics and oxygen metabolism indices in these patients.[48] The manipulations in hemodynamics should aim to achieve a cardiac index of more than 4.5 L/min/m^2, oxygen delivery more than 700 mL/min/m^2, oxygen consumption more than 170 mL/min/m^2, and a systemic vascular resistance index of more than 700 dynes/s/cm^5.[109]

Although cardiac arrhythmia is said to be common in fulminant hepatic failure, it usually is due to a definable precipitating event, such as hypokalemia or hyperkalemia, acidosis, hypoxia, or cardiac irritation by a catheter, especially Swan-Ganz catheters. Thus, the primary treatment should be directed at correction of any underlying cause before antiarrhythmic drugs are administered. Progressive bradycardia over a period of hours is a common terminal event, with the pulse rate falling in steady increments until asystole occurs.

RESPIRATORY COMPLICATIONS

Hyperventilation is commonly observed in association with other signs of cerebral edema, causing hypocapnea and contributing to the alkalosis described previously. Advanced cerebral edema may result in respiratory depression and finally apnea. In this situation, assisted mechanical ventilation may be indicated either for fatigue complicating hyperventilation or for respiratory depression.

Arterial hypoxemia is also common and often has a multifactorial cause. Aspiration of gastric contents is a particular risk in encephalopathic patients who are vomiting, and the need for airway protection may precipitate early endotracheal intubation. Radiologic evidence of bacterial infection was found in 24% of one series of patients,[105] while pathogens were cultured from sputum in 46% of patients in a different series.[91] Pulmonary edema was diagnosed in 37% of patients, including almost half of those with radiologic evidence of pneumonia.[105] The pulmonary edema is largely noncardiogenic in origin (pulmonary capillary wedge pressure corrected for serum albumin less than 18 mmHg) and is especially frequent in patients after an acetaminophen overdose. Intrapulmonary hemorrhage and basal atelectasis are other factors that may contribute to the arterial hypoxemia. In some patients, the hypoxemia occurs in association with a normal chest radiograph and is attributed to a ventilation–perfusion mismatch consequent on intrapulmonary vascular shunting. Assisted mechanical ventilation is usually required once hypoxemia develops. Bronchoscopy and lavage may be beneficial in selected cases to establish the cause of infection and to direct antibiotic therapy. The restrictions on physiotherapy in patients with coexisting cerebral edema were discussed previously.

COAGULOPATHY

Considering the central role of the liver in the synthesis of the coagulation factors and some of the inhibitors of coagulation and fibrinolysis, it is not surprising to find a complex coagulopathy in fulminant hepatic failure. The hepatocyte synthesizes most of the coagulation factors other than factor VIII, and in fulminant hepatic failure, circulating levels of fibrinogen, prothrombin, and factors V, VII, IX, and X are reduced. The prothrombin time is used widely as an indicator of the severity of liver damage, although in France, the measurement of factor V levels is preferred for this purpose.[6] Circulating levels of antithrombin III, an inhibitor of coagulation, are also reduced in fulminant hepatic failure, and this has the clinical effect of shortening the half-life of heparin. A controlled trial of antithrombin III supplementation (3000 IU) before hemodialysis showed an improvement in heparin kinetics and a reduction in platelet losses during dialysis in the active treatment group.[63] In addition to decreased synthesis of factors by the liver, there is also evidence of increased peripheral consumption. Although overt disseminated intravascular coagulation is unusual, sensitive techniques point to the presence of a low-grade process in most patients.[53] Both quantitative and qualitative defects in platelet function are well described in fulminant hepatic failure. In one study, platelet counts of less than 100 × 10^9/L were documented in 69% of patients.[37] Platelet aggregation is impaired, but there is an increase in platelet adhesiveness, a pattern that may be due to increased levels of circulating of von Willebrand's factor in fulminant hepatic failure.[92]

In an early study, hemorrhage was documented in 73% of 132 patients with fulminant hepatic failure and was described as severe in 30%.[37] The clinical impact of the coagulopathy, however, has been reduced by the use of fresh frozen plasma, cryoprecipitate, and platelet concentrates. The deficiency of coagulation factors alone does not correlate with the risk of bleeding, and hemorrhage is most likely when there is an associated thrombocytopenia, especially in the minority of patients with frank disseminated intravascular coagulation syndrome. Gastrointestinal hemorrhage is common and is related to the development of gastric erosions, although the incidence and severity has been decreased by the prophylactic use of H_2 antagonists.[68] More recently, the use of H_2 antagonists has been linked with an increased incidence of nosocomial respiratory infections, and advantages have been suggested for using cytoprotective agents, such as sucralfate, that do not inhibit gastric acid secretion. The other main sites include nasopharynx, lungs, kidneys, retroperitoneum, and skin puncture sites. The prophylactic administration of fresh frozen plasma limits the prognostic contribution of coagulation studies and was not associated with a reduction in either morbidity or mortality in one study.[35] Because of the combined quantitative and qualitative defects in platelet function, platelet transfusions are indicated in patients with severe hemorrhage, and to maintain levels higher than $50 \times 10^9/L$ before invasive procedures are performed.

SEPSIS

Patients with fulminant hepatic failure are at increased risk of infection because of broadly compromised immune functions, including impaired neutrophil and Kupffer cell functions[15] and deficiency of opsonins (eg, complement components and fibronectin).[44,117] One early study in fulminant hepatic failure demonstrated a bacteremia rate of 22%, which was calculated as twice the expected rate for similarly ill patients without liver disease.[116] Covert infection, however, may be difficult to detect, and a high index of suspicion for sepsis is necessary. In a recent prospective study of infections in 50 patients with fulminant hepatic failure and at least grade 2 encephalopathy, bacterial infection was diagnosed in 40 patients (80%) on the basis of positive cultures.[91] In a further 5 patients, bacterial infection was suspected. The source of positive culture was blood in 14 (isolated bacteremia in 6), urine in 12, sputum in 25, and indwelling cannulas in 2 patients. The predominant isolated organisms were *Staphylococcus aureus*, *Streptococcus* sp, and coliform bacteria. In the same series, fungi were cultured from 16 (32%) patients, most of which were *Candida* sp, usually later in the hospital course. These infections were particularly difficult to diagnose and were detected antemortem in only half of cases. The coexistence of renal failure results in an increased risk of developing both bacterial and fungal sepsis.

Daily cultures of all available specimens are indicated to maintain tight surveillance for emerging infection. Positive cultures should be treated with appropriate antibiotics, but the question of prophylactic administration of broad-spectrum antibiotics has not yet been resolved. Controlled studies are also in progress to assess the value of selective small bowel decontamination in reducing the incidence of infections. Antibiotics and possibly antifungal agents should be commenced in patients who appear to be recovering from fulminant hepatic failure but in whom a downward trend in prothrombin time is arrested before normal values are attained. This pattern in our experience is almost invariably associated with underlying sepsis.

NUTRITIONAL SUPPORT

Patients with fulminant hepatic failure tend to be well nourished at the time of presentation. Hypercatabolic states either due to infection or after orthotopic liver transplantation are common, however, and patients surviving the first few days may lose weight and muscle bulk rapidly. Glucose supplementation to prevent hypoglycemia provides about 400 kcal/d. More aggressive nutritional support has been restricted by a number of actual or perceived problems. Enteral nutrition is impractical because of ileus, pancreatitis in some patients, and the reluctance to introduce protein into the gastrointestinal tract. Renal failure also limits the options with respect to volume and protein load. Although conventional wisdom suggests that lipid emulsions should not be given to patients with fulminant hepatic failure, a pilot study has demonstrated the clearance of lipids from serum in these patients and that positive energy and nitrogen balance could be attained with parenteral nutrition.[32] There is a theoretic advantage to using branched-chain amino acids, but this has not yet been established in clinical trials.

Specific Therapies

A number of treatment modalities have been used in fulminant hepatic failure, directed at either reducing the toxin load or promoting hepatocyte regeneration. There is no role for corticosteroid therapy in fulminant hepatic failure, and data available from controlled studies suggest that this treatment is contraindicated.[30] Although some patients with late-onset hepatic failure are steroid-responsive, they are not yet readily identifiable on the basis of serologic markers, and the use of corticosteroids increases the risk of sepsis.

Insulin and glucagon have been used to promote hepatic regeneration, and in one uncontrolled series, an increase in survival from 14.4% to 22.6% was noted in a subgroup of patients whose encephalopathy developed between 11 and 30 days after the onset of symptoms.[102] Two controlled studies, however, failed to show any benefit with insulin and glucagon infusions.[46,112] Circulating interferon levels were found to be reduced markedly in one study of 15 patients with fulminant hepatic failure of viral cause, and 7 of 9 patients treated with interferon for 3 or more days survived.[66] In another series, only 2 of 12 patients treated with α-interferon survived,[93] and no controlled studies have been reported to date.

The first enthusiastic report of prostaglandins in the treatment of fulminant hepatic failure concerned 17 patients with viral fulminant or subfulminant hepatitis who were given prostaglandin E_1 (PGE_1) at a rate of 0.2 to 0.6 μg/k/h for up to 28 days.[98] Two of these patients underwent liver transplantation, and 12 of the remainder (80%) survived. All 5 patients with non-A, non-B hepatitis relapsed after cessation of treatment, but a further remission was obtained with resumed infusion followed by oral administration of PGE_2 for up to 12 months. Two other groups, however, failed to reproduce these results; one achieved a spontaneous recovery in 4 of 10 patients given PGE_1,[5] while the second had only one survivor out of 10 patients without resorting to liver transplantation.[62] Once again, evaluation of this treatment by controlled trials is awaited.

The most recent interest has focused on N-acetylcysteine. Although the efficacy of this drug when administered within 15 hours of ingestion of acetaminophen is well established, a retrospective study of 100 patients developing acetaminophen-induced fulminant hepatic failure showed that N-acetylcysteine given 10 to 36 hours after drug ingestion was associated with a significant decrease in the development of advanced encephalopathy (51% versus 75%) and death (37% versus 58%) despite the development of comparable prolongations in prothrombin time.[47] These observations were confirmed in a prospective controlled trial of 50 patients with fulminant hepatic failure from acetaminophen overdose.[57] The probable mechanisms of action of N-acetylcysteine were outlined previously. The observation that the hemodynamic benefits were also seen in other causes[48] awaits controlled evaluation.

Charcoal hemoperfusion is the most extensively assessed of the proposed systems to reduce circulating toxins in fulminant hepatic failure. Charcoal is an effective absorbent of a wide range of water-soluble molecules, and significant reductions in the circulating levels of mercaptans, GABA, middle molecules, aromatic amino acids, and inhibitors of Na^+-K^+-ATPase have been demonstrated in patients with fulminant hepatic failure. A biocompatible system for charcoal hemoperfusion was perfected using prostacyclin,[40] and a subsequent study in 76 patients suggested a significant increase in survival with hemoperfusion when it was commenced while the patient was in grade 3 rather than grade 4 encephalopathy.[39] Subsequently, controlled trials to assess the efficacy and optimal duration of hemoperfusion were carried out in 137 patients.[79] Seventy-five patients with grade 3 encephalopathy were randomly assigned to receive 5 or 10 hours of hemoperfusion daily, and there was no difference in survival between the two groups (51.3% versus 50%). Sixty-two patients with grade 4 encephalopathy were randomized to receive either no hemoperfusion or 10 hours of hemoperfusion daily, and survival rates were also similar in the two groups (39.3% versus 34.5%). Preliminary studies with an albumin-coated resin column (Amberlite XAD-7) designed to remove protein toxins have established its biocompatibility in serial perfusions, and further evaluation is awaited.[54] Plasmapheresis and exchange transfusions have also been used, and although temporary improvement in encephalopathy may be observed, no sustained benefits have been established for these techniques.

Liver Transplantation

The successful use of orthotopic liver transplantation in fulminant hepatic failure has had the single greatest impact on the management of this condition, with survival rates ranging from 50% to 72%.[9,12,29,34,56,78,85,90,94,108] The optimization of the results requires the identification of suitable candidates as soon as possible in the disease process. Although orthotopic liver transplantation has been proposed as a primary therapy,[90] most centers select patients who are considered to have a poor prognosis. The development of encephalopathy in association with a progressive coagulopathy is the most commonly used selection criterion. In France, the coagulation criteria are age-adjusted factor V levels. In cognizance of the

fact that survival rates of 39% to 67% are achieved with medical management in some cases,[79] however, and in view of the urgency with which patients with a poor prognosis need to be identified, a model for selecting patients on the basis of early simple clinical indicators has been proposed.[77]

In non–acetaminophen-overdose cases, age, cause, and the duration between the onset of jaundice and the development of encephalopathy are the static variables used to assess prognosis (Table 39-5). These are combined with two commonly used dynamic parameters, serum bilirubin and prothrombin time, to complete the model. In acetaminophen-overdose cases, the pH of arterial blood has the strongest predictive value,[77] and a pH less than 7.3 suggests a poor prognosis. In patients who did not develop acidosis, the coexistence of a prothrombin time of more than 100 seconds (INR 6.7), serum creatinine higher than 300 μmol/L, and grade 3 encephalopathy was necessary to be reasonably certain of a poor prognosis. Despite the prompt identification of patients with a poor prognosis after an acetaminophen overdose, however, liver transplantation could only be achieved in 21% of cases because of rapid progression of the disease.[81]

Technically, the transplantation operation is considerably easier than anticipated, probably because of the lack of collateral circulations as a consequence of long-standing portal hypertension. Repletion with coagulation factors, and platelets when necessary, before surgery adequately reverses the clinical coagulopathy in most cases, and intraoperative blood losses are remarkably low. Cerebral edema persists during and up to 12 hours after a successful transplantation,[58] and continuous monitoring of intracerebral pressure during this period in susceptible patients is strongly advised. Failure of recovery of neurologic function, or persistent deficits, has been documented after transplantation.[9,56,94] The risk of sepsis, including fungal infection, also persists after transplantation, and the management policy described previously should be extended into this period.

The characteristics of the first 10 reported series of patients who underwent liver transplantation for fulminant hepatic failure are outlined in Table 39-6. Non-A, non-B hepatitis accounted for over half of all cases, and most were in grade 3 or 4 encephalopathy at the time of transplantation. The

TABLE 39-5   *Model Used at King's College Hospital to Select Patients With Fulminant Hepatic Failure for Liver Transplantation*

Acetaminophen Overdose
Arterial pH < 7.3 *or* all three of following:
   Prothrombin time > 100 seconds
   Creatinine > 300 μmol/L
   Grade 3 or 4 encephalopathy

Other Causes
Prothrombin time > 100 seconds or INR > 6.7 *or* any three of following:
   Unfavorable cause (non-A, non-B hepatitis, halothane hepatitis, or drug reaction)
   Jaundice > 7 days before encephalopathy
   Age < 10 or > 40 years
   Prothrombin time > 50 seconds or INR > 4
   Serum bilirubin > 300 μmol/L

INR, international normalized ratio.

TABLE 39-6 *Orthotopic Liver Transplantation for Fulminant Hepatic Failure*

	Reference									
	9	78	85	108	94	29	56	34	12	90
Patients	17	31	13	16	24	19	42	21	6	8
FHF/LOHF ratio	10:7	16:15	6:7	16:0	24:0	19:0	42:0	9:12	6:0	?
Age range of patients (y)	12–49	3–54	16–37	1–56	0–57		0–62	1–44	2–58	4–52
Hepatitis A	1	4	0	0	4	0	0	0	1	0
Hepatitis B	5	0	1	1	4	?	8	2	1	0
Non-A, non-B hepatitis	6	18	3	11	12	?	24	13	2	7
Drug-related	5	7	4	1	1	?	7	1	0	0
Acetaminophen overdose	0	0	0	0	0	0	2	0	1	0
Wilson's disease	0	2	5	0	0	?	0	2	0	0
Other causes	0	0	0	3	3	?	1	3	1	0
Encephalopathy grade 3 or 4	12	20	?	16	20	16	27	17	3	7
Cerebral edema	10	11	?	4	12	6	?	?	?	?
Survival rate (%)	71	61	55	56	58	58	50	72	67	63

FHF, fulminant hepatic failure; LOHF, late-onset hepatic failure.

overall survival figures did not match those obtained concurrently for elective transplantations,[94] despite the younger age of the recipients. The worst results were seen in patients with grade 4 encephalopathy, with survival figures of only 28.6% and 30% reported in two of the larger series.[34,56] Other series, however, found no correlation between the grade of encephalopathy and outcome.[78,94] Other factors that correlated with a poor outcome included a high serum bilirubin level before transplantation,[78] clinical bleeding,[56] and renal failure.[56]

Heterotopic auxiliary liver transplantation has interesting potential for cases that have the capacity to regain normal liver function after recovery from fulminant hepatic failure. One such case has been described in a patient with Wilson's disease.[101] The theoretic advantage of this approach is that immunosuppression can be withdrawn after the native liver has recovered, sparing the patient the need for lifelong immunosuppressive therapy.

References

1. Almdal T, Schroeder T, Ranek L. Cerebral blood flow and liver function in patients with encephalopathy due to acute and chronic liver disease. Scand J Gastroenterol 24:299–303, 1989
2. Arankalle VA, Ticehurst J, Sreenivasan MA, et al. Aetiological association of a virus-like particle with enterically transmitted non-A, non-B hepatitis. Lancet 1:550–554, 1988
3. Basile AS, Hughes RD, Harrison PM, et al. Elevated brain concentrations of 1,4-benzodiazepines in fulminant hepatic failure. N Engl J Med 325:473–478, 1991
4. Berman DH, Leventhal RI, Gavaler JS, Cadoff EM, Van Thiel DH. Clinical differentiation of fulminant Wilsonian hepatitis from other causes of hepatic failure. Gastroenterology 100:1129–1134, 1991
5. Bernuau J, Babany G, Bezeaud A, et al. Does prostaglandin E1 (PGE1) prevent further aggravation in severe, or early fulminant, hepatitis? A preliminary open trial. (Abstract) J Hepatol 9:S114, 1989
6. Bernuau J, Rueff B, Benhamou J-P. Fulminant and subfulminant liver failure: definitions and causes. Semin Liver Dis 6:97–106, 1986
7. Bihari DJ, Gimson AES, Williams R. Cardiovascular, pulmonary and renal complications of fulminant hepatic failure. Semin Liver Dis 6:119–128, 1986
8. Bird GLA, Smith H, Portmann B, Alexander GJM, Williams R. Acute liver decompensation on withdrawal of cytotoxic chemotherapy and immunosuppressive therapy in hepatitis B carriers. Q J Med 73:895–902, 1989
9. Bismuth H, Samuel D, Gugenheim, et al. Emergency liver transplantation for fulminant hepatitis. Ann Intern Med 107:337–341, 1987
10. Boyer JL, Klatskin G. Pattern of necrosis in acute viral hepatitis: prognostic value of bridging (subacute hepatic necrosis). N Engl J Med 12:1063–1071, 1970
11. Brechot C, Bernuau J, Thiers V, et al. Multiplication of hepatitis B virus in fulminant hepatitis B. Br Med J 288:270–271, 1984
12. Brems JJ, Hiatt JR, Ramming KP, et al. Fulminant hepatic failure: the role of liver transplantation as primary therapy. Am J Surg 154:137–141, 1987
13. Brunt EM, White H, Marsh JW, Holtmann B, Peters MG. Fulminant hepatic failure after repeated exposure to isoflurane anesthesia: a case report. Hepatology 13:1017–1021, 1991
14. Canalese J, Gimson AES, Davis C, et al. Controlled trial of dexamethasone and mannitol for the cerebral oedema of fulminant hepatic failure. Gut 23:625–629, 1982
15. Canalese J, Gove CD, Gimson AES, et al. Reticuloendothelial system and hepatocyte function in fulminant hepatic failure. Gut 23:265–269, 1982
16. Carman WF, Fagan EA, Hadziyannis S, et al. Association of a precore genomic variant of hepatitis B virus with fulminant hepatitis. Hepatology 14:219–222, 1991
17. Connor RW, Lorts G, Gilbert DN. Lethal herpes simplex virus type 1 hepatitis in a normal adult. Gastroenterology 76:590–594, 1979
18. Davenport A, Will EJ, Davison AM. Effect of posture on intracranial pressure and cerebral perfusion in patients with fulminant hepatic and renal failure after acetaminophen self-poisoning. Crit Care Med 18:286–289, 1990
19. Davies MH, Morgan-Capner P, Portmann B, Wilkinson SP, Williams R. A fatal case of Epstein-Barr virus infection with jaundice and renal failure. Postgrad Med J 56:794–795, 1980
20. Davies MH, Wilkinson SP, Hanid MA, et al. Acute liver disease with encephalopathy and renal failure in late pregnancy and the early puerperium: a study of fourteen patients. Br J Obstet Gynecol 87:1005–1014, 1980
21. Davies SE, Williams R, Portmann B. Hepatic morphology and histochemistry of Wilson's disease presenting as fulminant

hepatic failure: a study of 11 cases. Histopathology 15:385–394, 1989

22. Davis M. Protective agents for paracetamol overdose. Semin Liver Dis 6:138–147, 1986

23. Dawson DJ, Babbs C, Warnes TW, Neary RH. Hypophosphatemia in acute liver failure. Br Med J 295:1312–1313, 1987

24. Desmet VJ, De Groote J, Van Damme B. Acute hepatocellular failure: a study of 17 patients treated with exchange transfusion. Hum Pathol 3:167–182, 1972

25. Dienstag JL. Non-A, non-B hepatitis. I. Recognition, epidemiology and clinical features. Gastroenterology 85:439–462, 1983

26. Dirix LY, Polson RJ, Richardson A, Williams R. Primary sepsis presenting fulminant hepatic failure. Q J Med 73:1037–1043, 1989

27. Ede RJ, Gimson AES, Bihari D, Williams R. Controlled hyperventilation in the prevention of cerebral oedema in fulminant hepatic failure. J Hepatol 2:43–51, 1986

28. Ede RJ, Williams R. Hepatic encephalopathy and cerebral edema. Semin Liver Dis 6:107–118, 1986

29. Emond JC, Aran PP, Whitington PF, Broelsch CE, Baker AL. Liver transplantation in the management of fulminant hepatic failure. Gastroenterology 96:1583–1588, 1989

30. European Association for the Study of the Liver. Randomised trial of steroid therapy in acute liver failure. Gut 20:620–623, 1979

31. Forbes A, Alexander GJM, O'Grady JG, et al. Thiopental infusion in the treatment of intracranial hypertension complicating fulminant hepatic failure. Hepatology 10:306–310, 1989

32. Forbes A, Wicks C. Fulminant hepatic failure, nutrition and fat clearance. Recent Adv Nutriol 1:67A–69A, 1990

33. Forbes A, Williams R. Increasing age: an important adverse prognostic factor in hepatitis A virus infection. J R Coll Physicians Lond 22:237–239, 1988

34. Gallinger S, Greig PD, Levy G, et al. Liver transplantation for acute and subacute fulminant hepatic failure. Transplant Proc 21:2435–2438, 1989

35. Gazzard BG, Henderson JM, Williams R. Early changes following a paracetamol overdose and a controlled trial of fresh frozen plasma therapy. Gut 16:617–620, 1975

36. Gazzard BG, Portmann B, Murray-Lyon IM, Williams R. Causes of death in fulminant hepatic failure and relationship to quantitative histological assessment of parenchymal damage. Q J Med 44:615–626, 1975

37. Gazzard BG, Rake MO, Flute PT, Williams R. Bleeding in relation to the coagulation defect of fulminant hepatic failure. In: Williams R, Murray-Lyon IM, eds. Artificial liver support. London, Pitman Medical Publishing, 1975, pp 63–67

38. Gerber MA, Thung SN, Shen S, Stromeyer FW, Ishak KG. Phenotypic characterization of hepatic proliferation: antigenic expression of proliferating epithelial cells in fetal liver, massive hepatic necrosis and nodular transformation of the liver. Am J Pathol 110:70–74, 1983

39. Gimson AES, Braude S, Mellon PJ, et al. Earlier charcoal haemoperfusion in fulminant hepatic failure. Lancet 2:681–683, 1982

40. Gimson AES, Langley PG, Hughes RD, et al. Prostacyclin to prevent platelet activation during charcoal haemoperfusion in fulminant hepatic failure. Lancet 1:173–175, 1980

41. Gimson AES, O'Grady J, Ede RJ, et al. Late-onset hepatic failure: clinical, serological and histological features. Hepatology 6:288–294, 1986

42. Gimson AES, Tedder RS, White YS, Eddleston ALWF, Williams R. Serological markers in fulminant hepatitis B. Gut 24:615–617, 1983

43. Goertz J, Williams R. Histological appearance in fulminant hepatic failure with references to aetiology, time of survival and role of immunological processes. Digestion 8:68–79, 1973

44. Gonzales-Calvin J, Scully MF, Sanger Y, et al. Fibronectin in fulminant hepatic failure. Br Med J 285:1231–1232, 1982

45. Govindarajan S, Chin KP, Redeker AG, Peters RL. Fulminant B viral hepatitis: role of delta agent. Gastroenterology 86:1417–1420, 1984

46. Harrison PM, Hughes RD, Forbes A, et al. Failure of insulin and glucagon to stimulate liver regeneration in fulminant hepatic failure. J Hepatol 10:332–336, 1990

47. Harrison PM, Keays R, Bray GP, Alexander GJM, Williams R. Late N-acetylcysteine administration improves outcome for patients developing paracetamol-induced fulminant hepatic failure. Lancet 1:1572–1573, 1990

48. Harrison PM, Wendon JA, Gimson AES, Alexander GJM, Williams R. Improvement by N-acetylcysteine of hemodynamics and oxygen transport in fulminant hepatic failure. N Engl J Med 324:1853–1857, 1991

49. Hart GK, Thompson WR, Schneider J, Davis J, Oh TE. Fulminant hepatic failure and fatal encephalopathy associated with Epstein-Barr virus infection. Med J Aust 141:112–113, 1984

50. Hassanein T, Perper JA, Tepperman L, Starzl TE, Van Thiel DH. Liver failure occurring as a component of exertional heatstroke. Gastroenterology 100:1442–1447, 1991

51. Henson DE, Crimley PM, Strano AJ. Postnatal cytomegalovirus hepatitis: an autopsy and liver biopsy study. Hum Pathol 5:93–103, 1974

52. Horney JT, Galambos JT. The liver during and after fulminant hepatitis. Gastroenterology 73:639–645, 1977

53. Hughes RD, Lane DA, Ireland H, Langley PG, Gimson AES, Williams R. Fibrinogen derivatives and platelet activation products in acute and chronic liver disease. Clin Sci 68:701–707, 1985

54. Hughes R, Williams R. Clinical experience with charcoal and resin hemoperfusion. Semin Liver Dis 6:164–173, 1986

55. Ishak KG. Viral hepatitis: the morphologic spectrum. In: Gall EA, Mostofi FK, eds. The liver. Baltimore, Williams & Wilkins, 1973, pp 218–268

56. Iwatsuki S, Stieber AC, Marsh JW, et al. Liver transplantation for fulminant hepatic failure. Transplant Proc 21:2431–2434, 1989

57. Keays R, Harrison PM, Wendon JA, et al. Intravenous acetylcysteine in paracetamol induced fulminant hepatic failure: a prospective controlled trial. Br Med J 303:1026–1029, 1991

58. Keays R, Potter D, O'Grady J, et al. Intracranial and cerebral perfusion changes before, during and immediately after orthotopic liver transplantation for fulminant hepatic failure. Q J Med 79:425–433, 1991

59. Khuroo MS. Study of an epidemic of non-A, non-B hepatitis: possibility of another human hepatitis virus distinct from posttransfusion non-B type. Am J Med 68:818–824, 1980

60. Kosaka Y, Takase K, Kojima M, et al. Fulminant hepatitis B: induction by hepatitis B virus mutants defective in the precore region and incapable of encoding e antigen. Gastroenterology 100:1087–1094, 1991

61. Koukoulis G, Rayner A, Tan KC, Williams R, Portmann B. Immunolocalization of regenerating cell after submassive liver necrosis using PCNA staining. J Pathol 166:359–368, 1992

62. Kramer DJ, Aggarwal S, Martin M, et al. Management options in fulminant hepatic failure. Transplant Proc 23:1895–1898, 1991

63. Langley PG, Keays R, Hughes RD, Forbes A, Delvos U, Williams R. Antithrombin III supplementation reduces heparin requirement and platelet loss during hemodialysis of patients with fulminant hepatic failure. Hepatology 14:251–256, 1991

64. Lefkowitch JH. Bile ductular cholestasis: an ominous histopathologic sign related to sepsis and "cholangitis lenta." Hum Pathol 13:19–24, 1982

65. Lemon SM. Type A viral hepatitis: new developments in an old disease. N Engl J Med 313:1059–1067, 1985

66. Levin S, Hahn T. Interferon deficiency syndrome. Clin Exp Immunol 60:267–273, 1985

67. Liang TJ, Hasegawa K, Rimon N, Wands JR, Ben-Porath E. A hepatitis B virus mutant associated with an epidemic of fulminant hepatitis. N Engl J Med 324:1705–1709, 1991

68. Macdougall BRD, Williams R. H₂-receptor antagonist in the prevention of acute upper gastrointestinal hemorrhage in fulminant hepatic failure. Gastroenterology 74:164–165, 1978

69. McNeil M, Hoy JF, Richards MJ, et al. Aetiology of fatal viral hepatitis in Melbourne: a retrospective study. Med J Aust 141:637–640, 1984

70. Milandri M, Gaub J, Ranek L. Evidence for liver cell proliferation during fatal hepatic failure. Gut 21:423–427, 1980

71. Mori W, Shiga J, Irie H. Shwartzman reaction as a pathogenetic mechanism in fulminant hepatitis. Semin Liver Dis 6:267–276, 1986

72. Morishita K, Kodo H, Asano S, Fujii H, Miwa S. Fulminant varicella hepatitis following bone marrow transplantation. JAMA 253:511, 1985

73. Mullen KD, Martin JV, Mendelson, WB, et al. Could an endogenous benzodiazepine ligand contribute to hepatic encephalopathy? Lancet 1:457–459, 1988

74. Munoz SJ, Robinson M, Northrup B, et al. Elevated intracranial pressure and tomography of the brain in fulminant hepatic failure. Hepatology 13:209–212, 1991

75. Neuberger J, Gimson A, Davis M, Williams R. Specific serological markers in the diagnosis of fulminant hepatic failure following halothane anaesthesia. Br J Anaesth 55:15–19, 1983

76. O'Brien CJ, Wise RJS, O'Grady JG, Williams R. Neurological sequelae in patients following fulminant hepatic failure. Gut 28:93–95, 1987

77. O'Grady JG, Alexander GJM, Hallyar KM, Williams R. Early indicators of prognosis in fulminant hepatic failure. Gastroenterology 97:439–445, 1989

78. O'Grady JG, Alexander GJM, Thick M, Potter D, Calne RY, Williams R. Outcome of orthotopic liver transplantation in the aetiological and clinical variants of acute liver failure. Q J Med 69:817–824, 1988

79. O'Grady JG, Gimson AES, O'Brien CJ, et al. Controlled trials of charcoal hemoperfusion and prognostic factors in fulminant hepatic failure. Gastroenterology 94:1186–1192, 1988

80. O'Grady JG, Smith HM, Sutherland S, Sheron N, Williams R. Low detection of hepatitis C antibodies in serum after liver transplantation. (Abstract) J Hepatol 11:S47, 1990

81. O'Grady JG, Wendon J, Tan KC, et al. Indications and results of liver transplantation following paracetamol overdose. Br Med J 303:221–223, 1991

82. Omata M, Ehata T, Yokosuka O, Hosoda K, Ohto M. Mutations in the precore region of hepatitis B virus DNA in patients with fulminant and severe hepatitis. N Engl J Med 324:1669–1704, 1991

83. Osano Y, Yoshikawa T, Suga S, Yazaki T, Kondo K, Yamanishi K. Fatal fulminant hepatitis in an infant with human herpesvirus-6 infection. Lancet 335:862–863, 1991

84. Papaevangelou G, Tassopoulos N, Roumeliotou-Karayannis A, Richardson C. Etiology of fulminant viral hepatitis in Greece. Hepatology 4:369–372, 1984

85. Peleman RR, Gavaler JS, Van Thiel D, et al. Orthotopic liver transplantation for acute and subacute hepatic failure in adults. Hepatology 7:484–489, 1987

86. Peters RL, Omata M, Aschavai M, Liew CT. Protracted viral hepatitis with impaired regeneration. In: Vyas GN, Gohen SN, Schmid R, eds. Viral hepatitis. Philadelphia, Franklin Institute Press, 1978, pp 79–84

87. Phillips MJ, Poucell S. Modern aspects of the morphology of viral hepatitis. Hum Pathol 12:1060–1084, 1981

88. Portmann B, Talbot IC, Day DW, Davidson AR, Murray-Lyon IM, Williams R. Histopathological changes in the liver following a paracetamol overdose: correlation with clinical and biochemical parameters. J Pathol 117:169–181, 1975

89. Powell-Jackson PR, Ede RJ, Williams R. Budd-Chiari syndrome presenting as fulminant hepatic failure. Gut 27:1101–1105, 1986

90. Rakela J, Perkins JD, Gross JB, et al. Acute hepatic failure: the emerging role of orthotopic liver transplantation. Mayo Clin Proc 64:424–428, 1989

91. Ronaldo N, Harvey FAH, Brahm J, et al. Prospective study of bacterial infection in acute liver failure: an analysis of fifty patients. Hepatology 11:49–53, 1990

92. Rubin MH, Weston MJ, Bullock G, et al. Abnormal platelet function and ultrastructure in fulminant hepatic failure. Q J Med 183:339–352, 1977

93. Sanchez-Tapias JM, Mas A, Costa J, et al. Recombinant a₂c-interferon therapy in fulminant viral hepatitis. J Hepatol 5:205–210, 1987

94. Schafer DF, Shaw BW. Fulminant hepatic failure and orthotopic liver transplantation. Semin Liver Dis 9:189–194, 1989

95. Schenker S, Breen KJ, Heimberg M. Pathogenesis of tetracycline induced fatty liver. In: Gerok W, Sickinger K, eds. Drugs and the liver. Stuttgart, FK Schattauer Verlag, 1975, pp 269–280

96. Scheuer PJ. Viral hepatitis. In: MacSween RNM, Anthony PP, Scheuer PJ, eds. Pathology of the Liver, ed 2. Edinburgh, Churchill Livingstone, 1987, pp 202–223

97. Sette H, Hughes RD, Langley PG, Gimson AES, Williams R. Heparin response and clearance in acute and chronic liver disease. Thromb Haemost 54:591–594, 1985

98. Sinclair SB, Greig PD, Blendis LM, et al. Biochemical and clinical response of fulminant viral hepatitis to administration of prostaglandin E. J Clin Invest 84:1063–1069, 1989

99. Smedile A, Farci P, Verme G, et al. Influence of delta infection on severity of hepatitis B. Lancet 2:945–947, 1982

100. Smilkstein MJ, Knapp GL, Kulig KW, Rumack BH. Efficacy of oral N-acetylcysteine in the treatment of acetaminophen overdose. N Engl J Med 319:1557–1562, 1988

101. Stampfl DA, Munoz SJ, Moritz M, et al. Heterotopic liver transplantation for fulminant Wilson's disease. Gastroenterology 99:1834–1836, 1990

102. Takahashi Y. Acute hepatic failure: in special relation to treatment. Jpn J Med 22:140–145, 1983

103. Terblanche J, Starzl TE. Hepatic regeneration: implications in fulminant hepatic failure. Int J Artif Organs 2:49–52, 1979

104. Trepo CG, Robert D, Motin J, Trepo D, Sepetjian M, Prince AM. Hepatitis B antigen (HBsAg) and/or antibodies (anti-HBs and anti-HBc) in fulminant hepatitis: pathogenic and prognostic significance. Gut 17:10–13, 1976

105. Trewby PN, Warren S, Contini S, et al. Incidence and pathophysiology of pulmonary edema in fulminant hepatic failure. Gastroenterology 74:859–865, 1978

106. Trey C, Davidson LS. The management of fulminant hepatic failure. In: Popper H, Schaffner F, eds. Progress in liver disease. New York, Grune & Stratton, 1970, pp 282–298

107. Vallbracht A, Gabriel P, Maier K, et al. Cell-mediated cytotoxicity in hepatitis A virus infection. Hepatology 6:1308–1314, 1986

108. Vickers C, Neuberger J, Buckels J, McMaster P, Elias E. Transplantation of the liver in adults and children with fulminant hepatic failure. J Hepatol 7:143–150, 1988

109. Wendon J, Gimson AE, Potter D. Oxygen uptake and delivery in fulminant hepatic failure. Care Crit Ill 5:55–59, 1989

110. Wendon JA, Harrison PM, Keays R, Gimson AE, Alexander GJM, Williams R. The effects of vasopressor agents and prostacyclin on systemic haemodynamics and oxygen transport in patients with fulminant hepatic failure. Hepatology 15:1067–1071, 1992

111. Wilkinson SP, Weston MJ, Parsons V, Williams R. Dialysis in the treatment of renal failure in patients with liver disease. Clin Nephrol 8:287–292, 1977

112. Woolf GM, Redeker AG. Treatment of fulminant hepatic failure with insulin and glucagon: a randomised controlled trial. Dig Dis Sci 36:92–96, 1991

113. Woolf I, Sheikh N, Cullens H, et al. Enhanced HBsAb production in pathogenesis of fulminant viral hepatitis type B. Br Med J 2:669–671, 1976

114. Wong DC, Purcell RH, Sreenivasan MA, et al. Epidemic and endemic hepatitis in India: evidence for a non-A, non-B virus aetiology. Lancet 2:876–879, 1980

115. Wright T, Hsu H, Donegan E, et al. Hepatitis C virus not found in fulminant non-A, non-B hepatitis. Ann Intern Med 115:111–113, 1991

116. Wyke RJ, Canalese JC, Gimson AES, Williams R. Bacteraemia in patients with fulminant hepatic failure. Liver 2:45–52, 1982

117. Wyke RJ, Rajkovic IA, Eddleston ALWF, Williams R. Defective opsonisation and complement deficiency in serum from patients with fulminant hepatic failure. Gut 21:643–649, 1981

118. Zimmerman H. Even enflurane. (Editorial) Hepatology 13:1251–1253, 1991

119. Zimmerman HJ, Ishak KG. Valproate-induced hepatic injury: analysis of 23 fatal cases. Hepatology 2:591–597, 1982

Diseases of the Liver, Seventh Edition, edited by
Leon Schiff and Eugene R. Schiff. J.B. Lippincott Company, Philadelphia © 1993.

40

Budd-Chiari Syndrome

Telfer B. Reynolds

The Budd-Chiari syndrome is an uncommon disorder caused by obstruction to hepatic venous outflow. The first published clinical description is attributed to Budd in 1845,[9] and Chiari[13] added the first pathologic description of a liver with "obliterating endophlebitis of the hepatic veins" in 1899. Parker[47] summarized the literature in 1959 and was able to find accounts of 164 symptomatic cases with autopsy confirmation, including 18 from his own hospital. There are several reviews of relatively large series of cases. [14,17,36,41,49,67]

There are a number of known causes of the Budd-Chiari syndrome. Tumors such as hepatocellular carcinoma, hypernephroma, adrenal carcinoma, and leiomyosarcoma may obstruct major hepatic veins directly or in company with a blood clot.[39,61] The hepatic portion of the inferior vena cava often is occluded with the hepatic veins when the cause is tumor. A hepatic abscess or cyst may cause occlusion of neighboring hepatic veins, although this rarely results in the full clinical expression of the Budd-Chiari syndrome. In many instances of hepatic vein thrombosis, an underlying hypercoagulable state may be responsible. These now include the myeloproliferative syndrome,[68] paroxysmal nocturnal hemoglobinuria,[26,69] presence of the lupus anticoagulant,[57] and deficiencies of antithrombin III,[16] protein C,[6] and protein S, blood constituents that are protective against thrombosis. Valla and associates[68] believe that many patients with idiopathic hepatic vein thrombosis actually have a latent primary myeloproliferative syndrome, based on the finding of normal or low serum erythropoietin and spontaneous erythroid colony formation on bone marrow culture. Behcet's disease is associated with hepatic vein thrombosis,[5] usually in conjunction with vena caval thrombosis. Relations of hepatic vein thrombosis to pregnancy[31,56] and trauma[12] have been postulated but not proved. A causal relation with oral contraceptives has been assumed by some on the basis of reports of cases in oral contraceptive users.[38,75] In contrast with the definite increase in incidence of hepatic adenomas since the advent of oral contraceptives, my own experience and the published literature do not suggest an obvious increase in the frequency of hepatic vein thrombosis. In reviewing articles describing larger series of cases published between 1967 and 1983, and, including our own material, reporting a total of 172 cases,[54] the frequency of oral contraceptive use in female patients 15 to 50 years of age was low, approximately 25%

(not all reports listed the ages of the women), and less than some estimates for use in the general population of the United States.[43] In the only case control study published, however, Valla and colleagues[70] surveyed 33 French women between the ages of 15 and 45 years who had a diagnosis of hepatic vein thrombosis, and found the frequency of oral contraceptive use at the time of diagnosis to be 54.5%. This compared with a frequency of 31.4% among the 128 case-matched controls for a relative risk of 2.37 (95% confidence interval of 1.05 to 5.34, $P < .02$). Because 11 of the 18 birth control pill users with hepatic vein thrombosis had hematologic disorders known to be associated with hepatic vein thrombosis (paroxysmal nocturnal hemoglobinuria or primary myeloproliferative disease), they concluded that oral contraceptive use increased the risk of thrombosis by adding a thrombogenic tendency to that of an underlying disorder.

An important cause of the Budd-Chiari syndrome from the therapeutic standpoint is a fibrous diaphragm or web across the upper vena cava at or just above the entrance of the left and middle hepatic veins. This lesion appears to be more common in South Africa and in Asia than in the United States,[4,32,55,63,66,76] although we have encountered 10 cases in Los Angeles in the last 25 years.[53] In some cases, the membrane is thick and the fibrosis involves one or more of the major hepatic veins. This lesion has been considered by some to be congenital, related to closure of the ductus venosus.[32] Okuda[15] has argued, convincingly it seems to me, that it is an acquired lesion resulting from thrombosis. He points out the apparently late age of onset in some patients, the inconsistent involvement of the hepatic veins, and the lack of associated congenital anomalies.

More common than any of the known causes of hepatic vein occlusion is an unexplained partial or complete fibrous obliteration of the major hepatic veins or their ostia. This was found at autopsy in 44% of Parker's series,[47] and can be viewed either as a proliferative inflammation or as a result of partial organization of preceding thrombosis. Safouh and colleagues[58] report this type of pathologic process to be particularly common in Egyptian children with the Budd-Chiari syndrome. With increasing awareness of factors that predispose to a hypercoagulable state, the frequency of unexplained hepatic vein occlusion should decline.

Our experience with the Budd-Chiari syndrome in the Liver Unit at the Los Angeles County–University of Southern California Medical Center includes 47 cases, the presumed causes of which are listed in Table 40-1.

Robert L. Peters, MD, recently deceased Professor of Pathology at the University of Southern California, contributed importantly to the material.

TABLE 40-1 *Causes of Budd-Chiari Syndrome*

Cause	Cases	Cases With Vena Caval Occlusion	Clinical Course			Death	Autopsy
			Acute	Subacute	Chronic		
Thrombosis							
Myeloproliferative disease	5*	—	—	5	—	3	3
Paroxysmal nocturnal hemoglobinuria	3	1	1	1	1	2	1
Lupus anticoagulant	1	—	—	1	—	—	—
Unknown cause	2*	1	—	1	1	2	2
Tumor							
Adrenal carcinoma	2	2	—	2	—	2	2
Hypernephroma	2	2	—	2	—	2	2
Hepatocellular carcinoma	2	1	—	2	—	2	2
Choriocarcinoma	1	—	—	1	—	1	1
Breast carcinoma	1	—	1	—	—	1	—
Unknown primary	1	1	—	1	—	1	—
Fibrous obliteration of unknown cause	3	—	—	—	3	3	3
Vena caval web	10*	10	—	—	10	3	1
Radiation	2	—	—	2	—	2	2
Amebic abscess	2	—	2	—	—	2	2
Undetermined cause	10†	—	2	4	4	1	—

*One patient used oral contraceptives.
†Two patients used oral contraceptives.

Pathology

The Budd-Chiari syndrome, produced by any of the processes that impede egress of blood from the liver, is associated in the acute stage with a swollen, blunt-edged, red–purple liver. Cut surface of such a liver reveals the pale, undamaged, periportal tissue regularly demarcating the lobular units and the perivenular, darkened, depressed areas of congestion.

When the obstruction to venous flow is the result of a mechanical process such as a membranous diaphragm or a tumor involving the ostia of hepatic veins, the microscopic pattern during the acute stage is that of severe acute congestion. The sinusoids are engorged with blood, and the centrolobular hepatocytes undergo marked atrophy, often disappearing, with the endothelial processes remaining as a loose stromal network (Fig. 40-1). With continued obstruction, the central veins become obliterated by collapse of the stroma and a small amount of production of new collagen. Fibrin deposition and thrombosis are not prominent features.

The more mysterious primary endophlebitis, which represents the disease originally described by Chiari, is characterized by thrombosis or fibrin deposition in the central veins in the earliest stages of the process. The congestion may be so severe as to preclude evaluation of the stromal pattern of the liver. In many instances, however, the striking perivenular pool of blood and fibrin is surrounded by radiating dilated sinusoids devoid of erythrocytes that alternate with thin cords of hepatocytes surrounded by erythrocytes in the space of Disse. On casual inspection, the liver appears congested, but it actually has extravasation of blood into the space of Disse (Figs. 40-2 and 40-3). This may be a fundamental aspect of the pathogenesis of the Budd-Chiari syndrome, in contrast to those conditions that produce only passive congestion of the liver. Leopold and coworkers[37] describe extravasation of blood into the space of Disse in liver biopsy specimens taken from patients who have tumor masses occluding the hepatic veins. Other conditions that produce secondary severe venous stasis may be associated with extravasation of erythrocytes into the trabecula. Confluent necrosis of hepatocytes resulting from a hepatotoxic agent may be associated with a minor degree of dissection of erythrocytes into the trabecular structures.

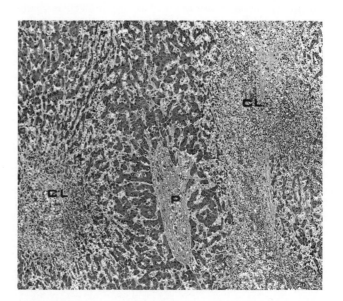

FIGURE 40-1 Low-power photomicrograph of the liver of a patient with Budd-Chiari syndrome showing the portal area in the center (P) with congested centrolobular areas (CL) to either side. Note that the liver cells have disappeared centrally (H&E, × 100).

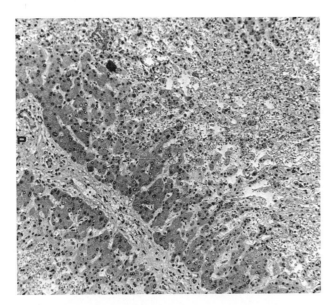

FIGURE 40-2 A portal area surrounded by intact hepatocytes. At the margin between collapsed liver cell stroma and intact hepatocytes, the sinusoids are dilated but not filled with erythrocytes, which are more localized in the space of Disse (see Fig. 40-3) (H&E, × 165).

As the disease moves into chronicity, the fibrin thrombi organize, each producing a fibrous core (Fig. 40-4). Extending in an arachnoid fashion from the central core, thin collagen strands replace the liver cords and the collapsed stroma. The congestion of the sinusoids becomes somewhat less uniform from one area to another. The larger hepatic vein radicles, not usually included in needle biopsy specimens, are sclerotic, usually to the ostia of the hepatic veins into the inferior vena cava (Fig. 40-5). Although it usually has been

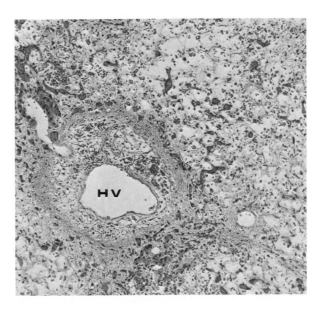

FIGURE 40-4 After a prolonged time, the sublobular hepatic veins (HV) may be thrombosed and recanalized with extensive loss of hepatocytes (H&E, × 160).

presumed that the thrombosclerotic process had its origin at the outlets of the hepatic veins, thereafter progressing into the liver, there is as much reason to believe that the process may begin in central veins and progress into the large vessels.

After 1 to 3 years, when the liver is studied at autopsy, the ostia of the hepatic veins are filled by sclerotic tissue (Fig. 40-6) that extends to the lobular level. Often, the inferior vena cava has a plastic thickening in its intrahepatic portion. On occasion, the caudate lobe may not be involved in the process and may enlarge as the major functioning unit. In this advanced stage, the liver becomes smaller, irregular, and tough.

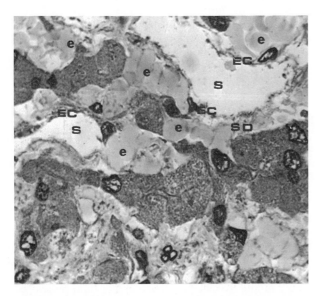

FIGURE 40-3 Higher-power photomicrograph showing the shrunken hepatocytes surrounded by erythrocytes (e) bloating the space of Disse (SD). The SD is separated from the empty sinusoids (S) by the endothelial cell processes (EC) (H&E, × 900).

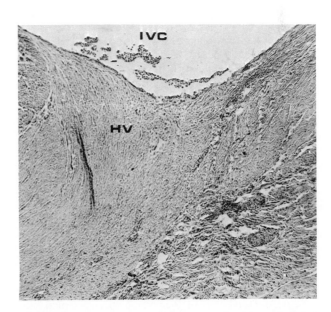

FIGURE 40-5 Low-power photomicrograph of an occluded site of entry of the hepatic vein (HV) into the inferior vena cava (IVC) (H&E, × 45).

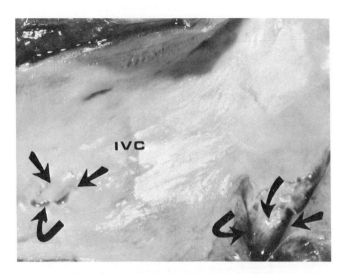

FIGURE 40-6 Intrahepatic portion of the inferior vena cava (IVC) in a fatal case of Budd-Chiari disease. Note the hyalinized thrombotic occlusion of two major hepatic vein radicles (*arrows*).

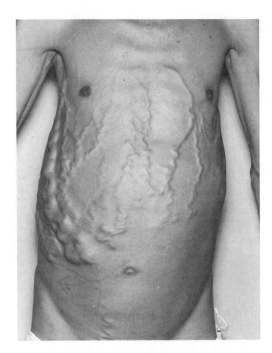

FIGURE 40-7 Collateral venous circulation on the abdomen of a patient with the Budd-Chiari syndrome caused by blockage of the inferior vena cava by a web lesion cephalad to the hepatic vein orifices.

Radiation administered to the liver may produce a nearly identical hepatic lesion, but unless the entire liver or the entire zone of entrance of hepatic veins into the vena cava is irradiated, the venoocclusive change involves only a part of the liver and the Budd-Chiari syndrome may not result. Radiation may induce other changes, including sclerotic thickening and even hyalinization of the hepatic arterioles in the portal regions, permitting its identification as the cause of hepatic vein sclerosis. The dissection of erythrocytes into the trabecula of the liver, in contrast to simple congestion of the sinusoids, has been pointed out in Jamaican venoocclusive disease[8] as well as in experimental monocrotaline poisoning in monkeys.[2] Only Leopold and colleagues,[37] however, have pointed out this feature in idiopathic Budd-Chiari syndrome. Budd-Chiari and venoocclusive diseases may be similar in etiology and pathogenesis.

A condition pathologically indistinguishable from the Budd-Chiari lesion occasionally occurs in felines housed in zoos in the United States. We have seen examples in a Bengal tiger and two cheetahs. The animals also manifest ascites and die in what appears to be hepatic coma.

An interesting association of Budd-Chiari syndrome with hepatocellular carcinoma has been pointed out by Simson[63] in patients with membranous obstruction of the inferior vena cava. Two of our 10 patients with the inferior vena cava web lesion had hepatocellular cancer.

Clinical Manifestations

The most important clinical manifestation are abdominal pain, hepatomegaly, and ascites. Seldom is the diagnosis made from the clinical picture alone; clinicians tend to ignore the abdominal pain and to ascribe the ascites and hepatomegaly to cirrhosis.

Astute interpretation of the liver biopsy specimen often provides the clue that results in a correct diagnosis. Clinical features in the Budd-Chiari syndrome vary with the extent and rapidity of onset of the venous occlusion and with the manifestations, if any, of the underlying disease. Rarely, acute illness with abdominal pain, hepatomegaly, and shock occurs and has a rapid course resulting in death. More commonly, there is a vague illness with abdominal distress weeks or months in duration followed by the appearance of ascites and an enlarged liver. Jaundice may be present but is usually mild. In a few patients, gradual development of hepatomegaly and ascites occurs without prominent abdominal pain; such patients are most likely to receive an erroneous diagnosis of cirrhosis. Portal hypertension develops in all patients with the Budd-Chiari syndrome and may be responsible eventually for hematemesis from esophageal varices.

When there is vena caval occlusion accompanying the Budd-Chiari syndrome and the patient survives long enough, collateral veins often appear on the abdomen or back (Fig. 40-7). Other findings suggesting vena caval involvement include protracted ankle edema, stasis ulceration, or episodes of pulmonary embolization. We described one patient with complete vena caval occlusion and severe hepatic congestion who had no symptoms or findings other than hepatomegaly and episodes of mild abdominal pain.[18]

Investigations

There is nothing distinctive about the biochemical test pattern in patients with the Budd-Chiari syndrome. Hepatic test abnormalities are variable in degree and are similar to those in any chronic liver disease. High ascitic fluid protein content has been said to be characteristic of the Budd-Chiari syndrome,[22,74] but, in my experience, protein levels more often have been in the range usually seen in cirrhosis of the liver. In 15 patients, I found a range of 0.5 to 4.5 g/dL, with a mean of 2.4 g/dL. In three patients, the value was greater than 50% of the serum protein level. Clain and colleagues[14] found values of 0.9 to 2.8 g/dL (mean, 1.8 g/dL) in six cases. Rarely, the ascitic fluid is blood-stained (in one of our cases and in one of those reported by Clain and associates[14]). Liver scan sometimes shows a marked increase in isotope uptake centrally,[14,67] possibly because of hypertrophy of the caudate lobe related to its venous drainage directly into the vena cava. This pattern was evident in 6 of the 17 patients in our series who had scans performed (Fig. 40-8).

Splenoportography and celiac angiography usually show portal collateral flow and failure of or minimal opacification of the main portal trunk.[19] Presumably, the portal vein often serves as an outflow vessel when the major hepatic veins are occluded, accounting for the lack of portal visualization with these procedures. Also, portal vein thrombosis sometimes accompanies hepatic vein thrombosis.[14,47]

Hepatic parenchymal contrast injection has been used in the diagnosis and localization of hepatic venous obstruction.[7,14,17,51] Pollard and Nebesar[48] found retrograde portal flow on selective hepatic artery contrast injection in one patient. Rector and Redeker[52] used transhepatic needling of hepatic veins to demonstrate abnormal pressure and abnormal direction of blood flow in three patients. Computed tomography and ultrasonography can be useful adjuncts by showing enlargement of the caudate lobe, absence of major hepatic vein images, and prolonged hepatic opacification after contrast injection.[3,40]

Few reports have been made of attempted hepatic vein catheterization in patients with suspected Budd-Chiari syndrome. One would anticipate difficulty with this procedure; however, Clain and associates[14] and Kreel and coworkers[34] were able to place a catheter at least a short distance into one hepatic vein in five of six patients. The main vessels appeared narrowed and partly occluded, and an unusual pattern of fine interlacing communicating vessels, interpreted as collaterals, was seen on wedged injection of contrast. We found a similar pattern in six of our patients (Fig. 40-9). A technically satisfactory wedged hepatic vein pressure is difficult to obtain in these patients; Clain and colleagues[14] found elevated levels

in two of four patients, and we found such levels in three of four.

Two relatively new procedures, both noninvasive, are extremely useful in evaluation of patients with suspected hepatic vein occlusion. Magnetic resonance imaging is capable of depicting the hepatic veins, portal vein, and inferior vena cava.[21,65] In Budd-Chiari syndrome, the hepatic veins are absent or poorly seen (Fig. 40-10), and there may be irregular intrahepatic collateral vessels.[42,64] A bonus of this procedure is visualization of the portal vein and vena cava, both of which may be abnormal. Duplex Doppler ultrasonography, particularly in the color mode, is another satisfactory method for examining the hepatic veins.[23,45] Portal and vena caval flow can be evaluated at the same examination. In addition to absence of the normal hepatic vein images, abnormalities that may be found include reversed flow in hepatic vein branches, intrahepatic anastomotic vessels, and in cases with high vena caval occlusion, reversed flow in the vena cava.

Evaluation of the inferior vena cava by magnetic resonance imaging, ultrasonography, or catheterization with angiography is important in patients being investigated for the Budd-Chiari syndrome. Only if this is done routinely will all cases associated with vena caval occlusion be identified. As emphasized by the case reported from this Liver Unit in 1968,[18] the vena cava may be completely obstructed without the appearance of collateral veins, ankle edema, or stasis ulcers. It is particularly important to examine the vena cava in patients with collateral veins visible on the back, because portal hypertension rarely causes collaterals to appear in this area. Vena caval pressure measurement is important in deciding about portosystemic shunt surgery for hepatic decompression.

Treatment

Treatment for hepatic vein occlusion is difficult and limited. Surgery to attempt removal of thrombus from hepatic veins is unlikely to be successful because of the extent of the pro-

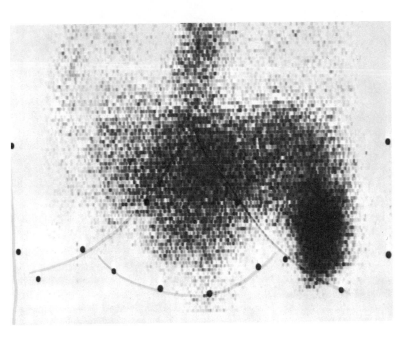

FIGURE 40-8 Increased central uptake of isotope in the liver scan of a patient with the Budd-Chiari syndrome caused by hepatic vein thrombosis related to myeloproliferative disease.

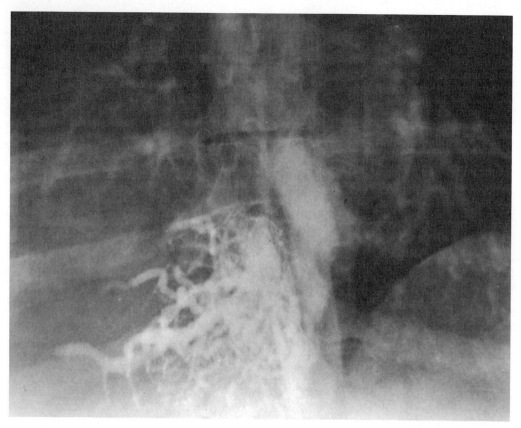

FIGURE 40-9   An unusual pattern of numerous interlacing vessels is seen after the injection of 7 mL of contrast medium through a catheter wedged in the right hepatic vein of a patient with Budd-Chiari syndrome caused by idiopathic hepatic vein occlusion. The catheter could not be passed more than a few centimeters into the hepatic vein.

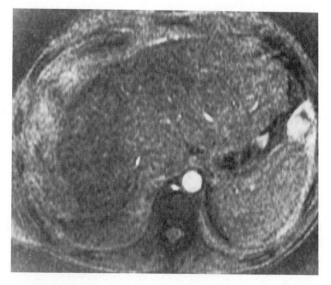

FIGURE 40-10   MRI scan (T2 phase) of liver in a patient with Budd-Chiari syndrome of uncertain cause. Note the slit-like inferior vena cava and the absence of any well-defined hepatic veins.

cess and the difficulty of exposure of the hepatic veins. Thrombolytic therapy has been attempted with at least temporary good results.[24] Decompression of the liver by any of the several existing types of side-to-side portacaval shunt may be helpful if the inferior vena cava is not occluded.[20,29,36,46,50,60] Often, the vena cava is narrowed by caudate lobe hypertrophy, causing pressure increase in the vessel below the point of narrowing. Theoretically, this could reduce flow through a side-to-side shunt and render the procedure ineffective. Some surgeons have proceeded with side-to-side shunt in this setting, regardless of this finding, seemingly with good results,[71] whereas others have turned to mesoatrial shunt.[1,10,33,72] Long-term patency of the mesoatrial shunt is a problem because of its length and relatively small caliber. Theoretically, after mesoatrial shunt and hepatic decompression, caudate lobe hypertrophy might regress, allowing conversion to a side-to-side shunt at a later time. Jennings and colleagues[30] described two patients in whom partial vena caval occlusion became complete after mesoatrial shunt, however, suggesting the original abnormality was a fibrotic process rather than compression from hepatic hypertrophy.

Long-term anticoagulant therapy generally is indicated after mesoatrial shunt or if there is evidence for a hypercoagulable state.

Liver transplantation is a consideration for fulminant or end-stage Budd-Chiari syndrome. The most recently published series shows a 45% 5-year survival rate.[25] The importance of long-term anticoagulation after transplantation was stressed in the two largest series reported.[11,25,62]

Surgical treatment may be particularly helpful when the Budd-Chiari syndrome is due to a fibrous diaphragm or web in the vena cava just below the right atrium. The presence and thickness of the web can be assessed when one catheter is placed in the right atrium and another one passed up the inferior vena cava from below. Transcardiac membranotomy has been performed successfully by several groups.[27,32,35,59,66,76] Other surgeons have resected the membrane under cardiopulmonary bypass[66,73] or used bypass grafts.[44,76] One of our patients with an incomplete membrane had successful balloon membranotomy,[28] and membrane resection was successful in three of our four patients in whom it was attempted.

Extensive hepatic vein occlusion usually is fatal within weeks or months of the onset of symptoms. Some patients, usually those with gradual onset of the syndrome, survive for extended periods with chronic ascites and portal hypertension and a course resembling that of idiopathic cirrhosis of the liver. Early diagnosis is important, with consideration of a portosystemic shunting procedure to decompress the liver. For end-stage disease or patients who fail to improve with surgical shunt, liver transplantation is the optimal therapy.

References

1. Ahn SS, Yellin A, Sheng FC, Colonna JO, Goldstein LI, Busuttil RW. Selective surgical therapy of the Budd-Chiari syndrome provides superior survivor rates than conservative medical management. J Vasc Surg 5:28, 1987
2. Allen JR, Carstens LA. Monocrotaline-induced Budd-Chiari syndrome in monkeys. Dig Dis 16:111, 1971
3. Baert AL, Fevery J, Marchal G, et al. Early diagnosis of Budd-Chiari syndrome by computed tomography and ultrasonography: report of 5 cases. Gastroenterology 84:587, 1983
4. Bennet I. A unique case of obstruction of the inferior vena cava. Bulletin of the Johns Hopkins Hospital 87:290, 1950
5. Bismuth E, Hadenque A, Hammel P, Benhamou J-P. Hepatic vein thrombosis in Behcet's disease. Hepatology 11:969, 1990
6. Bourliere M, LeTreut YP, Arnoux D, et al. Acute Budd-Chiari syndrome with hepatic failure and obstruction of the inferior vena cava as presenting manifestations of hereditary protein C deficiency. Gut 31:949, 1990
7. Brink AJ, Botha D. Budd-Chiari syndrome: diagnosis by hepatic venography. Br J Radiol 28:330, 1955
8. Brooks SEH, Miller CG, McKenzie K, Audretsch JJ, Bras G. Acute veno-occlusive disease of the liver. Arch Pathol 89:507, 1970
9. Budd G. On diseases of the liver. London, Churchill, 1845, p 147
10. Cameron JL, Maddrey WC. Mesoatrial shunt: a new treatment for the Budd-Chiari syndrome. Ann Surg 187:402, 1978
11. Campbell DA, Rolles K, Jamieson N, et al. Hepatic transplantation with perioperative and long-term anticoagulation as treatment for the Budd-Chiari syndrome. Surg Gynecol Obstet 166:511, 1988
12. Chamberlain DW, Walter JB. The relationship of Budd-Chiari syndrome to oral contraceptives and trauma. Can Med Assoc J 101:97, 1969
13. Chiari H. Ueber die selbständige Phlebitis obliterans der Hauptstämme der Vanae hepaticae als Todesursache. Beitr Z Pathol Anat 26:1, 1899
14. Clain D, Freston J, Kreel L, Sherlock S. Clinical diagnosis of the Budd-Chiari syndrome. Am J Med 43:544, 1967
15. Clinical-Pathological Conference. Aetiology of membranous obstruction of the inferior vena cava: congenital or acquired? Gastroenterol Int 3:70, 1990
16. Das M, Carroll SF. Antithrombin III deficiency; an etiology of Budd-Chiari syndrome. Surgery 97:242, 1985
17. Datta DV, Vashishta S, Samanta AK, Chhuttani PN. Diagnostic value of combined transhepatic venography and inferior vena cava cavography in chronic Budd-Chiari syndrome. Am J Dig Dis 23:1031, 1978
18. Davis M, Peters R, Reynolds T. Budd-Chiari syndrome due to inferior vena cava obstruction. Gastroenterology 54:1142, 1968
19. Deutsch V, Rosenthal T, Adar R, Mozes M. Budd-Chiari syndrome: study of angiographic findings and remarks on etiology. AJR 116:430, 1972
20. Erlik D, Shramek A, Brandstaetter S, Bassan H. Surgical cure of primary hepatic vein occlusion syndrome by side-to-side portacaval shunt. Surg Gynecol Obstet 114:368, 1962
21. Fisher MR, Wall SD, Hricak H, McCarthy S, Kerlan RK. Hepatic vascular anatomy on magnetic resonance imaging. AJR 144:739, 1985
22. Gibson JB. Chiari's disease and the Budd-Chiari syndrome. J Pathol Bacteriol 79:381, 1960
23. Grant EG, Perrella R, Tessler FN, Lois J, Busuttil R. Budd-Chiari syndrome: the results of duplex and color Doppler imaging. AJR 152:377, 1989
24. Greenwood LH, Yrizarry JM, Hallett JW, Scoville GS. Urokinase treatment of the Budd-Chiari syndrome. AJR 141:1057, 1983
25. Halff G, Todo S, Tzakis AG, Gordon RD, Starzl TE. Liver-transplantation for the Budd-Chiari syndrome. Ann Surg 211:43, 1990
26. Hartmann RC, Luther AB, Jenkins DE Jr, Tenorio LE, Saba HI. Fulminant hepatic venous thrombosis (Budd-Chiari syndrome) in paroxysmal nocturnal hemoglobinuria: definition of a medical emergency. Johns Hopkins Med J 146:247, 1980
27. Hirooka M, Kimura C. Membranous obstruction of the hepatic portion of the vena cava. Arch Surg 100:656, 1970
28. Horisawa M, Yokoyama T, Juttner H, Reynolds TB. Incomplete membranous obstruction of the inferior vena cava: hemodynamic measurements and correction by balloon membranotomy and surgical resection. Arch Surg 111:599, 1976
29. Huguet C, Liegeois A, Levy VG, Caroli J. Interposition mesocaval shunt for chronic primary occlusion of the hepatic veins. Surg Gynecol Obstet 148:691, 1979
30. Jennings RH, Henderson JM, Millikan WJ Jr, Warren WD. Two stage surgical management of Budd-Chiari syndrome with obstruction of the inferior vena cava. Surg Gynecol Obstet 169:501, 1989
31. Khuroo MS, Datta DV. Budd-Chiari syndrome following pregnancy. Am J Med 68:113, 1980
32. Kimura C, Shirotani H. Hirooka M, Terada M, Iwahashi K, Maetani S. Membranous obliteration of the inferior vena cava in the hepatic portion. J Cardiovasc Surg 4:87, 1963
33. Klein AS, Sitzmann JV, Coleman J, Herlong FH, Cameron JL. Current management of the Budd-Chiari syndrome. Ann Surg 212:144, 1990
34. Kreel L, Freston JW, Clain D. Vascular radiology in the Budd-Chiari syndrome. Br J Radiol 40:755, 1967
35. Lam CR, Green E, Gale H. Transcardiac membranotomy, for obstruction of the hepatic portion of the inferior vena cava. Circulation 31 and 32(Suppl):1, 1965
36. Langer B, Stone RM, Colapinto RF, et al. Clinical spectrum of the Budd-Chiari syndrome and its surgical management. Am J Surg 129:137, 1975
37. Leopold JG, Parry TE, Storring FK. A change in the sinusoid-trabecular structure of the liver with hepatic venous outflow block. J Pathol 100:87, 1970
38. Lewis JH, Tice HL, Zimmerman HJ. Budd-Chiari syndrome associated with oral contraceptive steroids: review of treatment of 47 cases. Dig Dis Sci 28:673, 1983

39. McMahon HE, Ball HG. Leiomyosarcoma of hepatic vein and the Budd-Chiari syndrome. Gastroenterology 61:239, 1971

40. Menu Y, Alison D, Lorphelin J-M, Valla D, Belghiti J, Nahum H. Budd-Chiari syndrome: U.S. evaluation. Radiology 157:761, 1985

41. Mitchell MC, Boitnott JK, Kaufman S, Cameron JL, Maddrey WC. Budd-Chiari syndrome: etiology, diagnosis and management. Medicine 61:199, 1982

42. Murphy FB, Steinberg HV, Shires GT, Martin LG, Bernardino ME. The Budd-Chiari syndrome: a review. AJR 147:9, 1986

43. National Center for Health Statistics. Contraceptive utilization among currently married women 15–44 years of age: United States, 1973. Monthly Vital Stat Report 25(Suppl):1, 1976

44. Ohara I. A bypass operation for occlusion of the hepatic inferior vena cava. Surg Gynecol Obstet 117:151, 1963

45. Ohnishi K, Terabayashi H, Tsunoda T, Nomura F. Budd-Chiari syndrome: diagnosis with duplex sonography. Am J Gastroenterol 85:165, 1990

46. Orloff MJ, Johansen KH. Treatment of Budd-Chiari syndrome by side-to-side portacaval shunt: experimental and clinical results. Ann Surg 188:494, 1978

47. Parker RGF. Occlusion of the hepatic veins in man. Medicine 38:369, 1959

48. Pollard JJ, Nebesar RA. Altered hemodynamics in the Budd-Chiari syndrome demonstrated by selected hepatic and selective splenic angiography. Radiology 89:236, 1967

49. Powell-Jackson PR, Melia W, Canalese J, Pickford RB, Portmann B, Williams R. Budd-Chiari syndrome: clinical patterns and therapy. Q J Med 51:79, 1982

50. Prandi D, Rueff B, Benhamou JP. Side-to-side portacaval shunt in the treatment of Budd-Chiari syndrome. Gastroenterology 68:137, 1975

51. Ramsay GC, Britton RC. Intraparenchymal angiography in the diagnosis of hepatic veno-occlusive diseases. Radiology 90:716, 1968

52. Rector WG Jr, Redeker AG. Direct transhepatic assessment of hepatic vein pressure and direction of flow using a thin needle in patients with cirrhosis and the Budd-Chiari syndrome. Gastroenterology 86:1395, 1984

53. Rector WG Jr, Xu YH, Goldstein L, Peters RL, Reynolds TB. Membranous obstruction of the inferior vena cava in the United States. Medicine 64:134, 1985

54. Reynolds TB. Budd-Chiari syndrome. In: Schiff L, Schiff ER, eds. Diseases of the liver, ed 6. Philadelphia, JB Lippincott, 1987, p 1466

55. Rogers MA, Chesler E, DuPlessis L. Membranous obstruction of the hepatic segment of the inferior vena cava. Br J Surg 54:221, 1967

56. Rosenthal T, Shani M, Deutsch V, Shamra H. The Budd-Chiari syndrome after pregnancy: report of two cases and a review of the literature. Am J Obstet Gynecol 113:789, 1972

57. Roudot-Thoraval F, Gouault-Heilmann M, Zafrani ES, Barge J, Dhumeaux D. Budd-Chiari syndrome and the lupus anticoagulant. Gastroenterology 88:605, 1985

58. Safouh M, Shehata A, Elwi A. Hepatic vein occlusion disease in Egyptian children. Arch Pathol 79:505, 1965

59. Schaffner F, Gadboys HL, Safran AP, et al. Budd-Chiari syndrome caused by a web in the inferior vena cava. Am J Med 42:838, 1967

60. Schramek A, Better OS, Brook JS, et al. New observations in the clinical spectrum of the Budd-Chiari syndrome. Ann Surg 180:368, 1974

61. Schraut WH, Chilcote RR. Metastatic Wilms' tumor causing acute hepatic vein occlusion (Budd-Chiari syndrome). Gastroenterology 88:576, 1985

62. Seltman HJ, Dekker A, Van Thiel DH, Boggs DR, Starzl TE. Budd-Chiari syndrome recurring in a transplanted liver. Gastroenterology 84:640, 1983

63. Simson IW. Membranous obstruction of the inferior vena cava and hepatocellular carcinoma in South Africa. Gastroenterology 82:171, 1982

64. Stark DD, Hahn PF, Trey C, et al. Budd-Chiari syndrome associated with obstruction of the inferior vena cava. Am J Med 51:11, 1971

65. Stark DD, Hahn PF, Trey C, Clouse ME, Ferruci JT Jr. MRI of the Budd-Chiari syndrome. AJR 146:1141, 1986

66. Takeuchi J, Takada A, Hasamura Y, et al. Budd-Chiari syndrome associated with obstruction of the inferior vena cava. Am J Med 51:11, 1971

67. Tavill AS, Wood EJ, Kreel L, et al. The Budd-Chiari syndrome: correlation between hepatic scintigraphy and the clinical radiological and pathological findings in nineteen cases of hepatic venous outflow obstruction. Gastroenterology 68:509, 1975

68. Valla D, Casadevall N, Lacombe N, et al. Primary myeloproliferative disorder and hepatic vein thrombosis. Ann Intern Med 103:329, 1985

69. Valla D, Dhumeaux D, Babany G, et al. Hepatic vein thrombosis in paroxysmal nocturnal hemoglobinuria. Gastroenterology 93:569, 1987

70. Valla D, Le MG, Poynard T, Zucman N, Rueff B, Benhamou J-P. Risk of hepatic vein thrombosis in relation to recent use of oral contraceptives: a case-control study. Gastroenterology 90:807, 1986

71. Vons C, Smadja C, Bourstyn E, Szekely A-M, Bonnet P, Franco D. Results of portal systemic shunts in Budd-Chiari syndrome. Ann Surg 203:366, 1986

72. Warren WD, Potts JR, Fulenwider JT, Millikan WJ Jr, Henderson JM. Two stage surgical management of the Budd-Chiari syndrome associated with obstruction of the inferior vena cava. Surg Gynecol Obstet 159:101, 1984

73. Watkins E Jr, Fortin CL. Surgical correction of a congenital coarctation of the inferior vena cava. Ann Surg 159:536, 1964

74. Witte MH, Witte CL, Dumont AE. Progress in liver disease: physiological factors involved in the causation of cirrhotic ascites. Gastroenterology 61:742, 1971

75. Wu S-M, Spurny OM, Klotz AP. Budd-Chiari syndrome after taking oral contraceptives. Dig Dis 22:623, 1977

76. Yamamoto S, Yokoyama Y, Takeshige K, et al. Budd-Chiari syndrome with obstruction of the inferior vena cava. Gastroenterology 54:1070, 1968

Diseases of the Liver, Seventh Edition, edited by
Leon Schiff and Eugene R. Schiff. J.B. Lippincott Company, Philadelphia © 1993.

41

Liver Disease in Infancy and Childhood

William F. Balistreri

William K. Schubert

The emergence and rapid growth of pediatric hepatology as a specific and focused field of interest may be attributed to an appreciation of the importance of the dramatic physiologic variables that occur in the maturing liver as well as to the recognition of the unique nature of the liver diseases that affect infants and children. In fact, these two features may well be closely related; several of the pathophysiologic disturbances noted specifically in early life may be a direct result of delayed or faulty maturation.

The liver must undergo major maturational changes in the perinatal period during the transition from an intrauterine existence; the efficiency with which these anatomic and physiologic adaptations are established governs the ability of the newborn to cope with the new environment. The multiple clinical and research implications attendant to a clear understanding of these dynamic events have focused attention on the discipline of pediatric hepatology. Determination of the ontogenic expression of specific hepatic functions has served as a probe of liver physiology and has provided insight into certain disease processes.[60,62,80,351,1008] "Experiments of nature," namely, inborn errors of hepatic structure and function initially manifested in this period of life, also offer an opportunity to understand liver function more clearly. Physiologic variations or limitations may render the immature liver vulnerable to injury by exogenous factors; for example, infants are subject to complications of severe transplacental and postnatal infection by agents that may cause insignificant disease in adults. The marked, age-related changes in hepatic structure and function must be kept in mind during the clinical evaluation of infants or children suspected of having liver disease.[38,60,80,82,98,292,371,426] In addition, the postnatal variables in liver and gallbladder size and function, as well as transitory differences in drug absorption, distribution, biotransformation, and excretion, must all be considered when planning (and monitoring) any therapeutic regimen for infants. The common *acquired* diseases of the liver seen in adults are uncommon in the pediatric age group; therefore, the clinician must develop an entirely new algorithm for the differential diagnosis of problems such as jaundice. Finally, standard methods of investigation of liver disease in adults, such as percutaneous transhepatic cholangiography and endoscopic cannulation of the bile duct, are seldom of value in the pediatric population. The use of percutaneous needle biopsy, however, has proved to be a safe and useful procedure in infants and children, providing for histologic, biochemical, and ultrastructural definition and management of liver disease.[487,1094] The availability of tissue for analysis has allowed for precise investigation, which in turn has permitted the field to progress rapidly. These factors have combined to create a fascinating field of study—pediatric hepatology—that is only in its early stage of development.[75] Further refinement of the discipline will emerge from a more precise understanding of hepatobiliary embryogenesis and molecular biology and an intensified focus on the clinical aspects of liver diseases in infants and children.

Hepatic Embryogenesis

The morphologic development and the embryonic derivation of the liver and the intrahepatic and extrahepatic bile ducts have been extensively studied (Table 41-1). In the fetus (3 to 4 weeks of gestation), the hepatic diverticulum of endodermal epithelium arises as a cluster of cells emerging from the cranial–ventral margin of the junction of the yolk sac with the posterior foregut. These progenitor cells (hepatoblasts, immature hepatocytes, prehepatocytes, or type I liver cells) merge into the mesodermal mesenchymal cells of the septum transversum (primordial anterior diaphragm).[537,564,925] The hepatocytes align as cords, separated by nascent sinusoids; the capillary plexus between the vitelline veins within the septum gives rise to the liver sinusoids. The undifferentiated nature of human fetal hepatocytes at 4 to 6 weeks of gestation is evidenced by a scant cytoplasmic constituency, large nuclei, and a proportionally minute, inactive secretory apparatus (rough endoplasmic reticulum and Golgi bodies). Canalicular domains of several adjacent hepatocytes juxtapose to form bile canaliculi for export of biliary components at about 6 weeks of gestation.[357] The requirement for rapid growth and differentiation is met by abundant free ribosomes and receptors for growth factors, such as insulin-like growth factor I (IGF-I).[205] α-Fetoprotein synthesis is characteristic.[534] Protein degradation seems to be a lower priority as evidenced by a paucity of lysosomes and receptors for proteins involved in catabolism, for example, the asialoglycoprotein receptor.[176,565,566,811] The acquisition of apical–basal polarity, each with a specific profile of transport proteins and receptors, at about 6 to 8 weeks of gestation, signals the evolution of mature liver cells (type II hepatocytes). After the first trimester, liver growth proceeds in an orderly linear fashion until well after birth.[682] The formation of the intrahepatic ducts occurs in close approximation to the branches of the portal vein and the surrounding mesenchyme. There is strong evidence that

TABLE 41-1   *Origins of Cells in the Liver*

Cell Type	Primordial Source
Hepatocytes	Foregut endoderm
Bile duct cells	Foregut endoderm
Endothelial cells	Septum transversum mesenchyma
Kupffer cells	Yolk sac or bone marrow
Ito cells	Septum transversum mesenchyma
Hematopoietic cells	? Septum transversum

(Modified from Kaufman SS. Organogenesis and histologic development of the liver. In: Fox W, Polin RA, eds. Fetal and neonatal physiology. Philadelphia, WB Saunders, 1992)

these intrahepatic bile ducts develop from hepatocytes, and in the earliest stages of embryonic development, biopotential progenitor cells are present.[930,931,998,1068,1069] Intrahepatic bile duct development is initiated when a ring of prehepatocytes, which surround branches of the portal vein, transform into bile duct cells; there is then concentric and sequential differentiation, which results in the *ductal plate*—a double walled cylinder containing a narrow lumen.[536,537] Remodeling of the ductal plate results in the mature bile duct structure.[281,282,1068,1069] The coalescence of these prehepatocytes and the mesenchymal cells signals a specific phase of organogenesis. This process of intrahepatic bile duct development is dynamic throughout embryogenesis and continues until sometime after birth, as evidenced by cytokeratin expression patterns and morphology.[541,930,931,1068,1069]

Modulation of intrahepatic bile duct development has been attributed to the effect of bile flow or specific bile acids, liver cell–adhesion molecule, or basement membrane glycoprotein (laminin).[564-566,665,851] Reif and colleagues[853] have suggested that differential expression of extracellular matrix proteins, namely an increase in fibronectin content coupled with a decrease in laminin levels, modulates the terminal differentiation of hepatocytes during development. During various situations of liver injury, ductular metaplasia occurs, and hepatocytes express bile duct–type cytokeratins, suggesting a recapitulation of the sequence of events that occurs during normal development of the intrahepatic bile ducts.[1068,1069]

The origin of the extrahepatic biliary ductal system is less clearly defined; it is believed that the extrahepatic bile ducts and gallbladder arise from the caudal aspect of the hepatic diverticulum; however, in the mouse embryo, the most proximal bile ducts may be derived from the cranial aspects.[939] There also appears to be a specific sequence in the development of gallbladder contractility; this has been extensively studied in the developing guinea pig.[244,276]

Development of Hepatic Metabolic and Excretory Function

The fetus is critically dependent on the maternal liver for diverse needs; bidirectional flow across the placenta serves to deliver nutrients, to provide a route of elimination of metabolic end products, and to expedite biotransformation reactions. After delivery, adaptation to an extrauterine existence must be rapidly accomplished through differentiation of tissue function (de novo synthesis and enzymatic differentiation).

These specific enzymatic processes emerge in clusters, each of which correlates with dynamic alterations in functional requirement.[139,236,239,424,658] For example, fetal liver metabolism is devoted to production of plasma proteins to allow cell proliferation; near birth, the primary needs are production and storage of essential nutrients, excretion of bile, and establishment of processes of elimination. Overall modulation or induction of these developmental processes in the fetus is presumably through substrate and hormonal input by means of the placenta. Among other candidates, IGF and its receptor have been assigned a role in the regulation of growth of the fetal and neonatal liver.[432] Similarly, in the postnatal period, dietary and hormonal factors (such as epidermal growth factor) are thought to affect neonatal hepatic growth and development.[119,478,673] Kohno and colleagues[590] have demonstrated that human milk stimulates DNA synthesis by neonatal rat hepatocytes in primary cultures, suggesting the importance of growth-promoting substances ingested in early life. There are also intrinsic timing mechanisms inherent to the expression of certain transport processes.[173,410]

The fetal liver is active metabolically, with high blood flow and oxygen consumption rates; gluconeogenesis does not occur, while processes later assumed by other organs, such as hematopoiesis (yolk sac) and immunocytogenesis, do occur; therefore, a large amount of hematopoietic tissue is localized to the fetal liver.[377,424,1151] The liver of the newborn, in contrast, has a lower blood flow and oxygen delivery as a result of hemodynamic alterations occurring at birth with the loss of the oxygen-enriched umbilical venous supply.[101,403,1047] In addition, the carbohydrate-rich placental nutrient flux is discontinued and replaced by a low-carbohydrate, high-lipid content milk intake. Thereafter, the newborn liver must produce, through gluconeogenesis, the glucose required for rapid utilization in the immediate postnatal period. Fatty acid oxidation, which also provides energy in early life, complements gluconeogenesis and glycogenolysis.[397] There is a restricted capacity for hepatic ketogenesis in the immediate postnatal period, and the newborn tolerates prolonged periods of fasting poorly.[193] In the first postnatal months, during the period of rapid growth, galactose serves as a major substrate for energy production and carbohydrate storage.[581] Additional stresses, such as intrauterine growth retardation or malnutrition, may exert an additional deleterious impact on hepatocellular function and result in a further reduction in hepatic metabolic capacity.[136,780]

The major electron transport components of the monooxygenase system, such as cytochrome P-450, NADPH, and cytochrome *c* reductase, are present in low concentrations in fetal liver microsomal preparations. The zonal heterogeneity characteristic of hepatocytes of the mature liver is *not* apparent during embryonic development; instead, there is homogeneity of function across the acinus.[35,561] The attainment of an adult pattern of gene expression in the developing liver occurs through specific regulatory steps, each with varying modulatory influences. The microenvironment surrounding fetal hepatocytes has an influence on expression of metabolic processes, such as cytochrome P-450 genes[206,1034]; this is, in part, related to the disparate derivation of blood flow to the left and right lobe of the fetal liver. In fetal life, the left and medial segments are supported almost exclusively by flow from the umbilical vein (well saturated with oxygen); right lobe perfusion is by the portal vein (low oxygen content), combined with the right branch of the umbilical vein; the hepatic artery contributes minimally to total liver flood flow.[887]

The variation of both oxygen content and the hormonal profile of blood supplying the right and left lobes of the liver may be responsible for the lobular heterogeneity. Many of the changes that occur after placental separation may be related to alterations in the hepatic circulation and oxygen delivery resulting from the discontinuation of blood flow through the umbilical vein and the dependence of liver perfusion on the portal vein and hepatic artery.[887] There are multiple examples of hepatic *metabolic* immaturity. Numerous studies have documented an impairment in hepatic xenobiotic metabolism in the newborn, with a decreased capacity to detoxify certain drugs, and age-related difference in pharmacokinetics.[5,426,1082] A dramatic example was the "gray baby" syndrome associated with altered chloramphenicol metabolism.[668] The sequence of the postnatal development appearance of hepatic enzymes involved in the antioxidant pathway was studied by Pittschieler and colleagues,[818] who documented that levels of copper–zinc superoxide dismutase (SOD) increased 10-fold to reach adult levels at 3 weeks; manganese—SOD content matured more rapidly (less than 1 week).

Evidence also exists of immaturity of the hepatic *excretory* function—"physiologic immaturity of the enterohepatic circulation"[80]—manifest by inefficient lipid digestion, delayed hepatic clearance and metabolism of exogenous compounds (drugs) and endogenous substrates (bile acids and bilirubin), and a cholestatic phase of liver development.[60,80,297,1008] In early fetal life, bile acid pools are localized primarily to an intrahepatic site, a finding that correlates with morphologic and histochemical evidence of perinatal changes in bile canalicular development in the rat.[80,82,291,292,424] Gallbladder and ductular bile water reabsorption, canalicular secretion, and hormone-induced choleresis are inefficient in the newborn dog and develop rapidly during postnatal life.[1033]

The age-related inefficiency of mechanisms that determine the rate of bile flow is directly correlated with hepatic bile acid secretion.[80,1008] Hepatic excretory function is subservient to placental excretory function in utero; however, after birth, gradual maturation occurs in this functional capacity. In fact, recent studies suggest that the placenta effectively modulates fetal bile acid metabolism. A carrier-mediated bile acid transport system, analogous to that localized to hepatic canalicular membranes, has been demonstrated in human placental membrane vesicles.[316,669]

Experimental data document inefficient hepatocyte transport and metabolism of bile acids in the postnatal period (Table 41-2). This was initially suggested by an elevation of serum bile acid concentrations,[80,98,969,1009] which was an indirect indicator of impaired hepatic clearance, and confirmed in experimental models in which decreased uptake of bile acids by hepatocytes and membrane vesicles isolated from immature animals was noted.[1006,1010] Recent studies have focused on the expression of bile acid transport proteins during liver development[760,1086]; decreased expression of the transporter may contribute to reduced bile flow. A hepatic lobular (periportal to central) gradient for bile acid uptake is noted in the adult rat, indicating that bile acids are efficiently extracted in the periportal area.[82,1007,1012] Inefficient transport,

TABLE 41-2 *Factors Responsible for Physiologic Cholestasis: Evidence That Bile Acid Transport and Metabolism Are Underdeveloped in Early Life*

Increased serum bile acid levels[98,969,1009]
Decreased hepatic uptake of bile acids (isolated hepatocytes, membrane vesicles)[969,1010]
Increased efflux of bile acids[82,97]
Absence of a lobular gradient for bile acid uptake[82,1007,1012]
Decreased conjugation, decreased sulfation, and decreased glucuronidation of bile acids[81,1008,1011]
Altered bile acid synthesis
  Qualitative[53,1000]
  Quantitative[80,82]
Decreased bile acid pool size
Decreased secretion of bile acids
Decreased intraluminal bile acid concentrations
Decreased ileal active transport of bile acids[1008]

namely decreased uptake and increased efflux of bile acids by the developing liver, results in the absence of a lobular distribution for bile acid uptake.[97,1007,1008]

The intracellular transport and metabolism (binding, translocation, and synthesis) of bile acids is inefficient in early life. The specific activity of the enzymes involved in bile acid conjugation, sulfation, and glucuronidation is low[81,1008,1011]; the overall capacity to conjugate cholic acid by suckling rat liver was found to be about 30% of the adult capacity.[1011] As a direct reflection of these intracellular events, there is a gradual increase in bile acid pool size in humans and in various animal models.[80,82] In addition to progressive quantitative changes in bile acid synthetic rate, there are qualitative differences, namely, the formation of atypical bile acids.[53,80,82,435,926,1000,1093] The detection of qualitatively abnormal bile acids suggests the existence of a fetal biosynthetic pathway as well as a delay in the establishment of a mature synthetic sequence. The physiologic importance and pathophysiologic effects are unknown. There may be a direct effect on bile flow as a result of the absence of choleretic and trophic primary bile acids. Certain of the resultant atypical bile acids, such as monohydroxy compounds (3β-hydroxy-5-cholenoic acid), are intrinsically hepatotoxic and may initiate or exacerbate cholestasis. Conversely, the polyhydroxylated bile acids (tetrahydroxycholanic acids), found in the urine of normal infants,[1000] are more soluble compounds; this may provide for an efficient alternative route of elimination.

Interrelated observations provide a morphologic basis for "physiologic cholestasis," demonstrating cytoskeletal and canalicular structural immaturity in developing rat liver with rapid perinatal differentiation.[290–292] A correlation exists between actin filament distribution, cellular development, and functional maturation of the liver cell.[565,566] In fetal rat hepatocytes, bile canalicular structure, motility characteristics, and actin filament distribution differ from that seen in mature liver cells.[713] Spontaneous canalicular contractions, which play a role in canalicular bile flow, are not seen.

Therefore, the morphologic and functional differences that exist between the neonatal and the mature liver create the potential for a decrease in bile flow and the production of abnormal bile acids. Exogenous insults to the unique vulnerable developing liver, such as *Escherichia coli* sepsis with endotoxemia, the intravenous administration of amino acids during nutritional support, hypoxia, hypoperfusion, and administration of medications to the low-birthweight infant, may result in marked cholestasis.[72,74,779]

Neonatal Jaundice Associated With Elevation of Unconjugated Bilirubin

PHYSIOLOGIC JAUNDICE

The most thoroughly studied reflection of immature hepatic function is the phenomenon of "physiologic jaundice." Most normal newborns exhibit a mild elevation of serum bilirubin in cord blood, a gradual rise to a maximum of 8 to 9 mg/dL on the third to fifth day, and a fall to normal values in the second week of life. In the premature infant, the peak serum bilirubin levels may be 3 to 5 mg/dL higher, occur later, vary inversely with gestational age, and last somewhat longer. The challenge for the clinician is to distinguish between physiologic hyperbilirubinemia, which is thought to be benign, and nonphysiologic (pathologic) hyperbilirubinemia, in which case further investigation to determine the basis for the elevated bilirubin levels and prompt management are indicated.[666,752,753]

Physiologic jaundice is a diagnosis of exclusion; an alternative cause of unconjugated hyperbilirubinemia should be considered when (1) the jaundice is of early onset (within 24 hours of birth), (2) an extremely elevated level of unconjugated bilirubin is present (more than 11 to 12 mg/dL in a formula-fed infant or more than 14 to 15 mg/dL in a breastfed infant), (3) a conjugated component (more than 2 mg/dL) is detected, or (4) jaundice is persistent (longer than 2 weeks). By definition, physiologic unconjugated hyperbilirubinemia occurs in the absence of hemolytic disease.

Mechanism

The cause of physiologic jaundice is multifactorial; the neonate is burdened by specific functional defects, of varying degree, that result in delivery of an excess load of unconjugated bilirubin to an inefficient hepatic excretory system (Table 41-3).

After delivery, the newborn can no longer rely on placental or maternal detoxification of unconjugated bilirubin; therefore, until induction of intrinsic metabolic and excretory processes occurs, there is an accumulation of unconjugated bilirubin. Perinatal physiologic alterations in hepatic blood flow may further raise serum unconjugated bilirubin levels. Portal venous blood flow, which normally provides 80% of the hepatic blood flow, may be shunted through the ductus venosus, away from the sinusoidal bed of the liver, thereby bypassing the mechanism for hepatic clearance of bilirubin.[887] Red cell survival is shortened compared with that in the adult; this effect, which increases the bilirubin preload, is even more pronounced in the premature infant.[800] In view of the normal plethoric state of the infant, an increased red cell mass must be degraded (1 g of hemoglobin yields 35 mg of bilirubin). Shunt bilirubin, from nonhemoglobin sources, is higher (over 20%) than that found in adults.[529]

Physiologic hyperbilirubinemia can also be attributed, in part, to immaturity of many of the processes involved in the transfer of bilirubin from plasma to bile (uptake into the liver

TABLE 41-3 *Factors Responsible for Initiation and Perpetuation of Physiologic Jaundice in the Normal Neonate*

Separation from placental *transport* function and maternal *detoxification* mechanism
Perinatal hepatic blood flow patterns that shunt bilirubin away from the sinusoid[887]
Enhanced *production* of unconjugated bilirubin due to:
  Larger RBC mass
  Shorter RBC life span (about 80 days)[800]
  Inefficient erythropoiesis[529]
  Increased heme oxygenase activity
Decreased albumin *binding* of unconjugated bilirubin due to:
  Lower serum albumin concentration
  Decreased binding capacity
  Stress (eg, sepsis, acidosis, hypoxia)
Decreased hepatic Y *protein* levels (therefore decreased uptake and decreased intracellular binding)[430]
Decreased capacity for bilirubin *conjugation* (due to decreased activity of uridine diphosphate, glucose dehydrogenase, and uridine diphosphate glucuronyl transferase)[164,319,335,384]
Impaired bile *secretion*[80,82,291,292]
Altered *enterohepatic circulation* of unconjugated bilirubin:
  Decreased bacterial flora leading to decreased formation of urobilinogen
  Hydrolysis of conjugated bilirubin to unconjugated bilirubin, mediated by intestinal β-glucuronidase, with subsequent reabsorption

cell, intracellular binding and conjugation, and secretion into the bile canaliculus). Of the factors contributing to defective bilirubin kinetics in the newborn and to the pathogenesis of physiologic jaundice in the nonhuman primate, defective bilirubin conjugation is central.[384] A distinctive pattern of bilirubin conjugate formation in human newborn infants was detected by Rosenthal and colleagues,[876] using high performance liquid chromatography. During the first 24 to 48 hours, two isomeric monoconjugates of bilirubin appeared in the serum; the diconjugate was noted on the third day of life. Very low levels of glucuronyltransferase activity are detectable in the young of certain animals and in human fetal and newborn liver.[164,319] Variant observations may be related to species or to methodologic differences or to the presence of activators or inhibitors of glucuronyl transferase, such as progestational steroids.[161,1002]

Deficiency of conjugating ability alone is unlikely to account for physiologic jaundice. Impaired hepatic uptake is suggested by studies in fetal and newborn guinea pigs and monkeys of the content of the two hepatic intracellular proteins, Y and Z, which specifically bind organic anions such as bilirubin.[633,634] In the monkey liver, Z protein reaches adult levels during fetal development and is normal at birth. Y protein, which has the greatest anion-binding capacity, is absent at birth and reaches adult levels at 10 days of age.[43] Levels of Y protein correlate inversely with the magnitude and duration of physiologic jaundice and of impaired anion excretion and delayed plasma clearance found in newborn monkeys. The subsequent return of bilirubin levels and anion excretion to normal is associated with increased binding protein.[633] Similarly, impaired hepatic secretion of bilirubin and organic anions is present in other fetal and neonatal animals and in humans.[117,426,901,1111] Conjugation is essential for secretion under normal (adult) conditions; however, secretion may be the rate-limiting step in the transfer of bilirubin from blood to bile by an immature liver. Impairment in the blood-to-bile transfer of bilirubin in the human infant appears to result from a combination of varying degrees of alteration of uptake, conjugation, and secretion.

The existence of an enterohepatic circulation of bilirubin may contribute significantly to the genesis of physiologic jaundice.[762,820] The intestine of the fetus and newborn possesses β-glucuronidase activity and an absence of the bacterial flora that in the adult reduces bilirubin glucuronide to urobilinogen.[160,527] Bilirubin diglucuronide secreted into the intestine in the neonatal period can be hydrolyzed to the unconjugated form, which is more readily absorbed.[395,629,631] In utero, if conjugated bilirubin is hydrolyzed to the unconjugated state, it is reabsorbed and excreted through the placenta; after birth, the reabsorbed unconjugated bilirubin may elevate the level in serum. Interruption of the enterohepatic circulation, by feeding bilirubin-binding agents such as charcoal, cholestyramine, or agar to infants,[270,630,680,764,820,1058] reduces the maximal level of serum bilirubin attained during the first week in full-term infants.

Any delay in feeding of newborn infants may exaggerate the degree of physiologic jaundice. Fasted newborn Gunn rats have a greater degree of hyperbilirubinemia and increased activity of hepatic heme oxygenase. Early feeding has been shown to lower the maximal bilirubin level in full-term and premature infants as well as in infants of diabetic mothers.[1109] The relation of the mechanism of an increased level of jaundice in infants in whom feeding is delayed to the hyperbilirubinemia induced by fasting in Gilbert's disease is unclear.[356] Serum bilirubin elevation is associated with fasting in both conditions; however, in the infant, the maximal serum bilirubin level can be reduced equally well by water and glucose-water feedings.

Implications: Kernicterus (Bilirubin Encephalopathy)

The implications of an elevated serum bilirubin level are only partially understood. The major concern is classic neonatal neurotoxicity (kernicterus) attributed to an elevated unconjugated bilirubin level; however, there may be a wider range of toxicities and possibly an antianabolic bioactivity.[1076] Conversely, there is recent evidence that unconjugated bilirubin may provide important beneficial physiologic functions, serving as an antioxidant or as a substrate for induction of critical processes.[666,995]

Kernicterus, classically defined as bilirubin staining of the basal ganglia, pons, or cerebellum, was most often noted in postmortem examination of infants who had severe unconjugated hyperbilirubinemia associated with Rh isoimmune hemolysis.[159,195,758,552] The incidence of this postmortem finding has decreased with the decrease in Rh disease and with the introduction of better methods to control serum bilirubin levels in early life. At present, the most frequent setting for the detection of kernicterus is in autopsies of critically ill, low-birthweight infants.[195] Confounding variables noted in these low-birthweight infants are the presence of respiratory distress, hypoxia, acidosis, intraventricular hemorrhage, sepsis, and extreme prematurity.[335] These insults may open the blood–brain barrier[635] and thereby cause bilirubin encephalopathy to occur at levels of serum unconjugated bilirubin less than 20 mg/dL.[152,153]

Clinical manifestations of kernicterus vary from lethargy, hypotonia, and poor feeding due to loss of the suck reflex to opisthotonos, spasticity, and death.[1072] Survivors may show high-frequency deafness, chorioathetosis, and dental dysplasia. Physiologic monitoring, such as assessment of changes in auditory-evoked brain-stem responses, may provide a noninvasive measure of bilirubin encephalopathy.[7,210,288,526,1083,1084] In long-term follow-up of apparently normal infants with unconjugated hyperbilirubinemia, subtle neurologic abnormalities, impaired motor performance, hearing loss, and psychological dysfunction have been documented.[531,900] Van de Bor and colleagues[1065] have described a dose-response relation between the peak total serum bilirubin concentration and the documentation of a neurologic handicap at 2 years of age; they noted an increase in risk of about 30% for each 2.9 mg/dL increment in bilirubin concentration. It remains to be determined, however, whether rapid, meaningful intervention, with successful reduction of the maximal bilirubin concentrations, will diminish the risk of neurologic injury.[753]

In plasma, lipid-soluble unconjugated bilirubin is bound to albumin, which provides an efficient biologic buffer; however, the binding capacity is limited and can be easily exceeded.[8,195,763,862] Albumin-bound bilirubin is in equilibrium with a small amount of unbound bilirubin (less than 0.5 mg/dL).[763,765,766] The ratio of available binding sites to true binding capacity may be lowered in the presence of other substances that compete directly with bilirubin or that alter binding sites by attaching to alternate albumin sites.[624] In theory, only free bilirubin can diffuse into cells and exert toxic metabolic effects. There is the possibility, however, of reversible opening of the blood–brain barrier to albumin as well as to bilirubin in the presence of altered vascular permeability, hyperosmolarity, hypoxia, or acidosis.[152,153,522,623,635,805] Subsequent dissociation of bilirubin from albumin allows passage from serum into the cell. Unbound bilirubin interacts with cell membranes and is toxic to membrane-associated metabolic processes.[902] This is abetted by the fact that bilirubin demonstrates an affinity for cell membrane phospholipids and is relatively insoluble at physiologic pH. Unconjugated bilirubin, when present at certain concentrations in the brain tissue, may also alter the rate of uptake and consumption of cerebral oxygen, glucose, and lactate.[149] Diffusion into mitochondria, with subsequent uncoupling of oxidative phosphorylation, may be a mechanism of toxicity; unconjugated bilirubin inhibits oxidative processes in isolated mitochondria, thereby exerting a cytotoxic effect by means of a decrease in local adenosine triphosphate (ATP) levels and impairment of energy-dependent cerebral metabolism.[32,729] Unconjugated bilirubin also causes specific changes in electrophysiology.[451] Bilirubin toxicity may be initiated by modulation of cerebral-protein phosphorylation. A direct effect on membrane function is suggested by the toxicity of free bilirubin on the non–mitochondria-containing renal papillae of Gunn rats.[763,765] The peculiar vulnerability of the central nervous system to free bilirubin toxicity may be related to the low albumin concentration in brain interstitial fluid, which is 1/10 that of plasma.

Any condition that reduces plasma bilirubin binding capacity predisposes to higher tissue bilirubin levels and kernicterus. Factors of clinical importance in the neonate are hypoalbuminemia, acidosis, and the presence of organic anions that bind to albumin, such as sulfonamides, salicylates, heparin, caffeine, sodium benzoate, nonesterified fatty acids, and hematin.[195,363] Plasma free fatty acid (FFA), present in low concentrations, can compete with bilirubin for binding at the primary (high-affinity) site on albumin. This displaces bilirubin and shifts most of it to secondary (low-affinity) binding sites, from which it is easily displaced into tissue. If the FFA concentration increases (molar ratio of FFA to albumin more than 5:1), there is competition for the secondary sites as well.[763] Bilirubin neurotoxicity is exaggerated in the presence of anoxia; the resultant tissue acidosis may further impair mitochondrial oxidation of bilirubin.[158] In the Gunn rat, there are dramatic strain differences in susceptibility to kernicterus with mortality; this implies that additional factors may modulate the vulnerability to bilirubin toxicity, both in this species and perhaps in humans.[993]

These observations suggest that blood levels of bilirubin are not a reliable predictor of toxicity: if drugs displace bilirubin, plasma levels are low, while tissue levels are high; conversely, after albumin infusion, blood levels increase as bilirubin exits from tissue. Therefore, monitoring and therapy must be individualized, taking these variables into account.

NONPHYSIOLOGIC JAUNDICE

The differential diagnosis of unconjugated hyperbilirubinemia in early life is outlined in Table 41-4.

Increased Bilirubin Production

Increased bilirubin production results from erythrocyte hemolysis, breakdown of blood in enclosed hematomas, and any condition that further increases red cell mass before or at parturition.

Incompatibility

RH ISOIMMUNIZATION.   Rh disease is primarily of historic interest. Prevention of isoimmunization is achieved by administration of potent anti-D γ-globulin to the mother after each delivery, abortion, or miscarriage; this destroys fetal Rh-positive red cells that enter the maternal circulation at parturition.[228] In women already sensitized, amniocentesis allows diagnosis before 30 weeks of gestation. Rh isoimmunization may result in the onset of jaundice in the first 24 hours of life, with a rapid increase to levels that require treatment. The most severely affected infants are pale, edematous, and suffer circulatory collapse related to the anemia, or they are stillborn with hydrops fetalis. The diagnosis is usually anticipated on the basis of prenatal Rh testing. The definitive diagnosis depends on demonstration of maternal antibody coating fetal red cells; 93% of affected mothers have anti-D antibody despite the large number of antigens on the red cell, which theoretically could cause isoimmunization. In Rh disease, the Coombs' test is strongly positive, as opposed to the weakly positive reaction characteristic of ABO incompatibility. Cord blood hemoglobin concentration is reduced, and bilirubin levels are elevated in direct proportion to the severity of the hemolytic process.

Affected infants may have elevated levels of conjugated (25% to 30% of the total) as well as of unconjugated bilirubin in cord blood; this may be due to in utero substrate activation of uptake and conjugation by the large load of bilirubin or a relative failure of excretion.[1121] In infants who died of Rh disease within 48 hours, liver histology was the same whether or not conjugated bilirubin levels were elevated.[463] Extramedullary hematopoiesis, hemosiderin deposits, and iron

TABLE 41-4   *Differential Diagnosis of Unconjugated Hyperbilirubinemia in Infants*

Increased Bilirubin Production
Hemolytic disease: isoimmune
    Rh incompatibility
    ABO incompatibility
    Other (Lewis, M,S, Kidd, Kell, Duffy)
Congenital spherocytosis
Hereditary eliptocytosis
Infantile pyknocytosis
Erythrocyte enzyme defects
    Glucose-6-phosphate
    Pyruvate kinase
    Hexokinase
Infection
Enclosed hematoma (cephalohematoma, ecchymoses)
Polycythemia
    Diabetic mother
    Fetal transfusion (maternal, twin)
    Delayed cord clamping
Drugs
    Vitamin K
    Maternal oxytocin[170]
    Phenol disinfectants[1134]
Total parenteral nutrition

Decreased Bilirubin Uptake, Storage, or Metabolism
Crigler-Najjar (I) or Arias (II) syndrome
Gilbert's syndrome
Lucey-Driscoll syndrome
Drug inhibition
Hypothyroidism or hypopituitarism
Congestive heart failure
Portacaval shunt
Hypoxia
Acidosis
Sepsis

Enterohepatic Recirculation
Breast-milk jaundice
Intestinal obstruction
    Ileal atresia
    Hirschsprung's disease
    Cystic fibrosis
Antibiotic administration

pigment in hepatic and Kupffer cells were present, but there was no hepatic cell necrosis, giant cell change, or cholestasis. After severe Rh incompatibility, especially before widespread use of exchange transfusion, persistent elevation of conjugated bilirubin levels with acholic stools lasting 4 to 8 weeks was not uncommon. *Inspissated bile syndrome*, the term used to designate posterythroblastotic jaundice, originally referred to obstructive jaundice in infancy due to bile plugs in a stenotic or narrowed common duct.[603] The histology (disruption of liver cell cords, hepatocyte necrosis, giant cell transformation, extramedullary hematopoiesis, and portal fibrosis and inflammation of varying degree) was similar to that of neonatal hepatitis.[289] It is possible that short incubation posttransfusion hepatitis was involved in some cases. Therefore, the possibility of mechanical obstruction by bile plugs implied by the term may be incorrect, and the term has largely been discarded.

ABO INCOMPATIBILITY. In view of the declining incidence of Rh hemolytic disease, the most common cause of newborn hemolytic disease is ABO incompatibility (maternal alloantibody reacting with fetal red cells).[315] Twenty percent of pregnancies are heterospecific for A, B, and O blood groups. About 5% to 40% are sensitized as shown by the direct Coombs' test; the higher incidence is associated with maternal group O; half of sensitized infants have hemolysis, and in about half of these, peak bilirubin exceeds 10 mg/dL. The major problem is the risk of kernicterus; hydrops is rare, anemia is mild. Microspherocytosis on peripheral blood smear is characteristic. Although the direct Coombs' test is not as strongly positive as in Rh disease, the indirect Coombs' test against adult erythrocytes of the infant's type is positive when either infant serum or antibody eluted from the infant's cells is used.[315,1148] Amniocentesis is not indicated. First pregnancies may be involved; in subsequent pregnancies, the severity of hemolysis is increased, unchanged, or decreased in about equal proportions.

OTHER HEMOLYTIC ANEMIAS. Less commonly, other hemolytic anemias due to structural and enzymatic red cell defects may produce jaundice and anemia in the first 2 days of life. Congenital *spherocytosis* may be confused with ABO hemolytic disease, but in at least 60% of cases, one parent is affected and serologic studies are negative.[181] Hereditary *elliptocytosis*, which has variable clinical manifestations and striking morphologic alterations visible on blood smear, may cause severe neonatal jaundice.[257] Infantile *pyknocytosis*, limited to premature infants, is associated with peculiar small red cells with spiny projections and produces jaundice in the first few days of life.

Multiple genetically determined erythrocyte enzyme defects resulting in *nonspherocytic* hemolytic anemia have been described.[1063] Glucose-6-phosphate dehydrogenase (G6PD) deficiency is capable of causing marked jaundice. In infants of Asian and Mediterranean descent, the enzyme may be completely absent, and hemolysis may occur even in the absence of drugs recognized to cause hemolysis in this condition.[626,1060] In African Americans with G6PD deficiency, hemolysis in the absence of drug exposure is rare except in premature neonates. Pyruvate kinase deficiency, second in frequency, may cause significant jaundice or anemia.[1063] Generally, hemoglobinopathies do not present in the newborn period, presumably because of the normal presence of large amounts of fetal hemoglobin. Homozygous α-chain thalassemia has been associated with hydrops fetalis and stillbirths,[543] and γ-β-thalassemia has been associated with hemolytic disease in the newborn.[544]

Enclosed Hematoma. Blood separated from the circulation (cephalohematoma or extensive bruising of the skin) is degraded promptly and may contribute to the bilirubin load imposed on the neonatal liver.[843] A similar mechanism may occur with subdural hematoma, large vein thrombosis, and ingestion of maternal blood at delivery.[323]

Polycythemia. Senescence of an increased red cell mass, which is physiologic in utero, increases the bilirubin load to be excreted after birth. A further increase in the red cell mass may occur in infants of diabetic mothers (increased birthweight, hypoglycemia, and respiratory distress), in fetal transfusion in utero from either mother or a twin fetus, from overly aggressive stripping of the umbilical cord at birth, and in congenital adrenal hyperplasia.[702,844] The clinical appearance of excessive plethora may mask the degree of hyperbilirubinemia; treatment is by partial exchange transfusion.

Drugs. Drugs in excessive doses, such as water-soluble vitamin K, may produce hemolysis, Heinz bodies, and jaundice in premature infants without predisposing erythrocyte enzyme defects.[700] The appropriate dose of 1 mg is harmless. Neonatal hyperbilirubinemia occurred after oxytocin-induced labor as a result of a vasopressin-like effect leading to osmotic swelling, decreased deformability, and rapid destruction of red cells.[170]

Total Parenteral Nutrition. Parenteral infusion of amino acid, carbohydrate, and lipid is frequently used in the support of the low-birthweight and ill neonate. Amino acids and lipid in solution apparently do not interfere with bilirubin transport; they have no discernible effect on bilirubin kinetics; therefore, this mode of nutrition may be used in jaundiced neonates.[1041,1108] Emulsified fat, given intravenously, may serve as a sink to prevent flux of bilirubin into tissue. Further investigation with prospective studies of low-birthweight infants managed in this manner is needed.

Decreased Bilirubin Uptake, Storage, or Conjugation

Crigler-Najjar Syndrome. This form of familial nonhemolytic jaundice occurs in association with deficient hepatic microsomal bilirubin uridine-diphosphate-glucuronosyl-transferase (UDPGT) activity. This human condition is analogous to that found in the Gunn rat.[44,250,906] At least two genetic subtypes (I and II) have been described,[44,906] with liver histology being normal in both types. Type I, originally described by Crigler and Najjar, is defined as recessively inherited complete deficiency of UDPGT activity.[44,250,906,1067] Serum levels of unconjugated bilirubin are high (20 to 40 mg/dL), and kernicterus, which is frequent, may occur at any age.[129,131] Bile is colorless and contains no bilirubin diglucuronide. Despite the lack of bilirubin in bile in type I, stools are of normal color and fecal urobilinogen content is only slightly reduced, presumably because of transfer of unconjugated bilirubin across the intestinal mucosa. Serum bilirubin is maintained at relatively constant levels by this mechanism as well as by excretion of water-soluble derivatives.[906] Phenobarbital administration has no effect on serum bilirubin levels.[44,131,411] Type II patients generally have lower serum bilirubin levels (9 to 17 mg/dL), no neurologic disease, and bile that is slightly pigmented but contains bilirubin monoglucuronide in levels only slightly below the normal range.[41,44,131,249,411,1112] Phenobarbital administration results in a prompt fall in serum bilirubin to near-normal levels.[44,249,596,1112,1137] A precise differential of type I from type II may be difficult; however, assessment of bilirubin fractions by sensitive methods such as high-performance liquid chromatography, before and after treatment with phenobarbital, may help to discriminate.[810] The parents of affected children are anicteric in both types but may exhibit differences in glucuronide formation. Dominant inheritance of type II with incomplete penetrance is postulated.[44] Kernicterus, reported occasionally in patients otherwise conforming to the type II definition, can be attributed to multiple factors influencing serum bilirubin concentration in the neonatal period, such as hypoxia, acidosis, and drug administration. Rarely, patients with severe type I disease survive to their teens, emphasizing the importance of alternative excretory pathways and the use of bilirubin-binding agents and phototherapy.[517,551] In the future, the use of pharmacologic agents that block heme degradation to bilirubin may prove to be of benefit,[311-314] either alone or as an adjunct to phototherapy.[884] Restoration of glucuronyl transferase activity can be accomplished experimentally through the use of transplanted microencapsulated hepatocytes[301] or clinically through liver transplantation.[569] In view of the potential for progressive, devastating bilirubin encephalopathy, liver transplantation should be considered when phototherapy is unable to contain the serum unconjugated bilirubin levels in an acceptable range.[936]

Gilbert's Syndrome. A presumably heterogeneous condition characterized by low-grade elevation of unconjugated bilirubin, with mean levels ranging from 2 to 3 mg/dL, Gilbert's syndrome is often not diagnosed until puberty.[829] Scleral icterus is the only physical finding. Liver function and histology are normal except for minor alterations noted on electron microscopy. Subjective symptoms, such as fatigue, vague abdominal pain, and nausea, associated with the disease in the older child may be related primarily to anxiety.

A simple presumptive test is provided by the observation that caloric deprivation (400 cal/d) increases serum bilirubin levels two-fold to three-fold in adults with Gilbert's syndrome.[846] Because mild compensated hemolytic states[41,110] and posthepatitic liver dysfunction[41] may produce similar levels of unconjugated bilirubin, the diagnosis is restricted to patients with normal red cell survival and absence of histologic and functional abnormalities of the liver.[829] Within this definition, Gilbert's disease is presumably due to either defective transport of unconjugated bilirubin from blood to bile,[388] decreased membrane uptake, or altered conjugation of bilirubin. Bilirubin overproduction (dyserythropoiesis) may be a contributing coincident factor.[698] Attempts at demonstration of defective conjugation in vitro have yielded conflicting results; in reports in which decreased enzymatic activity was found, the decrease was only partial and insufficient to account for the hyperbilirubinemia.[41,127] Decreased hepatic uptake of bilirubin is suggested by alterations in bilirubin disappearance curves; organic anion clearance is normal, suggesting that Y and Z proteins are normal.[110,829] A familial incidence has been reported in 15% to 40% of cases[829] and would probably be higher if repeated bilirubin levels and the effects of fasting were determined. Available data suggest an autosomal dominant inheritance (varying penetrance), with males affected more frequently than females.[829,846]

Transient Familial Neonatal Hyperbilirubinemia. In 1961, Lucey and Driscoll observed infants with severe hyperbilirubinemia beginning on the first day of life; in untreated patients, the bilirubin levels exceeded 60 mg/dL, and kernicterus resulted.[46] After vigorous exchange transfusion, affected infants were anicteric without liver disease and were neurologically normal after the newborn period. Serum and urine from the apparently healthy mothers of affected infants inhibited glucuronyl transferase activity in vitro.

Drugs. Various compounds can result in bilirubin levels that are three times normal in term infants, presumably because of inhibition of glucuronyl transferase[496,1016] or displacement of bilirubin.[363]

Hypothyroidism. Prolonged elevation of indirect bilirubin may be the first clinical sign of congenital hypothyroidism.[12,213] In an analysis of infants with hypothyroidism, 20% had abnormal and prolonged (up to 7 weeks) jaundice; 33% had hyperbilirubinemia as a presenting sign.[1104]

Altered Enterohepatic Circulation

Breast Milk Jaundice. Breastfed infants have a higher incidence of elevated serum unconjugated bilirubin values in the first week of life (10% to 25% versus 4% to 7% in formula-fed infants).[615,909] This unconjugated hyperbilirubinemia also lasts longer and reaches higher peak values than in formula-fed infants.[42,380,580] In a small percentage of infants, hyperbilirubinemia is prolonged.[45,46,992] Typically, the infant is well, and the jaundice develops slowly, reaching a peak at about the second or third week. Peak bilirubin levels over 20 mg/dL may occur, but the usual range is 10 to 20 mg/dL. Despite the elevated serum bilirubin levels, weight gain continues, and neurologic damage does not occur. Interrupting breastfeeding for 24 hours may result in a fall in the serum bilirubin level, confirming the diagnosis and allowing resumption of breastfeeding. In the absence of breast milk feeding restriction, bilirubin levels gradually fall to normal. There is no sex predominance; succeeding infants may be affected.

Jaundice that occurs in infants fed breast milk has been proposed to be of two types, based on the age of onset: (1) *early-onset breast milk jaundice*, also called *breastfeeding jaundice* (or exaggerated physiologic jaundice), and (2) *late-onset breast milk jaundice*, the classic breast milk–induced jaundice syndrome that develops after the first week of life.[381,615] The mechanisms are also proposed to be disparate—the early-onset form may be related to the fact that neonates receive fewer calories in the first 3 to 5 days of life while receiving human milk. The mechanism by which breast milk from certain mothers induces a higher incidence of unconjugated hyperbilirubinemia (late-onset) in infants has been the subject of much study. Investigations by Arias and coworkers[45] demonstrated that breast milk from mothers of affected infants had an inhibitory effect on glucuronide formation in liver slices; they subsequently isolated 3α,20β-pregnanediol from the milk and found that this compound had an inhibitory effect on conjugation. Because ingestion of the steroid caused jaundice in two of four infants, the investigators concluded that it was the cause of jaundice.[45] Although the inhibitory effect of breast milk on glucuronyl transferase has been confirmed in vitro and in vivo, there is not uniform agreement that the inhibitor is 3α,20β-pregnanediol.[225,462,742] Other investigations have implicated FFA, lipase, and other components of breast milk. Numerous studies have suggested that reabsorption of unconjugated bilirubin from meconium occurs in neonates and that jaundiced infants have a lower output of bilirubin in the feces. The successful use of agar feedings to inhibit bilirubin reabsorption complements experimental studies that suggest that an exaggerated intestinal reabsorption of unconjugated bilirubin occurs.[270,764] Gartner and coworkers[382] demonstrated an increased enterohepatic circulation of bilirubin after ingestion of milk from mothers whose infants developed breast milk jaundice, suggesting that a constituent of milk fostered intestinal bilirubin absorption. In contrast, cow-milk formulas and normal human breast milk inhibit absorption of unconjugated bilirubin from the intestine.[18] Gourley and associates[414,415] have detected significant amounts of β-glucuronidase (which hydrolyses glucuronic acid from bilirubin glucuronides) in breast milk of women whose babies developed jaundice; they postulate that intraluminal hydrolysis by this enzyme liberates unconjugated bilirubin, which is then efficiently reabsorbed and contributes to the circulating pool of unconjugated bilirubin.

Management is problematic, especially when the serum bilirubin level exceeds 15 mg/dL.[666,667] While kernicterus has not been reported in infants with breast milk–induced jaundice, marked elevations of serum unconjugated bilirubin may pose a risk to the developing nervous system.[615] The minimal diagnostic and therapeutic endeavor, therefore, should be to temporarily interrupt breastfeeding; this should be associated with a rapid (24- to 72-hour) decrease in the serum bilirubin level.[381] This maneuver can be reassuring; with resumption of feedings, bilirubin levels may rise only slightly.

Bacterial Flora and Transit Time. Alteration of the enterohepatic circulation may lead to elevated serum levels of unconjugated bilirubin in other clinical situations. Fifteen percent of infants with pyloric stenosis have significant elevation of unconjugated bilirubin levels, which fall to normal 5 to 10 days after surgery.[137,355] An increase in unconjugated bilirubin may also occur in the presence of duodenal stenosis or atresia if the obstruction is above the ampulla of Vater. Late feeding of infants (after 48 hours) results in higher levels of bilirubin whether or not the feeding contains glucose.[497,1109] Antibiotic administration may exacerbate unconjugated hyperbilirubinemia. In these situations, movement of intestinal contents through the gut is decreased, or introduction of bacterial flora to the intestine is delayed. In the relative absence of intestinal bacteria, which function to reduce bilirubin to urobilinogen, reabsorption of unconjugated bilirubin produced in the gut by intestinal β-glucuronidase is possible.

TREATMENT OF UNCONJUGATED HYPERBILIRUBINEMIA

In the absence of hemolysis, the term infant with unconjugated hyperbilirubinemia may require no therapy[1096]; however, in the presence of confounding variables or any of the exaggerative conditions indicated previously, intervention *may* be required.

The goal of any therapeutic approach to unconjugated hyperbilirubinemia is to lower serum bilirubin levels and prevent toxicity (bilirubin encephalopathy). Current approaches are directed toward removal or degradation of bilirubin: (1) physical removal of unconjugated bilirubin by exchange transfusion or intraluminal binding in the gut, (2) photoconversion of bilirubin (formation of polar derivatives) or augmented excretion of unconjugated bilirubin, (3) stimulation of hepatic excretion of bilirubin (eg, with phenobarbital), and (4) blockage of heme conversion to bilirubin.

Exchange Transfusion
Initially applied in the management of Rh disease, exchange transfusion has been used to treat persistent hyperbilirubinemia in nonsensitized infants because kernicterus can occur in jaundiced infants in the absence of hemolytic disease.[293] Exchange transfusion removes bilirubin, corrects hypoalbuminemia, supplies albumin-binding sites, and may remove endogenous metabolites that have saturated potential albumin-binding sites. It can be supplemented with additional albumin to improve the efficiency of bilirubin removal.[765] Fortunately, this procedure is rarely indicated.

A serum unconjugated bilirubin level of 20 mg/dL has been widely used as a criterion for exchange or repeat exchange in hemolytic disease and for exchange transfusion in full-term infants with nonhemolytic hyperbilirubinemia. Bilirubin-binding capacity tests may have an improved predictive value over serum bilirubin levels, but their ultimate value in the usual clinical laboratory situation remains to be determined.[195,766] The occurrence of kernicterus at lower serum bilirubin levels in association with drug administration, hypoalbuminemia, hypoxia, acidosis, and in premature infants[152,153,383,572,635,766] emphasizes the need to consider all factors in deciding when to treat. The use of whole blood exchange may be obviated after further development and refinement of techniques, such as enzymatic (bilirubin oxidase) removal of bilirubin from blood.[620] Refinement of this technique, in which a reactor containing the immobilized enzyme is incorporated into an extracorporeal circuit, may allow a safe and effective alternative.[741]

Bilirubin-Binding Agents
Oral administration of bilirubin binding agents decrease absorption and increase fecal excretion of unconjugated bilirubin.[270,764,820,1058] Activated charcoal or agar feedings result in significantly lower mean bilirubin levels during the first 5 days of life in healthy infants.[820,1058] The potential therapeutic value is not known; Schmid and colleagues[908] found no beneficial effect from cholestyramine feeding begun on the third day of life in premature infants.

Phototherapy
Cremer and coworkers[248] reported the successful treatment of jaundiced infants by exposure to visible bright light. Photoenhanced excretion of bilirubin became widely used after controlled trials demonstrated efficiency in controlling serum bilirubin levels and in decreasing the need for exchange transfusion in neonatal jaundice.[656,687]

The mechanism of phototherapy has been extensively studied both in the Gunn rat model, which may not absolutely reflect the in vivo human situation, and in jaundiced neonates. Bilirubin is known to be photolabile. In the Gunn rat, phototherapy was noted to cause an accelerated turnover of bilirubin by increased appearance of unconjugated bilirubin in bile and by enhanced excretion of polar derivatives of bilirubin in bile and urine.[785,786]

Bilirubin undergoes several photoreactions in vivo and in vitro, whereby polar photoproducts are formed; these are readily excreted in bile or in urine. In the Z,Z state, intramolecular hydrogen bonds can form, rendering bilirubin insoluble in aqueous solutions. Therefore, a major mechanism of in vivo bilirubin photocatabolism is rapid nonoxidative photoisomerization, which occurs in the skin[6,220,524,686,687,784,785] (Fig. 41-1). This causes the formation

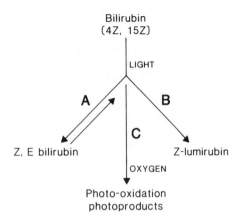

FIGURE 41-1 Photochemical reactions of bilirubin that occur in vivo after exposure to incident light in the 400- to 500-nm spectral range. The products are less lipophilic than bilirubin and do not require conjugation before excretion. (**A**) Configurational (geometric) isomerization. (**B**) Structural isomerization (intramolecular cyclization). (**C**) Photooxidation. Lumirubin is the major bilirubin species in bile of premature infants undergoing phototherapy.[331] Photooxidation photoproducts can be excreted in urine.[687]

of a series of polar photoisomers that partition into plasma, bind to albumin, and undergo hepatic clearance and secretion into bile. There, the less stable photobilirubin reverts spontaneously to the parent compound (bilirubin IX-α), especially in the presence of bile acids. This process accounts for the enhanced excretion of unconjugated bilirubin that is observed.[587,642] Lumirubin formation is an important route for bilirubin elimination.[331] Bilirubin is activated by a narrow spectrum of blue light; the most effective wavelengths are those near 450 nm, with secondary peaks at 410 nm and 490 nm.[333,334] Although blue light is most effective in reducing serum bilirubin levels, daylight fluorescent lamps supplying 200 to 400 foot-candles are adequate and may be safer.[332–334]

Despite the obvious efficacy of phototherapy in reducing serum bilirubin, caution is warranted in view of multiple postulated risks; however, there is little conclusive data regarding harmful long-term effects. The major concerns are overuse or inappropriate use—failure to recognize instances of cholestasis including sepsis; use in severe hemolysis, thereby delaying definitive management; and use in healthy but mildly jaundiced infants, where the net effect is to prolong the nursery stay.

Potential biologic ill effects of phototherapy include indirect effects due to toxicity of photoisomers (eg, diarrhea, tissue damage, possible neurotoxicity) and direct phototoxic reactions (light-mediated effects on membranes, lipid peroxidation) such as retinal damage, hemolysis, photodecomposition of proteins, amino acids and vitamins, and alteration of endocrine function and growth. Exposure of cells to light induces breaks in DNA strands, sister chromatid exchange, and mutations. Bilirubin acts as a photosensitizing agent, thereby enhancing the level of DNA damage in cells exposed to light.[875]

Direct injuries to body tissues, including retinal injury, have been observed in rats and piglets[757,950] but not in human infants.[542] Other postulated hazards are denaturation of albumin with resultant diminished bilirubin-binding capacity; platelet or red cell injury with hemolysis, especially in premature neonates; and a decrease in riboflavin in

plasma.[593,763,885] In vitro photooxidation products may not be cytotoxic[438,943]; in vivo products, although rapidly excreted, could have a different toxic potential. A significant portion of these products, which partition into chloroform at neutral pH, might diffuse into the brain. Although clinical and laboratory evidence is reassuring, further study of purified, isolated in vivo photodegradation products is needed.

Insensible water losses may be significant in low-birth-weight infants. Diarrhea may be suggested by large green stools occurring during phototreatment.[433,656,899] Overheating may occur from improper light units. The effects on cardiac output and peripheral vascular resistance need to be defined. Eye damage is a potential hazard if eye shields are not properly placed or are dislodged. Jaundice cannot be assessed clinically because the skin is decolorized; therefore, serum bilirubin must be measured before and after phototherapy. Clinical experience in over 4800 infants has shown no side effects on growth or endocrine status.[480,656,899] A controlled trial of phototherapy for neonatal hyperbilirubinemia, carried out by the National Institute of Child Health and Human Development, randomly assigned 1339 newborns to receive either phototherapy or to serve as a control group.[899] This study documented that phototherapy could effectively control unconjugated hyperbilirubinemia without evidence of adverse outcome at 6 years of age. Phototherapy 10 hours nightly for 3 years in one patient with Crigler-Najjar syndrome has been without ill effect on growth, development, intelligence quotient, or circadian rhythm.[551,680]

The bronze baby syndrome may occur in premature infants with *conjugated* hyperbilirubinemia treated with phototherapy.[593,693,885] Hemolysis and a gray-brown discoloration of the skin, serum, and urine are present, presumably as a result of retention of photooxidation products; this may reflect the effect of light on porphyrins.[885]

Phototherapy has also been used successfully in most of the unconjugated hyperbilirubinemic conditions described previously. In hyperbilirubinemia due to hemolytic disease, especially ABO incompatibility, phototherapy reduces but does not eliminate the need for exchange transfusions.[546,951] Perhaps the greatest controversy surrounds the use of prophylactic phototherapy in premature infants. Prophylactic treatment would result in 95% of infants being treated unnecessarily if 15 mg/dL is accepted as a critical level for kernicterus.[400] This approach is not recommended until further clinical experience confirms the apparent lack of toxicity. Increase in nursery illumination to 90 foot-candles at the infant's skin, which significantly reduces bilirubin levels in the premature infant and facilitates clinical observation, had been strongly recommended; however, this issue also needs to be clarified in view of the reported deleterious effect of environmental light.

Phenobarbital

Under various circumstances, phenobarbital is capable of inducing microsomal enzymes and hepatic transport, thereby increasing bilirubin uptake, conjugation to glucuronide by the microsomal enzyme cascade, and secretion into bile canaliculus.[44,197,221,763,865,1137] Phenobarbital has also been shown to decrease the efflux of bilirubin as a result of an increase in intracellular binding protein.[1131] Prospective controlled studies have shown phenobarbital to be effective in lowering serum bilirubin levels in neonates.[987,1052,1061,1079,1142] When barbiturates are administered to infants prophylactically from birth, serum bilirubin levels fall within 48 hours; if administered after jaundice has occurred, serum bilirubin levels require 4 to 5 days to fall. If given to the mother for 14 days before delivery, a decrease in cord bilirubin levels can be demonstrated.[681,1061] Phenobarbital administration results in a three-fold increase of glucuronyl transferase activity and decreases peak bilirubin concentration during the first 3 days of life in normal full-term neonates; it is less effective in premature infants.[191,384]

Potential undesirable barbiturate effects include accelerated drug (or vitamin D) metabolism, with loss of drug effectiveness; altered steroid metabolism, with a consequent potential effect on growth (including brain growth) and development; and depressed vitamin K–dependent clotting factors if administered to the mother.[294,1120] Furthermore, early-labeled pigment production may be increased because of increased hepatic heme synthesis.[1038] In female rats treated with phenobarbital, diminished litter size and increased neonatal mortality have been reported.[440] In human infants, a decreased sucking response and respiratory depression may occur.[1120] The availability of phototherapy in the United States has obviated routine phenobarbital prophylaxis. Controlled trials comparing agar feeding, intermittent phototherapy, continuous phototherapy, and phenobarbital administration have shown that continuous phototherapy is the most effective method in lowering serum bilirubin levels in premature infants and that phenobarbital is not additive.[48,680,681,1061]

In geographic areas with less access to intensive newborn care facilities and a high incidence of idiopathic hyperbilirubinemia or G6PD deficiency,[1142] prophylaxis both for mother and infant may be of public health value.

Blockage of Heme Conversion to Bilirubin

The therapeutic modalities used to date for infants with unconjugated hyperbilirubinemia have been directed at enhancing the metabolic disposition of bilirubin; a more effective strategy might be to prevent bilirubin formation.[688,787] Drummond and Kappas[312,313,314] used the principle of competitive enzyme inhibition of heme oxygenase to block the degradation of heme. Administration of a synthetic metalloporphyrin, tin-protoporphyrin (which has a high affinity for the catalytic site on heme oxygenase), inhibited the enzyme, reduced bilirubin levels, and increased the biliary excretion of unmetabolized heme.[549,945] A reduction in serum bilirubin levels was noted in clinical trials of this synthetic protoporphyrin in humans.[109,547,548,884,991] However, dermal and ocular photosensitivity, undesirable side effects of tin-protoporphyrin administration, limit the application of this therapeutic modality.[311,608] Acceptable options include the use of analogues with a lower potential for phototoxicity[274,311,1088,1089] or the development of alternative strategies, such as increasing the efficacy of heme oxygenase inhibition by encapsulation into liposomes.[609]

Prolonged Conjugated Hyperbilirubinemia (Neonatal Cholestasis)

Prolonged conjugated hyperbilirubinemia, or neonatal cholestasis, may be the initial manifestation of a heterogenous group of diseases[62,66] (Table 41-5); this creates a challenge in the evaluation and management of affected infants. Although

TABLE 41-5 *Classification of Disorders Associated With Neonatal Cholestasis*

Cholestasis Associated With Infection
Bacterial Infection
Generalized bacterial sepsis
Syphilis
Toxoplasmosis
Tuberculosis
Listeriosis
Congenital Viral Infection
Cytomegalovirus
Herpesvirus
Rubella virus
Coxsackievirus
Echovirus
Hepatitis B virus (? hepatitis C and other non-A, non-B viruses)
Human immunodeficiency virus
Parvovirus B19

Metabolic Disorders
Metabolic Diseases in Which the Defect Is Uncharacterized
α_1-Antitrypsin deficiency
Cystic fibrosis
Familial erythrophagocytic lymphohistiocytosis
Endocrine disorders
   Idiopathic hypopituitarism
   Hypothyroidism
Neonatal iron storage disease (perinatal hemochromatosis)
Infantile copper overload
Multiple acyl-CoA dehydrogenation deficiency (glutaric aciduria type II)[138]
Disorders of Bile Acid Synthesis and Metabolism
Primary enzyme deficiencies
   3β-Hydroxysteroid Δ^5-C_{27} steroid dehydrogenase isomerase[215]
   Δ4-3-oxosteroid 5β-reductase[928]
Secondary (peroxisomal disorders)
   Zellweger's syndrome (cerebrohepatorenal syndrome)
   Specific peroxisomal enzymopathies
Disorders of Carbohydrate Metabolism
Galactosemia
Fructosemia
Glycogen storage disease type IV
Disorders of Amino Acid Metabolism
Tyrosinemia
Hypermethioninemia
Disorders of Lipid Metabolism
Wolman's disease
Cholesterol ester storage disease
Niemann-Pick disease
Gaucher's disease

Toxic or Drug Related
Cholestasis associated with total parenteral nutrition
Sepsis with possible endotoxemia (urinary tract infection, gastroenteritis)
Chloral hydrate[607]

Genetic or Chromosomal
Trisomy E
Down's syndrome
Donahue's syndrome (leprechaunism)

Anatomic
Infantile polycystic disease or congenital hepatic fibrosis
Caroli's disease (cystic dilatation of intrahepatic ducts)

continued

TABLE 41-5 *(continued)*

Miscellaneous
Histiocytosis X
Shock or hypoperfusion
Intestinal obstruction
Polysplenia syndrome (with extrahepatic biliary atresia)
Neonatal lupus erythematosus[621]
Dubin-Johnson syndrome[937]
Arthrogryposis, cholestatic pigmentary disease, renal dysfunction syndrome[754]

Extrahepatic (Anatomic) Disorders
Choledochal cyst
Spontaneous bile duct perforation
Obstruction associated with cholelithiasis, bile or mucous plug, or mass or neoplasia
Neonatal sclerosing cholangitis[952]
Bile duct stenosis
Anomalous choledochopancreaticoductal junction
Biliary atresia or agenesis*

Idiopathic Obstructive Cholangiopathies
Extrahepatic biliary atresia*
Idiopathic neonatal hepatitis

Intrahepatic Cholestasis
Persistent
    With intrahepatic bile duct paucity
        Arteriohepatic dysplasia (Alagille's syndrome)
        Nonsyndromic paucity
    Progressive familial intrahepatic cholestasis
        Byler's disease
        Nielsen's syndrome (Greenland Eskimo)
        Microfilament dysfunction (North American Indian)
    Benign familial chronic intrahepatic cholestasis[338]
Recurrent
    Familial benign *recurrent* cholestasis
    Hereditary cholestasis with lymphedema (Aagenaes)[1,2]

*There may be various types of biliary atresia: biliary atresia or agenesis may represent a congenital *malformation*, whereas extrahepatic biliary atresia may represent an idiopathic postnatal *obliterative* cholangiopathy. (Modified from Balistreri WF. Neonatal cholestasis: lessons from the past, issues for the future. [Foreword] Semin Liver Dis 7, 1987; and Balistreri WF. Interrelationship between the infantile cholangiopathies and paucity of the intrahepatic bile ducts. In: Balistreri WF, Stocker JT, eds. Pediatric hepatology. Washington, DC, Hemisphere, 1990, pp 1–18)

the list of potential causes of cholestasis in the neonatal period is extensive and diverse, the relative frequency of *idiopathic neonatal hepatitis* and *extrahepatic biliary atresia* far exceeds that of any other entity. These two disorders account for about 60% to 70% of all cases of neonatal cholestasis (Table 41-6).

Neonatal jaundice associated with elevated serum levels of conjugated bilirubin is never physiologic and almost always signifies disease of the liver or biliary tract. Exceptions are certain rare diseases, such as Dubin-Johnson or Rotor's syndrome, which may represent pure defects in bilirubin excretion.[110]

The neonate presenting with cholestasis offers an interesting exercise in differential diagnosis. Neonatal cholestasis can be the result of infectious, metabolic, toxic, genetic, anatomic, or undefined abnormalities that result in either mechanical obstruction to bile flow or functional impairment of any of the myriad processes involved in hepatic excretory

function and bile secretion. An example of mechanical obstruction is obliterative cholangiopathy of the common bile duct, as is seen in the prototypic abnormality, extrahepatic biliary atresia. An example of a functional impairment is an inborn error of bile acid metabolism associated with significant hepatic disease. Functional impairment of bile secretion can also result from generalized damage to liver cells or injury to a specific organelle involved in the bile secretory process. Our conceptual approach is to divide neonates with cholestasis into those with primary extrahepatic disease and those with primary intrahepatic disease (Fig. 41-2). Within this framework, there are multiple areas of potential overlap (clinical, histologic, biochemical).

It is critical that a diagnosis be made promptly, so that patients with infectious causes are rapidly managed, those with metabolic or genetic diseases are appropriately counseled and treated, and those with surgical lesions are expeditiously operated. This chapter first reviews the known causes of cholestasis and then presents an overview of the idiopathic infantile obstructive cholangiopathies, namely, extrahepatic biliary atresia and idiopathic neonatal hepatitis.

INTRAHEPATIC DISEASE

Cholestasis Associated With Infection
Bacterial Sepsis. Bacterial infection is a frequent cause of an increase in conjugated bilirubin; in one series, 23 of 104 infants had sepsis as the cause of jaundice.[266] *E coli* has been the most common organism reported.[37,266] The mechanism of production of cholestasis may be endotoxin-mediated canalicular dysfunction.[1059,1147] Other gram-negative rods and, less often, staphylococci and streptococci have been associated.[114,447,838] Histologic studies of autopsy material have shown bile stasis and liver cell necrosis as the most striking findings.[114,447] The association of jaundice with bacterial infection in infants who are not clinically ill is emphasized by a report of 22 infants with positive blood or urine cultures, 9 of whom were active and well, with hyperbilirubinemia as the only finding.[871] Urinary tract infection with bacteremia has been emphasized in several series as a cause of neonatal jaundice, especially in male infants.[49,449,755,922,1023] In these patients, there were no associated genitourinary tract anomalies, and the disease occurred in clusters or epidemics. Thus, urine culture and sediment examination, along with blood, nasopharyngeal, stool, and cerebrospinal fluid cultures, should be obtained routinely to evaluate infection as a cause of neonatal jaundice. This will allow immediate initiation of antibiotic therapy in an infant suspected to have sepsis.

Syphilis. The recent increase in the incidence of congenital syphilis reemphasizes that this treatable disorder should be considered in the differential diagnosis of neonatal cholestasis.[306] As part of the multisystem syphilitic disease, which includes the characteristic diffuse rash, fever, anemia, and aseptic meningitis, hepatomegaly with increased aminotransferase and alkaline phosphatase levels may be noted. Syphilitic hepatitis is associated with enlargement of the liver and spleen, similar to other intrauterine infections, such as toxoplasmosis and cytomegalovirus (CMV) infection. Small granulomatous lesions, diffuse chronic inflammatory cell infiltration, and widespread portal fibrosis may be observed in biopsy samples. Paucity of the intrahepatic bile ducts has also been reported.[1013]

TABLE 41-6 *Relative Frequency of the Various Clinical Forms of Neonatal Cholestasis**

Clinical Form	Cumulative Percentage	Estimated Frequency (per 10,000 Live Births)
Idiopathic neonatal hepatitis	35–40	1.25
Extrahepatic biliary atresia	25–30	0.70
α_1-Antitrypsin deficiency	7–10	0.25
Intrahepatic cholestasis (with or without paucity)	5–6	0.14
Bacterial sepsis	2	<0.1
Cytomegalovirus hepatitis	3–5	<0.1
Rubella, herpes hepatitis	1	<0.1
Endocrine disorders (hypothyroidism, panhypopituitarism)	1	<0.1
Galactosemia	1	<0.1

*Based on more than 500 cases.
(Modified from Balistreri WF. Neonatal cholestasis: lessons from the past, issues for the future. [Foreword] Semin Liver Dis 7, 1987; and Balistreri WF. Neonatal cholestasis: medical progress. J Pediatr 106:171, 1985)

Assessment of the cord blood serology, which is obligatory in every infant, usually allows prompt diagnosis; placental morphology may be abnormal.[27] An infant with unexplained jaundice should have suitable serologic tests for syphilis repeated regardless of the cord blood result. If positive, prompt treatment should be instituted before the classic picture of congenital syphilis develops.

Toxoplasmosis. When infection with *Toxoplasma gondii* occurs during pregnancy, the parasite may cause severe congenital toxoplasmosis.[259]

Forty percent of infants with other clinical manifestations of congenital toxoplasmosis have conjugated hyperbilirubinemia, and 60% have hepatomegaly.[186,283] The severe classic illness, with hydrocephalus, chorioretinitis, and intracranial calcification, may not be present; the infant may appear normal at birth and develop hepatosplenomegaly and jaundice later.[240,442,707] Rarely, severe hemolysis is present and produces an erythroblastosis-like illness. Serum aminotransferase levels are elevated, and progressive liver dysfunction with ascites may occur. Parasites are almost never demonstrated in the liver; extramedullary hematopoiesis, hemosiderosis, canalicular bile stasis, and a scattered periportal mononuclear cell reaction are present.[186,240,707] Multinucleated giant cells may be detected.[66,163] Diagnosis may be made by demonstration of the organism in Wright-stained smears

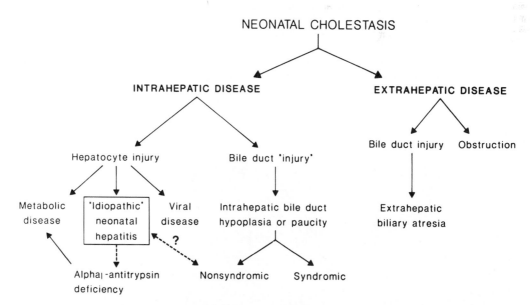

FIGURE 41-2 Conceptual scheme of the various forms of neonatal cholestasis. Most cases are classified as either extrahepatic biliary atresia or idiopathic neonatal hepatitis. The latter may include early *nonsyndromic* forms of intrahepatic cholestasis. Certain disorders (α-antitrypsin deficiency and inborn errors of bile acid metabolism), formerly included in the idiopathic category, have been delineated as specific metabolic disorders, decreasing the idiopathic category.

of spinal fluid sediment.[354] Demonstration of high-titer immunoglobulin M (IgM)-specific antibody in the infant may be helpful. The IgM fluorescent antibody test may be useful, although false-negative results have been reported, and an absence of IgM antibody does not rule out the diagnosis.[854] Serologic studies of both mother and child using the Sabin-Feldman dye test show high titers (1:1024) in the presence of active infection. If positive, the tests should be repeated at 3 to 4 months of age; persistence of elevated titers in both mother and child confirms the infection.[354]

T gondii organisms are present in the placenta of infected infants; therefore, study of this organ may be highly productive and lead to early positive morphologic diagnosis.[26,95] Treatment with a combination of sulfadiazine and pyrimethamine given with leucovorin and fresh bakers' yeast for 1 month may prevent further progression of tissue damage. Spiramycin has also been used, but a consistent benefit of treatment has not been proved. Prevention should be directed toward avoidance of ingestion of infective cysts and contact with sporulated oocysts.

Congenital Viral Infection

Herpes virus (CMV, herpes simplex virus [HSV], human herpes virus type 6 [HHV-6],[50,1025] and varicella zoster virus) may infect a pregnant woman and be transmitted to the fetus or newborn; the resultant infection may be asymptomatic or may be associated with severe acute symptoms. The potential for permanent sequelae, such as developmental impairment, is high.[977,978] The implications of the diagnosis of congenital infection are significant, therefore rapid recognition is important—this will allow appropriate therapeutic and preventive measures to be instituted.

Cytomegalovirus. CMV causes a spectrum of liver diseases in infants and in older children.[452,453,685,977,978] In view of the ubiquitous nature of CMV, the tendencies of latency, and the ability to be reactivated with stress, it is difficult to implicate this agent in the cause of neonatal cholestasis.

The overall prevalence of CMV infection is high—50% to 85%, depending on socioeconomic background. One in every 50 to 500 live births is infected; 10% are symptomatic at birth.[124,452,983,1105] Severely affected infants may present a classic syndrome shortly after birth, with jaundice (conjugated bilirubin elevation), hemolytic anemia, thrombocytopenic purpura, hepatosplenomegaly, and microcephaly uniformly present. This group has a high (20% to 30%) mortality rate, and more than 90% of the survivors have late complications (eg, hearing loss, mental retardation).[1106] Chorioretinitis and periventricular calcification are present in about one third of affected infants.[1106] Of the 90% who are asymptomatic at birth, 5% to 15% are at risk for late sequelae, especially sensorineural hearing loss. This may be related to continuous viral replication.

Affected infants may also present with the neonatal hepatitis syndrome of prolonged jaundice and hepatomegaly.[226,453,685,977,978,985,1106,1139] Prospective studies have demonstrated hepatomegaly without alteration of liver function tests.[124,977,978] The liver histology is also variable; there may be focal portal inflammatory infiltration with round cells and neutrophils and focal necrosis of hepatocytes with bile stasis and no giant cell formation or extensive giant cell transformation indistinguishable. Extramedullary hematopoiesis is uniformly noted. Significant portal or interstitial fibrosis may be present[372,685]; however, these changes are reversible, and follow-up studies have demonstrated normal liver size and function or mild residual portal fibrosis.[107,685] Characteristic swollen cells with intranuclear inclusions may be scanty, even in liver specimens from which the virus is cultured. Inclusions are found in bile duct epithelium but rarely in hepatocytes[59,685,985] (Fig. 41-3). Bile ductule obstruction may occur during CMV infection.[329,434] A possible relation of the biliary epithelial changes to extrahepatic biliary atresia has been suggested by the histologic findings in one case.[781] Obliterative cholangitis due to CMV has been postulated as a precursor of paucity of the intrahepatic bile ducts.[362] Electron microscopy of the liver in CMV infection shows degenerative changes of bile canaliculi with dilation and loss of microvilli as well as bile pigment in hepatocytes.[59,1119] The frequency of neonatal infection with CMV and the resemblance to idiopathic neonatal hepatitis have suggested that CMV is a major cause of idiopathic obstructive cholangiopathy (discussed later).[452,453,1106] Attempts to isolate the virus from large groups of infants with idiopathic neonatal hepatitis and biliary atresia, without any other manifestation of congenital infection, have not been productive.[632,985]

The diagnosis may be made by culture of fresh urine for virus since viruria persists for many months after birth.[452,685,1105,1106] The fluorescent antibody test for CMV-specific IgM antibody is rapid and sensitive and is positive in diseased infants and negative in the asymptomatic excretor.

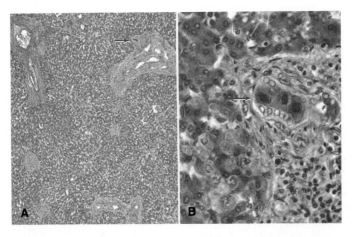

FIGURE 41-3 Cytomegalovirus infection (cytomegalic inclusion disease) in a premature infant who died at 5 days of age. (**A**) Extensive inflammatory exudate in all portal areas. (**B**) High-power view of area shows three enlarged bile duct epithelial cells with characteristic large intranuclear inclusions (*arrows*).

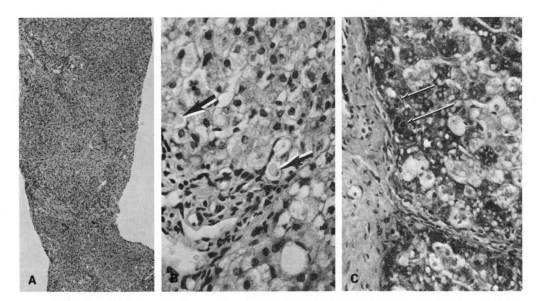

FIGURE 41-4 α_1-Antitrypsin deficiency. (**A**) Biopsy at age 1 year shows early cirrhosis (low power). (**B**) Spherical eosinophilic hyaline bodies resembling erythrocytes, but larger and not biconcave, are visible in periportal hepatocytes at higher power (*arrow*). (**C**) Periodic acid–Schiff stain shows positive staining, diastase-resistant globules adjacent to portal connective tissue.

are over 40 years of age; further detailed evaluation of this concept is needed.

Hepatic Pathology. Similar to the variable clinical manifestations, heterogenous patterns of liver injury may be noted. Lesions noted in the homozygous deficient neonate include (1) hepatocellular damage, giant cell transformation, minimal inflammation, and bile stasis; (2) portal fibrosis with bile duct proliferation; and (3) ductular hypoplasia (paucity).[437]

Hepatocyte inclusions can be seen on routine hematoxylin and eosin sections, where they appear as round to oval, slightly eosinophilic, hyaline-like globules (1 to 40 µm in diameter), localized predominantly to periportal hepatocytes (Fig. 41-4). Periodic acid–Schiff (PAS) stain, followed by diastase treatment, highlights these glycoprotein-rich inclusions. Bile duct inclusions may also be noted in α_1-AT–deficient patients with liver disease.[1149] Inclusions vary in size with both zygosity and age of the affected person; therefore, they may be difficult to identify in liver tissue from heterozygotes and from infants.[65] Composition of the hepatic inclusions has been demonstrated by immunochemistry to be α_1-AT immunoreactive material.

Immunohistochemistry remains a reliable method for identification and confirmation of the deficiency state. The ultrastructure of the liver inclusions is characteristic, namely, membrane-bound masses of electron-dense material (Fig. 41-5). Electron microscopy has demonstrated the presence of amorphous material localized within markedly dilated rough endoplasmic reticulum saccules in the liver in both homozygous (PiZZ) and heterozygous (PiMZ) deficient subjects without liver disease, some of whom were normal and some of whom had emphysema.[641,934] In heterozygous people, there are no specific ultrastructural changes; however, in homozygotes, an association of cell death in periportal cells with dilatation of the endoplasmic reticulum by accumulated α_1-AT was noted.[507]

The histologic evolution of the early lesions has been well documented; there may be complete histologic resolution, persisting liver disease, or the development of cirrhosis.[823,933,1027]

Diagnosis. The diagnosis of α_1-AT deficiency is best made by determination of the α_1-AT phenotype (isoelectric focusing on agarose electrophoresis at acid pH) and confirmed by liver biopsy. The level of α_1-AT measured immunochemically may be deceptive, especially in premature infants, in whom low levels may be found despite the normal PiMM genotype, and in heterozygous (PiMZ) patients, in

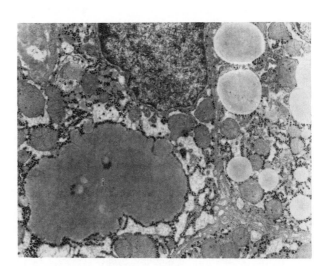

FIGURE 41-5 Ultrastructural findings in the liver of a patient with *homozygous α_1-antitrypsin deficiency* include large electron-dense, membrane-bound, amorphous inclusions (i), along with a mild degree of fat accumulation.

whom a rise of 60% to 80% may occur with inflammation, estrogen therapy, or pregnancy. Precise detection of specific α_1-AT variants can be carried out using the polymerase chain reaction to amplify genomic DNA or by monoclonal antibody.[157,279]

Proper study of the family thus requires determination of Pi phenotypes.[339,346] The estimated frequency of these conditions (PiMZ, 3% of the population; PiZZ, 0.07%) dictates that all children with liver disease be evaluated for α_1-AT deficiency.[65,346] Family screening and genetic counseling of affected patients can then be carried out.

Pathogenesis. Altered biosynthesis of the α_1-AT protein leads to production of an abnormal (misfolded) α_1-AT molecule, which in turn interferes with excretion of the protein from endoplasmic reticulum to the Golgi apparatus. Altered transport of the mutant α_1-AT molecules encoded by the Z allele has been demonstrated in other cells (monocytes and macrophages) from PiZZ subjects.[728,807] After injection with liver mRNA from PiMM and PiZZ subjects, *Xenopus* oocytes synthesize α_1-AT; the M protein is secreted, but the Z protein remains in the cell.[370,807,1078] Relentless accumulation of α_1-AT in the endoplasmic reticulum ensues, and serum protease inhibitor levels are low.

The association between low serum levels of α_1-AT, intrahepatic accumulation of the protein, and either pulmonary or hepatic disease is not completely understood[641,823]; however, recent studies of the molecular and cellular biology of α_1-AT have provided insight.[806] An inability to neutralize proteolytic enzymes (eg, elastase) released by leukocytes or bacteria in response to environmental challenge has been suggested as a mechanism for pulmonary disease.[339,616] Therefore, infusion of α_1-AT has been suggested in the therapy of α_1-AT deficiency–associated pulmonary disease. The cause (and treatment) of liver disease is less certain. The fact that liver involvement is not universal, occurring in 5% to 20% of homozygote-deficient subjects, has led to the suggestion of coexistent factors unique to this neonatal age group, environmental factors, or a functional defect of the Z-type α_1-AT.[773] Three theories have been proposed to account for hepatic injury in people with α_1-AT deficiency (PiZZ)—the decreased protease inhibitor theory, the immune-mediated injury theory, and the accumulation theory.

Decreased protease inhibition, or uptake of intact proteins from the gut into the systemic circulation, occurs frequently in newborns. Udall and coworkers[1055] have shown that luminal enzymes (proteases) are absorbed intact from the neonatal gut into the systemic circulation; in the absence of circulating protease inhibitors, as in α_1-AT–deficient patients, hepatic inflammation and fibrosis can be initiated. This theory was used to account for the fact that breastfeeding seemed to offer some protection against severe liver disease and early death in infants with α_1-AT deficiency. Udall and colleagues reasoned that antiproteases present in breast milk complex with luminal proteases to neutralize their activity and thereby offer a protective effect. They next identified infants with α_1-AT deficiency and investigated their early feeding histories.[1055] Severe liver disease was present in 40% of bottle-fed infants and in 8% of breastfed infants. This pattern was also noted in the population studied by Sveger[1018]; 26% of the infants breastfed for less than 1 month had clinical signs of liver disease, and 11% of the 71 infants breastfed for more than 1 month had liver disease. Early feeding practices may

therefore offer a confounding variable in the genesis of liver disease.[65] Deficiency of α_1-AT alone, however, is not sufficient to cause liver disease; subjects with the null–null phenotype (no circulating α_1-AT) do not have liver disease.[255,806]

Immune-mediated injury, or cytotoxic injury to hepatocytes related to an abnormal immune response to liver antigens, may initiate hepatic injury. It has been postulated that an immunoregulatory gene may influence the clinical outcome in PiZZ patients. Recent studies have noted an association of α_1-AT deficiency and liver disease with the uncommon HLA phenotype DR3-Dw25.[302] No conclusive pathogenetic link, however, has been made to an abnormal immune response. There is no difference in class II major histocompatibility complex antigen expression in the liver of α_1-AT deficient patients with liver disease.[650]

The *accumulation theory* holds that liver disease in α_1-AT–deficient patients is restricted to those alleles in which intrahepatocytic accumulation of nascent protein occurs.[256] Experiments conducted using transgenic mice, which carry the mutant Z allele of the human α_1-AT gene, have bolstered the theory that liver injury is a consequence of the intracellular accumulation of the mutant PiZZ α_1-AT molecule.[192,194,320,806] In this model, intracellular accumulation of the altered α_1-AT gene product occurred, globules appeared, a histologic pattern of neonatal hepatitis developed, and growth failure ensued.[320] Because serum levels of α_1-AT were normal, the liver injury was ascribed to the presence of the accumulated protein; in fact, the degree of liver damage correlated with the amount of accumulated PiZ α_1-AT in the liver. Perlmutter[808] has postulated that the alteration in folding of the mutant (Z) α_1-AT molecule permits an interaction (eg, with heat shock/stress proteins) that is responsible for specific retention of α_1-AT in the endoplasmic reticulum. In fact, the synthesis of stress proteins can be activated by the presence of misfolded proteins. This conceptual model requires the addition of a genetic or environmental factor to exacerbate the accumulation or to decrease the degradation of α_1-AT.[806] This theory was strengthened by the finding of an increased net synthesis of proteins in the heat shock/stress gene family only in the subset of PiZZ patients with liver disease.[808]

Treatment. No specific therapy has been found successful for the consequences of liver disease associated with α_1-AT deficiency. Breastfeeding of an affected neonate is advocated, but supplementation with vitamin K is recommended until all biochemical evidence of cholestasis has resolved. If the accumulation theory is correct, then replacement of the deficient protein by infusion of purified plasma α_1-AT could be injurious; the complex of α_1-AT and elastase might actually stimulate α_1-AT synthesis.[806] Liver transplantation has been performed and has been curative. Conversion of the α_1-AT phenotype to that of the donor occurs.[488,837,1070] In our series, liver transplantation has been performed in 10 patients with α_1-AT–associated cirrhosis; all are currently alive and well.[10,65] Somatic gene therapy is a theoretic possibility[255]; however, more precise understanding of the defect and the intracellular events that occur in α_1-AT deficiency must be a prelude to application of this strategy.[150]

Prenatal diagnosis of α_1-AT deficiency by direct analysis of the mutation site in the gene using specific oligonucleotide probes for the various alleles and direct analysis of fetal DNA is possible.[65,241,472,576,828] There is little to justify intervention, however, since no methodology available predicts which people with PiZZ will develop liver disease. Similarly, widespread screening for α_1-AT deficiency, in the absence of an effective intervention for liver disease, is not recommended since identification could produce a considerable adverse psychological effect.[691]

Other Endoplasmic Reticulum Storage Diseases

α_1-Antitrypsin deficiency is a prototype for other genetically determined endoplasmic reticulum storage diseases. In each of these disorders, a defect in the export of a secretory protein results in hepatocyte storage and plasma deficiency. Lindmark and colleagues[648] described chronic liver disease in a patient with selective and exclusive hepatocyte endoplasmic reticulum storage of α_1-antichymotrypsin in the form of granules; these features suggested the presence of an export block similar to that seen in PiZZ α_1-AT deficiency. Similarly, in patients with hereditary hypofibrinogenemia, there is hepatic storage of fibrinogen, with the development of cirrhosis.[187]

Cystic Fibrosis

As the life expectancy for patients with cystic fibrosis (CF) is extended, the incidence of recognized hepatobiliary complications increases.[782,790,834,883,1036,1064] As we gain an increased understanding of the basic defect in CF,[870] early diagnosis and novel therapy may be possible.

TABLE 41-9 *Hepatobiliary Diseases Reported in Patients With Cystic Fibrosis*

Specific to Cystic Fibrosis
Hepatic
Focal biliary cirrhosis with inspissation
Multilobular cirrhosis with inspissation
Biliary
Microgallbladder
Mucous hyperplasia of gallbladder
Mucocele

Secondary to Extrahepatic Disease
Lesions Associated With Cardiopulmonary Disease
Centrilobular necrosis
Cirrhosis
Lesions Associated With Pancreatic Disease
Pancreatic duct sludge (obstruction)
Pancreatic fibrosis (leading to bile duct compression or stricture)

Lesions That Occur With Higher Frequency in Patients With Cystic Fibrosis
Hepatic
Fatty liver
Neonatal cholestasis
Drug hepatotoxicity
Endotoxemia
Viral hepatitis[856]
Biliary
Biliary sludge
Cholelithiasis
Sclerosing cholangitis
Cholangiocarcinoma

(Modified from Balistreri WF. Spectrum of liver disease in patients with cystic fibrosis. Pediatr Pulmonol S5:71–73, 1990)

Incidence of Hepatobiliary Lesions. In her initial description in 1938 of postmortem findings of 49 patients with "cystic fibrosis of the pancreas," D.H. Andersen[36] noted a fatty liver in 39%, biliary cirrhosis in 6%, and a small atretic gallbladder in 16% of patients; several had "slight" portal fibrosis. Bile duct obstruction by inspissated eosinophilic material was reported in 1944 by Farber,[347] and focal biliary cirrhosis (FBC) was reported in 1952 by Bodian[134] in patients with CF. FBC was found in 25% of 62 patients at autopsy; Bodian described eosinophilic material obstructing dilated intrahepatic bile ducts surrounded by fibrous tissue in a nonuniform and focal distribution.[134] In 1956, Di Sant'Agnese and Blanc[299] described multilobular biliary cirrhosis (MBC) in 22% of CF patients at autopsy.

The incidence of these specific lesions and of other lesions, which are secondary to cardiopulmonary or pancreatic disease or occur with higher frequency in patients with CF, has been reported in subsequent series[67,790,883] (Table 41-9).

LESIONS SPECIFIC TO CYSTIC FIBROSIS. FBC may be asymptomatic and associated with normal liver function studies, but however it appears to be a progressive liver disease (Fig. 41-6). The pathogenesis has been ascribed to the accumulation (inspissation) of amorphous eosinophilic material in the intrahepatic ducts; this material blocks the duct, causing a chronic inflammatory infiltrate, bile duct proliferation, and fibrosis with extension and coalescence, culminating in FBC. It is likely that the pathogenesis is complex and that multiple interrelated factors are operant (Table 41-10). The incidence of FBC is poorly defined since there is no simple or reliable method for detection. FBC was found in 10% of infants who died before reaching 3 months of age.[782]

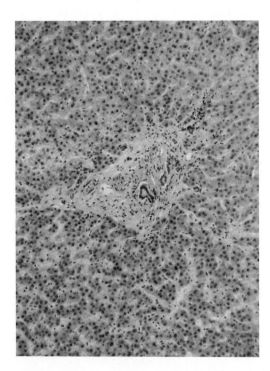

FIGURE 41-6 Biopsy specimen of a patient with cystic fibrosis demonstrates changes typical of focal biliary cirrhosis.

TABLE 41-10 *Factors Involved in the Pathogenesis of Hepatobiliary Diseases in Cystic Fibrosis*

Bile Duct Obstruction
Abnormal viscous secretions
  Mucous plugs
  Sludge
Lithogenic bile (due to bile acid malabsorption)
Stones (extrahepatic, intrahepatic)
Stenosis of common bile duct
Meconium ileus (?)

Nonhepatic Disease
Hypoperfusion or hypoxemia
Cor pulmonale
Pancreatic fibrosis

Nutritional Deficiencies
Taurine
Essential fatty acids
Vitamin E (oxidant imbalance)

Hepatotoxicity
Bile acids
Drugs
  Antibiotics (eg, carbenicillin, erythromycin)
  N-acetylcysteine

Immune Mechanisms (Sensitization)

(Modified from Balistreri WF. Spectrum of liver disease in patients with cystic fibrosis. Pediatr Pulmonol S5:71–73, 1990)

MBC (Fig. 41-7) may present as hepatomegaly, splenomegaly, variceal bleeding or pain due to perisplenitis or to abdominal distention.[299,1054] The pathogenesis of MBC seems to be related to an extension of the factors that cause FBC, with development of multilobular cirrhosis. The true incidence is similarly undefined.

LESIONS SECONDARY TO EXTRAHEPATIC DISEASE. Common bile duct stenosis, secondary to intrapancreatic strictures, has been postulated as a causative factor in the development of biliary cirrhosis in patients with CF.[385] With relief of the obstruction, clinical symptoms were relieved and hepatobiliary scans normalized. The incidence of extrahepatic strictures in patients with CF is not known; this deserves further study.[122,744,798]

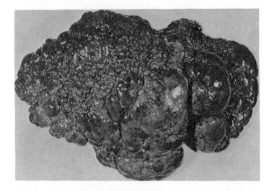

FIGURE 41-7 Autopsy of a patient with cystic fibrosis showing severe multinodular biliary cirrhosis.

LESIONS THAT OCCUR WITH HIGHER FREQUENCY IN CYSTIC FIBROSIS PATIENTS. *Fatty liver* is frequently reported in patients with CF; in published series, the extent is highly variable, and there are no reliable clinical or biochemical harbingers. Although there is no apparent correlation with age, the incidence seems to decrease with improved nutrition. The cause of steatosis is most likely multifactorial and possibly related to (1) poor nutritional status of the patient, with decreased hepatic secretion of triglyceride as very-low-density lipoprotein (VLDL) due to decreased apolipoprotein synthesis; (2) the existence of a specific deficiency, such as carnitine,[1049] essential fatty acids, or choline; or (3) toxin-induction of steatosis. The relation of fatty liver to other hepatic lesions in CF is not known.

Neonatal cholestasis is present in up to 30% of patients with CF.[790,883] The biopsy specimen resembles either neonatal hepatitis (presence of giant cells) or extrahepatic biliary atresia (bile plugs and bile duct proliferation). Paucity of interlobular bile ducts has also been reported.[376] The incidence of neonatal cholestasis in patients with CF increases several-fold in the presence of meconium ileus.[679] In a series of 74 patients with CF, 4 presented as neonatal hepatitis; conjugated bilirubin levels were elevated, and jaundice persisted from 20 days to 6 months.[834] Meconium ileus was present in half of infants presenting with cholestasis; this is about five times the incidence expected in patients with CF. Other series also have emphasized the high rate of neonatal cholestasis in association with meconium ileus and bowel obstruction.[883,1064] In certain cases, accumulation of thick, viscid bile was noted at laparotomy and was thought to have caused extrahepatic obstruction[1064]; flushing of the obstructed extrahepatic ducts was reported to be beneficial in two cases.

Sclerosing cholangitis, with typical cholangiographic findings, has been described in patients with CF.[102,999] It is unclear whether this lesion is secondary to choledocholithiasis or suppurative cholangitis or whether sclerosing cholangitis constitutes part of the CF–liver disease syndrome.

Gallbladder abnormalities have been noted in 20% of children with CF who are under 5 years of age and in up to 60% of older patients (5 to 15 years of age). Microgallbladder is found in 15% to 20% of CF patients. Cholesterol gallstones are a frequent finding; most are asymptomatic, but calculous cholecystitis may occur. Cholesterol supersaturation of bile may be related to (1) interruption of the enterohepatic circulation due to bile acid loss in feces; (2) alteration in cholesterol secretion into bile, with an uncoupling from bile acid output; or (3) the presence of mucin, which serves as a nucleation factor. Ultrasonography is a useful monitor of biliary tract disease in patients with CF.

Evaluation.   Because the abnormalities are insidious and the patient is often asymptomatic, it is difficult to screen for or monitor liver disease in patients with CF. In addition, liver function abnormalities are intermittent, and the histologic lesions may be heterogeneous, leading to biopsy sampling error.[67,353,790,883,911] Many evaluation methods have been used,[67] including (1) clinical examination to determine hepatosplenomegaly, (2) assessment of damage using standard enzymatic determinations, (3) specific function tests gauging synthetic activity, metabolic activity, or clearance (bile acids), and (4) analysis of hepatic structure using ultrasound and imaging.

Therapy. Intervention for variceal bleeding, using sclerotherapy or shunts, has been extensively used for patients with CF and cirrhosis. Surgical dilation of intrapancreatic biliary strictures was associated with a relief of pain.[385] Reports have been made of the successful use of orthotopic liver transplantation in CF patients with end-stage liver disease[243,1114]; this deserves further exploration.

The presumed underlying pathogenesis focuses on abnormal hyperviscid secretions with bile stasis; this suggests a rationale for therapy, namely to attempt to decrease the viscosity of bile or to replace or displace hepatotoxic bile acids. Ursodeoxycholic acid, a nontoxic, choleretic bile acid, has shown promise in preliminary studies of patients with CF-associated liver disease.[227,238,246,834] In these studies, ursodeoxycholic acid therapy was associated with an improvement in biochemical parameters and nutritional status. This drug deserves further study. The role of supplemental taurine in ameliorating gastrointestinal complications in CF must be similarly investigated.[883]

Familial Erythrophagocytic Lymphohistiocytosis

Familial erythrophagocytic lymphohistiocytosis is an autosomal recessive disease characterized by lever hepatosplenomegaly, jaundice, thrombocytopenia, liver dysfunction, and a rapidly progressive fatal course.[365,394] Lymphohistiocytic infiltration with marked erythrophagocytosis is noted in multiple organs. Affected patients have a characterized immunodeficiency with altered immunoregulatory activity and hyperlipidemia. Analysis of hepatic lipids revealed disproportionate concentrations of most of the major hepatic gangliosides, suggesting a role for abnormal lipid metabolism in the cause of the syndrome.[1133] Various treatment regimens have been attempted.[365]

Endocrine Disorders: Idiopathic Hypopituitarism and Cholestasis

There exists a unique association of congenital hypopituitarism secondary to hypothalamic hypophysiotropic hormonal deficiency or aplasia of the pituitary, hypoglycemia, microphallus, and neonatal cholestasis.[473,562,597,310]

Affected infants present with cholestasis and various symptoms of hypopituitarism, such as hypoglycemia or hypothyroidism. Patients with the full-blown constellation, which includes septooptic dysplasia (DeMosier's syndrome) or optic nerve hypoplasia, can be easily discerned clinically; the diagnosis is suggested on physical examination by the presence of wandering nystagmus.[562] Patients with hypopituitarism and cholestasis may have low levels of thyroid hormone, cortisol, and growth hormone. The histologic changes are those of nonspecific neonatal hepatitis. The cause of the liver injury in the face of the endocrinopathy is unknown; this feature may be primarily associated, that is, related to the occurrence of a common viral or toxic insult in perinatal life to both organs. Conversely, the liver disease may be a secondary feature: in the absence of the trophic hormones that modulate or stimulate bile canalicular development and bile acid synthesis, conjugation, and secretion, there may be inadequate development of the hepatobiliary secretory apparatus with resultant cholestasis. It is important to recognize this entity since hypoglycemia, hypothyroidism, and the endocrine imbalance can be effectively treated.[562,597] Appropriate treatment of the endocrinopathy usually results in resolution of the hepatic dysfunction.

Neonatal Hemochromatosis

In the past few years, the entity of neonatal hemochromatosis has been more clearly delineated. Neonatal hemochromatosis is a severe, often familial, disorder of iron metabolism characterized by massive iron accumulation in multiple nonreticuloendothelial tissues. Attendant cellular injury and reactive fibrosis are limited to the liver.[405,585,720,944]

Hemochromatosis in the newborn had been described in sporadic cases reports for many years,[237,361,585] dating back as far as 1957, when Cottier[237] ascribed a distinct form of neonatal cirrhosis with diffuse iron distribution to excessive placental uptake of iron. In another case description, the iron overload was attributed to altered ferritin kinetics.[361] In 1981, Goldfischer and colleagues[405] reported autopsy findings of two infants with neonatal liver failure and what they termed *idiopathic neonatal iron storage*. This clinicopathologic entity, which was distinct from Zellweger's syndrome or other metabolic diseases, was manifest as intrauterine growth retardation and premature birth, followed by the onset of hepatic failure in the immediate postnatal period, with rapid progression to death.[405]

With the emergence of additional clinical and histologic data, rigid criteria for the diagnosis of neonatal hemochromatosis have been defined: (1) a rapidly progressive clinical course with death in utero or in the early neonatal period; (2) increased iron deposition in multiple organs (liver, pancreas, heart, and endocrine glands), with the extrahepatic reticuloendothelial system relatively unaffected; and (3) no evidence for hemolytic disease or syndromes associated with hemosiderosis or exogenous iron overload from transfusions.[585] No causative agent for the hepatocellular injury has been identified. The disease, which affects both sexes equally, has a high recurrence rate in siblings, suggesting an inherited metabolic disease transmitted in an autosomal recessive manner.[585]

Biochemical changes include an elevated serum ferritin level and a serum iron/iron-binding capacity ratio near unity. Liver biopsy has been reported to show pseudoacinar and giant cell transformation or advanced siderotic cirrhosis, or central lobular diffuse hepatic fibrosis with hepatocellular necrosis and nodular regeneration.[585,944] It has been postulated that the massive hepatic necrosis commences in mid-fetal life.[944] Abundant stainable iron is present in the liver (pericanalicular hemosiderin, lysosomal granules, and biliary epithelial iron) as well as in various epithelia and in mesenchymal-derived tissues, with sparing of Kupffer cells and fixed macrophages of the spleen, lymph nodes, and bone marrow.[585,586] Oral mucosal biopsy may be of help in confirming the diagnosis by documenting siderosis of the acinar and ductular epithelium of the submucosal glands in the oral–hypopharyngeal–respiratory tract.[586] The syndrome of neonatal hemochromatosis has morphologic similarities to hereditary hemochromatosis, as manifested in later life, including early-onset (juvenile) forms.[271,340] A relation to hereditary hemochromatosis had been suggested by the detection of the disease in parents of affected siblings.[617] In addition, the HLA$_3$ alloantigen, which has been linked to hereditary hemochromatosis, has been detected in several affected infants.[944] Hardy and coworkers,[461] however, found no evidence for linkage of neonatal hemochromatosis to HLA serotypes.

The pathogenesis is undefined; it is unclear as to whether iron overload initiates the liver injury or whether siderosis is a result of the liver injury.[583,584] The postulated excessive transplacental uptake of iron, which would not explain the selective partitioning of iron into parenchymal cells with sparing of reticuloendothelial cells, does not seem likely.[585] Neonatal hemochromatosis may thus represent the end result of a variety of hepatic injuries that occur in the perinatal period; there are several postulates: (1) deranged or immature fetal iron transport or metabolism may play a role[944]; (2) the developing liver may be susceptible to excessive iron toxicity, in view of immature defense mechanisms[818]; or (3) an infective agent may cause hepatic injury with secondary iron accumulation.[589] In one of our patients with liver disease, massive transfusion of erythrocytes produced the same organ distribution of iron deposition, suggesting the possibility that defective processing of iron by reticuloendothelial cells may play a role.[144]

The specificity of this disorder was examined by Witzleben and Uri,[1126] who concluded that in severe subacute or chronic infantile liver disease due to recognized specific causes, it was unusual to detect prominent stainable iron accumulation in multiple organs. This observation, along with the early onset of injury, appears to confirm that the disorder termed *perinatal* or *neonatal hemochromatosis* represents a unique clinicopathologic phenotype but not necessarily one specific entity. Recognition of affected infants may allow further delineation of the precise pathogenesis of the disorder. Early recognition is also critical since in all reported cases, there was rapid deterioration; death occurred in early infancy as a result of severe liver disease. These patients might have benefitted from liver transplantation. Alternative therapeutic strategies, such as the use of chelation therapy, have been unsuccessful.[532] Liver transplantation therefore must be an early consideration. In view of the potential for recurrence of this catastrophic clinical illness in siblings, genetic counseling should be carried out.

Defects of Bile Acid Synthesis and Metabolism

Considerable attention has been directed toward documentation of the existence of possible defects in bile acid synthesis or metabolism in the pathogenesis of cholestasis.[66,344,454] These may be primary enzyme deficiencies or disorders of bile acid synthesis or metabolism that arise secondary to specific organelle dysfunction (eg, peroxisomal disorders; Table 41-11). The true incidence is not known, but the prospect of targeted bile acid replacement therapy should focus attention on more widespread screening.

Primary Defects. Defective bile acid synthesis or metabolism may be an initiating or perpetuating factor in neonatal cholestatic disorders[61,62,76,77]; the working hypothesis has been that primary inborn errors in bile acid biosynthesis, as a result of an inherited enzymopathy, may lead to either underproduction of the normal trophic and choleretic primary bile acids (cholic acid) or overproduction of potentially hepatotoxic primitive bile acid metabolites (monohydroxy bile acids). Application of technologic advances, specifically fast atom bombardment–mass spectrometry (FAB-MS) and gas chromatography–mass spectrometry (GC-MS), have allowed for specific delineation of disorders of bile acid synthesis that are associated with idiopathic neonatal hepatitis. FAB-MS, in which nonvolatile compounds can be rapidly analyzed directly in small volumes of biologic samples or simple extracts, has been used in screening and GC-MS in precisely identifying specific defects.[215,927,928]

TABLE 41-11   *Inborn Errors of Bile Acid Biosynthesis and Metabolism*

Primary Enzymopathies
Defective degradation of cholesterol side chain
   Cerebrotendinous xanthomatosis
Defective transformation of steroid nucleus
   3β-hydroxy-Δ⁵-C₂₇ steroid dehydrogenase/isomerase deficiency[215]
   Δ⁴-3-oxosteroid 5β-reductase deficiency[928]

Secondary Defects
Peroxisomal disorders[915]
   Disorders of peroxisome biogenesis with *general* loss of
      peroxisomal function
      Zellweger's (cerebrohepatorenal) syndrome
      Neonatal adrenoleukodystrophy
      Infantile Refsum's disease[175]
      Hyperpipecolic acidemia
      Leber's congenital amaurosis[326]
   Disorders with loss of *limited* number of peroxisomal functions
      (structure intact)
      Rhizomelic chondrodysplasia punctata
      Zellweger-like syndrome[1017]
   Disorders with loss of a *single* peroxisomal function (structure
      intact)
      Adrenoleukodystrophy (X-linked)
      Thiolase deficiency (pseudo-Zellweger's syndrome)[406]
      Bifunctional protein deficiency[1097]
      Acyl-CoA oxidase deficiency (pseudo-neonatal
         adrenoleukodystrophy)[196]
      Hyperoxaluria type I
      Acatalasemia
Hepatic synthetic dysfunction
   Tyrosinemia
   Fulminant hepatic failure

3β-HYDROXY-Δ⁵-C₂₇ STEROID DEHYDROGENASE DEFICIENCY. Before 1989, the only known inborn error of bile acid biosynthesis involved defective degradation of the cholesterol side chain—cerebrotendinous xanthomatosis.[927] Clayton and coworkers[215] described the first inborn error of metabolism affecting transformation in the steroid nucleus. They reported that a 3-month-old boy with neonatal cholestasis, one of three siblings with familial giant cell hepatitis, excreted monosulfates of 3β,7α-dihydroxy- and 3β,7α,12α-trihydroxy-5-cholenoic acids and their glycine conjugates in urine; cholic and chenodeoxycholic acid were undetectable. The biochemical profile and family history suggested the presence of an inborn error affecting 3β-hydroxysteroid dehydrogenase/isomerase, the second step in bile acid synthesis from cholesterol. Because the natural substrate for the enzyme is 7α-hydroxy cholesterol, there was a marked elevation of unesterified 7α-hydroxy cholesterol in serum. The presumed defect was later confirmed by Buchmann and colleagues,[171] who used cultured skin fibroblasts from the patient and documented complete absence of 3β-hydroxy-Δ⁵-C₂₇ steroid dehydrogenase/isomerase activity. Fibroblasts obtained from the parents exhibited *reduced* activity, suggesting a heterozygous genotype. This patient demonstrated clinical improvement after institution of oral bile acid therapy (chenodeoxycholic acid).[513]

Δ⁴-3-OXOSTEROID 5β-REDUCTASE DEFICIENCY. This disorder was described in monochorionic male twins born with marked cholestasis; a previous male sibling with neonatal hepatitis died of liver failure at 4 months of age.[928] Liver function tests at admission indicated elevated serum aminotransferase levels, marked conjugated hyperbilirubinemia, and severe coagulopathy. Liver biopsy revealed marked lobular disarray, pseudoacinar transformation of hepatocytes, hepatocellular and canalicular bile stasis, and extramedullary hematopoiesis (Fig. 41-8). Electron microscopy demonstrated bile canalicular abnormalities (diverticula, unconnected lumens, and lattice-shaped malformations filled with fine, granular, electron-dense material).[269] Initial FAB-MS analysis of urine samples from both infants indicated the presence of elevated amounts of taurine conjugates of hydroxyoxocholenoic and dihydroxyoxocholenoic acids.[928] Detailed analysis by GC-MS confirmed the copredominance of 3-oxo-7α-hydroxy-4-cholenoic and 3-oxo-7α,12α-dihydroxy-4-cholenoic acids. Gallbladder bile contained only trace amounts (under 2 μM) of bile acids, and Δ^4-3-oxo bile acids represented the major urinary bile acid. The bile acid synthetic rate, estimated from the daily urinary excretion, indicated markedly *reduced* total bile acid synthetic rates (less than 3 mg/d). These findings indicated a primary defect in bile acid synthesis that affected the conversion of the 3-oxo intermediates to the corresponding 3α-hydroxy-5β(H) structures. This reaction is normally catalyzed by an NADPH-dependent Δ^4-3-oxosteroid 5β-reductase enzyme[928] (Fig. 41-9). The cholestasis and liver injury were attributed to the lack of synthesis of adequate amounts of cholic acid, which would normally provide the major driving force for bile secretion, combined with the accumulation of Δ^4-3-oxo- and allo-bile acids, which are potentially hepatotoxic. Structural immaturity of the hepatocyte excretory pole suggested that maturation of the canalicular membrane and the transport system for bile acid secretion may require exposure to primary bile acids in early development.[61,76,269] In an attempt to specifically treat this disorder and reverse the hepatic injury, we initiated oral bile acid therapy. A combination of cholic acid (to suppress endogenous bile acid synthesis and prevent the further accumulation of the potentially hepatotoxic Δ^4-3-oxo- and allo-bile acids that arose in the presence of the enzyme deficiency) and ursodeoxycholic acid (a potent choleretic) was given orally to these patients.[76] Suppression of Δ^4-3-oxo and allo-bile acids occurred, and normalization of liver function tests and bile canalicular morphology was also noted during bile acid therapy.[76,927] These infants, and a similarly affected younger sibling in whom treatment was initiated at 6 days of age, are alive and well at 3½ years and 1 year of age.

Secondary Defects

PEROXISOMAL DISORDERS. Peroxisomes are essential for cellular metabolism, including bile acid β-oxidation; therefore, defective bile acid metabolism had been described as a secondary feature of peroxisomal disorders[196,212,216,731, 915,947,1017] (see Table 41-11).

ZELLWEGER'S SYNDROME. Infants with Zellweger's (cerebrohepatorenal) syndrome have defects in bile acid biosynthesis and metabolism that have been correlated with altered organelle function and morphology.[455] Clinical manifestations include profound psychomotor retardation, hypotonia, a characteristic facies (narrow cranium, prominent forehead, hypertelorism, and epicanthic folds), cortical cysts of the kidney, and intrahepatic cholestasis.[796,960] Hepatomegaly is usually present at birth, and jaundice appears at 2 to 3 weeks of life. Death occurs in most patients by 6 months of age. A diffuse micronodular cirrhosis is noted at autopsy. The premorbid histologic features of the liver include variable cholestasis, lobular disarray, focal necrosis, and in some cases, paucity of intrahepatic ducts.[396,796,960] Mitochondrial disarrangement, with twisting of cristae, and angulate lysosomes are visible.[407,723] Zellweger's syndrome is characterized by the virtual absence of peroxisomes in the liver. These microbodies, which are normally the site of catalases and oxidases, play an important role in β-oxidation of fatty acids and chain-shortening of bile acids.[559] Altered organelle function is suggested by the excessive urinary excretion of trihydroxycoprostanic acid (THCA), dihydroxycoprostanic acid (DHCA), and varanic acid, all precursors of primary bile acids that have not undergone complete side-chain oxidation.[454] In addition, increased concentrations of C-27 bile acid intermediates have been found in serum and bile of infants with Zellweger's syndrome.[125,268,343,476] THCA and other bile acid precursors may contribute to the hepatic pathology. Infusion of THCA into rats induces hemolysis and hepatic injury; the ultrastructural lesions consist of focal dilatation of vesicles within the lumina of the endoplasmic reticulum, decreased matrix density and elongated internal cristae in mitochondria, and filamen-

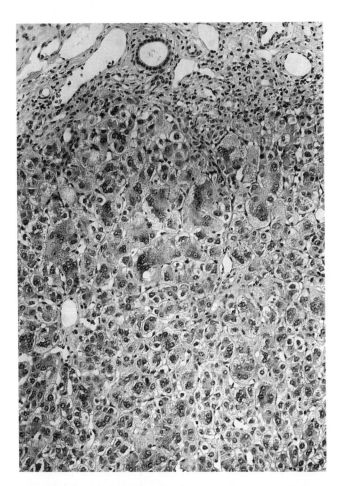

FIGURE 41-8 Initial (pretreatment) liver biopsy, obtained at 6 weeks of age, from a patient with Δ^4-3-oxosteroid 5β-reductase deficiency. The hepatic histology is that of idiopathic neonatal hepatitis, with giant cell transformation, lobular disarray, extramedullary hematopoiesis, and normal bile ductule (× 200).

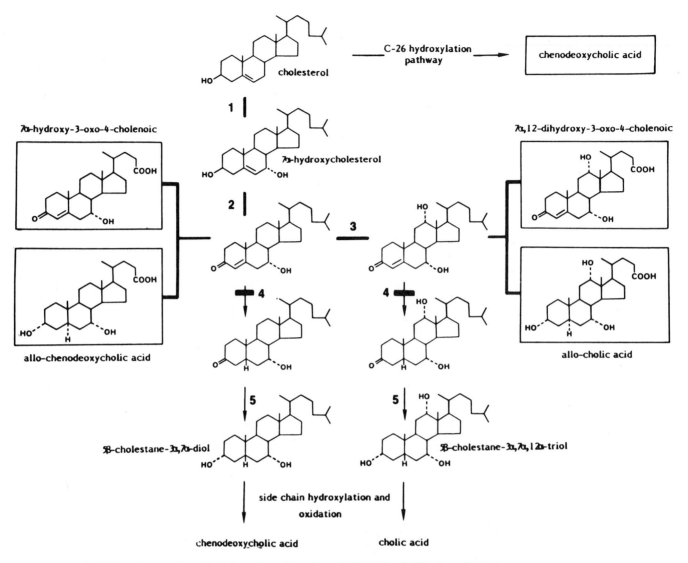

FIGURE 41-9 Biosynthetic pathway for bile acid synthesis from cholesterol; solid blocks indicate the site of the defect in synthesis (Δ^4-3-oxosteroid 5β-reductase). The numbers indicate the key enzymes: (1) cholesterol 7α-hydroxylase; (2) 3β-hydroxysterol dehydrogenase/isomerase; (3) 12α-hydroxylase; (4) Δ^4-3-oxosteroid 5β-reductase; (5) 3α-hydroxysteroid dehydrogenase. The defect in Δ^4-3-oxosteroid 5β-reductase activity was associated with an *increased* production of Δ^4-3-oxosteroids; there was subsequent metabolism of these precursors (side-chain oxidation) to yield Δ^4-3-oxo-bile acids and allo-bile acids (*boxes*). (Setchell KDR, Suchy FJ, Welsh MB, Zimmer-Nechemias L, Heubi J, Balistreri WF. Δ^4-3-Oxosteroid 5B-reductase deficiency described in identical twins with neonatal hepatitis: a new inborn error in bile acid synthesis. J Clin Invest 82:2148–2157, 1988)

tous material and vesicles within bile canaliculi.[456] The presence of these bile acid precursors, which are characterized by the partially oxidized side chain, suggest an important role for peroxisomes in bile acid metabolism.[558] These observations have led to a clearer elucidation of the class of diseases known as *peroxisomal disorders*[406–408,560,730,732,948] (see Table 41-11).

Altered peroxisomal metabolism also accounts for the other biochemical abnormalities that have been noted in patients with Zellweger's syndrome, such as impaired oxidation of phytanic acid, the presence of pipecolic acid (a product of lysine metabolism that accumulates because of deficient peroxisomal oxidase activity), and the accumulation of very-long-chain fatty acids (hexacosanoic acid C26:0 and hexa-

cosenoic acid C26:1) in the absence of peroxisomal oxidation.[416,912,913]

Precise biochemical diagnosis and differentiation of Zellweger's syndrome from other causes of hypotonia are important to provide genetic counseling. Characteristic dysmorphic, radiologic, biochemical, and pathologic findings have been described in four affected fetuses.[830] Prenatal diagnosis of Zellweger's syndrome is possible, based on the detection of increased levels of very-long-chain fatty acids (hexacosanoic acid and hexacosenoic acid) in amniotic fluid and in cultured amniocytes.[730,732,872]

The primary defect in Zellweger's syndrome has been postulated to be an inability to import matrix proteins into peroxisomes[895]; however, further studies are required.[379] At-

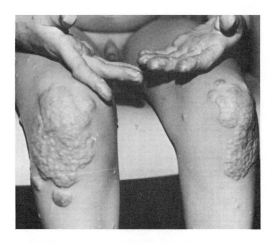

FIGURE 41-20 Characteristic skin xanthomas can be seen on hands and knees of a 5-year-old patient with intrahepatic cholestasis; serum cholesterol is above 500 mg/dL.

may persist after the neonatal period, and intense pruritus is usually noticed by 4 to 6 months of age. Hepatomegaly is a consistent feature. Extrahepatic anomalies are distinctive, but there is considerable variability in phenotypic expression[739,740,859]: unusual *facial* characteristics may be recognized in infancy, the forehead is broad and the chin pointed, giving the face a triangular appearance; there is also mid-facial hypoplasia, the eyes are deeply set and somewhat widely spaced, and the nose is elongated with a flattened tip; *vertebral arch defects* (butterfly vertebrae, hemivertebrae, and

TABLE 41-15 *Alagille's Syndrome (Arteriohepatic Dysplasia)*[16]

Criteria and Features	Incidence (%)
Major Features	
Bile duct paucity (decreased number of interlobular ducts and chronic cholestasis)	91
Extrahepatic anomalies (variable expression)	
Unusual facies (broad forehead; deeply set, widely spaced eyes; long straight nose)	95
Vertebral arch defects (butterfly vertebrae; hemivertebrae)	87
Cardiovascular abnormalities (peripheral pulmonic stenosis)	70
Posterior embryotoxon	89
Associated Features*	
Renal abnormalities	68
Growth retardation	50
Mental retardation	16
Hypogonadism	<10
Bone disease	<10
High-pitched voice	<10

*Many of the associated features may be secondary to chronic cholestasis, for example, vitamin E deficiency with attendant neuromuscular disease. (Alagille D, et al. Syndromic paucity of interlobular bile ducts. [Alagille syndrome or arteriohepatic dysplasia]: review of 80 cases. J Pediatr 110:195–200, 1987)

a decrease in the interpedicular distance) are present in most patients; ophthalmologic examination may reveal the presence of *posterior embryotoxon* (prominent Schwalbe's line); and *peripheral pulmonic stenosis*, the most common cardiovascular defect, is present in over 90% of these cases.[1098]

Short stature and renal abnormalities, most commonly tubulointerstitial nephropathy, are frequently associated. Hypercholesterolemia, often of an extreme degree (more than 1000 mg/dL), associated with cutaneous xanthoma formation (see Fig. 41-20) may also be noted.[318] Porphyria cutanea tarda–like blistering, fragility, and scarring of light-exposed skin, possibly related to coproporphyrin abnormalities, have recently been reported.[819]

Paucity or absence of the intrahepatic intralobular ducts, cholestasis, and an absence of significant fibrosis or cirrhosis may be noted in infancy, but these findings are not universal. The liver biopsy specimens obtained during infancy may resemble any other form of neonatal hepatitis, and evolution to classic findings of paucity may occur over time.[262] Ballooning of hepatocytes, bile ductular proliferation, portal inflammation, and giant cell transformation may be prominent during the first months of life. Mild periportal fibrosis may result, but progression to cirrhosis has not been described.[13,859] Portal tracts are reduced in size and number.[13,14,262,1062] The extrahepatic ductule systems in patients with arteriohepatic dysplasia are patent but are often hypoplastic.[262,670] The ultrastructural features suggest distinctive changes[1062]; bile regurgitation into the intercellular space is nearly universal, although the bile canaliculi appear normal. Bile pigment retention in the cytoplasm is seen, especially in lysosomes and in vesicles of the outer convex face of the Golgi apparatus, suggesting a block in the Golgi apparatus or in the pericanalicular cytoplasm. In addition, there is a lack of the ultrastructural pericanalicular changes noted in many forms of cholestasis, such as thickened ectoplasm, an absence of canalicular bile plugs, and bile canalicular dilatation; there is no microvillus atrophy.[1062] These features led the authors to postulate the existence of a bile secretory defect at a precanalicular site within the hepatocyte, possibly occurring at the level of the Golgi apparatus[1062]; this remains to be demonstrated.[1122]

The histopathologic diagnosis of arteriohepatic dysplasia may not be obvious in infancy.[278] Dahms and colleagues[262] have stressed an evolution of the characteristic pathology. Biopsies were performed on five patients during infancy (ie, younger than 6 months); the histologic features suggested intrahepatic cholestasis and portal inflammation. The infants did not have an absence of IBDs, and only two of the five had paucity (less than 0.5 IBD per triad). Six biopsies were performed later in life, at 3 to 20 years of age; all these patients had documented paucity or absence of bile ducts, and the cholestasis and inflammation had resolved. If biopsies are evaluated longitudinally, with increasing age, portal triads may be noted to contain fewer bile ducts; the progression of the lesion is not associated with inflammation or fibrosis. The pathogenesis of bile duct paucity is unknown; however, the progressive nature, from the early features of bile duct inflammation to the later observation of paucity, suggests immunologic injury, similar to other syndromes of disappearing intrahepatic bile ducts. Other postulated mechanisms include alterations in bile acid metabolism, intrauterine or postnatal infection, and chromosomal abnormalities. Partial deletion of the short arm of chromosome 20 has been noted in a small proportion (perhaps a subset) of affected individuals.[33,1152] This observation begs the issue of the role of chromosome 20 in the regulation of morphogenesis. The pathophysiologic importance of the postulated failure of the hepatocyte to secrete bile and bile acids into the canaliculus (discussed previously) also requires further investigation.[1062]

This form of intrahepatic cholestasis carries a relatively good prognosis. Most patients have survived the first decade, and several adults have been reported with this disorder. In most cases, parents are not obviously affected, but typical features have been noted in parents and siblings of affected children.[859,860] La Brecque and associates[601] have documented the presence of arteriohepatic dysplasia in four successive generations of a single kindred. Of 24 members, 15 had at least some of the characteristics of the arteriohepatic dysplasia syndrome. This and related observations strongly support an autosomal dominant mode of inheritance, with reduced penetrance and variable expressivity.[64,601,739,740,1152]

Although the prognosis for prolonged survival is good, patients with Alagille's syndrome are at high risk for morbidity due to pruritus, xanthomas, and complications secondary to vitamin deficiency, such as degenerative neurologic disease (ataxia and ophthalmoplegia) due to vitamin E deficiency. In addition, there are reports of hepatocellular carcinoma occurring in patients with Alagille's syndrome.[568,622] The good prognosis emphasizes the need for prompt and precise diagnosis and the avoidance of surgical procedures that alter the narrow, but patent, biliary tract (eg, hepatoportoenterostomy).[670]

Nonsyndromic Paucity. The term *nonsyndromic paucity* has been applied to those patients whose liver biopsy shows an absence or reduction of IBDs yet in whom none of the classic features of Alagille's syndrome is present. This most likely represents an eclectic group of diseases,[390,450,458,540] which is now more readily appreciated. In 31 cases of nonsyndromic paucity reported by Alagille and colleagues[16] in 1987, 21 had become manifested in the neonatal period, whereas 10 were diagnosed later in life. Of the neonatal-onset group, 7 were documented to have α_1-AT deficiency; in the other 14 patients and in all 10 in the delayed-onset group, the paucity was of unknown origin. The prognosis for patients with nonsyndromic forms of paucity is less favorable than for syndromic paucity; of the 15 cases of nonsyndromic paucity described by Alagille and colleagues,[16] 11 died with cirrhosis.

A seemingly related disorder, *idiopathic biliary ductopenia* (often familial), has been recognized with increasing frequency in young adults.[345,458,657,1150] Whether these cases represent a late manifestation of infantile obstructive cholangiopathy or ongoing obliteration of an unknown nature is not known. In the adults with idiopathic biliary ductopenia, progression to severe liver disease and the need for liver transplantation was common.[657,1150]

Hereditary Cholestasis With Lymphedema. Aagenaes and associates[1] have described patients of Norwegian extraction with intrahepatic cholestasis and lymphedema of the legs. Jaundice is consistently present during the neonatal period but occurs episodically in older children. Lymphedema in the lower extremities begins in later childhood and has been attributed to lymphatic vessel hypoplasia. The relation between the peripheral lymphatic obstruction and liver disease is uncertain. Aagenaes postulates a hepatic lymph-hypoplasia or a functional defect in lymphatic flow leading to cholestasis. Study of reported cases supports an autosomal recessive mode of inheritance of this disorder. Liver histology shows giant cell transformation and cholestasis in infancy. Cirrhosis has been found in several adult patients.[2]

Byler's Disease (Progressive Familial Intrahepatic Cholestasis). Severe forms of intrahepatic cholestasis with progressive hepatocellular damage occur sporadically or on a familial basis[535,771]; paucity of intrahepatic ducts is not a consistent finding. The clinical features and natural progression have been variable in these reports, implying significant heterogeneity among this group of patients. The most completely defined group includes members of several Amish sibships, each named Byler.[217] In these children, loose, foul-smelling stools appeared during the first weeks of life. The onset of jaundice was noted later during the first year and was initially episodic but became persistent between 1 and 4 years of age. Growth retardation and hepatosplenomegaly were regular features.[539] Moderate hyperbilirubinemia, elevation of aminotransferase levels, and elevated serum bile acid concentrations were present. Laboratory evaluation reflects the marked cholestasis, with an extreme elevation in serum bile acid concentrations and with elevated serum alkaline phosphatase and bilirubin levels. Paradoxically, serum cholesterol values and γ-glutamyl transpeptidase levels may be normal to low; this feature has been associated with a poor prognosis and may be a relatively specific feature of Byler's disease.[211,661,662] The pathogenesis is unknown.

Liver histology shows severe cholestasis. Slight proliferation of interlobular bile ducts was recorded in the description by Clayton and associates.[217] Progressive intrahepatic cholestasis and cirrhosis are present on subsequent biopsies. Electron microscopy shows dilatation of the canalicular lumen, which is filled with coarse, particulate, amorphous, granular material; reduction in the number of microvilli; and focal interruption of the canalicular membrane.[217] Particularly striking in one report were numerous microfilamentous structures in the pericanalicular ectoplasm and in the hepatocyte cytoplasm. The authors postulate a relation between the hyperplasia of microfilamentous structures in the liver and a defect in hepatic excretory function.[287]

Death from cirrhosis and liver failure is likely in childhood or early adolescence. Liver transplantation has been successfully performed, with no recurrence.[970] Twin brothers with a Byler-like illness died during their teen-age years of hepatocellular carcinoma.[260] The presence of consanguinity and liver dysfunction in parents of some affected children suggests an autosomal recessive inheritance.

Similar inherited syndromes with progressive intrahepatic cholestasis have been reported by others.[535,539,1101]

North American Indian Cholestasis. Weber[1101] described 14 North American Indian children with a severe form of familial cholestasis. In nine, the onset resembled neonatal cholestasis; however, in all, progressive deterioration with the development of portal fibrosis and neoductule proliferation developed. The electron microscopic changes were unique—marked widening of the pericanalicular ectoplasm with abundant pericanalicular microfilaments. Because these contractile proteins make up the hepatocyte cytoskeleton and are involved in bile acid transport and the generation of bile flow, the authors suggest microfilament dysfunction as the underlying disorder.

Fatal Familial Cholestasis Syndrome in Greenland Eskimo Children.   An analogous form of fatal familial cholestasis occurring in Greenland Eskimo patients was recently described.[756,783] The clinical features include jaundice, bleeding, pruritus, malnutrition, growth retardation, and steatorrhea. Despite the marked cholestasis, serum cholesterol levels are low to normal. Of these 16 patients, half died by 3 years of age.[783] The reported early histologic features were variable—canalicular cholestasis with rosette formation of the hepatocytes around dilated canaliculi and centrilobular fibrosis. Ultrastructural examination revealed granular material in bile canaliculi with a band-like condensation of microfilaments.[756,783]

Familial Benign Chronic Intrahepatic Cholestasis.   An unusual form of chronic, slowly progressive intrahepatic cholestasis was recently described in adults. Associated features were dermal hypertrichosis, increased pigmentation, and predisposition to autoimmune conditions, such as chronic thyroiditis with polyneuropathy.[338] High serum levels of α-lipoprotein were found. Prekeratin is an important component of the intermediate filaments in hepatocytes. The authors postulate that a defect in prekeratin–keratin metabolism might be operative, accounting for the hepatic as well as other manifestations.[338]

Benign Recurrent Intrahepatic Cholestasis.   Benign recurrent intrahepatic cholestasis most likely represents a variety of defects in hepatic excretory function. This poorly defined group of diseases is mentioned briefly here since onset is usually noted during childhood.[277,1014] About 20% of patients experience their first attack by 1 year of age. The illness may initially be confused with the more common progressive forms of infantile intrahepatic cholestasis and may represent related variants. Complete clinical and biochemical resolution followed by recurrent attacks establishes the diagnosis. Because many of the cases in the literature are inadequately documented, specific criteria have been suggested for this disorder: several episodes of pronounced jaundice with intense pruritus and biochemical evidence of cholestasis; bile plugs on liver biopsy; apparently normal intrahepatic and extrahepatic bile ducts on cholangiography; absence of factors (eg, drugs) known to produce cholestasis; and symptom-free intervals of months or years.[277] An increase in serum bile acid levels and a mild elevation in aminotransferase levels are characteristic of attacks. Benign recurrent intrahepatic cholestasis has been postulated to be due to an intrinsic abnormality in hepatic bile acid secretion.[710] The goal of treatment is the relief of symptoms, specifically pruritus, but this is generally unsatisfactory.

Medical Management of Chronic Cholestasis.   After diagnostic evaluation of the infant with neonatal cholestasis or prolonged hyperbilirubinemia, several possibilities exist—specific treatment (eg, dietary restriction of galactose), surgical attempt at palliation (eg, hepatoportoenterostomy), and nonspecific management of the consequences of cholestasis (Fig. 41-21). The clinical consequences of prolonged

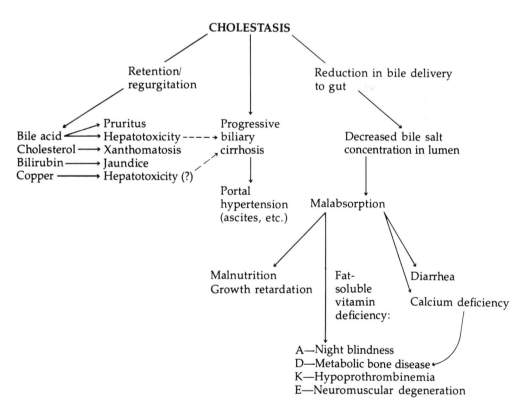

FIGURE 41-21   The clinical consequences of prolonged cholestasis result from (1) retention by the liver of substances normally excreted in bile with regurgitation into serum and into tissue, (2) a progressive biliary cirrhosis with complications such as portal hypertension, and (3) a reduction in bile acid delivery to the proximal intestine with inefficient micellar solubilization of dietary lipid and malabsorption.

cholestasis attributable directly or indirectly to diminished bile flow must be addressed: retention by the liver of substances normally excreted in bile, namely bile acids, bilirubin, cholesterol, and trace elements; decreased delivery of bile acids to the proximal intestine, with decreased intraluminal bile acid concentrations, resulting in malabsorption of fat and fat-soluble vitamins; and progressive liver damage, with biliary cirrhosis, portal hypertension, and liver failure. Cholestasis, liver damage, and malnutrition interact to alter the metabolism of hormones, somatomedins, or other factors required for growth, and thus result in marked growth failure. [62,66,69,78,172,966]

Therefore, for patients with idiopathic neonatal hepatitis, intrahepatic cholestasis, or extrahepatic biliary atresia in whom surgery is unsuccessful, management becomes an effort to minimize growth failure and to reduce discomfort, often while awaiting liver transplantation. The limiting factors remain the residual functional capacity of the liver and the rate of progression of the liver disease. Our recommendations for management of cholestasis (Table 41-16) are empiric; individualization and careful monitoring serve as the most reliable guides.

Impaired bile secretion can lead to malabsorption and

TABLE 41-16 *Medical Management of the Effects of Chronic Cholestasis in Children*

Malabsorption and Malnutrition
Supply medium-chain triglycerides
  Formula
  Oil
Decrease the percentage of dietary long-chain triglycerides
Ensure adequate protein intake

Vitamin Deficiency
Supplement
  Vitamin A as Aquasol A, up to 25,000 IU/d orally
  Vitamin D as D₁, up to 5000 IU/d, or as 25-
    hydroxycholecalciferol, 3–5 µg/kg/d PO
  Vitamin K as water-soluble derivative of menadione, 2–5 mg/d
  Vitamin E as Aquasol E, up to 400 IU/d; consider TPGS,
    15–25 IU/kg/d[965]
  Elemental calcium, 50–200 mg/kg/d, and elemental phosphorus,
    25–50 mg/kg/d

Pruritus and Xanthomas
Ursodeoxycholic acid, 15–30 mg/kg/d[71]
Cholestyramine, 8 g (2 packets) per day or more, given before and
  after the first meal of the day
Phenobarbital, 5 mg/kg/d[130]
Other potential modalities
  Chlorpromazine
  Carbamazepine
  Phototherapy
  Plasmaperfusion
  Biliary diversion

Ascites and Liver Failure
Decrease sodium intake (1–2 mEq/kg/d)
Diuretics
  Spironolactone, 3–5 mg/kg/d in four doses (adjust based on
    urinary electrolyte levels)
  Furosemide, 1–2 mg/kg/dose as needed
Transplantation

malnutrition due to ineffective intraluminal long-chain triglyceride lipolysis and absorption; therefore, medium-chain triglycerides administered in formula or as oil may be beneficial. [567,759] Oral nutrition alone may be insufficient to improve the nutritional status of children with prolonged cholestasis. Nocturnal enteral feeding should therefore be considered as a supplement to oral nutrition in a patient who fails to thrive. This has been shown to improve nutritional indices in patients with chronic cholestatic disease. [726,1114] Similarly, fat-soluble vitamin deficiency may occur in patients with chronic cholestasis and may be associated with significant symptoms, most prominently rickets caused by vitamin D deficiency and neuromuscular disease associated with vitamin E deficiency. [78,759,967,968] Malabsorption of these vitamins may be exacerbated by coadministration of cholestyramine. Chronic deficiency of vitamin E (α-tocopherol) results in the development of a progressive, disabling, degenerative neuromuscular syndrome composed of areflexia, cerebellar ataxia, ophthalmoplegia, posterior column dysfunction, and peripheral neuropathy. [78,874,964,967,968] The diagnosis of vitamin E deficiency in children with chronic cholestasis has been based on low serum levels; however, elevated lipid values allow vitamin E to partition into plasma lipoproteins and falsely raise the serum vitamin E concentration, often into the normal range. [967,968] Therefore, a more accurate reflection of vitamin E status in patients with chronic cholestasis is the vitamin E/lipid ratio. [968] The neurologic syndrome is partially reversible, so early attempts at repletion should be initiated. The marked improvement of vitamin E absorption may not be overcome, even after the administration of massive oral doses (50 to 200 IU/kg/d) of the α_1-tocopherol form of the vitamin. [66,78,967,968] An effective alternative is to administer a water-soluble form of vitamin E—tocopherol polyethylene glycol-1000 succinate (TPGS). [965] TPGS is capable of forming micelles in the absence of bile acids, thereby allowing tocopherol to traverse the unstirred water layer of the intestinal mucosa. TPGS was effective in normalizing serum vitamin E levels in patients with chronic cholestasis. [965]

Pruritus and xanthomas, which may cause significant morbidity, are difficult to treat. Compounds such as phenobarbital and cholestyramine may be effective if there is adequate biliary drainage to allow bile acids to reach the gut lumen. [78,130,759] Phenobarbital, a known choleretic agent, may also enhance the rate of formation of polar tetrahydroxylated bile acids, which can be readily excreted by the kidney. [62,66,130,1000]

Our preliminary results suggest that ursodeoxycholic acid (15 to 30 mg/kg/d) may be beneficial in ameliorating pruritus. [71] In patients refractory to all antipruritic therapy, partial external diversion of bile has provided effective relief. [1115] Ursodeoxycholic acid therapy, in our pilot trial, also reduced markedly elevated cholesterol levels and diminished the density of cutaneous xanthomas[71]; this observation requires further follow-up.

Patients with liver failure associated with chronic cholestasis are candidates for orthotopic liver transplantation. The major indication for liver transplantation in pediatric patients is extrahepatic biliary atresia, which accounts for about half of all recipients. [10,890,892,1114] High success rates have been reported for children; therefore, liver transplantation may offer the hope of long-term survival for patients with end-stage liver disease. [10,890,891,1114]

Metabolic Diseases of the Liver

Hepatic synthetic, degradative, and regulatory pathways are essential to carbohydrate, lipid, protein, trace element, and vitamin metabolism. Hepatic dysfunction therefore may be primarily or secondarily associated with enzymatic deficiencies or metabolic abnormalities. Hepatic involvement may manifest as hepatocyte *injury*, with secondary alteration in metabolic function and progression of the injury to cirrhosis; *storage* of lipid or glycogen; or absence of true histologic alteration but profound *clinical effects* of the enzyme deficiency (eg, in urea cycle defects). In the presence of a metabolic block, a normal nutrient or substrate may become a nonmetabolizable hepatotoxin. Rapid and precise recognition of inherited enzymopathies permits institution of one or more of the following treatment methods:

• Dietary restriction of the offending substrate
• Replacement of a deficient end product
• Depletion of a stored substance
• Administration of metabolic inhibitors
• Amplification of enzyme activity
• Replacement or modification of the mutant protein or gene
• Organ transplantation

The use of amniotic fluid, fibroblasts, and white cells in diagnosis or in screening may have important genetic implications.

Inherited metabolic diseases of the liver have protean clinical manifestations often mimicking infections, intoxications, or other systemic diseases; therefore, a high index of suspicion is required. Multiple clinical features should suggest the possibility of metabolic disease of the liver, including jaundice, hepatomegaly, splenomegaly, hepatic failure, hypoglycemia, organic acidemia, hyperammonemia, hypoprothrombinemia, recurrent vomiting, failure to thrive or short stature, dysmorphic features, developmental delay or psychomotor retardation, hypotonia, progressive neuromuscular deterioration, seizures, unusual odors, rickets, or cataracts. Information obtained from the family or dietary history, as well as clinical and laboratory examination, can be complemented by analysis of tissue obtained by liver biopsy. This confirms the suspicion or alerts the clinician to new possibilities and allows enzyme assay as well as qualitative and quantitative assay of stored material.

DISORDERS OF TYROSINE METABOLISM

Several distinct causes of hypertyrosinemia have been described. *Transient neonatal tyrosinemia* (TNT) has been described in premature infants[51,858]; this must be differentiated from classic hereditary tyrosinemia. In TNT, immaturity of tyrosine aminotransferase or deficiency of dietary ascorbic acid may be responsible for this mild elevation of serum levels; the liver is normal morphologically. Elevated tyrosine levels in blood may also be an *acquired* disorder secondary to any form of severe liver injury; therefore, this biochemical finding may be present in infants with galactosemia or neonatal hepatitis. This heterogeneity of symptoms suggests that hypertyrosinemia per se does *not* cause neurologic or hepatic damage.

Hereditary tyrosinemia type I is characterized by hepatic dysfunction, eventuating in liver failure or in cirrhosis; renal tubular dysfunction; and abnormal tyrosine metabolism.[921]

There are two apparent forms (acute or chronic), which may occur in the same family. Autosomal recessive inheritance has been suggested, with an especially high incidence in the providence of Quebec.[599,921] The disease may present in infancy as acute hepatic failure, failure to thrive, ascites, hypoprothrombinemia, bleeding, or jaundice; it may appear later in childhood as progressive cirrhosis and rickets.[921]

Recurrent episodes of severe, acute peripheral neuropathy are common and are an important cause of morbidity (pain) and mortality (respiratory insufficiency) in patients with hereditary tyrosinemia.[711] These episodes, which are associated with amino levulinic acid (ALA) excretion, may be responsive to infusion of hematin, which suppresses ALA synthase activity.[842]

The laboratory features of acute tyrosinemia often indicate disproportionate abnormalities of hepatic synthetic function versus biochemical indices of liver injury. This is evidenced by hypoalbuminemia and a decrease in vitamin K–dependent clotting factors, with only a mild to moderate rise in aminotransferase values. There is also a variable rise in total and direct bilirubin; hypophosphatemic rickets; marked elevation of serum tyrosine (to levels much higher than those seen in other liver diseases); hypermethioninemia; urinary excretion of phenolic acid by-products of tyrosine (*p*-hydroxyphenyl lactic acid, *p*-hydroxyphenyl pyruvic acid, and *p*-hydroxyphenyl acetic acid), which can be screened for with Nitrosonaphthol; succinylacetone and succinylacetoacetate in urine; and increased urinary excretion of δ-ALA. Affected patients are often anemic with evidence of hemolysis, are hypoglycemic, and have renal tubular dysfunction (Fanconi's syndrome), which can manifest as hyperphosphaturia, glucosuria, proteinuria, and aminoaciduria. In the acute phase, there may be generalized aminoacidemia with a disproportionate elevation of serum levels of tyrosine and methionine; in the older child, aminoacidemia is usually limited to tyrosine, but aminoaciduria is generalized, with tyrosine predominating.

The presence of greatly increased amounts of α-fetoprotein, in the presence of normal levels of tyrosine in cord blood of affected infants, suggests that hypertyrosinemia develops postnatally and that liver disease has a prenatal onset.[490] In the acute form, there is fatty infiltration of the liver; iron deposition; varying degrees of liver cell necrosis, which may be extreme; and fine diffuse fibrosis with formation of pseudoacini.[889,921] In the older child, there is a gross multilobular cirrhosis, and bile duct proliferation is often present. In some patients, regenerative nodules resembling a neoplasm may be present, and hepatoma may in fact occur in the older patient.[972,1103,273]

The primary site of metabolic block in hereditary tyrosinemia has been localized to the level of fumarylacetoacetate hydrolase,[647] the final step in the oxidative degradation of phenylalanine and tyrosine. Defective activity of this enzyme accounts for the secondary enzymatic and biochemical defects encountered in tyrosinemia. Accumulated metabolites, such as succinylacetoacetate, fumarylacetoacetate, and maleylacetoacetate, are found in blood and urine.[409,429] These reactive compounds are capable of binding to sulfhydryl groups and are toxic. Succinylacetone, derived from succinylacetoacetate, is a potent inhibitor of ALA-dehydratase activity and heme formation in humans and may account for the acute porphyria-like symptoms present in these patients.[896,897] Identification of succinylacetone in the amniotic fluid or assay of fumarylacetoacetate hydrolase activity in cultured amniotic fluid cells[598] of at-risk pregnancies allows for prenatal diagnosis.

Treatment with dietary restriction of phenylalanine and tyrosine is beneficial in some patients and is especially effective in improving renal tubular dysfunction.[56] The benefit of dietary treatment in patients with the acute infantile disease is unclear; its effect on the progression to cirrhosis is unknown. Presumably, if a metabolic block occurs at the step mediated by fumarylacetoacetate hydrolase, therapy in addition to phenylalanine and tyrosine restriction might include the administration of sulfhydryl-containing compounds, such as glutathione or penicillamine.[997] In view of the success of orthotopic liver transplantation in reversing the metabolic derangements and in preventing further neurologic disease or neoplastic degeneration, this option should be an early consideration for patients with hereditary tyrosinemia.[703,789,984,1073]

Sporadic reports have been made of what has been termed *hypermethioninemia*, with clinical and biochemical features of hereditary tyrosinemia, but the specificity of this entity has been questioned. Labrune and colleagues[602] recently described three siblings with hypermethioninemia and absolute methionine intolerance. These patients exhibited several unique clinical features, including failure to thrive, mental and motor retardation, facial dysmorphism with abnormal hair and teeth, and myocardiopathy. Hepatic *s*-adenosyl homocysteine hydrolase activity was decreased. Whether this or other reported cases of hypermethioninemia represents a primary or secondary defect remains to be determined.

DISORDERS OF CARBOHYDRATE METABOLISM

Degradation and synthesis of glycogen and the interconversion of glucose, fructose, and galactose are carried out by hepatocytic enzymes of the Embden-Meyerhof-Parnas-Cori pathway (Fig. 41-22). Deficient activity of a specific enzyme results in the hepatic involvement characteristic of galactosemia, fructose intolerance, and the multiple types of glycogen storage disease (GSD). In galactosemia and fructosemia, the early course may include cholestasis (discussed previously).

Galactosemia

Classic *transferase-deficient galactosemia* is a toxicity syndrome characterized by progressive liver and brain injury caused by the ingestion of galactose. The clinical presentation is in the neonatal period, within a short period after starting milk feedings, with vomiting, diarrhea, failure to thrive, hepatomegaly, cholestasis, aminoaciduria, and cataracts.[518] Affected infants have deficient activity of galactose-1-phosphate uridyl transferase[518] (see Fig. 41-22). Persistent elevation of conjugated bilirubin levels occurs in over 80% of untreated infants[743]; mental retardation and cirrhosis can occur in untreated patients.

Transferase deficiency results in accumulation of galactose-1-phosphate and galactose in tissue, with resultant toxicity to various organs.[304] Galactose may be reduced to the alcohol galactitol, and the development of cataracts is related to accumulation and toxicity of galactitol in the lens.[399] The liver, kidney, ovarian, and brain abnormalities are less well explained but seem related to galactose-1-phosphate or galac-

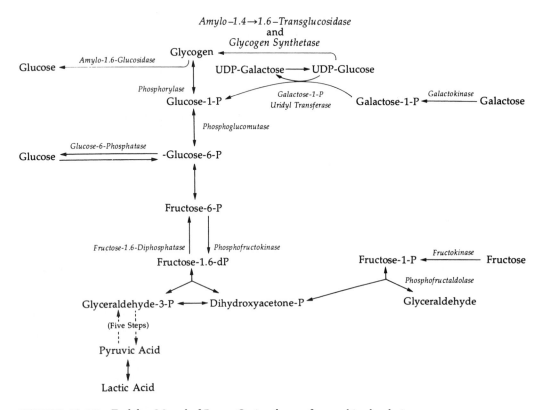

FIGURE 41-22   Embden-Meyerhof-Parnas-Cori pathway of anaerobic glycolysis.

tosamine accumulation.[563,1037,1135] In a related inherited disorder, galactokinase deficiency, accumulation of galactose and galactitol is associated with cataracts; however, there is no liver, brain, or renal disease.[563,1037] Hypoglycemia has been related to high tissue levels of galactose-1-phosphate, which interfere with phosphoglucomutase, the enzyme that catalyzes conversion of glucose-1-phosphate to glucose-6-phosphate; therefore, there is an inability to release glucose from glycogen.

The presence of reducing substance in the urine of cholestatic infants suggests the diagnosis. Testing the urine with both Clinitest (total reducing substance) and Clinistix or glucose oxidase paper (glucose) allows a tentative identification of the sugar at the bedside, which can be confirmed by chromatography. Conversely, routine use of glucose oxidase paper misses the diagnosis. Vomiting or poor intake of lactose at the time the urine is collected may also result in a false-negative test result. The resemblance of galactosemia to sepsis in the small infant is striking; indeed, gram-negative bacterial sepsis may complicate the disease.[636,743] Specific diagnosis depends on assay of galactose-1-phosphate uridyl transferase activity in erythrocytes, leukocytes, or liver.[514,571] Homozygotes have complete absence of red cell enzymatic-specific activity, and heterozygotes have intermediate values. Prenatal diagnosis is possible.[485] The galactose tolerance test is unnecessary for diagnosis and may be harmful. Even a remote suspicion of galactosemia is an indication to discontinue dietary lactose feedings until confirmatory tests can be done.

Other laboratory signs of liver injury (serum aminotransferase elevation and prolonged prothrombin time) are present in varying degrees. Hemolytic anemia and erythroid hyperplasia, occasionally severe and resembling erythroblastosis, occur in 40% of patients.[743] Renal tubular dysfunction may be manifest by aminoaciduria and proteinuria as well as galactosuria.

The histopathology of the liver depends on the age of the child and duration of galactose ingestion. In the first month of life, the liver is grossly fatty. Hepatocytes contain large droplets of neutral lipid and refractile material viewed with polarized light on frozen section.[957] Bile duct proliferation and early pseudoglandular proliferation of hepatic cells around bile canaliculi is present, but lobular architecture is preserved.[957] From 1 to 6 months of age, progressive formation of pseudoacini occurs, and lipid in hepatocytes decreases (Fig. 41-23). In older infants and children, progressive regen-

erative pseudolobules replace normal liver parenchyma, and portal cirrhosis ensues.[957] Strict dietary elimination of galactose, using commercial formulas, such as Nutramigen or Pregestimil, and no milk or milk products, results in remission. Dietary restriction should be continued for several years and possibly for life.[374,923] Erythrocyte galactose-1-phosphate levels may be monitored to gauge adherence to the diet.[305] Optimally, mothers of homozygous infants should be placed on a galactose-free diet during a subsequent pregnancy. Despite the relative rarity of this autosomal recessive disease (1 in 20,000 to 50,000 live births), it should be considered in any jaundiced infant because of the disastrous effects of delayed diagnosis.[1092]

Hereditary Fructose Intolerance

In the presence of an inherited enzyme deficiency, acute and chronic liver injury and metabolic illness can be caused by the ingestion of fructose. Of the three known defects in fructose metabolism, only *fructose-1-phosphate aldolase deficiency* leads to significant hepatic injury.

Fructose-1-Phosphate Aldolase Deficiency.

A syndrome resembling galactosemia, with vomiting, colic, hypoglycemia, diarrhea, hepatomegaly, jaundice, failure to thrive, and aminoaciduria, occurs in infants who have deficient activity of fructose-1-phosphate aldolase[253,375] (phosphofructaldolase; see Fig. 41-22). The onset is later in infancy, occurring when fructose is added to the diet either as fruit, cane sugar (sucrose, which hydrolyzes to glucose and fructose), or a sucrose-containing commercial infant formula.[375] The enzyme deficiency has been demonstrated in liver, kidney, and jejunal mucosa. The incidence is about 1 in 20,000 newborns,[54,772] and the transmission is autosomal recessive. Hypoglycemia and hypophosphatemia occur after fructose ingestion, and fructose appears in the urine. Intravenous fructose, injected rapidly in a single dose, reproduces these findings, but results may be negative if there is severe liver dysfunction.[375] In homozygotes, liver injury occurs within 3 hours of fructose feeding, as evidenced by elevations in serum aminotransferase levels and changes in the hepatocyte ultrastructure.[814] Fructose and fructose-1-phosphate accumulate in hepatocytes to a considerable degree, with eventual depletion of ATP and inorganic phosphorus. There is an increased rate of purine degradation, with resultant hyperuricemia and increased urate excretion. Phosphorylase is

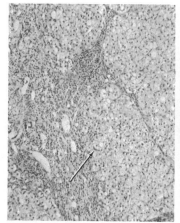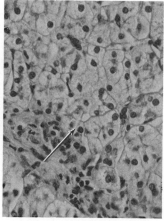

FIGURE 41-23 Galactosemia in a 9-week-old infant. Inflammatory portal exudate, fibrosis, and mild bile duct proliferation, as well as pseudoacinus (*arrow*), can be seen.

inhibited, impairing glycogenolysis and resulting in hypoglycemia. Hyperchloremic acidosis, hyperlactatemia, and hypokalemia are present. Light microscopy is normal at this time, but peculiar glycogen-associated membranous arrays occur in the cytoplasm, with rarefaction of a central core of hyaloplasm as evidence of liver cell injury.[814] Prolonged fructose ingestion produces diffuse fatty infiltration, hepatocellular necrosis, and bile duct proliferation (Fig. 41-24). Progressive liver disease and cirrhosis have been described. Deficiency of liver-dependent coagulation factors resembling hemorrhagic disease of the newborn may occur, and bleeding may be a presenting sign.

Treatment is by lifelong exclusion of all sources of fructose (eg, fruit, vegetables) and sucrose from the diet. Aversion to sugar may develop as a self-protective mechanism in older children and adults.[375,717,814] Hepatic lesions may be reversible, but persistent and variable steatosis is present in some patients, probably because of hidden sources of dietary fructose and sucrose, or possibly the ingestion of sorbitol, which is metabolized to fructose. Isolated reversible growth failure due to disordered adenine nucleotide metabolism may also be associated with chronic low levels of fructose ingestion.[717]

Fructose-1,6-Diphosphatase. Deficiency of fructose 1,6-diphosphatase results in hepatomegaly and hypoglycemia with acidosis precipitated by stress, fasting, or fructose ingestion.[58] The liver biopsy shows only ballooning of hepatic cells with large fat vacuoles. Episodes of hypoglycemia decrease with advancing age, confirming the favorable prognosis.[327]

Fructokinase. Deficiency of hepatic fructokinase results in a harmless asymptomatic condition, essential fructosuria, in which fructose is present in the urine after ingestion of fructose-containing foods.

Glycogenoses

The multiple forms of GSD (Table 41-17) produce diffuse hepatomegaly in all types described, except those that involve skeletal muscle.[499,907] GSD is considered to exist when the hepatic glycogen concentration (normal is 2% to 6%) or the molecular structure of glycogen is abnormal as the result of an inborn error of metabolism.[499] Classification, as first suggested by Cori,[232] is based on the specific enzymatic deficiency. Specific diagnosis depends on demonstration of the deficiency of enzyme activity in biopsy specimens of liver and muscle. The prognosis is highly variable.[958]

GSD type O, a deficiency of hepatic glycogen synthetase, has been reported in twins and in an unrelated child.[52,499] There is no response in blood glucose after glucagon administration since liver glycogen stores are depleted. The presentation is that of idiopathic or ketotic hypoglycemia.

GSD type I, due to dysfunction of any of the steps in the microsomal glucose-6-phosphatase system (Fig. 41-25), leads to glycogen accumulation in various organs (liver, kidney, and intestine). The glucose-6-phosphatase system consists of a multimetric complex of at least five polypeptides: the catalytic subunit of glucose-6-phosphatase with its active site situated in the lumen of the endoplasmic reticulum; a regulatory calcium-binding protein (stabilizing protein [SP]); and three transport proteins (translocases T_1, T_2, and T_3), which allow, respectively, glucose-6-phosphate, phosphate, and glucose to traverse the endoplasmic reticulum.[177] The ability of the liver to regulate the blood glucose level is related to the processes of gluconeogenesis and glycogenolysis, which permit release of glucose in times of need. Glucose-6-phosphatase catalyzes the terminal steps of each of these pathways; therefore, any deficiency that lowers the activity of this enzyme results in impaired regulation of blood glucose levels.[177]

In infants, GSD type I (also termed *GSD type Ia*) produces recurrent severe hypoglycemia, lactic acidemia, hyperlipidemia and hyperuricemia with massive hepatomegaly, growth failure, platelet dysfunction, asymptomatic renal enlargement, and a pot belly.[499] Instances of sudden infant death have been reported.[178] These clinical and biochemical features are attributable to chronic "glucose deprivation"; all reverse with maintenance of normoglycemia.[203,204,358] If untreated, patients with GSD type I are subject to hepatic adenoma formation[224]; malignant transformation is possible.[646,976] Glomerulosclerosis, osteoporosis, and gouty arthritis also may occur.[203] Autosomal recessive inheritance has been demonstrated.

The hepatic histologic changes in GSD type I are nonspecific. Fat-droplet deposition, marked irregular enlargement of hepatocytes, and prominent nuclear hyperglycogenosis are present. The ultrastructural changes are characteristic (Fig. 41-26). The severity of the hypoglycemia varies; some infants with GSD type I are severely hypoglycemic but have few symptoms. With increasing age, symptoms moderate, and the liver becomes smaller and abdominal protuberance less evident, despite deficient glucose-6-phosphatase activity.[233,499] The decrease in blood sugar is due to impaired glucose production.[1053] There is, therefore, an overproduction of glucose-6-phosphate due to continuous stimulation of glycogen breakdown; this increases glycolysis, which in turn results in a net increase in the production of lactate, triglyceride, cholesterol, and uric acid.[223] Avoidance of hypoglycemia and the attendant compensatory hormonal flux is the key to management. Treatment modalities are based on the rationale that a constant availability of exogenous glucose inhibits excess glycogenolysis, corrects the metabolic abnormalities, and alleviates clinical symptoms.[422,423] This can be accomplished by use of nocturnal intragastric feedings of a high-glucose elemental formula through a nasogastric tube or by frequent oral administration of uncooked cornstarch.[204,359,467,733,920,959,1129,1130] Successful maintenance of

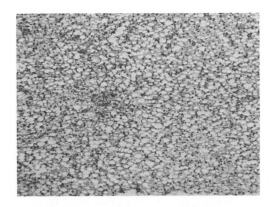

FIGURE 41-24 Fructosemia in a 3-month-old infant. All hepatocytes contain large fat droplets that displace the nucleus. Institution of a fructose-free diet resulted in normalization of liver morphology.

TABLE 41-17   *Glycogen Storage Diseases*

Type	Enzyme Deficiency	Tissue Involved	Clinical Symptoms	Synonyms/Notes
0	Glycogen synthetase[52,499]	Liver, muscle	Fasting hypoglycemia; prolonged hyperglycemia after glucose administration; mental retardation (hypoglycemic). Treatment by frequent protein-rich meals improves normal psychomotor development	A-glycogenosis; defect convincingly demonstrated in two unrelated families[499]
Ia	Glucose-6-phosphatase[233]	Liver, kidney, intestine	Enlarged liver and kidneys; "doll face," stunted growth, normal mental development; tendency to hypoglycemia, lactic (and pyruvic) acidosis, hyperlipidemia, hyperuricacidemia, gout, bleeding; no rise in blood glucose after IV glucagon.[499] Prognosis fair to good with treatment[204,422,423]	Von Gierke's disease (hepatorenal glycogenosis)
Ib	Translocase (T₁) responsible for movement of glucose-6-phosphate across intracellular membranes	Glucose-6-phosphatase activity is normal in homogenate made of frozen liver but is deficient in isotonic homogenate made of fresh (unfrozen) liver	Same as in type I; in addition, neutropenia may occur[29,94]	
Ic	Translocase (T₂, the microsomal phosphate/pyrophosphate transport protein); note that defects in other transport proteins (T₂ + T₃) could present a similar clinical picture[177]			
IIa Infantile[499] IIb Adult[330,499]	Lysosomal acid α-glucosidase (deficient activity of acid α-1,4- and of α-1,6-glucosidase)	In the fatal, infantile, classic form (IIa), glycogen concentration excessive in all organs examined; acid α-glucosidase deficiency may be generalized. Cardiac muscle in IIb normal but deficient in α-glucosidase activity; cardiac glycogen concentration normal	Clinically normal at birth but with minimal cardiomegaly, abnormal ECG, increased tissue glycogen; abnormal lysosomes in liver and skin, and acid α-glucosidase deficiency demonstrable at birth; within a few months, marked hypotonia, severe cardiomegaly, moderate hepatomegaly; normal mental development; death usually in infancy (IIa). Cases with involvement of muscle and liver but without cardiomegaly described in children and adults (IIb). Normal blood glucose response to glucagon	Pompe's disease (generalized glycogenosis, cardiac glycogenosis)
III	Amylo-1,6-glucosidase ("debrancher" enzyme)[232]; affects liver only or is generalized	Liver, muscle, heart, etc, in various combinations	Moderate to marked hepatomegaly; possibly moderate hypotonia or cardiomegaly; no hypoglycemia; no hyperlipidemia; glucagon produces a normal rise in blood glucose after a meal but not after fasting[499]; normal mental development. Prognosis fair to good	Limit dextrinosis (debrancher glycogenosis); Cori's disease; Forbes' disease
IV	Amylo-1,4 →1,6-transglucosidase ("brancher enzyme")[165]	Generalized (?); low to normal levels of abnormally structured glycogen (amylopectin-like) molecules	Hepatosplenomegaly, ascites, cirrhosis, liver failure; normal mental development; death in early childhood	Amylopectinosis (brancher glycogenosis); Andersen's disease
V	Muscle phosphorylase deficiency (congenital absence of skeletal muscle phosphorylase; phosphorylase-activating system intact)[907]	Skeletal muscle only	Temporary weakness and cramping of skeletal muscle after exercise; no rise in blood lactate during ischemic exercise; normal mental development. Fair to good prognosis	McArdle's syndrome (liver and smooth muscle phosphorylase not affected)

TABLE 41-17 *(continued)*

Type	Enzyme Deficiency	Tissue Involved	Clinical Symptoms	Synonyms/Notes
VI	Liver phosphorylase deficiency (phosphorylase-activating system intact)[501]	Liver; skeletal muscle normal	Marked hepatomegaly; no splenomegaly; no hypoglycemia; no acidosis; no hyperlipemia; no rise of blood glucose after IV glucagon; normal mental development. Good prognosis	Lack of glucagon-induced hyperglycemia distinguishes GSD VI from GSD IX; the latter shows a normal glucagon response
VII	Phosphofructokinase[445,1031]	Skeletal muscle, erythrocytes	Temporary weakness and cramping of skeletal muscle after exercise; no rise in blood lactate during ischemic exercise. Normal mental development (symptoms identical to those of type V glycogenosis). Good prognosis	Tauri's disease; reduction of phosphofructokinase activity severe in skeletal muscle, mild in erythrocytes, not established in other tissues
VIII	No enzymatic deficiency demonstrated (total liver phosphorylase normal, but most in the inactive form; phosphorylase-activating system intact)[499]	Liver, brain, skeletal muscle normal; cerebral glycogen increased	Hepatomegaly; truncal ataxia, nystagmus, "dancing eyes" may be present; neurologic deterioration progressing to spasticity, decerebration, and death. Urinary epinephrine increased acutely	
IX	Liver phosphorylase-kinase deficiency (total liver phosphorylase normal, but most in the inactive form because of deficient endogenous kinase)[499]	Liver only. Muscle tissue normal biochemically and microscopically	Marked hepatomegaly, no splenomegaly; no hypoglycemia or acidosis; normal rise in blood glucose after IV glucagon. Prognosis good; treatment may not be necessary	Liver phosphorylase can be activated in vitro by addition of exogenous kinase to the homogenate
IXa	Autosomal recessive			
IXb	X-linked recessive			
IXc	Liver and muscle phosphorylase kinase deficiency			
X	Loss of activity of cyclic 3′,5′-AMP–dependent kinase in muscle and presumably liver (total phosphorylase content of liver and skeletal muscle normal, but the enzyme completely deactivated in both organs; phosphorylase kinase activity half of normal, possibly due to loss of cAMP-dependent kinase activity)[502]	Liver and muscle	Marked hepatomegaly; patient otherwise clinically healthy. No cardiomegaly or hypoglycemia; no rise in blood glucose after IV glucagon or epinephrine	In vitro activation of phosphorylase occurs under assay conditions not requiring cAMP-dependent kinase
XI	All enzymatic activities measured to date normal (adenyl cyclase, cAMP-dependent kinase, phosphorylase kinase, phosphorylase, debrancher, brancher, glucose 6-phosphatase)	Liver, or liver and kidney	Tendency for acidosis; markedly stunted growth; vitamin D–resistant rickets (may be cured with high doses of vitamin D and oral supplementation of phosphate); hyperlipidemia, generalized aminoacidura, galactosuria, glucosuria, phosphaturia; normal renal size; no rise in blood glucose after IV glucagon	May include patients with varying enzymatic defects

blood glucose levels higher than 70 mg/dL decreases the hormonal stimulus to the liver to produce glucose. The initiation of either cornstarch therapy or continuous nasogastric feedings has been associated with normalization of biochemical parameters and enhanced growth. Chen and coworkers[203] also documented amelioration of the commonly associated proximal renal tubular dysfunction after the initiation of strict dietary therapy, including oral cornstarch (1.75 to 3 g/kg every 6 hours). This modality is not without risk,

however, in that it can abolish the tolerance for hypoglycemia. As mentioned, it has been noted by several investigators that before the initiation of therapy, children with GSD type I often tolerate hypoglycemia without clinical symptoms. This may be attributable in part to a dependence on lactate as an alternate cerebral metabolic fuel.[360] After initiation of therapy, hypoglycemia may be symptomatic and associated with central nervous system signs; therefore, total suppression of lactate is inadvisable.

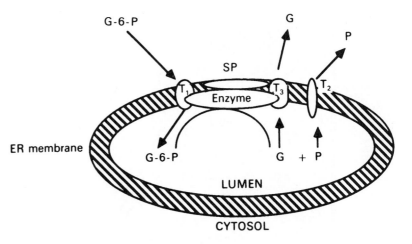

FIGURE 41-25 The hepatic microsomal glucose-6-phosphatase system. Glucose-6-phosphate (G-6-P) enters the lumen of the endoplasmic reticulum (ER) by the transport protein, translocase T_1. The enzyme glucose-6-phosphatase, composed of a catalytic subunit (enzyme and a regulatory protein [SP, stabilizing protein]) hydrolyzes G-6-P to glucose (G) and phosphate (Pi); these products exit the ER by transport proteins (translocases T_3 and T_2, respectively).[1090]

Recent observations have suggested that a similar clinical picture can occur in patients with deficiency of the 21-kd regulatory SP of hepatic microsomal glucose-6-phosphate (type I_aSP).[179]

A variant of GSD type I, GSD type Ib, also presents in a clinical manner identical to GSD type I; in addition, these patients are often neutropenic and are prone to recurrent infection and bleeding.[29,94,578,826] This subset is clearly distinguishable from patients with classic GSD type I. Confusion initially arose because of the fact that glucose-6-phosphatase activity in the liver homogenate was normal when the assay was run in hypotonic homogenate or when the liver tissue had been frozen before the assay. If the homogenate is prepared from fresh liver in isotonic buffer, however, then the assay for glucose-6-phosphatase will reveal defective activity. This is explained by deficiency of a hepatic translocase (T_1) system in patients with GSD type Ib.[177,1024] This enzyme serves to transport the substrate glucose-6-phosphate across intracellular membranes, permitting access to the enzyme glucose-6-phosphatase. Freezing or disruption abolishes intracellular membrane barriers and thus the need for translocase activity.

GSD type II, the first documented lysosomal storage disease, is associated with deficient activity of lysosomal acid α-glucosidase.[474] There are two subtypes (IIa and IIb), each associated with a specific clinical picture.[499] The most frequently recognized form is IIa, or Pompe's disease, in which profound hypotonia, cardiomegaly, and death in infancy occur. The liver is moderately enlarged until congestive heart failure occurs. Type IIb disease presents as progressive hypotonic muscular dystrophy, and prolonged survival has been observed. The heart is often normal in size, but respiratory failure may eventually occur.[330] The ultrastructural correlates of acid α-glucosidase deficiency are typical large vacuoles filled with monoparticulate glycogen[86,500] (Fig. 41-27A). Although equally severe deficiency of enzyme activity is present in both types, type IIa shows a marked increase in glycogen concentration and many large abnormal lysosomes. Type IIb has normal to slightly elevated glycogen content with fewer and smaller lysosomes.[499] In GSD type IIa, the amount of α-glucosidase is normal, but the structure of the enzyme molecule is altered, suggesting that it was catalytically incompetent.[106] In GSD type IIb, the amount of α-glucosidase is reduced, but the enzyme molecule is structurally normal.

In type II disease, hepatocytes are slightly enlarged and pale-staining without disturbance of lobular architecture (see Fig. 41-27B). They contain a myriad of 1- to 2-μm vacuoles, dispersed evenly throughout the cell, that are PAS-positive and digest with malt diastase.[683] They represent the enlarged lysosomes seen by electron microscopy. Nuclear glycogenosis is not prominent, and fibrosis does not occur. The increased frequency of the disease in males is unexplained, although autosomal recessive inheritance is commonly postulated.[499]

Treatment of type IIa patients with multiple agents has been unsuccessful.[499] Prenatal diagnosis of GSD type IIa is feasible.[499,503,938]

GSD type III is due to deficiency of amylo-1,6-glucosidase or debrancher enzyme activity[232] (Fig. 41-28). The liver, muscle, and heart may be involved in various combinations.[733] Hepatomegaly, which may be massive, is the most striking symptom; fasting hypoglycemia (due to a diminished ability to mobilize glucose from stored glycogen), myopathy, acidosis, and hyperlipidemia are often present.[427,499] Although hypotonia and cardiomegaly may be present, cardiac symptoms are rare. When the patient is in the fed state,

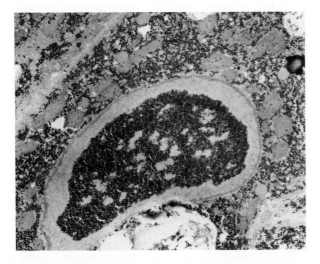

FIGURE 41-26 The liver in glycogen storage disease type I. Characteristic changes shown by electron microscopy include marked accumulation of glycogen in the nucleus, abundant glycogen in the cytosol, and the presence of lipid.

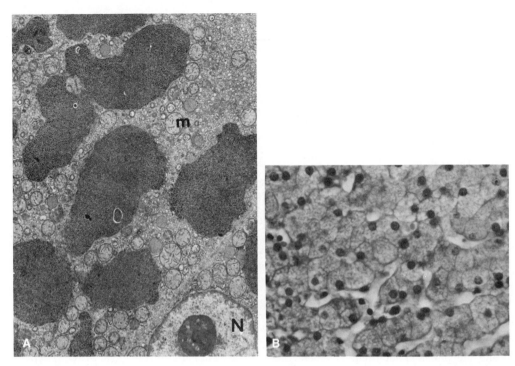

FIGURE 41-27 (**A**) Type II glycogenosis, liver ultrastructure (× 8000). Typical large vacuoles filled with monoparticulate glycogen. Compare size to nucleus (N) and mitochondria (m). In this postmortem specimen, nonlysosome-bound glycogen is absent, a finding seen after starvation and prolonged epinephrine administration. (**B**) Type II glycogenosis (× 250). The hepatocytes are slightly enlarged. A myriad of small vacuoles evenly dispersed throughout the cell are visible by light microscopy.

administration of glucagon activates hepatic phosphorylase and degrades the outer branches of the glycogen molecule to the 1,6 branch points, with a resultant rise in blood glucose; after a 12-hour fast, the outer branches have been degraded endogenously, and no rise in glucose occurs after glucagon administration.[499] The liver may be indistinguishable from that with type I disease.[500,683] Liver dysfunction with jaundice, aminotransferase elevation, and septal fibrosis may occur.[148,499] Family studies suggest an autosomal recessive inheritance.[148] Skin biopsy may be diagnostic[893]; prenatal diagnosis is possible.[298,938,1140] As in GSD type I, cornstarch therapy has been suggested.[733,1057] We administered oral cornstarch, 1.75 g/kg every 6 hours, to three children with GSD type III; this therapy was effective in maintaining nor-

moglycemia, in accelerating growth velocity, in decreasing liver size, and in decreasing aminotransferase levels.[427]

GSD type IV is associated with deficiency of amylo-1,4→1,6-transglucosidase, or brancher enzyme, activity (see Fig. 41-28) in liver and leukocytes and storage of an abnormal glycogen with fewer branch points and longer chains than normal.[165] Inheritance appears to be autosomal recessive. The abnormal glycogen is colorless in hematoxylin and eosin; stains positively with PAS, Best's carmine; and colloidal iron; and is diastase-resistant.[847] The accumulation of this insoluble, abnormal glycogen is associated with progressive liver injury. The onset of symptoms is noted in infancy, with failure to thrive, gastroenteritis, hepatosplenomegaly, and coagulopathy, followed by progressive cirrhosis with the onset

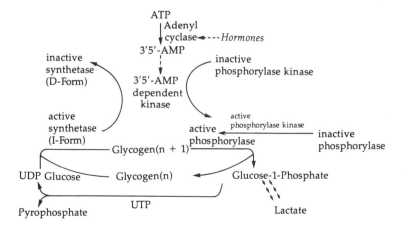

FIGURE 41-28 The enzymatic cascade of biologic amplification that results in activation or inactivation of phosphorylase. Inactivation of active phosphorylase *kinase* or active *phosphorylase* is mediated by the respective phosphatase. Glycogen storage disease (GSD) type III results from deficiency of debrancher (active *phosphorylase*) activity; GSD type IV results from deficient activity of the brancher (active synthetase) enzyme.

of ascites and liver failure. Death is usually in the second to fourth year, although prolonged survival[499] and nonprogressive liver disease[420] have been reported. The liver shows a uniform cirrhosis, with broad bands of fibrous tissue extending around and into lobules. Hepatocytes have eccentric nuclei and contain cytoplasmic deposits of the polysaccharide described previously.[847] Electron microscopy demonstrates large irregular areas of low-electron density in the cytoplasm. These consist of fibrils and finely granular material and are bordered by normal-appearing α particles or glycogen rosettes.[847] Blood glucose response to glucagon is normal, indicating that at least some glycogen is available for glycolysis.[847] The fact that a branched polysaccharide accumulates in the liver in the absence of branching enzyme is yet to be explained, as is the mechanism by which liver damage occurs, although a toxic effect of the abnormal carbohydrate is postulated.[847] Aggressive nutritional management has been reported to control hypoglycemia,[421] but liver transplantation should be contemplated in the presence of progressive cirrhosis.[10,924] Selby and associates[924] have reported normal growth and development, with an apparent diminution in the amount of stored glycogen in the heart and muscle, in five patients with GSD type IV after liver transplantation.

GSD types V, VI, VIII, IX, and X have been related to defects occurring in the phosphorylase system.[499,501,907] Figure 41-28 reviews the complex enzymatic cascade by which inactive phosphorylase is converted to active phosphorylase and glycogen is degraded. Reciprocal inactivation of glycogen production results from inactivation of glycogen synthetase, and blood glucose rises. It is apparent that deficiency of the phosphorylase enzyme, of phosphorylase kinase, of cyclic 3'5'-AMP-dependent kinase, and of adenylate cyclase could all potentially result in deficient phosphorylase activity in either liver or muscle tissue.

GSD type V results from inactivity of muscle phosphorylase.[907] Liver phosphorylase is normal, as is the activating system in the muscle.[499]

GSD type VII is due to deficiency of phosphofructokinase (see Fig. 41-22) in muscle; however, symptoms are identical to those of type V.[1031] Excess purine degradation occurs in the exercising muscle in both types, suggesting that the ATP pool is deranged because of the defective glycogenolysis or glycolysis.[709] The liver has not been studied.

GSD type VI is due to inactivity of the hepatic phosphorylase enzyme.[501] The activating system is normal as tested against exogenous phosphorylase, and the addition of phosphorylase kinase to the liver homogenate of the patient does not increase the phosphorylase activity of the patient's liver.[501] Glycogen content in the liver is increased, muscle is normal, and the major clinical manifestation is hepatomegaly. Patients with low hepatic phosphorylase activity previously designated as type VI should have activation studies done to define the enzyme defect.[501]

GSD type VIII presents as progressive neurologic deterioration and hepatomegaly.[499] Hepatic phosphorylase activity is low but can be brought to normal with the addition of ATP and $MgCl_2$. During the active phase of the disease, there is excess urinary excretion of catecholamines, and cerebral biopsy specimens demonstrate excess numbers of α-glycogen particles or rosettes, which are normally present only in liver. In vivo glucagon or epinephrine activates the patient's liver phosphorylase. Thus, the disease results from defective control of phosphorylase activation, although phosphorylase and its activating system are intact.

GSD type IX is characterized by asymptomatic hepatomegaly, low hepatic phosphorylase activity, and normal muscle phosphorylase activity.[499,1118] Total liver phosphorylase content is normal but is deactivated because of apparent inactivity of phosphorylase kinase. Addition of exogenous phosphorylase kinase results in normal activation of phosphorylase. Genetic subtypes have been described on the basis of determination of apparent k_m of hepatic phosphorylase kinase.[499] Autosomal recessive inheritance is present in GSD type IXa, in which the apparent k_m of the patient's enzyme is close to normal. In GSD IXb, the patient's apparent k_m is significantly higher than normal, and sex-linked recessive inheritance is suggested.[499] The k_m studies suggest that GSD type IXa may be a deficiency of regulation, whereas GSD type IXb may be due to a structural gene abnormality. This point is of biologic interest because sex-linked deficiency of muscle phosphorylase kinase has been observed in mice, and isoenzymes for phosphorylase exist in liver and muscle that may be affected independently by genetic defects.[499,659]

GSD type X is represented by a patient with increased glycogen and deactivated phosphorylase in liver and muscle and asymptomatic hepatomegaly.[502] Total phosphorylase was normal, but only 1% was in the active form; phosphorylase kinase activity was present. Type X disease is apparently due to deficient activity of the cyclic 3'5'-AMP-dependent kinase.[499,502]

GSD type XI, characterized by increased glycogen concentration in the liver and kidney, is without known enzymatic deficiency. Clinical manifestations include hepatomegaly and the presence of Fanconi's syndrome (with increased urinary excretion of phosphate, amino acids, glucose, and galactose) and growth failure. Florid rickets, resistant to vitamin D, may also be present.

Light microscopy of the liver in GSD types VI, VIII, IX, and X is similar to that of types I and III, with irregular enlargement of hepatocytes due to stored glycogen. Nuclear glycogenosis is less prominent than in type I. Similarly, the ultrastructural appearance of all hepatic glycogenoses, except type II, is similar (Fig. 41-29). There is crowding of endoplasmic reticulum by glycogen particles. Lipid droplets are frequent.[499,683] Intranuclear glycogen is more prominent in type I, and α particles have a fractured or splintered appearance in the four types involving the phosphorylase system.

DISORDERS OF LIPID METABOLISM

Abetalipoproteinemia

In the familial disorder of lipid transport abetalipoproteinemia, there is absence of apolipoprotein B from serum and an inability to form chylomicrons, the exogenous triglyceride transport particles, and VLDL, the endogenous triglyceride transport particle.[519] This defect in endogenous triglyceride transport often results in significant hepatomegaly. The well-known features of this syndrome are steatorrhea, acanthocytosis, retinitis, and an ataxic neuropathy due to vitamin E deficiency. The basic defect is impaired synthesis of the apolipoprotein, which is a major constituent of chylomicrons, low-density lipoprotein, and VLDL.[412]

Grossly, the liver is yellow-white.[795] Microscopically, hepatocytes are distended, with fat droplets ranging from 5 to 35 μm in diameter. In frozen sections, the lipid forms one or two large fat droplets in each cell, displacing the nucleus (Fig. 41-30). The lipid is triglyceride chemically and histochemically. Electron microscopy demonstrates a majority of

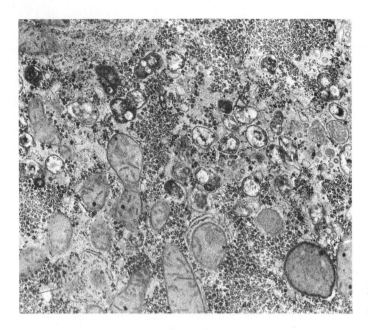

FIGURE 41-29 Liver in type IX glycogenosis (× 20,000). There is crowding of endoplasmic reticulum by numerous glycogen particles that have a splintered appearance.

non–membrane-bound fat droplets, an absence from the Golgi apparatus of the budding saccules normally associated with VLDL formation, and defective smooth endoplasmic reticulum formation adjacent to the Golgi apparatus.[795]

Vitamin E supplementation has been shown to retard the progression of the neurologic disease, the myopathy, and the retinopathy; there may be regression of symptoms.[570] Large oral doses of vitamin E have therefore been recommended. Supplemental vitamin A and K and carotene should also be considered. Micronodular cirrhosis was noted in two brothers who had received medium-chain triglycerides as a nutritional supplement;[795] this observation should suggest caution in the use of medium-chain triglycerides in this condition.

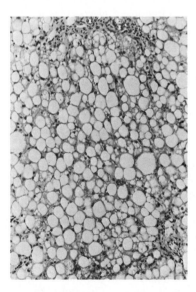

FIGURE 41-30 Abetalipoproteinemia at liver biopsy in a patient at age 10 months shows mild septal fibrosis with large fat-droplet accumulation in each hepatocyte.

Lysosomal Storage Disease

Lysosomes, which contain acid hydrolases (hydrolytic enzymes that exhibit a pH optima of 3.5 to 5.5), are bound by a single lipoprotein membrane. This organelle can therefore maintain an acidic intralysosomal pH and thereby allow full enzymatic hydrolytic activity. Substrates for acid hydrolases may be *endogenous* (autophagic), as during normal cell turnover when lysosomes degrade material produced by the cell, or *exogenous*.

Most hydrolases contained within lysosomes are exolytic and mediate cleavage of sulfates, fatty acids, or sugar moieties from larger molecules. Deficiency of a lysosomal enzyme results in inability to degrade the substrate within the autophagic vacuole, accumulation of the substrate, enlargement of these secondary lysosomes in cells, and organ enlargement. Many of the lysosomal hydrolases are composed of phosphorylated mannose residues; therefore, the possibility of altered mannose-phosphate recognition must be considered in addition to absence of enzyme activity.

Secondary lysosomes often have characteristic ultrastructural appearances; in some conditions, characteristic lysosomes may be present, although liver size and function are normal. Cultured skin fibroblasts usually demonstrate the enzymatic defect, accumulation of the substrate, and the secondary lysosomes by electron microscopy, permitting the option of the intrauterine diagnosis.

More than 40 inherited defects involving the intralysosomal enzymes have been described, many of which affect the liver.[404,594] These enzymes function to degrade waste macromolecules and enhance elimination; therefore, their failure is associated with the accumulation of the offending compound or abnormal metabolite within the hepatocyte. The net effect is that the hepatocyte is structurally and functionally destroyed by the accumulated waste material. A detailed understanding of biochemistry and transport mechanisms has brought us closer to treatment of lysosomal diseases by either organ replacement or replacement of the defective gene. Table 41-18 is a partial list of the lysosomal storage disorders of various classes that have been associated with hepatic in-

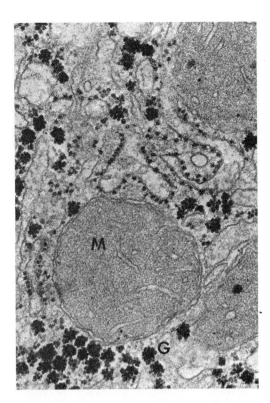

FIGURE 41-45   Reye's syndrome in the same patient as in Figure 41-44 four days after recovery. Mitochondrial morphology (M) is nearly normal, glycogen rosettes (G) are normal in number and form, and smooth endoplasmic reticulum is distended with lipid particles (*upper left*) (× 23,000).

tion of hypoglycin, a toxin found in the unripe fruit of the Ackee tree.[162] Hypoglycin ingestion produces vomiting, hypoglycemia, depletion of liver glycogen, fatty infiltration of the liver, coma, and death in up to 80% of cases. The incidence is higher in young children, especially in those with poor nutritional status. Hypoglycin, or α-aminomethylenecycloproprionic acid, must be converted to methylenecyclopropylacetic acid (MCPA) to exert toxicity. MCPA toxicity results from inhibition of fatty acid oxidation, causing increased glucose use and a block in gluconeogenesis, with resultant hypoglycemia. The inhibition of fatty acid oxidation causes accumulation of an acyl-CoA derivative of MCPA that is slowly metabolized in tissue, with consequent lowering of tissue levels of CoA and carnitine, cofactors needed for fatty acid oxidation.[155] Hypoglycin induces isovaleric and α-methylbutyric acidemia by its interaction with isovaleryl-CoA dehydrogenase.[1028] A possible relation of the neurotoxicity to accumulation of these branched-chain pentanoic acids, both of which are central nervous system depressants, has been suggested. Although hypoglycin ingestion is not the cause of Reye's syndrome, compounds of similar structure possessing a carbon–carbon double bond separated by two carbon atoms from the carboxyl group can have a similar effect. Ingestion of margosa oil, which contains a variety of fatty acids, may also produce a Reye-like illness.[949]

In experiments in which rat liver mitochondria were incubated with Reye's syndrome serum, a markedly unusual oxidative activity with stimulation of state 4 respiration and morphologic alterations—mitochondrial swelling and dis-

ruption—was seen.[39] An endogenous factor may be activated by the presence of a virus or an additional toxin and may precipitate the cascade responsible for the mitochondrial dysfunction.[545]

The finding of a factor in Reye's syndrome serum that is capable of uncoupling oxidative phosphorylation and impairing the formation of ATP led to the search for candidate uncouplers. Tonsgard and Getz[1045] demonstrated that dicarboxylic acids, which are known uncouplers, are present in the serum and urine of patients with Reye's syndrome; these may be responsible for the generalized impairment of mitochondrial function. Corkey and associates documented the accumulation of large amounts of hepatic acyl-CoA metabolites of lipid oxidation in patients with Reye's syndrome.[235] This observation suggested that mitochondrial β-oxidation was blocked at multiple acyl-CoA dehydrogenases. These investigators also detected elevated concentrations of cytokines (which inhibit mitochondrial β-oxidation) in plasma of patients acutely ill with Reye's syndrome.[235] Correlating these observations, they proposed a genetic defect in cytokine receptor–modulated signal transduction and suggested that the coexistence of three conditions eventuates in Reye's syndrome: (1) a viral illness that stimulates local cytokine production by circulating monocytes; (2) aspirin, which further amplifies cytokine production; and (3) a genetic or acquired loss of the protective inhibitory component of the response to high cytokine levels.[234] Cell damage due to inhibition of fatty acid oxidation ensues. This model might explain the clinical observation that provision of glucose (a substrate not requiring flavin-linked enzymes) might be of therapeutic value during the acute phase of the illness.[234] The more global implication is the delineation of diseases highlighted by defects of β-oxidation and the accumulation of dicarboxylic acids, especially long-chain dicarboxylic acids, which are clinically similar to Reye's syndrome. These include medium-chain acyl-CoA dehydrogenase deficiency (MCAD), long-chain acyl-CoA dehydrogenase deficiency (LCAD), and systemic carnitine deficiency.

Aspirin and Reye's Syndrome.   The epidemiologic link between aspirin and Reye's syndrome was initially established by the finding in case-control studies of a higher frequency of aspirin usage in patients with Reye's syndrome than in controls. In 97 cases of Reye's syndrome in an Ohio study, 97% were reportedly recipients of aspirin; a control group of 156 children had a lower exposure rate (71%).[446] Similar data emerged from the case-control studies performed in Arizona and Michigan. In each study, the proportion of Reye's syndrome cases exposed to salicylate was significantly higher than the portion of controls exposed to salicylate. The association of salicylates and Reye's syndrome is a reasonable one since salicylates may compromise mitochondrial function directly by uncoupling oxidative phosphorylation. Salicylates are also capable of inducing mitochondrial swelling in vitro, displacing bound fatty acids and dicarboxylic acids from serum albumin and causing aberrations in the immune response.[672,1144,1145] A genetic susceptibility to salicylate-induced metabolic injury might be operant, with Reye's syndrome occurring in the subset of people with impaired oxidative metabolism of salicylate.[692]

An increased incidence of Reye's syndrome may occur in children with juvenile rheumatoid arthritis who require chronic aspirin therapy. Not all children with Reye's syndrome, however, are exposed to aspirin, and the number of children exposed to aspirin is extremely high compared with the number of cases of Reye's syndrome. Nevertheless, in 1982, the Surgeon General advised against the use of salicylates, and a task force was appointed to carry out a pilot study to address the question of a link between aspirin and Reye's syndrome. The pilot study demonstrated that of 30 patients with Reye's syndrome, 93% had been exposed to salicylates, whereas in 143 controls selected from emergency room patients, inpatients, and schoolmates chosen at random, the exposure rate to salicylates ranged from 23% to 59%.[509] These observations suggested a strong association between Reye's syndrome and the use of aspirin, with an estimated odds ratio of 25:1. The main study of aspirin use in Reye's syndrome, which was expeditiously carried out, confirmed the association.[508] Of 27 cases of Reye's syndrome, 96% reported a history of salicylate administration during the antecedent illness. Of the total group of 140 controls, only 38% had received salicylate. The authors concluded that most Reye's syndrome cases may be attributable to salicylate usage.[508] Subsequent to this study, there was a mandate for warning labels on all aspirin products and a decline in the purchase of children's aspirin—this was coincident with a dramatic and persistent decline in the number of cases of Reye's syndrome in all reporting centers.[47,63,84,824,855,942]

Treatment. Successful management of Reye's syndrome is based on two key factors:

1. Early diagnosis is essential; therefore, the illness should be suspected in any child with unexplained neurologic symptoms with or without vomiting.
2. Control of increased intracranial pressure, since cerebral edema appears to be the major factor contributing to the high mortality rate. In the brain, there is a loss of the ability to maintain water and electrolyte homeostasis, and marked edema occurs.[285] As intracranial pressure approaches systemic arterial pressure, brain perfusion becomes inadequate, with resultant brain damage or death. It is imperative that cell swelling be counteracted and that aerobic metabolism be maintained; vasoconstriction must be induced without further impairment of perfusion. Thus, the primary goal of therapy is to decrease intracranial pressure; a secondary goal would be to reverse the metabolic injury.

Several studies have demonstrated the value of close monitoring of intracranial pressure.[935] This modality allows for more rational decisions regarding osmotherapy and other modalities since clinical signs may not be reliable.

Outcome. An association exists between the severity of the encephalopathy of Reye's syndrome and the behavioral outcome. In the Cincinnati study, the length of the period of disordered central nervous system function during the acute stage of the illness was the best predictor of eventual neuropsychological outcome.[914] In those patients with grade I disease, recovery is rapid and complete. With increasing severity and duration of illness, there may be an apparently normal recovery with subsequent subtle neuropsychological defects noted. The Cincinnati study documented defects in measured intelligence, school achievement, visual-motor integration, and concept formation.

Diseases That Resemble Reye's Syndrome

Based on recent studies, it is reasonable to suggest that it is more likely that a child with suspected Reye's syndrome will be found to be affected with a *specific metabolic illness*.[63,419,882] Multiple diseases present a clinicopathologic picture that resembles Reye's syndrome (see Table 41-20). Therefore, the spectrum of Reye's syndrome has been expanded and separated into (1) idiopathic cases, with the classic clinical features described previously, and (2) Reye-like illnesses (or Reye's syndrome mimickers), which are identifiable metabolic illnesses.[63] The biochemical alterations found in patients with idiopathic Reye's syndrome—namely, perturbed mitochondrial function due to an endogenously produced substance and a urinary metabolite profile reflective of a pronounced catabolic state (excessive lipolysis, inefficient mitochondrial β-oxidation of fatty acids, and an increased excretion of carnitine)[868]—resemble those seen in patients with known defects in hepatic fatty acid oxidation, such as the acyl-CoA dehydrogenase deficiencies MCAD and LCAD.[235,716,981,1032,1050,1051] In each of these diseases, and in patients with idiopathic Reye's syndrome, there is disruption of intramitochondrial processes. As a result, the patient is unable to use fatty acids for energy or ketone body production, and intracellular energy depletion occurs when glycogen stores are exhausted. These patients manifest a *hypoketotic hypoglycemia*. A major difference is that the ultrastructural findings that were stated to be characteristic for idiopathic Reye's syndrome are *not* found in MCAD or LCAD deficiency.[1051] Therefore, any patient suspected to have Reye's syndrome, especially those who exhibit a recurrent, familial, infantile, or atypical pattern, should undergo biopsy, and studies should be initiated to recognize these metabolic diseases.[63]

Defects in Fatty Acid Oxidation

In the presence of defective β-oxidation, fatty acids are metabolized by hydroxylation pathways leading to dicarboxylic acid, fatty acids with carboxylic acid moieties at each end of the molecule, which are then excreted in urine.[716,1051] Inadequate oxidation of fatty acids results in fasting nonketotic hypoglycemia.[981,1032,1051] The disease spectrum in which defective fatty acid oxidation occurs is shown in Table 41-20.[821,981]

Medium-Chain and Long-Chain Acyl-CoA Dehydrogenase Deficiencies. MCAD and LCAD deficiencies are specific inborn errors of fatty acid oxidation that are recognized as causes of catastrophic illnesses that closely resemble idiopathic Reye's syndrome. Clinical features of the acyl-CoA dehydrogenase deficiencies help to differentiate these disorders from idiopathic Reye's syndrome. Patients with MCAD or LCAD deficiencies are generally younger at presentation and often have a history of unexplained sibling death or of a previous episode of lethargy, decreased blood sugar, or acidosis that is precipitated by stress, such as fasting.[31,63,441] In patients suspected of having MCAD or LCAD deficiency, it is critical to document the characteristic organic aciduria when the patient is ill. It may be necessary to perform a liver biopsy, which will exhibit panlobular steatosis, either macro- or microvesicular, and unique ultrastructural changes (crystalloids in a condensed matrix).[31,142,1032,1051]

The biochemical changes in patients with MCAD deficiency were first described in 1982 by Kolvraa[591]; this was followed by detailed clinical studies. Since that time, multiple cases have been reported, and the incidence may be as high as 1 in 10,000 births.[980,1143] The incidence of MCAD deficiency, therefore, is among the highest of inborn errors of metabolism.[861] A specific transition in the human MCAD gene appears to be the most prevalent mutation.[1143]

Stanley and colleagues studied three children in two families presenting in early childhood with episodes of coma, hypoglycemia, hyperammonemia, and fatty liver associated with fasting.[980] In one case, fatal cerebral edema occurred. These children manifested an absence of ketosis on fasting, despite elevated serum levels of FFA, suggesting that hepatic fatty acid oxidation was impaired. Urinary dicarboxylic acid levels were increased during fasting, and a secondary carnitine deficiency was noted. The authors documented that the mid-portion of the intramitochondrial β-oxidation pathway at the MCAD step was defective.[980]

Children with MCAD exhibit many of the features of idiopathic Reye's syndrome, such as altered neurologic status and episodic vomiting with rapid deterioration. This disorder may also mimic sudden infant death syndrome. Laboratory abnormalities present during the acute episode consists of elevated ammonia, decreased blood glucose, and an absence of ketosis; serum carnitine levels are secondarily decreased. As mentioned previously, during the acute illness, microvesicular or macrovesicular fatty infiltration of the liver and ultrastructural abnormalities are present.[1032,1051] Between episodes, in the absence of fasting or acute illness, affected children appear to be healthy. The diagnosis can be confirmed by analysis of the urine, which shows the typical dicarboxylic aciduria,[867,868,869] octanoyl carnitine,[121,235] and acylglycine excretion.[861] Prompt recognition of patients with MCAD deficiency allows institution of a relatively effective treatment strategy—during the acute phase, glucose infusion can correct the metabolic aberration. It is then possible to prevent further episodes. Patients with MCAD cannot tolerate fasting; thus, chronic management consists of avoidance of fasting, ingestion of a carbohydrate-enriched diet, and modest dietary fat restriction with carnitine supplementation.[867,868,981]

Carnitine Deficiency.   Carnitine is an essential cofactor in that it allows β-oxidation of fatty acids by facilitating their transfer across the inner mitochondrial membrane. In the presence of carnitine deficiency, there is impaired metabolism of long-chain fatty acids, tissue accumulation of fatty acyl derivatives that inhibit gluconeogenesis, and inadequate production of energy in tissues dependent on oxidative metabolism.[201,393]

Several clinical forms of primary and secondary carnitine deficiency are recognized.[201,275,393] These have been attributed to altered synthesis, transport, or excretion of carnitine. In all reported conditions, there is hypoglycemia with an absence of ketonuria; plasma and tissue carnitine levels are low. There are two forms of deficiency of the enzyme carnitine palmitoyl transferase, which controls long-chain fatty acid transport into mitochondria: the *myopathic* form results in muscular necrosis, and the *hepatic* form resembles Reye's syndrome.[201,275] There is extensive fine lipid droplet accumulation in the liver, proliferation of the endoplasmic reticulum, and an increased number of peroxisomes and lipid vacuoles in carnitine palmitoyl transferase deficiency.[201,393]

Carnitine deficiency may be a secondary feature of defects in fatty oxidation described previously as well as mitochondrial diseases and disorders of organic acid metabolism. Replacement therapy with L-carnitine has been reported to be effective in treatment of the myopathic form.

Hepatitis in Children
ACUTE VIRAL HEPATITIS

Recent advances in the diagnosis and management of human infection with the hepatitis viruses have had a major impact on the pediatric patient.[68] Early tracking of hepatitis A virus (HAV) through daycare center clientele and personnel has led to effective measures to prevent further spread throughout the entire community. Perinatal transmission of HBV remains a major source of spread; early detection and the use of improved methods of immunoprophylaxis, including universal vaccination, will dramatically reduce the incidence and impact of this form of hepatitis. The implications of the discovery of the hepatitis C virus (HCV) on the pediatric population is unknown, but the benefit for patients who require frequent transfusions or receive large volumes of blood is obvious. Efforts to control HBV and HCV may lead to a decrease in the incidence of hepatocellular carcinoma. These and other aspects of hepatitis are covered elsewhere in this text.

Hepatitis A
Non–toilet-trained infants serve as hosts as well as vectors in the spread of HAV infection. Several studies have traced outbreaks of HAV infection to daycare centers. The high rate of transmission is due to the hygienic condition (overcrowded, understaffed, sharing of fomites such as toys, nonwashed hands, and diaper-changing surfaces) present in implicated centers.[68,439] Daycare center–associated outbreaks of HAV infection have an impact not only on attendees but also on caretakers and parents or siblings of the often asymptomatic yet infected infant. Management consists of identification, suspension of new admissions to the center, exclusion of documented infected infants until fecal viral excretion has ceased, and administration of standard immunoglobulin to employees and children. The use of immunoglobulin is an effective means of controlling HAV infection both within the daycare center and in the community.[439]

Hepatitis B
Transmission of HBV from infected mothers to infants in the perinatal period is responsible for maintenance of a worldwide pool of hepatitis B surface antigen (HBsAg) carriers. If the mother is a chronic carrier of HBsAg or if she develops HBsAg-positive hepatitis during late pregnancy, HBsAg may be found in the cord blood or in the serum of the infant during the first year of life in up to 90% of cases, unless prophylaxis is successfully accomplished.[715,989] Several factors, in addition to geographic and ethnic variations, predispose the infant to antigenemia—high maternal HBsAg titer, maternal hepatitis B e antigen (HBeAg) positivity, cord blood HBsAg antigenemia, and documented sibling antigenemia.[92,989] Almost all the offspring of HBeAg-positive mothers were found to be infected with HBV; over 85% became chronic HBsAg carriers. Children of mothers who had antibody to HBeAg rarely were found to be infected with HBV,

and none developed the carrier state.[777,989] The most common outcome of perinatal infection with HBV is the onset of a mild icteric hepatitis followed by chronic persistent hepatitis and the development of the carrier state. Rare cases of fulminant hepatitis have been described[1040] (Fig. 41-46).

Interruption of perinatal transmission is possible by immunization. High-titer hepatitis B immunoglobulin (HBIG) has been administered to infants of HBsAg-positive mothers in hope of achieving prophylaxis.[848,990,1044,1136] Beasley[90,91] administered 0.5 mL of HBIG at birth and at 3 to 6 months of age to Taiwanese infants; this treatment decreased the HBV infection rate from 94% to 75% and decreased the chronic carrier rate from 91% to 22%. Recent data suggest that combined administration of HBIG and hepatitis B vaccination can reduce the rate of chronic carriage to 5%.[68,70,990] Therefore, recommendations are for early (within 12 hours of birth) administration of HBIG for infants born to HBsAg-positive women; this should be coupled with the initiation of the series of hepatitis B vaccinations.[715] A proposed policy of universal vaccination of all infants against HBV infection has received widespread support.

Another group at high risk for acquisition of HBV infection and the development of HBsAg carrier state are residents of institutions for the mentally retarded. The risk of spread of infection to clients and staff is attributable to improper hygiene, interpersonal contact, and behavioral or medical conditions.[156] Supplemental vaccinations may be necessary in this special group of patients to achieve protective levels of antibody to HBsAg.[470] In a series of autopsies of all (138) deaths that occurred in one such institution, three cases of hepatocellular carcinoma were found; all were carriers of HBsAg without cirrhosis.[651] Serial monitoring of α-fetoprotein levels may allow early detection of carcinoma in this setting.

A unique clinical manifestation of HBV infection in childhood is infantile papular acrodermatitis (Gianotti-Crosti disease), which presents as a diffuse macular or maculopapular rash with arthritis[1042]; this is often associated with HBsAg subtype ayw. There is a high incidence of HBsAg in children with membranous glomerulonephropathy, another immune complex–mediated extrahepatic manifestation of HBV infection.[971] Serologic evidence of infection with HBV-associated delta agent has been found in Italian children; the prevalence increased in parallel with the activity of the liver disease and was maximal in the presence of cirrhosis.[348]

Cytomegalovirus Infection in the Older Child

The syndrome of congenital CMV infection was described previously; however, acquired CMV infection must also be considered in the differential diagnosis of unexplained hepatomegaly in older children. Associated splenomegaly occurs in about one third of these patients; mild abnormalities in liver function are common, but serum aminotransferase and total bilirubin levels may be within the normal range.[452,671] Rare inclusion-bearing cells, characteristic of CMV infection, may be seen in the liver. Other histologic changes vary from minimal hepatocellular unrest to granulomatous hepatitis. A child with hepatomegaly and a positive CMV culture or serology requires complete evaluation since this agent can be isolated from normal children and may not be related etiologically to the liver disease in the patient. Conversely, definitive diagnosis of CMV infection as causative of liver disease provides epidemiologic as well as prognostic information. In the immunocompromised patient, antiviral therapy with ganciclovir and immunoglobulin may be beneficial.

Herpes Simplex Hepatitis in the Older Child

Hepatitis due to HSV in the nonneonatal age group is uncommon and is most often observed in patients with postulated defects in cell-mediated immunity, in patients with severe malnutrition, in organ transplantation patients, and in patients with malignancy, burns, and skin diseases. HSV hepatitis has been associated with pregnancy and the postmeasles state. HSV infection should be considered in the differential diagnosis of fulminant hepatic failure.[719] With the introduction of relatively safe and effective antiviral therapy, early diagnosis is important.[978,1035] The associated clinical and laboratory features include localized oral or genital herpetic lesions, fever, enlarging hepatomegaly, deteriorating pneumonia, and leukopenia, along with elevations in levels of aminotransferase. Characteristic intranuclear inclusions can be seen on routine light microscopy, usually in the setting of focal coagulative necrosis surrounded by degenerating liver cells, with hemorrhage.[840] The inflammatory response is minimal.

The prognosis for affected adult patients is poor; of 23 patients, 21 sustained a fatal outcome.[1035] The outcome of HSV

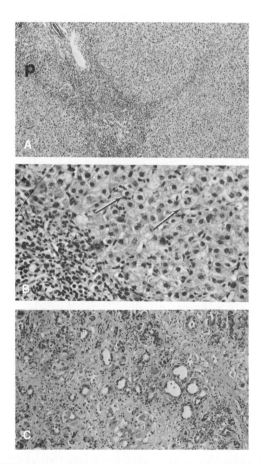

FIGURE 41-46 Fulminant viral hepatitis in a 4-year-old patient. (**A**) Initial biopsy specimen at low power shows extensive portal inflammatory infiltrate (p) extending into parenchyma of lobule. (**B**) Higher power shows liver cell necrosis and mitosis (*arrow*). (**C**) Second biopsy 6 weeks later, shortly before death, showed collapsed reticulum, free of normal hepatocytes, containing proliferating pseudoductules.

hepatitis has not been well defined in children. Five children aged 2 to 48 months who were at risk for disseminated herpes infection were given antiviral agents; one recovered, two survived with cerebral sequelae, and two died.[1035]

WILSON'S DISEASE

In every child with unexplained acute or chronic liver disease, Wilson's disease should be considered because of the potential benefits of early treatment.[905,988,1095] The disease may present with or without jaundice and without Kayser-Fleischer rings or neurologic involvement. This disease is reviewed elsewhere in this text.

CHRONIC HEPATITIS

As in adults, *chronic hepatitis* is defined by biochemical and histologic features. In children, the term chronic hepatitis encompasses a wide spectrum of disorders that differ in respect to cause, natural history, and response to treatment.[141,770,1005] The spectrum of severity is also broad, ranging from asymptomatic biochemical abnormalities to chronic symptomatic liver disease and liver failure. In this age group, it is especially important to consider treatable disorders, such as Wilson's disease,[905] autoimmune CAH, or other metabolic liver diseases in the differential of chronic hepatitis; α_1-AT deficiency should also be considered. CAH related to drug administration should be promptly recognized so that alternative therapy can be used. In view of the clinical and biochemical overlap between chronic persistent hepatitis and CAH, as in the adult, liver biopsy is essential.[1005]

With the exception of the treatable disorders mentioned, there is no specific therapy for pediatric patients with CAH. Therefore, the absence of controlled trials and a unclear understanding of the natural history precludes an accurate statement regarding management; this is especially true of CAH-B. Progression to cirrhosis has been suggested to be uncommon in pediatric patients with chronic HBV infection,[140] but in one study of patients with autoimmune CAH, the incidence of cirrhosis was high.[1074] This may also be true of chronic hepatitis C since in one study of 13 hemophiliac patients with abnormal biochemical values, biopsies performed at 2 to 9 years of age revealed chronic persistent hepatitis in 4 children and CAH in 2, including 1 with cirrhosis.[689] The role of α-interferon therapy in both chronic hepatitis B and chronic hepatitis C in pediatric patients remains to be determined.

AUTOIMMUNE CHRONIC ACTIVE HEPATITIS

Autoimmune (steroid-responsive) CAH in pediatric patients, as in adults, is most often manifest as malaise, anorexia, nausea, vomiting, and jaundice. Other patients may have an insidious onset, and the diagnosis is suspected by the physical finding of hepatosplenomegaly or stigmata of chronic liver disease, such as spider telangiectasia, palmar erythema, or manifestations of portal hypertension.[1005] This histologic feature is similar to those found in adults with autoimmune CAH. There is a wide variety of extrahepatic manifestations, including arthritis, thyroiditis, vasculitis, and nephritis.[1005] Autoimmune CAH is seen in association with inflammatory bowel disease, but the differentiation from sclerosing cholangitis may be difficult.[73] Hyperglobulinemia (polyclonal) may be noted, and non–organ-specific antibodies, antinu-

clear antibodies (ANA), anti–smooth muscle antibodies (SMA), and anti-mitochrondrial antibodies may be found.[1005]

Two subgroups of autoimmune CAH have been identified based on autoantibody pattern: (1) SMA (with or without ANA)–antibody-positive and (2) anti–liver-kidney microsome–antibody-positive.[486,660,770] There are distinct differences between these subgroups with regard to clinical features and response to therapy; the latter is frequently associated with extrahepatic autoimmune manifestations (diabetes, vitiligo, thyroiditis).[219,660,770,822] Although controlled trials of pharmacologic management of CAH in pediatric patients have not been carried out, several studies suggest that immunosuppressive therapy can be of benefit.[40,664,1077] Prednisone, often combined with azathioprine, has been shown to induce clinical, biochemical, and histologic remission. Early institution of therapy is essential since the outcome is less favorable if a delay occurs.[1005,1077] The initial daily dose of prednisone, 2 mg/kg/d, up to a maximum of 40 mg/d, should be continued until biochemical and clinical symptoms improve.[40,664,770,1077] The dose of prednisone can then be tapered over a 4- to 6-week period to the lowest maintenance dose possible. Azathioprine, 1 mg/kg/d, up to a maximum 50 mg/d, can be added to exert a steroid-sparing effect. If biochemical, clinical, and histologic improvement occurs, withdrawal of treatment may be possible; this has been successful in about half of reported cases. In patients who progress to cirrhosis or liver failure, however, orthotopic liver transplantation should be an early consideration.

Primary Sclerosing Cholangitis

The spectrum of etiologically obscure inflammatory disorders of the hepatobiliary tract includes the infantile obstructive cholangiopathies (biliary atresia and neonatal hepatitis) and PSC, which affects patients of all ages, particularly those with chronic inflammatory bowel disease.[73] Although these disorders differ somewhat in clinical expression and possibly in etiology, they have substantial overlap in morphologic features.

PSC is a chronic hepatobiliary disorder characterized by inflammation of the intrahepatic or extrahepatic ducts or both, with local dilatation, narrowing, or obliteration, accompanied by local periductal fibrosis.[73] Progression to biliary cirrhosis may occur. The abnormalities in bile duct structure can be documented by cholangiography, which has been considered essential to establish the diagnosis. The histologic changes may be less specific because of the progressive, dynamic nature of the lesions, which range from nonspecific portal edema or fibrosis and subtle pericholangitis to severe pericholangiolar edema and sclerosis with frank obliteration (Fig. 41-47).

In the pediatric age group, the number of reported cases of PSC is low[328,428,952,975,1110]; however, there is increasing recognition of the entity, due in part to the increased use of cholangiography in this group as well as appreciation of the gamut of manifestations. As in adults with PSC, most case reports discuss PSC in relation to inflammatory bowel disease[73,750]; the wide spectrum of hepatobiliary lesions recognized in adults is present in children with ulcerative colitis and Crohn's disease. Recent reports, however, emphasize that PSC may occur in the *absence* of any definable associated disease or develop in association with a wide variety of disorders (Table 41-22). In a review of 78 pediatric cases of

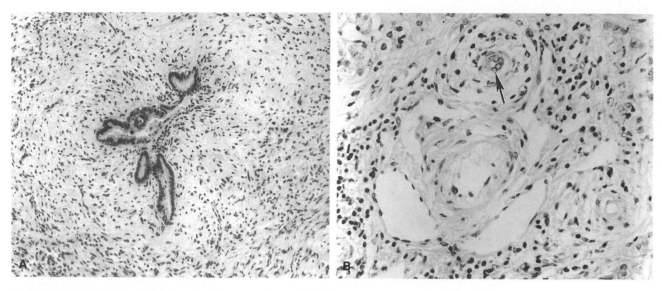

FIGURE 41-47 Primary sclerosing cholangitis in a 4-year-old child with a 6-week history of jaundice, pruritus, and hepatomegaly; the diagnosis was confirmed by operative cholangiography and biopsy. (**A**) Large interlobular bile duct lined by intact epithelium is compressed and distorted by surrounding fibroblastic stoma, which are sparsely infiltrated by lymphocytes (× 140). (**B**) Small interlobular bile duct (*arrow*) has a reduced lumen and reactive epithelial cells; it is surrounded by fibrosis, edema, and lymphoid cells in a laminar concentric pattern (× 400).

TABLE 41-22   *Recognized Forms of Cholangitis in Childhood*

Primary Sclerosing Cholangitis
In association with inflammatory bowel disease
In association with congenital or acquired immunodeficiency[428]
    Cytomegalovirus
    Cryptosporidium
    Cryptococcus neoformans
    Idiopathic
Inflammatory pseudotumor and retroperitonitis[19]
Idiopathic primary sclerosing cholangitis
Neonatal sclerosing cholangitis[952]

Idiopathic Cholangiopathy of Infancy With Bile Duct Obliteration
Biliary atresia (extrahepatic and possibly intrahepatic ducts)
Neonatal hepatitis (intrahepatic ducts)
Alagille's syndrome (intrahepatic ducts)
Postportoenterostomy (intrahepatic ducts)

Cholangitis Due to Stasis or Obstruction, With or Without Superimposed Bacterial Infection
Choledocholithiasis (sludge)
    Sickle cell anemia
    Total parenteral nutrition associated
Polycystic disease
Anomalous ducts
Cystic fibrosis[102,999]
Ductal carcinoma
Histiocytosis X
Status after biliary surgery

(Modified from Balistreri WF, Bove K. Primary sclerosing cholangitis and related hepatobiliary lesions. In: Balistreri WF, Vanderhoof J, eds: Pediatric gastroenterology. Chapman Hall, 1990, pp 196–123)

PSC, Sisto and coworkers found 47% to be in association with chronic inflammatory bowel disease.[952] About one fourth of cases were *not* associated with an underlying disorder; these patients presented with prolonged cholestasis, often originating in infancy[30,952] (see previous section on neonatal sclerosing cholangitis). The relation of this entire spectrum of diseases to extrahepatic biliary atresia is not clear; the bile duct lesions in biliary atresia are also inflammatory, progressive, obliterative, and segmental and may involve the intrahepatic ducts as well as the extrahepatic system.[73] Similarly, the relation of PSC to syndromic and nonsyndromic forms of bile duct paucity or ductopenia due to progressive destruction or loss of intrahepatic bile ducts needs to be defined.[657,1150]

The clinical and laboratory manifestations of PSC in children are similar to those reported in adults, often with the additional unique features of poor growth and delayed puberty. El-Shabrawi and colleagues[328] reported the constellation of findings in 13 children with PSC (age range, 2½ to 13½ years); the diagnosis had been documented by cholangiography. Nine patients had confirmed accompanying inflammatory bowel disease; the symptoms of bowel disease had been present for variable periods (ages 8 months to 13 years). The presenting manifestations of PSC in these children were hepatomegaly, pruritus, fever, or biochemical abnormalities. The aminotransferase activity was elevated in 12 patients, the alkaline phosphatase in 8, IgG in 12, and bilirubin in 3; 12 were ANA- or SMA-positive. The histologic findings were highly variable, periductal fibrosis was universal, but the presence of piecemeal necrosis in four patients suggested the diagnosis of CAH.

No controlled treatment trials in pediatric PSC have been reported. In the series of El-Shabrawi and colleagues,[328] 12 patients received immunosuppressive therapy, either prednisone or azathioprine, or both, and all showed symptomatic improvement. Preliminary reports have been made of a beneficial effect of ursodeoxycholic acid therapy.[202]

Cystic Disease of the Liver

Multiple hepatic ductal cysts may occur in patients with cystic lesions in other viscera, especially the kidney. In these heritable conditions, the cysts may be diffuse or localized and may or may not communicate directly with the biliary excretory tract. An increase in fibrous tissue and biliary ducts can also be noted in certain subsets. These cystic conditions may resemble other conditions, such as Caroli's disease, in which other visceral involvement is not demonstrable. The heterogeneity suggests a variable etiopathogenesis.

The associated renal abnormalities, infectious complications, or hepatic fibrosis may dominate the clinical picture. Affected patients may share common organ involvement and histologic abnormalities yet demonstrate inheritance patterns that support a presumed heterogenous etiology.

Morphometric analyses by Landing and associates[612] of liver lesions in children with various forms of cystic diseases of the liver have led to our conceptualization. They demonstrated that various entities previously termed congenital, perinatal, and infantile forms of polycystic disease[132] produce the same liver lesion and recommended that the name *infantile polycystic disease* (IPCD) of the liver and kidney be used to describe all patients with this autosomal recessive disorder. They associated the entity previously termed the juvenile form of polycystic disease with a liver lesion similar to that classically termed congenital hepatic fibrosis (CHF); these patients present in later childhood with portal hypertension. The authors[612] also suggest that the morphologic features remain constant, and therefore CHF is not IPCD seen at an advanced age. This remains conjectural, however. They have also stressed differences in the patterns of renal lesions between IPCD and CHF.

INFANTILE POLYCYSTIC DISEASE OF THE LIVER AND KIDNEYS

Infantile polycystic disease is a rare, autosomal recessive, hepatorenal malformation complex.[378,640] Gang and Herrin[378] have suggested that IPCD represents a continuum of renal and hepatic disease with a spectrum of phenotypic expression; prognostic implications are derivable from tissue analysis in the individual patient.

Massive enlargement of both organs may be present at birth and may produce respiratory difficulty in the newborn period. Acidosis, azotemia, hypertension, and congestive heart failure may be severe and cause death in the first month of life. The kidneys may decrease in size with age in survivors, but the urine-specific gravity remains low, and progression of renal insufficiency is variable, with prolonged survival reported.[378,640] Hepatomegaly is present in all types, but liver function is not impaired. In reported cases, serum aminotransferase levels and bromsulphalein excretion were normal. Grossly, the liver is firm, and cysts are not visible; microscopically, the liver shows cystic dilatation of ductules at the periphery of the portal zone, cystic Hering's ductules within lobules, and portal fibrosis that increases with age[640] (Fig. 41-48). Microdissection studies have shown that the hepatic cysts affect the Hering and interlobular ducts (ie, the terminal

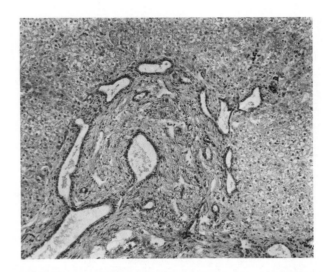

FIGURE 41-48   Infantile polycystic disease of the liver and kidneys. Characteristic features, shown here, include cystic dilatation of ductules located at the periphery of the portal area and portal fibrosis.

duct system), a finding parallel to the cystic dilation in the kidney, which involves the terminal branches of the collecting tubules.[612] The relation to the ductal plate malformation is unclear.[537] Portal hypertension may occur, but the manifestations of renal insufficiency predominate.[640]

CONGENITAL HEPATIC FIBROSIS

Congenital hepatic fibrosis, a recessive genetic disease, presents in later childhood with hepatomegaly, normal liver function, and portal hypertension with esophageal varices[573–575,612] (Fig. 41-49). There is a relatively characteristic histology— parenchymal lobules separated by broad bands of diffuse periportal or perilobular fibrous tissue. This often is associated with multiple distorted bile duct–like structures that do not connect to the biliary tract and portal vein anomalies. CHF has been associated with a wide variety of renal abnormalities, most commonly autosomal recessive polycystic kidney disease.[218,286,612,1039] Lesions resembling medullary sponge kidney disease of adults, in which segmental dilation of the bile ducts also occurs, have been reported in CHF; the identity of the two diseases is suggested despite the different clinical manifestations.[574] Recent reports have documented an association of CHF with autosomal dominant polycystic kidney disease; it was generally thought that CHF did not accompany this disease.[218,286,1039] Polycystic liver disease, with a different histologic picture, is commonly reported in autosomal dominant polycystic kidney disease.

Treatment of patients with CHF is directed at control of variceal hemorrhage, which may be managed by standard methods, including endoscopic sclerotherapy. These patients have basically normal liver function; therefore, after more severe recurrent hemorrhage, they are candidates for relief of portal hypertension by a portacaval anastomosis. The prognosis is good after a successful shunting procedure; however, survival in some patients may be limited by renal failure.

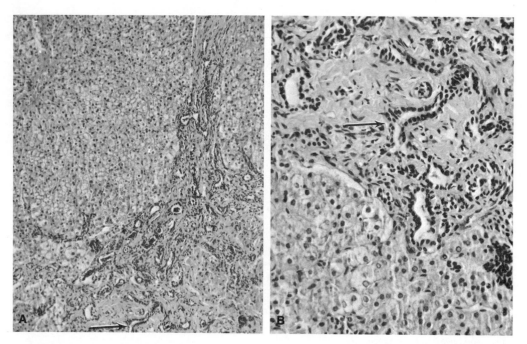

FIGURE 41-49   Congenital hepatic fibrosis, liver biopsy specimen in a patient 6 years of age. (**A**) Liver shows portal fibrosis and dilated cystic bile ductules (*arrow*) at the periphery of the lobule. (**B**) High-power view of the same ductule adjacent to normal liver parenchyma. Intravenous pyelogram was normal.

Progressive renal disease with pathologic features, namely nephrophthisis, which differs from IPCD, has been noted to occur in patients whose hepatic lesion resembles CHF.[1125] In these patients, the mortality due to renal disease is high.

Another diverse group of diseases in which hepatic cystic lesions are encountered includes the following[113,128,132,477,575,612,640,1125]:

Meckel's syndrome—characterized by encephalocele, polydactyly, and distinctive cystic renal disease

Jeune's syndrome (asphyxiating thoracic dystrophy)—characterized by skeletal dysplasia and late-onset renal disease

Secretory diarrhea—characterized by protein-losing enteropathy, enterocolitis cystica superficialis, intestinal lymphangiectasia, and CHF[802]

Miscellaneous disorders (vaginal atresia, Ellis–van Creveld syndrome, Ivemark's syndrome, and tuberous sclerosis)—characterized by hepatic ductular polycystic disease

CYSTIC DILATION OF THE INTRAHEPATIC BILE DUCTS (CAROLI'S DISEASE)

Cystic dilation of the intrahepatic bile ducts is a diverse spectrum of diseases that may include such variants as Caroli's disease, in which nonobstructive saccular dilation of the intrahepatic bile ducts, alternating with areas of stenosis, is present.[612,1125] Multiple segments of the biliary tract may be involved. The dilated intrahepatic biliary ducts, which are usually contiguous with the unaffected biliary system, are lined by typical cuboidal epithelium. The major complications include recurrent cholangitis with a predisposition to stone or abscess formation.

Cirrhosis

Cirrhosis is the end stage of many of the childhood liver diseases discussed previously.[460,748] Defining the cause of cirrhosis is of importance for genetic counseling, even if the severity of the lesion precludes specific treatment. Hepatic fibrosis has been documented to occur in infants born to alcoholic women (the fetal alcohol syndrome); the histologic lesion resembles adult alcoholic liver disease.[627] Management of the complications of cirrhosis is similar in children and adults. Cases of familial cirrhosis suggest the existence of other undefined infectious or metabolic diseases.[589]

PROGRESSIVE NEURONAL DEGENERATION AND CHILDHOOD CIRRHOSIS

This unique multisystem entity with degenerative disease of the cerebral gray matter was initially described in 1931 by Alpers[21]; subsequent reports documented the coexistence of cirrhosis.[459,510,747] The syndrome, transmitted in an autosomal recessive manner, is characterized by cerebral cortical degeneration leading to developmental delay, intractable seizures, and progressive neuromuscular deterioration.[21,459,747] The initial presentation may occur any time within the first 2 years of life with rapid progressive hypotonia, ataxia, seizures, vomiting, and failure to thrive. The liver disease, manifest as hepatomegaly, coagulopathy, and hypoalbuminemia, is often noted subsequently, raising the question whether anticonvulsant hepatotoxicity is the cause.[747] Death is usually due to hepatic failure. The hepatic histologic findings consist of microvesicular steatosis, lobular disarray, periportal inflammation, hepatocyte necrosis, bile duct proliferation, and cirrhosis. In the brain, astrocytic proliferation and spongy degeneration, with progressive involvement of deeper cortical layers and profound loss of neural cells, is noted. It is possible that this represents a specific metabolic disorder, such as a defect in mitochondrial or peroxisomal function.

INDIAN CHILDHOOD CIRRHOSIS

A unique familial form of cirrhosis, Indian childhood cirrhosis (ICC), confined primarily to the Indian subcontinent, affects Hindu children under the age of 3 years. ICC is progressive and results in hepatocellular failure and death.[538] Affected children present with hepatomegaly, abnormal stools, and behavioral changes, such as increased appetite, excessive irritability, and disturbed sleep patterns. Jaundice is uncommon; liver tissue obtained at an early stage reveals only vacuolization of hepatocytes, possibly with focal reticulum condensation. The disease progresses to an intermediate stage in which firm hepatomegaly, with splenomegaly and abdominal distention, occurs. Liver biopsy at this time shows progressive fibrosis. In the advanced stage, signs of liver failure dominate, with a histopathologic pattern of disorganized liver architecture, widespread necrosis with Mallory's hyaline bodies, and interstitial fibrosis with minimal evidence of regeneration. The suggestion of the proliferative nature of ICC has been complemented by the finding in serum and liver tissue of an oncodevelopmental protein, the Regan isoenzyme, which is a developmental phenotype of alkaline phosphatase isoenzyme.[788] Introduction of copper-contaminated milk feeding can explain the epidemiologic features and possibly the cause.[120,1030] Penicillamine therapy has been attempted.[1029]

HEPATIC COPPER OVERLOAD

Lefkowitch and coworkers[628] described four white American siblings who died in early childhood of an unknown form of cirrhosis. The children presented in the third to fourth year of life with progressive lethargy, abdominal swelling, jaundice, and fever. Hepatic histopathology resembled ICC—severe panlobular liver cell swelling, pericellular fibrosis, cirrhosis, and marked copper deposition. The authors[628] suggest that this represents a genetically determined disturbance in copper metabolism. Muller-Hocker and associates[738] described a progressive hepatic disease, resembling ICC and hepatic copper overload in American children, in three German children; two were siblings. The onset of symptoms was at 5 to 9 months of age; death occurred in two at 10 and 13 months. The liver biopsy in one was characterized by severe ballooning of hepatocytes, cell necrosis, Mallory body formation and venoocclusive changes. Micronodular cirrhosis was present in the two siblings. There was massive hepatic storage of copper. Copper intoxication in early life appeared to be causative. An unaffected sibling had not been exposed to copper-contaminated drinking water in the first 9 months of life.

BACTERIAL PERITONITIS

Spontaneous bacterial peritonitis, a well-recognized complication of cirrhosis in adults, has been documented with increasing frequency in children with cirrhosis and ascites. The illness is characterized by increased abdominal distention, fe-

ver and abdominal pain often with vomiting, and rapid progression of symptoms. Bowel sounds are reduced, and abdominal tenderness is apparent. The episode may precipitate encephalopathy. Leukocyte counts are elevated, and serum bilirubin and aminotransferase levels are also increased. The ascitic fluid contains an increased concentration of leukocytes, with polymorphonuclear leukocytes predominating. In a series by Larcher and coworkers,[613] *Streptococcus pneumoniae* was isolated in 8 of 12 episodes; *Klebsiella pneumoniae* and *Haemophilus influenzae* were noted in other cases. In this series, despite antibiotic therapy, 7 of the 11 patients died. Nevertheless, the importance of early diagnostic paracentesis, with early institution of therapy in hope of lowering the mortality rate, must be emphasized. In view of the high frequency of pneumococcal infection and the apparent association with complement deficiency, future studies should evaluate prophylactic use of pneumococcal vaccine and plasma infusion.

Fulminant Hepatic Failure

The causes and principles of management of children with fulminant hepatic failure in children parallel those reported in adults. There are, however, certain unique, age-related differences in liver metabolism and in etiology (Table 41-23) that require special attention when evaluating and treating liver failure in the pediatric population.[963] Fulminant hepatic failure may be the presenting feature not only of acute liver injury but also chronic liver disease that has remained quiescent for long periods of time.[888,963]

Tumors

Primary tumors of the liver and tumor-like lesions affecting the liver (Table 41-24) are discussed elsewhere in this text. These are uncommon in infants and children.[214,272,373,515,994,1102] Thus, only certain features of hepatic tumors unique to this age group are discussed here. About 60% to 70% of all hepatic masses found in children are of a malignant nature, especially in the male population. Solitary cysts, focal nodular hyperplasia, and hemangioendothelioma are more commonly found in females. The white/black ratio for all tumors is 10:1. The estimated incidence of malignant neoplasms in American white children under 15 years of age is 1.9 cases per million according to the Third National Cancer Survey.[1146] The major malignant tumors, hepatoblastoma and hepatocellular carcinoma, have an incidence of about 0.2 and 0.7 cases per million, respectively.

Hepatoblastoma usually appears in children younger than 2 years of age (60% of all cases) but may occur at any age.[516,675,994] The tumor is usually without symptoms and presents on routine examination as a progressively enlarging, nontender, nodular abdominal mass.[516,675,994] Liver function tests are normal, but 80% to 90% of patients have α-fetoprotein detectable in serum.[23,994] Most (80%) are single masses involving the right lobe. Associated findings were hemihypertrophy, macroglossia, and sexual precocity presumably due to ectopic gonadotropin production.[96,516,675] Microscopically, at least two patterns were noted—epithelial and mesenchymal. The epithelial elements consist of small, dark-staining, elongated embryonal-type cells and polyhed-

TABLE 41-23   *Age-Related Differential of Acute Hepatic Failure in the Pediatric Population*

***Early (<1 Week) Perinatal Period*[888]**
Herpes simplex[100]
Echovirus[118,734]
Hepatitis B[70]
Adenovirus
Perinatal hemochromatosis[585,944]

Late Perinatal Period
Tyrosinemia
Fructosemia (after introduction of sucrose- or fructose-containing feedings)
Galactosemia
Epstein-Barr virus
Zellweger's syndrome
Inborn errors of bile acid metabolism[61]
α_1-Antitrypsin deficiency[65,391,392]

Childhood/Adolescent Period

Viral Infection
Hepatitis A
Hepatitis B (with or without delta virus)
Hepatitis C
Hepatitis E
Hepatitis P (paramyovirus)[813]
Coxsackievirus
Leptospirosis

Drugs
Acetaminophen
Sodium valproate
Methyldopa

Toxins
Amanita phalloides
Phosphorus
Carbon tetrachloride

Metabolic Disorders
Wilson's disease
α_1-Antitrypsin deficiency
Hemochromatosis[271]

Vascular Insufficiency
Pericarditis
Myocarditis
Hypoperfusion and hypoxemia

Miscellaneous Disorders
Chronic hepatitis (fulminant presentation)[663]

TABLE 41-24   *Primary Hepatic Tumors and Tumor-Like Lesions of Infancy and Childhood*

Malignant Group
Tumors of hepatic cell origin (entodermal)
    Hepatoblastoma
        Epithelial
            Embryonal
            Fetal
            Mixed
    Hepatocellular carcinoma
    Cholangiocarcinoma
    Adenocarcinoma
Tumors of supporting structure (mesodermal)
    Angiosarcoma
    Rhabdomyosarcoma
    Mesenchymoma
    Myxosarcoma
    Fibrosarcoma
Secondary tumors
    Wilms' tumor
    Neuroblastoma

Benign Group
Tumor-like epithelial lesions
    Focal nodular hyperplasia
    Multiple nodular hyperplasia (with antecedent liver disease)
    Accessory lobe
Benign epithelial tumors
    Adenoma
    Adrenal rest tumor
Cysts and tumor-like mesenchymal lesions
    Mesenchymal hamartoma
    Nonparasitic cyst
Benign mesenchymal tumors
    Cavernous hemangioma
    Infantile hemangioendothelioma
    Lymphangioma
    Fibroma
Teratomas

(Modified from Edmondson HA. Differential diagnosis of tumor and tumor-like lesions in infancy and children. Ann Surg 142:214, 1955)

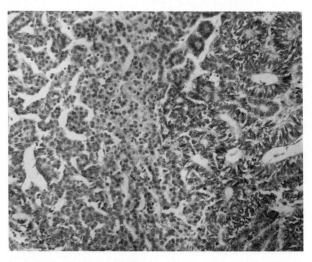

FIGURE 41-50   Hepatoblastoma. Tissue present in the right half of this biopsy section contains *embryonal*-type cells with rosette formation; the left half contains typical *fetal*-type cells.

ral, glycogen-containing, larger fetal-type cells that form canalicular and sinusoidal complexes (Fig. 41-50). The mesenchymal element may be represented by fibrous connective tissue, osteoid, and cartilage. Aggressive surgery, with hepatic lobectomy after multidrug chemotherapy to shrink local masses, is the treatment of choice; these tumors are resistant to radiation and chemotherapy. Liver transplantation should be considered for nonmetastatic unresectable hepatoblastoma.[592]

Hepatocellular carcinoma usually occurs in people over 3 years of age, who often have a cirrhotic liver in the presence of α_1-AT deficiency, tyrosinemia, and HBV infection.[200,994,1103] It also presents as an abdominal mass (75%), and abdominal pain is frequent (67%). Microscopically, the tumor is identical to the adult type of carcinoma of the liver.[555] Total excision offers the only chance of survival.

Benign tumors include hamartoma, cavernous hemangioma, focal nodular hyperplasia, and infantile hemangioendothelioma.[199,325,994] Although most cases of *focal nodular hyperplasia* are noted during the third to fifth decades, about 10% present in the first 15 years of life, most frequently between 6 and 10 years of age.[994] There is a clear female predominance.[994] The tumor is usually asymptomatic and discovered incidentally, but it has been detected during serial monitoring of patients with GSD type I.[994] Ultrasonography may demonstrate focal nodular hyperplasia, documenting the echogenic central core and surrounding areas of low amplitude echoes.[994] Selective angiography displays the hypervascular mass. Diagnostic imaging may be of help in diagnosis since radionucleotide uptake, which is decreased in most liver tumors, is normal in patients with focal nodular hyperplasia.

Mesenchymal hamartoma is a benign multicystic lesion, consisting of loose mesenchymal tissue containing small bile ducts and variable sizes of unlined spaces filled with serous fluid.[849,994] Cystic mesenchymal hamartoma typically occurs in boys younger than 2 years of age. Affected patients usually present with asymptomatic abdominal enlargement or an abdominal mass. In infancy, the abdominal mass may lead to respiratory distress. The cystic nature of the lesion can be documented by ultrasonography, computed tomography, or magnetic resonance imaging (Fig. 41-51). Microscopically, there are irregular strands of biliary epithelium in a myoid stoma. Mesenchymal hamartoma may represent a developmental anomaly rather than a true neoplasm. Resection of the lesion with drainage of the cyst and marsupialization of the walls is curative.

Hemangioma is the most frequent benign tumor of the liver in childhood; most of these tumors are asymptomatic.[199,325]

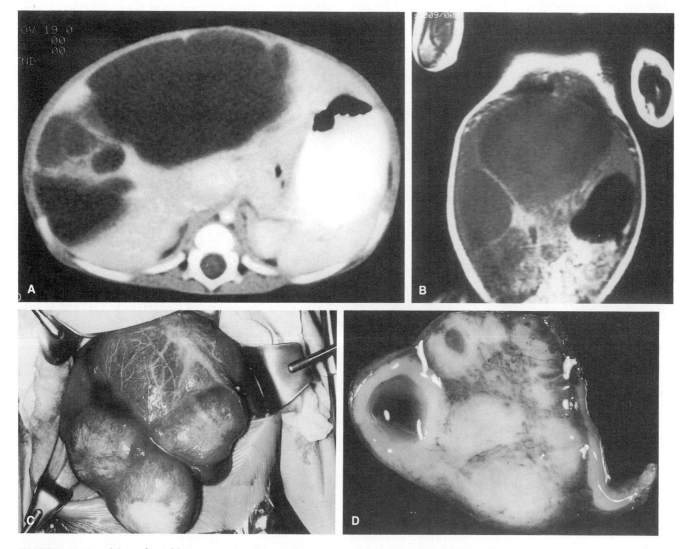

FIGURE 41-51   Mesenchymal hamartoma in a 10-month-old infant with hepatomegaly. (**A**) Axial CT images show multiloculated cysts of varying sizes in both lobes of the liver. Some cysts have sharply defined walls, while others are less well defined. (**B**) Coronal T1-weighted image shows global extent of low-density cysts. (**C**) Preresection multiloculated cysts. (**D**) Resected, transected cyst.

Hemangioendothelioma is frequently associated with multiple strawberry hemangiomas. There is a 2:1 female predominance. The tumor often involves the entire liver and, grossly, produces solitary or multiple red-purple to gray pulsatile, nonencapsulated nodules of various sizes, which have been mistaken for metastatic neuroblastoma.[252,863,982] Microscopically, the lesion has highly cellular endothelial-lined channels (angiosarcoma-like; Fig. 41-52). Although histologically benign, there are possible life-threatening complications. The classic presentation includes the triad of congestive failure in the absence of heart disease, hepatomegaly with a systolic bruit over the liver due to arteriovenous fistulas and cutaneous hemangiomas, often with thrombocytopenia; however, isolated hepatomegaly is the most common presentation. In a series described by McLean,[690] there was a high (70%) mortality rate, due in most cases to severe high-output cardiac failure. Recent series report much lower mortality rates. Initial evaluation should include sonography of the abdomen; the diagnosis can be confirmed by angiography or computed tomography[803,1046] (Fig. 41-53). Localized lesions, if symptomatic, can be resected with care because of a risk of hypotensive complications.[1091] In diffuse disease (or if the patient's condition prohibits surgery), treatment with prednisone, diuretics, and digoxin should be used initially. Surgery may then be performed safely in 10 to 14 days. Confirmation of the lesion must first be obtained by open biopsy of nodules.[183,880] Hepatic artery ligation or embolization of the lesion has replaced radiation therapy. Treatment should be vigorous because complete regression and cure are possible. Cavernous hemangioma is rare and presents as a mass lesion to be distinguished from other tumors only at laparotomy.[322] Surgical resection should be attempted since rupture with fatal intraperitoneal hemorrhage is frequent.[322,832]

Neuroblastoma may present after widespread metastasis, especially in infancy. All patients with liver tumors, therefore, should have catecholamine studies, ultrasound, computed tomography, and renal imaging performed before surgery. There is a high rate of spontaneous regression in infants with stage IV disease. If bone metastasis has not occurred, a high cure rate can be expected with removal of the primary tumor and radiation therapy to the liver.[804]

Portal Hypertension

Portal hypertension in infants and children can occur as a result of obstruction to flow at several sites, with a disease spectrum similar to that seen in adults. There are, however, several unique features of portal hypertension as it occurs in the pediatric age group.

EXTRAHEPATIC (PRESINUSOIDAL) BLOCK

Extrahepatic (presinusoidal) block, as is seen in cavernous transformation of the portal vein, is more commonly seen in children than in adults.[28,705,932,1100] Portal hypertension may be manifest by splenomegaly with or without hypersplenism, hematemesis, or ascites. A predisposing illness, such as intraabdominal sepsis, omphalitis, or dehydration, can be documented in up to 40% of cases. Variceal bleeding has been reported as a late complication of neonatal umbilical vein catheterization; however, the true incidence of this sequela is unknown.[619] The occurrence of congenital anomalies—cardiovascular and biliary malformations—in some cases of idiopathic extrahepatic block suggests that a developmental defect underlies the association.[767] Hematemesis is the most common presentation, and ascites occurs in about 35% of children, an incidence that is lower than that in adults. Diagnosis is by ultrasound or angiography and by exclusion of liver disease by appropriate function tests, liver biopsy, and screening for known causes of cirrhosis. This is followed by attempts to visualize the portal vein anatomy and the varices (Fig. 41-54A). Direct splenoportography may result in significant hemorrhage and require immediate splenectomy and shunting. In the young child, this may produce a suboptimal shunt, less than 1 cm in diameter, which may subsequently undergo thrombosis.

In review of 69 patients with extrahepatic portal venous obstruction, Fonkalsrud and coworkers[369] documented 338 episodes of bleeding. This and several other series, however, have suggested that portal-system shunting is often avoidable in this condition. Advocates of a conservative approach have emphasized that (1) the initial episode is rarely life-threatening and has a low mortality rate; (2) there is a decreased frequency of bleeding with age, and in many patients, bleeding has been noted to cease spontaneously; (3) shunts undertaken at a young age have poor long-term patency rates, often requiring multiple revisions after the initial operative procedure[369,1100]; and (4) there is a higher long-term mortality rate and possible adverse neuropsychiatric consequences in

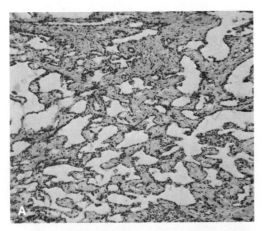

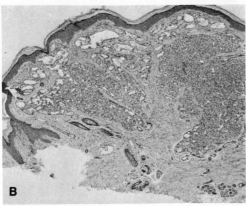

FIGURE 41-52 (A) Hemangioendothelioma, liver. (B) Strawberry skin hemangioma from same patient. The liver lesion, part of a gray nodule obtained at laparotomy, contains multiple cellular endothelium-lined channels similar to those of the skin lesion.

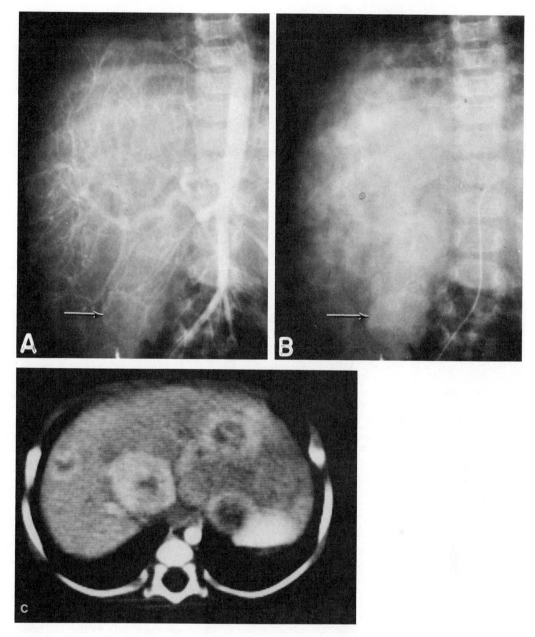

FIGURE 41-53 Hemangioendothelioma, aortogram. (**A**) Arterial phase shows increased liver vascularity and stretching of small arteries around the hemangiomatous nodules (*arrow*). (**B**) Late phase shows similar-sized, multiple large nodules retaining contrast material (*arrow*). (**C**) Three-month-old girl with hepatomegaly in whom ultrasonography demonstrated multiple, intrahepatic, echo-free nodules. CT examination of the abdomen with rapid bolus injection of contrast material revealed nodular densities with a donut-like appearance, subsequently shown to represent hemangioendothelioma.

those subjected to shunt procedures.[15] Despite a concern for the physiologic consequences of portal diversion, sequelae are uncommon in patients with normal liver function. Variceal bleeding usually responds to nasogastric lavage and transfusion of fresh blood. Vasopressin (Pitressin) may be infused intravenously if necessary; sclerotherapy is highly effective.[494,736] Balloon tamponade is rarely needed. When a definitive shunt procedure is needed after repeated hemorrhagic episodes, it should be delayed until late childhood. There is a high incidence of shunt thrombosis if the patient is under

10 years of age or if the portovenous anastomosis is less than 10 mm in diameter. A standard end-to-side portacaval shunt often cannot be constructed. In these patients, the portal vein usually is free of thrombosis for a distance of 1.5 to 2 cm beyond the junction of the superior mesenteric and splenic vein, and it is possible to anastomose this segment end-to-side to the vena cava or to the central portion of the left renal vein.[674] Alvarez and coworkers[28] have advocated a more aggressive approach. They have demonstrated that a portal diversion procedure can be successful in young patients with

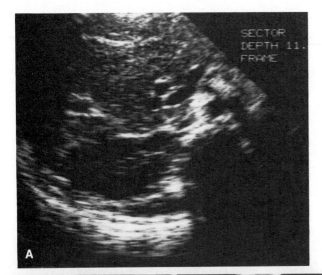

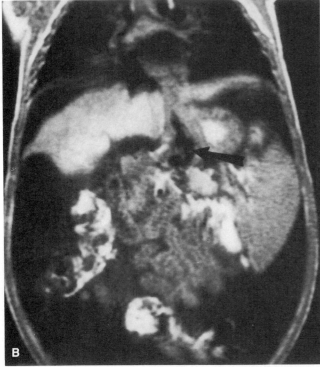

FIGURE 41-54 (**A**) A 15-month-old boy presenting with splenomegaly. Ultrasound examination (transverse scan) demonstrates round echolucent structures in the hilum of the liver corresponding to collateral vessels. (**B**) A 4-month-old child with α_1-antitrypsin deficiency. T1-weighted coronal MRI scan demonstrates small nodular liver, massive ascites, prominent esophageal varices (*arrow*), and splenomegaly.

portal vein thrombosis; adverse sequelae were minimal in their series. Greater than 90% of shunts in their series remained patent.

INTRAHEPATIC (SINUSOIDAL) BLOCK

Portal hypertension may be associated with CHF or cystic disease of the liver in which liver function is apparently normal despite hepatomegaly and variceal bleeding[573,575] (see

Fig. 41-54*B*). If, as in adults, cirrhosis underlies the altered flow, the nature of the primary disease should be established since treatment may improve hepatic function in certain metabolic diseases, such as Wilson's disease, and genetic counseling can be accomplished. In patients with recurrent bleeding refractory to sclerotherapy, esophageal transection with paraesophagogastric devascularization may be safe and effective. In contrast to patients with extrahepatic block, this group may derive significant benefit from a shunt procedure.[25] The distal splenorenal shunt for selective decompression of the esophageal plexus with maintenance of portal venous flow has been employed successfully in children.[866]

POSTSINUSOIDAL BLOCK

Postsinusoidal block (suprahepatic obstruction) is rare in the pediatric group but may occur as a primary or secondary phenomenon and should be ruled out in children with unexplained hepatomegaly and ascites. Hepatic vein occlusion most often is associated with vasculitis, sickle cell anemia, polycythemia, leukemia, or tumor masses obliterating the lumen. The obstruction may occur at any level above the liver up to and including the heart, as in heart failure or constrictive pericarditis (Fig. 41-55). Primary pulmonary hypertension may present as suprahepatic portal hypertension.

Membranous obstruction of the inferior vena cava at the level of the diaphragm may cause a Budd-Chiari–like syndrome.[184] This entity is successfully treated by transcardiac membranotomy. Occlusion of central and sublobular hepatic veins by intimal fibrosis or edema or by venoocclusive disease in association with immunodeficiency has been well recognized.[694] We have noted occlusive disease of the hepatic venous outflow pathway in patients who are bone marrow transplant recipients, in hypervitaminosis A, and in infants who received an intravenous vitamin E supplement.[144]

Gentil-Kocher and colleagues[387] reviewed 22 cases of Budd-Chiari syndrome in children; 3 patients presented with refractory ascites, all others had firm hepatomegaly. Liver tests were normal. The diagnosis was suggested by ultrasound or biopsy and confirmed by angiography, which demonstrated partial or total obstruction of the hepatic veins. In only 5 of the 22 cases was a cause identified (liver tumor, hepatic vein malformation, and 3 with membranous obstruction). Eighteen patients underwent shunt surgery (mesocaval or mesoatrial); in the 13 survivors, follow-up biopsies demonstrated disappearance or regression of centrilobular hemorrhagic infiltration.

Liver Transplantation

The development of improved methods of immune suppression, organ preservation, and surgical technology have made liver transplantation a realistic therapeutic option for an increasing number of pediatric patients with end-stage liver disease.[10,182,341,1114] The remaining factor that limits widespread application and prevents access by all pediatric candidates to transplantation is the scarcity of adequate size-matched donor organs. This is compounded by the fact that the most common indication for liver transplantation in the pediatric population is biliary atresia; in these patients, liver replacement is most often required at a very young age and small size in view of the rapid progression of the hepatic disease and poor nutritional status.[10,890,891] This creates an epidemiologic dis-

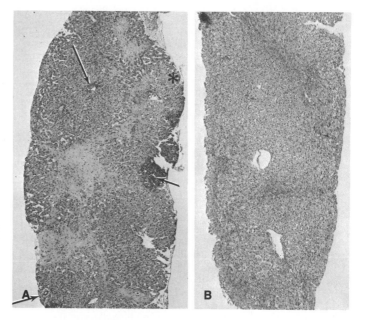

FIGURE 41-55 Suprahepatic venous obstruction. An infant aged 6 months had constrictive pericarditis with protein-losing enteropathy. (**A**) Liver biopsy shows three portal tracts (*arrows*), ectasia of sinusoids and central veins (*asterisk*), and fibrosis around other central veins. (**B**) Biopsy specimen 6 months after pericardiectomy shows resolution of the connective tissue and normal sinusoids.

parity since most pediatric donors are of school age or older. Consequently, there may be an increased death rate in pediatric patients awaiting liver transplantation; alternatively, suboptimal donor organs may be accepted in a desperate attempt to address recipient needs.[891] Recent studies have suggested that the use of segmental orthotopic hepatic transplantation is an effective strategy to improve patient survival and decrease waiting-list mortality.[890] Since the institution of segmental transplantation at Cincinnati Children's Hospital Medical Center, no child has died while awaiting donor organ availability, the incidence of hepatic artery thrombosis has been reduced, and segmental liver transplantation survival has been equivalent to that of whole-organ graft recipients.[890,891] These results suggest that successful liver transplantation may be available to a greater number of pediatric candidates with end-stage liver disease.

Acknowledgments

This original work was supported by National Institutes of Health Grant RR00123 (General Clinical Research Centers Program, Division of Research Resources, NIH, FDA Grant FD-R-000357-03), and the Pediatric Liver Care Center, Children's Hospital Medical Center. The invaluable assistance of Drs. George Hug, Janet E. Strife, Kevin E. Bove, Cynthia Daugherty, and Fred Ryckman, and of Patti Gubser and Anthony Balistreri of the Children's Hospital Research Foundation is acknowledged.

References

1. Aagenaes O. Hereditary recurrent cholestasis with lymphoedema: two new families. Acta Paediatr Scand 63:465, 1974
2. Aagenaes O, et al. Hereditary neonatal cholestasis combined with vascular malformations. In: Berenberg SR, ed. Liver diseases in infancy and childhood. Baltimore, Williams & Wilkins, 1976, pp 199–206
3. Abad-Lacruz A, Gonzalez-Huix F, Esteve M, et al. Liver function test abnormalities in patients with inflammatory bowel disease receiving artificial nutrition: a prospective randomized study of total enteral nutrition vs. total parenteral nutrition. J Parenter Enter Nutr 14:618–621, 1990
4. Abramov A, et al. Generalized xanthomatosis with calcified adrenals. Am J Dis Child 91:282, 1956
5. Adamson GM, Papadimitriou JM, Harman AW. Postnatal mice have low susceptibility to paracetamol toxicity. Pediatr Res 29:496–499, 1991
6. Agati G, Fusi F. New trends in photobiology: recent advances in bilirubin photophysics. J Photochem Photobiol [B] 7:1–4, 1990
7. Ahlfors CE, Bennett SH, Shoemaker CT, et al. Changes in the auditory brainstem response associated with intravenous infusion of unconjugated bilirubin into infant rhesus monkeys. Pediatr Res 20:511–515, 1986
8. Ahlfors CE, DiBiasio-Erwin D. Rate constants for dissociation of bilirubin from its binding sites in neonatal (cord) and adult sera. J Pediatr 108:295–298, 1986
9. Ahrens EH Jr, et al. Atresia of the intrahepatic bile ducts. Pediatrics 8:628, 1951
10. A-Kader HH, Ryckman FC, Balistreri WF. Liver transplantation in the pediatric population: indications and monitoring. Clin Transplant 5:161–167, 1991
11. A-Kader HH, Zeldis JB, Kuramoto IK, Balistreri WF. Hepatitis C serology (anti-HCV) in patients with neonatal cholestasis (neonatal hepatitis and extrahepatic biliary atresia). Hepatology 12:844, 1990
12. Akerren Y. Prolonged jaundice in newborn associated with congenital myxedema. Acta Paediatr 43:411, 1954
13. Alagille D. Cholestasis in the first three months of life. In: Popper H, Schaffner F, eds. Progress in liver disease. New York, Grune & Stratton, 1979, p 471
14. Alagille D, et al. Hepatic ductular hypoplasia associated with characteristic facies, vertebral malformations, retarded physical, mental, and sexual development, and cardiac murmur. J Pediatr 86:63, 1975
15. Alagille D, Carlier JC, Chiva M, et al. Long-term neuropsychological outcome in children undergoing portal-systemic shunts for portal vein obstruction without liver disease. J Pediatr Gastroenterol Nutr 5:861–866, 1986
16. Alagille D, Estrada A, Hadchouel M, Gautier M, Odievre M, Dommergues JP. Syndromic paucity of interlobular bile ducts (Alagille syndrome or arteriohepatic dysplasia): review of 80 cases. J Pediatr 110:195–200, 1987
17. Alford CA Jr, et al. Subclinical central nervous system dis-

ease of neonates: a prospective study of infants born with increased levels of IgM. J Pediatr 75:1167, 1969

18. Alonso EM, Whitington PF, Whitington SH, Rivard WA, Given G. Enterohepatic circulation of nonconjugated bilirubin in rats fed with human milk. J Pediatr 118:425–430, 1991

19. Alonso EM, Zdunek TM, Brown MR, Yousefzadeh DK, Whitington PF. Fibroinflammatory tumor of the liver causing biliary cirrhosis in an infant. J Pediatr Gastroenterol Nutr 12:283–287, 1991

20. Alonso-Lej, et al. Congenital choledochal duct cyst, with a report of 2, and an analysis of 94 cases. Int Abstr Surg 108:1, 1959

21. Alpers BJ. Diffuse degeneration of the cerebral grey matter. Neurol Psychiatr 25:469, 1931

22. Alpert LI, et al. Neonatal hepatitis associated with trisomy 17–18 syndrome. N Engl J Med 280:16, 1969

23. Alpert ME, et al. Alpha-1-fetoglobulin in the diagnosis of human hepatoma. N Engl J Med 278:984, 1968

24. Altman RP. The portoenterostomy procedure for biliary atresia: a five year experience. Ann Surg 188:351, 1978

25. Altman RP, Potter BM. Portal decompression in infants and children with the interposition mesocaval shunt. Am J Surg 135:65, 1978

26. Altshuler G. Toxoplasmosis as a cause of hydranencephaly: case report including a description of the placenta. Am J Dis Child 125:251, 1973

27. Altshuler G, McAdams AJ. The role of the placenta in fetal and perinatal pathology. Am J Obstet Gynecol 113:616, 1972

28. Alvarez F, et al. Portal obstruction in children. I. Clinical investigation and hemorrhage risk. II. Results of surgical portosystemic shunts. J Pediatr 103:696, 703, 1983

29. Ambruso DR, et al. Infectious and bleeding complications in patients with glycogenosis Ib. Am J Dis Child 139:691, 1985

30. Amedee-Manesme O, Bernard O, Brunelle F, et al. Sclerosing cholangitis with neonatal onset. J Pediatr 111:225–229, 1987

31. Amendt BA, Rhead WJ. Catalytic defect of medium-chain acylco-enzyme A dehydrogenase deficiency: lack of both cofactor responsiveness and biochemical heterogeneity in eight patients. J Clin Invest 76:963, 1985

32. Amit Y, Chan G, Fedunec M, Poznansky J, Schiff D. Bilirubin toxicity in a neuroblastoma cell line N-115. I. Effects on Na$^+$K$^+$ ATPase, (^{3}H)-thymidine uptake, L-(^{35}S)-methionine incorporation, and mitochondrial function. Pediatr Res 25:364–368, 1989

33. Anad F, Burn J, Matthews D, et al. Alagille syndrome and deletion of 20p. J Med Genet 27:729–737, 1990

34. Anand A, Gray ES, Brown T, Clewley JP, Cohen BT. Human parvovirus infection in pregnancy and hydrops fetalis. N Engl J Med 316:183–186, 1987

35. Andersen B, Zierz S, Jungermann K. Perinatal development of the distributions of phosphoenolypyruvate carboxykinase and succinate dehydrogenase in rat liver parenchyma. Eur J Cell Biol 30:126–131, 1983

36. Andersen DH. Cystic fibrosis of the pancreas and its relation to celiac disease. Am J Dis Child 56:344–399, 1938

37. Andres JM. Frequency and characteristics of hyperbilirubinemia associated with bacteremia. J Pediatr Gastroenterol Nutr 7:149, 1988

38. Andres JM, et al. Liver disease in infants. I. Developmental hepatology and mechanisms of liver function. J Pediatr 90:686, 1977

39. Aprille JR. Reye's syndrome: patient serum alters mitochondrial function and morphology in vitro. Science 197:908, 1977

40. Arasu TS, et al. Management of chronic aggressive hepatitis in children and adolescents. J Pediatr 95:514, 1979

41. Arias IM. Chronic unconjugated hyperbilirubinemia without overt signs of hemolysis in adolescents and adults. J Clin Invest 41:2233, 1962

42. Arias IM, Gartner LM. Breast-milk jaundice. Br Med J 4:177, 1970

43. Arias IM, Jansen P. Protein binding and conjugation of bilirubin in the liver cell. In: Goresky CA, Fischer MM, eds. Jaundice. New York, Plenum Press, 1975, pp 175–188

44. Arias IM, et al. Chronic nonhemolytic unconjugated hyperbilirubinemia with glycuronyl transferase deficiency: clinical, biochemical, pharmacologic and genetic evidence for heterogeneity. Am J Med 47:395, 1969

45. Arias IM, et al. Prolonged neonatal unconjugated hyperbilirubinemia associated with breast feeding and a steroid (pregnane-3-α, 20-β-diol), in maternal milk that inhibits glucuronide formation in vitro. J Clin Invest 43:2037, 1964

46. Arias IM, et al. Transient familial neonatal hyperbilirubinemia. J Clin Invest 44:1442, 1965

47. Arrowsmith JB, Kennedy DL, Kuritsky JN, et al. National patterns of aspirin use and Reye's syndrome reporting, United States, 1980 to 1985. Pediatrics 79:888, 1987

48. Arrowsmith WA, et al. Comparison of treatments for congenital nonobstructive nonhemolytic hyperbilirubinemia. Arch Dis Child 50:197, 1975

49. Arthur AB, Wilson BDR. Urinary infection presenting with jaundice. Br Med J 1:539, 1967

50. Asano Y, Yoshikawa T, Suga S, Yazaki T, Kondo K, Yamanshi K: Fatal fulminant hepatitis in an infant with human herpesvirus-6 infection. Lancet 335:862–863, 1990

51. Avery ME, et al. Transient tyrosinemia of the newborn. Pediatrics 38:378, 1967

52. Aynsley-Green A, et al. Hepatic glycogen synthetase deficiency: definition of the syndrome from metabolic and enzyme studies on a nine year old girl. Arch Dis Child 52:573, 1977

53. Back P, Walter K. Developmental pattern of bile acid metabolism as revealed by bile acid analysis of meconium. Gastroenterology 78:671, 1980

54. Baerlocher K, et al. Hereditary fructose intolerance in early childhood: a major diagnostic challenge. Helv Paediatr Acta 33:465, 1978

55. Bailey PV, Connors RH, Tracy TF, Sotelo-Avila C, Lewis JE, Weber TR. Changing spectrum of cholelithiasis and cholecystitis in infants and children. Am J Surg 158:585–588, 1989

56. Bain MD, Purkiss P, Jones M, Bingham P, Stacey TE, Chalmers RA. Dietary treatment eliminates succinylacetone from the urine of a patient with tyrosinaemia type 1. Eur J Pediatr 149:637–639, 1990

57. Baker AL, Rosenberg IH. Hepatic complications of total parenteral nutrition. Am J Med 82:489–497, 1987

58. Baker L, Winegrad AI. Fasting hypoglycaemia and metabolic acidosis associated with deficiency of hepatic fructose-1,6-diphosphatase activity. Lancet 2:13, 1970

59. Balazs M. Electron microscopic examination of congenital cytomegalovirus hepatitis. Virchows Arch Pathol Anat 405:119, 1984

60. Balistreri WF. Anatomic and biochemical ontogeny of the gastrointestinal tract and liver. In: Tsang RC, Nichols BL, eds. Nutrition during infancy. Philadelphia, Hanley & Belfus, 1987, pp 33–57

61. Balistreri WF. Fetal and bile acid synthesis and metabolism: clinical implications. J Inherit Metab Dis 14:459–477, 1991

62. Balistreri WF. Neonatal cholestasis: lessons from the past, issues for the future. (Foreword) Semin Liver Dis 7, 1987

63. Balistreri WF. Idiopathic Reye's syndrome and its metabolic mimickers. In: Balistreri WF, Stocker JT, eds. Pediatric hepatology. Washington, DC, Hemisphere, 1990, pp 183–202

64. Balistreri WF. Interrelationship between the infantile cholangiopathies and paucity of the intrahepatic bile ducts. In:

Balistreri WF, Stocker JT, eds. Pediatric hepatology. Washington, DC, Hemisphere, 1990, pp 1–18

65. Balistreri WF. Liver disease associated with α_1-antitrypsin deficiency. In: Balistreri WF, Stocker JT, eds. Pediatric hepatology. Washington, DC, Hemisphere, 1990, pp 159–176

66. Balistreri WF. Neonatal cholestasis: medical progress. J Pediatr 106:171, 1985

67. Balistreri WF. Spectrum of liver disease in patients with cystic fibrosis. Pediatr Pulmonol S5:71–73, 1990

68. Balistreri WF. Viral hepatitis: implications to pediatric practice. In: Barness LA, ed. Advances in pediatrics. Chicago, Year Book Medical Pub, 1985, pp 287–320

69. Balistreri WF. The effects of liver disease on nutrition and growth. In: Cohen SA, ed. The underweight infant, child, and adolescent. Norwalk CT, Appleton-Century-Crofts, 1986, pp 121–130

70. Balistreri WF. Viral hepatitis. Pediatr Clin North Am 35:375–407, 637–689, 1988

71. Balistreri WF, A-Kader HH, Ryckman FC, Whitington PF, Heubi JE, Setchell KD. Biochemical and clinical response to ursodeoxycholic acid administration in pediatric patients with chronic cholestasis. In: Proceedings of XI International Bile Acid Meeting: bile acids as therapeutic agents. Lancaster, UK, Kluwer, 1991, pp 323–333

72. Balistreri WF, Bove K. Hepatobiliary consequences of parenteral nutrition. In: Progress in liver disease, vol 9. 1989, pp 567–601

73. Balistreri WF, Bove K. Primary sclerosing cholangitis and related hepatobiliary lesions. In: Balistreri WF, Vanderhoof J, eds: Pediatric gastroenterology. London, Chapman Hall, 1990, pp 196–123

74. Balistreri WF, Farrell MK, Bove KE. Lessons from the E-ferol[R] tragedy. Pediatrics 78:503–506, 1986

75. Balistreri WF, Fjellstedt TA, Go VLW, et al. Mechanisms and management of pediatric hepatobiliary disease: a report of a conference. J Pediatr Gastroenterol Nutr 10:138–147, 1990

76. Balistreri WF, Hofmann AF, A-Kader HH, Setchell KDR. Successful bile acid therapy in 3 siblings with neonatal hepatitis due to an inborn error of bile acid biosynthesis. Pediatr Res 29:99A, 1991

77. Balistreri WF, Setchell KDR. Clinical implications of bile acid metabolism. In: Silverberg M, Daum F, eds. Textbook of pediatric gastroenterology. Chicago, Year Book Medical Publ, 1987, pp 72–89

78. Balistreri WF, Sokol RJ. Nutritional consequences of chronic cholestasis in childhood: vitamin E deficiency. In: Proceedings of Falk Symposium No. 41 on Nutrition. Freiburg, Germany, MTP Press Limited, 1985, pp 181–189

79. Balistreri WF, et al. Absence of an association between hepatitis A or B virus and biliary atresia or neonatal hepatitis. Pediatrics 66:269, 1980

80. Balistreri WF, et al. Immaturity of the enterohepatic circulation in early life: factors predisposing to "physiologic" maldigestion and cholestasis. J Pediatr Gastroenterol Nutr 2:346, 1983

81. Balistreri WF, et al. Bile salt sulfotransferase: alterations during maturation and non-inducibility during substrate ingestion. J Lipid Res 25:228, 1984

82. Balistreri WF, et al. Immaturity of the enterohepatic circulation of bile acids in early life: factors responsible for increased peripheral serum bile acid concentrations. In: Proceedings of Falk Symposium No. 42, Eighth International Bile Acid Meeting. Berne, Switzerland, MTP Press Limited, 1985, pp 87–93

83. Barlow B, et al. Choledochal cyst: a review of 19 cases. J Pediatr 89:934, 1976

84. Barrett MJ, Hurwitz ES, Schonenberger LB, et al. Changing epidemiology of Reye syndrome in the United States. Pediatrics 77:598, 1986

85. Barton NW, Furbish FS, Murray GJ, Garfield M, Brady RO. Therapeutic response to intravenous infusions of glucocerebrosidase in a patient with Gaucher disease. Proc Nat Acad Sci 87:1913–1916, 1990 (see also: N Engl J Med 324:1464–1470, 1991)

86. Barudhuin P, et al. An electron microscopic and biochemical study of type II glycogenosis. Lab Invest 13:1139, 1964

87. Bathurst JC, Travis J, George PM, et al. Structural and functional characterization of the abnormal Z α_1-antitrypsin isolated from human liver. FEBS Lett 177:179, 1984

88. Batshaw ML, Msall M, Beaudet AL, Trojak J. Risk of serious illness in heterozygotes for ornithine transcarbamylase deficiency. J Pediatr 108:236–241, 1986

89. Beale EF, et al. Intrahepatic cholestasis associated with parenteral nutrition in premature infants. Pediatrics 64:342, 1979

90. Beasley RP, et al. Efficacy of hepatitis B immune globulin (HBIG) for prevention of perinatal transmission of the hepatitis B virus carrier state: final report of a randomized double-blind placebo-controlled trial. Hepatology 3:135, 1983

91. Beasley RP, et al. Prevention of perinatally transmitted hepatitis B virus infections with hepatitis B immune globulin and hepatitis B vaccine. Lancet 2:1099, 1983

92. Beasley RP, et al. The e antigen and vertical transmission of hepatitis B surface antigen. Am J Epidemiol 105:94, 1977

93. Beau P, Chammartin F, Matuchansky C. Biological hepatic abnormalities, cholestatic jaundice and hospital artificial nutrition: a comparative study in adults with cyclic total parenteral nutrition and enteral nutrition. Gastroenterol Clin Biol 12:326–331, 1988

94. Beaudet AL, et al. Neutropenia and impaired neutrophil migration in type Ib glycogen storage disease. J Pediatr 97:906, 1980

95. Beckett RS, Flynn FJ Jr. Toxoplasmosis: report of two new cases, with classification and with demonstration of organisms in human placenta. N Engl J Med 249:345, 1953

96. Behrle FC, et al. Virilization accompanying hepatoblastoma. Pediatrics 32:265, 1963

97. Belknap WM, Zimmer-Nechemias L, Sucy FJ, Balistreri WF. Bile acid efflux from suckling hepatocytes. Pediatric Res 23:364–367, 1988

98. Belknap WM, et al. Physiologic cholestasis. II. Serum bile acid levels reflect the development of the enterohepatic circulation in rats. Hepatology 1:613, 1981

99. Bell H, Schrumpf E, Fagerhol MK. Heterozygous MZ alpha-1-antitrypsin deficiency in adults with chronic liver disease. Scand J Gastroenterol 25:788–792, 1990

100. Benador N, Mannhardt W, Schranz D, et al. Three cases of neonatal herpes simplex virus infection presenting as fulminant hepatitis. Eur J Pediatrs 149:555–559, 1990

101. Bendeck JL, Noguchi A. Age-related changes in the adrenergic control of glycogenolysis in rat liver: the significance of changes in receptor density. Pediatr Res 19:862, 1985

102. Benett I, Salh B, Haboubi NY. Sclerosing cholangitis with hepatic microvesicular steatosis in cystic fibrosis and chronic pancreatitis. J Clin Pathol 42:466–469, 1989

103. Bengoa JM, Hanauer SB, Sitrin MD, et al. Pattern and prognosis of liver function test abnormalities during parenteral nutrition in inflammatory bowel disease. Hepatology 5:79–84, 1985

104. Benjamin DR. Cholelithiasis in infants: the role of total parenteral nutrition and gastrointestinal dysfunction. J Pediatr Surg 17:386–389, 1982

105. Benjamin DR. Hepatobiliary dysfunction in infants and children associated with long-term total parenteral nutrition: a clinicopathologic study. Am J Clin Pathol 76:276, 1981

106. Beratis NG, et al. Characterization of the molecular defect in infantile and adult acid alpha-glucosidase deficiency fibroblasts. J Clin Invest 62:1264, 1978

107. Berenberg W, Nankervis G. Long-term follow up of cytomegalic inclusion disease. Pediatrics 46:403, 1970

108. Berg NO, Eriksson S. Liver disease in adults with alpha$_1$-antitrypsin deficiency. N Engl J Med 287:1264–1267, 1972

109. Berglund L, Angelin B, Blomstrand R, et al. Sn-protophorphyrin lowers serum bilirubin levels, decreases biliary bilirubin output, enhances biliary heme excretion and potently inhibits hepatic heme oxygenase activity in normal human subjects. Hepatology 8:625–631, 1988

110. Berk PD, et al. Inborn errors of bilirubin metabolism. Med Clin North Am 59:803, 1975

111. Berkovich S, Smithwick EM. Transplacental infection due to ECHO virus type 22. J Pediatr 72:94, 1968

112. Bernard O, Hadchouel M, Scotto J, Odievre M, Alagille D. Severe giant cell hepatitis with autoimmune hemolytic anemia in early childhood. J Pediatr 99:704–711, 1981

113. Bernstein J. Hepatic involvement in hereditary renal syndromes. Birth Defects 23:115–130, 1987

114. Bernstein J, Brown AK. Sepsis and jaundice in early infancy. Pediatrics 29:873, 1962

115. Bernstein J, et al. Bile plug syndrome: correctable cause of obstructive jaundice in infants. Pediatrics 43:273, 1969

116. Bernstein J, et al. Conjugated hyperbilirubinemia in infancy associated with parenteral alimentation. J Pediatr 90:361, 1977

117. Bernstein RB, et al. Bilirubin metabolism in the fetus. J Clin Invest 48:1678, 1969

118. Berry PF, Nagington J. Fatal infection with echovirus 11. Arch Dis Child 57:22–29, 1982

119. Berseth CL, Go VLW. Enhancement of neonatal somatic hepatic growth by orally administered epidermal growth factor in rats. J Pediatr Gastroenterol Nutr 7:889–893, 1988

120. Bhave SA, Pandit AN, Tanner MS. Comparison of feeding history of children with indian childhood cirrhosis and paired controls. J Pediatr Gastroenterol Nutr 6:562–567, 1987

121. Bhuiyan AKMJ, Watmough NJ, Turnbull DM, et al. A new simple screening method for the diagnosis of medium chain acyl-CoA dehydrogenase deficiency. Clin Chim Acta 165:39, 1987

122. Bilton D, Fox R, Webb AK, Lawler W, McMahon RFT, Howat JMT. Pathology of common bile duct stenosis in cystic fibrosis. Gut 31:236–238, 1990

123. Binder ND, Buckmaster JW, Benda GI. Outcome for fetus with ascites and cytomegalovirus infection. Pediatrics 82:100–103, 1988

124. Birnbaum G, et al. Cytomegalovirus infections in newborn infants. J Pediatr 75:789, 1969

125. Bjorkhem I, et al. Urinary excretion of dicarboxylic acids from patients with the Zellweger syndrome: importance of peroxisomes in beta-oxidation of dicarboxylic acids. Biochim Biophys Acta 795:15, 1984

126. Bjorkhem I, et al. Unsuccessful attempts to induce peroxisomes in two cases of Zellweger disease by treatment with clofibrate. Pediatr Res 19:590, 1985

127. Black M, Billing BH. Hepatic bilirubin UDP-glucuronyl transferase activity in liver disease and Gilbert's syndrome. N Engl J Med 280:1266, 1969

128. Blankenberg TA, Ruebner BH, Ellis WG, et al. Pathology of renal and hepatic anomalies in Meckel syndrome. Am J Med Genet 3:395–410, 1987

129. Blaschke TF, Berk PD, Scharschmidt BF, et al. Crigler-Najjar syndrome: an unusual course with development of neurologic damage at age eighteen. Pediatr Res 8:573–590, 1974

130. Bloomer JR, Boyer JL. Phenobarbital effects in cholestatic liver disease. Ann Intern Med 82:310, 1975

131. Blumenschein SD, et al. Familial onset of nonhemolytic jaundice with late onset of neurologic damage. Pediatrics 42:786, 1968

132. Blyth H, Ockenden BG. Polycystic disease of kidneys and liver presenting in childhood. J Med Genet 8:257, 1971

133. Bobo RC, et al. Reye syndrome: treatment by exchange transfusion with special reference to the 1974 epidemic in Cincinnati, Ohio. J Pediatr 87:881, 1975

134. Bodian M. Fibrocystic disease of the pancreas: a congenital disorder of mucus production. New York, Grune & Stratton, 1952

135. Body JJ, Bleiberg H, Bron D, et al. Total parenteral nutrition-induced cholestasis mimicking large bile duct obstruction. Histopathology 6:787–792, 1982

136. Boehm G, Muller DM, Teichmann B, Krumbiegel P. Influence of intrauterine growth retardation on parameters of liver function in low birth weight infants. Eur J Pediatr 149:396–398, 1990

137. Boggs TR, Bishop H. Neonatal hyperbilirubinemia associated with high obstruction of the small bowel. J Pediatr 66:349, 1965

138. Bohm N, et al. Multiple acyl-CoA dehydrogenation deficiency (glutaric aciduria type II), congenital polycystic kidneys and symmetric warty dysplasia of the cerebral cortex in two newborn brothers. II. Morphology and pathogenesis. Eur J Pediatr 139:60, 1982

139. Bohme JH, Sparmann G, Hofmann E. Biochemistry of liver development in the perinatal period. Experimentia 39:473–483, 1983

140. Bortolotti F, Calzia R, Cadrobbi P, et al. Liver cirrhosis associated with chronic hepatitis B infection in childhood. J Pediatr 108:224–227, 1986

141. Bortolotti F, Calzia R, Vegnente A, et al. Chronic hepatitis in childhood: the spectrum of the disease. Gut 29:659–664, 1988

142. Bougneres PF, et al. Medium-chain acyl-CoA dehydrogenase deficiency in two siblings with a Reye-like syndrome. J Pediatr 106:918, 1985

143. Bove KE, et al. The hepatic lesion in Reye's syndrome. Gastroenterology 69:685, 1975

144. Bove KE, et al. Vasculopathic hepatotoxicity associated with E-ferol syndrome in low-birth-weight infants. JAMA 254:2422, 1985

145. Bower RH. Hepatic complications of parenteral nutrition. Semin Liver Dis 3:216–224, 1983

146. Brady RO, et al. Demonstration of a deficiency of glucocerebrosidase cleaving enzyme in Gaucher's disease. J Clin Invest 45:112, 1966

147. Brady RO, et al. The metabolism of sphingomyelin. II. Evidence of an enzymatic block in Niemann-Pick disease. Proc Natl Acad Sci USA 55:366, 1966

148. Brandt IK, DeLuca VA Jr. Type III glycogenosis: a family with an unusual tissue distribution of the enzyme lesion. Am J Med 40:779, 1966

149. Brann BS, Stonestreet BS, Oh W, Cashore WJ. The in vivo effect of bilirubin and sulfisoxazole on cerebral oxygen, glucose, and lactate metabolism in newborn piglets. Pediatr Res 22:135–141, 1987

150. Brantly M, Courtney M, Crystal RG. Repair of the secretion defect in the Z form of α_1-antitrypsyin by addition of a second mutation. Science 242:1700–1702, 1988

151. Brantly M, Nukiwa T, Crystal RG. Molecular basis of α_1-antitrypsin deficiency. Am J Med 84:13–31, 1988

152. Bratlid D, et al. Effect of serum hyperosmolality on opening of blood–brain barrier to bilirubin in rat brain. Pediatrics 71:909, 1983

153. Bratlid D, et al. Effect of acidosis on bilirubin deposition in rat brain. Pediatrics 73:431, 1984

154. Brent RL. Persistent jaundice in infancy. J Pediatr 61:111, 1962

155. Bressler R, et al. Hypoglycin and hypoglycin-like compounds. Pharmacol Rev 21:105, 1969

156. Breuer B, et al. Transmission of hepatitis B virus to class-

room contacts of mentally retarded carriers. JAMA 254:3190, 1985

157. Brind AM, McIntosh I, Brock DJH, James OFW, Bassendine MF. Polymerase chain reaction for detection of the alpha-1-antitrypsin Z allele in chronic liver disease. J Hepatol 10:240–243, 1990

158. Brodersen R. Prevention of kernicterus, based on recent progress in bilirubin chemistry. Acta Pediatr Scand 66:625, 1977

159. Brodersen R. Bilirubin transport in the newborn infant, reviewed with relation to kernicterus. J Pediatr 96:349, 1980

160. Brodersen R, Hermann LS. Intestinal reabsorption of unconjugated bilirubin: a possible contributing factor in neonatal jaundice. Lancet 1:1242, 1963

161. Brodersen R, et al. Bilirubin conjugation in the human fetus. Scand J Clin Lab Invest 20:41, 1967

162. Brooks SEH, Audretsch JJ. Studies on hypoglycin toxicity in rats. I. Changes in hepatic ultrastructure. Am J Pathol 59:161, 1970

163. Brough AJ, Bernstein J. Conjugated hyperbilirubinemia in early infancy. Hum Pathol 5:507, 1974

164. Brown A, Zuelzer W. Studies on the neonatal development of the glucuronide conjugating systems. J Clin Invest 37:332, 1958

165. Brown BI, Brown DH. Lack of an alpha-1,4-glucan; alpha-1,4-glucan 6-glycosyl transferase in a case of type IV glycogenosis. Proc Natl Acad Sci USA 56:725, 1966

166. Brown WR, Sokol RJ, Levin MJ, et al. Lack of correlation between infection with reovirus 3 and extrahepatic biliary atresia or neonatal hepatitis. J. Pediatr 113:670–676, 1988

167. Brusilow SW. Arginine, an indispensable amino acid for patients with inborn errors of urea synthesis. J Clin Invest 74:2144, 1984

168. Brusilow SW. Phenylacetylglutamine may replace urea as a vehicle for waste nitrogen excretion. Pediatr Res 29:147–150, 1991

169. Brusilow SW, et al. Treatment of episodic hyperammonemia in children with inborn errors of urea synthesis. N Engl J Med 310:1630, 1984

170. Buchan P. Pathogenesis of neonatal hyperbilirubinaemia after induction of labour with oxytocin. Br Med J 2:1255, 1979

171. Buchmann MS, Kvittingen EA, Nazer H, et al. Lack of 3β-hydroxy-Δ^5-C_{27}-steroid dehydrogenase/isomerase in fibroblasts from a child with urinary excretion of 3β-hydroxy-Δ^5-bile acids: a new inborn error of metabolism. J Clin Invest 86:2034–2037, 1990

172. Bucuvalas JC, Cutfield W, Horn H, et al. Resistance to the growth-promoting and metabolic effects of growth hormone in children with chronic liver disease. J Pediatr 117:397–402, 1990

173. Bucuvalas JC, Goodrich AL, Suchy FJ. Enhanced uptake of taurine by basolateral plasma membrane vesicles isolated from developing rat liver. Pediatr Res 23:172–175, 1988

174. Bucuvalas JC, et al. Amino acids are potent inhibitors of bile acid uptake by liver plasma membrane vesicles isolated from suckling rats. Pediatr Res 19:1298, 1985

175. Budden SS, Kennaway NG, Phil D, Buist NRM, Poulos A, Weleber RG. Dysmorphic syndrome with phytanic acid oxidase deficiency, abnormal very long chain fatty acids, and pipecolic acidemia: studies in four children. J Pediatr 108:33–39, 1986

176. Bujanover Y, Amarri S, Lebenthal E, et al. The effect of dexamethasone and glucagon on the expression of hepatocyte plasma membrane proteins during development. Hepatology 8:722–727, 1988

177. Burchell A. Molecular pathology of glucose-6-phosphatase. FASE B J 4:2978–2988, 1990

178. Burchell A, Bell JE, Busuttil A, Hume R. Hepatic microsomal glucose-6-phosphatase systems and sudden infant death syndrome. Lancet 2:291–193, 1989

179. Burchell A, Waddell ID. Diagnosis of a novel glycogen storage disease: type 1aSP. J Inherit Metab Dis 13:247–249, 1990

180. Burke JA, Schubert WK. Deficient activity of hepatic acid lipase in cholesterol ester storage disease. Science 176:309, 1972

181. Burman D. Congenital spherocytosis in infancy. Arch Dis Child 33:335, 1958

182. Busuttil RW, Seu P, Millis JM, et al. Liver transplantation in children. Ann Surg 213:48–57, 1991

183. Byard RW, Burrows PE, Izakawa T, Silver MM. Diffuse infantile haemangiomatosis: clinicopathological features and management problems in five fatal cases. Eur J Pediatr 150:224–227, 1991

184. Cabrera J, et al. Budd-Chiari syndrome due to a membranous obstruction of the inferior vena cava in a child. J Pediatr 96:435, 1980

185. Callahan WP, Lorincz AE. Hepatic ultrastructure in the Hurler syndrome. Am J Pathol 48:277, 1966

186. Callahan WP Jr, et al. Human toxoplasmosis: a clinicopathologic study with presentation of five cases and review of the literature. Medicine 25:343, 1946

187. Callea F, Devos R, Pinackat J, Torri A, Desmet VJ. Hereditary hypofibrinogenemia with hepatic storage of fibrinogen: a new endoplasmic reticulum storage disease. In: Lowe GDO, et al., ed. Fibrinogen: 2. biochemistry, physiology and clinical relevance. Amsterdam: Elsevier, 1987, pp 75–78

188. Campos AC, Oler A, Meguid MM, Chen TY. Liver biochemical and histological changes with graded amounts of total parenteral nutrition. Arch Surg 125:447–450, 1990

189. Campra JL, Craig JR, Peters RL, et al. Cirrhosis associated with partial deficiency of alpha$_1$-antitrypsin in an adult. Ann Intern Med 78:233, 1973

190. Cano N, Cicero F, Ranieri F, et al. Ultrasonographic study of gallbladder motility during total parenteral nutrition. Gastroenterology 91:313–317, 1986

191. Cao A, et al. Phenobarbital effect on serum bilirubin levels in underweight infants. Helv Paediatr Acta 28:231, 1973

192. Carlson JA, Rogers BB, Sifers RN, et al. Accumulation of PiZ α$_1$-antitrypsin causes liver damage in transgenic mice. J Clin Invest 83:1183–1190, 1989

193. Carr BR, Simpson ER. Cholesterol synthesis in human fetal tissues. J Clin Endocrinol Metab 55:447–452, 1982

194. Carrell RW. α$_1$-Antitrypsin: molecular pathology, leukocytes and tissue damage. J Clin Invest 78:1427–1431, 1986

195. Cashore WJ. Kernicterus and bilirubin encephalopathy. Semin Liver Dis 8:163–167, 1988

196. Casteels M, Schepers L, Van Veldhoven PP, Eyssen HJ, Mannaerts GP. Separate peroxisomal oxidases for fatty acyl-CoAs and trihydroxycoprostanoyl-CoA in human liver. J Lipid Res 31:1865–1872, 1990

197. Catz C, Yaffe SJ. Barbiturate enhancement of bilirubin conjugation and excretion in young and adult animals. Pediatr Res 2:361, 1968

198. Chandra RS, Altman RP. Ductal remnants in extrahepatic biliary atresia: a histopathologic study with clinical correlation. J Pediatr 93:196, 1978

199. Chandra RS, et al. Benign hepatocellular tumors in the young: a clinicopathologic spectrum. Arch Pathol Lab Med 108:168, 1984

200. Chang MW, Chen PJ, Chen JY, et al. Hepatitis B virus integration in hepatitis B virus-related hepatocellular carcinoma in childhood. Hepatology 13:316–320, 1991

201. Chapoy PR, et al. Systemic carnitine deficiency: a treatable inherited lipid-storage disease presenting as Reye's syndrome. N Engl J Med 303:1389, 1980

202. Chazouilleres O, Poupon R, Capron, et al. Is ursodeoxycholic acid an effective treatment for primary sclerosing cholangitis? Gastroenterology 96:A583, 1989

203. Chen YT, Scheinman JI, Park HK, Coleman RA, Roe CR.

Amelioration of proximal renal tubular dysfunction in type i glycogen storage disease with dietary therapy. N Engl J Med 323:590–592, 1990

204. Chen YT, et al. Cornstarch therapy in type I glycogen storage disease. N Engl J Med 310:171, 1984
205. Chernausek DS, Beach DC, Banach W, et al. Characteristics of hepatic receptors for somatomedin-c/insulin-like growth factor i and insulins in the developing human. J Clin Endocrinol Metabol 64:737–743, 1987
206. Chianale J, Dvorak C, Farmer DL, Michaels L, Gumucio JJ. Cytochrome p-450 gene expression in the functional units of the fetal liver. Hepatology 8:318–326, 1988
207. Chiba T, Kasai M. Differentiation of biliary atresia from neonatal hepatitis by routine clinical examination. Tohoku J Exp Med 115:327, 1975
208. Chiba T, Ohi R, Uchida T, Hayashi T, Mochizuki I. Persistent jaundice after hepatic portojejunostomy in biliary atresia: are the patients' prognoses determined within 3 months after surgery? Tohoku J Exp Med 154:149–156, 1988
209. Chilukuri S, Bonet V, Cobb M. Antenatal spontaneous perforation of the extrahepatic biliary tree. Am J Obstet Gynecol 163:1201–1202, 1990
210. Chin KC, Taylor MJ, Perlman M. Improvement in auditory and visual evoked potentials in jaundiced preterm infants after exchange transfusion. Arch Dis Child 60:714–717, 1985
211. Chobert MN, Bernard O, Bulle F, Lemonnier A, Guellaen G, Alagille D. High hepatic b-glutamyltransferase (b-GT) activity with normal serum b-GT in children with progressive idiopathic cholestasis. J Hepatol 8:22–25, 1989
212. Christensen E, Van Eldere J, Brandt NJ, Schutgens RBH, Wanders RJA, Eyssen HJ. A new Peroxisomal disorder: di- and trihydroxycholestanaemia due to a presumed trihydroxycholestanoyl-CoA oxidase deficiency. J Inherit Metab Dis 13:363–366, 1990
213. Christensen JF. Prolonged icterus neonatorum and congenital myxedema. Acta Paediatr 45:367, 1956
214. Clatworthy HW, et al. Primary liver tumors in infancy and childhood. Arch Surg 109:143, 1974
215. Clayton PT, Leonard JV, Lawson AM, et al. Familial giant cell hepatitis associated with synthesis of 3β, 7α-dihydroxy- and 3β, 7α, 12α-trihydroxy-5-cholenoic acids. J Clin Invest 79:1031–1038, 1987
216. Clayton PT, Patel E, Lawson AM, Carruthers RA, Collins J. Bile acid profiles in peroxisomal 3-oxoacyl-coenzyme A thiolase deficiency. J Clin Invest 85:1267–1273, 1990
217. Clayton RJ, et al. Byler disease: fatal familial intrahepatic cholestasis in an Amish kindred. Am J Dis Child 117:112, 1969
218. Cobben JM, Breuning MH, Schoots C, Ten Kate LP, Zerres K. Congenital hepatic fibrosis in autosomal-dominant polycystic kidney disease. Kidney Int 38:880–885, 1990
219. Codoner-Franch P, Bernard O, Maggiore G, Alagille D, Alvarez F. Clinical and immunological heterogeneity of anti-liver-kidney microsome antibody-positive autoimmune hepatitis in children. J Pediatr Gastroenterol Nutr 9:436–440, 1989
220. Cohen AN, Ostrow JD. New concepts in phototherapy: photoisomerization of bilirubin IX alpha and potential toxic effects of light. Pediatrics 65:740, 1980
221. Cohen AN, et al. Effects of phenobarbital on bilirubin metabolism and its response to phototherapy in the jaundiced Gunn rat. Hepatology 5:310, 1985
222. Cohen C, Olsen MM. Pediatric total parenteral nutrition: liver histopathology. Arch Pathol Lab Med 105:152, 1981
223. Cohen JL, Vinik A, Faller J, Fox IH. Hyperuricemia in glycogen storage disease type I: contributions by hypoglycemia and hyperglucagonemia to increased urate production. J Clin Invest 75:251–257, 1985
224. Coire C, Qizilbash A, Castelli M. Hepatic adenomata in type Ia glycogen storage disease. Arch Pathol Lab Med 111:166–169, 1987
225. Cole AP, Hargreaves T. Conjugation inhibitors and early neonatal hyperbilirubinemia. Arch Dis Child 47:415, 1972
226. Collaborative study. Cytomegalovirus infection in the northwest of England: a report on a two-year study. Arch Dis Child 45:513, 1970
227. Colombo C, Setchell KDR, Podda M, Crosignani A, Roda A, Curcio L, Ronchi M, Giunta A. Effects of ursodeoxycholic acid therapy for liver disease associated with cystic fibrosis. J Pediatr 117:482–489, 1990
228. Combined study. Prevention of Rh hemolytic disease: final results of the "high risk" clinical trial: a combined study from centers in England and Baltimore. Br Med J 2:607, 1971
229. Cooper A, Betts JM, Pereira GR, et al. Taurine deficiency in the severe hepatic dysfunction complicating total parenteral nutrition. J Pediatr Surg 19:462–466, 1984
230. Corey L, et al. A nationwide outbreak of Reye's syndrome: its epidemiologic relationship to influenza B. Am J Med 61:615, 1976
231. Corey L, et al. Reye's syndrome: clinical progression and evaluation. Pediatrics 60:708, 1977
232. Cori GT. Biochemical aspect of glycogen deposition disease. Mod Probl Paediatr 3:344 1958
233. Cori GT, Cori CF. Glucose-6-phosphatase of liver in glycogen storage disease. J Biol Chem 199:661, 1952
234. Corkey BE, Geschwind JF, Deeney FJ, Hale DE, Douglas SD, Kilpatrick L. Ca²⁺ responses to interleukin 1 and tumor necrosis factor in cultured human skin fibroblasts: possible implications for Reye syndrome. J Clin Invest 87:778–786, 1991
235. Corkey BE, Hale DE, Glennon MC, et al. Relationship between unusual acyl-coenzyme A profiles and the pathogenesis of Reye's syndrome. J Clin Invest 82:782, 1988
236. Cornelius CE. Hepatic ontogenesis. Hepatology 5:1213–1221, 1985
237. Cottier H. Ueber Ein Der Hamochromatose Vergleichbares Krankheitsbild bei Neugeborenen. Schweiz Med Wochenschr 37:39–53, 1957
238. Cotting J, Lentze MJ, Reichen J. Effects of ursodeoxycholic acid treatment on nutrition and liver function in patients with cystic fibrosis and longstanding cholestasis. Gut 31:918–921, 1990
239. Coufalik AH, Monder C. Regulation of the tyrosine oxidizing system in fetal rat liver. Arch Biochem Biophys 199:67–75, 1980
240. Couvreu J, Desmonts G. Congenital and maternal toxoplasmosis: review of 300 congenital cases. Dev Med Child Neurol 4:519, 1962
241. Cox DW, Mansfield T. Prenatal diagnosis of α₁-antitrypsin deficiency and estimates of fetal risk for disease. J Med Genet 24:52–59, 1987
242. Cox DW, Smyth S. Risk for liver disease in adults with alpha₁-antitrypsin deficiency. Am J Med 74:221, 1983
243. Cox KL, Ward RE, Furgiuele TL, et al. Orthotopic liver transplantation in patients with cystic fibrosis. Pediatrics 80:570–574, 1987
244. Cox KL, Cheung ATW, Lohse CL, et al. Biliary motility: postnatal changes in guinea pigs. Pediatric Res 21:170–175, 1987
245. Craig JM, Landing BH. Form of hepatitis in neonatal period simulating biliary atresia. Arch Pathol 54:321, 1952
246. Craig JM, et al. The pathological changes in the liver in cystic fibrosis of the pancreas. Am J Dis Child 93:357, 1957
247. Craig RM, Neumann T, Jeejeebhoy KN, et al. Severe hepatocellular reaction resembling alcoholic hepatitis with cirrhosis after massive small bowel resection and prolonged total parenteral nutrition. Gastroenterology 79:131–137, 1980
248. Cremer RJ, et al. Influence of light on the hyperbilirubinemia of infants. Lancet 1:1094, 1958

249. Crigler JF, Gold NI. Sodium phenobarbital induced decrease in serum bilirubin in an infant with congenital nonhaemolytic jaundice and kernicterus. J Clin Invest 45:998, 1966

250. Crigler JF, Najjar VA. Congenital familial nonhemolytic jaundice with kernicterus. Pediatrics 10:169, 1952

251. Crocker AC, Forbes S. Neimann-Pick disease: a review of 18 patients. Medicine 37:1, 1958

252. Crocker DW, Cleland RS. Infantile hemangioendothelioma of liver: report of three cases. Pediatrics 19:596, 1957

253. Cross NCP, deFranchis R, Sebastio G, et al. Molecular analysis of aldolase B genes in hereditary fructose intolerance. Lancet 335:306–309, 1990

254. Crowley JJ, Sharp HL, Freier E, et al. Fatal liver disease associated with α_1-antitrypsin deficiency PiM$_l$/PiM$_{duarte}$. Gastroenterology 93:242–244, 1987

255. Crystal RG. Alpha-1-antitrypsin deficiency, emphysema and liver disease: genetic basis and strategies for therapy. J Clin Invest 85:1343–1352, 1990

256. Curiel DT, Holmes MD, Okayama H, et al. Molecular basis of the liver and lung disease associated with the α_1-antitrypsin deficiency allele M$_{malton}$as. J Biol Chem 264:13938–13945, 1989

257. Cutting HO, et al. Autosomal dominant hemolytic anemia characterized by ovalocytosis: a family study of seven involved members. Am J Med 39:21, 1965

258. Cutz E, Cox DW. Alpha-1-antitrypsin deficiency: the spectrum of pathology and pathophysiology. Perspect Pediatr Pathol 5:1, 1979

259. Daffos F, Forestier F, Capella-Pavlovsky M, et al. Prenatal management of 746 pregnancies at risk for congenital toxoplasmosis. N Engl J Med 318:271–275, 1988

260. Dahms BB. Hepatoma in familial cholestatic cirrhosis of childhood. Arch Pathol Lab Med 103:30, 1979

261. Dahms BB, Halpin TC. Serial liver biopsies in parenteral nutrition-associated cholestasis of early infancy. Gastroenterology 81:136, 1981

262. Dahms BB, et al. Arteriohepatic dysplasia in infancy and childhood: a longitudinal study of six patients. Hepatology 2:350, 1982

263. Dalinka MK, et al. Metachromatic leukodystrophy: a cause of cholelithiasis in childhood. Am J Dig Dis 14:603, 1969

264. Danks D, Bodian M. A genetic study of neonatal obstructive jaundice. Arch Dis Child 38:378, 1963

265. Danks DM, Campbell PE. Extrahepatic biliary atresia: comments on the frequency of potentially operable cases. J Pediatr 69:21, 1966

266. Danks DM, et al. Studies of the aetiology of neonatal hepatitis and biliary atresia. Arch Dis Child 52:360, 1977

267. Danks DM, et al. Prognosis of babies with neonatal hepatitis. Arch Dis Child 52:368, 1977

268. Datta NS, et al. Deficiency of enzymes catalyzing the biosynthesis of glycerol-ether lipids in Zellweger syndrome. N Engl J Med 311:1080, 1984

269. Daugherty CC, Setchell KD, Balistreri WF. Bile canalicular abnormalities in an inborn error of bile acid (BA) metabolism (Δ^4-3-oxosteroid 5β-reductase deficiency). Soc Pediatr Pathol, 1990

270. Davis DR, et al. Activated charcoal decreases plasma bilirubin levels in the hyperbilirubinemic rat. Pediatr Res 17:208, 1983

271. DeBont B, Walker AC, Carter FR, Oldfield RK, Davidson GP. Idiopathic hemochromatosis presenting as acute hepatitis. J Pediatr 110:431–433, 1987

272. Dehner LP. Hepatic tumors in the pediatric age group: a distinctive clinicopathologic spectrum. Perspect Pediatr Pathol 4:217, 1978

273. Dehner LP, Snover DC, Sharp HL, Ascher N, Nakhleh R, Day DL. Hereditary tyrosinemia type I (chronic form): pathologic findings in the liver. Hum Pathol 20:149–158, 1989

274. Delaney JK, Mauzerall D, Drummond GS, Kappas A. Photophysical properties of Sn-porphyrins: potential clinical implications. Pediatrics 81:498–504, 1988

275. Demaugre F, Bonnefont JP, Colonna M, et al. Infantile form of carnitine palmitoyltransferase II deficiency with hepatomuscular symptoms and sudden death. J Clin Invest 87:859–864, 1991

276. Denehy CM, Ryan JR. Development of gallbladder contractility in the guinea pig. Pediatric Res 20:214–217, 1986

277. De Pagter AGF, et al. Familial benign recurrent intrahepatic cholestasis: interrelation with intrahepatic cholestasis of pregnancy and from oral contraceptives? Gastroenterology 71:202, 1976

278. Deprettere A, Portmann B, Mowat AP. Syndromic paucity of the intrahepatic bile ducts: diagnostic difficulty; severe morbidity throughout early childhood. J Pediatr Gastroenterol Nutr 6:865–871, 1987

279. Dermer SJ, Johnson EM. Methods in laboratory investigation: rapid DNA analysis of α_1-antitrypsin deficiency. Lab Invest 59:403–408, 1988

280. Descos B, et al. Pigment gallstones of the common bile duct in infancy. Hepatology 4:678, 1984

281. Desmet VJ. Cholangiopathies: past, present and future. Semin Liver Dis 7:67–76, 1987

282. Desmet VJ. Intrahepatic bile ducts under the lens. J Hepatol 1:545–559, 1985

283. Desmonts G, Couvreur J. Congenital toxoplasmosis. N Engl J Med 290:1110, 1974

284. Deutsch J, et al. Long term prognosis for babies with neonatal liver disease. Arch Dis Child 60:447, 1985

285. DeVivo DC, Keating JP. Reye's syndrome. Adv Pediatr 22:175, 1976

286. DeVos M, Barbier F, Cuvelier C. Congenital hepatic fibrosis. J Hepatol 6:222–228, 1988

287. DeVos R, et al. Progressive intrahepatic cholestasis (Byler's disease): case report. Gut 16:943, 1975

288. de Vries LS, et al. Relationship of serum bilirubin levels to ototoxicity and deafness in high-risk low-birth-weight infants. Pediatrics 76:351, 1985

289. DeWolf-Peeters C, et al. Conjugated bilirubin in foetal liver in erythroblastosis. Lancet 1:471, 1969

290. DeWolf-Peeters C, et al. Histochemical evidence of a cholestatic period in neonatal rats. Pediatr Res 5:704, 1971

291. DeWolf-Peeters C, et al. Electron microscopy and histochemistry of canalicular differentiation in fetal and neonatal rat liver. Tissue Cell 4:379, 1976

292. DeWolf-Peeters C, et al. Electron microscopy and morphometry of canalicular differentiation in fetal and neonatal rat liver. Exp Mol Pathol 21:339, 1974

293. Diamond LK. Replacement transfusion as a treatment for erythroblastosis fetalis. Pediatrics 2:520, 1948

294. Diaz J, Schain RJ. Phenobarbital: effects of long-term administration on behavior and brain of artificially reared rats. Science 199:90, 1978

295. DiBisceglie AM, Ishak DG, Rabin L, Hoeg JM. Cholesteryl ester storage disease: hepatopathology and effects of therapy with lovastatin. Hepatology 11:764–772, 1990

296. Dick MC, Mowat AP. Hepatitis syndrome in infancy: an epidemiological survey with 10 year follow up. Arch Dis Child 60:512, 1985

297. Dijkstra M, Kuipers F, Havinga R, Smit EP, Vonk RJ. Bile secretion of trace elements in rats with a congenital defect in hepatobiliary transport of glutathione. Pediatr Res 28:339–343, 1990

298. Ding JH, deBarsy T, Brown BI, Coleman RA, Chen YT. Immunoblot analyses of glycogen debranching enzyme in different subtypes of glycogen storage disease type III. J Pediatr 116:95–100, 1990

299. di Sant'Agnese PA, Blanc WA. A distinctive type of biliary cirrhosis of the liver associated with cystic fibrosis of the pancreas. Pediatrics 18:387–409, 1956

300. Dische MR. Metachromatic leukodystrophic polyposis of the gallbladder. J Pathol 97:388, 1969

301. Dixit V, Darvasi R, Arthur M, Brezina M, Lewin K, Gitnick G. Restoration of liver function in Gunn rats without immunosuppression using transplanted microencapsulated hepatocytes. Hepatology 12:1342–1349, 1990

302. Doherty DG, Donaldson, PT, Whitehouse DB, et al. HLA phenotypes and gene polymorphisms in juvenile liver disease associated with α₁-antitrypsin deficiency. Hepatology 12:218–223, 1990

303. Donn SM, Thoene JG. Prospective prevention of neonatal hyperammonaemia in argininosuccinic aciduria by arginine therapy. J Inherit Metab Dis 8:18, 1985

304. Donnell GN, et al. Galactose-1-phosphate in galactosemia. Pediatrics 31:802, 1963

305. Donnell GN, et al. Observations on results of management of galactosemic patients. In: Hsia D Y-Y, ed. Galactosemia. Springfield IL, Charles C Thomas, 1969, pp 247–268

306. Dorfman DH, Glaser JH. Congenital syphilis presenting in infants after the newborn period. N Engl J Med 323:1299–1302, 1990

307. Dorvil NP, et al. Taurine prevents cholestasis induced by lithocholic acid sulfate in guinea pigs. Am J Clin Nutr 37:221, 1983

308. Dosi PC, et al. Perinatal factors underlying neonatal cholestasis. J Pediatr 106:471, 1985

309. Driscoll SG. Histopathology of gestational rubella. Am J Dis Child 118:49, 1969

310. Drop SLS, et al. Hyperbilirubinemia and idiopathic hypopituitarism in the newborn period. Acta Paediatr Scand 68:227, 1979

311. Drummond GS, Galbraith RA, Sarbana MK, Kappas A. Reduction of the C₂ and C₄ vinyl groups of Sn-protoporphyrin to form Sn-mesoporphyrin markedly enhances the ability of the metalloporphyrin to inhibit in vivo heme catabolism. Arch Biochem Biophys 255:64–74, 1987

312. Drummond GS, Kappas A. An experimental model of postnatal jaundice in the suckling rat: suppression of induced hyperbilirubinemia by Sn-protoporphyrin. J Clin Invest 74:142, 1984

313. Drummond GS, Kappas A. Chemoprevention of neonatal jaundice: potency of tin-protoporphyrin in an animal model. Science 217:1250–1252, 1982

314. Drummond GS, Kappas A. Sn-protoporphyrin inhibition of fetal and neonatal brain heme oxygenase. J Clin Invest 77:971–976, 1986

315. Dufour DR, Monoghan WP. ABO hemolytic disease of the newborn: a retrospective analysis of 254 cases. Am J Clin Pathol 73:369, 1980

316. Dumaswala R, Ananthanarayanan M, Suchy FJ. Characterization of a specific transport mechanism for bile acids on the brush border membrane of human placenta. Hepatology 8:1260, 1988

317. Dunn L, Hulman, Weiner J, et al. Beneficial effects of early hypocaloric enteral feeding on neonatal gastrointestinal function: preliminary report of a randomized trial. J Pediatr 112:622–629, 1988

318. Dupont J, Raulin J, Gautier M, et al. Cholesterol and prostaglandin synthesis by cultured human skin fibroblasts in the Alagille syndrome involving paucity of interlobular bile ducts. J Inherit Metab Dis 12:436–444, 1989

319. Dutton GJ. Glucuronide synthesis in foetal liver and other tissues. Biochem J 71:141, 1959

320. Dycaico JM, Grant SGN, Felts K, et al. Neonatal hepatitis induced by α₁-antitrypsin: a transgenic mouse model. Science 242:1409–1412, 1988. (see also: Geller SA, Nichols WS, Dycaico MJ, Felts KA, Sorge JA. Histopathology of α₁-antitrypsin liver disease in a transgenic mouse model. Hepatology 12:40–47, 1990)

321. Ecoffey C, Rothman E, Barnard O, et al. Bacterial cholangitis after surgery for biliary atresia. J Pediatr 111:824–829, 1987

322. Edmondson HA. Differential diagnosis of tumor and tumor-like lesions in infancy and children. Ann Surg 142:214, 1955

323. Egan WA II, et al. Neonatal hyperbilirubinemia associated with ingestion of maternal blood. Pediatrics 43:894, 1969

324. Eggermont E, et al. Angiographic evidence of low portal liver perfusion in transient neonatal hyperammonemia. Acta Pediatr Belg 33:163, 1980

325. Ehren H, et al. Benign liver tumors in infancy and childhood: report of 48 cases. Am J Surg 145:325, 1983

326. Ek J, Kase BF, Reith A, Bjorkhem I, Pedersen JI. Peroxisomal dysfunction in a boy with neurologic symptoms and amaurosis (Leber disease): clinical and biochemical findings similar to those observed in Zellweger syndrome. J Pediatr 108:19–24, 1986

327. Elpeleg ON, Hurvitz, H, Branski D, et al. Fructose-1, 6-diphosphatase deficiency: a 20-year follow-up. Am J Dis Child 143:140–141, 1989

328. El-Shabrawi M, Wilkinson ML, Portmann B, et al. Primary sclerosing cholangitis in childhood. Gastroenterology 92:1226–1235, 1987

329. Embil JA, et al. Congenital cytomegalovirus infection in two siblings from consecutive pregnancies. J Pediatr 77:417, 1970

330. Engel AG. Acid maltase deficiency in adults: studies in four cases of a syndrome which may mimic muscular dystrophy or other myopathies. Brain 93:599, 1970

331. Ennever JF, Costarino AT, Polin RA, Speck. WT. Rapid clearance of a structural isomer of bilirubin during phototherapy. J Clin Invest 79:1674–1678, 1987

332. Ennever JF, Knox I, Speck WT. Differences in bilirubin isomer composition in infants treated with green and white light phototherapy. J Pediatr 109:119–122, 1986

333. Ennever JF, et al. Phototherapy for neonatal jaundice: in vivo clearance of bilirubin photoproducts. Pediatr Res 19:205, 1985

334. Ennever JF, et al. Phototherapy for neonatal jaundice: in vitro comparison of light sources. Pediatr Res 18:667, 1984

335. Epstein MF, Levinton A, Kuban KCK, et al. Bilirubin, intraventricular hemorrhage, and phenobarbital in very low birth weight babies. Pediatrics 82:350–354, 1988

336. Eriksson S. α₁-Antitrypsin deficiency and liver cirrhosis in adults: an analysis of 35 Swedish autopsied cases. Acta Med Scand 221:461–467, 1987

337. Eriksson S, Carlson J, Velez R. Risk of cirrhosis and primary liver cancer in alpha₁-antitrypsin deficiency. N Engl J Med 314:736–739, 1986

338. Eriksson S, Larsson C. Familial benign chronic intrahepatic cholestasis. Hepatology 3:391, 1983

339. Eriksson SL. Studies in alpha-1-antitrypsin. Acta Med Scand (suppl) 432:177, 1965

340. Escobar GJ, Heyman MB, Smith WB, Thaler MM. Primary hemochromatosis in childhood. Pediatrics 80:549–554, 1987

341. Esquivel CO, Koneru B, Karer F, et al. Liver transplantation before 1 year of age. J Pediatr 110:545–548, 1987

342. Esterly JR, et al. Hepatic lesions in the congenital rubella syndrome. J Pediatr 71:676, 1976

343. Eyssen H, Eggermont E, Van Eldere J, Jaeken J, Parmentier G, Janssen G. Bile acid abnormalities and the diagnosis of cerebro-hepato-renal syndrome (Zellweger syndrome). Acta Paediatr Scand 74:539–544, 1985

344. Eyssen H, et al. Trihydroxycoprostanic acid in the duodenal bile of two children with intrahepatic bile duct anomalies. Biochim Biophys Acta 273:212, 1972

345. Faa G, Van Eyken P, Demelia L. Idiopathic adulthood ductopenia presenting with chronic recurrent cholestasis. J Hepatol 12:14–20, 1991

346. Fagerhol M. Genetics of the Pi system. In: Pulmonary Emphysema and Proteolysis. New York, Academic Press, 1972, pp 123–133

347. Farber S. Pancreatic function and disease in early life. V. Pathologic changes associated with pancreatic insufficiency in early life. Arch Pathol 37:238–250, 1944

348. Farci P, et al. Infection with the delta agent in children. Gut 26:4, 1985

349. Farrell DF, MacMartin MP. Gm₁ gangliosidosis: enzymatic variation in a single family. Ann Neurol 9:232, 1981

350. Farrell MK, et al. Serum-sulfated lithocholate as an indicator of cholestasis during parenteral nutrition in infants and children. J Parenter Enter Nutr 6:30, 1982

351. Fausto N, Mead JE. Regulation of liver growth: protooncogenes and transforming growth factors. Lab Invest 60:4–13, 1989

352. Fechner RE, et al. Coxsackie B virus infection of the newborn. Am J Pathol 42:493, 1963

353. Feigelson J, Peccau Y, Cathelineau L, et al. Additional data on hepatic function tests in cystic fibrosis. Acta Paediatr Scand 64:337–344, 1975

354. Feldman HA. Toxoplasmosis. N Engl J Med 279:1370, 1431, 1968

355. Felsher BF, et al. Hepatic bilirubin glucuronidation in neonates with unconjugated hyperbilirubinemia and congenital gastrointestinal obstruction. J Lab Clin Med 83:90, 1974

356. Felsher BF, et al. The reciprocal relation between caloric intake and the degree of hyperbilirubinemia in Gilbert's syndrome. N Engl J Med 283:170, 1970

357. Feracci H, Connolly TP, Margolis RN, et al. The establishment of hepatocyte cell surface polarity during fetal liver development. Dev Biol 123:73–84, 1987

358. Fernandes J, Berger R. Urinary excretion of lactate, 2-oxoglutarate, citrate, and glycerol in patients with glycogenosis type I. Pediatr Res 21:279–282, 1987

359. Fernandes J, Leonard JW, Moses SW, et al. Glycogen storage disease: recommendations for treatment. Eur J Pediatr 147:226–228, 1988

360. Fernandes J, et al. Lactate as a cerebral metabolic fuel for glucose-6-phosphatase deficient children. Pediatr Res 18:335, 1984

361. Fienberg R. Perinatal idiopathic hemochromatosis: giant cell hepatitis interpreted as an inborn error of metabolism. Am J Clin Pathol 33:480–491, 1960

362. Finegold MJ, Carpenter RJ. Obliterative cholangitis due to cytomegalovirus: a possible precursor of paucity of intrahepatic bile ducts. Hum Pathol 13:662, 1982

363. Fink S, Karp W, Robertson A. Ceftriaxone effect on bilirubin-albumin binding. Pediatrics 80:873–875, 1987

364. Finkelstein JE, Hauser ER, Leonard CO, Brusilow SW. Late-onset ornithine transcarbamylase deficiency in male patients. J Pediatr 117:897–902, 1990

365. Fischer A, Virelizier JL, Arenzana-Seisdedos F, Perez N, Nezelof C, Griscelli C. Treatment of four patients with erythrophagocytic lymphohistiocytosis by a combination of epipodophyllotoxin, steroids, intrathecal methotrexate, and cranial irradiation. Pediatrics 76:263–268, 1985

366. Fisher RL, et al. Alpha-1-antitrypsin deficiency in liver disease: the extent of the problem. Gastroenterology 71:646, 1976

367. Flannery DB, et al. Current status of hyperammonemic syndromes. Hepatology 2:495, 1982

368. Fonkalsrud EW, Boles T. Choledochal cysts in infancy and childhood. Surg Gynecol Obstet 121:733, 1965

369. Fonkalsrud EW, et al. Management of extrahepatic portal hypertension in children. Ann Surg 180:487, 1974

370. Foreman RC. Disruption of the LYS-290-GLU-342 salt bridge in human α₁-antitrypsin does not prevent its synthesis and secretion. FEBS Lett 216:79, 1987

371. Forestier F, Daffos F, Rainaut M, Bruneau M, Trivien F. Blood chemistry of normal human fetuses at midtrimester of pregnancy. Pediatr Res 21:579–583, 1987

372. Frank DJ, et al. Fetal ascites and cytomegalic inclusion disease. Am J Dis Child 112:604, 1966

373. Fraumeni JF, et al. Primary carcinoma of the liver in childhood: an epidemiologic study. J Natl Cancer Inst 40:1087, 1968

374. Friedman JH, Levy HL, Boustany RM. Late onset of distinct neurologic syndromes in galactosemic siblings. Neurology 39:741–742, 1989

375. Froesch ER, et al. Hereditary fructose intolerance: an inborn defect of hepatic fructose-1-phosphate splitting aldolase. Am J Med 34:151, 1963

376. Furuya KN, Roberts EA, Canny GJ, Phillips MJ. Neonatal hepatitis syndrome with paucity of interlobular bile ducts in cystic fibrosis. J Pediatr Gastroenterol Nutr 12:127–130, 1991

377. Gale RP. Development of the immune system in human fetal liver. Thymus 10:45–56, 1987

378. Gang DL, Herrin JT. Infantile polycystic disease of the liver and kidneys. Clin Nephrol 25:28–36, 1986

379. Gartner J, Chen WW, Kelley RI, Mihalik SJ, Moser HW. The 22-kD peroxisomal integral membrane protein in Zellweger syndrome: presence, abundance, and association with a peroxisomal thiolase precursor protein. Pediatr Research 29:141–146, 1991

380. Gartner LM, Arias IM. Studies of prolonged neonatal jaundice in the breast-fed infant. J Pediatr 68:54, 1966

381. Gartner LM, Auerbach KG. Breast milk and breast feeding jaundice. Adv Pediatr 34:249–275, 1987

382. Gartner LM, et al. Effect of milk feeding on intestinal bilirubin absorption in the rat. J Pediatr 103:464, 1983

383. Gartner LM, et al. Kernicterus: high incidence in premature infants with low serum bilirubin concentrations. Pediatrics 45:906, 1970

384. Gartner LM, et al. Development of bilirubin transport and metabolism in the newborn rhesus monkey. J Pediatr 90:513, 1977

385. Gaskin KJ, Waters DLM, Howman-Giles R, et al. Liver disease and common-bile-duct stenosis in cystic fibrosis. N Engl J Med 318:340–346, 1988

386. Gautier M, et al. Morphologic study of 98 biliary remnants. Arch Pathol Lab Med 105:397, 1981

387. Gentil-Kocher S, Bernard O, Brunelle F, et al. Budd-Chiari syndrome in children: report of 22 Cases. J Pediatr 113:30–38, 1988

388. Gentile S, Persico M, Tiribelli C. Abnormal hepatic uptake of low doses of sulfobromophthalein in Gilbert's syndrome: the role of reduced affinity of the plasma membrane carrier of organic anions. Hepatology 12:213–217, 1990

389. Gerhold JP, et al. Diagnosis of biliary atresia with radionuclide hepatobiliary imaging. Radiology 146:499, 1983

390. Gherardi GH, MacMahon HE. Hypoplasia of terminal bile ducts: occurrence in two jaundiced male siblings. Am J Dis Child 120:151, 1970

391. Ghishan FK, Gray GF, Greene HL. Alpha-1-antitrypsin deficiency presenting with ascites and cirrhosis in the neonatal period. Gastroenterology 85:435, 1983

392. Ghishan FK, Greene HL. Liver disease in children with PiZZ α₁-antitrypsin deficiency. Hepatology 8:307–310, 1988

393. Gilbert EF. Carnitine deficiency. Pathology 17:161, 1985

394. Gilbert EF, et al. Familial hemophagocytic lymphohistiocytosis. Pediatr Pathol 3:59, 1985

394a. Gillam GL, Stokes KB, McLellan J, Smith AL. Fulminant hepatic failure with intractable ascites due to an echovirus 11 infection successfully managed with a peritoneo-venous (LeVeen) shunt. J Pediatr Gastroenterol Nutr 5:476–480, 1986

395. Gilbertson AS, et al. Enteropathic circulation of unconjugated bilirubin in man. Nature 196:141, 1962

396. Gilchrist KW, et al. Studies of malformation syndromes of

man: XIB. the cerebro-hepato-renal syndrome of Zellweger: comparative pathology. Eur J Pediatr 121:99, 1976

397. Girard J. Control of fetal and neonatal glucose metabolism by pancreatic hormones. Baillieres Clin Endocrinol Metab 3:817–836, 1989

398. Gitlin N, et al. Fulminant neonatal hepatic necrosis associated with echovirus type 11 infection. West J Med 138:260, 1983

399. Gitzelmann R, et al. Galactitol and galactose-1-phosphate in the lens of a galactosemic infant. Exp Eye Res 6:1, 1967

400. Giunta F. A one year experience with phototherapy for jaundice of prematurity. Pediatrics 47:123, 1971

401. Glaser JH, Morecki R. Reovirus type 3 and neonatal cholestasis. Semin Liver Dis 7:100–107, 1987

402. Glaser JH, et al. The role of reovirus type 3 in persistent infantile cholestasis. J Pediatr 105:912–915, 1984

403. Gleason CA, et al. Hepatic oxygen consumption, lactate uptake, and glucose production in neonatal lambs. Pediatr Res 19:1235, 1985

404. Glew RH, et al. Biology of disease: lysosomal storage diseases. Lab Invest 53:250, 1985

405. Goldfischer S. Idiopathic neonatal iron storage involving the liver, pancreas, heart and endocrine and exocrine glands. Hepatology 1:58, 1981

406. Goldfischer S, Collins J, Rapin I, et al. Pseudo-Zellweger syndrome: deficiencies in several peroxisomal oxidative activities. J Pediatr 108:25–32, 1986

407. Goldfischer S, et al. Peroxisomal and mitochondrial defects in the cerebro-hepato-renal syndrome. Science 182:62, 1973

408. Goldfischer S, et al. Peroxisomal defects in neonatal-onset and X-linked adrenoleukodystrophies. Science 227:67, 1985

409. Goodman SI. Screening for metabolic liver disease. In: Balistreri WF, Stocker JT, eds. Pediatric hepatology. Washington, DC, Hemisphere, 1990, pp 177–181

410. Goodrich AL, Suchy FL. Na$^+$ – H$^+$ exchange in basolateral plasma membrane vesicles from neonatal rat liver. Am J Physiol 259:G334–G339, 1990

411. Gorodischer R, et al. Congenital nonobstructive jaundice: effect of phototherapy. N Engl J Med 282:375, 1970

412. Gotto AM, et al. On the protein defect in abetalipoproteinemia. N Engl J Med 284:813, 1971

413. Gottrand F, Bernard O, Hadchouel M, Pariente D, Gauthier F, Alagille D. Late cholangitis after successful surgical repair of biliary atresia. Am J Dis Child 145:213–215, 1991

414. Gourley GR, Arend RA. β-Glucuronidase and hyperbilirubinemia in breast-fed and formula-fed babies. Lancet 1:644–646, 1986

415. Gourley GR, Gourley MF, Arend R, Palta M. The effect of saccharolactone on rat intestinal absorption of bilirubin in the presence of human breast m6ilk. Pediatr Res 25:234–238, 1989

416. Govaerts LCP, van den Berg GA, Theeuwes A, Muskiet FAJ, Monnens LAH. Urinary polyamine and metabolite excretion by children with Zellweger's syndrome. Clin Chim Acta 192:61–68, 1990

417. Graham MF, et al. Inhibition of bile flow in the isolated perfused rat liver by a synthetic parenteral amino acid mixture. Hepatology 4:69, 1984

418. Gray OP, Saunders RA. Familial intrahepatic jaundice in infancy. Arch Dis Child 41:320, 1966

419. Greene CL, Blitzer MG, Shapira E. Inborn errors of metabolism and Reye's syndrome: Differential diagnosis. J Pediatr 113:156–159, 1988

420. Greene HL, Brown BI, McClenathan DT, et al. A new variant of type IV glycogenosis: deficiency of branching enzyme activity without apparent progressive liver disease. Hepatology 8:302–306, 1988

421. Greene HL, Ghishan FK, Brown B, et al. Hypoglycemia in type IV glycogenosis: hepatic improvement in two patients with nutritional management. J Pediatr 112:55–58, 1988

422. Greene HL, et al. Continuous nocturnal intragastric feeding for management of type I glycogen-storage disease. N Engl J Med 294:423, 1976

423. Greene HL, et al. Type I glycogen storage disease: a metabolic basis for advances in treatment. Adv Pediatr 26:63, 1979

424. Greengard O. Enzymatic differentiation in mammalian liver. Science 163:891, 1969

425. Greenwood RD, et al. Syndrome of intrahepatic biliary dysgenesis and cardiovascular malformations. Pediatrics 58:243, 1976

426. Gregus Z, Klaassen CD. Hepatic disposition of xenobiotics during prenatal and early postnatal development. In: Fow W, Polin RA, eds. Fetal and neonatal physiology. Philadelphia, WB Saunders, 1992

427. Gremse DA, Bucuvalas JC, Balistreri WF. Efficacy of cornstarch therapy in type III glycogen storage disease. Am J Clin Nutr 52:671–674, 1990

428. Gremse DA, Bucuvalas, JC, Bongiovanni GI. Papillary stenosis and sclerosing cholangitis in an immunodeficient child. Gastroenterology 96:1600–1603, 1989

429. Grenier A, et al. Detection of succinylacetone and the use of its measurement in mass screening for hereditary tyrosinemia. Clin Chim Acta 123:93, 1982

430. Grodsky GM, et al. Effect of age of rat on development of hepatic carriers for bilirubin: a possible explanation for physiologic jaundice and hyperbilirubinemia in the newborn. Metabolism 19:246, 1970

431. Grosfeld JL, Fitzgerald JF, Predaina R, West KW, Vane DW. The efficacy of hepatoportoenterostomy in biliary atresia. Surgery 106:692–701, 1989

432. Gruppuso PA, Walker TD, Carter PA. Ontogeny of hepatic type I insulin-like growth factor receptors in the rat. Pediatr Res 29:226–230, 1991

433. Guandalini S, Fasano A, Albini F, et al. Unconjugated bilirubin and the bile from light exposed Gunn rats inhibit intestinal water and electrolyte absorption. Gut 29:366–371, 1988

434. Guburn-Salisachs L. La maladie atresiante des coies biliares extrahepatiques. Arch Fr Pediatr 25:415, 1968

435. Gustafsson J. Bile acid synthesis during development: mitochondrial 12-hydroxylation in human fetal liver. J Clin Invest 75:604, 1985

436. Hadchouel M. Immunoglobulin deposits in the biliary remnants of extrahepatic biliary atresia: a study by immunoperoxidase staining in 128 infants. Histopathology 5:217, 1981

437. Hadchouel M, Gautier M. Histopathologic study of the liver in the early cholestatic phase of alpha-1-antitrypsin deficiency. J Pediatr 89:211, 1976

438. Haddock JH, Nadler HL. Bilirubin toxicity in human cultivated fibroblasts and its modification by light treatment. Proc Soc Exp Biol Med 134:45, 1970

439. Hadler SC, et al. Effect of immunoglobulin on hepatitis A in day-care centers. JAMA 249:48, 1983

440. Halac E Jr, Sicignano C. Re-evaluation of the influence of sex, age, pregnancy and phenobarbital in the activity of UDP-glucuronyl transferase in rat liver. J Lab Clin Med 73:677, 1969

441. Hale DE, et al. Long-chain acyl coenzyme A dehydrogenase deficiency: an inherited cause of nonketotic hypoglycemia. Pediatr Res 19:666, 1985

442. Hall EG, et al. Congenital toxoplasmosis in the newborn. Arch Dis Child 28:117, 1953

443. Hall RI, Grant JP, Ross LH, et al. Pathogenesis of hepatic steatosis in the parenterally fed rat. J Clin Invest 74:1658–1668, 1989

444. Haller JO, Condon VR, Berdon WE, et al. Spontaneous perforation of the common bile duct in children. Radiology 172:621–624, 1989

445. Haller RG, Lewis SF. Glucose-induced exertional fatigue in

muscle phosphofructokinase deficiency. N Engl J Med 324:364–369, 1991

446. Halpin TJ, et al. Reye's syndrome and medication use. JAMA 248:687, 1982

447. Hamilton JR, Sass-Kortsak A. Jaundice associated with severe bacterial infection in young infants. J Pediatr 63:121, 1963

448. Hammoudi SM, Alauddin A. Idiopathic perforation of the biliary tract in infancy and childhood. J Pediatr Surg 23:185–187, 1988

449. Handel D, Kitlak W. Jaundice as chief symptom of pyuria during infancy. Dtsch Med Wochenschr 91:1781, 1966

450. Hano H, Takasaki S, Ishikawa E. Intrahepatic biliary hypoplasia (non-syndromatic) with special reference to the three dimensional structure of the intrahepatic biliary system. Acta Hepatol Jpn 28:1340, 1987

451. Hansen TWR, Paulsen O, Gjerstad L, et al. Short term exposure to bilirubin reduces synaptic activation in rat transverse hippocampal slices. Pediatr Res 23:453–456, 1988

452. Hanshaw JB. Congenital cytomegalovirus infection: a fifteen year perspective. J Infect Dis 123:355, 1971

453. Hanshaw JB, et al. Acquired cytomegalovirus infection: associated with hepatomegaly and abnormal liver function tests. N Engl J Med 272:602, 1965

454. Hanson RF, et al. The metabolism of 3 alpha, 7 alpha, 12 alpha, trihydroxy-5 beta-cholestan-26-oic acid in two siblings with cholestasis due to intrahepatic bile duct anomalies. J Clin Invest 56:577, 1975

455. Hanson RF, et al. Defects of bile acid synthesis in Zellweger's syndrome. Science 203:1107, 1979

456. Hanson RF, et al. Hepatic lesions and hemolysis following administration of 3 alpha, 7 alpha, 12 alpha-trihydroxy-5 beta-cholestan-26 oyl taurine in rats. J Lab Clin Med 90:536, 1977

457. Haraguchi Y, Aparicio JM, Takiguchi M, et al. Molecular basis of argininemia: identification of two discrete frame-shift deletions in the liver-type arginase gene. J Clin Invest 86:347–350, 1990

458. Haratake J, et al. Familial intrahepatic cholestatic cirrhosis in young adults. Gastroenterology 89:202, 1985

459. Harding BN, Egger J, Portman B, Erdohazi A. Progressive neuronal degeneration of childhood with liver disease. Brain 109:181, 1986

460. Hardwick DF, Dimmick JE. Metabolic cirrhoses of infancy and early childhood. Perspect Pediatr Pathol 3:103, 1976

461. Hardy L, Hansen JL, Kushner JP, Knisely AS. Neonatal hemochromatosis: genetic analysis of transferrin-receptor, H-apoferritin, and L-apoferritin loci and of the human leukocyte antigen class I region. Am J Pathol 137:149–153, 1990

462. Hargreaves T, Piper RF. Breast milk jaundice: effect of inhibitory breast milk and 3 alpha, 20 beta-pregnanediol on glucuronyl transferase. Arch Dis Child 46:195, 1971

463. Harris LE, et al. Conjugated serum bilirubin in erythroblastosis fetalis: an analysis of 38 cases. Proc Staff Meet Mayo Clin 37:574, 1962

464. Hart MH, Kaufman SS, Vanderhoof JA, et al. Neonatal hepatitis and extrahepatic biliary atresia associated with cytomegalovirus infection in twins. Am J Dis Child 145:302–305, 1991

465. Hass GM. Hepatoadrenal necrosis with intranuclear inclusions: report of a case. Am J Pathol 11:127, 1935

466. Hauser ER, Finkelstein JE, Valle D, Brusilow SW. Allopurinol-induced orotidinuria: a test for mutations at the ornithine carbamoyltransferase locus in women. N Engl J Med 322:1641–1645, 1990

467. Hayde M, Widhalm K. Effects of cornstarch treatment in very young children with type I glycogen storage disease. Eur J Pediatr 149:630–633, 1990

468. Hays DM, et al. Diagnosis of biliary atresia: relative accuracy of percutaneous liver biopsy, open liver biopsy and operative cholangiography. J Pediatr 71:598, 1967

469. Heathcote J, et al. Intrahepatic cholestasis in childhood. N Engl J Med 295:801, 1976

470. Heijtink RA, et al. Hepatitis B vaccination in Down's syndrome and other mentally retarded patients. Hepatology 4:611, 1984

471. Heird WC, Dell RB, Helms RA, et al. Amino acid mixture designed to maintain normal plasma amino acid patterns in infants and children requiring parenteral nutrition. Pediatrics 80:401–408, 1987

472. Hejtmancik JF, et al. In vitro amplification of the α_1-antitrypsin gene: application to prenatal diagnosis. Prenat Diagn 9:177–186, 1989

473. Herman SP, et al. Liver dysfunction and histologic abnormalities in neonatal hypopituitarism. J Pediatr 87:892, 1975

474. Hers HG. Alpha-glucosidase deficiency in generalized glycogen storage disease (Pompe's disease). Biochem J 86:11, 1963

475. Heubi JE, et al. Grade I Reye's syndrome: outcome and predictors of progression to deeper coma grades. N Engl J Med 311:1539, 1984

476. Heymans HSA, et al. Severe plasmalogen deficiency in tissues of infants without peroxisomes (Zellweger syndrome). Nature 306:69, 1983

477. Hiraoka K, Haratake J, Horie A, Miyagawa T. Bilateral renal dysplasia, pancreatic fibrosis, intrahepatic biliary dysgenesis, and situs inversus totalis in a boy. Hum Pathol 19:871–873, 1988

478. Hoath SB, Pickens WL, Bucuvalas JC, Suchy FJ. Characterization of hepatic epidermal growth factor receptors in the developing rat. Biochim Biophys Acta 930:107–113, 1987

479. Hodes JE, Grosfeld JL, Weber TR, et al. Hepatic failure in infants on total parenteral nutrition (TPN): clinical and histopathologic observations. J Pediatr Surg 17:463–468, 1982

480. Hodgeman JE, Teberg A. Effect of phototherapy on subsequent growth and development of the premature infant. Birth Defects 6:75, 1970

481. Hodges JR, et al. Heterozygous MZ alpha-1-antitrypsin deficiency in adults with chronic active hepatitis and cryptogenic cirrhosis. N Engl J Med 304:557, 1981

482. Hoeg JM, et al. Characterization of neutral and acid ester hydrolase in Wolman's disease. Biochim Biophys Acta 711:59, 1982

483. Holcomb GW, Holcomb GW. Cholelithiasis in infants, children, and adolescents. Pediatr Rev 11:268–274, 1990

484. Holder TM. Atresia of the extrahepatic bile duct. Am J Surg 107:458, 1964

485. Holton JB, Allen JT, Gillett MG. Prenatal diagnosis of disorders of galactose metabolism. J Inherit Metab Dis 12:202–206, 1989

486. Homberg JC, Abuaf N, Bernard O, et al. Chronic active hepatitis associated with anti-liver kidney microsome antibody type 1: a second type of "autoimmune" hepatitis. Hepatology 7:1333–1339, 1987

487. Hong R, Schubert WK. Menghini needle biopsy of the liver. Am J Dis Child 100:42, 1960

488. Hood JM, et al. Liver transplantation for advanced liver disease with alpha-1-antitrypsin deficiency. N Engl J Med 302:272, 1980

489. Hoogstraten J, deSa DJ, Knisely AS. Fetal liver disease may precede extrahepatic siderosis in neonatal hemochromatosis. Gastroenterology 98:1699–1701, 1990

490. Hostetter MK, et al. Evidence for liver disease preceding amino acid abnormalities in hereditary tyrosinemia. N Engl J Med 308:1265, 1983

491. Houwen RJH, Zwierstra RP, Severijnen RSVM, et al. Prognosis of extrahepatic biliary atresia. Arch Dis Child 64:214–218, 1989

492. Hovig DE, et al. Herpes virus hominis infection in the new-

born with recurrences during infancy. Am J Dis Child 115:438, 1968

493. Howard ER, et al. Spontaneous perforation of common bile duct in infants. Arch Dis Child 51:883, 1976

494. Howard ER, et al. Management of esophageal varices in children by injection sclerotherapy. J Pediatr Surg 19:2, 1984

495. Hsia D Y-Y, et al. Prolonged obstructive jaundice in infancy. V. The genetic components of neonatal hepatitis. Am J Dis Child 95:485, 1958

496. Hsia D Y-Y, et al. Inhibitors of glucuronyl transferase in the newborn. Ann NY Acad Sci 111:326, 1963

497. Hubbell JP, et al. "Early" vs. "late" feeding of infants of diabetic mothers. N Engl J Med 265:835, 1961

498. Hudak ML, et al. Differentiation of transient hyperammonemia of the newborn and urea cycle enzyme defects by clinical presentation. J Pediatr 107:712, 1985

499. Hug G. Glycogen storage disease. In: Kelly VC, ed. Practice of pediatrics, chap 30. Philadelphia, Harper & Row, 1985

500. Hug G, Schubert WK. Glycogenosis type II: glycogen distribution in tissues. Arch Pathol 84:141, 1967

501. Hug G, et al. Type VI glycogenosis: biochemical demonstration of liver phosphorylase deficiency. Biochem Biophys Res Commun 41:1178, 1970

502. Hug G, et al. Loss of cyclic 3′,5′-AMP dependent kinase and reduction of phosphorylase kinase in skeletal muscle of a girl with deactivated phosphorylase kinase and glycogenosis of liver and muscle. Biochem Biophys Res Commun 40:982, 1970

503. Hug G, et al. Rapid prenatal diagnosis of glycogen storage disease type II by electron microscopy of uncultured amniotic-fluid cells. N Engl J Med 310:1018, 1984

504. Hughes CA, Talbot IC, Ducker DA, et al. Total parenteral nutrition in infancy: effect on the liver and suggested pathogenesis. Gut 24:241–248, 1981

505. Hughes JR, et al. Echovirus 14 infection associated with fatal neonatal hepatic necrosis. Am J Dis Child 123:61, 1972

506. Hultcrantz R, Jelf E, Nilsson LH. Minimal liver disease in young persons with homozygous and heterozygous α₁-antitrypsin deficiency. Scand J Gastroenterol 19:389, 1984

507. Hultcrantz R, Mengarelli S. Ultrastructural liver pathology in patients with minimal liver disease and α₁-antitrypsin deficiency: a comparison between heterozygous and homozygous patients. Hepatology 4:937, 1984

508. Hurwitz ES, Barrett MJ, Bregman D, et al. Public health service study of Reye's syndrome and medications: report of the main study. JAMA 257:1905–1911, 1987

509. Hurwitz ES, et al. Public health service study on Reye's syndrome and medications: report of the pilot phase. N Engl J Med 313:849, 1985

510. Huttenlocher PR, Solitare GB, Adams G. Infantile diffuse cerebral degeneration with hepatic cirrhosis. Arch Neurol 33:186–192, 1976

511. Hyams JS, et al. Discordance for biliary atresia in two sets of monozygotic twins. J Pediatr 107:420, 1985

512. Ibarguen E, Gross CR, Savik SK, Sharp HL. Liver disease in alpha-1-antitrypsin deficiency: prognostic indicators. J Pediatr 117:864–870, 1990

513. Ichimiya H, Nazer H, Gunasekaran T, Clayton P, Sjovall J. Treatment of chronic liver disease caused by 3β-hydroxy-Δ⁵-C₂₇-steroid dehydrogenase deficiency with chenodeoxycholic acid. Arch Dis Child 65:1121–1124, 1990

514. Inouye T, et al. Galactose-1-phosphate uridyl transferase in red and white blood cells. Clin Chim Acta 19:169, 1968

515. Ishak KG. Primary hepatic tumors in childhood. In: Popper H, Schaffner F, eds. Progress in liver diseases. New York, Grune & Stratton, 1976, pp 636–667

516. Ishak KG, Glunz PR. Hepatoblastoma and hepatocarcinoma in infancy and childhood: report of 47 cases. Cancer 20:396, 1967

517. Israel JB, Arias IM. Inheritable disorders of bilirubin metabolism. Adv Intern Med 21:77, 1976

518. Isselbacher KJ, et al. Congenital galactosemia, a single enzymatic block in galactose metabolism. Science 123:635, 1956

519. Isselbacher KJ, et al. Congenital betalipoprotein deficiency: an hereditary disorder involving a defect in the absorption and transport of lipids. Medicine 43:347, 1964

520. Ito T, et al. Intrahepatic bile ducts in biliary atresia: a possible factor determining the prognosis. J Pediatr Surg 18:124, 1983

521. Ivemark BI, et al. Niemann-Pick disease in infancy: report of two siblings with clinical, histologic and biochemical studies. Acta Paediatr 52:391, 1963

522. Ives NK, Gardiner RM. Blood–brain barrier permeability to bilirubin in the rat studied using intracarotid bolus injection and in situ brain perfusion techniques. Pediatr Res 27:436–441, 1990

523. Jacir NN, Anderson KD, Eichelberger M, et al. Cholelithiasis in infancy: resolution of gallstones in three of four infants. J Pediatr Surg 21:567–569, 1986

524. Jaehrig K, Ballke EH, Koenig A, Meisel P. Transepithelial electric potential difference in newborns undergoing phototherapy. Pediatr Res 21:283–284, 1987

525. James SP, et al. Liver abnormalities in patients with Gaucher's disease. Gastroenterology 80:126, 1981

526. Jirka JH, et al. Effect of bilirubin on brainstem auditory evoked potentials in the asphyxiated rat. Pediatr Res 19:556, 1985

527. Jirsova V, et al. Beta-glucuronidase activity in different organs of human fetuses. Biol Neonate 8:23, 1965

528. Johnson G, et al. A study of sixteen fatal cases of encephalitis-like disease in North Carolina children. NC Med J 24:464, 1963

529. Johnson JD. Neonatal nonhemolytic jaundice. N Engl J Med 292:197, 1975

530. Johnston JH. Spontaneous perforation of the common bile duct in infancy. Br J Surg 48:532, 1961

531. Johnston WH, et al. Erythroblastosis fetalis and hypebilirubinemia: a five year follow-up with neurological, psychological and audiological evaluation. Pediatrics 39:88, 1967

532. Jonas MM, Kaweblum YA, Fojaco R. Neonatal hemochromatosis: failure of deferoxamine therapy. J Pediatr Gastroenterol Nutr 6:984–988, 1987

533. Jonas A, Yahav J, Fradkin A, et al. Choledocholithiasis in infants: diagnostic and therapeutic problems. J Pediatr Gastroenterol Nutr 11:513–517, 1990

534. Jones CT, Rolph TP. Metabolism during fetal life: a functional assessment of metabolic development. Physiol Rev 65:357–430, 1985

535. Jones EA, et al. Progressive intrahepatic cholestasis of infancy and childhood: a clinicopathological study of a patient surviving to the age of 18 years. Gastroenterology 71:675, 1976

536. Jorgensen MJ. The ductal plate malformation: a study of the intrahepatic bile-duct lesion in infantile polycystic disease and congenital hepatic fibrosis. Acta Pathol Microbiol Immunol Scand (A) (Suppl) 257:33–44, 1976

537. Jorgensen MJ. The ductal plate malformation. Acta Pathol Microbiol Scand (A) (Suppl) 257:1, 1977

538. Joshi V. Indian childhood cirrhosis. Perspect Pediatr Pathol 11:175–192, 1987

539. Juberg RC, et al. Familial intrahepatic cholestasis with growth retardation. Pediatrics 38:819, 1966

540. Kahn E, Daum F, Markowitz J, et al. Nonsyndromatic paucity of interlobular bile ducts: light and electron microscopic evaluation of sequential liver biopsies in early childhood. Hepatology 6:890–901, 1986

541. Kahn E, Markowitz J, Aiges H, Daum F. Human ontogeny of the bile duct to portal space ratio. Hepatology 10:21–23, 1989

542. Kalina RE, Forrest GL. Ocular hazards of phototherapy for hyperbilirubinemia. J Pediatr Ophthalmol 8:116, 1971

543. Kan YW, et al. Hydrops fetalis with alpha thalassemia. N Engl J Med 276:18, 1967

544. Kan YW, et al. Gamma-beta thalassemia as a cause of hemolytic disease of the newborn. N Engl J Med 286:129, 1972

545. Kang ES, Galloway MS, Ellis J, et al. Hepatic steatosis during convalescence from influenza B infection in ferrets with postprandial hyperinsulinemia. J Lab Clin Med 116:335–344, 1990

546. Kaplan E, et al. Phototherapy in ABO hemolytic disease of the newborn infant. J Pediatr 79:911, 1971

547. Kappas A, Drummond GS. Control of heme metabolism with synthetic metalloporphyrins. J Clin Invest 77:335–339, 1986

548. Kappas A, Drummond GS, Manola T, Petmezaki S, Valaes T. Sn-protoporphyrin use in the management of hyperbilirubinemia in term newborns with direct Coombs-positive ABO incompatibility. Pediatrics 81:485–497, 1988

549. Kappas A, et al. The liver excretes large amounts of heme into bile when heme oxygenase is inhibited competitively by SN-protoporphyrin. Proc Natl Acad Sci 82:896, 1985

550. Karjoo M, et al. Choledochal cyst presenting as recurrent pancreatitis. Pediatrics 51:289, 1973

551. Karon M, et al. Effective phototherapy in congenital nonobstructive, nonhemolytic jaundice. N Engl J Med 282:377, 1970

552. Karp WB. Biochemical alterations in neonatal hyperbilirubinemia and bilirubin encephalopathy: a review. Pediatrics 64:361, 1979

553. Kasai M. Treatment of biliary atresia with special reference to hepatic portoenterostomy and its modification. Prog Pediatr Surg 6:6, 1974

554. Kasai M, Mochizuki I, Ohkohchi N, Chiba T, Ohi R. Surgical limitations for biliary atresia: indication for liver transplantation. J Pediatr Surg 24:851–854, 1989

555. Kasai M, Watanabe I. Histologic classification of liver cell carcinoma in infancy and childhood: clinical evaluation. Cancer 25:551, 1970

556. Kasai M, et al. Follow-up studies of long-term survivors after hepatic portoenterostomy for "noncorrectable" biliary atresia. J Pediatr Surg 10:173, 1975

557. Kasai M, et al. Surgical treatment of biliary atresia. J Pediatr Surg 3:665, 1968

558. Kase BF, Pedersen JI, Wathne JO, Gustafsson J, Bjorkhem I. Importance of peroxisomes in the formation of chenodeoxycholic acid in human liver: metabolism of 3α, 7α-dihydroxy-5β-cholestanoic acid in Zellweger syndrome. Pediatr Res 29:64–69, 1991

559. Kase BF, Pedersen JI, Strandvik B, Bjorkhem I. In vivo and in vitro studies on formation of bile acids in patients with Zellweger syndrome. J Clin Invest 76:2393–2402, 1985

560. Kase BF, et al. Defective peroxisomal cleavage of the C_{27} steroid side chain in the cerebro-hepato-renal syndrome of Zellweger. J Clin Invest 75:427, 1985

561. Katz N, Teutsch HF, Jungermann K, Sasse D. Perinatal development of the metabolic zonation of hamster liver parenchyma. FEBS Letters 69:23–26, 1976

562. Kaufman FR, et al. Neonatal cholestasis and hypopituitarism. Arch Dis Child 59:787, 1984

563. Kaufman FR, et al. Hypergonadatropic hypogonadism in female patients with galactosemia. N Engl J Med 304:994, 1981

564. Kaufman SS. Organogenesis and histologic development of the liver. In: Fow W, Polin RA, eds. Fetal and neonatal physiology. Philadelphia, WB Saunders, 1992

565. Kaufman SS, Blain PL, Park JHY, Tuma DJ. Altered role of microtubules in asialoglycoprotein trafficking in developing liver. Am J Physiol 258:G129–G137, 1990

566. Kaufman SS, Blain PL, Park JHY, Tuma DJ. Role of microfilaments in asialoglycoprotein processing in adults and developing liver. Am J Physiol 259:G639–G645, 1990

567. Kaufman SS, Murray ND, Wood RP, Shaw BW, Vanderhoof JA. Nutritional support for the infant with extrahepatic biliary atresia. J Pediatr 110:679–686, 1987

568. Kaufman SS, Wood R, Shaw B, et al. Hepatocarcinoma in a child with the Alagille syndrome 141:698–700, 1987

569. Kaufman SS, Wood RP, Shaw BW, et al. Orthotopic liver transplantation for type I Crigler-Najjar syndrome. Hepatology 6:1259–1262, 1986

570. Kayden HJ, Traber MG. Clinical, nutritional, and biochemical consequences of apolipoprotein B deficiency. Adv Exp Med Biol 201:67, 1986

571. Kelley RI, Feinberg DM, Segal S. Galactose-1-phosphate uridyl transferase in density-fractionated erythrocytes. Hum Genet 82:99–103, 1989

572. Keenan WK, et al. Kernicterus in small sick premature infants receiving phototherapy. Pediatrics 49:652, 1972

573. Kerr DNS, et al. Congenital hepatic fibrosis. Q J Med 30:91, 1961

574. Kerr DNS, et al. A lesion resembling medullary sponge kidney in patients with congenital hepatic fibrosis. Clin Radiol 13:85, 1962

575. Kerr DNS, et al. Congenital hepatic fibrosis: the long-term prognosis. Gut 19:514, 1978

576. Kidd VJ, et al. Prenatal diagnosis of alpha-1-antitrypsin deficiency by direct analysis of the mutation site in the gene. N Engl J Med 310:639, 1984

577. Kilbrick S, Benirschke K. Severe generalized disease occurring in the newborn period and due to infection with coxsackie virus group B. Pediatrics 22:857, 1958

578. Kilpatrick L, Garty BZ, Lundquist KF, et al. Impaired metabolic function and signaling defects in phagocytic cells in glycogen storage disease type 1b. J Clin Invest 86:196–202, 1990

579. King DR, Ginn-Pease ME, Lloyd TV, et al. Parenteral nutrition with associated cholelithiasis: another iatrogenic disease of infants and children. J Pediatr Surg 22:593–596, 1987

580. Kivlahan C, James EJP. The natural history of neonatal jaundice. Pediatrics 74:364, 1984

581. Kliegman RM, Sparks JW. Perinatal galactose metabolism. J Pediatr 107:831–841, 1985

582. Knisely AS. Parvovirus B19 infection in the fetus. Lancet 336:443, 1990

583. Knisely AS, Grady RW, Kramer EE, Jones RL. Cytoferrin, maternofetal iron transport, and neonatal hemochromatosis. Am J Clin Pathol 92:755–759, 1989

584. Knisely AS, Harford JB, Klausner RD, Taylor SR. Neonatal hemochromatosis: the regulation of transferrin-receptor and ferritin synthesis by iron in cultured fibroblastic-line cells. Am J Pathol 134:439–445, 1989

585. Knisely AS, Magid MS, Dische MR, Cutz E. Neonatal hemochromatosis. Birth Defects 23:75–102, 1987

586. Knisely AS, O'Shea PA, Stocks JF, Dimmick JE. Oropharyngeal and upper respiratory mucosal-gland siderosis in neonatal hemochromatosis: an approach to biopsy diagnosis. J Pediatr 113:871, 1988

587. Knox I, et al. Urinary excretion of an isomer of bilirubin during phototherapy. Pediatr Res 19:198, 1985

588. Kobayashi A. Ascending cholangitis after successful surgical repair of biliary atresia. Arch Dis Child 48:697, 1973

589. Kocak N, Ozsoylu S. Familial cirrhosis. Am J Dis Child 133:1160, 1979

590. Kohno Y, Shiraki K, Mura T. The effect of human milk on DNA synthesis of neonatal rat hepatocytes in primary culture. Pediatr Res 29:251–255, 1991

591. Kolvraa S, Gregersen N, Christensen E, Hobolth N. In vitro fibroblast studies of a patient with C_6-C_{10}-dicarboxylic aciduria: evidence for a defect in general acyl-CoA dehydrogenase. Clin Chim Acta 126:53–67, 1982

592. Koneru B, Flye MW, Busuttil RW, et al. Liver transplantation for hepatoblastoma. Ann Surg 213:118–121, 1991

593. Kopelman AE, et al. The "bronze baby" complication of phototherapy. Pediatr Res 5:642, 1971

594. Kornfeld S, Sly WS. Lysosomal storage defects. Hosp Pract August:71, 1985
595. Korones SB, et al. Congenital rubella syndrome: study of 22 infants. Am J Dis Child 110:434, 1965
596. Kreek MJ, Sleisenger M. Reduction of serum-unconjugated bilirubin with phenobarbitone in adult congenital non-haemolytic unconjugated hyperbilirubinemia. Lancet 1:73, 1968
597. Kumura D, Miller JH, Sinatra FR. Septo-optic dysplasia: recognition of causes of false-positive hepatobiliary scintigraphy in neonatal jaundice. J Nucl Med 28:966–972, 1987
598. Kvittingen EA, et al. Prenatal diagnosis of hereditary tyrosinemia by determination of fumarylacetoacetase in cultured amniotic fluid cells. Pediatr Res 19:334, 1985
599. Laberge C, Grenier A, Valet JP, Morissette J. Fumarylacetoacetase measurement as a mass-screening procedure for hereditary tyrosinemia type I. Am J Hum Genet 47:325–328, 1990
600. LaBrecque DR, Latham PS, Riely CA, Hsia YE, Klatskin G. Heritable urea cycle enzyme deficiency-liver disease in 16 patients. J Pediatr 94:580–587, 1979
601. LaBrecque DR, et al. Four generations of arteriohepatic dysplasia. Hepatology 4:467, 1982
602. Labrune P, Perignon JL, Rault M, et al. Familial hypermethioninemia partially responsive to dietary restriction. J Pediatr 117:220–226, 1990
603. Ladd WE. Congenital obstruction of bile ducts. Ann Surg 102:242, 1935
604. Lake BD, Patrick AD. Wolman's disease: deficiency of E 600-resistant acid esterase with storage of lipids in lysosomes. J Pediatr 76:262, 1970
605. Lally KP, Kanegaye J, Matsumura M, Rosenthal P, Sinatra F, Atkinson JB. Perioperative factors affecting the outcome following repair of biliary atresia. Pediatrics 83:723–726, 1989
606. Lambert MA, Marescau B, Desjardins M, et al. Hyperargininemia: intellectual and motor improvement related to changes in biochemical data. J Pediatr 118:420–424, 1991
607. Lambert GH, Muraskas J, Anderson CL, Myers TF. Direct hyperbilirubinemia associated with chloral hydrate administration in the newborn. Pediatrics 86:277–281, 1990
608. Land EJ, McDonagh AF, McGarvey DJ, Truscott TG. Photophysical studies of tin(IV)-protoporphyrin: potential phototoxicity of a chemotherapeutic agent proposed for the prevention of neonatal jaundice. Proc Natl Acad Sci USA 85:5249–5253, 1988
609. Landaw SA, Drummond GS, Kappas A. Targeting of heme oxygenase inhibitors to the spleen markedly increases their ability to diminish bilirubin production. Pediatrics 84:1091–1096, 1989
610. Landing BH. Consideration of the pathogenesis of neonatal hepatitis, biliary atresia and choledochal cyst: the concept of infantile obstructive cholangiopathy. Prog Pediatr Surg 6:113, 1974
611. Landing BH, et al. Familial neurovisceral lipidosis. Am J Dis Child 108:503, 1964
612. Landing BH, et al. Morphometric analysis of liver lesions in cystic diseases of childhood. Hum Pathol 11:549, 1980
613. Larcher VF, et al. Spontaneous bacterial peritonitis in children with chronic liver disease: clinical features and etiologic features. J Pediatr 106:907, 1985
614. Larsson C. Natural history and life expectancy in severe α_1-antitrypsin deficiency, PiZ. Acta Med Scand 204:345, 1978
615. Lascari AD. "Early" breast-feeding jaundice: clinical significance. J Pediatr 108:156–158, 1986
616. Laurell CB, Eriksson S. The electrophoretic alpha-1-globulin pattern of serum in alpha-1-antitrypsin deficiency. Scand J Clin Lab Invest 15:132, 1963
617. Laurendeau T, Hill JE, Manning GB. Idiopathic neonatal hemochromatosis in siblings: an inborn error of metabolism. Arch Pathol 72:410–423, 1961
618. Laurent J, Gauthier F, Bernard O, et al. Long-term outcome after surgery for biliary atresia: study of 40 patients surviving for more than 10 years. Gastroenterology 99:1793–1797, 1990
619. Lauridsen UB, et al. Oesophageal varices as a late complication to neonatal umbilical vein catheterization. Acta Paediatr Scand 67:663, 1978
620. Lavin A, et al. Enzymatic removal of bilirubin from blood: a potential treatment for neonatal jaundice. Science 230:543, 1985
621. Laxer RM, Roberts EA, Gross KR, et al. Liver disease in neonatal lupus erythematosus. J Pediatr 116:238–242, 1990
622. LeBail B, Bioulac-Sage P, Arnoux R, Perissat J, Saric J, Balabaud C. Late recurrence of a hepatocellular carcinoma in a patient with incomplete Alagille syndrome. Gastroenterology 99:1514–1516, 1990
623. Lee C, Oh W, Stonestreet B, Cashore WJ. Permeability of the blood brain barrier for 125 I-albumin-bound bilirubin in newborn piglets. Pediatr Res 25:452–456, 1989
624. Lee KS, Gartner LM. Bilirubin binding by plasma proteins: a critical evaluation of methods and clinical implications. Rev Perinatol Med 2:319, 1978
625. Lee SS, et al. Choledochal cyst: a report of nine cases and review of the literature. Arch Surg 99:19, 1969
626. Lee T, et al. Increased incidence of severe hyperbilirubinemia among newborn Chinese infants with G-6-PD deficiency. Pediatrics 37:994, 1968
627. Lefkowitch JH, et al. Hepatic fibrosis in fetal alcohol syndrome: pathologic similarities to adult alcoholic liver disease. Gastroenterology 85:951, 1983
628. Lefkowitch JH, et al. Hepatic copper overload and features of Indian childhood cirrhosis in an American sibship. N Engl J Med 307:271, 1982
629. Lester R, Schmid R. Intestinal absorption of bile pigments. I. The enterohepatic circulation of bilirubin in the rat. J Clin Invest 42:736, 1963
630. Lester R, et al. A new therapeutic approach to unconjugated hyperbilirubinaemia. Lancet 2:1257, 1962
631. Lester R, et al. Intestinal absorption of bile pigments. II. Bilirubin absorption in man. N Engl J Med 269:178, 1963
632. Le Tan V, et al. Associate de malformation congenitale et de cytomegalie: etude de 18 observations anatomocliniques. Nouv Presse Med 2:1411, 1973
633. Levi AJ. Two hepatic cytoplasmic protein fractions, Y and Z, and their possible role in the hepatic uptake of bilirubin sulfobromophthalein and other anions. J Clin Invest 48:2156, 1969
634. Levi AJ, et al. Deficiency of hepatic organic anion-binding protein, impaired organic anion uptake by liver and "physiologic" jaundice in newborn monkeys. N Engl J Med 283:1136, 1970
635. Levine RL, et al. Clearance of bilirubin from rat brain after reversible osmotic opening of the blood–brain barrier. Pediatr Res 19:1040, 1985
636. Levy HL, et al. Sepsis due to *Escherichia coli* in neonates with galactosemia. N Engl J Med 297:823, 1977
637. Li S, Nussbaum MS, McFadden DW, et al. Addition of L-glutamine to total parenteral nutrition and its effects on portal insulin and glucagon and the development of hepatic steatosis in rats. J Surg Res 48:421–426, 1990
638. Li S, Nussbaum MS, McFadden DW, Dayal R, Fischer JE. Reversal of hepatic steatosis in rats by addition of glucagon to total parenteral nutrition (TPN). J Surg Res 46:557–566, 1989
639. Lichtensten PK, et al. Grade I Reye's syndrome: a frequent cause of vomiting and liver dysfunction after varicella and upper-respiratory-tract infections. N Engl J Med 309:133, 1983

640. Lieberman E, et al. Infantile polycystic disease of the kidneys and liver: clinical, pathological and radiological correlations and comparison with congenital hepatic fibrosis. Medicine 50:277, 1971

641. Lieberman J, et al. Alpha-1-antitrypsin in the livers of patients with emphysema. Science 175:63, 1972

642. Lightner DA, et al. Bilirubin photooxidation products in the urine of jaundiced neonates receiving phototherapy. Pediatr Res 18:696, 1984

643. Lilly JR, Altman RP. Hepatic portoenterostomy (the Kasai operation) for biliary atresia. Surgery 78:76, 1975

644. Lilly JR, Karrer FM, Hall RJ, et al. The surgery of biliary atresia. Ann Surg 210:289–296, 1989

645. Lilly JR, et al. Spontaneous perforation of the extrahepatic bile ducts and bile peritonitis in infancy. Surgery 75:664, 1974

646. Limmer J, Fleig WE, Leupold D, et al. Hepatocellular carcinoma in type I glycogen storage disease. Hepatology 8:531–537, 1988

647. Lindblad B, et al. On the enzymic defects in hereditary tyrosinemia. Proc Natl Acad Sci USA 74:4641, 1977

648. Lindmark B, Millward-Sadler H, Callea F, Eriksson S. Hepatocyte inclusions of α_1-antichymotrypsin in a patient with partial deficiency of α_1-antichymotrypsin and chronic liver disease. Histopathology 16:221–225, 1990

649. Lindor KD, Fleming CR, Abrams A, et al. Liver function values in adults receiving total parenteral nutrition. JAMA 241:2398–2400, 1979

650. Lobo-Yeo A, Senaldi G, Portmann B, et al. Class I and class II major histocompatibility complex antigen expression on hepatocytes. Hepatology 12:224–232, 1990

651. Lohiya G, et al. Hepatocellular carcinoma in young, mentally retarded HBsAg carriers without cirrhosis. Hepatology 5:824, 1985

652. Lough J, et al. Wolman's disease: an electron microscopic, histochemical and biochemical study. Arch Pathol 89:103, 1970

653. Lowry SF, Brennan MF. Abnormal liver function during parenteral nutrition: relation to infusion excess. J Surg Res 26:300–307, 1979

654. Lucas A, Bloom SR, Aynsley-Green A. Gut hormones and minimal enteral feeding. Acta Paediatr Scand 75:719–723, 1986

655. Lucas A, et al. Metabolic and endocrine consequences of depriving preterm infants of enteral nutrition. Acta Pediatr Scand 72:245, 1983

656. Lucey JF, et al. Prevention of hyperbilirubinemia of prematurity by phototherapy. Pediatrics 41:1047, 1968

657. Ludwig J, Wiesner RH, LaRusso NF. Idiopathic adulthood ductopenia: a cause of chronic cholestatic liver disease and biliary cirrhosis. J Hepatol 7:193–199, 1988

658. Luzzatto AC. Hepatocyte differentiation during early fetal development in the rat. Cell Tissue Res 215:133–142, 1981

659. Lyon JB Jr, Porter J. The effect of pyridoxine deficiency on muscle and liver phosphorylase of two inbred strains of mice. Biochim Biophys Acta 58:348, 1962

660. Maggiore G, Bernard O, Homberg JC, et al. Liver disease associated with anti-liver-kidney microsome antibody in children. J Pediatr 108:399–404, 1986

661. Maggiore G, Bernard O, Hadchouel M, Lemmonnier A, Alagille D. Diagnostic value of serum b-glutamyl transpeptidase activity in liver diseases in children. J Pediatr Gastroenterol Nutr. 12:21–26, 1991

662. Maggiore G, Bernard O, Riely CA, Hadchouel M, Lemonnier A, Alagille D. Normal serum β-glutamyl-transpeptidase activity identifies groups of infants with idiopathic cholestasis with poor prognosis. J Pediatr 111:251–252, 1987

663. Maggiore G, Porta G, Bernard O, et al. Autoimmune hepatitis with initial presentation as acute hepatic failure in young children. J Pediatr 116:280–282, 1990

664. Maggiore G, et al. Treatment of autoimmune chronic active hepatitis in childhood. J Pediatr 104:839, 1984

665. Maher JJ, Friedman SL, Roll FJ, et al. Immunolocalization of laminin in normal rat liver and biosynthesis of laminin by hepatic lipocytes in primary culture. Gastroenterol 94:1053–1062, 1988

666. Maisels MJ. Neonatal jaundice. Semin Liver Dis 8:148–162, 1988

667. Maisels MJ, Gifford K, Antle CE, Leib GR. Jaundice in the healthy newborn infant: a new approach to an old problem. Pediatrics 81:505–511, 1988

668. Mannering GJ. Drug metabolism in the newborn. Fed Proceed 44:2302, 1985

669. Marin JJG, Serrano MA, El-Mir MY, Eleno N, Boyd CAR. Bile acid transport by basal membrane vesicles of human term placental trophoblast. Gastroenterology 99:1431–1435, 1990

670. Markowitz J, et al. Arteriohepatic dysplasia. I. Pitfalls in diagnosis and management. Hepatology 3:74, 1983

671. Marshall GS, Starr SE, Witzleben CL, Gonczol E, Plotkin SA. Protracted mononucleosis-like illness associated with acquired cytomegalovirus infection in a previously healthy child: transient cellular immune defects and chronic hepatopathy. Pediatrics 87:556–562, 1991

672. Martens ME, Lee CP. Reye's syndrome: salicylates and mithochondrial functions. Biochem Pharmacol 33:2869, 1984

673. Marti U, Burwen SJ, Jones AL. Biological effects of epidermal growth factor, with emphasis on the gastrointestinal tract and liver: an update. Hepatology 9:126–138, 1989

674. Martin LW. Changing concepts in the management of portal hypertension in childhood. J Pediatr Surg 7:559, 1972

675. Martin LW, Woodman KS. Hepatic lobectomy for hepatoblastoma in infants and children. Arch Surg 98:1, 1969

676. Marwick TH, Cooney PT, Kerlin P. Cirrhosis and hepatocellular carcinoma in a patient with heterozygous (MZ) alpha-1-antitrypsin deficiency. Pathology 17:649, 1985

677. Matos C, Avni EF, Van Gansbeke D, et al. Total parenteral ntrition (TPN) and gallbladder diseases in neonates. J Ultrasound Med 6:243–248, 1987

678. Matsui A, et al. Serum bile acid levels in patients with extrahepatic biliary atresia and neonatal hepatitis during the first 10 days of life. J Pediatr 107:255, 1985

679. Maurage C, Lenaerts C, Weber A, Brochu P, Yousef I, Roy CC. Meconium ileus and its equivalent as a risk factor for the development of cirrhosis: an autopsy study in cystic fibrosis. J Pediatr Gastroenterol 9:17–20, 1989

680. Maurer HM, et al. Controlled trial comparing agar, intermittent phototherapy and continuous phototherapy for reducing neonatal hyperbilirubinemia. J Pediatr 82:73, 1973

681. Maurer HM, et al. Reduction in concentration of total serum bilirubin in offspring of women treated with phenobarbitone during pregnancy. Lancet 2:122, 1968

682. Mauro F, Takamori H, Aoki S, et al. Ultrasonographic measurement of the human fetal liver *in utero*. Gynecol Obstet Invest 24:145–150, 1987

683. McAdams AJ, Wilson HE. The liver in generalized glycogen storage disease: light microscopic observations. Am J Pathol 49:99, 1966

684. McClement JW, et al. Results of surgical treatment for extrahepatic biliary atresia in United Kingdom 1980–2. Br Med J 290:345, 1985

685. McCracken GH Jr, et al. Congenital cytomegalic inclusion disease: a longitudinal study of 20 patients. Am J Dis Child 117:522, 1969

686. McDonagh AF. Blue light and bilirubin excretion. Science 208:145, 1980

687. McDonagh AF, Ramonas LM. Jaundice phototherapy: micro flow-cell photometry reveals rapid biliary response of Gunn rats to light. Science 201:829, 1978

688. McDonagh AF. Purple versus yellow: preventing neonatal jaundice with tin-porphyrins. J Pediatr 113:777–781, 1988

689. McGrath KM, et al. Liver disease complicating severe hemophilia in childhood. Arch Dis Child 55:537, 1980

690. McLean RH, et al. Multinodular hemangiomatosis of the liver in infancy. Pediatrics 49:563, 1972

691. McNeil TF, Sveger T, Thelin T. Psychosocial effects of screening for somatic risk: the Swedish α_1-antitrypsin experience. Thorax 43:505–507, 1988

692. Meert KL, Kauffman RE, Deshmukh DR, Sarnaik AP. Impaired oxidative metabolism of salicylate in Reye's syndrome. Dev Pharmacol Ther 15:57–60, 1990

693. Meisel P, Jahrig D, Meisel M. Detection of photobilirubin in urine of jaundiced infants supporting the diagnosis of "bronze baby syndrome." Clin Chim Acta 166:61–65, 1987

694. Mellis C, et al. Familial hepatic venoocclusive disease with probable immune deficiency. J Pediatr 88:236, 1976

695. Merritt RJ, et al. Cholestatic effect of intraperitoneal administration of tryptophan to suckling rat pups. Pediatr Res 18:904, 1984

696. Messing B. Gallbladder sludge and lithiasis: complications of bowel rest. Nutrition 6:190, 1990

697. Messing B, Bories C, Kunstlinger F, et al. Does total parenteral nutrition induce gallbladder sludge formation and lithiasis? Gastroenterology 84:1012–1019, 1983

698. Metreau JM, et al. Role of bilirubin overproduction in revealing Gilbert's syndrome: is dyserythropoiesis an important factor? Gut 19:838, 1978

699. Metzman R, Anand A, DeGiulio PA, Knisely AS. Hepatic disease associated with intrauterine parvovirus B19 infection in a newborn premature infant. J Pediatr Gastroenterol Nutr 9:112–114, 1989

700. Meyer TC, Angus J. The effect of large doses of "Synkavit" in the newborn. Arch Dis Child 31:212, 1956

701. Meythaler JM, Varma PR. Reye's syndrome in adults. Arch Intern Med 147:61–64, 1987

702. Michael AF Jr, Mauer AM. Maternal–fetal transfusion as a cause of plethora in the neonatal period. Pediatrics 28:458, 1961

703. Mieles LA, Esquivel CO, Van Thiel DH, et al. Liver transplantation for tyrosinemia: a review of 10 cases from the University of Pittsburgh. Dig Dis Sci 35:153–157, 1990

704. Mieli-Vergani G, Howard ER, Portmann B, Mowat AP. Late referral for biliary atresia: missed opportunity for effective surgery. Lancet 1:421–423, 1989

705. Mikkelsen WP. Extrahepatic portal hypertension in children. Am J Surg 111:333, 1966

706. Miller DR, et al. Fatal disseminated herpes simplex virus infection and hemorrhage in the neonate: coagulation studies in a case and a review. J Pediatr 76:409, 1970

707. Miller MJ, et al. Clinical spectrum of congenital toxoplasmosis: problems in recognition. J Pediatr 70:714, 1967

708. Millis JM, Brems JJ, Hiatt JR, et al. Orthotopic liver Transplantation for Biliary Atresia. Arch Surg 123:1237–1239, 1988

709. Mineo I, et al. Excess purine degradation in exercising muscles of patients with glycogen storage disease types V and VII. J Clin Invest 76:556, 1985

710. Minuk GY, Shaffer EA. Benign recurrent intrahepatic cholestasis: evidence for an intrinsic abnormality in hepatocyte secretion. Gastroenterology 93:1187–1193, 1987

711. Mitchell G, Larochelle J, Lambert M, et al. Neurologic crises in hereditary tyrosinemia. N Engl J Med 322:432–437, 1990

712. Mitchell JE, McCall FC. Transplacental infection by herpes simplex virus. Am J Dis Child 106:207, 1963

713. Miyairi M, et al. Cell motility of fetal hepatocytes in short-term culture. Pediatr Res 19:1226, 1985

714. MMWR. Reye's syndrome surveillance: United States, 1989. 40:88–90, 1991

715. MMWR. Protection against viral hepatitis: recommendations of the immunization practice advisory committee. 39:RR-2, 1990

716. Mock DM. Fatty acids and Reye's syndrome. Hepatology 6:1414, 1986

717. Mock DM, et al. Chronic fructose intoxication after infancy in children with hereditary fructose intolerance: a cause of growth retardation. N Engl J Med 309:764, 1983

718. Modlin JF. Fatal echovirus II disease in premature neonates. Pediatrics 66:775, 1980

719. Moedy A, et al. Fatal disseminated herpes simplex virus infection in a healthy child. Am J Dis Child 135:45, 1981

720. Moerman P, Pauwels P, Vandenberghe K, et al. Neonatal haemochromatosis. Histopathology 17:345–351, 1990

721. Moniff GRG, et al. Postmortem isolation of rubella virus from three children with rubella syndrome defects. Lancet 1:723, 1965

722. Montgomery CK, Ruebner BH. Neonatal hepatocellular giant cell transformation: a review. Perspect Pediatr Pathol 3:85, 1976

723. Mooi WJ, et al. Ultrastructure of the liver in cerebrohepatorenal syndrome of Zellweger. Ultrastruct Pathol 5:135, 1983

724. Morecki R, et al. Biliary atresia and reovirus type 3 infection. N Engl J Med 307:481, 1982

725. Morecki R, et al. Detection of reovirus type 3 in the porta hepatis of an infant with extrahepatic biliary atresia: ultrastructural and immunocytochemical study. Hepatology 4:1137, 1984

726. Moreno LA, Gottrand F, Hoden S, et al. Improvement of nutritional status in cholestatic children with supplemental nocturnal enteral nutrition. J Pediatr Gastroenterol Nutr 12:213–216, 1991

727. Morin T, et al. Heterozygous alpha 1-antitrypsin deficiency and cirrhosis in adults: a fortuitous association. Lancet 1:250, 1985

728. Mornex JF, Chytil-Weir A, Martinset Y, et al. Expression of the alpha-1-antitrypsin gene in mononuclear phagocytes of normal and alpha-1-antitrypsin-deficient individuals. J Clin Invest 77:1952–1961, 1986

729. Morphis L, et al. Bilirubin-induced modulation of cerebral protein phosphorylation in neonate rabbits in vivo. Science 218:156, 1982

730. Moser AE, et al. The cerebrohepatorenal (Zellweger) syndrome: increased levels and impaired degradation of very-long-chain fatty acids and their use in prenatal diagnosis. N Engl J Med 310:1141, 1984

731. Moser HW. Peroxisomal diseases. Adv Pediatr 36:1–38, 1989

732. Moser HW, et al. Adrenoleukodystrophy: survey of 303 cases: biochemistry, diagnosis and therapy. Ann Neurol 16:628, 1984

733. Moses SW. Pathophysiology and dietary treatment of the glycogen storage disease. J Pediatr Gastroenterol Nutr 11:155–174, 1990 (see also: Moses SW, Wanderman KL, Myroz A, Frydman M. Cardiac involvement in glycogen storage disease type III. Eur J Pediatr 148:764–766, 1989)

734. Mostoufizadel M, Lack EE, Gang DL, Perez-Atayde AR, Driscoll SP. Post mortem manifestations of echovirus 11 sepsis in five newborn infants. Hum Pathol 9:818–823, 1983

735. Mowat AP, et al. Extrahepatic biliary atresia versus neonatal hepatitis: review of 137 prospectively investigated infants. Arch Dis Child 51:763, 1976

736. Mowat AP. Prevention of variceal bleeding. J Pediatr Gastroenterol Nutr 5:679–681, 1986

737. Msall M, et al. Neurologic outcome in children with inborn errors of urea synthesis: outcome of urea cycle enzymopathies. N Engl J Med 310:1500, 1984

738. Muller-Hocker J, Meyer U, Wiebecke B. Copper storage disease of the liver and chronic dietary copper intoxication in two further German infants mimicking Indian childhood cirrhosis. Pathol Res Pract 183:39–45, 1988

739. Mueller RF. The Alagille syndrome. J Med Genet 24:621–626, 1987

740. Mueller RF, Pagan RA, Pepin MB, et al. Arteriohepatic dysplasia: phenotypic features and family studies. Clin Genet 25:323–331, 1984

741. Mullon CJP, Tosone CM, Langer R. Simulation of bilirubin detoxification in the newborn using an extracorporeal bilirubin oxidase reactor. Pediatr Res 26:452–457, 1989

742. Murphy JF, Hughes I, Verrier-Jones ER, et al. Pregnanediols and breast milk jaundice. Arch Dis Child 56:474–476, 1981

743. Nadler HL, et al. Congenital galactosemia: a study of 55 cases. In: Hsia D Y-Y, ed. Galactosemia. Springfield IL, Charles C Thomas, 1969, pp 127–139

744. Nagel RA, Javaid A, Meire HB, et al. Liver disease and bile duct abnormalities in adults with cystic fibrosis. Lancet 2:1422–1425, 1989

745. Nahmias AJ, et al. Newborn infection with herpes virus hominis types 1 and 2. J Pediatr 75:1194, 1969

746. Nahmias AJ, et al. Neonatal herpes simplex infection: role of genital infection in mother as the source of virus in the newborn. JAMA 199:164, 1967

747. Narkewicz MR, Sokol RJ, Beckwith B, Sondheimer J, Silverman A. Liver involvement in Alpers disease. J Pediatr 119:260–267, 1991

748. Nayak NC, Ramalingaswami V. Childhood cirrhosis. In: Beck FF, Dekker M, eds. The liver, part B. 1975, pp 851–882

749. Nebbia G, Hadchouel M, Odievre M, et al. Early assessment of evolution of liver disease associated with α_1-antitrypsin deficiency in childhood. J Pediatr 102:661, 1983

750. Nemeth A, Ejderhamn J, Glaumann H, Strandvik B. Liver damage in juvenile inflammatory bowel disease. Liver 10:239–248, 1990

751. Nemeth A, et al. Alpha-1-antitrypsin deficiency and juvenile liver disease: ultrastructural observations compared with light microscopy and routine liver tests. Virchows Arch [A] 44:15, 1983

752. Newman TB, Easterling J, Goldman ES, Stevenson DK. Laboratory evaluation of jaundice in newborns. Am J Dis Child 144:364–368, 1990

753. Newman TB, Maisels MJ. Bilirubin and brain damage: what do we do now? Pediatrics 83:1062–1065, 1989

754. Nezelof C, Dupart MC, Joubert F, et al. A lethal familial syndrome associating arthrogryposis multiplex congenita, renal dysfunction and a cholestatic and pigmentary liver disease. J Pediatr 94:258–260, 1979

755. Ng SH, Rawstron JR. Urinary tract infection presenting with jaundice. Arch Dis Child 46:173, 1971

756. Nielsen IM, Ornvold K, Jacobsen BB, Ranek L. Fatal familial cholestatic syndrome in Greenland Eskimo children. Acta Paediatr Scand 75:1010–1016, 1986

757. Noell WK, et al. Retinal damage by light in rats. Invest Ophthalmol 5:450, 1966

758. Notter M, Kendig J. Differential sensitivity of neural cells to bilirubin toxicity. Exp Neurol 94:670–682, 1986

759. Novak, DA, Balistreri WF. Management of chronic cholestasis. Pediatr Ann 14:488, 1985

760. Novak DA, Suchy FJ. Postnatal expression of the canalicular bile acid transport system in rat liver. Hepatology 7:1037, 1987

761. O'Brien JS. Generalized gangliosidosis. J Pediatr 75:167, 1969

762. Odell GB. "Physiologic" hyperbilirubinemia in the neonatal period. N Engl J Med 277:193, 1967

763. Odell GB, et al. The influence of fatty acids on the binding of bilirubin to albumin. J Lab Clin Med 89:295, 1977

764. Odell GB, et al. Enteral administration of agar as an effective adjunct to phototherapy of neonatal hyperbilirubinemia. Pediatr Res 17:810, 1983

765. Odell GB, et al. Administration of albumin in the management of hyperbilirubinemia by exchange transfusion. Pediatrics 30:613, 1962

766. Odell GB, et al. Studies in kernicterus. III. The saturation of serum proteins with bilirubin during neonatal life and its relationship to brain damage at five years. J Pediatr 76:12, 1970

767. Odievre M, et al. Congenital abnormalities associated with extrahepatic portal hypertension. Arch Dis Child 52:383, 1977

768. Odievre M, et al. Long-term prognosis for infants with intrahepatic cholestasis and patent extrahepatic biliary tract. Arch Dis Child 56:373, 1981

769. Odievre M, et al. Alpha-1-antitrypsin deficiency and liver disease in children: phenotypes, manifestations, and prognosis. Pediatrics 57:226, 1976

770. Odievre M, et al. Seroimmunologic classification of chronic hepatitis in 57 children. Hepatology 3:407, 1983

771. Odievre M, et al. Severe familial intrahepatic cholestasis. Arch Dis Child 48:806, 1973

772. Odievre M, et al. Hereditary fructose intolerance in childhood. Am J Dis Child 132:605, 1978

773. Ogushi F, Fells GA, Hubbard RC, et al. Z-type α 1-antitrypsin is less competent than M1-type α 1-antitrypsin as an inhibitor of neutrophil elastase. J Clin Invest 80:1366, 1987

774. Ohi R, et al. Reoperation in patients with biliary atresia. J Pediatr Surg 20:256, 1985 (see also: Ohi R, et al. Progress in the treatment of biliary atresia. World J Surg 9:285, 1985)

775. Ohya T, Miyano T, Kimura K. Indication for portoenterostomy based on 103 patients with suruga II modification. J Pediatr Surg 25:801–804, 1990

776. Okada A, Nakamura T, Higaki J, Okumura K, Kamata S, Oguchi Y. Congenital dilatation of the bile duct in 100 instances and its relationship with anomalous junction. Surg Gynecol Obstet 171:291–298, 1990

777. Okada K, et al. E antigen and anti-e in the serum of asymptomatic carrier mothers as indicators of positive and negative transmission of hepatitis B virus to their infants. N Engl J Med 294:746, 1976

778. Okada S, et al. Ganglioside GM_2 storage diseases: hexosaminidase deficiencies in cultured fibroblasts. Am J Hum Genet 23:55, 1971

779. Okayasu T, Nagano S, Takada K, Tomita M, Arashima S, Matsumoto S. Cytotoxicity of galactose, tyrosine and methionine in cultured suckling rat hepatocytes: relation to liver immaturity. Acta Paediatr Scand 78:930–934, 1989

780. Opleta K, Butzner JD, Shaffer EA, et al. The effect of protein-calorie malnutrition on the developing liver. Pediatr Res 23:505–508, 1988

781. Oppenheimer E, Esterly JR. Cytomegalovirus infection: a possible cause of biliary atresia. Am J Pathol 72:2a, 1973

782. Oppenheimer EH, Esterly JR. Hepatic changes in young infants with cystic fibrosis: possible relation to focal biliary cirrhosis. J Pediatr 86:683–689, 1975

783. Ornvold K, Nielsen IM, Poulsen H. Fatal familial cholestatic syndrome in Greenland Eskimo children. Virchows Arch [A] 415:275–281, 1989

784. Ostrow JD. Photocatabolism of labeled bilirubin in the congenitally jaundiced (Gunn) rat. J Clin Invest 50:707, 1971

785. Ostrow JD. Effect of phototherapy on hepatic excretory function in normal and Gunn rats. Gastroenterology 62:168, 1972

786. Ostrow JD, et al. Effect of phototherapy on bilirubin excretion in man and the rat. In: Bergsma E, Blondheim SH, eds. Bilirubin metabolism in the newborn, vol 2. New York, American Elsevier, 1976

787. Ostrow JD. Therapeutic amelioration of jaundice: old and new strategies. Hepatology 8:683–689, 1988

788. Pakekh SR, et al. Detection of Regan variant type of alkaline phosphatase isoenzyme in liver tissue of Indian childhood cirrhosis. Hepatology 3:572, 1983

789. Paradis K, Weber A, Seidman EG, et al. Liver transplanta-

tion for hereditary tyrosinemia: the Quebec experience. Am J Hum Genet 47:338–342, 1990

790. Park RW, Grand RJ. Gastrointestinal manifestations of cystic fibrosis: a review. Gastroenterology 81:1143, 1981

791. Partin JC. Reye's syndrome: diagnosis and treatment. Gastroenterology 69:511, 1975

792. Partin JC, Schubert WK. Small intestinal mucosa in cholesterol ester storage disease: a light and electron microscopy study. Gastroenterology 57:542, 1969

793. Partin JC, et al. Brain ultrastructure in Reye's syndrome (encephalopathy and fatty alteration of the viscera). J Neuropathol Exp Neurol 34:425, 1975

794. Partin JC, et al. Mitochondrial ultrastructure in Reye's syndrome (encephalopathy and fatty degeneration of the viscera). N Engl J Med 285:1339, 1971

795. Partin JS, et al. Liver ultrastructure in abetalipoproteinemia evolution of micronodular cirrhosis. Gastroenterology 67:107, 1974

796. Passarge E, McAdams AJ. Cerebro-hepato-renal syndrome. J Pediatr 71:691, 1967

797. Patrick AD, Lake BD. Deficiency of an acid lipase in Wolman's disease. Nature 222:1067, 1969

798. Patrick MK, Howman-Giles R, De Silva M, et al. Common bile duct obstruction causing right upper abdominal pain in cystic fibrosis. J Pediatr 108:101–102, 1986

799. Patterson K, Kapur SP, Chandra RS. Hepatocellular carcinoma in a noncirrhotic infant after prolonged parenteral nutrition. J Pediatr 106:797–800, 1985

800. Pearson HA. Life span of fetal red cells. J Pediatr 70:166, 1967

801. Peden VH, et al. Total parenteral nutrition. J Pediatr 78:180, 1971

802. Pelletier VA, Galeano N, Brochu P, Morin CL, Weber AM, Roy CC. Secretory diarrhea with protein-losing enteropathy, enterocolitis cystica superficialis, intestinal lymphangiectasia, and congenital hepatic fibrosis: a new syndrome. J Pediatr 107:61–65, 1985

803. Pereyra R, et al. Management of massive hepatic hemangiomas in infants and children: a review of 13 cases. Pediatrics 70:254, 1982

804. Perez CA, et al. Treatment of malignant sympathetic tumors in children: clinicopathologic correlation. Pediatrics 41:452, 1968

805. Perlman M, Frank JW. Bilirubin beyond the blood–brain barrier. Pediatrics 81:304–315, 1988

806. Perlmutter DH. The cellular basis for liver injury in α_1-antitrypsin deficiency. Hepatology 13:172–185, 1991

807. Perlmutter DH, Kay RM, Cole FS, Rossing TH, Van Thiel DH, Colten HR. The cellular defect in α_1-antitrypsin inhibitor deficiency is expressed in human monocytes and in xenopus oocytes injected with human liver mRNA. Proc Natl Acad Sci USA 82:6918–6921, 1985

808. Perlmutter DH, Schlesinger MJ, Pierce JA, Punsal PI, Schwartz AL. Synthesis of stress proteins is increased in individuals with homozygous PiZZ α_1-antitrypsin deficiency and liver disease. J Clin Invest 84:1555–1561, 1989

809. Perlmutter DH, Travis J, Punsal PI. Elastase regulates the synthesis of its inhibitor α_1-proteinase inhibitor, and exaggerates the defect in homozygous PiZZ α_1-proteinase inhibitor deficiency. J Clin Invest 81:1774–1780, 1988

810. Persico M, Romano M, Muraca M, Gentile S. Responsiveness to phenobarbital in an adult with Crigler-Najjar disease associated with neurological involvement and skin hyperextensibility. Hepatology 13:213–215, 1991

811. Petell JK, Doyle D. Developmental regulation of the hepatocyte receptor for galactose-terminated glycoproteins. Arch Biochem Biophys 241:550–560, 1985

812. Philip AGS, Larson EJ. Overwhelming neonatal infection with ECHO 19 virus. J Pediatr 82:391, 1973

813. Phillips JM, Blendis LM, Poucell S, et al. Syncytial giant-cell hepatitis: sporadic hepatitis with distinctive pathological features, a severe clinical course, and paramyxoviral features. N Engl J Med 324:455–460, 1991

814. Phillips MJ, et al. Subcellular pathology of hereditary fructose intolerance. Am J Med 44:910, 1968

815. Piccoli DA, Witzleben CL, Guico CJ, Morrison A, Rubin DH. Synergism between hepatic injuries and a nonhepatotrophic reovirus in mice: enhanced hepatic infection and death. J Clin Invest 86:1038–1045, 1990

816. Pitkanen O, Hallman M, Anderson S. Generation of free radicals in lipid emulsion used in parenteral nutrition. Pediatr Res 29:56–59, 1991

817. Pittschieler K. Liver disease and heterozygous alpha-1-antitrypsin deficiency. Acta Pediatr Scand 80:323–327, 1991

818. Pittschieler K, Lebenthal E, Bujanover Y, Petell JK. Levels of Cu-Zn and Mn superoxide dismutases in rat liver during development. Gastroenterology 100:1062–1068, 1991

819. Poh-Fitzpatrick MB, Zaider E, Sokol RJ, et al. Cutaneous photosensitivity and co-proporphyrin abnormalities in the Alagille syndrome. Gastroenterology 99:831–835, 1990

820. Poland RL, Odell GB. Physiologic jaundice: the enterohepatic circulation of bilirubin. N Engl J Med 284:1, 1971

821. Pollitt RJ. Disorders of mitochondrial B-oxidation: prenatal and early postnatal diagnosis and their relevance to Reye's syndrome and sudden infant death. J Inherit Metab Dis 12:215–230, 1989

822. Porta G, da Costa Gayotto LC, Alvarez F. Anti-liver-kidney microsome antibody-positive autoimmune hepatitis presenting as fulminant liver failure. J Pediatr Gastroenterol Nutr 11:138–140, 1990

823. Porter CA, et al. Alpha-1-antitrypsin deficiency and neonatal hepatitis. Br Med J 3:435, 1972

824. Porter JDH, Robinson PH, Glasgow JFT, Banks JH, Hall SM. Trends in the incidence of Reye's syndrome and the use of aspirin. Arch Dis Child 65:826–829, 1990

825. Postuma R, Trevenen CL. Liver disease in infants receiving total parenteral nutrition. Pediatrics 63:110, 1979

826. Potashnik R, Moran A, Moses SW, Peleg N, Bashan N. Hexose uptake and transport in polymorphonuclear leukocytes from patients with glycogen storage disease Ib. Pediatr Res 28:19–23, 1990

827. Poulos A, Whiting MJ. Identification of 3 alpha, 7 alpha, 12 alpha-trihydroxy-5 beta-cholestan-26-oic acid, an intermediate in cholic acid synthesis, in the plasma of patients with infantile Refsum's disease. J Inherit Metab Dis 8:13, 1985

828. Povey S. Genetics of α_1-antitrypsin deficiency in relation to neonatal liver disease. Mol Biol Med 7:161–162, 1990

829. Powell LW, et al. Idiopathic unconjugated hyperbilirubinemia (Gilbert's syndrome): a study of 42 families. N Engl J Med 277:1108, 1967

830. Powers JM, et al. Fetal cerebrohepatorenal (Zellweger) syndrome: dysmorphic, radiologic, biochemical, and pathologic findings in four affected fetuses. Hum Pathol 16:610, 1985

831. Prober CG, Hensleigh PA, Boucher FD, Yasukawa LL, Au DS, Arvin AM. Use of routine viral cultures at delivery to identify neonates exposed to herpes simplex virus. N Engl J Med 318:887–891, 1988

832. Pryles CV, Heggestad GE. Large cavernous hemangioma of the liver. Am J Dis Child 88:759, 1954

833. Psacharopoulos HT, Howard ER, Portmann B, Mowat AP. Extrahepatic biliary atresia: preoperative assessment and surgical results in 47 consecutive cases. Arch Dis Child 55:851–856, 1980

834. Psacharopoulos HT, et al. Hepatic complications of cystic fibrosis. Lancet 2:78, 1981

835. Psacharopoulos HT, et al. Outcome of liver disease associated with alpha-1-antitrypsin deficiency (PiZ): implications for genetic counselling and antenatal diagnosis. Arch Dis Child 58:882, 1983

836. Pugh RCB, et al. Hepatic necrosis in disseminated herpes simplex. Arch Dis Child 29:60, 1954

837. Putnam CW, Porter KA, Peters RL, et al. Liver replacement for alpha₁-antitrypsin deficiency. Surgery 81:258, 1977

838. Quale JM, Mandel LJ, Bergasa NV, Straus EW. Clinical significance and pathogenesis of hyperbilirubinemia associated with Staphylococcus aureus septicemia. Am J Med 85:615–618, 1988

839. Quilligan JJ Jr, Wilson JL. Fatal herpes simplex infection in a newborn infant. J Lab Clin Med 38:742, 1951

840. Raga J, et al. Usefulness of clinical features and liver biopsy in diagnosis of disseminated herpes simplex infection. Arch Dis Child 59:820, 1984

841. Rakela J, Goldschmiedt M, Ludwig J. Late manifestations of chronic liver disease in adults with α_1-antitrypsin deficiency. Dig Dis Sci 32:1358, 1987

842. Rank JM, Pascual-Leone A, Payne W, Glock M, Freeese D, Sharp H, Bloomer JR. Hematin therapy for the neurologic crisis of tyrosinemia. J Pediatr 118:136–139, 1991

843. Rausen AR, Diamond LK. Enclosed hemorrhage and neonatal jaundice. Am J Dis Child 101:164, 1961

844. Rausen AR, et al. Twin transfusion syndrome: a review of 19 cases studied at one institution. J Pediatr 66:613, 1965

845. Raweily EA, Gibson AAM, Burt AD. Abnormalities of intrahepatic bile ducts in extrahepatic biliary atresia. Histopathology 17:521–527, 1990

846. Redeker AG, et al. The reciprocal relationship between caloric intake and degree of hyperbilirubinemia in Gilbert's syndrome. Gastroenterology 58:303, 1970

847. Reed GB Jr, et al. Type IV glycogenosis. Lab Invest 19:546, 1968

848. Reesink HW, et al. Prevention of chronic HBsAg carrier state in infants of HBsAg-positive mothers by hepatitis B immunoglobulin. Lancet 2:436, 1979

849. Reffensberger JG, Gonzalez-Crussi F, Skeehan T. Mesenchymal hamartoma of the liver. J Pediatr Surg 18:585, 1983

850. Reid CL, Wiener GJ, Cox DW, et al. Diffuse hepatocellular dysplasia and carcinoma associated with the Malton variant of α_1-antitrypsin. Gastroenterology 93:181, 1987

851. Reif S, Lebenthal E. Extracellular matrix modulation of liver ontogeny. J Pediatr Gastroenterol Nutr 12:1–4, 1991

852. Reif S, Sloven DG, Lebenthal E. Gallstones in children: characterization by age, etiology and outcome. Am J Dis Child 145:105–108, 1991

853. Reif S, Terranova VP, El-Bendary M, Lebenthal E, Petell JK. Modulation of extracellular matrix proteins in rat liver during development. Hepatology 12:519–525, 1990

854. Remington JS, Desmonts G. Congenital toxoplasmosis: variability in the IgM fluorescent antibody response and some pitfalls in diagnosis. J Pediatr 88:27, 1973

855. Remington PL, Rowley D, McGee H, et al. Decreasing trends in Reye syndrome and aspirin use in Michigan, 1979 to 1984. Pediatrics 77:93, 1986

856. Resti M, Adami Lami C, Tucci F, et al. False diagnosis of non-A/non-B hepatitis hiding two cases of cystic fibrosis. Eur J Pediatr 150:97–99, 1990

857. Reye RDK, et al. Encephalopathy and fatty degeneration of the viscera. Lancet 2:749, 1963

858. Rice DN, Houston IB, Lyon ICT, et al. Transient neonatal tyrosinaemia. J Inherit Metab Dis 12:13–22, 1989

859. Riely CA. Familial intrahepatic cholestatic syndromes. Semin Liver Dis 7:119–126, 1987

860. Riely CA, et al. A father and son with cholestasis and peripheral pulmonic stenosis. J Pediatr 92:406, 1978

861. Rinaldo P, O'Shea JJ, Coates PM, Hale DE, Stanley CA, Tanaka K. Medium-chain acyl-CoA dehydrogenase deficiency: diagnosis by stable-isotope dilution measurement of urinary N-hexanoylglycine and 3-phenylpropionylglycine. N Engl J Med 319:1308–1313, 1988 (see also: Bennett, et al. J Inherit Metab Dis 13:707–715, 1990)

862. Ritter DA, Kenny JD. Bilirubin binding in premature infants from birth to 3 months. Arch Dis Child 61:352–356, 1986

863. Robbins BH, Castle RF. Hemangiomas, hepatic involvement, congestive failure. Pediatrics 35:868, 1965

864. Roberts EA, et al. Occurrence of alpha-1-antitrypsin deficiency in 155 patients with alcoholic liver disease. Am J Clin Pathol 82:424, 1984

865. Robinson SH, et al. Bilirubin excretion in rats with normal and impaired bilirubin conjugation: effect of phenobarbital. J Clin Invest 50:2606, 1971

866. Rodgers BM, Talbert JL. Distal spleno-renal shunt for portal decompression in childhood. J Pediatr Surg 14:33, 1979

867. Roe CR, Millington DS, Maltby DA. Identification of 3-methylglutarylcarnitine: a new diagnostic metabolite of 3-hydroxy-3-methylglutaryl-coenzyme A lyase deficiency. J Clin Invest 77:1391, 1986

868. Roe CR, Millington DS, Maltby DA, et al. Diagnostic and therapeutic implications of medium-chain acylcarnitines in medium-chain acyl CoA dehydrogenase deficiency. Pediatr Res 19:459, 1985

869. Roe CR, Millington DS, Maltby DA, et al. Recognition of medium-chain acyl CoA dehydrogenase deficiency in asymptomatic siblings of children dying of sudden infant death or Reye-like syndrome. J Pediatr 108:13, 1986

870. Rommens JM, Iannuzzi MC, Kerem BS, et al. Identification of the cystic fibrosis gene: chromosome walking and jumping. Science 245:1059–1065, 1989

871. Rooney JC, et al. Jaundice associated with bacterial infection in the newborn. Am J Dis Child 122:39, 1971

872. Roscher A, et al. The cerebrohepatorenal (Zellweger) syndrome: an improved method for the biochemical diagnosis and its potential value for prenatal detection. Pediatr Res 19:930, 1985

873. Rosenberg DP, et al. Extrahepatic biliary atresia in a rhesus monkey (*Macaca mulatta*). Hepatology 3:577, 1983

874. Rosenblum JL, et al. A progressive neurologic syndrome in children with chronic liver disease. N Engl J Med 304:503, 1981

875. Rosenstein BS, Ducore JM. Enhancement by bilirubin of DNA damage induced in human cells exposed to phototherapy light. Pediatr Res 18:3, 1984

876. Rosenthal P, Blanckaert N, Kabra PM, et al. Formation of bilirubin conjugates in human newborns. Pediatr Res 20:947–950, 1986

877. Rosenthal P, Liebman WM, Thaler MM, et al. Alpha₁-antitrypsin deficiency and severe infantile liver disease. Am J Dis Child 133:1195, 1979

878. Roslyn JJ, Berquist WE, Pitt HA, et al. Increased risk of gallstones in children receiving total parenteral nutrition. Pediatrics 71:784–789, 1983

879. Roslyn JJ, et al. Gallbladder disease in patients on long-term parenteral nutrition. Gastroenterology 84:148, 1983

880. Rotman M, et al. Radiation treatment of pediatric hepatic hemangiomatosis and coexisting cardiac failure. N Engl J Med 302:852, 1980

881. Rowe PC, Newman SL, Brusilow SW. Natural history of symptomatic partial ornithine transcarbamylase deficiency. N Engl J Med 314:541–547, 1986

882. Rowe PC, Valle D, Brusilow SW. Inborn errors of metabolism in children referred with Reye's syndrome (a changing pattern). JAMA 260:3167, 1988

883. Roy CC, Weber AM, Morin CL, et al. Hepatobiliary disease in cystic fibrosis: a survey of current issues and concepts. J Pediatr Gastroenterol Nutr 1:469–478, 1982

884. Rubaltelli FF, Guerrini P, Reddi E, Jori GL. Tin-protoporphyrin in the management of children with crigler-najjar disease. Pediatrics 84:728–730, 1989

885. Rubaltelli FF, et al. Bronze baby syndrome: new insights in bilirubin-photosensitization of copper-porphyrins. In: Rub-

altelli FF, Jori G, eds. Neonatal jaundice: new trends in phototherapy. New York, Plenum Press, 1984, p 265

886. Rubella surveillance. National Communicable Disease Center, United States Department of Health, Education and Welfare, June 1969, p 11

887. Rudolph AM. Hepatic and ductus venosus blood flows during fetal life. Hepatology 3:254, 1983

888. Russell GJ, Fitzgerald JF, Clark JH. Fulminant hepatic failure. J Pediatr 111:313–319, 1987

889. Russo P, O'Regan S. Visceral pathology of hereditary tyrosinemia type I. Am J Hum Genet 47:317–324, 1990

890. Ryckman FC, Fisher RA, Pedersen S, et al. Optimal surgical management for biliary atresia: sequential portoenterostomy and segmental liver transplantation yields excellent survival. Gastroenterology 100:A791, 1991

891. Ryckman FC, Flake AW, Fisher RA, Tchervenkov JI, Pedersen SH, Balistreri WF. Segmental orthotopic hepatic transplantation as a means to improve patient survival and diminish waiting-list mortality. J Pediatr Surg 26:422–428, 1991

892. Ryckman FC, Noseworthy J. Neonatal cholestatic conditions requiring surgical reconstruction. Semin Liver Dis 7:134–154, 1987

893. Sancho S, Navarro C, Fernandez JM, et al. Skin biopsy findings in glycogenosis. III. Clinical, biochemical, and electrophysiological correlations. Ann Neurol 27:480–486, 1990

894. Sandhoff K. Variation of beta-N-acetylhexosaminidase pattern in Tay-Sachs disease. Fed Eur Biochem Soc Lett 4:351, 1969

895. Santos MJ, Imanaka T, Shio H, Small GM, Lazarow PB. Peroxisomal membrane ghosts in Zellweger syndrome: aberrant organelle assembly. Science 239:1536–1538, 1988

896. Sassa S, Fujita H, Kappas A. Succinylacetone and b-aminolevulinic acid dehydratase in hereditary tyrosinemia: immunochemical study of the enzyme. Pediatrics 86:84–86, 1990

897. Sassa S, Kappas A. Hereditary tyrosinemia and the heme biosynthetic pathway. J Clin Invest 71:625, 1983

898. Scheele PM, Bonar MJ, Zumwalt R, Ray MB. Bile duct adenomas in heterozygous (MZ) deficiency of α_1-protease inhibitor. Arch Pathol Lab Med 112:945–947, 1988

899. Scheidt PC, Bryla DA, Nelson KB, Hirtz DG, Hoffmann HJ. Phototherapy for neonatal hyperbilirubinemia: six-year follow-up of the National Institute of Child Health and Human Development Clinical Trial. Pediatrics 85:455–463, 1990 (see also: Pediatrics 87:787–805, 1991)

900. Scheidt PC, et al. Toxicity to bilirubin in neonates: infant development during first year in relation to maximum neonatal serum bilirubin concentration. J Pediatr 91:292, 1977

901. Schenker S, et al. Bilirubin metabolism in the fetus. J Clin Invest 43:32, 1964

902. Schiff D, et al. Bilirubin toxicity in neural cell lines N 115 and NBR 10A. Pediatr Res 19:908, 1985

903. Schiff L, et al. Effects of clofibrate in cholesterol ester storage disease. Gastroenterology 56:414, 1969

904. Schiff L, et al. Hepatic cholesterol ester storage disease: a familial disorder. I. Clinical aspects. Am J Med 44:538, 1968

905. Schilsky ML, Scheinberg H, Sternlieb I. Prognosis of Wilsonian chronic active hepatitis. Gastroenterology 100:762–767, 1991

906. Schmid R, Hammaker L. Metabolism and distribution of bilirubin in congenital nonhemolytic jaundice. J Clin Invest 42:1720, 1963

907. Schmid R, Mahler R. Chronic progressive myopathy with myoglobinuria: demonstration of a glycogenolytic defect in the muscle. J Clin Invest 348:2044, 1959

908. Schmid R, et al. Lack of effect of cholestyramine resin on the hyperbilirubinemia of premature infants. Lancet 2:938, 1963

909. Schneider AP. Breast milk jaundice in the newborn: a real entity. JAMA 255:3270–3274, 1986

910. Schneider PB, Kennedy EB. Sphingomyelinase in normal human spleens and in spleens from subjects with Niemann-Pick disease. J Lipid Res 8:202, 1967

911. Schoenau E, Boeswald W, Wanner R, et al. High-molecular-mass ("biliary") isoenzyme of alkaline phosphatase and the diagnosis of liver dysfunction in cystic fibrosis. Clin Chem 35:9, 1989

912. Schrakamp G, et al. Alkyl dihydroxyacetone phosphate synthase in human fibroblasts and its deficiency in Zellweger syndrome. J Lipid Res 26:867, 1985

913. Schrakamp G, et al. The cerebro-hepato-renal (Zellweger) syndrome: impaired de novo biosynthesis of plasmalogens in cultured skin fibroblasts. Biochim Biophys Acta 833:170, 1985

914. Schubert WK, et al. Encephalopathy and fatty liver (Reye's syndrome). In: Popper H, Schaffner E, eds. Progress in liver diseases, ed 4. New York, Grune & Stratton, 1972, pp 489–510

915. Schutgens RBH, Schrakamp G, Wanders RJA, Heymans HSA, Tager JM, van den Bosch H. Prenatal and perinatal diagnosis of peroxisomal disorders. J Inherit Metab Dis 12:118–134, 1989 (see also: J Inherit Metab Dis 13:4–36, 1990)

916. Schwarz KB, Larroya S, Vogler C, et al. Role of influenza B virus in hepatic steatosis and mitochondrial abnormalities in a mouse model of Reye syndrome. Hepatology 13:96–103, 1991

917. Schwartz MZ, Hall RJ, Reubner B, Lilly JR, Brogen T, Toyama WM. Agenesis of the extrahepatic bile ducts: report of five cases. J Pediatr Surg 25:805–807, 1990

918. Schweizer P. Treatment of extrahepatic bile duct atresia: results and long-term prognosis after hepatic portoenterostomy. Pediatr Surg 1:30–36, 1986

919. Schweizer P, Kerremans J. Discordant findings in extrahepatic bile duct atresia in 6 sets of twins. Z Kinderchir 43:72–75, 1988

920. Schwenk WF, Haymond MW. Optimal rate of enteral glucose administration in children with glycogen storage disease type I. N Engl J Med 314:682–685, 1986

921. Scriver CR, et al. Hereditary tyrosinemia and tyrosyluria in a French Canadian geographic isolate. Am J Dis Child 113:41, 1967

922. Seeler RA, Hahn K. Jaundice in urinary tract infection in infancy. Am J Dis Child 118:553, 1969

923. Segal S, et al. The metabolism of galactose by patients with congenital galactosemia. Am J Med 38:62, 1965

924. Selby R, Starzl TE, Yunis E, et al. Liver transplantation for type IV glycogen storage disease. N Engl J Med 324:39–42, 1991

925. Sell S. Is there a liver stem cell? Cancer Res 40:3811–3815, 1990

926. Setchell KDR, Dumaswala R, Colombo C, Ronchi M. Hepatic bile acid metabolism during early development revealed from the analysis of human fetal gall-bladder bile. J Biol Chem 263:16637–16644, 1988

927. Setchell KDR, Street JM. Inborn errors of bile acid synthesis. Semin Liver Dis 7:85–99, 1987 (see also: Setchell KDR. Disorders of bile acid synthesis. Pediatric gastrointestinal disease, vol 2. 1991, pp 992–1013)

928. Setchell KDR, Suchy FJ, Welsh MB, Zimmer-Nechemias L, Heubi J, Balistreri WF. Δ^4-3-Oxosteroid 5β-reductase deficiency described in identical twins with neonatal hepatitis: a new inborn error in bile acid synthesis. J Clin Invest 82:2148–2157, 1988

929. Shaffer EA, Zahavi I, Gall DG. Postnatal development of hepatic bile formation in the rabbit. Dig Dis Sci 30:558–562, 1985

930. Shah RD, Gerber MA. Development of intrahepatic bile ducts in humans: immunohistochemical study using monoclonal cytokeratin antibodies. Arch Pathol Lab Med 113:1135–1138, 1989

931. Shah RD, Gerber MA. Development of intrahepatic bile ducts in humans: possible role of laminin. Arch Pathol Lab Med 114:597–600, 1990

932. Shaldon S, Sherlock S. Obstruction to the extrahepatic portal system in childhood. Lancet 1:63, 1963

933. Sharp HL, et al. Cirrhosis associated with alpha-1-antitrypsin deficiency: a previously unrecognized inherited disorder. J Lab Clin Med 73:934, 1969

934. Sharp HL, et al. The liver in noncirrhotic alpha-1-antitrypsin deficiency. J Lab Clin Med 78:1012, 1971

935. Shaywitz B, et al. Prolonged continuous monitoring of intracranial pressure in Reye's syndrome. Pediatrics 59:595, 1977

936. Shevell MI, Bernard B, Adelson JW, Doody DP, Laberge JM, Guttman FM. Crigler-Najjar syndrome type I: treatment by home phototherapy followed by orthotopic hepatic transplantation. J Pediatr 110:429–431, 1987

937. Shieh CC, Chang MH, Chen CL. Dubin-Johnson syndrome presenting with neonatal cholestasis. Arch Dis Child 65:898–899, 1990

938. Shin YS, Rieth M, Tausenfreund J, Endres W. First trimester diagnosis of glycogen storage disease type II and type III. J Inherit Metab Dis 12:289–291, 1989

939. Shiojiri N, Katayama H. Secondary joining of the bile ducts during the hepatogenesis of the mouse embryo. Anat Embryol 177:153–163, 1987

940. Shirak K. Liver in congenital bile duct atresia: histological changes in relation to age. Paediatr Univ Tokyo 12:68, 1966

941. Sieber OF Jr, et al. In utero infection of the fetus by herpes simplex virus. J Pediatr 69:30, 1966

942. Sienko DG, Ando RF, McGee HB, et al. Reye's syndrome-salicylates. JAMA 258:3119, 1987

943. Silberberg DH, et al. Effects of photodegradation products of bilirubin on myelinating cerebellum cultures. J Pediatr 77:613, 1970

944. Silver MM, Beverly DW, Valberg LS, Cutz E, Phillips JH, Shaheed WA. Perinatal hemochromatosis: clinical, morphologic, and quantitative iron studies. Am J Pathol 128:538–554, 1987

945. Simionatto CS, et al. Studies on the mechanism of Sn-protoporphyrin suppression of hyperbilirubinemia: inhibition of heme oxidation and bilirubin production. J Clin Invest 75:513, 1985

946. Singer DB, et al. Pathology of the congenital rubella syndrome. J Pediatr 71:665, 1967

947. Singh I, Johnson GH, Brown FR. Peroxisomal disorders. Am J Dis Child 142:1297–1301, 1988

948. Singh I, et al. Adrenoleukodystrophy: impaired oxidation of very long chain fatty acids in white blood cells, cultured skin fibroblasts, and amniocytes. Pediatr Res 18:286, 1984

949. Sinniah D, et al. Investigation of an animal model of a Reye-like syndrome caused by margosa oil. Pediatr Res 19:1346, 1985

950. Sisson TRC, et al. Retinal changes produced by phototherapy. J Pediatr 77:221, 1970

951. Sisson TRC, et al. Phototherapy of jaundice in newborn infants. I. ABO blood group incompatibility. J Pediatr 79:904, 1971

952. Sisto A, Feldman P, Garel L, et al. Primary sclerosing cholangitis in children: study of five cases and review of the literature. Pediatrics 80:818–823, 1987

953. Sitzman JV, Pitt HA, Steinborn PA, Pasha ZR, Sanders RC. Cholecystokinin prevents parenteral nutrition induced biliary sludge in humans. Surg Gynecol Obstet 170:25–31, 1990

954. Slagle TA, Gross SJ. Effect of early low-volume enteral substrate on subsequent feeding tolerance in very low birth weight infants. J Pediatr 113:526–531, 1988

955. Sloan HR, et al. Deficiency of sphingomyelin cleaving enzyme activity in tissue cultures derived from patients with Niemann-Pick disease. Biochem Biophys Res Commun 34:582, 1969

956. Sloan HR, et al. Enzyme deficiency in cholesterol ester storage disease. J Clin Invest 51:1923, 1972

957. Smetana HF, Olen E. Hereditary galactose disease. Am J Clin Pathol 38:3, 1962

958. Smit GPA, Fernandes J, Leonard JV, et al. The long-term outcome ǿf patients with glycogen storage diseases. J Inherit Metab Dis 13:411–418, 1990

959. Smit GPA, et al. The dietary treatment of children with type I glycogen storage disease with slow release carbohydrate. Pediatr Res 18:879, 1984

960. Smith DW, et al. A syndrome of multiple developmental defects including polycystic kidneys and intrahepatic biliary dysgenesis in 2 siblings. J Pediatr 67:617, 1965

961. Smith EI, et al. Improved results with hepatic portoenterostomy: a reassessment of its value in the treatment of biliary atresia. Ann Surg 195:746, 1982

962. So SKS, et al. Bile ascites during infancy: diagnosis using disofenin Tc 99m sequential scintiphotography. Pediatrics 71:402, 1983

963. Sokol RJ. Fulminant hepatic failure. In: Balistreri WF, Stocker JT, eds. Pediatric hepatology. Washington, DC, Hemipshere, 1990, pp 316–362

964. Sokol RJ. Medical management of the infant or child with chronic liver disease. Semin Liver Dis 7:155–167, 1987

965. Sokol RJ, Heubi JE, Butler-Simon N, McClung HJ, Lilly JR. Treatment of vitamin E deficiency during chronic childhood cholestasis with oral tocopheryl polyethylene glycol-1000. Gastroenterology 93:975–985, 1987

966. Sokol RJ, Stall C. Anthropometric evaluation of children with chronic liver disease. Am J Clin Nutr 52:203–208, 1990

967. Sokol RJ, et al. Mechanism causing vitamin E deficiency during chronic childhood cholestasis. Gastroenterology 85:1172, 1983

968. Sokol RJ, et al. Vitamin E deficiency with normal serum vitamin E concentrations in children with chronic cholestasis. N Engl J Med 310:1209, 1984

969. Sondheimer JM, et al. Cholestatic tendencies in premature infants on and off parenteral nutrition. Pediatrics 62:984, 1978

970. Soubrane O, Gauthier F, DeVictor D, et al. Orthotopic liver transplantation for Byler disease. Transplantation 50:804–806, 1990

971. Southwest Pediatric Nephrology Study Group. Hepatitis B surface antigenemia in North American children with membranous glomerulonephropathy. J Pediatr 106:571, 1985

972. Sovik O, Kvittingen EA, Steen-Johnson J, Halvorsen S. Hereditary tyrosinemia of chronic course without rickets and renal tubular dysfunction. Acta Paediatr Scand 79:1063–1068, 1990

973. Spence JE, Maddalena A, O'Brien WE, et al. Prenatal diagnosis and heterozygote detection by DNA analysis in ornithine transcarbamylase deficiency. J Pediatr 114:582–588, 1989

974. Spivak W, Sarkar S, Winter D, Glassman M, Donlon E, Tucker KJ. Diagnostic utility of hepatobiliary scintigraphy with ^{99m}Tc-DISIDA in neonatal cholestasis. J Pediatr 110:855–861, 1987

975. Spivak W, et al. A case of primary sclerosing cholangitis in childhood. Gastroenterology 82:129, 1982

976. Spycher MS, Gitzelmann R. Glycogenosis type I (glucose-6-phosphatase deficiency): ultrastructural alterations of hepatocytes in a tumor bearing liver. Virchows Arch Cell Pathol 8:133, 1971

977. Stagno S. Congenital cytomegalovirus infection. N Engl J Med 306:945, 1982

978. Stagno S, Whitley RJ. Herpesvirus infections of pregnancy. I. Cytomegalovirus and Epstein-Barr virus infections. II. Herpes simplex virus and varicella-zoster virus infections. N Engl J Med 313:1270, 1327, 1985

979. Stanko RT, Nathan G, Mendelow H, Adibi SA. Development of hepatic cholestasis and fibrosis in patients with mas-

sive loss of intestine supported by prolonged parenteral nutrition. Gastroenterology 92:197–202, 1987

980. Stanley CA, Hales DE, Coates PM, et al. Medium-chain acyl-CoA dehydrogenase deficiency in children with nonketotic hypoglycemia and low carnitine levels. Pediatr Res 17:877, 1983

981. Stanley CA, Hale DE, Coates PM. Medium-chain acyl-CoA dehydrogenase deficiency. In: Fatty acid oxidation: clinical, biochemical and molecular Aspects. New York, Alan R Liss, 1990, pp 291–302

982. Stanley P, Geer GD, Miller JH, et al. Infantile hepatic hemangiomas. Cancer 64:936–949, 1989

983. Starr JG, et al. Inapparent cytomegalovirus infection: clinical and epidemiologic characteristics in early infancy. N Engl J Med 282:1075, 1970

984. Starzl TE, et al. Changing concepts: liver replacement for hereditary tyrosinemia and hepatoma. J Pediatr 106:604, 1985

985. Stern H. Isolation of cytomegalovirus and clinical manifestations of infection at different ages. Br Med J 1:665, 1968

986. Stern H, Williams BM. Isolation of rubella virus in a case of neonatal giant-cell hepatitis. Lancet 1:293, 1966

987. Stern L, et al. Effect of phenobarbital on hyperbilirubinemia and glucuronide formation in newborns. Am J Dis Child 120:26, 1970

988. Sternlieb I. Perspectives on Wilson's disease. Hepatology 12:1234–1239, 1990

989. Stevens CE, et al. Vertical transmission of hepatitis B antigen in Taiwan. N Engl J Med 292:771, 1975

990. Stevens CE, et al. Perinatal hepatitis B virus transmission in the United States: prevention by passive-active immunization. JAMA 253:1740, 1985

991. Stevenson DK, Rodgers PA, Vreman JH. The use of metalloporphyrins for the chemoprevention of neonatal jaundice. Am J Dis Child 143:353–356, 1989

992. Stiehm RE, Ryan J. Breast fed jaundice. Am J Dis Child 109:212, 1965

993. Stobie PE, Hansen CT, Hailey JR, Levine RL. A difference in mortality between two strains of jaundiced rats. Pediatrics 87:88–93, 1991

994. Stocker JT. Hepatic tumors. In: Balistreri WF, Stocker JT, eds. Pediatric hepatology. Washington, DC, Hemisphere, 1991, pp 399–488

995. Stocker R, Yamamoto Y, McDonagh AF, Glazer AN, Ames BN. Bilirubin is an antioxidant of possible physiological importance. Science 235:1043–1046, 1987

996. Stokes J Jr, et al. Viral hepatitis in the newborn: clinical features, epidemiology and pathology. Am J Dis Child 82:213, 1951

997. Stoner E, et al. Biochemical studies of a patient with hereditary hepatorenal tyrosinemia: evidence of glutathione deficiency. Pediatr Res 18:1332, 1984

998. Stosiek P, Kasper M, Karsten U. Expression of cytokeratin 19 during human liver organogenesis. Liver 10:59–63, 1990

999. Strandvik B, Hjelte L, Gabrielsson N, et al. Sclerosing cholangitis in cystic fibrosis. Scand J Gastroenterol 23:121–124, 1988

1000. Strandvik B, Wikstrom SA. Tetrahydroxylated bile acids in healthy human newborns. Eur J Clin Invest 12:301, 1982

1001. Strauss L, Bernstein J. Neonatal hepatitis in congenital rubella: a histopathological study. Arch Pathol 86:317, 1968

1002. Strebel L, Odell GB. UDP glucuronyl transferase in rat liver: genetic variation and maturation. Pediatr Res 3:351, 1969

1003. Strickland AD, et al. Biliary atresia in two sets of twins. J Pediatr 107:418, 1985

1004. Su T-S, et al. Molecular analysis of argininosuccinate synthetase deficiency in human fibroblasts. J Clin Invest 70:1334, 1982

1005. Suchy FJ. Chronic hepatitis. In: Balistreri WF, Stocker Jt, eds. Pediatric hepatology. Washington, DC, Hemisphere, 1990, pp 273–284

1006. Suchy FJ, Balistreri WF. Taurocholate uptake in hepatocytes from developing rats. Pediatr Res 16:282, 1982

1007. Suchy FJ, Balistreri WF, Breslin JS, Dumaswala R, Setchell KDR, Garfield SA. Absence of an acinar gradient for bile acid uptake in developing rat liver. Pediatr Res 21:417–421, 1987

1008. Suchy F, Bucuvalas J, Novak D. Determinants of bile formation during development: ontogeny of hepatic bile acid metabolism and transport. Semin Liver Dis 7:77–84, 1987

1009. Suchy FJ, et al. Physiologic cholestasis: elevations of the primary serum bile acid concentrations in normal infants. Gastroenterology 80:1037, 1981

1010. Suchy FJ, et al. Taurocholate transport by basolateral plasma membrane vesicles isolated from developing rat liver. Am J Physiol 248:G648, 1985

1011. Suchy FJ, et al. Ontogeny of hepatic bile acid conjugation in the rat. Pediatr Res 19:97, 1985

1012. Suchy FJ, et al. Absence of a hepatic lobular gradient for bile acid uptake in the suckling rat. Hepatology 3:847, 1983

1013. Sugiura H, Hayashi M, Koshida R, Watanabe R, Nakanuma Y, Ohta G. Nonsyndromic paucity of intrahepatic bile ducts in congenital syphilis: a case report. Acta Pathol Jpn 38:1061–1068, 1988

1014. Summerskill WJH, Walshe JM. Benign recurrent intrahepatic "obstructive" jaundice. Lancet 2:686, 1959

1015. Suruga K, et al. A clinical and pathological study of congenital biliary atresia. J Pediatr Surg 71:655, 1972

1016. Sutherland J, Keller WH. Novobiocin and neonatal hyperbilirubinemia. Am J Dis Child 101:447, 1961

1017. Suzuki Y, Shimozawa N, Ori T, et al. Zellweger-like syndrome with detectable hepatic peroxisomes: a variant form of peroxisomal disorder. J Pediatr 113:841–845, 1988

1018. Sveger T. Breast-feeding, α_1-antitrypsin deficiency, and liver disease? JAMA 254:3036, 1985

1019. Sveger T. Liver disease in alpha-1-antitrypsin deficiency detected by screening of 200,000 infants. N Engl J Med 294:1316, 1976

1020. Sveger T. Prospective study of children with alpha-1-antitrypsin deficiency: eight-year-old follow-up. J Pediatr 104:91, 1984

1021. Sveger T. The natural history of liver disease in α_1-antitrypsin deficient children. Acta Paediatr Scand 77:847–851, 1988

1022. Sveger T, Thelin T. Four-year-old children with α_1-antitrypsin deficiency. Acta Paediatr Scand 70:171–177, 1981

1023. Sweet AY, Wolinsky E. An outbreak of urinary tract and other infections due to E coli. Pediatrics 33:865, 1964

1024. Tada K, et al. Glycogen storage disease type IB: a new model of genetic disorders involving the transport system of intracellular membrane. Biochem Med 33:215, 1985

1025. Tajiri H, Nose O, Baba K, Okada S. Human herpesvirus-6 infection with liver injury in neonatal hepatitis. Lancet 335:863, 1990

1026. Takiff H, Fonkalsrud EW. Gallbladder disease in childhood. Am J Dis Child 138:565–568, 1984

1027. Talamo RC, Feingold M. Infantile cirrhosis with hereditary alpha-1-antitrypsin deficiency. Am J Dis Child 125:843, 1973

1028. Tanaka K, et al. Isovaleric and alpha-methylbutyric acidemias induced by hypoglycin A: mechanism of Jamaican vomiting sickness. Science 175:69, 1972

1029. Tanner MS, Bhave SA, Pradhan AM, et al. Clinical trials of penicillamine in indian childhood cirrhosis. Arch Dis Child 62:1118–11124, 1987

1030. Tanner MS, et al. Early introduction of copper-contaminated animal milk feeds as possible cause of Indian childhood cirrhosis. Lancet 2:992, 1983

1031. Tarui S, et al. Phosphofructokinase deficiency in skeletal muscle: a new type of glycogenosis. Biochem Biophys Res Commun 19:517, 1965

1032. Taubman B, Hale DE, Kelley RI. Familial Reye-like syndrome: a presentation of medium-chain acyl-coenzyme A dehydrogenase deficiency. Pediatrics 79:382, 1987

1033. Tavoloni N. Bile secretion and its Control in the newborn puppy. Pediatr Res 20:203–208, 1986

1034. Tavoloni N. Postnatal changes in hepatic microsomal enzyme activities in the puppy. Biol Neonate 47:305–316, 1985

1035. Taylor RJ, et al. Primary disseminated herpes simplex infection with fulminant hepatitis following renal transplantation. Arch Intern Med 141:1519, 1981

1036. Taylor WF, Quaquandah BY. Neonatal jaundice associated with cystic fibrosis. Am J Dis Child 123:161, 1972

1037. Tedesco TA, Miller KL. Galactosemia: alterations in sulfate metabolism secondary to galactose-1-phosphate uridyl-transferase deficiency. Science 205:1395, 1979

1038. Tephly TR, et al. Effect of drugs on heme synthesis in the liver. Metabolism 20:200, 1971

1039. Terada T, Nakanuma Y. Congenital biliary dilatation in autosomal dominant adult polycystic disease of the liver and kidneys. Arch Pathol Lab Med 112:1113–1116, 1988

1040. Terazawa S, Kojima M, Yamanaka T, et al. Hepatitis B virus mutants with precore-region defects in two babies with fulminant hepatitis and their mothers positive for antibody to hepatitis B e antigen. Pediatr Res 29:5–9, 1991

1041. Thaler MM, et al. Influence of intravenous nutrients on bilirubin transport. II. Emulsified lipid solutions. III. Emulsified fat solutions. Pediatr Res 11:167, 171, 1977

1042. Toda G, et al. Infantile papular acrodermatitis (Gianotti's disease) and intrafamilial occurrence of acute hepatitis B with jaundice: age dependency of clinical manifestations of hepatitis B virus infection. J Infect Dis 138:211, 1978

1043. Tondeur M, Loeb H. Etude ultrastructurelle du foie dans la maladie de Morquio. Pediatr Res 3:19, 1969

1044. Tong MJ, et al. Prevention of hepatitis B infection by hepatitis B immune globulin in infants born to mothers with acute hepatitis during pregnancy. Gastroenterology 89:160, 1985

1045. Tonsgard JH, Getz GS. Effect of Reye's syndrome serum on isolated chinchilla liver mitochondria. J Clin Invest 76:816, 1985

1046. Touloukian RJ. Hepatic hemangioendothelioma during infancy: pathology, diagnosis and treatment with prednisone. Pediatrics 45:71, 1970

1047. Townsend SF, Rudolph CD, Rudolph AM. Changes in ovine hepatic circulation and oxygen consumption at birth. Pediatr Res 25:300–304, 1989

1048. Treem WR, Malet PF, Gourley GR, Hyams JS. Bile and stone analysis in two infants with brown pigment gallstones and infected bile. Gastroenterology 96:519–523, 1989

1049. Treem WR, Stanley CA. Massive hepatomegaly, steatosis, and secondary plasma carnitine deficiency in an infant with cystic fibrosis. Pediatrics 83:993, 1989

1050. Treem WR, Stanley CA, Hale DE, et al. Hypoglycemia, hypotonia, and cardiomyopathy: the evolving clinical picture of long-chain acyl-CoA dehydrogenase deficiency. Pediatrics 87:328–333, 1991

1051. Treem WR, Witzleben CA, Piccoli DA, et al. Medium-chain and long-chain acyl CoA dehydrogenase deficiency: clinical, pathologic and ultrastructural differentiation from Reye's syndrome. Hepatology 6:1270, 1986

1052. Trolle D: Decrease of total serum bilirubin concentration in newborn infants after phenobarbitone treatment. Lancet 2:705, 1968

1053. Tsalikian E, et al. Glucose production and utilization in children with glycogen storage disease type I. Am J Physiol 247:E513, 1984

1054. Tyson KRT, et al. Portal hypertension in cystic fibrosis. J Pediatr Surg 3:271, 1968

1055. Udall JN, et al. Liver disease in alpha-1-antitrypsin deficiency: a retrospective analysis of the influence of early breast- vs. bottle-feeding. JAMA 253:2679, 1985

1056. Ullrich D, Rating D, Schroter W, et al. Treatment with ur-

sodeoxycholic acid renders children with biliary atresia suitable for liver transplantation. Lancet 2:1324, 1987

1057. Ullrich K, Schmidt H, van Teeffelen-Heithoff A. Glycogen storage disease type I and III and pyruvate carboxylase deficiency: results of long-term treatment with uncooked cornstarch. Acta Paediatr Scand 77:531–536, 1988

1058. Ulstrom RA, Eisenklam E. The enterohepatic shunting of bilirubin in the newborn infants. I. Use of oral activated charcoal to reduce normal serum bilirubin values. J Pediatr 65:27, 1964

1059. Utili R, et al. Inhibition of Na$^+$,K$^+$-ATPase by endotoxin: a possible mechanism for endotoxin-induced cholestasis. J Infect Dis 136:583, 1977

1060. Valaes T, et al. Incidence and mechanism of neonatal jaundice related to glucose-6-phosphate dehydrogenase deficiency. Pediatr Res 3:448, 1969

1061. Valdes OS, et al. Controlled clinical trial of phenobarbital and/or light in reducing neonatal hyperbilirubinemia in a predominantly Negro population. J Pediatr 79:1015, 1971

1062. Valencia-Mayoral P, et al. Possible defect in the bile secretory apparatus in arteriohepatic dysplasia (Alagille's syndrome): a review with observations on the ultrastructure of liver. Hepatology 4:691, 1984

1063. Valentine WN, Tanaka KR, Paglea DE. Pyruvate kinase and other enzyme deficiency disorders of the erythrocyte. In: Scrivner CR, Beaudot AL, Sly WS, Vale D, eds. The metabolic basis of inherited disease, ed 6, chap 94., New York, McGraw-Hill, 1989, pp 2341

1064. Valman HB, et al. Prolonged neonatal jaundice in cystic fibrosis. Arch Dis Child 46:805, 1971

1065. van de Bor M, van Zeben-Van der Aa TM, Verloove-Vanhorick SP, et al. Hyperbilirubinemia in very preterm infants and neurodevelopmental outcome at 2 years of age: results of a national collaborative survey. Pediatrics 83:915–920, 1989

1066. Vandenplas Y, Franckx J, Liebaers I, et al. Neonatal hepatitis with obstructive jaundice in SZ heterozygous alpha 1-antitrypsin-deficient boy and destructive lung disease in his SZ mother. Eur J Pediatr 144:391, 1985

1067. van Es HHG, Goldhoorn BG, Paul-Abrahamse M, Elferink RPJO, Jansen PLM. Immunochemical analysis of uridine disphosphate-glucuronosyltransferase in four patients with the Crigler-Najjar syndrome type I. J Clin Invest 85:1199–1205, 1990

1068. Van Eyken P, Sciot R, Callea F, Van Der Steen K, Moerman P, Desmet FJ. The development of intrahepatic bile ducts in man: a keratin-immunohistochemical study. Hepatology 8:1586–1595, 1988

1069. Van Eyken, Sciot R, Desmet V. Intrahepatic bile duct development in the rat: a cytokeratin-immunohistochemical study. Lab Invest 59:52–58, 1988

1070. Van Furth R, Kramps JA, Van Der Putten ABMM, et al. Change in α 1-antitrypsin phenotype after orthotopic liver transplant. Clin Exp Immunol 66:669, 1986

1071. Van Geet C, Vandenbossche L, Eggermont E, Devlieger H, Vermylen J, Jaeken J. Possible platelet contribution to pathogenesis of transient neonatal hyperammonaemia syndrome. Lancet 337:73–75, 1991

1072. Van Praagh R. Diagnosis of kernicterus in the neonatal period. Pediatrics 28:870, 1961

1073. van Spronsen FJ, Berger R, Smit GPA, et al. Tyrosinaemia type I: orthotopic liver transplantation as the only definitive answer to a metabolic as well as an oncological problem. J Inherit Metab Dis 12:339–342, 1989

1074. Varjo P, Hadchouel P, Hadchouel M, Bernard O, Alagille D. Incidence of cirrhosis in children with chronic hepatitis. J Pediatr 117:392–396, 1990

1075. Varma RR, et al. Reye's syndrome in nonpediatric age groups. JAMA 242:1373, 1979

1076. Vassilipoulou-Sellin R, Foster P, Oyedeji CO. Bilirubin and heme as growth inhibitors of chicken embryos in ovo. Pediatr Res 27:617–621, 1990

1077. Vegnente A, et al. Duration of chronic active hepatitis and the development of cirrhosis. Arch Dis Child 59:330, 1984

1078. Verbanac KM, Heath EC. Biosynthesis, processing, and secretion of M and Z variant human α_1-antitrypsin. J Biol Chem 261:9979, 1986

1079. Vest M, et al. A double blind study of the effect of phenobarbitone on neonatal hyperbilirubinemia and frequency of exchange transfusion. Acta Paediatr Scand 59:681, 1970

1080. Vileisis RA, Sorensen K, Gonzalez-Crussi F, et al. Liver malignancy after parenteral nutrition. J Pediatr 100:88–90, 1982

1081. Vileisis RA, et al. Prospective controlled study of parenteral nutrition-associated cholestatic jaundice: effect of protein intake. J Pediatr 96:893, 1980

1082. Vlessis AA, Mela-Riker L. Perinatal development of heart, kidney, and liver mitochondrial antioxidant defense. Pediatr Res 26:220–226, 1989

1083. Vohr BR, Karp D, O'Dea C, et al. Behavioral changes correlated with brain-stem auditory evoked responses in term infants with moderate hyperbilirubinemia. J Pediatr 117:288–291, 1990

1084. Vohr BR, Lester B, Rapisardi G, et al. Abnormal (brain-stem auditory evoked) response correlates with acoustic cry features in term infants with hyperbilirubinemia. J Pediatr 115:303–308, 1989

1085. Volk BJ, Wallace BJ. The liver in lipidosis: an electron microscopic and histochemical study. Am J Pathol 49:203, 1966

1086. von Dippe P, Levy D. Expression of the bile acid transport protein during liver development and in hepatoma cells. J Biol Chem 265:5942–5945, 1990

1087. Voorhies TM, et al. Acute hyperammonemia in the young primate: physiologic and neuropathologic correlates. Pediatr Res 17:970, 1983

1088. Vreman HJ, Rodgers PA, Stevenson DK. Zinc protoporphyrin administration for suppression of increased bilirubin production by iatrogenic hemolysis in rhesus neonates. J Pediatr 117:292–297, 1990

1089. Vreman HJ, Stevenson DK. Metalloporphyrin-enhanced photodegradation of bilirubin in vitro. Am J Dis Child 144:590–594, 1990

1090. Waddell ID, Gibb L, Burchell A. Calcium activates glucose-6-phosphatase in intact rat hepatic microsomes. Biochem J 267:549–551, 1990

1091. Wagget J, et al. Hemangioendothelioma of the liver in an infant: hypotensive crisis during resection. Surgery 65:352, 1969

1092. Waggoner DD, Buist NRM, Donnell GN: Long-term prognosis in galactosaemia: results of a survey of 350 cases. J Inherit Metab Dis 13:802–818, 1990

1093. Wahlen E, Egestad B, Strandvik B, Sjovall J. Ketonic bile acids in urine of infants during the neonatal period. J Lipid Res 30:1847–1857, 1989

1094. Walker WA, et al. Needle biopsy of the liver in infancy and childhood: a safe diagnostic aid in liver disease. Pediatrics 40:946, 1967

1095. Walshe JM. Wilson's disease presenting with features of hepatic dysfunction: a clinical analysis of eighty-seven patients. Q J Med 70:253–263, 1989

1096. Watchko JF, Oski FA. Bilirubin 20 mg/dl = viginitiphobia. Pediatrics 71:660–663, 1983

1097. Watkins PA, Chen WW, Harris CJ, et al. Peroxisomal bifunctional enzyme deficiency. J Clin Invest 83:771–777, 1989

1098. Watson GH, Miller V. Arteriohepatic dysplasia: familial pulmonary arterial stenosis with neonatal liver disease. Arch Dis Child 43:459, 1973

1099. Watson JRH. Hepatosplenomegaly as a complication of maternal rubella: report of two cases. Med J Aust 1:516, 1952

1100. Webb LJ, Sherlock S. The aetiology, presentation and natural history of extra-hepatic portal venous obstruction. Q J Med 192:627, 1979

1101. Weber A, et al. Severe familial cholestasis in North American Indian children: a clinical model of microfilament dysfunction? Gastroenterology 81:653, 1981

1102. Weinberg AG, Finegold MJ. Primary hepatic tumors of childhood. Hum Pathol 14:512, 1983

1103. Weinberg AG, et al. The occurrence of hepatoma in the chronic form of hereditary tyrosinemia. J Pediatr 88:434, 1976

1104. Weldon AP, Danks DM. Congenital hypothyroidism and neonatal jaundice. Arch Dis Child 47:469, 1972

1105. Weller TH. The cytomegalovirus: ubiquitous agents with protein clinical manifestations. N Engl J Med 285:203, 267, 1971

1106. Weller TH, Hanshaw JV. Virological and clinical observations on cytomegalic inclusion disease. N Engl J Med 266:1233, 1962

1107. Wenger DA, et al. Niemann-Pick disease: a genetic model in Siamese cats. Science 208:1471, 1980

1108. Wennberg RP, Thaler MM. Influence of intravenous nutrients on bilirubin transport. I. Amino acid solutions. Pediatr Res 11:163, 1977

1109. Wennberg RP, et al. Early versus delayed feeding of low birth weight infants: effects on physiologic jaundice. J Pediatr 68:860, 1966

1110. Werlin SL, Glicklich M, Jona J, et al. Sclerosing cholangitis in childhood. J Pediatr 96:433–435, 1980

1111. Whalen G, et al. Impaired biliary excretion of phenol 3,6-dibromophthalein disulfonate in neonatal guinea pigs. Proc Soc Exp Biol Med 137:598, 1971

1112. Whelton MJ, et al. Reduction in serum bilirubin by phenobarbital in adult nonconjugative hemolytic jaundice. Am J Med 45:160, 1968

1113. Whitington PF. Cholestasis associated with total parenteral nutrition in infants. Hepatology 5:693, 1985

1114. Whitington PF, Balistreri WF. Liver transplantation in pediatrics: indications, contraindications, and pre-transplant management. J Pediatr 118:169–177, 1991

1115. Whitington PF, Whitington GL. Partial external diversion of bile for the treatment of intractable pruritus associated with intrahepatic cholestasis. Gastroenterology 95:130–136, 1988

1116. Wilkinson EJ, Raab K, Browning CA, et al. Familial hepatic cirrhosis in infants associated with alpha$_1$-antitrypsin SZ phenotype. J Pediatr 85:159, 1974

1117. Wilkinson ML, Meili-Vergani G, Ball C, Portmann B, Mowat AP. Endoscopic retrograde cholangiopancreatography in infantile cholestasis. Arch Dis Child 66:121–123, 1991

1118. Willems PJ, Gerver WJM, Berger R, Fernandes J. The natural history of liver glycogenosis due to phosphorylase kinase deficiency: a longitudinal study of 41 patients. Eur J Pediatr 149:268–271, 1990

1119. Wills EJ. Electron microscopy of the liver in infectious mononucleosis, hepatitis and cytomegalovirus hepatitis. Am J Dis Child 123:301, 1972

1120. Wilson JT. Phenobarbital in the neonatal period. Pediatrics 43:324, 1969

1121. Winsnes A, Bratlid D. Effects of bilirubin loading of pregnant rats on hepatic UDP-glucuronyltransferase activity in the offspring. Biol Neonate 22:367, 1973

1122. Witzleben CL, Finegold M, Piccoli DA, Treem WR. Bile canalicular morphometry in arteriohepatic dysplasia. Hepatology 7:1262–1266, 1987

1123. Witzleben CL, Marshall GS, Wenner W, Piccoli DA, Barbour SD. HIV as a cause of giant cell hepatitis. Hum Pathol 19:603–605, 1988

1124. Witzleben CL, Palmieri MJ, Watkins JB, et al. Sphingomyelin lipidosis variant with cirrhosis in the pediatric age group. Arch Pathol Lab Med 110:508–512, 1986

1125. Witzleben CL, Sharp AR. Nephronophthisis-congenital hepatic fibrosis: an additional hepatorenal disorder. Hum Pathol 13:728, 1982

1126. Witzleben CL, Uri A. Perinatal hemochromatosis: entity or end result? Hum Pathol 20:335–340, 1989

1127. Wolfe HJ, Pictra G. The visceral lesions of metachromatic leukodystrophy. Am J Pathol 44:921, 1964

1128. Wolfe BM, Walker BK, Shaul DB, Wong L, Ruebner BH. Effect of total parenteral nutrition on hepatic histology. Arch Surg 123:1084–1090, 1988

1129. Wolfsdorf JI, Keller RJ, Landy H, Crigler JF. Glucose therapy for glycogenosis type 1 in infants: comparison of intermittent uncooked cornstarch and continuous overnight glucose feedings. J Pediatr 117:384–391, 1990

1130. Wolfsdorf JI, Plotkin RA, Laffel LMB, Crigler JF. Continuous glucose for treatment of patients with type 1 glycogen-storage disease: comparison of the effects of dextrose and uncooked cornstarch on biochemical variables. Am J Clin Nutr 52:1043–1050, 1051–1057, 1990

1131. Wolkoff AW, et al. Role of ligandin in transfer of bilirubin from plasma into liver. Am J Physiol 236:E638, 1979

1132. Wolman M, et al. Primary familal xanthomatosis with involvement and calcification of the adrenals. Pediatrics 28:742, 1961

1133. Wong CG, et al. Hepatic ganglioside abnormalities in a patient with familial erythrophagocytic lymphohistiocytosis. Pediatr Res 17:413, 1983

1134. Wysowski, et al. Epidemic neonatal hyperbilirubinemia and use of a phenolic disinfectant detergent. Pediatrics 61:165, 1978

1135. Xu YK, Ng WG, Kaufman FR, Lobo RA, Donnell GN. Galactose metabolism in human ovarian tissue. Pediatr Res 25:151–155, 1989

1136. Xu ZY, et al. Prevention of perinatal acquisition of hepatitis B virus carriage using vaccine: preliminary report of a randomized, double-blind placebo-controlled and comparative trial. Pediatrics 76:713, 1985

1137. Yaffe SJ, et al. Enhancement of glucuronide-conjugating capacity in a hyperbilirubinemic infant due to apparent enzyme induction by phenobarbital. N Engl J Med 275:1461, 1966

1138. Yamamoto K, et al. Hilar biliary plexus in human liver: a comparative study of the intrahepatic bile ducts in man and animals. Lab Invest 52:103, 1985

1139. Yamashita Y, Iwanaga R, Goto R, et al. Congenital cyto-megalovirus infection associated with fetal ascites and intrahepatic calcifications. Acta Paediatr Scand 78:965–967, 1989

1140. Yang BZ, Ding JH, Brown BI, Chen YT. Definitive prenatal diagnosis for type III glycogen storage disease. Am J Hum Genet 47:735–739, 1990

1141. Yen SSC, et al. Herpes simplex infection in female genital tract. Obstet Gynecol 25:479, 1965

1142. Yeung CY, et al. Phenobarbitone prophylaxis for neonatal hyperbilirubinemia. Pediatrics 48:372, 1971

1143. Yokota I, Indo Y, Coates PM, Tanaka K. Molecular basis of medium chain acyl-coenzyme A dehydrogenase deficiency: an A to G transition at position 985 that causes lysine-304 to glutamate substitution in the mature protein is the single prevalent mutation. J Clin Invest 86:1000–1003, 1990

1144. Yoshida Y, Fujii M, Brown FR, et al. Effect of salicylic acid on mitochondrial-peroxisomal fatty acid catabolism. Pediatr Res 23:338, 1988

1145. You K. Salicylate and mitochondrial injury in Reye's syndrome. Science 221:163, 1983

1146. Young JL, Miller RW. Incidence of malignant tumors in U.S. children. J Pediatr 86:254, 1975

1147. Young RSK, Woods C, Towfighi J. Hepatic damage in neonatal rat due to E. coli endotoxin. Dig Dis Sci 31:651–656, 1986

1148. Yunis E, Bridges R. The serologic diagnosis of ABO hemolytic disease of the newborn. Am J Clin Pathol 41:1964

1149. Yunis EJ, et al. Fine structural observations of the liver in alpha-1-antitrypsin deficiency. Am J Pathol 82:265, 1976

1150. Zafrani ES, Metreau JM, Douvin C, et al. Idiopathic biliary ductopenia in adults: a report of five cases. Gastroenterology 99:1823–1828, 1990

1151. Zamboni L. Electron microscopic studies of blood embryogenesis in humans. II. The hemopoietic activity in the fetal liver. J Ultrastruct Res 12:525–541, 1985

1152. Zhang F, Deleuze JF, Aurias A, et al. Interstitial deletion of the short arm of chromosome 20 in arteriohepatic dysplasia (Alagille syndrome). J Pediatr 116:73–77, 1990

1153. Zimmerman A, Bachmann C, Baumgartner R. Severe liver fibrosis in argininosuccinic aciduria. Arch Pathol Lab Med 110:136–140, 1986

1154. Zuelzer WW, Stulberg CS. Herpes simplex virus as the cause of fulminating visceral disease and hepatitis in infancy. Am J Dis Child 83:421, 1952

Diseases of the Liver, Seventh Edition, edited by Leon Schiff and Eugene R. Schiff. J.B. Lippincott Company, Philadelphia © 1993.

42

Congenital Hepatic Fibrosis and Caroli's Syndrome

Jean-Pierre Benhamou

CONGENITAL HEPATIC FIBROSIS

Congenital hepatic fibrosis is an inherited, congenital malformation characterized by large, fibrotic portal spaces that contain multiple bile ductules, the main consequence of which is portal hypertension. The disease was described as fibrocystic disease of the liver by Grumbach and coworkers[15] in 1954. The denomination of congenital hepatic fibrosis was introduced by Kerr and associates[17] in 1961.

Pathology and Pathogenesis

The lesion of congenital hepatic fibrosis consists of portal spaces markedly increased in size because of abundant connective tissue and numerous bile ductules, more or less ectatic, communicating with the biliary tree (Fig. 42-1). Congenital hepatic fibrosis is not simply fibrosis, and bile ductular proliferation is an essential component of the lesion. A few portal spaces remain normal, which explains why congenital hepatic fibrosis may be unrecognized at histologic examination of a small specimen taken by liver biopsy. Some clusters of multiple bile ductules surrounded with fibrosis may be present within the lobules, apart from the portal spaces. Some bile ductules are so markedly dilated that they form microcysts; the microcysts communicate with the biliary tree. Separation between the fibrotic portal spaces and the rest of the liver parenchyma is sharp. The architecture of the liver remains normal.

The primary disorder of congenital hepatic fibrosis is likely to be bile ductular proliferation, with fibrosis being secondarily induced by the multiple bile ductules. The initial lesion might be clusters of multiple bile ductules (ie, Meyenburg's complexes) that resemble the initial lesion of the liver cysts associated with adult polycystic kidney disease. In congenital hepatic fibrosis, the abnormal bile ductules maintain their communications with the biliary tree and, as a result, only microcysts are formed; in contrast, in adult polycystic kidney disease, the abnormal bile ductules lose their communication with the biliary tree and, as a result, dilate markedly and form large cysts.

The mechanism for the development of multiple bile ductules in congenital hepatic fibrosis is unknown. It has been suggested that bile ductular proliferation might result from a disproportionate overgrowth of the biliary epithelium.[26] A similar disorder that affects the epithelium of the large bile ducts might account for Caroli's syndrome associated with congenital hepatic fibrosis. A similar mechanism might explain the dilatation of the renal collecting tubules and the dilatation of pancreatic ducts, two extrahepatic malformations that may be associated with congenital hepatic fibrosis.

Etiology and Prevalence

Congenital hepatic fibrosis is an inherited malformation transmitted as an autosomal recessive trait.[1,9,17,33] The parents, presumably heterozygous, are phenotypically normal. Males and females are equally affected. Several siblings may be affected. Consanguinity increases the risk of congenital hepatic fibrosis.

The prevalence of congenital hepatic fibrosis has not been established, but it is low and might be of the same order of magnitude as that of another autosomal recessive liver disease, Wilson's disease (ie, about 1:100,000).[30] There is no ethnic predominance.

Clinical Manifestations and Diagnosis

The main consequence of congenital hepatic fibrosis is portal hypertension, which is likely to have been present since the patient's birth. In most patients, the disease is recognized at the first episode of gastrointestinal bleeding caused by ruptured esophageal or gastric varices, which usually occurs between 5 and 20 years, sometimes later. In a few patients, the disease is recognized before any episode of gastrointestinal bleeding because of blood disorders caused by hyperplenism, abdominal discomfort caused by an enlarged spleen, or the presence of abdominal collateral venous circulation. In a small number of patients, an episode of bacterial cholangitis is the presenting manifestation.[9] The disease may remain silent for the patient's entire life.[2]

At clinical examination, the liver often is enlarged. Splenomegaly is present in most patients. Abdominal collateral circulation (Cruveilhier-Baumgarten syndrome in some patients) often is visible. Ascites is absent. There is no symptom or sign indicating liver dysfunction, in particular jaundice or spiders. The liver tests are normal, except for moderately increased levels of alkaline phosphatase and γ-glutamyl transpeptidase in a few patients. Endoscopic or radiographic examination demonstrates esophageal varices. Ultrasonography and computed tomography (CT) commonly show that the liver is enlarged (often hyperechoic because of fibrosis and ductular proliferation), the portal vein is patent (which excludes extrahepatic portal hypertension), the spleen is en-

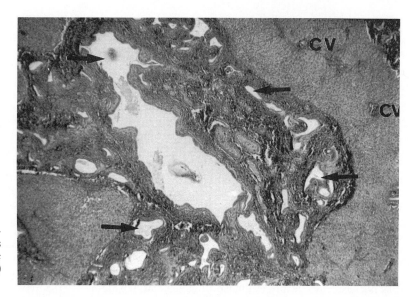

FIGURE 42-1 Congenital hepatic fibrosis. The portal space is markedly increased in size and contains abundant fibrosis and numerous, more or less ectatic bile ductules. (Some of them are indicated by arrows.) CV, centrilobular vein (H&E, × 70).

larged, and portacaval anastomoses are present; the venous phase of celiac and supramesenteric arteriographies provide similar information. Histologic examination of a hepatic tissue specimen taken by needle biopsy demonstrates the typical lesion in most patients; if the specimen is small, the lesion may be missed because, as mentioned above, some of the portal spaces may be normal.

Course and Complications

The course of the disease is dominated by recurrent episodes of gastrointestinal bleeding. The episodes of gastrointestinal bleeding usually are well tolerated and not followed by hepatic encephalopathy, ascites, or jaundice. The patient's death is due to massive bleeding but not to liver dysfunction. Thus, the course of congenital hepatic fibrosis resembles that of extrahepatic portal hypertension and differs from that of cirrhosis. Even in the absence of associated Caroli's syndrome, recurrent episodes of bacterial cholangitis affect a few patients.[1,9,11]

Associated Malformations

Congenital hepatic fibrosis often is associated with Caroli's syndrome, either clinically silent (demonstrated by ultrasonography or CT) or determining cholangitis (see later discussion).

Congenital hepatic fibrosis likewise often is associated with a renal malformation that consists of ectatic collecting tubules, resembling sponge kidney.[19] Dilatation affects the medullary and cortical portions of the collecting tubules in congenital hepatic fibrosis, whereas it is limited to the medullary portion of the collecting tubules in sponge kidney.[7,13] This renal malformation is clinically silent, except for hematuria or urinary infection in a few patients. Dilatation of the collecting tubules can be demonstrated by intravenous pyelography that shows enlarged kidneys and coarse streaking of the medulla (Fig. 42-2). These radiologic abnormalities are present in about two thirds of patients[1,19]; their presence

is good evidence for but their absence is not an argument against the diagnosis of congenital hepatic fibrosis. In some patients with normal intravenous pyelogram, histologic examination of the kidney may show ectatic collecting tubules.[7]

In most patients, dilatation of collecting tubules remains stable. In some, the ectatic segments lose their communications with the urinary tree and transform into large renal cysts[10]; the renal malformation then resembles adult polycystic kidney disease. This transformation accounts for the large

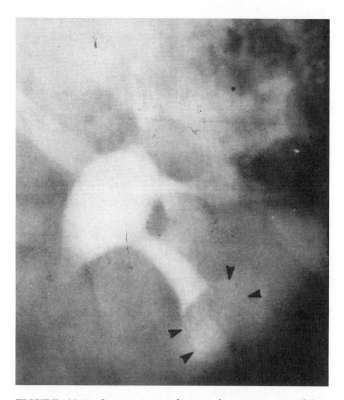

FIGURE 42-2 Intravenous pyelogram showing congenital hepatic fibrosis. Coarse streaking of the papilla (*arrowheads*) reflects ectatic collecting tubules.

renal cysts detectable by ultrasonography or intravenous pyelography in a number of patients with congenital hepatic fibrosis.[1,7,9,19] This transformation may take place early in infancy or later, with large renal cysts being formed over 30 to 40 years. In patients with large renal cysts, the renal malformation may cause renal failure or arterial hypertension.

Other associated malformations are uncommon and include duplication of the intrahepatic portal vein branches,[1,27] cystic dysplasia of the pancreas,[17] intestinal lymphangiectasia,[5] pulmonary emphysema,[40] cerebellar hemangioma,[38] aneurysms of renal and cerebral arteries,[17] and cleft palate.[17]

Treatment

Active bleeding from ruptured esophageal varices requires blood transfusions and esophageal tamponade. Endoscopic sclerotherapy of esophageal varices can be recommended for the prevention of recurrent bleeding, although this procedure has not been specifically evaluated in congenital hepatic fibrosis. The efficacy of sclerotherapy has been demonstrated, however, for prevention of variceal bleeding in cirrhosis and can be reasonably expected in congenital hepatic fibrosis.

In the few patients in whom sclerotherapy is inefficient, poorly tolerated, or not feasible, surgical portacaval shunt can be considered. Hepatic encephalopathy and liver failure after portal-systemic shunt would be less common in patients with congenital hepatic fibrosis than in patients with cirrhosis.[1,9,18]

Splenectomy does not prevent occurrence or recurrence of gastrointestinal bleeding and may be followed by portal vein thrombosis, preventing subsequent surgical portacaval shunt. Operations or invasive investigations on the biliary tree, such as cholecystectomy, choledochotomy, T-tube drainage, intraoperative cholangiography, and endoscopic retrograde cholangiography, must be avoided because of the risk of inducing bacterial cholangitis.

CAROLI'S SYNDROME

Caroli's syndrome is a congenital malformation characterized by multifocal dilatation of segmental bile ducts, the main consequence of which is recurrent bacterial cholangitis. This malformation was described by Caroli and coworkers[4] in 1958. It is not a single entity, and for this reason, the terms of Caroli's syndrome are more appropriate than those of Caroli's disease.

Pathology, Classification, and Etiology

The lesion of Caroli's syndrome consists of multifocal dilatation of the segmental bile ducts. The ectatic portions form cysts of various size, separated by portions of bile ducts that are normal or regularly dilated. Septa that contain portal veins protrude in the lumen of the ectatic bile ducts.[6] The multifocal dilatation may be diffuse, affecting the whole intrahepatic biliary tree (although it may be more marked in a part of the liver), or it may be confined in a part of the liver, commonly the left lobe or a segment of the left lobe.[3] The number of cysts is large in the diffuse form and smaller, usually fewer than 10, in the localized form.

Multifocal dilatation of the segmental bile ducts is not a single entity. In about half the cases, multifocal dilatation of the segmental bile ducts is associated with congenital hepatic fibrosis.[13,33] In this type of Caroli's syndrome, the distribution of multifocal dilatation is diffuse; as congenital hepatic fibrosis, the malformation is transmitted as an autosomal recessive trait and may be associated with a renal malformation.

In about half the cases, multifocal dilatation of the segmental bile ducts is not associated with congenital hepatic fibrosis.[9,33] In such cases, multifocal dilatation may be confined to a part of the liver, usually the left lobe.[3] This type of Caroli's syndrome is not inherited and usually not associated with a renal malformation, but it may be associated with other malformations of the biliary tree, in particular choledochal cyst.[21,33]

Manifestations and Diagnosis

Caroli's syndrome, which is likely to be present at birth, remains asymptomatic for the first 5 to 20 years of the patient's life (sometimes longer); in a few cases, it may remain asymptomatic during the patient's whole life. Asymptomatic Caroli's syndrome remains unrecognized except in patients in whom an imaging investigation of the liver is performed for unrelated reasons and in those in whom congenital hepatic fibrosis has been diagnosed and multifocal dilatation of the segmental bile ducts has been suspected and demonstrated by ultrasonography or CT.

In most patients, the first episode of bacterial cholangitis occurs in the absence of any apparent precipitating factor. In a few patients, the first episode of bacterial cholangitis is induced by a surgical operation or an invasive investigation on the biliary tree, such as cholecystectomy, choledochotomy, T-tube drainage, intraoperative cholangiography, and endoscopic retrograde cholangiography.[7,15]

The main and often the only symptom of bacterial cholangitis caused by Caroli's syndrome is fever without abdominal pain and jaundice, in contrast to bacterial cholangitis complicating common bile duct stones, in which fever usually is accompanied by pain or jaundice or both. As a consequence, the first episodes of fever may not be attributed to bacterial cholangitis.

At clinical examination, the liver usually is enlarged. There is no sign or symptom indicating liver dysfunction. In patients with Caroli's syndrome associated with congenital hepatic fibrosis, manifestations of portal hypertension are present. Liver tests are normal, except for alkaline phosphatase and γ-glutamyl transpeptidase levels, which may be moderately increased.

Ultrasonography and CT show cysts of various size that are distributed throughout the liver or confined to a part of the liver (Fig. 42-3); the cysts are associated or not associated with tubular dilatation of the segmental bile ducts. Ultrasonography and CT may show tiny dots within the dilated bile ducts, corresponding to intrahepatic portal veins protruding in the lumen of the cysts.[6]

The main characteristic of these cysts is their communication with the biliary tract. Communication of the cysts with the biliary tree may be obvious because the cysts clearly are in continuity with the large intrahepatic bile ducts or they contain biliary stones or air. These communications, when not obvious, can be demonstrated by several procedures: (1) hepatobiliary scintiscan shows cold areas at the early phase that become hot at the late phase[32]; (2) CT after intravenous

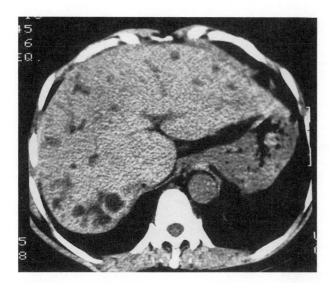

FIGURE 42-3   CT scan in a patient with Caroli's syndrome. Numerous water-density formations can be seen in the liver, predominantly in the right lobe, which indicates that they communicate with the liver.

injection of biliary contrast shows opacification of the cysts (Fig. 42-4); and (3) communication can be demonstrated by opacification of the cysts by endoscopic retrograde cholangiography or intraoperative cholangiography or postoperative cholangiography through a T-tube (Fig. 42-5). These invasive procedures can induce bacterial cholangitis and must be performed only in the few patients in whom communication of the cyst with the biliary cannot be demonstrated by a noninvasive method.

The intrahepatic cysts of Caroli's syndrome must be distinguished from (1) the multiple liver cysts and the liver cysts of adult polycystic kidney disease (these cysts do not communicate with the biliary tract), (2) dilated bile ducts caused by obstructed common bile duct, and (3) ectatic bile ducts caused by primary sclerosing cholangitis.[22,23,34] Most ectactic

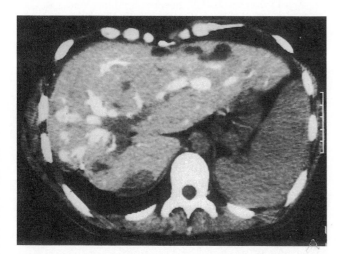

FIGURE 42-4   CT scan taken after intravenous injection of biliary contrast in a patient with Caroli's syndrome. Most of the ectatic bile ducts are opacified, which indicates that they communicate with the biliary tract.

bile ducts of primary sclerosing cholangitis are small; they are relatively large, however, in a few cases of sclerosing cholangitis[23,24] in whom an erroneous diagnosis of Caroli's syndrome has been made.[22,23]

Course and Complications

The course of Caroli's syndrome is dominated by recurrent episodes of bacterial cholangitis, the frequency of which varies widely: some patients experience 10 to 20, whereas others suffer only 1 or 2 episodes a year. In patients with frequent episodes of bacterial cholangitis, the prognosis is poor; most such patients die 5 to 10 years after the onset of cholangitis, usually of an uncontrolled biliary bacterial infection. Bacterial cholangitis may be complicated by liver abscesses, septicemia, extrahepatic abscesses, and secondary amyloidosis.[14]

Bacterial cholangitis often induces the formation of intracystic pigment stones,[24] which are easily recognized by ultrasonography but may be missed by CT when not calcified. These stones can migrate from the cysts into the common bile duct and then determine biliary pain, cholestasis, or acute pancreatitis.[29] Cholangiocellular carcinoma develops in some patients with Caroli's syndrome.[4,8,12,33] Hepatocellular carcinoma has been reported in association with Caroli's syndrome.[16]

Associated Malformations

In patients with Caroli's syndrome and congenital hepatic fibrosis, the malformations described in association with congenital hepatic fibrosis may be present. In patients afflicted by Caroli's syndrome with or, more often, without congenital hepatic fibrosis, associated choledocal cyst is relatively common.[21,33] Exceptionally, Caroli's syndrome is associated with Laurence-Moon-Biedl-Bardet syndrome.[36]

Treatment

Episodes of bacterial cholangitis are treated by appropriate antibiotics.

The prevention of recurrent bacterial cholangitis is difficult. Periodic administration of antibiotics is efficacious in some patients but inefficient in others. T-tube drainage is inefficacious and may be dangerous in patients with associated congenital hepatic fibrosis: large amounts of water and electrolytes secreted by the multiple bile ductules may be lost through the T-tube, which may result in severe dehydration.[37] Administration of chenodiol or ursodiol has been used for the prevention and treatment of intracystic stones; although chenodiol has induced the disappearance of intracystic stones in one patient,[20] this treatment has not been clearly efficacious in others.[24] Transhepatic intubation and drainage of the biliary tree have been used successfully in a small number of patients.[41] Surgical biliointestinal anastomoses or endoscopic papillotomy may facilitate the passage of stones from the common bile duct into the intestine; these procedures may increase the frequency and severity of the episodes of bacterial cholangitis[39] and, therefore, must be avoided in these patients. In the localized form of Caroli's syndrome, partial hepatectomy is indicated, and excellent results can be expected.[25,28,31,35] In the diffuse form, if the cysts predominate

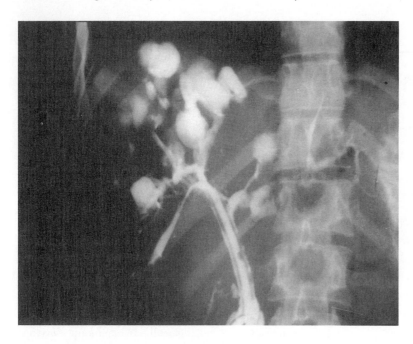

FIGURE 42-5 T-tube cholangiography in a patient with Caroli's syndrome. Cystic formations communicate with the biliary tree.

in a part of the liver, partial hepatectomy can likewise be envisaged; in such patients, partial hepatectomy is difficult because of associated congenital hepatic fibrosis and portal hypertension, and the long-term results may be compromised because multifocal dilatation affecting the remaining liver may be the source of recurrent bacterial cholangitis.[28] In the diffuse form without predominance of the cysts in any part of the liver, complicated by severe recurrent bacterial cholangitis, liver transplantation may be considered.

References

1. Alvarez F, Bernard O, Brunelle F, Brunelle F, Hadchouel M, Leblanc A, Odièvre M, Alagille D. Congenital hepatic fibrosis in children. J Pediatr 99:370–375, 1981
2. Averback P. Congenital hepatic fibrosis. Asymptomatic adults without renal anomaly. Arch Pathol Lab Med 101:260–261, 1977
3. Caroli J, Couinaud C, Soupault R, Porcher P, Eteve J. Une affection nouvelle, sans doute congénitale, des voies biliaires: la dilatation kystique unilobaire des canaux hépatiques. Semin Hôp Paris 34:136–142, 1958
4. Caroli J, Soupault R, Kossakowski J, Plocker L, Pardowska A. La dilatation polykystique congénitale des voies biliaires intra-hépatiques: essai de classification. Sem Hôp Paris 34:488–495, 1958
5. Chagnon JP, Barge J, Hay JM, Devars du Mayne JF, Richard JP, Hardouin JP. Fibrose hépatique congénitale, polykystose rénale et lymphangiectasies intestinales primitives. Gastroenterol Clin Biol 6:326–332, 1982
6. Choi BI, Yeon KM, Kim SH, Han MC. Caroli's disease: central dot sign in CT. Radiology 174:161–163, 1990
7. Clermont RJ, Maillard JN, Benhamou JP, Fauvert R. Fibrose hépatique congénitale. Can Med Assoc J 97:1272–1278, 1967
8. Dayton MT, Longmire WP, Tompkins RK. Caroli's disease: a premalignant condition? Am J Surg 145:41–48, 1983
9. De Vos M, Barbier F, Cuvelier C. Congenital hepatic fibrosis. J Hepatol 6:222–228, 1988
10. Dupond JL, Miguet JP, Carbillet JP, Saint-Hillier Y, Perol C, Leconte des Floris R. Kidney polycystic disease in adult congenital hepatic fibrosis. Ann Intern Med 88:514–515, 1978
11. Erlinger S, Sakellaridis A, Maillard JN, Benhamou JP. Les formes angiocholitiques de la fibrose hépatique congénitale. Presse Med 77:1189–1191, 1969
12. Etienne JC, Bouillot JL, Alexandre JH. Cholangiocarcinome développé sur maladie de Caroli: a propos d'un cas—revue de la littérature. J Chir (Paris) 124:161–164, 1987
13. Fauvert F, Benhamou JP. Congenital hepatic fibrosis. In: Schaffner F, Sherlock S, Leevy CM, eds. The liver and its diseases. New York, IMS, 1974, pp 283–288
14. Fevery J, Tanghe W, Kerremans R, Desmet V, De Groote J. Congenital dilatation of the intrahepatic bile ducts associated with the development of amyloidosis. Gut 13:604–609, 1972
15. Grumbach R, Bourillon J, Auvert JP. Maladie fibrokystique du foie avec hypertension portale chez l'enfant: deux observations. Arch Anat Pathol 30:74–77, 1954
16. Kchir N, Haouet S, Boubaker S, M'Kaouer R, Daghfous MH, Chatti S, Hadj Salah H, Zitouna MM. Maladie de Caroli associée à un hépatocarcinome: a propos d'une observation et revue de la littérature. Sem Hôp Paris 66:1962–1966, 1990
17. Kerr DNS, Harrison CV, Sherlock S, Milnes Walker R. Congenital hepatic fibrosis. Q J Med 30:91–117, 1961
18. Kerr DNS, Okonkwo S, Choa RG. Congenital hepatic fibrosis: the long-term prognosis. Gut 19:514–520, 1978
19. Kerr DNS, Warrick CK, Hart-Mercier J. Lesion resembling medullary sponge kidney in patients with congenital hepatic fibrosis. Clin Radiol 12:85–91, 1962
20. Kutz K, Mederer SE, Paumgartner G. Chenodesoxycholic acid therapy of intrahepatic radiolucent gallstones in a patient with Caroli's syndrome. Acta Hepatogastroenterol 25:398–401, 1978
21. Loubeau JM, Steichen FM. Dilatation of intrahepatic bile ducts in choledocal cyst: case report with follow-up and review of the literature. Arch Surg 111:1384–1390, 1976
22. Ludwig J, McCarty RL, LaRusso NF, Krom RAF, Wiesner RH. Intrahepatic cholangiectases and large-duct obliteration in primary sclerosing cholangitis. Hepatology 6:560–568, 1986
23. Ludwig J, Wiesner RH, LaRusso NF. Focal dilatation of intrahepatic bile ducts (Caroli's disease), cholangiocarcinoma, and sclerosis of intrahepatic bile ducts. J Clin Gastroenterol 4:53–57, 1982
24. Mathias K, Waldmann D, Daikeler G, Kauffmann G. Intrahepatic cystic bile duct dilatations and stone formation: a new case of Caroli's disease. Acta Hepatogastroenterol 25:30–34, 1978

25. Nagasue N. Successful treatment of Caroli's disease by hepatic resection: report of six patients. Ann Surg 200:718–723, 1984
26. Nakanuma Y, Terada T, Ohta G, Kurachi M, Matsubara F. Caroli's disease in congenital hepatic fibrosis and infantile polycystic disease. Liver 2:346–352, 1982
27. Odièvre M, Chaumont P, Montagne JP, Alagille D. Anomalies of the intrahepatic portal venous system in congenital hepatic fibrosis. Radiology 122:427–430, 1977
28. Ramond MJ, Huguet C, Danan G, Rueff B, Benhamou JP. Partial hepatectomy in the treatment of Caroli's disease: report of a case and review of the literature. Dig Dis Sci 29:367–370, 1984
29. Sahel J, Bourry J, Sarles H. Maladie de Caroli avec pancréatite aiguë et angiocholite: intérêt diagnostique et thérapeutique de la cholédoco-wirsungographie endoscopique. Nouv Presse Med 5:2067–2069, 1976
30. Scheinberg IH, Sternlieb IM. Wilson's disease. Philadelphia, WB Saunders, 1984
31. Serejo F, Velosa J, Carneiro de Moura M, Palhano MJ, Batista A, Diaz Gonçalves M. Caroli's disease of the left hepatic lobe associated with hepatic fibrosis. J Clin Gastroenterol 10:559–564, 1988
32. Stilman A, Earnest D, Woolfenden T. Hepatobiliary scanning in diagnosis and management of Caroli's disease. (Abstract) Gastroenterology 80:1295, 1981
33. Summerfield JA, Nagafuchi Y, Sherlock S, Cadafalch J, Scheuer PJ. Hepatobiliary fibropolycystic diseases: a clinical and histological review of 51 patients. J Hepatol 2:141–156, 1986
34. Theilmann L, Stiehl A. Detection of large intrahepatic cholangiectases in patients with primary sclerosing cholangitis by endoscopic retrograde cholangiography. Endoscopy 22:49–50, 1990
35. Thompson HH, Tompkins RK, Longmire WP. Major hepatic resection: a 25-year experience. Ann Surg 197:375–388, 1983
36. Tsuchiya R, Nishimura R, Ito T. Congenital cystic dilatation of the bile ducts associated with Laurence-Moon-Biedl-Bardet syndrome. Arch Surg 112:82–84, 1977
37. Turnberg LA, Jones EA, Sherlock S. Biliary secretion in a patient with cystic dilatation of the intrahepatic biliary tree. Gastroenterology 54:1155–1161, 1968
38. Wagenvoort CA, Baggenstoss AH, Love JG. Subarachnoid hemorrhage due to cerebellar hemangioma associated with congenital hepatic fibrosis and polycystic kidneys: report of a case. Proc Mayo Clin 37:301–306, 1962
39. Watts DR, Lorenzo GA, Beal JM. Congenital dilatation of the intrahepatic bile ducts. Arch Surg 108:592–608, 1974
40. Williams R, Scheuer P, Heard BE. Congenital hepatic fibrosis with an unusual pulmonary lesion. J Clin Pathol 17:135–142, 1964
41. Witlin LT, Gadacz TR, Zuidema GD, Kridelbangh WW. Transhepatic decompression of the biliary tree in Caroli's disease. Surgery 91:205–209, 1982

Diseases of the Liver, Seventh Edition, edited by
Leon Schiff and Eugene R. Schiff. J.B. Lippincott Company, Philadelphia © 1993.

43

Liver Transplantation

Robert D. Gordon

David H. Van Thiel

Thomas E. Starzl

During the past decade, liver transplantation advanced rapidly to the forefront of therapies available for patients with end-stage liver disease and has had a dramatic impact on the practice of hepatology. Advances in immunosuppression, refinement of surgical technique, new methods of organ procurement and preservation, improved perioperative patient care, new agents for prophylaxis and treatment of opportunistic infection, and wider public and professional acceptance of voluntary cadaveric organ donation have all contributed significantly to the progress in this field.

Figure 43-1 demonstrates the linear increase in case experience in Europe and the United States during the last 5 years of the 1980s. Since October 1, 1987, a national liver transplant registry has been maintained by the United Network for Organ Sharing, which operates under federal contract as the national organ sharing and procurement network. Through December 1989, 66 transplant centers had reported 4193 liver transplantations in 3610 patients (Fig. 43-2). During the same period, Western European centers reported to the European Liver Transplant Registry in Paris 2964 liver transplantations in 2706 patients[44] (Fig. 43-3).

Indications for Liver Transplantation

Liver transplantation is performed for many diseases that lead to irreversible acute and chronic liver failure, for which no reasonable medical or surgical alternative therapy exists. In both Europe and the United States, the leading indications for liver replacement are cirrhosis, cholestatic liver disease (primary biliary cirrhosis [PBC], sclerosing cholangitis, biliary atresia), inborn errors of metabolism, fulminant hepatic failure, and neoplasms (Fig. 43-4). Among the patients with cirrhosis, posthepatitic and alcoholic cirrhosis are the most common types for which liver transplantation is performed (Fig. 43-5). Patient survival rates after liver transplantation in the United States and Europe for common indications are summarized in Table 43-1.

PARENCHYMAL LIVER DISEASE

Postnecrotic Cirrhosis

Patient survival rates after liver transplantation for postnecrotic cirrhosis, excluding hepatitis B surface antigen (HBsAg)-positive patients, are 73% to 75% at 1 year and 67%

to 73% at 2 years (see Table 43-1). The hepatitis C virus (HCV), a ribonucleic acid virus recently cloned by Choo and associates,[19] is believed to be the agent responsible for most cases of transfusion-related non-A, non-B hepatitis. The precise incidence of posttransplantation HCV-related hepatitis is not known, but preliminary studies from the Mayo Clinic suggest that HCV is an important cause of posttransplantation chronic hepatitis and that a significant proportion of cases represent recurrent HCV-related disease.[119]

Reinfection after liver transplantation in HBsAg-positive patients is common, and overall patient and graft survival rates have not been as high as for other forms of cirrhosis. Although many patients enjoy a prolonged period of rehabilitation after liver transplantation for hepatitis B virus (HBV)–related cirrhosis, most retain the carrier state, and there is a high reinfection rate.[28,37,65,110,117,127] At the University of Pittsburgh, 1- and 2-year patient survival rates for postnecrotic cirrhosis in HBsAg-negative patients are 76% and 73%, respectively, but the same rates for HBsAg-positive patients are 58.8% and 48.6%, respectively.[47] Registry survival rates in Europe (68% at 2 years) have been better than survival rates reported in the United States (43% at 2 years) in HBsAg-positive patients for reasons that are not known but that may relate to differences in strategies used to alter the incidence and course of HBV infection.

Several approaches have been reported to alter the course of HBV reinfection of a liver allograft, including active immunization with hepatitis vaccine, passive immunization with hyperimmune globulin, and immunomodulation with α-interferon.[15,37,81,99,129,149] In all these reports, there was evidence that perioperative and postoperative therapy with hyperimmune globulin may delay the reappearance and, in some cases, provide long-term clearance of HBsAg. Further trials of long-term passive immunoprophylaxis appear warranted. On the other hand, treatment with α-interferon, which has shown some promise in altering the course of HBV infection in the nontransplantation situation, has yet to show any significant promise in transplant recipients.[37,122,149]

Alcoholic Cirrhosis

Alcoholic cirrhosis is the most common cause of chronic liver disease in Western society. Because of the hazards associated with surgery in such patients and a high risk of recidivism, Laennec's cirrhosis had been considered a contraindication to liver transplantation. In fact, recent experience has shown that patient survival rates after liver transplanta-

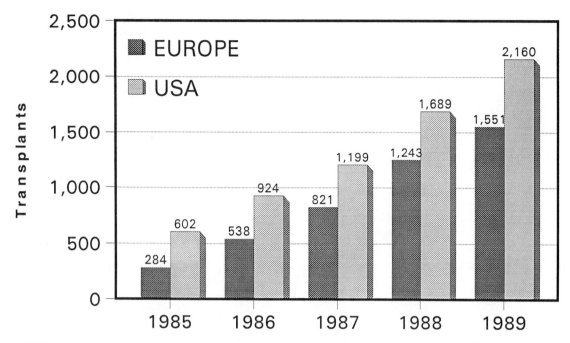

FIGURE 43-1 Liver transplantations performed per year in the United States and Europe, 1985 to 1989.

tion for alcoholic cirrhosis are comparable with patient survival rates after liver transplantation for postnecrotic cirrhosis and cholestatic liver disease[11,63,140] (see Table 43-1).

Actual rates of recidivism are difficult to determine, since patient denial is common but not always truthful and objective pathology is not always available. Recidivism rates are probably higher than those published so far, but it is clear that the patients at greatest risk are those who are actively drinking just before transplantation. It is difficult to justify demanding a prolonged period of abstinence before transplantation, since many patients are too ill to wait. The excellent patient survival rates that have been achieved must now be matched by similar improvements in methods of rehabilitation and behavior modification.

CHOLESTATIC LIVER DISEASE

Sclerosing Cholangitis

Cholestatic liver diseases, including sclerosing cholangitis, PBC, and biliary atresia, are among the best established indications for liver transplantation, but issues remain concerning patient selection, alternative surgical procedures, and timing of transplantation.

Primary sclerosing cholangitis (PSC) is a progressive disease with a substantial morbidity and mortality, even when it is detected in asymptomatic patients.[116] Although only a small percentage of patients with inflammatory bowel disease eventually develop PSC, as many as 70% of cases of sclerosing cholangitis have been associated with inflammatory

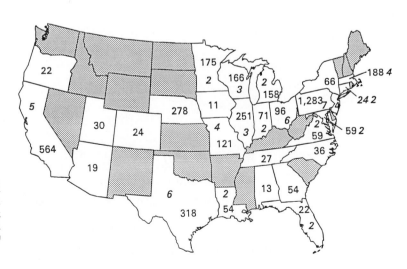

FIGURE 43-2 Liver transplantation in the United States, October 1987 to December 1989. Numbers in normal face are transplantations performed in each state; numbers in italics are transplant centers in each state. A total of 4193 transplantations were performed in 3610 patients in 66 centers.

bowel disease.[165] The disease is associated with an increased risk of cholangiocarcinoma. In patients with ulcerative colitis, there is also an increased risk of adenocarcinoma of the colon. Thus, the evaluation of patients with PSC should include a complete evaluation of the biliary tree and gastrointestinal tract. Multiple percutaneous or endoscopic brushings of the biliary tree are recommended. A negative brushing on one examination is insufficient, in our experience, to exclude the presence of biliary tract tumor.

Conventional biliary tract reconstructive surgery is advocated for cases that have not progressed to persistent jaundice, refractory cholangitis, secondary biliary cirrhosis, and portal hypertension, especially for patients in whom obstructive disease is limited to the hepatic duct bifurcation or extrahepatic biliary tree.[16,85] Only a minority of patients may qualify for such surgery, given the usual distribution of the disease and its progressive nature. In a series of 178 cases recently reviewed by the Lahey Clinic, 71% of patients had intrahepatic or diffuse disease. Although they reported some benefit of biliary surgery in 75% of cases, subsequent operations were associated with a higher morbidity and mortality.[91] Involvement of the extrahepatic bile ducts alone may be more common in patients without associated inflammatory bowel disease.[121]

Survival after liver transplantation for PSC in patients free of cancer is comparable with survival after liver transplantation for other cholestatic liver diseases and for postnecrotic cirrhosis (see Table 43-1). Given the excellent results that are attainable with this form of surgery,[80,90] we recommend conservative use of conventional biliary tract reconstructions, except in those patients without cirrhosis and portal hypertension and with distribution of disease that is easily approached. Reoperation should be avoided. Many patients who require biliary tract decompression but who probably will require

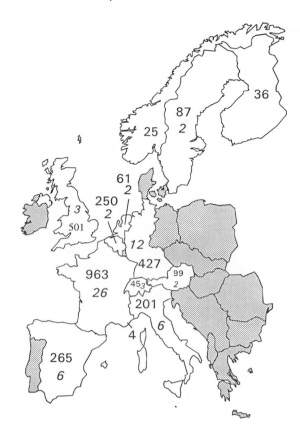

FIGURE 43-3   Liver transplantation in Europe, October 1987 to December 1989. Numbers in normal face are transplantations performed in each state; numbers in italics are transplant centers in each state. A total 2964 grafts were performed in 2706 patients and 67 centers in the registry as of December 1989.

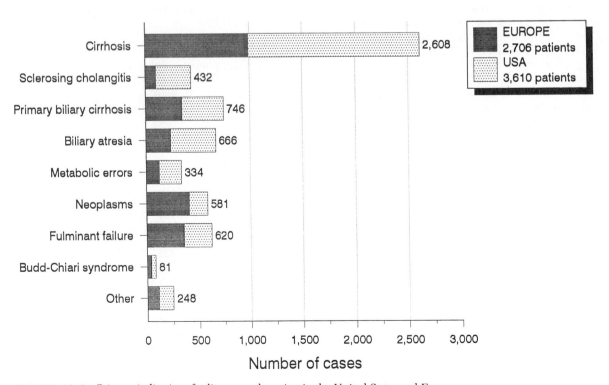

FIGURE 43-4   Primary indications for liver transplantation in the United States and Europe.

FULMINANT HEPATIC FAILURE

The management of fulminant hepatic failure (FHF) requires a high level of expertise. Early transfer to a liver unit where facilities for specialized monitoring, medical management, and transplantation services are available should be considered. Special precautions are necessary during patient transfer. Patients with encephalopathy above stage II level should be intubated to protect against aspiration. Survival depends on cause, expert care, and, in cases complicated by advanced stages of coma, cerebral edema, renal failure, or metabolic acidosis, prompt replacement of the liver.

The King's College Hospital Liver Unit found a strong correlation between survival (without transplantation) and the cause of FHF.[104] Survival by etiologic group was fulminant hepatitis A, 66.7%; acetaminophen toxicity, 52.9%; fulminant hepatitis B, 38.9%; non-A, non-B hepatitis, 20.0%; and halothane or idiosyncratic hepatitis, 12.5%. Outcome was also correlated with complications, especially cerebral edema, oliguric renal failure, and uncompensated metabolic acidosis. Uncompensated metabolic acidosis was associated with less than 10% survival. Only 37% of patients in stage 4 coma and 50% of patients in stage 3 coma survived. In subsequent studies, it has also been found that a continued increase in prothrombin time on day 4 or a peak prothrombin time of 180 seconds or greater is associated with less than 8% chance of survival in cases of acetaminophen overdose.[56] Arterial pH and serum creatinine levels also correlate with survival. In patients with viral hepatitis and drug reactions, age less than 11 years or more than 40 years, serum bilirubin level greater than 300 μmol/L (17.5 mg/dL), and prothrombin time greater than 50 seconds correlated with poor survival.

Of 42 patients who received liver transplants over a 7-year period for FHF in our Pittsburgh series, survival after transplantation for HBV-related disease was 87.5%; for non-A, non-B hepatitis, 63%; and for toxic hepatitis, 33.3%. Only 5 of 10 patients with stage IV encephalopathy who survived more than 1 week after transplantation had complete neurologic recovery.[67] Vickers and colleagues[161] also found a strong correlation between stage of encephalopathy and survival. Eighteen of 19 patients (95%) with stage I or II encephalopathy survived compared with only 13 of 38 patients (34%) with stage III or IV encephalopathy.

With prompt recognition of poor prospects for medical recovery and transfer to a liver transplant center, more than 50% of patients with FHF can be saved.[33,67,161] Although this is not as good as can be achieved for patients with chronic liver failure, the results are a significant achievement, given the circumstances.

PATIENT SELECTION AND PREOPERATIVE MANAGEMENT

Evaluation of the candidate for liver transplantation includes establishment of the primary diagnosis, stage of disease, and prognosis; assessment of liver size and portal vein patency; and, in the case of patients with (or suspected of having) hepatic tumors, determination of the extent of disease. Most patients are referred to the transplant center with an established diagnosis and a poor prognosis without transplantation. A major gastrointestinal bleed, a history of repeated bouts of encephalopathy, progressive neuropathy, refractory ascites, a recent precipitous deterioration in liver function (eg, a recent increase in the rate of rise of serum bilirubin level), rapid progression of bone disease, spontaneous bacterial peritonitis, poor hepatic synthetic function, loss of liver volume, and progressive muscle wasting are indications for early transplantation.

Portal vein patency usually can be determined by ultrasonography or magnetic resonance imaging (MRI), but occasionally arteriography is necessary. MRI is probably the most reliable of the noninvasive screening studies for determining portal vein patency, but it is not always readily available. Portal vein thrombosis is not an absolute contraindication to liver transplantation, and venous phase arteriography may be necessary for adequate study of the mesenteric venous circulation. Computed tomography (CT) scans are useful to detect the presence of tumors, with or without extrahepatic extension, and can be used to determine liver volume. Upper gastrointestinal endoscopy to check for varices is indicated in patients who have not had such an examination within the past 3 months. We do not recommend prophylactic sclerotherapy if esophageal varices are present but the patient has no history of bleeding.

Patients with sclerosing cholangitis should have multiple endoscopic or percutaneous brushings of the biliary tree to evaluate for the presence of cholangiocarcinoma. Patients with liver masses detected by ultrasonography or CT scan should have an appropriate diagnostic evaluation for extrahepatic spread of disease. This includes CT examinations of the abdomen and chest and a bone scan. Blood tumor markers, including carcinoembryonic antigen, vitamin B_{12} binding protein, ferritin, α-fetoprotein, and PIKVA-2, are also screened in our protocols for the management of suspected tumor. If a neuroendocrine lesion is suspected, appropriate tests for these neoplasms should be performed. Baseline studies in preparation for chemotherapy include electrocardiography, a multiple-gated acquisition heart scan, 24-hour creatinine clearance, and biopsy proof of tumor.

A complete serologic screen for hepatitis A, B, and C should be performed. All patients without demonstrable immunity to hepatitis B should receive a complete course of recombinant vaccine for HBV, before transplantation if feasible. As discussed previously, HBV carriers (HBsAg-positive) may benefit from administration of hyperimmune globulin beginning during surgery and continuing indefinitely.

Cytomegalovirus (CMV), varicella-zoster virus (VZV), and *Toxoplasma* immunoglobulin titers should be obtained as part of the pretransplantation evaluation. CMV infections, both primary infections and reactivation infections, are among the most common and most serious encountered after transplantation. Purified protein derivative (PPD) status must be known before transplantation. It is also important to know if the patient is anergic to other antigens, such as *Trichophyton*, *Candida*, or mumps. Antiviral and antitubercular prophylaxis are discussed in a later section.

Attention to the nutritional requirements of patients with liver failure is also important. Many such patients have severe deficiencies of fat-soluble vitamins and trace elements.

MANAGEMENT OF PORTAL HYPERTENSION

Ascites

Refractory ascites can be a challenging management problem and can lead to serious complications, including spontaneous bacterial peritonitis and ulcerating umbilical hernia. Judicious use of diuretics and colloid is required, and large-volume paracentesis is recommended for severe cases. Peritoneal-venous shunts (LeVeen shunt, Denver shunt) can be useful and can easily be removed at the time of transplantation. In our experience, the use of these shunts is associated with the formation of inflammatory intraabdominal adhesions, possibly from recurrent episodes of spontaneous bacterial peritonitis, which can make the transplantation procedure more difficult. Patients with previous failed shunts should have a Doppler ultrasound examination before transplantation to evaluate the patency of the jugular and subclavian veins. Thrombosis of these vessels is a complication of failed shunts and can make venous bypass access difficult or impossible during transplantation.

Variceal Hemorrhage

Before the availability of liver transplantation, the role of the surgeon in the management of variceal bleeding from portal hypertension was directed at prevention of rebleeding. Balloon tamponade, selective or peripheral infusion of vasopressin, transthoracic variceal ligation, and nonselective portosystemic shunts were the classic approaches taken. In the elective setting, the selective distal splenorenal shunt has become the operation of choice, and it may still be the preferred procedure in patients with good hepatic reserve (Child's class A patients). For most patients with significant underlying liver disease, transplantation is required, and shunt procedures should be reserved only for such patients whose hemorrhage cannot be controlled by conservative measures, such as balloon intubation or sclerotherapy, and for whom a liver cannot be found or for whom transplantation is contraindicated for other reasons.

Sclerotherapy is a preferred method for controlling acute variceal hemorrhage in patients with portal hypertension. Acute bleeding is reported to be controlled in 80% to 95% of patients by sclerotherapy performed by a skilled endoscopist, although eventual rebleeding can be expected in 38% to 60% of patients.[32]

In our experience, emergency sclerotherapy for acute bleeding in liver transplantation candidates has a high rate of complications (69.4%), including esophageal stricture (56.0%), bleeding esophageal ulcers (10.5%), and esophageal perforation (2.9%).[112] For this reason, in the acute setting, we prefer to first use balloon tamponade and peripheral vasopressin to stabilize the patient with massive hemorrhage. In the elective setting, the rate of complications is much lower (12.6%), including esophageal stricture (9.0%), bleeding esophageal ulcers (3.1%), and esophageal perforation (0.5%).

Esophageal transection and devascularization procedures should be avoided because severe scarring may result that can make liver transplantation extremely difficult. Some recent reports suggest that percutaneous transjugular placement of an intrahepatic stent-shunt may be a valuable technique in patients waiting for a liver transplant to control portal hypertension without invasive surgery.[124,125] If an emergency surgical shunt is needed to control persistent or recurrent hemorrhage, a mesocaval shunt is preferred, since this avoids dissection in the hepatic hilum, but even a portocaval shunt does not make liver transplantation prohibitive. Survival rates after liver transplantation in patients with or without a history of variceal hemorrhage and in those with or without a history of a shunt procedure are not significantly different.[1,66]

Finally, acutely bleeding patients can be managed by immediate liver transplantation. The transplant corrects the underlying liver disease and provides immediate portal decompression. Most patients stop bleeding once the graft is in place. Unfortunately, a suitable liver graft seldom is available on such an urgent basis.

CONTRAINDICATIONS TO LIVER TRANSPLANTATION

There are few absolute contraindications to liver transplantation. Severe systemic conditions, not also amenable to medical or surgical correction, may contraindicate liver transplantation if the ability of the patient to withstand the stress of operation is in serious doubt, the life expectancy of the patient would not be significantly prolonged, or a poor quality of life would not be improved. Uncontrolled sepsis outside the liver or biliary tree, acute hemodynamic instability with compromise of other vital organs, active substance abuse, extrahepatic or metastatic cancer (with some exceptions as noted previously), irreversible brain damage or neurologic dysfunction, and a history of behavioral or psychiatric disorders that would interfere with the patient's ability to comply with the necessary medical regimen are contraindications to liver transplantation. Spontaneous bacterial peritonitis should be treated for at least 48 hours and preferably for 7 days before liver transplantation is attempted.

Advanced age was once considered to be a contraindication, but excellent results have recently been reported for patients over age 60.[141] The oldest patient to receive a liver graft in Pittsburgh was 76 years old at the time of operation, and as of this writing, she is alive and well at age 81.

Most problematic is whether or not patients with positive serology for the human immunodeficiency virus (HIV) should be candidates for liver transplantation.[136] A retrospective survey of stored sera from patients given liver transplants between 1981 and 1986 revealed a 2.6% incidence of HIV.[30] HIV antibodies predated the transplantation in one third of these recipients, and the rest seroconverted afterward. Among the 10 children in the HIV-positive group, only 1 died of a complication related to HIV. Among the 16 adults in this series, the acquired immunodeficiency syndrome (AIDS)-related mortality was 37%.

It is clear that HIV positivity carries an increased risk of AIDS-related morbidity and mortality in the transplant population. Many patients who, despite evidence of past exposure to HIV, are still free of clinical manifestations of AIDS can receive substantial, prolonged benefit from liver transplantation. For these patients, the immediate threat is end-stage liver disease, not AIDS, and these patients can do well despite the risks of immunosuppression required for transplantation.

Intrapulmonary shunting with hypoxemia is a complication of advanced liver disease and sometimes has been considered a contraindication to liver transplantation. After transplantation, the shunts eventually close and the extrapulmonic manifestations reverse.[144] In severe cases, this can take several months, and an extended period of ventilatory support may be required. Patients with significant pulmonary artery hypertension, however, usually cannot tolerate operation. Therefore right-sided heart catheterization should be performed before surgery to measure pulmonary artery pressure.

Patients with the most advanced degrees of muscle wasting and nutritional deprivation may be unable to survive liver transplantation. If operation is attempted in severely debilitated patients, tracheostomy should be considered at the same time as transplantation, since these patients inevitably also require prolonged ventilatory as well as intensive nutritional support after surgery.

Organ Preservation

The University of Wisconsin (UW) preservation solution introduced in 1987 by Belzer and Southard[7,70,73] represents the first major advance in liver preservation since the original descriptions of slush preservation more than a decade earlier. Using this solution, it has been possible to extend liver preservation from a mean preservation time of about 5 hours to 12 hours and to extend the limits of preservation out to at least 18 hours with comparable quality of graft function and a low incidence of primary graft failure.[20,106,114,152] Although we have seen perfect liver function even with organs kept in cold storage in UW solution for 20 to 34 hours, the rate of retransplantation and the incidence of primary graft failure increase significantly with longer preservation times[42] (Fig. 43-6). It is, therefore, recommended that organs be used within 20 hours of storage.

The practical benefits of longer preservation time are significant, and this has changed liver transplantation from an urgent operation to a semielective procedure in many cases. Patients have more time to be called in to the transplant center for surgery, and thus, more patients can wait at home. Grafts can be sent to transplant centers from distant sources. Surgeons can explore patients and have time to arrange for a backup patient if the intended recipient proves to be inoperable.

The incidence of primary graft failure after liver transplantation is 5% to 10% in most reported series. There is no accepted and reliable test to predict which grafts will function and which will fail before implantation. Pretransplantation biopsies can be useful if certain findings are present. Signif-

icant fatty infiltration (macrovesicular steatosis),[25,148] extensive ballooning of hepatocytes (hydropic degeneration),[25] and pericentral and panlobular individual hepatocyte necrosis[88] are associated with a higher risk of primary graft failure. In postperfusion biopsies, the presence of zonal or severe focal necrosis and a severe neutrophilic exudate (findings that may suggest hyperacute rejection) have been associated with a difficult postoperative course but not with inevitable graft failure.[72] A normal pretransplantation biopsy is not a guarantee of graft viability, since irreversible subcellular ischemic damage may not be detectable with conventional histology.

Availability of a simple, rapid test for graft viability would significantly reduce the incidence of primary graft function. MEGX, a metabolite of lidocaine, has been compared favorably with other methods of assessment, such as indocyanine green clearance, and is easily and rapidly measured.[102] It has shown some promise as a test of pretransplantation graft viability, but prognostic sensitivity and specificity are only about 75%.[103] It may prove useful when used in combination with other parameters of graft quality.

Surgical Procedure

Details of the operative techniques of liver transplantation are beyond the intended scope of this chapter and have been addressed elsewhere.[46,137] In brief, the operation is performed in four stages. The first stage, recipient hepatectomy, can be formidable if the patient has had extensive previous surgery in the upper abdomen, has a severe, uncorrectable coagulopathy, or has a small contracted liver. The second, anhepatic phase, during which the recipient vessels are anastomosed to the vessels of the graft, has been greatly facilitated in larger children and adults by routine use of a partial veno-venous bypass. The bypass effectively decompresses the systemic and mesenteric venous drainage and maintains delivery of an adequate blood volume to the right side of the heart during the period of interruption of the suprarenal inferior vena cava and portal vein. This reduces mesenteric venous congestion, renal vein hypertension, and bleeding from the usually rich and fragile venous collateral bed in patients with long-standing portal hypertension. The third phase begins on revascularization of the new liver, when both surgical and medical bleeding commonly is encountered, and requires considerable skill on the part of both the surgical and the anesthesia teams to control. Once hemostasis has been achieved, the final stage of the procedure, a biliary reconstruction, is performed.

INFERIOR VENA CAVA

In the conventional reconstruction, the suprahepatic vena cava of the graft is anastomosed end to end to a cuff of infradiaphragmatic recipient inferior vena cava followed by anastomosis of the infrahepatic graft vena cava end to end to a cuff of suprarenal recipient inferior vena cava. The intrahepatic portion of the recipient vena cava is removed with the native liver. The right adrenal vein must be ligated, and this can lead to venous infarction of the gland with hemorrhage.

An alternative to the standard technique is to piggyback the suprahepatic portion of the graft vena cava to the confluence of the recipient hepatic veins and oversew the infrahepatic end of the graft vena cava.[153] The native liver is first

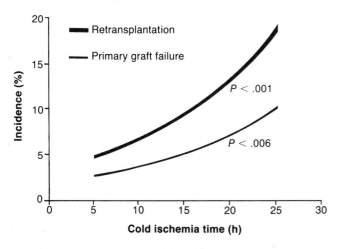

FIGURE 43-6 Logistic regression model to estimate the relation between cold ischemia time and rates of retransplantation and primary graft failure for liver grafts stored in UW solution. (Furukawa H, et al. Effect of cold ischemia time on the early outcome of human hepatic allografts preserved with UW solution. Transplantation 51:1000, 1991)

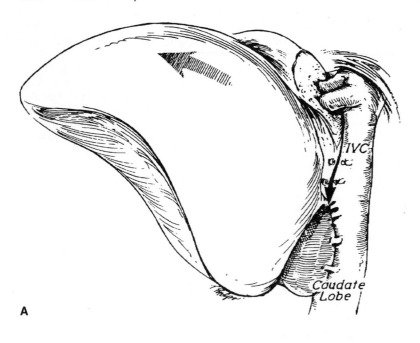

A

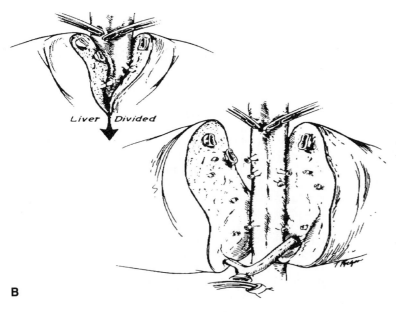

B

FIGURE 43-7 The piggyback technique for implantation of a liver allograft with preservation of the recipient inferior vena cava. (**A**) After completion of the hilar dissection, the left lobe is rotated, individual hepatic veins are ligated, and the main hepatic veins are exposed. (**B**) If difficulty is encountered in exposing the hepatic veins, the parenchyma can be split and the veins controlled from inside the liver. (**C**) The hepatic vein cuffs are prepared for anastomosis. The middle and left hepatic veins usually are used for anastomosis and the right hepatic vein is oversewn, as shown here. (**D**) The completed implant lying on the intact recipient vena cava. The infrahepatic portion of the graft vena cava has been oversewn. (Tzakis A, et al. Orthotopic liver transplantation with preservation of the inferior vena cava. Ann Surg 210:649, 1989)

carefully dissected off the recipient vena cava, which is left in place (Fig. 43-7). The right adrenal vein is, therefore, left intact. The end of the infrahepatic graft vena cava is simply oversewn.

The piggyback approach can be advantageous in selected cases in which the graft size is mismatched with the recipient or there is a large discrepancy in the diameter of the recipient and graft venae cavae. It provides an alternative to the use of the veno-venous bypass, since the recipient vena cava is left in continuity, and is, therefore, a method of choice in patients in whom venous bypass cannot be used, such as patients with thrombosis of the subclavian veins after failed peritoneal-venous shunts. Care must be taken to avoid excessive traction on the vena cava during dissection, which might obstruct blood flow. The longer period of portal vein obstruction endured with this approach may predispose to translocation of infectious organisms from the gut during a

period of splanchnic congestion and increase the risk of postoperative sepsis. The cuff of vena cava constructed from the recipient hepatic veins must be generous enough to provide for unobstructed outflow, and the liver must not be free to twist in the abdomen on the axis of the vena cava anastomosis.

Advanced cirrhosis may result in retrograde portal vein flow, which may progress to portal vein thrombosis. Thrombosis may involve only the main portal vein or may also involve the mesenteric or splenic veins (Fig. 43-8). This is also a potential complication of central or selective portosystemic shunting procedures. Cavernous transformation of the portal vein with generous venous collaterals in the hilum may develop, and ultrasonographers may mistake this high venous flow for a patent portal vein. Even if thrombosis of the portal vein does not occur, the vein wall may become diseased, rendering the vessel unsuitable for anastomosis.

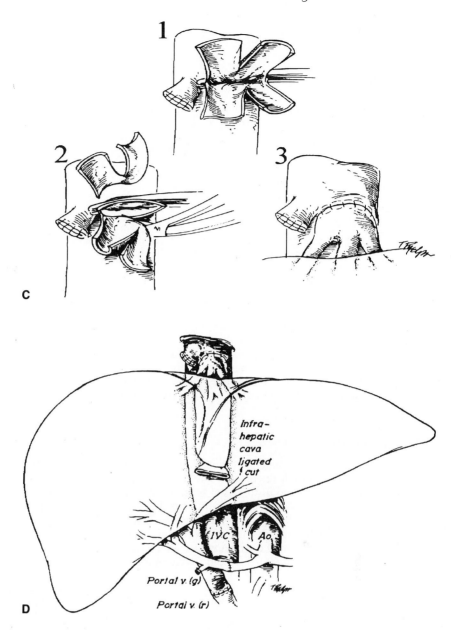

If the confluence of the mesenteric and splenic veins is suitable, a graft of iliac vein from the liver donor can be used to extend the recipient portal vein (Fig. 43-9). In rare cases, a large collateral vein, such as a coronary vein or a choledochal vein, has been used for anastomosis to the portal vein. In most patients, however, it is possible and preferable to construct a venous jump graft of donor iliac vein from either the superior mesenteric vein or one of its large branches, such as the right colic vein, to the graft portal vein[131,143,154] (Fig. 43-10). This graft can be tunneled through the transverse mesocolon, over the pancreas, and beneath the pylorus to emerge in an ideal location for anastomosis, a route also used for arterial grafts. If venous phase arteriography fails to visualize a suitable mesenteric vein in a patient with portal vein thrombosis, it may be necessary to explore the patient to determine if such revascularization is feasible and to have a backup patient available if it is not.

HEPATIC ARTERY

Hepatic artery thrombosis is one of the most common and dreaded technical complications after liver transplantation. It is best prevented by meticulous surgical technique and liberal use of alternative reconstruction techniques if there is any doubt about the integrity of a conventional anastomosis. In most adult patients, the celiac artery of the graft is sewn end to end to the common hepatic artery of the recipient. In young children, the anastomosis may be placed closer to the recipient aorta at the level of the celiac axis. In about 12% of adults and 50% of children, the native recipient artery is unsuitable for anastomosis and a new hepatic artery must be reconstructed.[151] This usually is performed by anastomosis of the donor hepatic or celiac artery to an iliac artery graft taken from the liver donor and placed on the anterior surface of the proximal infrarenal recipient aorta. The graft is tunneled

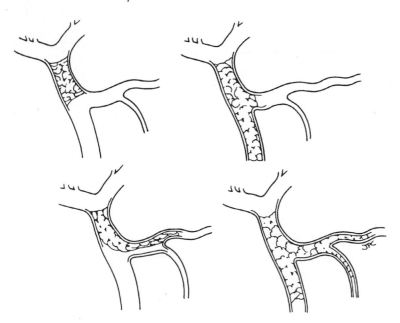

FIGURE 43-8   Patterns of thrombosis of the portal vein in advanced cirrhosis. (Stieber AC, et al. The spectrum of portal vein thrombosis in liver transplantation. Ann Surg 213:199, 1991)

through the transverse mesocolon, over the pancreas, and behind the pylorus[157] (Fig. 43-11) or posterior to the superior mesenteric artery, duodenum, and pancreas to emerge between the inferior vena cava posteriorly and the portal vein anteriorly.

BILIARY RECONSTRUCTION

When possible, direct end-to-end anastomosis of the recipient bile duct to the donor bile duct over a T-tube stent externalized through a stab wound in the distal recipient duct is the preferred method of biliary tract reconstruction (Fig. 43-12, *inset*). The ampulla of Vater is preserved and the T-tube permits monitoring of the quantity and quality of bile output and radiographic examination of the biliary tract. Progressive dilatation of the bile duct, presumably from spastic dysfunc-

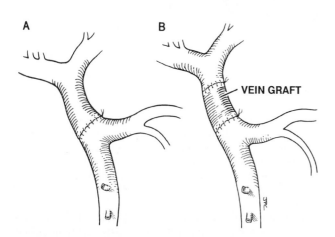

FIGURE 43-9   (**A**) Portal vein reconstruction using a long donor portal vein anastomosed to the splenic vein–superior mesenteric vein confluence. (**B**) Reconstruction of the portal vein using an interposition graft of donor iliac vein. (Stieber AC, et al. The spectrum of portal vein thrombosis in liver transplantation. Ann Surg 213:199, 1991)

tion of a denervated ampulla of Vater, is a common complication that can necessitate conversion to a Roux-en-Y choledochojejunostomy. Leaks and strictures are also important complications (discussed further under technical complications).

End-to-side anastomosis of the donor bile duct to a Roux-en-Y limb of proximal jejunum is the preferred alternative to duct-to-duct reconstruction and is the method of choice in patients with disease of the extrahepatic bile ducts (see Fig. 43-12). Although more complex, it has proved to be a durable and reliable method of reconstruction. Ascending cholangitis is uncommon after this reconstruction when properly performed. Bile leak after this reconstruction can be more serious than after duct-to-duct reconstruction because of open bowel contamination of the abdominal cavity. Contrast examination of the biliary tree requires percutaneous cholangiography.

Another technique of biliary reconstruction that uses the donor gallbladder as a conduit between the donor and the recipient bile ducts has a few advocates (Fig. 43-13). We have limited use of this reconstruction to highly selected cases when previous surgery has caused extensive scarring or previous extensive intestinal resection prohibits reconstruction of an appropriate Roux limb for choledochojejunostomy. In our experience, half of these reconstructions were complicated by biliary stones or sludge formation.[53] The King's College Hospital group reported abnormal cholangiograms in 80% of patients with this type of reconstruction who were observed for 3 years. Findings included biliary strictures, inspissated bile, bile leak, and malpositioned T-tubes.[36] This method has been used by Wall and associates[162] in London, Ontario, without a T-tube or internal stent with a reported complication rate of 13.6%.

Postoperative Care

Postoperative care of the liver transplant recipient is demanding and requires a lifelong commitment to the patient. Mistakes in management after surgery are just as dangerous as

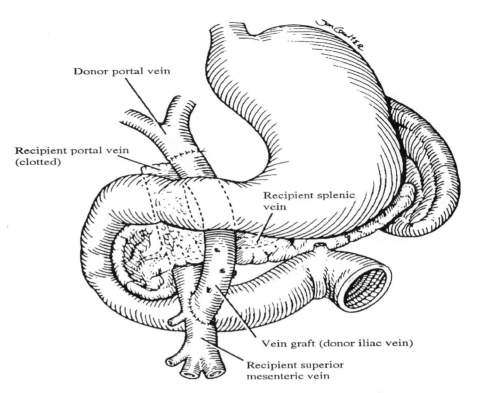

Donor portal vein

Recipient portal vein (clotted)

Recipient splenic vein

Vein graft (donor iliac vein)

Recipient superior mesenteric vein

FIGURE 43-10 Portal vein reconstruction using a jump graft of donor iliac vein from the superior mesenteric vein to the donor portal vein. The graft is passed through a tunnel in the base of the transverse mesocolon, superior to the pancreas and inferior to the distal stomach, to reach the hepatic hilum. This is the preferred method of reconstruction when the recipient portal vein and the confluence of the mesenteric and splenic veins are thrombosed but the main superior mesenteric vein is patent. (Tzakis AG, et al. Venous jump grafts for liver transplantation in patients with portal vein thrombosis. Transplantation 48:530, 1989)

technical misadventures in the operating room. Coordination of effort and continuous liaison between the transplant center staff and primary care providers are essential to the patient's welfare.

EARLY POSTOPERATIVE RECOVERY

In typical cases, if the graft functions well immediately after implantation and the recipient has no extraordinary risk factors, a prompt recovery with a 24- to 48-hour stay in the intensive care unit and a 14- to 21-day stay on the regular hospital floor can be anticipated. In many respects, the care of the postoperative liver transplant recipient resembles the care of other general surgical patients, but there are some important differences.

On leaving the operating room, the patients are always in a state of volume excess with considerable third spacing of fluid, but many patients are oliguric for 24 to 48 hours. Diuretics and colloid often are required, but crystalloid should be limited to modest maintenance requirements to avoid pulmonary edema. Potassium should be given as an intermittent infusion when needed rather than added to maintenance fluids. Graft necrosis (primary nonfunction, hepatic artery thrombosis, hyperacute rejection) can result in sudden increases in serum potassium levels. Hypertension is common and must be treated aggressively. The moderate prolongation of prothrombin time and the thrombocytopenia commonly seen early after liver transplantation when combined with hypertension leave the patient at significant risk of intracerebral bleeding.

Except in patients with active bleeding, a prothrombin time elevated within 15 to 20 seconds of control and platelet counts as low as 30,000/μL are not corrected. Inappropriate correction of moderate coagulation abnormalities may con-

tribute to hepatic artery thrombosis, especially in children. Patients at high risk of vascular thrombosis, such as young children, are anticoagulated with low-molecular-weight dextran (Dextran 40), 5 mL/h intravenously for 5 days, and given aspirin and dipyridamole (Persantine). Once the prothrombin time is less than 18 seconds, heparin, 50 IU/kg subcutaneously, is given every 12 hours. This regimen seldom is needed in adult patients.

Intraabdominal bleeding and primary graft failure are the two most common major problems seen in the immediate postoperative period. Reexploration is advised for the patient who bleeds significantly after surgery, even if the patient stabilizes. If the abdomen is distended with blood or noninvasive imaging studies show a significant volume of clot in the abdomen, it is best to evacuate the abdomen and check the integrity of all vascular anastomoses, lest one be faced with an infected hematoma or a false or mycotic aneurysm later. Patients who require blood should not be permitted to become hypotensive or anuric before reexploration is considered.

Primary graft failure may not be evident immediately because some grafts have partial function for a few days before it becomes evident that the liver cannot sustain the patient. Causes of immediate graft failure include ischemic preservation injury, vascular thrombosis, and hyperacute rejection. Persistent abnormal liver function tests, uncorrectable prolongation of the prothrombin time, elevated lactate levels, oliguria, and central nervous system (CNS) changes (lethargy, seizures) are the common early findings. Narcotics and sleep medications should be avoided early after liver transplantation, since they impair assessment of CNS status. Bedside Doppler ultrasound studies are useful in assessing the patency of the portal vein and hepatic artery. Coma, alkalosis, hyperkalemia, and hypoglycemia characterize the ad-

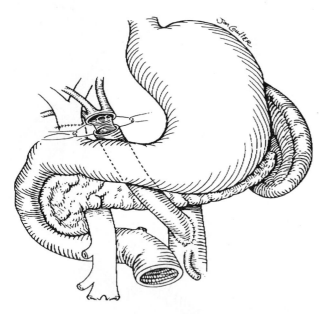

FIGURE 43-11 Route of a freestanding donor iliac arterial graft from the infrarenal abdominal aorta to the hepatic hilum. The graft passes through a rent in the transverse mesocolon (not shown) to pass anterior to the pancreas and behind the pylorus. Note the anomalous donor arterial supply to the liver graft with separate origins of hepatic arterial branches. Complex donor arterial anomalies are best handled by this method of reconstruction. (Tzakis AG, et al. The anterior route for arterial graft conduits in liver transplantation. Transplant Int 2:121, 1989)

vanced stage of primary graft failure. Potassium infusions must be avoided, and dextrose 10% in water may need to be given to support blood glucose levels. Ultimately, only urgent retransplantation before pneumonia or irreversible coma sets in can save the patient with primary graft failure.

COMPLICATIONS

Technical complications are common after liver transplantation and associated with an increase in postoperative mortality. Postoperative bleeding and biliary leak or obstruction are the most common complications that require reoperation.[83]

Intraabdominal bleeding early after surgery has already been discussed and usually is the result of technical problems. Another rare but important cause of hemorrhage is rupture of a preexisting splenic artery aneurysm.[3,13] These lesions may be identified on preoperative studies such as CT scans and ultrasonography. At the time of transplantation, the course of the splenic artery along the upper margin of the pancreas should be palpated. If a splenic artery aneurysm is present, the artery should be ligated.

Biliary Complications

Biliary leak or obstruction are among the most frequent complications after liver transplantation.[126,146] The most common site of biliary leakage after liver transplantation is from the exit site of the T-tube from the common bile duct in patients with a duct-to-duct reconstruction. The diagnosis is confirmed by cholangiography. If the leak is discovered incidentally on a routine cholangiogram and the patient is asymptomatic, no treatment may be necessary. Even most symptomatic leaks are minor and can be managed by retrograde endoscopic placement of a nasobiliary stent or simple suture repair.[107] Leaks from the duct-to-duct anastomosis are more serious, and most require reconstruction by conversion to a Roux-en-Y choledochojejunostomy. Simple suture repair usually fails. If the leak is the result of necrosis of the duct from hepatic artery thrombosis, external drainage of the biliary tree may be required until retransplantation can be performed.

Most T-tube stents are removed about 3 months after transplantation. This may be accompanied by bile leakage.

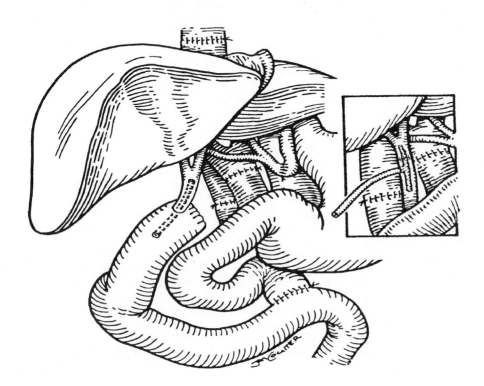

FIGURE 43-12 Methods of biliary reconstruction. Roux-en-Y choledochojejunostomy over an internal stent and choledochocholedochostomy over a T-tube stent (*inset*).

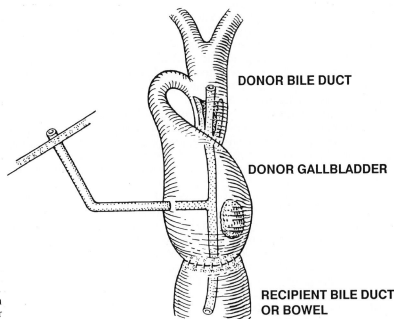

DONOR BILE DUCT

DONOR GALLBLADDER

RECIPIENT BILE DUCT OR BOWEL

FIGURE 43-13 Waddell-Calne biliary conduit. (Adapted from Halff G, et al. Late complications with gallbladder conduit biliary reconstruction after liver transplantation. Transplantation 48:537, 1989)

Patients complain of abdominal or shoulder pain, usually within 1 hour of T-tube removal. Symptomatic patients should be observed in the hospital and kept lying on the right side. If symptoms persist and signs of peritonitis progress, the patient should be explored and the T-tube exit site sutured to stop the leak.

Leaks from the choledochojejunostomy after a Roux-en-Y limb reconstruction are less common but more serious because of the violation of the intestinal tract. A fresh anastomosis to a less inflamed site on the Roux-en-Y limb should be performed when feasible. If severe infection is present, external drainage and deferred reconstruction may be required. Necrosis of the bile duct from hepatic artery thrombosis should be suspected.

Biliary strictures typically occur later in the postoperative course and may present insidiously with alterations in liver function similar to those seen with rejection, hepatitis, or drug toxicity. Liver biopsy, hepatitis serology, ultrasonography, and cholangiography are used to make the differential diagnosis. Patterns of biliary obstruction include anastomotic stricture, donor distal duct narrowing, multiple intrahepatic strictures, dilatation of the donor and recipient ducts without a demonstrable point of obstruction, iatrogenic obstruction by T-tubes or internal stents, and unusual causes, such as a mucocele of the cystic duct stump,[170] or recurrent biliary tract disease, such as sclerosing cholangitis or cancer.[58]

An indwelling catheter, which usually can be placed percutaneously by the interventional radiologist, should be left in patients with a demonstrable obstruction at cholangiography. If the obstruction is localized, balloon cholangioplasty may be tried. Obstructions with biliary stones or biliary dilatation without an obvious site of obstruction (as commonly is seen in patients with ampullary dysfunction after a duct-to-duct reconstruction) require surgical correction (usually conversion to a Roux-en-Y choledochojejunostomy) or endoscopic sphincterotomy. An obstructing mucocele is resected.

Multiple intrahepatic strictures present a more difficult problem. Hepatic artery thrombosis or stricture may be the

cause. Biliary stenting and, occasionally, balloon dilation may be useful in achieving some decompression of the biliary tree, but surgical correction by retransplantation usually is necessary. In those cases in which the strictures are confined to an appropriate anatomic distribution in the liver, subtotal hepatic resection can be done.

Vascular Complications

Hepatic artery thrombosis is one of the most serious complications after liver transplantation. It usually is the result of a technical error, but it can also result from preservation injury of the graft with ischemic injury to the hepatic microcirculation, inappropriate correction of coagulation parameters after operation, high hematocrit, a posttransplantation hypercoagulable state, and uncontrolled allograft rejection with increased intrahepatic vascular resistance and in association with pancreatitis.[4,92,134,169]

Arterial thrombosis should be suspected in any liver transplant recipient with a sudden high temperature and an elevation in liver function studies. Blood cultures that grow enteric organisms (*Klebsiella* sp, *Escherichia coli*, enterococci) are almost pathognomonic. Doppler ultrasonography is an effective noninvasive screening device,[40] but arteriography is necessary even if ultrasonography is negative when there is a high index of clinical suspicion.

Hepatic arterial thrombosis has three general presentations: (1) acute hepatic gangrene with fulminant liver failure, (2) delayed biliary leak with or without bile abscess, and (3) relapsing bacteremia with minimal, if any, liver dysfunction. Treatment depends on cause and presentation. If a technical flaw is quickly identified, immediate surgical correction sometimes is possible and can save the graft.[168] In a few cases, hepatic arterial thrombosis has been successfully treated with intravascular fibrinolytic therapy.[59] Acute hepatic gangrene requires urgent retransplantation. Bile duct necrosis also requires retransplantation but can be controlled with antibiotics and appropriate surgical drainage until a new graft can be found. Relapsing bacteremia is treated with intravenous antibiotics followed by a course of oral suppressive therapy. If the patient remains afebrile with satisfactory liver function, retransplantation may be avoided or only become necessary when chronic ischemic biliary strictures develop. Most patients with persistent bacteremia and most of those who develop intrahepatic abscesses require retransplantation. Percutaneous drainage of an intrahepatic biloma or abscess usually is only a temporizing maneuver.[74]

Portal vein thrombosis is much less common than hepatic artery thrombosis. It may result in fulminant graft failure, especially when it occurs soon after transplantation, but it should also be suspected in patients with severe ascites or a variceal hemorrhage after transplantation. In patients with a viable graft but complications of portal hypertension, a distal splenorenal shunt has been used successfully.[87,128]

Complications of the vena cava anastomoses are rare. Stenosis of the suprahepatic inferior vena cava anastomosis may impair venous drainage enough to cause a Budd-Chiari syndrome and should be considered in any patient with persistent, massive ascites after an otherwise successful liver transplantation. Percutaneous transluminal balloon dilatation has been successfully used in some cases as an alternative to surgical repair or retransplantation.[171]

Intestinal Complications

Bowel obstruction is uncommon after liver transplantation. Most adhesions are confined to the supracolic portion of the abdomen. If the base of the mesentery of a Roux-en-Y limb is not tacked down, the small bowel may herniate through and obstruct. Overuse of aluminum-containing antacids may result in inspissation and obstruction of the intestine. Pseudo-obstruction of the colon is much less common than after renal transplantation but must be treated aggressively to avoid disastrous colon perforation.

The gastrointestinal tract is one of the common sites for lymphoproliferative lesions in immunosuppressed patients, and these may obstruct or perforate the bowel. Segmental resection of involved bowel is recommended for localized lesions.

Most intestinal perforations that occur early after transplantation are anastomotic leaks, perforation in an area of denuded serosa, or perforation of bowel injured by electrocautery. Anastomotic leaks are more common in children and should be suspected whenever there is evidence of intraabdominal polymicrobial or candidal infection. Hematogenous or abdominal wound candidiasis is also suggestive of a violation of the gut. Prompt surgical exploration is indicated. Most late perforations are caused by diverticulitis, appendicitis, CMV enteritis, or lymphoproliferative lesions.

Gastrointestinal Bleeding

Bleeding may occur anywhere in the gastrointestinal tract after liver transplantation. Endoscopy, radionuclide scanning, and angiography are indicated to localize the bleeding site. A common site of bleeding after liver transplantation in patients with a Roux-en-Y biliary reconstruction is from the suture line of the jejunojejunostomy. The bleed typically is from a single arteriole and usually can be managed by opening the anterior portion of the anastomosis to find and repair the site. Less commonly, the bleeding is from the closed end of the Roux loop. Variceal hemorrhage after liver transplantation suggests either portal vein thrombosis or esophageal stricture.

Mucous ulceration of the esophagus, stomach, small bowel, or colon may result from opportunistic infection, such as in CMV gastroenteritis or colitis and *Clostridium difficile* pseudomembranous colitis, and present with bleeding. Management is red blood cell replacement, reduction of immunosuppression, and appropriate antibiotic therapy (eg, ganciclovir, metronidazole [Flagyl]). Total colectomy or subtotal gastrectomy is only necessary in unusually severe or persistent cases.

A rare but particularly dangerous cause of gastrointestinal bleeding after liver transplantation is a fistula between the gastrointestinal tract and a vascular anastomosis, either the hepatic arterial anastomosis or anastomosis of an iliac artery conduit to the aorta. Ligation of the involved vessel usually is required, since most of these fistulas are the result of an infected false aneurysm, often with *Candida*, and cannot be repaired primarily without a high risk of breakdown and hemorrhage. In some cases, the liver has tolerated arterial ligation and retransplantation has not been necessary.

Ascites

Ascites may persist for several weeks or months after liver transplantation. Technical faults, such as portal vein or suprahepatic inferior vena cava obstruction or thrombosis, should be ruled out. Ascites usually can be managed with salt restriction and diuretics and gradually diminishes with time. In some cases, placement of a peritoneal-venous shunt may be required. Late recurrence of ascites suggests cirrhosis and should be investigated to determine its cause (rejection, hepatitis, recurrence of original disease).

Pancreatitis

Many patients have a mild, asymptomatic pancreatitis with a mild ileus and modest hyperamylasemia (500 IU/dL) early after liver transplantation. This usually resolves without sequelae. Edema and enlargement of the pancreas on a CT scan or ultrasound are more ominous and may lead to abscess, pseudocyst, and, occasionally, frank hemorrhagic pancreatitis.

The cause of pancreatitis after liver transplantation is uncertain but may be multifactorial. Manipulation of the pancreas during dissection of the hepatic artery or creation of tunnels for vascular grafts, ischemic insult from ligation of the gastroduodenal artery, venous congestion of the pancreas during the anhepatic phase of the liver transplantation procedure, and use of high-dose steroids for induction of immunosuppression may contribute. Significant clinical pancreatitis is also more common in patients with active viral liver disease, particularly in patients with acute hepatitis B in the allograft.[2]

Aplastic Anemia

Patients undergoing liver transplantation for non-A, non-B hepatitis are at special risk of developing aplastic anemia.[155] In a series of 32 patients with acute non-A, non-B hepatitis, 9 patients developed aplastic anemia 1 to 7 weeks after transplantation. Four of these died of infectious complications. Two patients followed for at least 1 year developed recovery of marrow function.

Liver Biopsy Complications

Liver biopsy is the most common procedure performed on patients after liver transplantation. Complications include pneumothorax, hemothorax, intraperitoneal hemorrhage, intrahepatic or subcapsular hematoma, bacteremia, and pseudoaneurysm of an intrahepatic artery or arteriobiliary fistula with hematobilia.

Infection

Infections are the cause of most of the morbidity and mortality after organ transplantation. Organisms that normally colonize the gastrointestinal tract and skin can become dangerous pathogens in the immunosuppressed transplant recipient. Modern immunosuppressive regimens are more selective in their effects and have permitted less reliance on azathioprine and steroids. This has reduced the risk of bacterial infections and made them easier to manage, but 50% to 70% of organ recipients experience at least one bacterial infection. Latent viral infections often are present in otherwise sterile tissues, and immunosuppression may permit viral replication with clinical infection. About 30% to 60% of patients experience a symptomatic viral infection. Herpes simplex virus (HSV), CMV, Epstein-Barr virus (EBV), and VZV infections are the most frequently encountered. Invasive fungal infections are also more common.

EVALUATION OF FEVER

Fever is always an important clinical finding in a transplant recipient. All fevers over 38.5°C must be thoroughly investigated. The basic evaluation includes liver function tests, a chest film, urinalysis, Gram stain of sputum, and cultures of blood, sputum, urine, and all drains, indwelling tubes, and lines. Viral cultures should be taken of buffy coat blood, throat washes, and urine. An abdominal CT scan usually is indicated. Additional studies to be considered include acute-phase serum samples (including EBV, HSV, and CMV titers), arterial blood cultures for candidiasis, stool for ova and parasites, pelvic examination, head CT scan, skin tests for tuberculosis and mycoses, *Legionella* titers, spinal fluid examination, cholangiography, and hepatitis serology screens. Bronchoalveolar lavage and liver biopsy specimens should be stained and cultured for viruses and fungi when pneumonitis or hepatitis is suspected.

VIRAL INFECTIONS

Cytomegalovirus infections are the most common viral infections encountered in patients after liver transplantation. In a review of 121 liver transplantations at the University of Pittsburgh, the overall incidence of CMV infection was 59%, compared with 35% for HSV, 25% for EBV, and 7% for VZV.[133] Symptomatic and disseminated CMV infections are more common in primary CMV infection than with reactivation CMV infection. Infection may involve the urinary tract, gastrointestinal tract (esophagus, stomach, duodenum and small bowel, or colon), lungs, liver, and CNS. Transmission from the organ donor is the most important source of primary CMV infection. Disseminated primary CMV infection has been associated with prior treatment with monoclonal antibody but reactivation infection has not.

There is evidence that prophylactic high-dose acyclovir and intravenous immune globulin may be of value for CMV disease in transplant recipients.[145] High-dose acyclovir, 800 mg orally four times a day, is begun as soon as the patient has resumed oral intake. Patients are maintained on acyclovir for at least 6 months. Dosage should be adjusted for patients with impaired renal function, but doses of less than 800 mg/d are probably ineffective in preventing CMV infection. Patients who tend to have recurrent oral or genital herpes infections may be continued on acyclovir at a reduced dose (200 mg twice a day) beyond 6 months. High-risk patients, such as seronegative recipients who receive an organ from a seropositive donor, should also receive a course of CMV immune globulin.

HSV infections typically are limited to oral and genital herpes, but HSV may also produce pneumonitis or hepatitis. HSV hepatitis commonly occurs earlier (median, 18 days) than CMV hepatitis, which usually occurs 30 to 40 days after transplantation, and may be focal or diffuse in the liver.[78] Symptomatic reactivation of HSV in seropositive patients is more common in those who have received therapy for rejection with monoclonal antibody.[133] Disseminated HSV infection has a poor prognosis, and early therapy with high-dose acyclovir is essential. Prophylactic acyclovir may be effective in preventing disseminated HSV disease.

Exposure to VZV infection can have serious consequences. Seronegative patients should receive VZV immune globulin (VZIG) within 72 hours of exposure to an infected person. In cases of strong exposure, such as to a family member with chickenpox, it is advisable to give VZIG even to seropositive patients and to administer acyclovir to seronegative patients, since clinical disease has occurred in susceptible people even after administration of VZIG.[95] Disseminated VZV requires high-dose acyclovir therapy.

PNEUMOCYSTIS PNEUMONIA

Pneumocystis pneumonia has long been one of the dreaded complications of immunosuppression in organ transplantation patients. Oral prophylaxis with sulfamethoxazole-trimethoprim (one single-strength tablet per day) is highly effective in preventing this infection. Patients who are unable to be treated with sulfamethoxazole-trimethoprim can be treated with dapsone, 100 mg/d, or aerosolized pentamidine, 300 mg once a month.[61] Prophylaxis should be continued for life, but the frequency of sulfamethoxazole-trimethoprim can be reduced to three times per week. We have seen *Pneumocystis carinii* pneumonia develop shortly after withdrawal of suppressive therapy in patients 3 or more years after transplantation. Furthermore, suppressive prophylaxis may also afford protection from *Legionella*, *Nocardia*, and toxoplasmosis.

FUNGAL INFECTIONS

Candidal infections are common in immunosuppressed patients. Noninvasive overgrowth of oropharyngeal, esophageal, and vaginal cavities is most common and can be managed with topical therapy. Mycostatin suspension, 500,000 IU (5 mL) every 6 hours, is given orally or through a nasogastric tube beginning after surgery and continued for several months until the dosage of immunosuppression is reduced. It should be reinstituted whenever immunosuppression is increased, such as for treatment of rejection. Clotrimazole (Mycelex troche), which dissolves slowly in the mouth, can be used instead of mycostatin. Candidal infections are more common and often more troublesome in patients with diabetes. It is advisable to continue *Candida* prophylaxis longer and perhaps indefinitely in these patients.

Invasive candidal infection requires treatment with systemic therapy, such as amphotericin B or fluconazole. High-risk patients should be considered for pretransplantation prophylaxis to reduce *Candida* colonization of the gut. This may also be accomplished as part of a program of selective decolonization of the gut, which may reduce the incidence of gram-negative and candidal infections after transplantation.[5,164] We have used a combination of colistin, gentamicin, and nystatin or paste in Orabase (polymyxin 2%, gentamicin 2%, and nystatin 2%) for patients waiting for transplantation in a critical care setting.

Aspergillus infections may involve the lungs, upper respiratory tract, skin, soft tissues, or CNS. The disease commonly presents as a diffuse pneumonia with patchy infiltrates rather than as a fungus ball in the lungs. Blood vessel invasion with metastatic spread of infection occurs early. Development of brain abscess is insidious and cure is difficult. Definitive diagnosis requires intracranial biopsy. A long course of systemic therapy with amphotericin B is indicated in patients with aspergillus infections. Flucytosine may benefit patients with ophthalmic or CNS involvement. Itraconazole, a new agent, has shown promise for the treatment of aspergillosis in our limited experience with it.

Cryptococcal infections (lung, CNS, disseminated cutaneous infection) are another hazard in immunosuppressed patients. A spinal fluid examination with India ink stains and analysis for cryptococcal antigen should be considered in patients with persistent headache or signs of meningism and in all patients with pulmonary cryptococcal infection.

Infections with *Mucor* or *Rhizopus* species are rare but may produce severe CNS or soft tissue infections that are difficult to eradicate. Treatment requires reduction of immunosuppression, local excision, and a long course of systemic antifungal therapy.

ANTITUBERCULAR PROPHYLAXIS

Patients who are PPD-positive, especially those from areas with a high endemic rate of tuberculosis or those who travel to such areas, should receive antitubercular prophylaxis. Patients with a history of potential exposure and anergic skin reactivity should also be considered for prophylaxis with isoniazid (INH). INH prophylaxis usually is begun in the third week after liver transplantation and continued for at least 6 months.

EPSTEIN-BARR VIRUS AND LYMPHOPROLIFERATIVE DISORDERS

A ubiquitous DNA virus, EBV can produce a spectrum of syndromes in immunocompromised patients ranging from a typical mononucleosis syndrome to frank lymphoma. In addition to a classic mononucleosis presentation, the viral syndrome may be characterized by atypical findings such as jaw pain, arthralgias, joint space effusions, diarrhea, encephalitis, pneumonitis, mediastinal lymphadenopathy, ascites, and hepatitis.[123] Changes in the liver allograft in EBV infection range from findings typical of infectious mononucleosis to a distinctive histopathology characterized by a mixed mononuclear and sinusoidal infiltrate, lobular hepatitis, and mild duct damage not in proportion to the severity of the inflammatory infiltrate.

Lymphoproliferative disease is seen in patients with congenital and acquired immunodeficiency states, including transplantation patients receiving immunosuppressive medications. Most are associated with EBV infection. In some patients, EBV DNA cannot be found in tumor specimens.[166] Also, EBV is trophic for B cells and about 15% of lymphomas are of T-cell origin.[109] In our experience, lymphomas after transplantation have occurred in 4.6% of combined heart and lung recipients, 2.2% of liver recipients, 1.8% of heart recipients, and 1% of kidney recipients.[100] The higher incidence in extrarenal transplant recipients may be related to the higher levels of immunosuppression used in patients for whom there is no alternative artificial organ support if therapy for graft rescue fails.

Posttransplantation lymphomas are believed to be a consequence of overall levels of immunosuppression rather than treatment with any particular agent. The disease may present as a diffuse involvement of multiple organ systems with massive infiltration of many tissues with immunoblasts or mature plasma cells or as solid tumors that involve the tonsils, lungs, and spleen with spread to the liver, kidneys, lymph nodes, and brain. Most patients who survive this complication have evidence of primary or reactivated EBV infection, polyclonal lesions, solid tumors rather than diffuse disease, and B-cell hyperplasia rather than lymphoma. In liver recipients, the hepatic allograft is involved in one third of cases, and tonsils, kidneys, and small bowel often are involved.[21]

Early recognition, reduction, or withdrawal of immunosuppression and systemic antiviral therapy with acyclovir or ganciclovir are important for successful management of these lesions. Localized solid lesions in the gastrointestinal tract may obstruct or perforate and should be resected. α-Interferon has been used in an effort to prevent early lymphoma transformation.[79] Anti-CD21–specific and anti-CD24–specific (anti–B-cell) monoclonal antibodies have recently been shown to be effective in controlling diffuse, severe oligoclonal B-cell lymphoproliferative disease in patients without CNS involvement.[39] Sometimes more aggressive monoclonal lymphomas require conventional anticancer therapy.

Immunosuppression

Recent improvements in immunosuppression have been responsible for much of the success now being experienced in solid organ transplantation. We can expect further significant advances in the near future as another generation of agents is introduced into clinical practice. This section briefly reviews the immunosuppressive agents currently in use and the management strategies for induction immunosuppression and treatment of rejection.

CYCLOSPORINE

Cyclosporine was isolated from a fungus found growing in a soil sample taken from the largest highland plateau in Europe, the Hardanger Valda in southern Norway. Borel first described the immunosuppressive properties of cyclosporine in 1976, and clinical trials were begun by Calne in 1978. The systematic use of cyclosporine in combination with low-dose prednisone was begun by Starzl in 1980. The improved survival achieved by Starzl in his first trials with the drug in liver transplant recipients demonstrated that liver transplantation was a practical therapy for patients with end-stage liver disease. A National Institutes of Health Consensus Development conference held in 1983 supported this conclusion. The Health Care Financing Administration now provides Medicare reimbursement for some of the most common indications for pediatric and adult liver transplantation.

Cyclosporine is a highly lipid-soluble drug, and its absorption depends on the enterohepatic circulation. It is metabolized in the liver, and the major route of excretion is in bile. Toxicity is most commonly manifested by hypertension, tremulousness, gingival hyperplasia, and nephrotoxicity. Acute nephrotoxicity is characterized by hyperkalemic renal tubular acidosis and chronic cyclosporine nephrotoxicity, by a progressive interstitial fibrosis of the kidneys. A low serum magnesium level potentiates neurotoxicity, and this may result in seizures, especially when cyclosporine is administered intravenously. Cyclosporine can produce changes in personality, including paranoid delusions and hallucinations. Liver function may also be impaired by cyclosporine, but this is much less common than nephrotoxicity and other causes of liver dysfunction (rejection, hepatitis, technical complications) must be ruled out.

Cyclosporine initially is administered intravenously as a continuous infusion, usually at a dose of 3 to 5 mg/kg/d. As soon as patients are able to tolerate oral intake, oral cyclosporine, 12 to 15 mg/kg/d in two divided doses, is begun. Daily trough levels of serum or whole blood are monitored and levels adjusted to maintain an appropriate therapeutic range. Once oral dosage is well established and blood levels are stable, patients are weaned off the intravenous form.

Because of concern about the nephrotoxicity of cyclosporine, various cyclosporine-sparing protocols have been adopted by transplant centers during the induction phase of immunosuppression. In this approach, no cyclosporine is given during the first 2 to 7 days after transplantation until good urine output and creatinine clearance are demonstrated. During the period of cyclosporine sparing, patients may be treated with various combinations of azathioprine, prednisone, and either polyclonal or monoclonal antibody. Once good renal function is established, oral cyclosporine is started.

Drugs that affect hepatic enzyme systems, especially the cytochrome P-450 system, can alter the metabolism of cyclosporine. Two of the more common drugs that do this are phenytoin (Dilantin), which causes a fall in cyclosporine serum concentration, and erythromycin, which causes significant increases and may precipitate acute toxicity. These drugs must be used with caution and with careful attention to the monitoring of blood levels.

CORTICOSTEROIDS

Although cyclosporine has permitted a significant reduction in the amounts of steroid required to maintain a liver allograft, corticosteroids still have an important role in the induction and maintenance of immunosuppression in liver transplant recipients. At most centers, patients receive a 1-g bolus of methylprednisolone during surgery followed by a high-dose taper of steroids until a daily maintenance dose of 20 mg is reached (less in young children). In patients with diabetes, advanced osteoporosis, or refractory hypertension, an attempt usually is made to lower the dose of steroids further early in the course, but this is not always possible. Steroids are also important in the management of acute rejection. The lower maintenance doses of steroids able to be used

in combination with cyclosporine allows pediatric patients to resume normal growth and development after liver transplantation.[159]

AZATHIOPRINE

Azathioprine is widely used in transplantation to spare cyclosporine during the early recovery phase when renal function may be compromised, to provide an adjunctive agent in patients unable to tolerate usual doses of cyclosporine, or to augment immunosuppression in patients with persistent or recurrent rejection despite appropriate therapy with cyclosporine and steroids. Therapy usually is started at 1 mg/kg and may be gradually increased to 1.5 to 2 mg/kg as needed. If the peripheral leukocyte count falls below 5000/μL, the dose is reduced. If the count falls below 3000/μL, the drug is discontinued.

ANTIBODY THERAPY

Muromonab-CD3 (Orthoclone OKT3) is a mouse antihuman monoclonal antibody with activity against the CD3 determinant on human T cells. A highly effective immunosuppressive agent, it is used for induction immunosuppression as part of cyclosporine-sparing protocols; for induction immunoprophylaxis, especially in high-risk patients (patients with high titers of cytotoxic antibody or patients with a history of graft rejection); and for the treatment of steroid-resistant allograft rejection.[23,48,98] A recent report could find no long-term benefit to the routine use of prophylactic OKT3 and recommended that OKT3 be reserved for the treatment of steroid-resistant rejection and for cyclosporine intolerance.[93] OKT3 usually is administered as a 5-mL intravenous bolus over 5 minutes repeated daily for 10 to 14 days. Fluid overload should be corrected before OKT3 is given. Patients should be premedicated with steroids, antihistamine, and acetaminophen for the first few doses. Adverse effects such as headache, joint pains, fever, chills, tachycardia, nausea, and abdominal discomfort are common and probably a result of the sudden lysis of lymphocytes and release of cytokines with the first few administrations. Seizures may occur after administration and are potentiated by hypocalcemia or hyponatremia. Aseptic meningitis has been reported in less than 5% of patients. It causes fever and headache, and some patients experience nuchal rigidity and altered mentation. Polymorphonuclear leukocytes and lymphocytes may be present in spinal fluid, but spinal fluid cultures are negative. The syndrome is self-limited and does not require the drug to be stopped.

Other monoclonal agents directed against T-cell determinants and interleukin receptors are under investigation, but OKT3 is the only Food and Drug Administration–approved monoclonal antibody in use. Because OKT3 is a mouse protein, patients may develop antimurine antibodies that inactivate the drug. Most patients develop only low titers of antimurine antibody with a first course of treatment, and this titer decreases with time. Thus, many patients can be retreated with a second course of OKT3 if rejection recurs. It often is helpful to monitor CD3 cell counts and OKT3 levels in patients being retreated with OKT3, especially if there is a poor clinical response. The drug is ineffective if CD3 cell counts do not drop or effective serum levels cannot be achieved.[22,38,130]

Now that monoclonal therapy is available, there is much less use of polyclonal agents. These preparations are still used by some centers for cyclosporine-sparing during induction and as an alternative therapy to the monoclonal agents in patients with recurrent rejection or a poor response to OKT3.

FK 506 AND OTHER NEW AGENTS

FK 506 represents the first of a new generation of immunosuppressive agents. It is a macrolide antibiotic belonging to the same family of compounds as erythromycin and a potent immunosuppressive agent. Its actions on T cells are similar to those of cyclosporine, including suppression of interleukin-2 production, but it is many times more potent and acts on a different cell receptor.[55,132] In extensive clinical trials at the University of Pittsburgh, FK 506 has been found to be remarkably effective in preventing and controlling liver allograft rejection, and many patients can be weaned off steroids early in their course after transplantation.[150] Most patients who develop steroid-resistant rejection during therapy with FK 506 can be treated with a short, 3- to 5-day course of OKT3. FK 506 has also proved to be a highly effective rescue drug for patients who cannot be maintained on cyclosporine and those with failing grafts despite aggressive cyclosporine therapy.[41] The drug is more effective than any other available agent in reversing or decelerating the progression of chronic allograft rejection and in preventing acute vanishing bile duct syndrome.

The toxicity profile of FK 506 differs from that of cyclosporine. It is less nephrotoxic, and troublesome hypertension is less common. Gastrointestinal adverse effects, especially nausea and diarrhea, are common early complaints and may be related to an antibiotic action of the drug in the gut. Headache and insomnia are common complaints and are dose-related. Tremors are much less common than with cyclosporine, and the drug may cause mild hair loss rather than the hirsutism commonly experienced by patients on cyclosporine. The severest neurologic complications seen with FK 506 are seizures and central pontine myelinolysis with severe speech and motor disturbances. As with cyclosporine, these complications are most common early after transplantation, when the drug is being given intravenously. Metabolic disturbances, especially significant fluctuations in serum sodium levels, have also been associated with such neurologic disorders in transplant recipients.[10,35,167]

When FK 506 is given, much of it is cleared on the first pass through the liver. Therefore, graft function has a significant effect on drug activity and blood levels.[69] In the early period after transplantation, FK 506 levels may rise rapidly to toxic levels if graft function is poor. Appropriate monitoring of blood levels and adjustments in dosage must be made during periods of graft dysfunction.

In addition to its impressive immunosuppressive effects, FK 506 has a remarkable hepatotrophic effect that is stronger than that seen with cyclosporine. In an experimental animal model in which portal blood supply is diverted by an Eck fistula to the vena cava and FK 506 is selectively infused into one lobe of the liver, the size, anatomic quality, and replication of hepatocytes is enhanced in the FK 506–infused portion of the liver.[138] This effect of FK 506 on hepatic regeneration and repair may make it particularly advantageous for use in liver transplantation.

Several other interesting agents are under investigation and may become important for clinical practice in the near future. Among these are rapamycin, an antibiotic with some similarities to FK 506, and RS-61143, a guanine monophosphate inhibitor.

Allograft Rejection

Antibody-mediated hyperacute rejection of the liver has been demonstrated in animal models but is rare in the clinical setting. In kidney transplantation, hyperacute rejection usually occurs on the operating table because antibody deposition and accumulation of formed blood elements rapidly destroy the microcirculation of the kidney. In the case of a liver graft, the process may evolve over 24 to 48 hours after surgery and after a brief initial period of good graft function. It is most likely to occur in patients in whom an ABO incompatibility between donor and recipient has been crossed and occasionally occurs in a patient with a strongly positive antibody crossmatch. Hyperacute rejection usually is characterized by a severe hemorrhagic necrosis of the liver within hours or days of implantation. Submassive necrosis with a sparse polymorphonuclear infiltrate in the portal tracts and hepatic lobules has also been described in a patient with a high titer of lymphocytotoxic antibody.[9] Patchy deposits of immunoglobulin, C3 complement component, factor P, and fibrinogen are characteristic.[52] Accelerated acute cellular rejection can also occur in the first few days after transplantation. Liver biopsy is necessary to distinguish between early forms of rejection and ischemic graft injury.

Acute cellular rejection may occur at any time after liver transplantation and may be characterized by any or all of the following: malaise, fever, graft tenderness or enlargement, and diminished graft function with elevated levels of bilirubin and aminotransferase or canalicular enzymes. The presence of preformed antidonor lymphocytotoxic antibody is not predictive of hyperacute rejection but may be an important warning that the recipient is more likely to experience acute cellular rejection and that rejection may be more difficult to treat.

Acute cellular rejection is characterized by a portal infiltrate with damage to small bile ducts in the portal tracts. Inflammatory cells may also accumulate beneath the portal and terminal hepatic veins (central venulitis). An inflammatory arteritis may also be present, but the vessels involved typically are in the hilum and not accessible by liver biopsy. The hepatic lobule usually is spared, but in severe rejection, the inflammatory infiltrate may spill over into the hepatic lobule and be associated with hepatic necrosis. The histologic picture is different from the piecemeal necrosis seen with hepatitis.

Chronic rejection is an obliterative arteriopathy that results in an insidious and relentless loss of small bile ducts. It typically presents with elevated levels of canalicular enzymes and progressive jaundice. Hepatic synthetic function usually is well preserved, and most patients feel well until late in the course. In some cases, chronic rejection may progress rapidly, a syndrome that has been called the acute vanishing bile duct syndrome. Vanishing bile duct syndrome may be more commonly seen in patients with a positive lymphocytotoxic antibody crossmatch.[6] The syndrome has also been reported to be less frequent in patients treated with combination immunosuppressive regimens, such as triple therapy with cyclosporine, prednisone, and azathioprine or quadruple regimens including these agents and prophylactic antibody therapy.[113,160] Hepatic lobular changes of chronic rejection also reflect progressive ischemic damage and include centrolobular cholestasis, patchy acidophilic necrosis, centrolobular ballooning or atrophy of hepatocytes, perivenular sclerosis, and intrasinusoidal foam cells.

The differential diagnosis of allograft rejection commonly includes preservation injury, vascular compromise, biliary tract obstruction, viral or toxic hepatitis, systemic infection, and recurrent disease. Liver biopsy usually is required for definitive diagnosis, but Doppler ultrasonography, cholangiography, angiography, and CT scanning may be needed as well, depending on the clinical setting. Serologic screens for hepatitis and other infectious disease evaluations may also be required.

MANAGEMENT OF REJECTION

No effective therapy exists for hyperacute rejection of the liver other than urgent retransplantation of the liver. Acute cellular rejection usually is treated with steroids and, if there is an inadequate response, a course of antibody therapy. In cases of chronic rejection in which bile ducts are still present in some portal tracts on liver biopsy, conversion from cyclosporine to FK 506 may rescue the graft or significantly slow the progression of the rejection process. Otherwise, chronic rejection is refractory to further therapy. The inevitability of retransplantation should be accepted, and overtreatment of the patient should be avoided.

Timing of Transplantation

Outcome is related to patient condition at the time of transplantation. Liver grafts are allocated in the United States according to a point system that is based mainly on medical urgency, as defined by the required level of medical care, and waiting time. Patients with the highest urgency and longest waiting times receive the highest priority. Experience shows, however, that these patients also have the highest mortality after liver transplantation. Patients in the lowest urgency classes have 6-month survival rates approaching 90%, whereas those who go to the operating room from an intensive care unit to receive a liver transplant have only a 65% chance of survival.[45]

Liver transplantation is not experimental, and it is now widely available in North America, Europe, and Australia. It is not an option to be considered only for a patient with end-stage liver disease who has reached a desperate or debilitated state. Excellent results can be achieved if patients are referred before their condition deteriorates to the point at which survival is jeopardized. The severely ill deserve to be and can be served, but early referral is essential to further reduce morbidity, mortality, and cost.

References

1. AbouJaoude M, Grant D, Ghent C, Mimeault R, Wall WJ. Effect of portasystemic shunts on subsequent transplantation of the liver. Surg Gynecol Obstet 172:215, 1991
2. Alexander JA, Demetris AJ, Gavaler JS, et al. Pancreatitis following liver transplantation. Transplantation 45:1062, 1988
3. Ayalon A, Wiesner RH, Perkins JD, et al. Splenic artery aneurysms in liver transplant patients. Transplantation 45:386, 1988
4. Badger I, Buckels JA. Hepatic artery thrombosis due to acute pancreatitis following liver transplantation. Transplantation 48:526, 1989
5. Badger IL, Crosby HA, Kong JP, et al. Is selective decontamination of the digestive tract beneficial in liver transplant recipients? Interim results of a prospective, randomized trial. Transplant Proc 23:1460, 1991
6. Batts KP, Moore SB, Perkins JD, et al. Influence of positive lymphocyte crossmatch and HLA mismatching on vanishing bile duct syndrome in human liver allografts. Transplantation 45:376, 1988
7. Belzer FO, Southard JH. Principles of solid organ preservation by cold storage. Transplantation 45:673, 1988
8. Bilheimer DW, Goldstein JL, Grundy SM, Starzl TE, Brown MS. Liver transplantation to provide low density lipoprotein receptors and lower plasma cholesterol in a child with homozygous familial hypercholesterolemia. N Engl J Med 311:1658, 1984
9. Bird G, Friend P, O'Grady J, et al. Hyperacute rejection in liver transplantation: a case report. Transplant Proc 21:3742, 1989
10. Bird GL, Meadows J, Goka J, Polson R, Williams R. Cyclosporin-associated akinetic mutism and extrapyramidal syndrome after liver transplantation. J Neurol Neurosurg Psychiatry 53:1068, 1990
11. Bird GL, O'Grady JG, Harvey FA, Calne RY, Williams R. Liver transplantation in patients with alcoholic cirrhosis. Br Med J [Clin Res] 301:15, 1990
12. Bonsel GJ, Klompmaker IJ, Veer F, Habbema JD, Sloof MJ. Use of prognostic models for assessment of value of liver transplantation in primary biliary cirrhosis. Lancet 335:493, 1990
13. Brems JJ, Hiatt JR, Klein AS, Colonna JO, Busuttil RW. Splenic artery aneurysm rupture following orthotopic liver transplantation. Transplantation 45:1136, 1988
14. Broelsch CE, Emond JC, Thistlethwaite JR, Rouch DA, Whitington PF, Lichtor JL. Liver transplantation with reduced-sized organs. Transplantation 45:519, 1988
15. Bumhardt G, Neuhaus P, Bechstein R, et al. Liver transplantation in HBsAg-positive patients. Transplant Proc 22:1517, 1990
16. Cameron JL, Pitt HA, Zinner MJ, et al. Resection of hepatic duct bifurcation and transhepatic stenting for sclerosing cholangitis. Ann Surg 207:614, 1988
17. Campbell DA Jr, Rolles K, Jamieson N, et al. Hepatic transplantation with perioperative and long term anticoagulation as treatment for Budd-Chiari syndrome. Surg Gynecol Obstet 166:511, 1988
18. Casella JF, Lewis JH, Bontempo FA, Zitelli BJ, Markel H, Starzl TE. Successful treatment of protein C deficiency by hepatic transplantation. Lancet 1:435, 1988
19. Choo Q-L, Kuo G, Weiner AJ, et al. Isolation of a cDNA clone derived from a blood-borne non-A, non-B viral hepatitis genome. Science 244:359, 1989
20. Cofer JB, Klintmalm GB, Howard TK, et al. A comparison of UW with Euro-Collins preservation solution in liver transplantation. Transplantation 49:1088, 1990
21. Cohen JI. Epstein-Barr virus lymphoproliferative disease associated with acquired immunodeficiency. Medicine 70:137, 1991
22. Colonna JO, Millis JM, Martello J, et al. The successful use of repeated courses of OKT3 for hepatic allograft rejection using T3 cells to adjust dose. Transplant Proc 21:2247, 1989
23. Cosimi AB, Jenkins RL, Rohrer RJ, et al. A randomized clinical trial of prophylactic OKT3 monoclonal antibody in liver allograft recipients. Arch Surg 125:781, 1990
24. Cyes C, Millar AJ. Assessment of the nutritional status of infants and children with biliary atresia. S Afr Med J 77:131, 1990

25. D'Alessandro A, Kalayoglu M, Sollinger HW, et al. The predictive value of donor liver biopsies for the development of primary nonfunction after orthotopic liver transplantation. Transplantation 51:157, 1991

26. Dehner LP, Snover DC, Sharp HL, Ascher N, Nakhleh R, Day DL. Hereditary tyrosinemia type I (chronic form): pathologic findings in the liver. Hum Pathol 20:149, 1989

27. Delorme MA, Adams PC, Grant D, Ghent CN, Walker IR, Wall WJ. Orthotopic liver transplantation in a patient with combined hemophilia A and B. Am J Hematol 33:136, 1990

28. Demetris AJ, Jaffe R, Sheahan DG, et al. Recurrent hepatitis B in liver allografts: differentiation between viral hepatitis B and rejection. Am J Pathol 125:161, 1986

29. Dickson ER, Grambsch PM, Fleming TR, Fisher LD, Langworthy A. Prognosis in primary biliary cirrhosis: model for decision making. Hepatology 10:1, 1989

30. Dummer JS, Erb S, Breinig MK, et al. Infection with human immunodeficiency virus in the Pittsburgh transplant population: a study of 583 donors and 1043 recipients. Transplantation 47:134, 1989

31. Dzik WJ, Arkin CF, Jenkins RL. Transfer of congenital factor XI deficiency from donor to recipient as a result of liver transplantation. N Engl J Med 316:1217, 1987

32. Eckhauser F, Eggenberger J, Johnkoski J. Therapeutic options in portal hypertension. Surg Rounds 11:44, 1988

33. Emond JC, Aran PP, Whitington PF, et al. Liver transplantation in the management of fulminant hepatic failure. Gastroenterology 96:1583, 1989

34. Esquivel CO, Van Thiel D, Demetris AJ, et al. Transplantation for primary biliary cirrhosis. Gastroenterology 94:1207, 1988

35. Estol CJ, Faris AA, Martinez AJ, Ahdab-Barmada M. Central pontine myelinolysis after liver transplantation. Neurology 39:493, 1989

36. Evans RA, Raby ND, O'Grady JG, et al. Biliary complications following orthotopic liver transplantation. Clin Radiol 41:190, 1990

37. Ferla G, Colledan M, Doglia M, at al. B hepatitis and liver transplantation. Transplant Proc 20(Suppl 1):566, 1988

38. First MR, Schroeder TJ, Hurtubise PE, et al. Successful retreatment of allograft rejection with OKT3. Transplantation 47:88, 1989

39. Fischer A, Blanche S, Le Bidois J, et al. Anti-B-cell monoclonal antibodies in the treatment of severe B-cell lymphoproliferative syndrome following bone marrow and solid organ transplantation. N Engl J Med 324:1451, 1991

40. Flint EW, Sumkin JH, Zajko AB, Bowen A. Duplex sonography of hepatic artery thrombosis after liver transplantation. AJR 151:481, 1988

41. Fung JJ, Todo S, Jain A, et al. Conversion from cyclosporine to FK 506 in liver allograft recipients with cyclosporine related complications. Transplant Proc 22:6, 1990

42. Furukawa H, Todo S, Imventarza O, et al. Effect of cold ischemia time on the early outcome of human hepatic allografts preserved with UW solution. Transplantation 51:1000, 1991

43. Gibas A, Dienstag JL, Schafer AI, et al. Cure of hemophilia A by orthotopic liver transplantation. Gastroenterology 95:192, 1988

44. Gordon RD, Bismuth H. Liver transplantation registry report. Transplant Proc 23:58, 1991

45. Gordon RD, Hartner CN, Casavilla A, et al. The liver transplant waiting list: a single center analysis. Transplantation 51:128, 1991

46. Gordon RD, Teperman L, Iwatsuki S, Starzl TE. Orthotopic liver transplantation. In: Schwartz I, Ellis E, eds. Maingot's abdominal operations, ed 9. Norwalk, CT, Appleton & Lange, 1989, p 1291

47. Gordon RD, Todo S, Tzakis AG, et al. Liver transplantation under cyclosporine: a decade of experience. Transplant Proc 23:1393, 1991

48. Gordon RD, Tzakis AG, Iwatsuki S, et al. Experience with Orthoclone OKT3 monoclonal antibody in liver transplantation. Am J Kidney Dis 11:141, 1988

49. Gores GJ, Wiesner RH, Dickson ER, Zinsmeister AR, Jorgensen RA, Langworthy A. Prospective evaluation of esophageal varices in primary biliary cirrhosis: development, natural history, and influence on survival. Gastroenterology 96:1552, 1989

50. Grambsch PM, Dickson ER, Kaplan M, LeSage G, Fleming TR, Langworthy AL. Extramural cross-validation of the Mayo primary biliary cirrhosis model establishes its generalizability. Hepatology 10:846, 1989

51. Grosfeld JL, Fitzgerald JF, Predaina R, West KW, Vane DW, Rescorla FJ. The efficacy of portoenterostomy in biliary atresia. Surgery 106:692, 1989

52. Gubernatis G, Kemnitz J, Bornscheuer A, et al. Potential various appearances of hyperacute rejection in human liver transplantation. Langenbecks Arch Chir 374:240, 1989

53. Halff G, Todo S, Hall R. Late complications with gallbladder conduit biliary reconstruction after liver transplantation. Transplantation 48:537, 1989

54. Halff G, Todo S, Tzakis AG, Gordon RD, Starzl TE. Liver transplantation for the Budd-Chiari syndrome. Ann Surg 211:43, 1990

55. Harding MW, Galat A, Uehling DE, Schrieber SL. A receptor for the immunosuppressant FK 506 has a *cis-trans* peptidyl-prolyl isomerase. Nature 341:758, 1989

56. Harrison PM, O'Grady JG, Keays RT, et al. Serial prothrombin time as prognostic indicator in paracetamol induced fulminant hepatic failure. Br Med J [Clin Res] 301:964, 1990

57. Henderson JM, Warren WD, Millikan WJ Jr, et al. Surgical options, hematologic evaluation, and pathologic changes in Budd-Chiari syndrome. Am J Surg 159:41, 1990

58. Herbener T, Zaijko AB, Koneru B, Bron K, Campbell WL. Recurrent cholangiocarcinoma in the biliary tree after liver transplantation. Radiology 169:641, 1988

59. Hidalgo EG, Abad J, Cantarero JM, et al. High-dose intraarterial urokinase for the treatment of hepatic artery thrombosis in liver transplantation. Hepatogastroenterology 36:529, 1989

60. Higashi H, Yanaga K, Marsh JW, Tzakis A, Kakizoe S, Starzl TE. Development of colon cancer after liver transplantation for primary sclerosing cholangitis. Hepatology 11:477, 1990

61. Hirschel B, Lazzarin A, Chopard P, et al. A controlled study of inhaled pentamidine for primary prevention of *Pneumocystis carinii* pneumonia. N Engl J Med 324:1079, 1991

62. Hoffman MA, Celli S, Ninkov P, Rolles K, Calne RY. Orthotopic transplantation of the liver in children with biliary atresia and polysplenia syndrome: report of two cases. J Pediatr Surg 24:1020, 1989

63. Hotta S. Assessment of liver transplantation. Health Technology Assessment Report, Agency for Health Care Policy and Research, 1990, pp 1–43

64. Houwen RH, Zwierstra RP, Severijnen RS, et al. Prognosis of extrahepatic biliary atresia. Arch Dis Child 64:214, 1989

65. Iwatsuki S, Starzl TE, Todo S, et al. Experience with 1000 liver transplants under cyclosporine-steroid therapy: a survival report. Transplant Proc 20(Suppl 1):498, 1988

66. Iwatsuki S, Starzl TE, Todo S, et al. Liver transplantation in the treatment of bleeding esophageal varices. Surgery 104:697, 1988

67. Iwatsuki S, Stieber A, Marsh JW, et al. Liver transplantation for fulminant hepatic failure. Transplant Proc 21:2431, 1989

68. Iwatsuki SI, Gordon RD, Shaw BW Jr, Starzl TE. Role of liver transplantation in cancer therapy. Ann Surg 202:401, 1985

69. Jain AB, Venkataramanan R, Cadoff E, et al. Effect of hepatic dysfunction and T-tube clamping on FK 506 pharmacokinetics and trough concentrations. Transplant Proc 22:57, 1990

70. Jamieson NV, Sundberg R, Lindell S, et al. Preservation of

the canine liver for 24–48 hours using simple cold storage with UW solution. Transplantation 46:517, 1988

71. Jeffrey GP, Hoffman NE, Reed WD. Validation of prognostic models in primary biliary cirrhosis. Aust NZ J Med 20:107, 1990

72. Kakizoe S, Yanaga K, Starzl TE, Demetris AJ. Evaluation of protocol before transplantation and after reperfusion biopsies from human orthotopic liver allografts: considerations of preservation and early immunological injury. Hepatology 11:932, 1990

73. Kalayoglu M, Sollinger HW, Stratta RJ, et al. Extended preservation of the human liver for clinical transplantation. Lancet 1:617, 1988

74. Kaplan SB, Zajko AB, Koneru B. Hepatic bilomas due to hepatic artery thrombosis in liver transplant recipients: percutaneous drainage and clinical outcome. Radiology 174:1031, 1990

75. Kasai M, Mochizuki I, Ohkohchi N, Chiba T, Ohi R. Surgical limitation for biliary atresia: indication for liver transplantation. J Pediatr Surg 24:851, 1989

76. Koneru B, Casavilla A, Bowman J, Iwatsuki S, Starzl TE. Liver transplantation for malignant tumors. Gastroenterol Clin North Am 17:177, 1988

77. Koneru B, Flye MW, Busuttil RW, et al. Liver transplantation for hepatoblastoma. The American experience. Ann Surg 231:118, 1991

78. Kusne S, Schwartz M, Breinig MK, et al. Herpes simplex virus infections after solid organ transplantation in adults. J Infect Dis 163:1001, 1991

79. Langnas AN, Castaldo P, Markin RS, et al. The spectrum of Epstein-Barr virus infection with hepatitis following liver transplantation. Transplant Proc 23:1513, 1991

80. Langnas AN, Grazi GL, Stratta RJ, et al. Primary sclerosing cholangitis: the emerging role for liver transplantation. Am J Gastroenterol 85:1136, 1990

81. Lauchart W, Muller R, Pichlmayr R. Immunoprophylaxis of hepatitis B virus reinfection in recipients of human liver allografts. Transplant Proc 19:2387, 1987

82. Laurent J, Gauthier F, Bernard O, et al. Long-term outcome after surgery for biliary atresia: study of 40 patients surviving for more than 10 years. Gastroenterology 99:1793, 1990

83. Lebeau G, Yanaga K, Marsh JW, et al. Analysis of surgical complications after 397 liver transplantations. Surg Gynecol Obstet 170:317, 1990

84. Lewis JH, Bontempo FA, Spero JA, Ragni MJ, Starzl TE. Liver transplantation in a hemophiliac. N Engl J Med 312:1189, 1985

85. Lillemoe KD, Pitt HA, Cameron JL. Primary sclerosing cholangitis. Surg Clin North Am 70:1381, 1990

86. Lilly JR, Karrer FM, Hall RJ, et al. The surgery of biliary atresia. Ann Surg 210:289, 1989

87. Marino IR, Esquivel CO, Zajko AB, et al. Distal splenorenal shunt for portal vein thrombosis after liver transplantation. Am J Gastroenterol 84:67, 1989

88. Markin RS, Wood RP, Stratta RJ, et al. Predictive value of intraoperative liver biopsies of donor organs in patients undergoing orthotopic liver transplantation. Transplant Proc 22:418, 1990

89. Markus BH, Dickson ER, Grambsch PM, et al. Efficiency of liver transplantation in patients with primary biliary cirrhosis. N Engl J Med 320:1709, 1989

90. Marsh JW, Iwatsuki S, Makowka L, et al. Orthotopic liver transplantation for sclerosing cholangitis. Ann Surg 207:21, 1988

91. Martin FM, Rossi RL, Nugent FW, et al. Surgical aspects of sclerosing cholangitis: results in 178 patients. Ann Surg 212:551, 1990

92. Mazzaferro V, Esquivel CO, Makowka L, et al. Hepatic artery thrombosis after pediatric liver transplantation: a medical or surgical event? Transplantation 47:971, 1989

93. McDiarmid SV, Busuttil RW, Levy P, et al. The long-term outcome of OKT3 compared with cyclosporine prophylaxis after liver transplantation. Transplantation 52:91, 1991

94. McDonald JC, Landreneau MD, Rohr MS, Devault GA Jr. Reversal by liver transplantation of the complications of primary hyperoxaluria as well as the metabolic defect. N Engl J Med 321:1100, 1989

95. McGregor RS, Zitelli BJ, Urbach AH, et al. Varicella zoster in pediatric orthotopic liver transplant recipients. Pediatrics 83:256, 1989

96. Merion RM, Delius RL, Cambell DA, Turcotte JG. Orthotopic liver transplantation totally corrects factor IX deficiency in hemophilia B. Surgery 104:929, 1988

97. Merman MA, Burnham JA, Sheehan DG. Fibrolamellar carcinoma of the liver: an immunohistochemical study of nineteen cases and a review of the literature. Hum Pathol 29:784, 1988

98. Millis JM, McDiarmid SV, Hiatt JR, et al. Randomized prospective trial of OKT3 for early prophylaxis of rejection after liver transplantation. Transplantation 47:82, 1989

99. Mora NP, Klintmalm GB, Poplawski SS, et al. Recurrence of hepatitis B after liver transplantation. Transplant Proc 22:1549, 1990

100. Nalesnik MA, Makowka L, Starzl TE. The diagnosis and treatment of posttransplant lymphoproliferative disorders. Curr Probl Surg 25:367, 1988

101. Neuberger J, Portmann D, MacDougall BRD, et al. Recurrence of primary biliary cirrhosis after liver transplantation. N Engl J Med 306:1, 1982

102. Oellerich M, Burdelski M, Lautz HU, et al. Lidocaine metabolite formation as a measure of liver function in patients with cirrhosis. Ther Drug Monit 12:219, 1990

103. Oellerich M, Burdelski M, Ringe B, et al. Lignocaine metabolite formation as a measure of pretransplantation liver function. Lancet 1:640, 1989

104. O'Grady JG, Gimson AE, O'Brien CJ, et al. Controlled trials of charcoal hemoperfusion and prognostic factors in fulminant hepatic failure. Gastroenterology 94:1186, 1988

105. O'Grady JG, Polson RJ, Rolles K, Calne RY. Liver transplantation for malignant disease. Ann Surg 207:373, 1988

106. Olthoff KM, Millis JM, Imagawa DK, et al. Comparison of UW solution and Euro-Collins solution for cold preservation of human liver grafts. Transplantation 49:284, 1990

107. Ostroff JW, Roberts JP, Ring EJ, Ascher NL. The management of T-tube leaks in orthotopic liver transplant recipients with endoscopically placed nasobiliary catheters. Transplantation 49:922, 1990

108. Otte JB, Ville de Goyet J, Sokal E, et al. Size reduction of the donor liver is a safe way to alleviate the shortage of size-matched organs in pediatric liver transplantation. Ann Surg 211:146, 1990

109. Penn I. The enigma of posttransplant lymphomas: literature scan. Transplantation 7:1, 1991

110. Pichlmayr R, Ringe B, Lauchart W, Wonigeit K. Liver transplantation. Transplant Proc 19:103, 1987

111. Pichlmayr R, Ringe B, Wittekind C, et al. Liver grafting for malignant tumors. Transplant Proc 21:2403, 1989

112. Pillay P, Starzl TE, Van Thiel DH. Complications of sclerotherapy for esophageal varices in liver transplant candidates. Transplant Proc 22:2149, 1990

113. Pirsch JD, Kalayoglu M, Hafez GR, et al. Evidence that the vanishing bile duct syndrome is vanishing. Transplantation 49:1015, 1990

114. Ploeg RJ. Preliminary results of the European multicenter study on UW solution in liver transplantation. Transplant Proc 2:2185, 1990

115. Polson RJ, Portmann B, Neuberger J, Calne RY, Williams R. Evidence of disease recurrence after liver transplantation for primary biliary cirrhosis: clinical and histologic follow-up studies, Gastroenterology 97:715, 1989

116. Porayko MK, Wiesner RH, LaRusso NF, et al. Patients with asymptomatic primary sclerosing cholangitis frequently have progressive disease. Gastroenterology 98:1594, 1990
117. Portmann B, O'Grady J, Williams R. Disease recurrence following orthotopic liver transplantation. Transplant Proc 18:135, 1986
118. Portmann B, Wight DGD. Pathology of liver transplantation (excluding rejection). In: Calne RW, ed. Liver transplantation, ed 2. Orlando, Grune & Stratton, 1987, p 437
119. Poterucha J, Rakela J, Ludwig J, Taswll HF, Weisner RH. Hepatitis C antibodies in patients with chronic hepatitis of unknown etiology after orthotopic liver transplantation. Transplant Proc 23:1495, 1991
120. Poupon RE, Balkau B, Eschwège E, et al. A multi-center controlled trial of ursodiol for the treatment of primary biliary cirrhosis. N Engl J Med 324:1548, 1991
121. Rabinovitz M, Gavaler J, Schade R, Dindzans VJ, Chien M, Van Thiel D. Does primary sclerosing cholangitis occurring in association with inflammatory bowel disease differ from that occurring in the absence of inflammatory bowel disease? A study of sixty-six subjects. Hepatology 11:7, 1990
122. Rakela J, Wooten RS, Batts KP, et al. Failure of interferon to prevent recurrent hepatitis B infection in hepatic allograft. Mayo Clin Proc 64:429, 1989
123. Randhawa PS, Markin RS, Starzl TE, Demetris AJ. Epstein-Barr virus–associated syndromes in immunosuppressed liver transplant recipients. Am J Surg Pathol 14:538, 1990
124. Richter GM, Noeldge G, Palmasz JC, Roessle M. The transjugular intrahepatic portosystemic stentshunt (TIPPS): result of pilot study. Cardiovasc Intervent Radiol 13:200, 1990
125. Ring E, Lake JR, Sterneck M, Ascher NL. Intrahepatic portocaval shunt for variceal hemorrhage prior to liver transplantation. Transplantation 52:161, 1991
126. Ringe B, Oldhafer K, Bunzedahl H, et al. Analysis of biliary tract complications following orthotopic liver transplantation. Transplant Proc 21:2472, 1989
127. Rizetto R, Macagno S, Chiaberge E, et al. Liver transplantation in hepatitis delta virus disease. Lancet 2:469, 1987
128. Rouch DA, Emond JC, Ferrari M, et al. The successful management of portal vein thrombosis after hepatic transplantation with a splenorenal shunt. Surg Gynecol Obstet 166:311, 1988
129. Samuel D, Bismuth A, Serres C, et al. HBV infection after liver transplantation in HBsAg positive patients: experience with long-term immunoprophylaxis. Transplant Proc 23:1492, 1991
130. Schroeder TJ, First MR, Hurtubise PE, et al. Immunologic monitoring with Orthoclone OKT3 therapy. J Heart Transplant 8:371, 1989
131. Sheil AGR, Thompson JF, Stevens MS, Eyers AA, Graham JC, Bookallil MJ. Mesoportal graft for thrombosed portal vein in liver transplantation. Clin Transplant 1:18, 1987
132. Siekierka JJ, Hung SHY, Poe M, Lin CS, Sigal NH. A cytosolic binding protein for the immunosuppressant FK 506 has peptidyl-prolyl isomerase activity but is distinct from cyclophilin. Nature 341:755, 1989
133. Singh N, Dummer JS, Kusne S, et al. Infections with cytomegalovirus and other herpes viruses in 121 liver transplant recipients: transmission by donated organ and the effect of OKT3 antibodies. J Infect Dis 158:124, 1988
134. Stahl RL, Duncan A, Hooks MA, et al. A hypercoagulable state follows orthotopic liver transplantation. Hepatology 12:553, 1990
135. Starzl TE. Surgery for metabolic liver disease. In: McDermott WV, ed. Surgery of the liver, ed 2. Oxford, Blackwell Scientific Publications, 1986, p 127
136. Starzl TE, Demetris AJ, Van Thiel D. Medical progress: liver transplantation. N Engl J Med 321:1014, 1989
137. Starzl TE, Iwatsuki S, Esquivel CO, et al. Refinements in the technique of liver transplantation. Semin Liver Dis 5:349, 1985

138. Starzl TE, Porter KA, Mazzaferro V, Todo S, Fung J, Francavilla A. Hepatotrophic effect of FK 506 in dogs. Transplantation 51:67, 1991
139. Starzl TE, Todo S, Tzakis AG, et al. Abdominal organ cluster transplantation for treatment of upper abdominal malignancies. Ann Surg 210:118, 1989
140. Starzl TE, Van Thiel D, Tzakis A, et al. Orthotopic liver transplantation for alcoholic cirrhosis. JAMA 260:2542, 1988
141. Stieber AC, Gordon RD, Todo S, et al. Liver transplantation in patients over sixty years of age. Transplantation 51:271, 1991
142. Stieber AC, Marino IR, Iwatsuki S, Starzl TE. Cholangiocarcinoma in sclerosing cholangitis: the role of liver transplantation. Int Surg 74:1, 1989
143. Steiber AC, Zetti G, Todo S, et al. The spectrum of portal vein thrombosis in liver transplantation. Ann Surg 213:199, 1991
144. Stoller JK, Moodie D, Schiavone WA, et al. Reduction of intrapulmonary shunt and resolution of digital clubbing associated with primary biliary cirrhosis after liver transplantation. Hepatology 11:54, 1990
145. Stratta RJ, Schaefer MS, Cushing KA, et al. Successful prophylaxis of cytomegalovirus disease after primary exposure in liver transplant recipients. Transplantation 51:90, 1991
146. Stratta RJ, Wood RP, Langas AN, et al. Diagnosis and treatment of biliary tract complications after orthotopic liver transplantation. Surgery 106:675, 1989
147. Strong R, Ong TH, Pillay P, Wall D, Balderson G, Lynch S. A new method of segmental orthotopic liver transplantation in children. Surgery 104:104, 1988
148. Todo S, Demetris A, Makowka L, et al. Primary nonfunction of hepatic allografts with preexisting fatty infiltration. Transplantation 47:903, 1989
149. Todo S, Demetris AJ, Van Thiel D, Teperman L, Fung JJ, Starzl TE. Orthotopic liver transplantation for patients with hepatitis B virus–related liver disease. Hepatology 13:619, 1991
150. Todo S, Fung JJ, Starzl TE, et al. Liver, kidney, and thoracic organ transplantation under FK 506. Ann Surg 212:295, 1990
151. Todo S, Makowka L, Tzakis AG, et al. Hepatic artery in liver transplantation. Transplant Proc 19:2406, 1987
152. Todo S, Nery J, Yanaga K, et al. Extended preservation of human liver grafts with UW solution. JAMA 261:711, 1989
153. Tzakis A, Todo S, Starzl TE. Orthotopic liver transplantation with preservation of the inferior vena cava. Ann Surg 210:649, 1989
154. Tzakis A, Todo S, Stieber A, Starzl TE. Venous jump grafts for liver transplantation in patients with portal vein thrombosis. Transplantation 48:530, 1989
155. Tzakis AG, Arditi M, Whitington PF, et al. Aplastic anemia complication orthotopic liver transplantation for non-A, non-B hepatitis. N Engl J Med 319:393, 1988
156. Tzakis AG, Carcassonne C, Todo S, Makowka L, Starzl TE. Liver transplantation for primary biliary cirrhosis. Semin Liver Dis 9:144, 1989
157. Tzakis AG, Todo S, Starzl TE. The anterior route for arterial graft conduits in liver transplantation. Transplant Int 2:121, 1989
158. Tzakis AG, Todo S, Starzl TE. Upper abdominal exenteration with liver replacement: a modification of the "cluster" procedure. Transplant Proc 22:273, 1990
159. Urbach AH, Gartner JC, Malatack JJ, et al. Linear growth following pediatric liver transplantation. Am J Dis Child 141:547, 1987
160. Van Hoek B, Weisner RH, Ludwig J, et al. Combination immunosuppression with azathioprine reduces the incidence of ductopenic rejection and vanishing bile duct syndrome after liver transplantation. Transplant Proc 23:1403, 1991
161. Vickers C, Neuberger J, Buckels J, et al. Transplantation of the liver in adults and children with fulminant hepatic failure. J Hepatol 7:143, 1988

162. Wall WJ, Grant DR, Mimeault RE, et al. Biliary tract reconstruction in liver transplantation. Can J Surg 32:97, 1989
163. Watts RWE, Calne RY, Rolles K. Successful treatment of primary hyperoxaluria type I by combined hepatic and renal transplantation. Lancet 2:474, 1987
164. Weisner RH. The incidence of gram-negative bacterial and fungal infections in liver transplant recipients treated with selective decontamination of the gut. Infection 18(Suppl 1):S19, 1990
165. Wiesner RH, Grambsch PM, Dickson ER, et al. Primary sclerosing cholangitis: natural history, prognostic factors and survival analysis. Hepatology 10:430, 1989
166. Wilkinson AH, Smith J, Hunsicker L, et al. Increased frequency of posttransplant lymphomas in patients treated with cyclosporine, azathioprine, and prednisone. Transplantation 47:293, 1989
167. Wszolek ZK, McComb RD, Pfeiffer RF, et al. Pontine and extrapontine myelinolysis following liver transplantation. Relationship to serum sodium. Transplantation 48:1006, 1989
168. Yanaga K, Lebeau G, Marsh JW, et al. Hepatic artery reconstruction for hepatic artery thrombosis after orthotopic liver transplantation. Arch Surg 125:628, 1990
169. Yanaga K, Makowka L, Starzl TE. Is hepatic artery thrombosis after liver transplantation really a surgical complication? Transplant Proc 21:3511, 1989
170. Zajko AB, Bennett MJ, Campbell WL, Koneu B. Mucocoele of the cystic duct remnant in eight liver transplant recipients: findings at cholangiography, CT and US. Radiology 177:691, 1990
171. Zajko AB, Claus D, Clapuyt P, et al. Obstruction to hepatic venous drainage after liver transplantation: treatment with balloon angioplasty. Radiology 170:763, 1989

Diseases of the Liver, Seventh Edition, edited by Leon Schiff and Eugene R. Schiff. J.B. Lippincott Company, Philadelphia © 1993.

Neoplasms of the Liver

Kunio Okuda

Masamichi Kojiro

Hiroaki Okuda

Primary hepatic neoplasms are rare, and physicians encounter secondary liver tumors much more frequently in the western countries, whereas primary liver cell carcinoma or hepatocellular carcinoma (HCC) is prevalent and seen more often in the clinical setting than metastatic tumors in other parts of the world such as sub-Saharan Africa and the Far East. The recent progress in imaging diagnosis and disclosure of some of the causative factors have caused a recent surge of interest among clinicians as well as basic investigators in related fields. In this chapter, for these reasons, emphasis is placed on primary malignant tumors of the liver.

BENIGN TUMORS OF THE LIVER

Benign hepatic tumors are detected more frequently than in the past with modern imaging and excised. They are divided into three categories—hepatocellular, cholangiocellular, and nonepithelial.

Benign Epithelial Tumors and Tumor-Like Lesions

LIVER CELL ADENOMA

Liver cell adenoma (LCA) had been a rare tumor until the introduction of oral contraceptives, but in countries where oral contraceptives are not used, it is still uncommon. For instance, in Japan, only a few cases have been reported. Although there are several different causative factors, oral contraceptive–related LCA is the most common, and therefore, most patients are women in their reproductive years, ages 15 to 45. By contrast, anabolic steroid–induced LCA occurs in young men.

Grossly, LCAs are well demarcated, occasionally encapsulated, and yellow to tan (Fig. 44-1A). Although most LCAs have a fairly homogeneous appearance, unlike HCC, some may show subdivision of mass by fibrous septa; in such cases, each division varies in appearance, depending on the presence or absence of degenerative changes, necrosis, and hemorrhage. According to Edmondson and coworkers,[59] infarction and hemorrhage were seen only in women taking oral contraceptives. Regression and regressive enlargement of LCAs after withdrawal of oral contraceptives have been reported.[62,179] Histologically, LCAs consist of neoplastic hepatocytes that are slightly larger than normal and frequently have a pale cytoplasm because of glycogen or fat accumulation. The tumor cells typically are arranged in a cord pattern two to three cells thick with an occasional acinar structure. There are many vascular channels with or without muscular walls, but portal tracts are not found (see Fig. 44-1B). The tumor is found incidentally in 5% to 10% of cases; the patient notices an abdominal mass in 25% to 35%; there is chronic or mild abdominal pain in 20% to 25%; and the patient presents suddenly with acute abdominal pain caused by hemorrhage in 30% to 40%. The bleeding occurs within the mass in about one third of cases and into the free abdominal cavity in two thirds.[80] If the LCA is caused by an underlying metabolic disease, symptoms are associated with it. LCAs associated with glycogen storage disease are multiple in about half the patients. They may develop into HCC later. Colloid scintigraphy usually shows an LCA as a defect. On computed tomography (CT) scanning, it appears as a low-density mass, and on celiac angiography, it is seen as a round or ovoid hypervascular mass with hepatic arteries entering from its periphery.[79,258] In the late phase of angiography, a sharply demarcated tumor stain and a fine zone of relative radiolucency representing a fibrous capsule may be discerned.[37] The prognosis is related to the underlying causative factor and the clinical presentation. Acute abdominal catastrophe can only be treated by emergency surgery.

FOCAL NODULAR HYPERPLASIA

Focal nodular hyperplasia (FNH) is a solitary, nodular hepatic lesion of unknown pathogenesis. FNH used to be an incidental finding at autopsy or surgery. In recent years, increasing numbers of FNH have been detected and resected as a result of improved imaging diagnosis. This lesion affects people of all ages, but most are between ages 20 and 50. Female predominance has been noted, and the male/female ratio is around 1:2. It has been suggested that FNH is a hamartomatous lesion or a response to a vascular malformation rather than a neoplastic lesion.[373] In fact, many arteries and veins suggestive of vascular abnormalities are observed in both the fibrous stroma and the parenchyma.

Grossly, FNH is a well-demarcated, unencapsulated, solitary nodule. Most are smaller than 5 cm, and about 3% are larger than 10 cm.[80] The nodule commonly is located in the subcapsular portion and frequently protrudes with an umbilication or is pedunculated. On the cut surface, characteristic fibrous septa that subdivide the tumor into nodules are seen

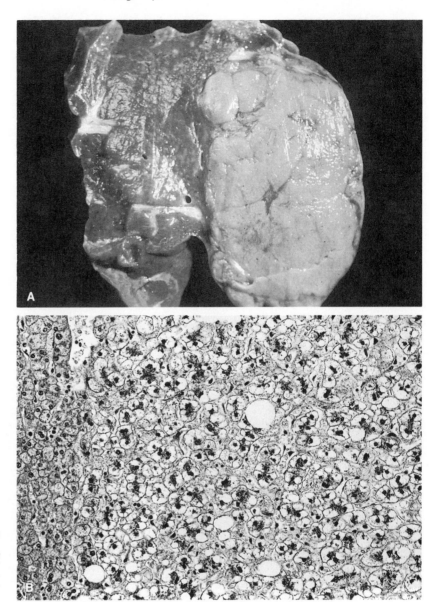

FIGURE 44-1 Liver cell adenoma. (**A**) Gross appearance. (**B**) Histology of liver cell adenoma. This tumor is not encapsulated and consists of neohepatocytes that show watery vacuolization and lipochrome-like pigment, growing in a compact pattern. (**A** courtesy of Dr. Kamal G. Ishak)

radiating from the center (central scar) (Fig. 44-2A). We have observed such characteristic septa even in a 1-cm FNH.

Histologically, a dense, central fibrous scar with radiating fibrosis contains many thick-walled arteries and veins. Ductular proliferation of varying degree, which is considered a result of hepatocyte metaplasia rather than of proliferation of bile ducts, is observed along the margin of the radiating fibrous bands and the parenchyma. Varying numbers of lymphocytes and plasma cells are also recognized in the fibrous septa. Hyperplastic hepatocytes are arranged in plates that are two or more cells thick with a distinct trabecular structure (see Fig. 44-2B). Acinar or glandular structures and cholestatic features occasionally are seen.

NODULAR REGENERATIVE HYPERPLASIA

Nodular regenerative hyperplasia (NRH) is also known as nodular transformation of the liver, nodular noncirrhotic liver, diffuse nodular hyperplasia of the liver, and hepatocel-

lular adenomatosis. Although the pathogenesis of this lesion is obscure, a possible pathogenetic relation with vascular lesions such as venous occlusion, arteritis, and collagen disease has been suggested.

Grossly, multiple miliary nodules are distributed throughout the cut surface of the liver (Fig. 44-3). Histologically, the nodules consist of hyperplasia of hepatocytes. Hepatic cords between each nodule are atrophied by the expanding nodules, but the basic lobular architecture is not obliterated. Fibrous septa are not seen at the boundaries of the nodules. Although the nodular pattern can be appreciated by routine hematoxylin–eosin stain, reticulin impregnation makes it more distinct. The hepatocytes of the nodules appear almost normal.

ADENOMATOUS HYPERPLASIA

Adenomatous hyperplasia (AH) of the liver has the following synonyms: adenomatoid hyperplasia, macroregenerative nod-

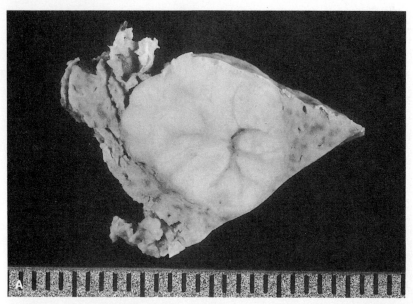

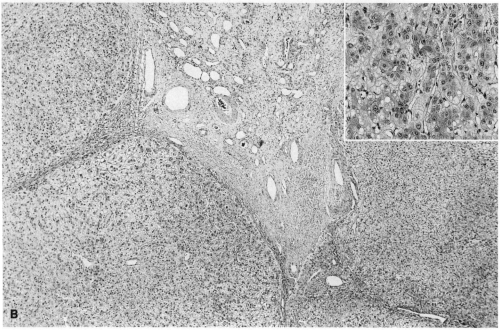

FIGURE 44-2 Focal nodular hyperplasia. (**A**) Small (1.2 × 1–cm) focal nodular hyperplasia with characteristic stellate fibrosis. (**B**) Dense central fibrous scar containing many arterial and venous vessels. Fine fibrous bands extend into the parenchyma (× 20; *inset* × 100).

ule, multiple nodular hyperplasia, and cirrhotic pseudotumor. The term *adenomatous hyperplasia* was first applied to the hyperplastic regenerative nodules seen in severe acute hepatic injury, such as submassive hepatic necrosis, and chronic liver diseases, particularly liver cirrhosis. AH in cirrhotic liver has recently attracted much interest from both clinicians and pathologists because it is now suspected to be a precursor lesion of HCC.

Grossly, AH is seen as a nodular lesion 1 to 2 cm in diameter in a cirrhotic liver (Fig. 44-4A). It frequently is multiple and often seen in the vicinity of small HCCs. Histologically, hepatocytes in AH show varying degrees of hyperplastic

change, such as increased cellularity and more distinct trabecular pattern (see Fig. 44-4B). Arakawa and coworkers[9] reported five cases of AH in which early malignant foci were seen as small nodule-in-nodule lesions and suggested that AH nodules in cirrhotic livers may be preneoplastic, already committed to malignant transformation. Increasing numbers of AH-containing cancerous foci have subsequently been reported in Japan.[330,336,356] According to Sugihara and associates,[330] the mean size of AH-containing cancerous foci is 16.2 mm, significantly larger than that (9.4 mm) of AHs without cancerous foci. Takayama and colleagues[336] clinically followed 17 patients with 20 biopsy-proven AHs for 1 to

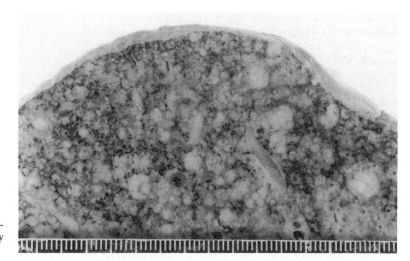

FIGURE 44-3 Nodular regenerative hyperplasia. Nodules of varying size, ranging up to 1 cm, are diffusely scattered in the liver.

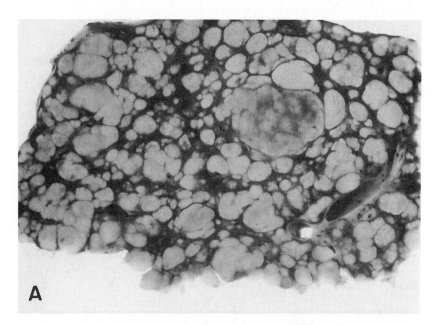

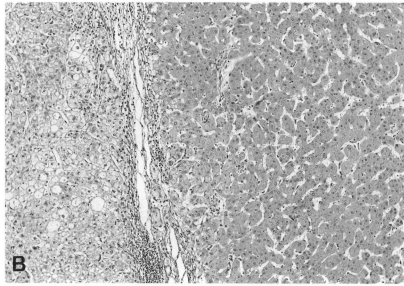

FIGURE 44-4 Adenomatous hyperplasia. (**A**) A 1.3 × 0.7–cm nodule stands out among mixed macronodules and micronodules of cirrhotic liver. (**B**) Histologically, it exhibits increased cellularity and a distinct trabecular arrangement (*right side*; × 50).

5 years and found transformation to HCC in 9 of 18 nodules within 6 to 50 months after biopsy. They concluded that AH is an absolute precursor of HCC because of the high risk of malignant transformation and stressed that it should be treated as a potential malignant lesion.

The characteristic feature of AH-containing cancerous foci is that it is almost always accompanied by some fatty changes (Fig. 44-5). Considering the high frequency of fatty changes in well-differentiated HCC in the early stage,[144] fatty changes in an AH or AH-like hyperplastic lesion may be a morphologic marker of malignant transformation.

BILE DUCT ADENOMA

Bile duct adenoma (BDA) is a small, solitary nodule, usually less than 1 cm, that occurs beneath the liver capsule. Ishak and Rabin[104] analyzed 68 cases of BDA at the Armed Forced Institute of Pathology. Forty-nine patients were male and 19 were female. Two thirds were over age 50, and only 3 were under age 30. There were no significant clinical signs attributable to this tumor. Grossly, BDAs are firm and gray-white. Histologically, the tumor consists of relatively small ductular structures with variable fibrous stroma. The ductular epithelium does not represent atypism and is similar to bile duct epithelium.

CYSTIC LESIONS OF THE LIVER

Simple Hepatic Cyst
A simple hepatic cyst is unilocular, single or multiple, and lined by a single layer of cuboidal epithelium. The reported incidence of simple hepatic cyst ranges from 1% to about 20%.[45] It usually can be detected by imaging techniques.

Biliary Cystadenoma
A relatively rare lesion, this multilocular cyst is lined by cuboidal or columnar epithelium. Despite the term *biliary cystadenoma*, its histogenesis remains unclear. This lesion occurs predominantly in middle-aged women.[105] About 70% of the tumors are multilocular, and the remainder contain intramural loculi on microscopic examination.[45] Locules of the cyst vary in size and are lined by mucin-secreting columnar epithelium. The cysts contain clear, cloudy, mucinous, or gelatinous fluid. In some tumors, the subepithelial layer consists of mesenchymal stroma that resembles ovarian stroma and is characterized by fibrous tissue with fibroblast-like round- to spindle-shaped cells. It is not uncommon to encounter the features of cystadenocarcinoma in part, and the transition from benign to malignant epithelium may be seen.

Meyenburg's Complex
Also called biliary microhamartoma, Meyenburg's complex is thought to be a hamartomatous malformation that results from arrested development or abnormal remodeling of the primitive ductal plate, which is the precursor of the normal bile duct.[51,80] The lesion is solitary or multiple and well demarcated. It consists of irregular cystic spaces lined by thin cuboidal epithelium and fibrous stroma. The lesion should not be mistaken for BDA or metastatic adenocarcinoma.

Benign Mesenchymal Tumors

CAVERNOUS HEMANGIOMA

Cavernous hemangioma is the most common benign mesenchymal tumor of the liver. Although this tumor occurs at any age, it is seen most frequently in adults. Grossly, hepatic hemangioma is a well-demarcated, reddish tumor ranging in size from a few millimeters to more than 20 cm (Fig. 44-6A). Most of these tumors are solitary, but multiple hemangiomas occur in about 10%.[101] Histologically, the tumor is composed of various size blood-filled spaces arranged in a cavernous pattern (see Fig. 44-6B). Although fibrous stroma is not large, the center of the tumor often is fibrotic or mucinous. The entire tumor occasionally is replaced by dense, often hyalinized fibrotic tissue with a few dilated cavernous spaces (sclerosed hemangioma).

When the liver is studied by ultrasonography, the tumor

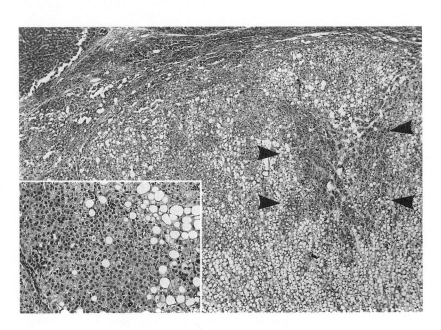

FIGURE 44-5 Adenomatous hyperplasia containing a cancerous focus (*arrowheads*) with diffusely fatty changes (× 20; *inset* × 200).

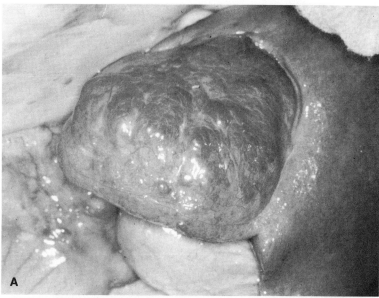

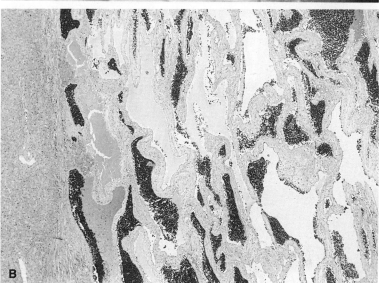

FIGURE 44-6 *Cavernous hemangioma.* (**A**) Medium-size hemangioma protruding from the liver surface above the gallbladder. (**B**) Tumor consisting of irregular vascular channels surrounded by fibrous stroma of low cellularity (× 20).

is shown as a hyperechoic lesion. In countries where HCC is endemic, hemangioma creates a serious problem because it can be mistaken for small HCC by imaging. The reported incidence in autopsies varies from 0.4% to as high as 20%, depending on the thoroughness of the examination.[45] Small hemangiomas do not produce any symptoms, but about 40% of hemangiomas larger than 4 cm are associated with such symptoms as pain, abdominal discomfort, and hepatic mass. Pain may be induced by intermittent thromboses. Consumption coagulopathy is a rare complication. The diagnosis relies mainly on imaging because needle biopsy entails a bleeding risk, particularly if the mass is large or located near the hepatic surface. For small hemangiomas, thin-needle biopsy may be necessary when the differential diagnosis from HCC cannot be made with certainty. The imaging and differential features are described later in the diagnosis of HCC. Angiography provides important information for differential diagnosis; the contrast medium remains in the mass much longer than it does in HCC, and the same phenomenon is observed with dynamic CT scan. Large hemangiomas may be en-

hanced on dynamic CT or stained on angiography only in its periphery because of the scarring of the tumor interior.

LIPOMATOUS TUMORS

Although lipomatous tumors, such as lipoma, angiomyolipoma, myelolipoma, and focal fatty change, are rare, as are other mesenchymal tumors of the liver, they are increasingly found with ultrasound examination; lipomatous lesions are hyperechoic.

Angiomyolipoma is grossly a well-defined, yellowish tumor with hemorrhagic areas and consists of adipose tissue that contains arteries, veins, bundles of smooth muscle admixed with fibrous tissue, and, occasionally, nerve fibers.

OTHER BENIGN MESENCHYMAL TUMORS

Infantile hemangioendothelioma, fibroma, leiomyoma, myxoma, and mesenchymal hamartoma are rare and have been sporadically reported.[92,101]

INFLAMMATORY PSEUDOTUMOR

Inflammatory pseudotumors typically are well-defined, solitary, tumor-like lesions (Fig. 44-7A) composed invariably of inflammatory cells, mostly plasma cells, and varying degrees of fibrosis[6,45] (see Fig. 44-7B). Clinically, there may be mild fever, malaise, weight loss, and other signs. The cause remains unknown. Craig and coworkers[45] have proposed a new term, inflammatory myofibroblastic tumor, for this lesion because of the presence of bland spindle cells (myofibroblasts). They suggest that if the cause for a solitary hepatic inflammatory mass is identified, such as a healing abscess or posttraumatic injury, then the term inflammatory myofibroblastic tumor does not apply, even though the histologic features may be similar.

MALIGNANT TUMORS OF THE LIVER

Primary malignant tumors of the liver are histogenetically either epithelial, mesenchymal, or mixed, but epithelial malignant tumors far exceed others in frequency. Of these, HCC is the most common worldwide. The clinical manifestations of primary hepatic neoplasms are more or less similar, with an enlarged liver bearing a large mass, weight loss, malaise, and emaciation, and except for cholangiocarcinoma (CCC), jaundice is not an early manifestation. Masses are seen as space-occupying lesions by imaging. The speed of tumor growth, frequency of extrahepatic metastases, and other clinicopathologic features vary with the individual tumor type and patient. The prognosis was poor in the past because of

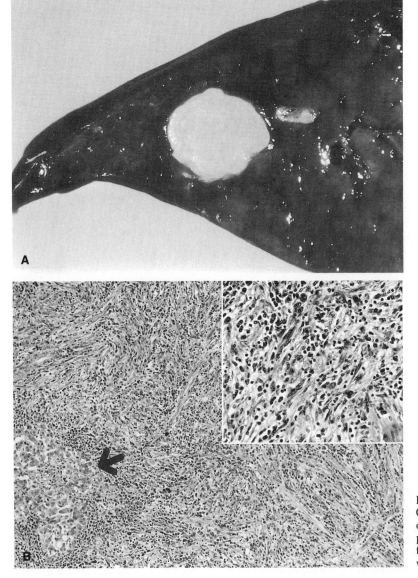

FIGURE 44-7 Inflammatory pseudotumor. (**A**) Gross appearance of pseudotumor on the cut surface of the liver. (**B**) Dense inflammatory infiltrate composed of plasma cells and lymphocytes is prominent in the fibrous stroma. An island of hepatocytes is seen within the lesion (*at arrow; × 50; inset × 100*).

late detection, but even with early detection of the tumor by modern imaging and the practice of surgical removal of the mass, improvement in survival has not been as impressive as expected. Clearly, prevention is the only solution. With the development of vaccines for hepatitis B and, it is hoped, C viruses, it seems that HCC may be prevented in large measure in the future.

Primary Malignant Epithelial Tumors

Primary malignant epithelial tumors are histopathologically divided into HCC, cholangiocellular carcinoma (CCC), combined hepatocellular and CCC (hepatocholangiocarcinoma), hepatoblastoma, and rare other tumors, such as squamous cell carcinoma. As shown in Table 44-1, HCC is by far the most frequent among primary liver cancers. There has been a semantic problem with epithelial tumors. The word hepatoma was coined by Yamagiwa[382] in 1911 to distinguish primary liver cell carcinoma from intrahepatic bile duct carcinoma. The term cholangioma was also created as its counterpart. Hepatoma came to be prefixed by benign and malignant, such as benign hepatoma, creating confusion in its definition. Furthermore, cholangioma often included carcinomas that arise from the extrahepatic bile duct system. Thus, in 1976, the International Association for the Study of the Liver formally adopted and recommended the terms *hepatocellular carcinoma* and *cholangiocarcinoma*, the latter applying only to intrahepatic bile duct carcinoma.[157]

Hepatocellular Carcinoma

Definition

HCC is a malignant tumor composed of cells that resemble or are derived from the hepatocyte. It usually occurs in association with chronic liver disease, most frequently with cirrhosis. There is a male predominance, and the incidence varies from area to area perhaps because of differences in the frequency of hepatitis virus infection and in the degree of exposure to hepatocarcinogens. Several histologic types with certain clinical characteristics are recognized. The prognosis usually is poor, depending not only on the extent of tumor invasion at diagnosis but also on the disease state of the noncancerous hepatic parenchyma.

Epidemiology

Geographic Prevalence. It has been established that the incidence of HCC varies considerably with the geographic region perhaps because of differences in the major causative factors and their frequencies. Whereas the incidence is low among whites in the United Kingdom, the United States, and Australia, it is much higher among the blacks in Mozambique, the sub-Saharan African natives, and in the Far East.

It is difficult to grasp the exact incidence rate of HCC because the vital statistics are based on the diagnoses made by physicians, most of which lack histologic confirmation and list HCC and CCC combined as primary liver cancer. Without histologic diagnosis, secondary liver cancer may be mistaken for primary or vice versa. Liver tumor associated with cirrhosis is almost invariably HCC in high-incidence areas. In our case control study based on autopsy, 369 of 391 liver cancers associated with cirrhosis were primary in Japan, contrasted by comparable figures of 88 of 226 cirrhosis-associated liver cancers being primary in Trieste in northern Italy.[186] Histologic diagnosis is reliable in autopsy studies, but only a relative frequency among all deaths or all cancers can be calculated; there is a certain bias at the time of hospital admission and autopsy because of the socioeconomic state of the society and the changing interest on the part of physicians. Well-established cancer registry with frequent histologic diagnosis may be more reliable, yet the statistics based on cancer registry are different from vital statistics, which depend on death certificates.

Berman[16] and later Higginson[95] called world attention to the extremely high incidence rate of HCC among the male black population (Shangaan tribe) in Mozambique. Table 44-2 gives the age-adjusted incidence rates of primary liver cancer per 100,000 persons per year in various countries, areas, and ethnic groups. The rates may be divided into the high-incidence areas and peoples (more than 20 per 100,000 per year), which include Mozambique, Zimbabwe, Senegal, Singapore Chinese, South African blacks, China, Taiwan,

TABLE 44-1   *Relative Frequency of Major Types of Primary Malignant Epithelial Tumors—Los Angeles and Japan*

Tumor Type	Los Angeles (Autopsies) 1918–1982 (720/96,625)*	Japan (National Study, Histology Confirmed)	
		1968–1977 (2829)†	1982–1985 (4755)‡
Hepatocellular carcinoma	642 (89.3%)	2411 (85.2%)	4354 (91.6%)
Hepatoblastoma	5 (0.7%)	69 (2.4%)	22 (0.5%)
Cholangiocarcinoma	71 (9.9%)	269 (9.5%)	256 (5.4%)
Combined type		58 (2.4%)	49 (1.0%)
Others	2 (0.3%)	23 (0.8%)§	74 (1.6%)§

*Craig JR, et al. Tumors of the liver and intrahepatic bile ducts. Fasc. 26. Washington, DC, Armed Forces Institute of Pathology 1989.
†Okuda K, et al. Primary liver cancers in Japan. Cancer 45:2663, 1980.
‡Liver Cancer Study Group of Japan. Primary liver cancer in Japan. Clinicopathologic features and results of surgical treatment. Ann Surg 211:277, 1990.
§Includes sarcomas.

TABLE 44-2 *Age-Adjusted Incidence Rates of Liver Cancer in Various Countries, Cities, and Ethnic Groups*

Country	Incidence Rate (per 100,000/y) Males	Females
Mozambique, Lourenco Marques	112.9	30.8
Zimbabwe, Bulawayo	64.6	25.4
Gambia	33.1	12.6
Senegal	25.6	9.0
Cape		
Bantu	26.3	8.4
Colored	1.5	0.7
White	1.2	0.6
Algeria	1.6	1.4
Nigeria, Ibadan	15.4	3.2
Argentina, Tandil	9.9	5.8
Brazil, Fortaleza	3.5	3.7
Peru, Lima	4.0	2.9
Jamaica	6.1	2.1
United States, San Francisco		
Chinese	19.1	3.6
Black	3.9	1.8
Japanese	3.0	0.4
White	2.9	1.1
Canada		
Eskimos	6.9	3.7
Alberta	1.3	0.5
Switzerland, Geneva	10.2	1.5
Italy, Parma	8.6	3.3
Spain, Zaragoza	7.2	5.5
France, Doubs	3.7	1.0
Germany, Hamburg	4.5	1.7
Denmark	3.6	2.3
Yugoslavia, Slovenia	2.0	1.2
Czechoslovakia, Slovakia	5.1	2.8
United Kingdom, England and Wales	1.6	0.8
Ireland	0.1	0.3
China, Shanghai	34.4	11.6
Singapore		
Chinese	31.6	7.2
Malay	15.6	5.3
Indian	14.1	2.8
Korea	13.8	3.2
Japan		
Miyagi	11.2	4.0
Nagasaki	25.8	7.9
India, Bombay	4.9	2.5
Philippines, Manila	19.9	6.2
Hong Kong	32.3	7.4
Pakistan	0.7	0.8
New Zealand		
Maori	11.2	4.2
Non-Maori	2.4	1.1
Pacific Polynesian Islands	26.6	2.3
Australia, South	2.0	0.7
Hawaii, Chinese	7.8	2.4

(Bosch FC, Munoz N. Hepatocellular carcinoma in the world: epidemiologic questions. In: Tabor E, et al, eds. Etiology, pathology and treatment of hepatocellular carcinoma in North America. Woodlands Portfolio, 1991, p 35; Munoz N, Bosch X. Epidemiology of hepatocellular carcinoma. In: Okuda K, Ishak KG, eds. Neoplasms of the liver. Tokyo, Springer, 1987, p. 3)

and Japan (after 1976); the intermediate-incidence areas and peoples (5 to 20 per 100,000 per year), which include Singapore Malay, Singapore Indians, Brazil (Recife), Nigeria, Indians in South Africa, Switzerland (Geneva), Poland, Spain, New Zealand Maori, American Indians, Jamaica, Cuba, and Canadian Inuits; and the low-incidence areas and peoples (less than 5 per 100,000 per year), such as New Zealand whites, Sweden, the United Kingdom, Ireland, Mauritius, Norway, whites and blacks in the United States, Australian whites, Algeria, Canadian whites, Israel, the area formerly known as West Germany, Denmark, Yugoslavia (Slovenia), Hungary, India (Bombay), and Pakistan.[198,199] The relative significance of this type of cancer among all cancers may be appreciated from the age-standardized cancer rates shown in Table 44-3. Within the same region or city, the incidence rate varies markedly with the ethnic group. Although the African blacks and the Chinese have high incidence rates, the rates are much lower among the blacks in the United States, who originally came from Africa, and a similar difference exists between the Chinese in Hawaii and those in the Far East. The Chinese in the San Francisco Bay area, who still have a relatively high incidence, may not have lived in the United States long enough to have as much reduction in incidence as the black population in the United States shows. These Chinese are known to have a high carrier rate for hepatitis B surface antigen (HBsAg), which may be an important causative factor among them. Even within the same ethnic group, the incidence differs because of differences in the living conditions. In Mozambique, for instance, there is a nine-fold difference between the coastal and the inland region.[89]

China has a unique history of cancer epidemiology study. During the period from 1972 to 1977, a huge number of medical personnel were mobilized in a mass survey on cancer incidence in 840 million people. It was found that the main endemic areas for liver cancer are along the southeast coast, particularly the deltas, valleys, and islands. The hyperendemic areas have a standardized mortality of more than 60 per 100,000 per year, whereas in low-incidence areas, it is less than one tenth this figure.[390]

Time Trends.   Studies on time trends are subject to errors because of changing diagnostic capability. Statistics based on autopsy give relative frequency of histologically proven HCC among all autopsies, and time trends may be studied when old and new data are available. In the National Registry of Autopsies published annually by the Japan Pathological Society, which records nearly 90% of all individual autopsy cases compiled by major hospitals throughout the country, HCC constituted 1.91% among 19,356 necropsies in 1958 to 1959 in Japan. This rate steadily increased in the ensuing 30 years to the current (1986 to 1987) 7.66%, demonstrating an indisputable increase. The same trend was verified by our study based on the cancer registry in the Osaka area.[257] In this study, the incidence rate was found to have risen from 16.3/100,000/yr in 1966 to 1968 to 40.9 in 1984 to 1986 among males, but peculiarly, the increase among females was much less. Thus, there is a distinct sex prevalence not only in the incidence rate but also in time trends. In Los Angeles, the rate of HCC among all autopsies was 0.15% in 1918 to 1953; it rose to 1.48% in 1964 to 1983,[45] again the increase being remarkable. In the Florence area of Italy, an eight-fold increase has been reported. A less dramatic but significant

TABLE 44-3 *Frequency of Primary Liver Cancer Among All Cancers and Relative to Other Major Cancers in Developed Countries*

Organ	Males (%)			Females (%)		
	Japan*	US[†]	England and Wales[‡]	Japan*	US[†]	England and Wales[‡]
Stomach	25.4	3.3	7.8	22.5	2.5	5.6
Lung	19.0	34.3	33.8	10.7	19.2	15.3
Liver	13.6	1.7	0.9	7.4	1.3	0.8
	(3rd)			(6th)		
Pancreas	5.7	4.5	4.1	6.5	5.5	4.6

*Vital statistics, 1987, Japan.
[†]Vital statistics of the United States, vol II, pt A, 1987.
[‡]Mortality statistics cause, 1987.

increase was also noted in western Scotland. According to the study of Saracci and Repetto[298] in 1980, based on cancer registries, there was an increase in the incidence rate among males in 24 of 37 countries and among females in 26 of 37 countries. Liver cancer mortality increased about two-fold from 1959 to 1976 in Shanghai, China.[390]

Sex and Age.   With practically no geographic exception, HCC is more common in males than in females, but the male/female ratio differs with the country as well as with the year of survey because of changing time trends. It appears that the male/female ratio is greater in the high-prevalence regions, such as Africa, China, and Japan, and lower in the low-incidence regions, such as Latin America and Europe. The ratio rises as the incidence rate increases, as is the case in Japan, because the increase mainly occurs in males.[257] The greater susceptibility of males may be related to hormones, genetics, or a greater exposure to carcinogenic environmental factors. The incidence rate of cancer increases in proportion to age with a tendency to level off in old age. In high-incidence areas, such as Mozambique and Zimbabwe, the age curve shifts toward the younger age groups. The crude incidence among Mozambican males aged 25 to 34 years is more than 500 times that of the equivalent white population of the United Kingdom or the United States because HCC under age 40 is rare in the latter. The difference becomes smaller (15 times) in the aged populations over age 65.[199,374] HCC can occur in childhood and adolescence, but primary liver cancer in the young often is fibrolamellar carcinoma,[44] a variant HCC, and under age 5, it is mostly hepatoblastoma.[252] The male/female ratio decreases with younger ages, and the frequency of underlying cirrhosis is also low.[254]

Relation to Cirrhosis.   Most patients with HCC have chronic liver disease, notably cirrhosis.[259] It is the underlying disease in 80% to 90% of patients with HCC in most countries, and nonalcoholic posthepatitic cirrhosis is more frequently associated with HCC than is alcoholic micronodular cirrhosis. Among African blacks who have a high incidence of HCC, the association of cirrhosis with HCC is less strong and cirrhosis is mild if present, whereas in low-incidence areas, cirrhosis is more frequently associated with HCC.[124,129,130,255,324] If one compares young and older patients with HCC, cirrhosis is less common and HBsAg much

more frequently positive in the former. Studies of Miyaji and associates[189] and Shikata[308] in Japan clearly showed that cirrhotic livers with large nodules and thin stromas are more commonly associated with HCC than livers with small nodules and thick stromas. The former type is assumed to have greater regenerative activities of hepatocytes with increased DNA synthesis, and hence more frequent rearrangements of DNA sequences in the chromosomes. In a study in London, there was a higher incidence of HCC among patients with alcoholic cirrhosis who had abstained and whose micronodular cirrhosis had turned macronodular.[156] With abstinence, there is a surge of regenerative activity, transforming small nodules to large ones. Clinically, patients with alcoholic cirrhosis seldom develop HCC while they are imbibing. Alcoholic cirrhosis is the predominant type in the western countries, whereas posthepatitic cirrhosis is much more common in the Far East,[194] and there is a considerable difference in the frequency of HCC and the age at which it develops.[359]

High death rates for cirrhosis are observed in Chile, Mexico, Portugal, France, Puerto Rico, Italy, Ireland, and Austria, which have low rates for HCC. By contrast, lower death rates for cirrhosis are reported in Thailand, Hong Kong, Greece, and Switzerland, which have relatively high rates for HCC.[380] It is thought that macronodular cirrhosis is more commonly associated with hepatitis B virus (HBV) infection and is more prone to hepatocarcinogenesis, but the association of HBV and HCC is even stronger among young HCC patients without cirrhosis in Japan. In Senegal, it was estimated that in 62% of HCC cases positive for HBsAg, cancer arose in noncirrhotic livers and that the degree of association with HBV was similar for HCC with and without cirrhosis.[285] In Japan, this association has been emphasized in HBV-positive cirrhosis up to 1980 or so,[218] but more recently, this trend has disappeared with increasing hepatitis C virus (HCV)-associated cirrhosis.[242] In high-incidence areas, cirrhosis terminates in HCC in more than half of patients. In Japan, death due to HCC was about 30% among patients with cirrhosis before 1970, but this rate has steadily increased to 80%.[257] The change has been attributed to various factors, such as prolongation of survival of patients as a result of improved management and an increase in non-A, non-B (C) virus–induced cirrhosis, which is a slowly progressive, mixed macronodular and micronodular cirrhosis.[212]

Under experimental conditions in animals, high doses of hepatocarcinogens induce cirrhosis and HCC,[68,379] but in humans, there is no evidence that aflatoxins or other hepatocarcinogens are responsible for the development of cirrhosis that underlies HCC.

Etiology

Hepatitis Virus

HBV INFECTION. Numerous epidemiologic and biologic studies have suggested an important role of HBV infection in hepatocarcinogenesis. When the close relation between HBV infection and HCC incidence was found, it was thought that the age-old enigma of its close association with cirrhosis was resolved: both cirrhosis and HCC were caused by HBV infection. It turned out that HBV is not an oncovirus. Worldwide, there is a certain parallelism between the HBsAg carrier rate and the incidence rate of HCC; the carrier rate is high in areas of high HCC incidence and low in areas of low HCC incidence (Table 44-4). There are exceptions to this geographic relation, such as in Latin America, Sri Lanka, and Greenland, where HCC is uncommon, yet the carrier rate is relatively high.

It has also been established that HBsAg is significantly more often positive in patients with HCC than in those without HCC and in controls. All the case control studies have demonstrated this correlation, and cohort studies showed that HBsAg carriers have a significantly higher risk of developing HCC (Table 44-5). The study conducted in Taiwan among male government employees is of particular significance because of the large cohort size and the long study period; it showed a relative risk greater than 100.[13] In Taiwan, about 90% of patients with HCC are positive for HBsAg. Our own study in Tokyo similarly came up with a relative risk of 30 among adult carriers compared with the controls.[295] Conversely, those who have anti-HBs antibody have a lower risk.[334]

Familial clustering of HBV-related diseases, including HCC, is common throughout the world. It is due to vertical transmission of HBV from a hepatitis B e antigen (HBeAg)-positive mother to her children. In a study in West Africa, there was no significant difference in the antigen detection rate between the mothers and fathers, but the mothers of patients with HCC were HBsAg-positive almost four times more frequently than their fathers.[155] Most such patients are assumed to have acquired HBV by vertical transmission from HBeAg-positive mothers, and there is evidence that vertical transmission of HBV occurs more frequently in areas of high-HCC incidence than in low-incidence areas. In our cohort study in Tokyo, it was found that HBeAg-positive carriers at entry had a higher risk of developing HCC than did negative carriers during the 8-year follow-up period.[295]

HBsAg can be stained in tissue by Shikata's orcein, immunoperoxidase, and other techniques. It is well known that the parenchyma of the liver bearing an HCC from an HBsAg-positive patient frequently contains stainable HBsAg in the hepatocytes.[214] The former may be recognized in hematoxylin–eosin-stained sections because it looks like ground glass.[87] Such stainable HBsAg is thought to be a result of excessive expression of the pre-S and S genes of the HBV genome integrated in the chromosomal DNA to form a large molecular protein.[35] Some HCC cells contain HBsAg and core antigen (HBcAg),[98] but replication of episomal DNA of HBV is less frequently demonstrable in the cytoplasm of HCC cells.

DNA extracted from HCC tissue taken from HBsAg-positive patients often contains HBV DNA demonstrable by the Southern blot hybridization technique, showing integration of HBV DNA into the chromosomal DNA of the host.[22,301] Whether most patients with alcoholic cirrhosis who have developed HCC with no seromarkers of HBV infection also have integrated HBV DNA, as emphasized by Brechot and associates,[23] who even used the polymerase chain reaction, is disputed.[271] Other studies[100,387] have not been able to confirm it.

A number of established cell lines derived from human HCC tissue, notably PLC/PRF/5 cell line, produce HBsAg in the culture medium, suggesting the expression of S-gene integrated in the chromosomal DNA of the cell. After the discovery in 1978 of the woodchuck hepatitis virus (WHV),[333] which is akin to HBV, similar DNA viruses have been found in other animal species in nature, such as ground

TABLE 44-4   *Correlation Between Prevalence of Primary Liver Cancer (Mortality) and HBsAg Carrier Rate*

Country	Primary Liver Cancer Mortality (per 100,000/y)	HBsAg Carrier Rate Among Population
High-Incidence Areas		
Mozambique	98.2	14.0
South African blacks	22.0	9.0
China	17	7.5–14.0
Intermediate-Incidence Areas		
India	—	2.5
Japan	15	2.6
Greece	12	5.0
Low-Incidence Areas		
United States	2.7–4.7	0.2
Scandinavia	2.1–3.5	0.1
Central Europe and United Kingdom	1–7	0.25

(Hadziyannis SJ. Hepatocellular carcinoma and type B hepatitis. Clin Gastroenterol 9:117, 1980)

TABLE 44-5 *Cohort Studies on HBsAg Carriers and HCC Risk*

| Area/Country | Cohort | | HCC Risk |
	Total	HBsAg-Positive	
Taiwan	22,707	3454	104.0
Japan	32,177	496	10.4
Japan, Tokyo (Sakuma88)	25,547	513	30.0
United States, New York	—	6850	9.7
England/Wales	—	3934	42.0

HCC, hepatocellular carcinoma.
(Modified from Munoz N, Bosch X. Epidemiology of hepatocellular carcinoma. In: Okuda K, Ishak KG, eds. Neoplasms of the liver. Tokyo, Springer, 1987, p 3)

squirrels[180] and Pekin ducks.[181] They are collectively referred to as hepadna viruses.[290] Although these viruses produce HCC in the host animals,[264] WHV is most oncogenic[281]; practically all virus-carrier woodchucks develop HCC, although there are still acute hepatitic changes in the liver without going through the stage of cirrhosis.[280] In the animals that have developed HCC, integration of the hepadna virus DNA has been demonstrated.[386]

HEPATITIS C VIRUS. Previously called non-A, non-B hepatitis virus, HCV has recently been isolated and identified by the cloning method at the Chiron Corporation Laboratories. At the time of this writing, most available data were based on C-100-3 antibody, the first commercial kit. Some sera from patients who are negative for this antibody may test positive for other types of anti-HCV antibodies or may be found to contain HCV if the polymerase chain reaction is used.[125] Early results may include false-positive tests as well. Therefore, the available data on the frequency of antibody positivity among patients with HCC in various parts of the world shown in Table 44-6 may be modified in the future. Nevertheless, it is clear from this table that many patients with HCC who are negative for HBsAg are positive for anti-HCV with a significant difference from the control values of about 1% or less throughout the world, except for South Africa, where involvement of HCV in liver cancer seems less important.

HCV is transmitted not only by blood transfusion but also by poorly understood routes and causes chronic hepatitis that ensues acute infection in most patients. In due time, cirrhosis develops in such patients, and after an average interval of 29 years or so from acute infection, HCC develops in Japan.[137] Some patients have been followed from acute posttransfusion hepatitis until the emergence of HCC in the liver (Fig. 44-8). The causative role of non-A, non-B hepatitis virus in HCC was first suspected in Japan[113,233] because many patients with cirrhosis negative for HBsAg who had had blood transfusions in the long past began developing HCC in the late 1970s. Even after the introduction of HBV screening tests for blood donors, posttransfusion hepatitis occurred in a considerable proportion of blood recipients in Japan. It has also been noted that the relative proportion of HBsAg-positive cases among all patients with HCC is steadily declining with increasing HBV-unrelated cases,[257] although the absolute number of HBsAg-positive cases remains rather constant. The data compiled by the Japan Liver Cancer Study Group showed the HBsAg positivity rate to be 40.7% in the period up to 1977,[252] and it has been steadily declining to 22.4%.[165]

The natural history of those patients with chronic non-A, non-B hepatitis is such that the disease looks deceivingly benign in the early stage but ends up with cirrhosis and HCC, as commonly experienced in Japan; the same does not seem to apply to comparable patients in the United States.[53,242] The HCV carrier rate among blood donors in Japan is about 1.2% and lower in the western countries; the difference is much less, compared with the difference in the prevalence of HCV-related HCC between these two regions, suggesting that ad-

TABLE 44-6 *Prevalence of Antibodies to HCV Among HCC Patients*

| Area/Country | Author | Overall Anti-HCV Positivity Rate | HBsAg | |
			Positive	Negative
Central Japan	Kiyosawa[137]	74% (61/83)	35%(10/29)	94% (51/54)
North Italy	Colombo[42]	65% (86/132)	54%(22/41)	70% (64/91)
North Italy	Levrero[158]	58% (97/167)	28%(15/53)	72% (82/114)
Sicily, Italy	Simonetti[314]	76% (152/200)	58%(18/31)	79% (134/169)
South Spain	Bruix[26]	75% (72/96)	56%(6/9)	77% (67/87)
Miami, United States	Hasan[90]	36% (35/97)	14%(4/28)	53% (31/59)
South Africa	Kew[134]	29% (110/360)	26%(47/184)	32% (63/196)
Taiwan	Chen[33]	33% (22/66)	17%(7/42)	63% (15/24)

HCV, hepatitis C virus; HCC, hepatocellular carcinoma.

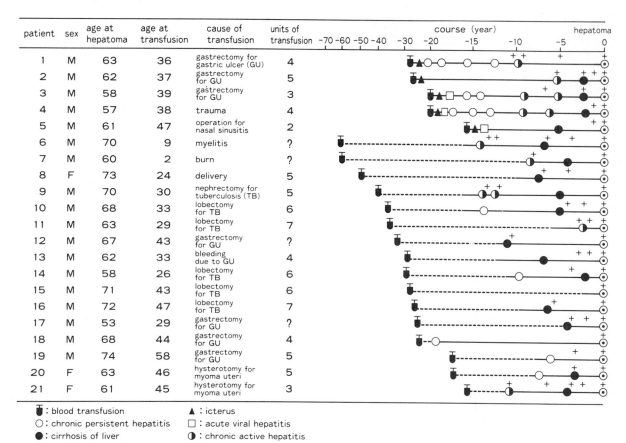

FIGURE 44-8 Interval in years from blood transfusion and date of diagnosis of chronic non-A, non-B hepatitis–related disease. (Kiyosawa K, et al. Interrelationship of blood transfusion, non-A, non-B hepatitis and hepatocellular carcinoma: analysis by detection of antibody to hepatitis C. Hepatology 12:671, 1990; courtesy of Dr. Kendo Kiyosawa)

ditional causative factors are operating in Japan. In several areas in Japan where anti-HCV screening was carried out in regional residents, the anti-C positivity rate was much higher among the elderly population (above age 50) compared with the younger population. Repeated use of poorly sterilized needles for mass vaccination in schoolchildren before the advent of disposable needles has been suspected as the cause of the high HCV infection rate among the aged and of the increase of C-related HCC in recent years in Japan. Certain differences exist between B-related and B-unrelated (mostly C-related) HCCs in Japan; the age group affected is older and the underlying cirrhosis more advanced in patients with B-unrelated HCC and the HCC tends to be small and expanding in growth pattern.[234,242] The detection of small HCCs by close follow-up with α-fetoprotein (AFP) measurement and abdominal ultrasonography is made more commonly in B-negative patients, perhaps because HCC grows slowly in such patients.

As long as HCV is a ribonucleic acid (RNA) virus that is not reverse transcribed to DNA, its oncogenic association is not explained by integration of genomic material into the host chromosome. It may act simply as a cause of cirrhosis, which in itself is a premalignant state with increased hepatocyte regeneration, hence increased DNA synthesis. Nevertheless, from the point of view of number of patients who develop HCC, this virus seems to be more important than HBV in some countries.

Chemical Carcinogens. With the progress of science and improving mode of life, various carcinogenic chemicals, mostly organic synthetic compounds, have been introduced into our lives and environment. A number of pesticides, such as DDT, once widely used, were found to be carcinogenic, and some are no longer produced. Many organic compounds may prove carcinogenic or cocarcinogenic under certain conditions, although they have gone through necessary tests for carcinogenicity and mutagenicity. The acute rise in the HCC incidence rate in Japan in recent years[257] cannot be explained by increased HCV infection alone as discussed. In Qidong County in China, north of Shanghai across the Yangtze River, farmers in the newly reclaimed coastal region had difficulty getting water from the ground. According to Su,[328] there was a crude HCC death rate of 62 to 101/100,000/yr among those who were drinking stagnant ditch water around their houses as contrasted with 0 to 11.9 deaths/100,000 among well-water drinkers. On government recommendation, many wells were dug, and the same survey made later showed a 20% to 30% reduction in HCC frequency. It was then suspected that pesticides used in farming had contaminated stagnant water. Subsequent analyses of fat tissues from

and the associated inflammatory and regenerative response constitute a preneoplastic process that inevitably evolves toward cancer if sufficient time is allowed to elapse. This hypothesis explains the fact that HCC develops in virtually every chronic liver disease in which there is continuous hepatocyte necrosis accompanied by compensatory regenerative activities.

Pathology

The gross feature of HCC varies, depending on the size of the tumor and the presence or absence of associated liver cirrhosis. Most cases of advanced HCC represent an expansile or infiltrative mass with varying numbers and sizes of intrahepatic metastases. Many of the HCCs associated with liver cirrhosis are found as a well-demarcated encapsulated tumor. Meanwhile, with increasing numbers of resected small HCCs detected by modern diagnostic imagings, it has become evident that most minute HCCs in an early stage are nodular or indiscretely nodular.[119]

The gross appearance of HCC varies in different geographic areas. According to Okuda and coworkers,[255] who compared the gross features of HCC in the United States, South Africa, and Japan, the most striking difference among these three countries was the high incidence of encapsulated HCC in Japan in contrast to that in the other countries. When one of us (M.K.) compared the gross features of HCC in Spain and Japan, no specific differences in the morphology of HCC, other than the type of associated cirrhosis, was evident; macronodular cirrhosis was predominant among Japanese cases and micronodular cirrhosis, among Spanish counterparts.[143]

Gross Pathology.

The gross anatomic classification of HCC proposed by Eggel[62a] in 1901 has been widely used up to the present time. He classified HCC into massive, nodular, and diffuse types. It has become difficult, however, to classify relatively small, surgically resected HCCs using Eggel's classification, which is based on autopsy cases with an extensively advanced tumor. Although several new classifications were proposed,[209,255] none of them has been widely accepted. The Liver Cancer Study Group of Japan[164] has recently subclassified Eggel's nodular type HCC into four types

to be adaptable to relatively small HCCs—single nodular with and without perinodular tumor growth, confluent multinodular, and multinodular. Nakashima and Kojiro[209] classified advanced HCC according to the difference in the growth pattern with consideration of capsule, cirrhosis, and portal vein tumor thrombus.

INFILTRATIVE TYPE. This type is virtually the same as the spreading type in the Okuda-Peters-Simson classification.[255] A typical infiltrative type is seen in HCC without liver cirrhosis, in which the tumor–nontumor boundary is irregular and indistinct (Fig. 44-9). In cases associated with liver cirrhosis, the tumor proliferates as if it were replacing the cirrhotic regenerative nodules. The infiltrative type of HCC accounts for about one third of autopsy cases of advanced HCC in Japan.

EXPANSIVE TYPE. The tumor mass is well demarcated, nodular, and, frequently, encapsulated. Most HCCs of this type are associated with liver cirrhosis. According to the number of tumor nodules, this type may be subclassified into single nodular and multinodular. The former is clearly demarcated and usually with a distinct fibrous capsule that is also called encapsulated HCC[250] (Fig. 44-10). The fibrous capsule is more distinct in HCCs with liver cirrhosis and seems to form when the tumor size reaches around 1.5 cm in diameter when studied in resected HCCs. This type of HCC accounts for 10% of advanced HCC. The multinodular type consists of more than two nodules of the expansive type, regardless of whether there are intrahepatic metastases or it is of unicentric or multicentric origin. Tumor nodules are nearly the same size, and it is difficult to determine whether they have arisen multicentrically and which are metastatic nodules (Fig. 44-11). This type of HCC accounts for about 8% of advanced HCCs.

MIXED EXPANSIVE AND INFILTRATIVE TYPE. The primary focus of the expansive type can be identified in association with infiltrative foci outside the capsule or intrahepatic metastases. This type of HCC constitutes about 33% of advanced HCCs.

DIFFUSE TYPE. Diffuse-type HCC almost always occurs in a cirrhotic liver and consists of numerous small tumor nodules, less than 1 cm in diameter, scattered throughout the liver, not fusing with one another (Fig. 44-12). It often is

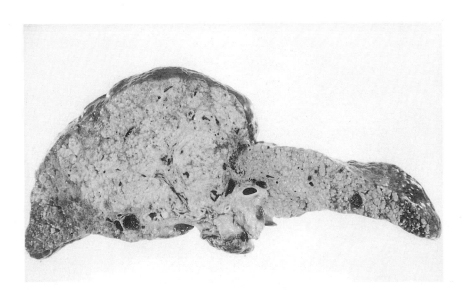

FIGURE 44-9 Hepatocellular carcinoma, infiltrative type. The tumor proliferates in an infiltrative manner without forming a distinct tumor mass or a clearly demarcated boundary with the nontumor parenchyma.

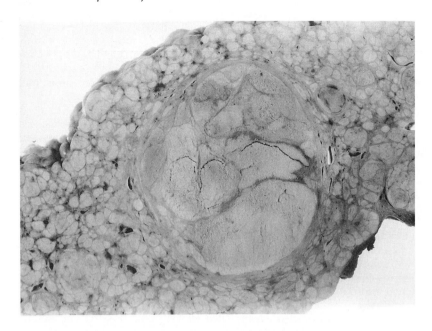

FIGURE 44-10 Encapsulated hepatocellular carcinoma. The tumor is surrounded by a thick fibrous capsule and subdivided by thin fibrous septa.

difficult to distinguish tumor nodules from regenerative nodules. Intrahepatic spreading of the tumor through the portal vein is thought to be the cause.[253] This type of HCC accounts for about 5% of advanced HCCs.

Despite the frequent intrahepatic metastases through the portal vein branches in the early stage, it is thought that extrahepatic metastases occur at a relatively late stage. The incidence of extrahepatic metastasis in HCC ranges from 50% to 70% in most reports from western countries.[58,173,273] Among our 439 autopsy cases of HCC, extrahepatic metastases were found in 63.3%. The incidence of extrahepatic metastases is slightly higher in HCC without cirrhosis than in HCC with cirrhosis. In the Los Angles series,[273] extrahepatic metastases occurred in 67% and 46.2% among HCCs without and with cirrhosis, respectively. The corresponding figures in our series are 76.1% and 60.1%. As described in the section on the growth pattern of HCC, extrahepatic me-

tastases are much more frequent in HCCs with a sinusoidal growth pattern. Hematogeneous metastases are much more common than lymphatic metastases in HCC, the frequency of the former being 48.7%, significantly higher than the 29.4% for the latter.

It is not uncommon to encounter unusual tumor growths in HCC, such as pedunculated growth, intra–bile duct growth, and intraatrial growth through the inferior vena cava. Although such unusual tumor growths were incidental findings at autopsy in the past, advances in diagnostic imaging now permit antemortem detection of them, and it is important to understand their pathomorphologic characteristics.

Pedunculated Type.   A massive extrahepatic tumor growth with little tumor invasion into the liver occasionally is encountered in advanced HCC. For some reason, a tumor that occurs in the subcapsular portion of the liver grows ex-

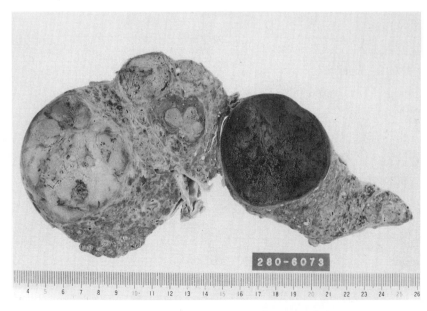

FIGURE 44-11 Hepatocellular carcinoma, multinodular type. Four well-demarcated and encapsulated tumors are seen, three in the right lobe and one in the left. The latter is dark brown, suggesting bilirubin production (green—hepatoma), and clearly of a different clone from the others.

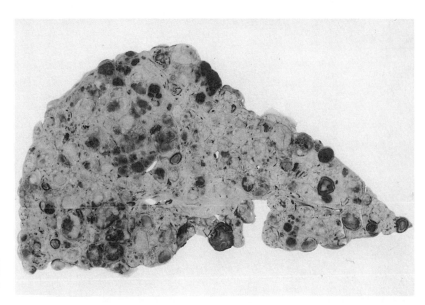

FIGURE 44-12 Hepatocellular carcinoma, diffuse type. Numerous small tumor nodules 1 to 2 cm in diameter are scattered throughout the liver with macronodular cirrhosis.

trahepatically with or without a pedicle. Also, some cases suggest tumor development in an accessory lobe.

Intra–Bile Duct Growth. Tumor invasion into the hepatic duct or common bile duct is not a rare phenomenon at autopsy, and it is seen in 2% to 6% of advanced HCCs.[139] In all patients with HCC who present with tumor invasion into a major bile duct, progressive obstructive jaundice is a major clinical sign. Patients with an HCC that is growing into the bile duct have a significantly shorter survival after diagnosis than other patients with HCC. We found a prominent tumor growth in the hepatic duct or common bile duct in 27 (6.1%) of the 439 autopsies, and progressive obstructive jaundice was the initial sign in 13 of them. Among the patients presenting with obstructive jaundice caused by intra–bile duct tumor growth, those with normal or low AFP levels were clinically thought to have bile duct carcinoma or stones. Intraductal growth is not merely one of the terminal events

in HCC but is mostly due to direct invasion of an infiltrative tumor located near the biliary tract; it seldom comes from a massive tumor thrombus in the portal vein. Massive hemorrhage into the bile duct (hemobilia) occurs occasionally (Fig. 44-13), causing hypovolemic shock that leads to death.

Intraatrial Growth. It is not uncommon to find a tumor growth in the right atrium in malignant neoplasms, such as HCC, renal cell carcinoma, pulmonary carcinoma, and pancreatic carcinoma. It is possible that recent prolongation of patients' survival has increased its frequency. Edmondson and Steiner[58] observed tumor extension into the right atrium in only 1 of 100 autopsy cases of primary liver cancer and MacDonald,[173] in 3 of 108 cases of HCC. In our series of 439 cases, tumor extended into the vena cava inferior in 48 (10.9%) and into the right atrium in 18 (4.8%) (Fig. 44-14). A tumor bolus crossed the tricuspid valves and entered the ventricle in five of them, and direct tumor inva-

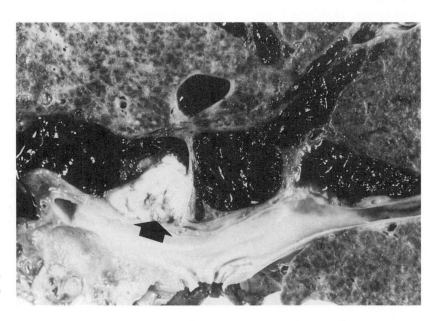

FIGURE 44-13 Bleeding in the major biliary tract (hemobilia) caused by tumor invasion into the hepatic duct (*arrow*).

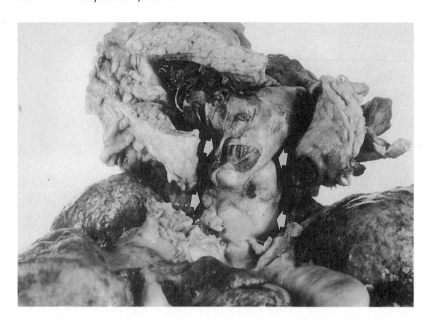

FIGURE 44-14 Intraatrial tumor growth (*arrows*) through the inferior vena cava.

sion into the myocardium was found in two. Most such patients have marked diuretic-resistant edema in the lower extremities and venous dilatation in the abdominal wall.[140] We have encountered only one patient who died of sudden cardiac arrest caused by tricuspid obstruction. It has been documented that intermittent tricuspid obstruction by a ball-shaped thrombus causes the so-called ball-valve thrombus syndrome, characterized by dyspnea of the oxygen hunger type, feeble or absent pulses during the attack, a changing heart murmur, and relief produced by changing the position.[88] Tumor extension into the right atrium was detected by angiography or ultrasonography 3 to 4 months before death in five of our cases, but none had serious cardiac symptoms.

Histology

The histologic structure of HCC resembles that of a normal liver, in that the tumor parenchyma comprises a liver cell cord-like (trabecular) structure and the stroma consists of a sinusoid-like blood space lined by a single layer of endothelial cells. The histology of HCC varies with a combination of the following features: the structural pattern (trabecular, pseudoglandular, solid, sclerosing), difference in the degree of cancer cell differentiation (well, moderately, poorly, undifferentiated), and cytologic variants (eg, bile production, clear cells, fatty change, cytoplasmic hyalin, ground-glass inclusion, pleomorphism, sarcomatoid; Fig. 44-15).

World Health Organization Classification. The histologic classification proposed by the World Health Organization (WHO) has been accepted worldwide.

TRABECULAR TYPE (SINUSOIDAL). The tumor cells grow in cords of variable thickness separated by flat endothelial cells. The endothelial cells, usually inconspicuous, sharply define the trabeculae. In well-differentiated HCC, the tumor cells are arranged in two- to three-cell thickness, presenting a thin trabecular pattern (Fig. 44-16A).

PSEUDOGLANDULAR TYPE (ACINAR). This type of HCC shows a variety of gland-like structures, but the basic trabecular structure remains recognizable (see Fig. 44-16B). Can-

aliculi, with or without bile, often are recognizable and may be dilated into gland-like spaces.

COMPACT TYPE. This is basically a trabecular pattern, but the tumor cells grow in an apparently solid mass and the blood spaces are rendered inconspicuous by compression (see Fig. 44-16C).

SCIRRHOUS TYPE. Areas with abundant fibrous stroma separating cords of tumor cells are most often seen after radiation, chemotherapy, or infarction (see Fig. 44-16D). This appearance should be distinguished from those of CCC and metastatic carcinoma. Furthermore, this type of HCC should not be confused with HCC of the fibrolamellar type.[44]

Histologic Variants. Fibrolamellar carcinoma is a variant of HCC with unique clinicopathologic characteristics. It mostly occurs in the noncirrhotic livers of adolescents or young adults.[44] Grossly, the tumor is well demarcated, but the boundary is irregular. Histologically, the tumor cells proliferate in small trabeculae with thick, lamellar, and, frequently, hyalinized collagen (Fig. 44-17). Calcification commonly is observed in the lamellar stroma. Tumor cells are large, have abundant eosinophilic cytoplasm, and typically contain cytoplasmic inclusions, such as eosinophilic globules, pale bodies, and Mallory bodies.

Sarcomatous features consisting of spindle-shaped or pleomorphic anaplastic tumor cells occasionally are found in part of the HCC with or without a transitional feature between trabecular HCC and the sarcomatous area.[142] Although it is difficult to determine whether the sarcomatous features are due to such changes occurring in a portion of HCC or to the coexistence of HCC and sarcoma, we believe that the former is the case. In fact, in the revised edition of *Histological Typing of Tumors of the Liver*, published by WHO, HCC with sarcomatous changes is listed as a sarcomatoid variant of HCC (Ishak KG, personal communication, March 1991). We found 14 HCC cases (3.9%) that exhibited a sarcomatous appearance among 355 consecutive autopsy cases. It is conceivable that a certain proportion of sarcomatous HCCs were caused by morphologic or phenotypic changes caused by anticancer therapy because the incidence of sarcomatous

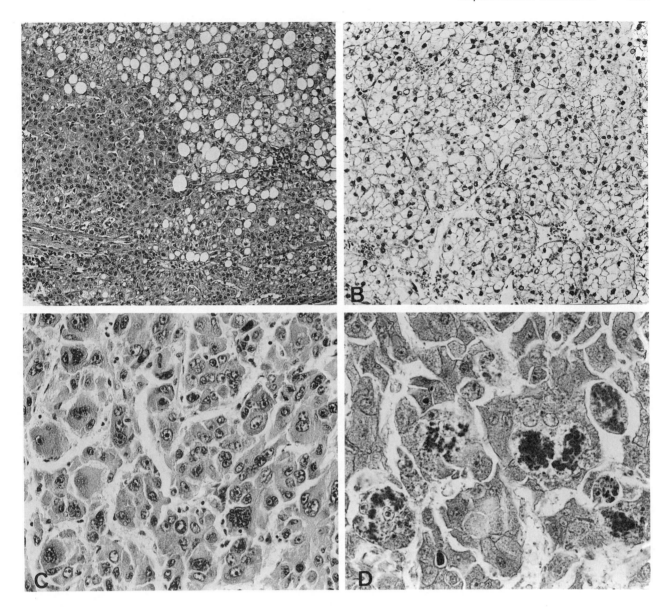

FIGURE 44-15 Cytologic variations of hepatocellular carcinoma. (**A**) Fatty changes seen in a well-differentiated carcinoma. (**B**) Clear cell carcinoma. (**C**) Giant cell carcinoma. (**D**) Mallory's bodies in hepatocellular carcinoma cells.

changes was significantly higher among HCC cases treated by transcatheter arterial embolization compared with non-treated cases.[142]

Histologic Growth Pattern. The histologic growth patterns at the tumor-nontumor boundary can be divided into two basic patterns—replacing and sinusoidal.[211]

REPLACING GROWTH PATTERN. This is considered to be the basic growth pattern in HCC, and almost all minute HCCs in the early stage grow in a replacing manner. In this pattern, tumor cells grow as if they were replacing the hepatocytes within the liver cell cords (Fig. 44-18A). When the tumor reaches a size of around 1.5 cm, it comes to grow expansively, and a fibrous capsule forms at the tumor-nontumor boundary. When the tumor grows beyond the capsule, it grows in a replacing pattern.

SINUSOIDAL GROWTH PATTERN. In the sinusoidal growth pattern, the tumor cells, which lack mutual cohesiveness, grow in the sinusoids at the boundary in an infiltrative manner; atrophied liver cell cords and hepatocytes are seen in the cancerous tissue around the boundary (see Fig. 44-18B). The incidence of extrahepatic metastasis is significantly higher in HCC with the sinusoidal growth pattern than in HCC with the replacing growth pattern.[313]

Pathomorphologic Characteristics of Minute Hepatocellular Carcinoma or Hepatocellular Carcinoma in the Early Stage

The most striking morphologic characteristics of small HCCs in the early stage is that most are well differentiated.[145] Those well-differentiated small HCCs are characterized by a various combination of the following features: (1) increased cellular-

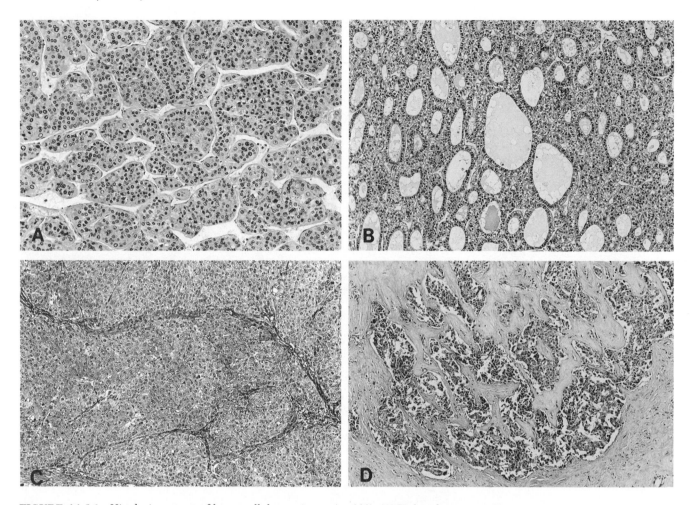

FIGURE 44-16   Histologic patterns of hepatocellular carcinoma (× 100). (**A**) Trabecular pattern. Tumor nests are covered by a single layer of endothelial cells. (**B**) Pseudoglandular (acinar) pattern. Glandular structures of varying size are prominent, but the trabecular pattern is still discerned. (**C**) Compact pattern. Tumor cells are arranged in a solid manner and divided by thin fibrous bands. (**D**) Scirrhous pattern. Blood spaces of the tumor are replaced by hyalinized connective tissue (stroma), and tumor nests are separated by the proliferating connective tissue.

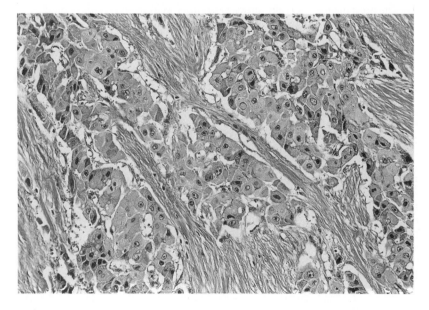

FIGURE 44-17   Fibrolamellar carcinoma. The tumor cells have abundant eosinophilic cytoplasm, and lamellar fibrous stroma is characteristic.

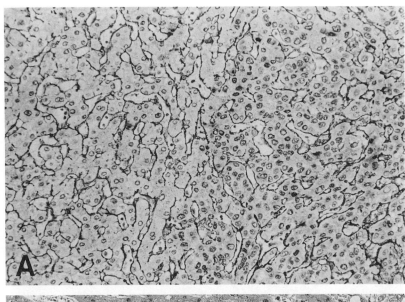

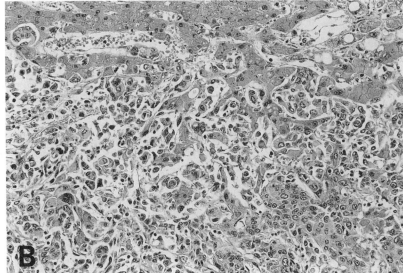

FIGURE 44-18 (**A**) Replacing growth pattern. Cancer cells (*right half*) are proliferating as if they were replacing adjacent hepatocytes within the liver cell cord. The reticulin framework is contiguous and not distorted or disrupted at the boundary (reticulin stain, × 200). (**B**) Sinusoidal growth pattern. Poorly differentiated cancer cells of the free-cell type or low cohesiveness are proliferating along the sinusoids in an infiltrative manner (× 200).

ity with an increased nucleus/cytoplasm ratio and increased staining affinity (eosinophilic or basophilic); (2) irregular, thin trabecular pattern with frequent pseudoglandular or acinar structures; and (3) frequent fatty changes (Fig. 44-19). In about one third of minute HCCs up to 2 cm in diameter, the tumor nodule consists of more than two cancerous tissues of different groups of cells of varying grades of differentiation, from well to moderately differentiated. Less differentiated cancerous tissues are almost always surrounded by well-differentiated ones, and the areas of well-differentiated cancerous tissues diminish in size as the tumor size increases.[128] The so-called slow-growing hepatoma, which grows slowly or expands little in a period from 1 to several years, occasionally has been encountered. Serial biopsy study of such tumors revealed that most were well differentiated, demonstrating a slow dedifferentiation or remaining in a well-differentiated state. Thus, it seems that the dedifferentiation phenomenon that occurs as a result of replacement of well-differentiated cancerous tissues by less differentiated cancerous tissue is responsible for tumor proliferation.[144]

Clinical Features

Past and Personal Histories. Many patients with HCC in developed countries in which adults often undergo a medical checkup have current or past histories of chronic liver disease. In a survey conducted by the Liver Cancer Study Group of Japan during the period of 1986 to 1987,[165] 339 of 2319 cases (23%) of HCC had a history of blood transfusion and about one third had an alcohol intake of more than 85 g/d ethanol for more than 10 years. About 60% were aware of having cirrhosis, and about 50% of them had past or ongoing chronic hepatitis. A history of acute hepatitis was elicited in about one sixth of these patients, but it could have been an acute exacerbation of chronic B hepatitis in HBsAg-positive cases. Past history of blood transfusion is perhaps related to HCV infection.

Presenting Symptoms. As shown in Table 44-8, general malaise, upper abdominal pain, anorexia, abdominal full sensation, weight loss, ascites, palpable mass, nausea,

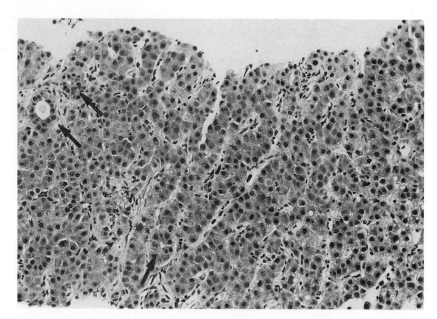

FIGURE 44-19   Well-differentiated hepatocellular carcinoma seen in a biopsy specimen taken under ultrasound guidance from a hypoechoic tumor 1.3 cm in diameter. It consists of tumor cells showing an irregular, thin trabecular pattern with occasional pseudogland structure (*arrows*; × 100).

vomiting, jaundice, fever, leg edema, hematemesis, and melena are the presenting symptoms among Japanese patients.[165] Among South African rural blacks, most patients present with abdominal pain and 35% have fever.[130] Symptoms mainly caused by cirrhosis, such as ascites, pedal edema, and jaundice, are more common among the former, and the differences seem to be due to more frequent advanced cirrhosis in Japanese patients. In one survey, the symptoms of HCC associated with cirrhosis were compared with those of HCC not associated with cirrhosis; it was found that abdominal pain and palpable mass were more frequent in patients without cirrhosis.[244] High fever often is associated with poorly differentiated HCC,[260] and in fact, liver pathology

shows frequent poorly differentiated HCC[324] in South African blacks, many of whom present with high fever. In a Hong Kong series, presenting symptoms included, beside the listed ones, hypoglycemia (2%), diarrhea (2%), encephalopathy, and dyspnea caused by pleural effusion.[152] Among the predominantly white patients seen in Spain, liver failure signs such as ascites (51.6%), jaundice (32.0%), and encephalopathy (17.1%) are much more common and abdominal pain is less frequent (26.1%).[30] These data are based on patients with advanced or overt HCC. Small HCCs, more frequently detected in recent years by improved imaging techniques and regular checkup of chronic liver disease, usually are not associated with any symptoms caused by tumor. In our study

TABLE 44-8   *Comparison of Early Symptoms in Patients With HCC*

	Occurrence (%)	
Symptom	*Japan (1986–1987)**	*South Africa (1982)†*
General malaise	59.4	34
Abdominal pain	45.3	95
Anorexia	43.8	25
Abdominal full sensation	43.3	
Weight loss	25.7	34
Ascites	22.7	
Palpable mass	21.7	43 (Abdominal swelling)
Nausea, vomiting	15.4	10
Jaundice	14.7	5
Fever	14.7	35
Leg edema	14.3	
Hematemesis, melena	5.4	2
Acute abdominal catastrophe		10
Bone pain		3

HCC, hepatocellular carcinoma.
*Taken from the 9th Report of the Japan Liver Cancer Study Group (2520 cases).
†Data from Kew MC, Geddes EW. Hepatocellular carcinoma in rural South African blacks. Medicine 61:98, 1982. (548 cases).

of 51 cases of HCC smaller than 5 cm, no abdominal pain was reported and only 13.7% of the cases complained of a full sensation of the abdomen after meals.[312]

Clinical Manifestations. When the patient is found to have a liver mass, which usually is the case in countries that have no early-detection program, the upper abdomen visibly protrudes. On auscultation, an arterial bruit commonly is heard over the mass, suggesting a hypervascular or an arterialized tumor. The right diaphgram often is elevated. Sometimes only the left lobe is enlarged by the mass. According to Kew and Geddes,[130] arterial bruit is audible over the liver in 23% of African black patients. Table 44-9 lists the frequency of major objective physical signs. Ascites and jaundice are mostly caused by preexisting cirrhosis and tumor invasion. Berman[16] divided his patients seen in Johannesburg into five clinical types: frank cancer (typical presentation), acute abdominal cancer (rupture and hemoperitoneum), febrile cancer, occult cancer (patients seen for other reasons and tumor found), and metastatic cancer (such as bone metastasis). This classification applies only to advanced cases. The size of cancer in patients seen at major gastrointestinal centers in Japan is smaller than 5 cm in more than half, and these patients have only the signs attributable to cirrhosis. Thus, a comparable classification in Japan should have an additional group that may be called cirrhotic type.[238] In our series of 376 cases, 11 (2.9%) were rushed to the hospital because of abdominal pain, rapidly progressing anemia, and enlarging abdominal girth. This acute abdominal type is much more common, occurring in 8%[16] to 10%[130] of patients in South Africa, perhaps because of rapid tumor growth. In Hong Kong, 42 of 207 patients with HCC seen at a surgical unit up to 1972 had a ruptured tumor.[265] In a Japanese series of 11 such cases, 7 were spontaneous and 4 were caused by a trivial traumatic injury.[201] Palpation of a large liver with suspected HCC should be done with utmost caution. Emergency celiac angiography may be carried out for arterial embolization, which stops the bleeding as shown in Figure 44-20. At autopsy, ascites typically is bloody, and hemoperitoneum without an acute sign is common in the preterminal stage. In a Bangkok series of 459 cases of primary liver cancer, 55 had hemoperitoneum on admission, and 53 of them had no dramatic symptoms; all had abdominal pain of varing degree, however.[276]

Some patients present with rapidly progressive jaundice with or without pain, suggestive of gallstones or obstructive jaundice. This type of presentation may be called cholestatic type.[238] In our series, 1.9% of the patients were of this type. It is due to cancer invasion into a major bile duct or to hemobilia, as described earlier (Fig. 44-21). Before the advent of direct cholangiography, such patients often were operated on for suspected stone disease. On opening the biliary tract, hemobilia, blood clots, or a frail material containing necrotized tumor tissue may be seen. Sometimes a separate clot is found lodged in the distal end of the common bile duct.

Because a considerable proportion of the patients have portal hypertension, variceal bleeding could be the first clinical presentation. In a national survey conducted in 1979 in Japan, esophageal varices were recorded in 23.1% of 2411 cases,[252] but this figure would have been much higher if endoscopy were done in all. In a Spanish series, 19.7% had gastrointestinal bleeding.[30] According to Nakashima,[208] 8.2% of patients with HCC not associated with cirrhosis had varices on autopsy, probably caused by tumor invasion into the hepatic and portal vein systems. Cooney and associates[43] described a patient without cirrhosis who developed portal hypertension as a result of microscopic tumor invasion in the central veins and small portal radicles. In HCC associated with cirrhosis, portal invasion of HCC does not cause a sudden, marked increase in portal pressure because of the preexisting portal hypertension. Although uncommon outside South Africa, fever may be the presenting symptom, and if there is marked leukocytosis, the clinical picture is exactly that of liver abscess. The tumor typically is anaplastic and may appear sarcomatous in places. In our series, it occurred in 2.1%, but about one third of South African black patients have fever.[16,130] In some patients, the presenting symptom is due to extrahepatic metastasis, such as a lump on the head.

Diagnosis
Although histologic diagnosis is ideal, biopsy entails a certain risk of bleeding, particularly when the target mass is near the liver surface. HCC is known for its frailty and arterial hypervascularity. The diagnosis of HCC is still possible without histologic confirmation if the liver is cirrhotic, space-occupying lesions are discerned by imaging, and serum levels of AFP or des-γ-carboxy prothrombin are high. The diagnosis of cirrhosis is not difficult with modern imaging. In areas

TABLE 44-9 *Physical Findings in HCC at Diagnosis*

Series	Physical Findings (%)				
	Hepatomegaly	Ascites	Splenomegaly	Jaundice	Others
South Africa, 1982[130]	92	51	42	28	Arterial bruit, 23; Dilated abdominal veins, 22
Japan, 1980[252]	67.2	43.6	14.4	30.6	Varices, 23
United States, Virginia, 1971[46]	92	27		33	Gastrointestinal bleed, 30
Spain, 1990[30]	92.3	51.6	40.6	17.1	Encephalopathy, 17; Gastrointestinal bleed, 20

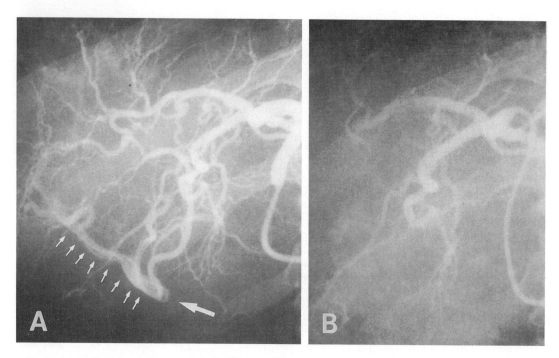

FIGURE 44-20   Acute hemoperitoneum. (**A**) Emergency celiac angiography demonstrated flow of contrast medium from one of the branches of the posterior hepatic artery into the abdominal cavity (*small arrows*). The large arrow points to the bleeding site. (**B**) Transcatheter arterial embolization using Gelfoam particles stopped bleeding.

where HCC is endemic, identification of a space-occupying lesion in a cirrhotic liver is highly diagnostic of HCC because metastasis from other organs to the liver is uncommon[186]; HCC evolves in the liver in such patients before any other type of carcinoma develops.

Laboratory Findings

Hematology.   Pancytopenia may be present as a result of splenomegaly caused by portal hypertension. Rapidly progressive anemia is suggestive of bleeding from the tumor into the peritoneal cavity. Erythrocytosis as a paraneoplastic syndrome is uncommon but does occur (see below). Leukocytosis is common,[238] and a count exceeding 20,000/μL could be due to elaboration of a G-CSF–like substance by the tumor tissue, although no such study has been made.

Blood Chemistry.   In the advanced stage, serum levels of aspartate aminotransferase (AST), alanine aminotransferase (ALT), lactate dehydrogenase (LDH), and alkaline phosphatase (ALP) are elevated. An important biochemical feature of HCC is a large difference between AST and ALT, the former being higher and the difference becoming greater with the progression of the disease.[309] In some patients, ALP levels are markedly elevated perhaps because of increased tumor-specific ALP. Isoenzyme LDH_5 usually is higher than LDH_4 in HCC, whereas the reverse is common with metastatic liver cancer.[238] Marked hypercholesterolemia is common in Ugandan patients, according to Alpert and colleagues,[5] but it is less common elsewhere.[153,238] In a study in Spain, 13 (5.2%) 249 patients had cholesterol levels higher than 300 mg/dL,[30] and 13.6% of rural black patients in Johannesburg showed cholesterol levels above 250 mg/dL.[130]

Tumor-Specific Proteins.   Tumor cells produce certain embryonic proteins because of chromosomal dedifferentiation, and some of these oncofetal proteins are used for diagnosis.

α-FETOPROTEIN.   α-Fetoprotein, a glycoprotein with an electrophoretic mobility of $α_1$-globulin, is produced in the fetal yolk sac, liver, and intestine. The biologic properties of AFP and albumin are similar, and the major control of AFP synthesis is at the level of gene transcription. After birth, production of AFP is almost totally repressed, and the serum concentration decreases to less than 20 ng/mL. Values above 1000 ng/mL are highly suggestive of HCC. Because levels above 400 ng/mL seldom are seen in benign liver diseases, values around 400 ng/mL often are used as the cutoff value to make the test specific for HCC.[238]

Although AFP is the most important diagnostic marker with a relatively high specificity and sensitivity and has been extensively used in the clinical setting,[131,246] it seldom proves diagnostic in small HCCs.[56,312] Radioimmunoassay is the most sensitive, and the reported positivity rates vary with the method used. Although the figures obtained in western countries were low, the material might have included fibrolamellar carcinoma, which does not produce AFP.

Serum AFP levels increase after massive or submassive hepatic necrosis in patients who survive, but it is not simply due to hepatocyte regeneration because no such increase occurs after hepatic resection.[346] In patients with chronic hepatitis and cirrhosis, serum AFP levels often fluctuate between 20 and 1000 ng/mL, reflecting necrosis and liver cell regeneration. One point value in this range is unreliable, and follow-up measurements are necessary. When AFP levels continuously rise at an exponential rate, the patient probably has HCC. AFP production by HCC is age-related, and younger

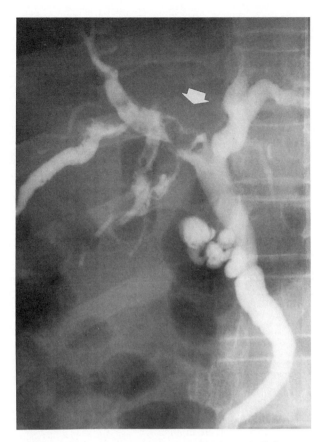

FIGURE 44-21 Intraductal invasion by hepatocellular carcinoma (*arrow*) seen in this percutaneous transhepatic cholangiogram.

patients are more likely to have elevated serum levels. Although AFP synthesis seems to be related to the degree of tumor cell differentiation in chemically induced HCC in mice, no such correlation is demonstrable in human HCC, nor are serum AFP levels shown to correlate with clinical and biochemical indices of HCC.[131] The number of carcinoma cells with stainable AFP is roughly proportional to serum AFP levels,[139] but other hepatocytes, particularly proliferating oval cells, may also contain stainable AFP.

FUCOSYLATED AFP. It has recently been shown that HCC-derived AFP is fucosylated at N-acetyl-glucosamine, whereas the AFP molecule derived from the yolk sac is not.[383] Binding of AFP to lentil can be used to distinguish HCC from benign liver diseases; a significantly higher proportion of AFP binds to lentil lectin in patients with HCC (45%) than in those with benign liver diseases (4%).[8] Similarly, binding to jack bean lectin (concanavalin A) may distinguish HCC from other AFP-producing tumors. Lentil lectin binding may be useful in identifying presymptomatic HCC in patients with a slightly or moderately elevated AFP concentration,[7] and concanavalin A–reactive AFP is more useful in assessing response to chemotherapy than are total serum AFP levels.[12] Taketa and coworkers[347] suggested that simultaneous analysis of lentil lectin A–reactive AFP-L$_3$ and erythroagglutinating phytohemagglutinin–reactive AFP-P$_4$ was effective in monitoring the evolution of HCC in patients with cirrhosis.

DES-γ-CARBOXY PROTHROMBIN. In the synthesis of prothrombin (factor II), vitamin K (K) is required in the γ-car-boxylation of the glutamic acid residue (Glu) of prothrombin precursors. In K deficiency or after ingestion of K antagonists, such as warfarin, the 10 Glu of the prothrombin molecule are not fully carboxylated. As a result, des-γ-carboxy prothrombin (DCP), which lacks the coagulant activity, appears in blood. This abnormal prothrombin is also called PIVKA-II (protein induced by vitamin K absence or antagonist-II).

The diagnostic significance of DCP was first demonstrated in 1984 by Liebman and associates.[161] Motohara and colleagues[197] developed an enzyme-linked immunosorbent assay for the diagnosis of pediatric K deficiency using a monoclonal antibody raised against DCP, and DCP measured by this method was positive in 59% of Japanese patients with HCC (Fig. 44-22). It has also been found that DCP elevation is more specific for HCC than AFP. There is no correlation between DCP and AFP levels in patients with HCC, and the combination of these two tests should improve nonimaging diagnosis of HCC.[235] The chromogenic assay that uses staphylocoagulase[322] or *Dispholidus typus* venom[135] gives the same results.

Hepatoma cells in culture produce DCP in the absence of K, but its production decreases on addition of this vitamin.[236] Plasma DCP levels also decline on administration of K to patients.[75] The exact mechanism for the production of DCP by HCC cells is not known.

The K-dependent plasma proteins include, besides prothrombin, many other coagulation factors. They all have 10 to 12 Gla in the structure. If not all of Glu change to Gla, the resultant des-γ-carboxy forms (PIVKAs) of these proteins appear in blood, such as PIVKA-PC and PIVKA-IX.[237] They may also serve as additional markers.

VARIANT ALKALINE PHOSPHATASE. There are several isoenzymes of ALP of which only variant ALP is known to appear in HCC. It has also been called hepatoma ALP and Kasahara isoenzyme, but the frequency with which this enzyme is demonstrated in HCC is low.

NOVEL γ-GLUTAMYLTRANSPEPTIDASE ISOENZYME. Experimental studies have shown that γ-glutamyltranspeptidase (γ-GTP) is strikingly activated during the course of tumorigenesis in animals and that it is significantly increased in liver cells both during the precancerous stage and when HCC develops.[364] Like AFP, γ-GTP activity is low in the adult liver, but it is high in the fetal liver and in HCC. Sawabu and coworkers[300] demonstrated three hepatoma-specific novel γ-GTP isoenzymes using a polyacrylamide gradient gel electrophoresis. They were present in 55% of patients with HCC in contrast to a near zero positivity in other liver diseases or cancers. Similar results have been reported from South Africa.[132] The activities of γ-GTP isoenzymes are low in serum, and a diagnostic kit has not been produced commercially.

CARCINOEMBRYONIC ANTIGEN. Carcinoembryonic antigen (CEA) is a useful but not infallible marker of advanced digestive tract cancers, particularly in colorectal cancer and extensive metastatic liver cancer. CEA usually is not elevated in HCC, and differential diagnosis between HCC and metastatic liver cancer becomes more accurate if both AFP and CEA are measured in serum. Aburano and associates[2] showed that the predictive value for HCC with positive AFP alone was 80% and rose to 91% when negative CEA was combined.

α-L-FUCOSIDASE. α-L-Fucosidase (AFU) is a lysosomal hydrolase, and a number of its isoenzymes have been identified in human tissues, including two hepatic forms. Deug-

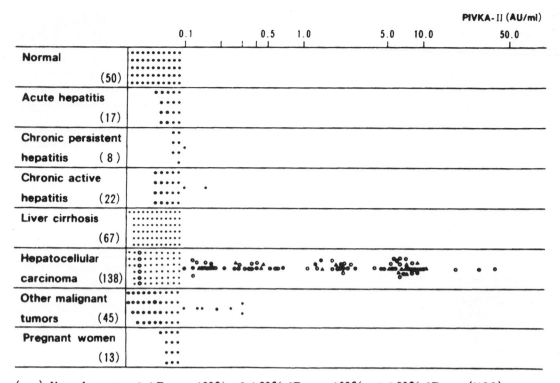

FIGURE 44-22 Plasma levels of des-γ-carboxy prothrombin (PIVKA-II) in hepatocellular carcinoma and other diseases. Specificity of this test is higher than that of α-fetoprotein, and high levels are mostly associated with large tumors. Percentages in the marginal note give tumor size on two-dimensional image.

nier and colleagues[52] first noted elevated serum AFU levels in patients with HCC and later reported a sensitivity of 75% and a specificity of 90% in European patients with HCC. The same sensitivity with a lower specificity rate of 70% subsequently was found in black patients.[27] The number of false-negative AFP results could be reduced from 13% to 5.5% if AFU and AFP were used together. Thus, AFU combined with AFP may be useful in regions with a low incidence of HCC.

THROMBIN–ANTITHROMBIN III COMPLEX. Although hypercoagulability in cancer has long been known, it has not been applied to the diagnosis. Thrombin that converts fibrinogen to fibrin is mainly inactivated by antithrombin III (ATIII), which forms a covalent, irreversible 1:1 complex in the physiologic state. Thus, thrombin–antithrombin III complex (TAT) is thought to be a sensitive parameter of thrombin generation even when hepatic dysfunction is present. Tomiya and Fujiwara[362] determined plasma levels of TAT in patients with cirrhosis with and without HCC using immunopurified polyclonal rabbit antibodies to human thrombin as the solid phase and antibodies to human ATIII as the liquid phase. The levels were above 2 ng/mL in 80% of patients with HCC but only in 12% of patients with cirrhosis but without HCC ($P < .01$). Levels over 2 ng/mL occurred in five of six patients with HCC with normal AFP levels and in two of three patients with HCC less than 2 cm in diameter. There was no correlation between plasma TAT levels and AFP or DCP levels.[362]

TRANSCOBALAMIN 1. In 1973, Waxman and Gilbert[375] noted marked elevation of vitamin B_{12} levels in serum in ad-

olescent patients with primary liver cancer. This was due to elevation of transcobalamin 1 (TC 1), a vitamin B_{12}–binding protein in serum. Subsequent studies indicated that these young patients with increased serum TC 1 levels had fibrolamellar carcinoma of the liver and that TC 1 was produced by fibrolamellar cancer cells.[270] This type of cancer also seems to be associated with increased levels of neurotensin, a gut hormone.[41]

OTHER TUMOR-SPECIFIC PROTEINS. Other biochemical markers suggested as being diagnostic or frequently increased in patients with HCC include ferritin, isoferritin, basic fetoprotein, tissue polypeptide antigen, aldolase isoenzyme-type A, glutathione S transferase isoenzyme type B, carbohydrate antigen 19-9, calcitonin, and the tumor-associated isoenzyme of 5-nucleotide phosphodiesterase. These markers do not seem to be of practical significance in the diagnosis of HCC.

Systemic Manifestations Related to Humoral Effects of Tumor

HCC occasionally is associated with an unusual symptom caused by metabolic effects of the tumor (paraneoplastic syndrome). The underlying mechanism for such clinical manifestations is thought to be either synthesis by the tumor of certain proteins, hormones, and hormone-like substances; altered metabolism as a result of loss of regulatory mechanism; increased utilization of normal constituents of plasma by the massive tumor tissue; or decrease in their production because of insufficient remaining liver tissue.

Erythrocytosis. Erythrocytosis is uncommon in HCC, expt for one study in Hong Kong reporting a 10% incidence. According to Ohta and coworkers,[226] there were 34 cases of HCC associated with erythrocytosis in the Japanese literature from 1974 to 1980. Considering the large number of patients seen in Japan, this number clearly suggests rarity of the syndrome. In a recent national survey in Japan, only 22 cases of erythrocytosis out of 2635 patients were studied (0.8%).[165] Such patients usually have underlying cirrhosis, and because of an expanded plasma volume, hematocrit values may be lower than they would be in the absence of cirrhosis; an increasing red blood cell count in cirrhosis may suggest HCC in endemic areas. Although erythropoietin levels commonly are elevated in serum, some patients have normal values, and the evidence that cancer is producing erythropoietin is still equivocal. An analysis of the reports in Japan has shown that erythropoietin was elevated in plasma in 13 of 17 cases, urinary erythropoietin increased in seven of eight cases and cancer tissue erythropoietin increased in two of seven cases.[226] Other mechanisms that elevate plasma erythropoietin levels in the absence of excess production have also been suggested.

Hypoglycemia. Hypoglycemia usually does not occur in patients with a small HCC. The reported prevalence varies up to 27%. Most Japanese studies suggest a prevalence of 3% to 8%,[226] but in a recent national survey (1986 to 1987), hypoglycemia was noted in only 20 of 2589 cases (0.8%).[165] According to the analysis of 75 cases reported in 1974 to 1980 in Japan, average liver weight was 3191 g, and the lowest blood glucose level ranged from 4 to 51 mg/dL (average, 21.9 mg/dL).[226] McFadzean and Yeung[184] divided HCC-associated hypoglycemia into two types based on clinical and pathologic features. Type A tumor, which constitutes 83%, is poorly differentiated histologically and fast-growing, patients rapidly develop wasting and profound muscle weakness, and hypoglycemia is a preterminal phenomenon. Type B tumor is well differentiated, slow-growing, weight loss and muscle weakness occur only preterminally, but hypoglycemia develops early and tumor cells contain large amounts of glycogen. Types A and B cannot be explained by the same mechanism. A number of biochemical derangements have been proposed. Production of insulin or insulin-like substances by the tumor is an attractive theory, but it has not been verified by immunologic means. Generation of hypoglycemic substances has also been suggested. Other possible mechanisms include increased utility of glucose by the tumor—neoplastic cells usually have a high rate of glycolysis and increased blood lactate levels are consistent with it; decrease of glucose production by the liver is another possibility, and reduced glycogenolysis is suggested in type B tumors.

In the reports made in Japan during the period of 1974 to 1980, blood immunoreactive insulin (IRI) levels were lower than normal in 46 of 52, tumor tissue was negative for IRI in 4 of 5 studied, glycogen was increased in liver tissue in 3 of 7 and in tumor tissue in 10 of 18, cancer cells contained glycogen granules in 10 of 18, and islet cells in the pancreas were hyperplastic in 5 of 35.[226] These results failed to come up with a single mechanism for explanation.

Hypercalcemia. Pseudoparathyroidism or hypercalcemia in the absence of bone destruction or parathyroid adenoma occasionally is observed in HCC, and the production of parathyroid hormone or like substances has been suspected. This theory is supported by the observations that tumor resection normalizes blood calcium levels and removal of the parathyroid gland does not improve hypercalcemia. Cochrane and Williams[40] measured parathyroid hormone in the hepatic and portal veins in one patient with HCC and demonstrated a large gradient; after liver transplantation, blood calcium and parathyroid hormone levels returned to normal. For reasons that are unclear, hypercalcemia is a relatively common feature in sclerosing carcinoma of the liver.[263]

Other Tumor-Associated Syndromes. Less common syndromes reported include dysfibrinogenemia,[370] increased fibrinolytic activity in plasma,[151] cryofibrinogenemia,[15] PCT with increased uroporphyrin,[357] hypertrophic pulmonary osteoarthropathy,[192] and carcinoid syndrome. The Japanese literature on HCC-associated biochemical and hematologic syndromes in the 1974 to 1980 period documented the following 30 cases: hyperfibrinogenemia in 6 patients, hypercalcemia in 5, thrombocythemia in 5, leukocytosis in 3, monoclonal gammopathy in 2, and hypergammaglobulinemia, thyroxin-binding globulinemia, hypercholine-esterasemia, hypergonadotropinemia, allylamidasemia, hyperkalemia, eosinophilia, porphyria, and citrullinemia in 1 patient each.[226]

Imaging Diagnosis

Plain Radiography. Chest films may demonstrate elevation of the right hemidiaphragm or coin lesions in the lung fields. Localized diaphragmatic elevation must be differentiated from partial eventration of the diaphragm, which is common among the aged in the Far East. In South African blacks with HCC, only 36% showed normal chest films. Hepatomegaly may be discerned on plain abdominal films, and displaced duodenal gas is an indirect sign of hepatomegaly.

Radionuclide Scanning. In the past, scintigraphy using radioactive colloids commonly was done[243] for the detection of space-occupying lesions, which are seen as cold (photopenic) areas. Even with single-photon emission computed tomography (SPECT)[24] or positron CT, the sensitivity is still inferior to ultrasonography and x-ray CT. Only half of hepatic lesions about 2 cm in size are visualized by SPECT. For these reasons, radionuclide scanning is much less frequently carried out for the diagnosis of hepatic tumors. In the recent national survey, it was found that radionuclide examination was carried out in only 37.1% of 2633 patients with HCC.[165] Instead of visualizing mass lesions as negative images, there are several ways to demonstrate them as positive hot images—intravenous administration of gallium-69, indium-111,[1] technetium-99m hepatobiliary imaging agents,[91] and subtraction of colloid scan from selenomethionine-75 scan.[39] Gallium-67 is taken up by HCC, but there are many false-positive scans; indium behaves like gallium. Selenomethionine-75 has a relatively long biologic half-life in humans[39] and is not a good radionuclide. HCC takes up organic anions such as hepatobiliary imaging agents, as do hepatocytes, but it is incapable of excreting them into bile and, therefore, retains the agent for a long period. If images are made several hours after intravenous administration of a biliary agent, HCC may be visualized as a hot lesion against the background of liver parenchyma, which by that time has cleared the agent. More than half the Japanese patients with HCC show such hot images by this technique,[91] and a similar figure is reported in Spain.[29] By contrast, no such imaging was obtained in South African blacks perhaps because HCC is more frequently poorly differentiated (see earlier discussion) and does not share the metabolic function with normal hepatocytes.[299]

Taking advantage of the hypervascularity of HCC, blood pool scanning may be done just to see whether the lesion seen as a defect on a colloid scan is vascular (tumor) or avascular (abscess). To that end, technetium-99m–colloid,[323] technetium-99m–labeled erythrocytes,[171] and indium-111– or indium-113m–chloride[83] may be used. Ionic indium is immediately bound to transferrin after intravenous injection.[83]

Ultrasonography. Real-time ultrasonography, using a linear, convex, or sector transducer, is a useful and practical method for detecting focal lesions within the liver. Diffuse liver disease, particularly liver cirrhosis, is also diagnosed by ultrasonography with relative ease from visible surface irregularity of the liver, size reduction or deformity of the liver, and presence of the changes attributable to portal hypertension (splenomegaly, dilated portal and gastric veins, or ascites). For these reasons, ultrasonography should be carried out on patients with suspected hepatobiliary disease before any diagnostic imaging is done.[239] A space-occupying lesion found in a cirrhotic liver is probably HCC, regardless of cause.[186] The echo pattern within the lesion varies with the tumor histology and usually is different from the parenchymal echo, or the lesion may be demarcated by a hypoechoic rim.[311] In metastatic cancer, the interior echo may be hyperechoic, less frequently mixed hyperechoic and hypoechoic, or hypoechoic with or without central and peripheral sonolucency.[20] Distinction of large HCCs and metastatic cancer by echo pattern alone may be difficult, but the latter is more often multiple. Small HCCs usually are distinguished from a metastatic lesion because they typically are hypoechoic (Fig. 44-23), whereas metastases of comparable sizes are isoechoic or hyperechoic.[311] As the tumor enlarges, the internal echo changes from hypoechoic to isoechoic or hyperechoic.[56]

For the detection of small HCC, ultrasonography is more sensitive than other imaging modalities, and without ultrasonography, early detection of HCC is not possible (see later discussion).[120,231,241] Small HCCs of less than 2 cm often are found as hyperechoic lesions[305] because fatty changes are common in extremely well differentiated early lesions, making differential diagnosis from hemangioma difficult. Benign hemangiomas are mostly hyperechoic, as previously discussed (Fig. 44-24), and do not change in echo pattern during the follow-up. In the case of a hyperechoic small HCC, the echo pattern changes to hypoechoic from the periphery as it enlarges. When the differential diagnosis is difficult, additional imaging modalities are required. In a special technique called angioechography, a small amount of carbon dioxide is injected into the hepatic artery; a small HCC is seen as a clearly demarcated hyperechoic lesion after several minutes from injection (Fig. 44-25). It may prove useful in differentiating an HCC and a benign nodule.[294]

An important merit of ultrasonography is its capability of demonstrating major portal and hepatic veins and intravascular tumor invasion[239] (Color Fig. 28). Cavernous transformation of the portal vein that follows portal occlusion by HCC[224] can also be readily recognized by ultrasonography as an irregular vascular structure in the hepatic hilum. Other merits of ultrasonography include its usefulness in assessing therapeutic effects and monitoring hepatic metastasis after chemotherapy. Intraoperative ultrasonography is considered a necessity during operation for hepatic resection.[176] Some sonographers advocate peritoneoscopic ultrasonography because it produces better images, although it is invasive. Diffuse-type HCC, in which multiple small tumor nodules are diffusely scattered among cirrhotic nodules, may escape recognition by ultrasonography.

Computed Tomography. Neoplastic lesions in the liver usually are seen as areas of decreased attenuation, but occasionally they are isodense or hyperdense because of calcification. The reported accuracy of CT for metastatic liver

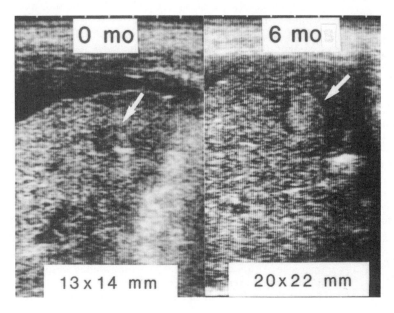

FIGURE 44-23 Hypoechoic 13 × 14-mm hepatocellular carcinoma (*arrow*) was found by ultrasonography in a cirrhotic liver with ascites (*left*). This lesion (*arrow*) grew to 20 × 22 mm in 6 months (doubling time, about 3 months) with the internal echo changing to high echo (*right*).

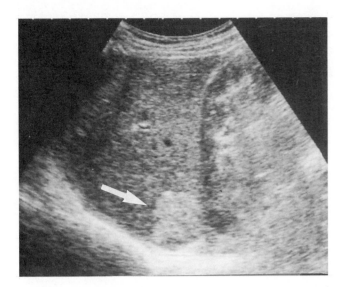

FIGURE 44-24 Hemangioma seen by ultrasonography (*arrow*). It usually is hyperechoic.

tumors has been about 90%, and for HCC, it is about the same. In the series of 47 cases of HCC studied by Itai and associates,[109] 11% were negative by plain CT, and our own experience in 116 HCC cases gave a similar incidence of isodensity. To increase the contrast, an iodized contrast medium is given for enhancement. In metastatic cancers, slow intravenous injection usually produces sufficient contrast with increased density in the parenchyma, but in the case of HCC, dynamic CT or intravenous bolus injection enhancement is most desirable. With this technique, an arterially supplied HCC is quickly enhanced before the parenchyma receives enough contrast medium to be enhanced, producing a strong and positive contrast. The contrast subsequently is

reversed, with the mass becoming lower in density relative to the parenchyma, which is now enhanced, because arterially enhanced HCC is quickly de-enhanced[10] (Fig. 44-26). Another important feature of HCC is its frequent encapsulation,[250] particularly in the Far East, and the capsule is enhanced later and remains enhanced for a prolonged period. In colorectal cancer metastasis, late scanning (3 to 5 minutes) after bolus injection produces an enhanced center because of fibrous connective tissue and a peripheral low-density area representing viable tumor tissue.

According to Itai and colleagues,[110] the major features that assist in differential diagnosis of HCC and metastatic cancer are HCC is suggested by the presence of an isodense mass, a narrow circular zone surrounding the mass (capsule), bulging of the tumor from the liver surface, decreased attenuation of an entire hepatic lobe (because of portal tumor thrombosis),[217] and diffuse homogeneous enhancement after bolus injection. The presence of cirrhotic changes favors the diagnosis. Most metastatic cancers show more than 10 lesions, masses with nodular margins showing a gradual decrease in density toward the center, multiple calcifications, and peripheral enhancement after bolus injection. A large HCC frequently demonstrates an interior with several different densities in a mosaic pattern or septa.[365] A tumor thrombus in the portal trunk may be recognized by plain CT or from lobar attenuation differences, but portal invasion is more readily diagnosed by dynamic CT, which opacifies peripheral portal branches during the arterial phase.[213]

Conventional dynamic CT is carried out in the fixed section in which a lesion was found by the prior plain CT scan. With improved faster CT scanners, without the knowledge of tumor location, one can slice the entire liver while contrast medium is being injected at a high speed, using either table incrementation technique or dynamic sequential CT. Better still, although invasive, one can catheterize the hepatic artery and carry out dynamic sequential CT to find an HCC enhanced during the arterial phase[345] (Fig. 44-27A). With the

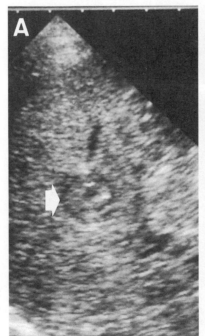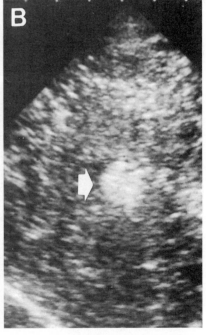

FIGURE 44-25 Angioechography. (**A**) Before injection of CO_2. A 2-cm low periphery lesion is seen (*arrow*). (**B**) Two minutes after injection of CO_2. The same lesion has become hyperechoic and better contrasted by the surrounding parenchyma. (Courtesy of Dr. Akiko Saito)

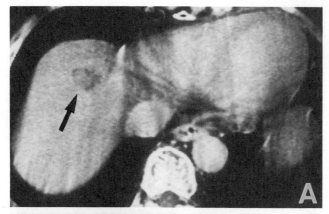

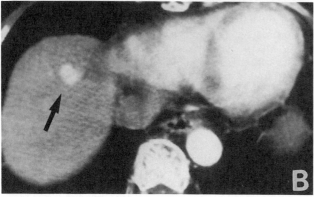

FIGURE 44-26   Dynamic CT scan. (**A**) Small, low-density lesion (*arrow*) is seen in segment 8 near the diaphragm on this plain CT scan. (**B**) On dynamic CT scan, the same lesion is immediately enhanced (*arrow*), whereas the contrast medium is still in the heart, a typical feature of hypervascular hepatocellular carcinoma.

catheter re-placed in the superior mesenteric artery, arterial portography is carried out and the liver is sliced while contrast medium is coming into the liver by way of the portal vein[182] (see Fig. 44-27B). This angiographic CT procedure is a sensitive technique for the small HCC.[345] CT is less sensitive than ultrasonography in the detection of HCCs smaller than 2 cm, and even with bolus injection, the sensitivity does not improve much[365] because small HCCs are not arterialized, but these angiographic CT techniques vastly increase sensitivity.

For differential diagnosis of HCC and hemangioma, dynamic CT is indispensable. In the latter, contrast medium first opacifies the periphery of the mass and then spreads in all directions as time elapses (Fig. 44-28); hyperdensity of the mass lasts for more than 3 minutes in large lesions. Small hemangiomas may show diffuse enhancement of a shorter duration, but it is still much longer than the enhancement of HCC.[108]

Lipiodol Computed Tomography.   In this technique, several milliliters of Lipiodol, an iodized oil contrast medium, is injected into the hepatic artery and a CT scan is made 10 days to 2 weeks later.[391] Lipiodol remains in the tumor for a long period while it is cleared from liver parenchyma, creating a distinct contrast. A lesion as small as 3 mm may be discerned, despite the partial volume phenomenon (Fig. 44-29). Lipiodol CT is perhaps the most sensitive of all imaging modalites for the diagnosis of small but overt HCC. Some small HCCs are not yet arterialized or have more fibrous tissue than tumor cells; such tumors are not well visualized by this technique. Some of the small, well-differentiated HCCs may not be visualized by Lipiodol CT. Small hemangiomas also take up Lipiodol and retain it. When hepatic resection is contemplated and investigation is required

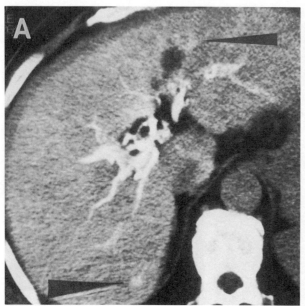

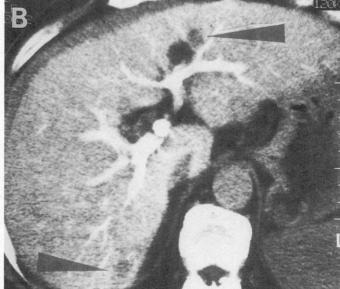

FIGURE 44-27   Angiographic CT scan. (**A**) Arterial CT scan demonstrates two 1-cm hepatocellular carcinoma lesions enhanced during the arterial phase (*arrowheads*). (**B**) On portal CT scan made during the portal phase after superior mesenteric arteriography, the same lesions are seen negatively contrasted (*arrowheads*).

population and subjected to screening—people who have a history of liver disease, blood transfusion, or a family member who has or had an HCC and who are HBsAg carriers. Ultrasonographic examination, serum AFP measurement, and several liver tests are carried out. In this program, 6104 persons were screened, and 353 were found to have cirrhosis. There were 64 cases of asymptomatic HCC (1.05%).

Clinical Course, Therapy, and Prognosis

The clinical course of advanced HCC is relentlessly progressive, and the patient succumbs within a few months (Fig. 44-35). The cure of HCC is not possible without total removal or complete destruction of the cancer. Even if this has been achieved, the underlying cirrhosis poses a constant threat of de novo emergence of HCC. A new HCC will develop from the cirrhotic nodules, which are preneoplastic themselves, one after another as the patient lives on. Posttreatment emergence of new lesions, often called recurrence, is common, making the prognosis poor even with successful treatment. In the Far East, the early lesion is more often single, permitting a surgical approach, but whether cancer occurs unicentrically or multicentrically is merely a question of how long or how short the interval is between the first tumor and the second, third, or fourth tumors. There has always been a doubt as to whether early detection and early resection afford a permanent cure or a significant prolongation of survival. The available data clearly show that those fortunate patients with less advanced cirrhosis who have undergone successful resection live much longer than those who did not have the same luck. A recent analysis made in Japan demonstrated that 1306 patients who had had curative hepatic resections (with a sufficient clean margin) had a median survival of 3.6 years and a 7-year survival rate of 46%.[166] Similarly, Tang[351] in Shanghai gives a 72.9% 5-year survival rate among subclinical patients after resection. They also analyzed 19 patients living more than 10 years postoperatively. Some of them had recurrence, for which reoperation was carried out.[394] The

world literature abounds with anecdotal case reports in which HCC did not grow, grew so slowly, or even regressed. Excluding such lucky cases, most patients have a poor prognosis, dying from either tumor growth, tumor recurrence, or hepatic failure as an end result of cirrhosis. Although there is pessimism about the virtue of early detection and positive therapeutic approach because of the low cost-effectiveness, we believe that it is unethical not to try to detect and treat HCC early because there are patients, although small in number, who benefit from successful treatment. The longest surviving patient in the Shanghai series lived 26 years and 7 months (living without disease).[394]

Primary liver cancer has not been listed as a major indication for orthotopic liver transplantation[369] because of the poor results owing to posttransplantation tumor recurrence.[221] Clearly, the transplanted patients were advanced cases already with extrahepatic metastases. In a limited number of recipients in whom a small HCC was found in the liver removed for other reasons, the results have been excellent.[114] We believe that patients with a small HCC found in a highly cirrhotic liver, experienced in large numbers in Japan, constitute good candidates for liver transplantation. Such patients eventually die of either cancer or advanced cirrhosis.

The prognosis of HCC largely depends on the size of tumor; growth speed, which can be assessed from tumor doubling time[232]; the degree of cirrhotic changes; and underlying diseases. There is no international staging system for assessing various treatment modalities. Unless the same staging scheme is used universally, no comparison of prognosis in relation to treatment is possible. When such a system was proposed by Primack and associates,[284] based on Ugandan patients, the median survival of least advanced cases (stage I) was 3 months and that of advanced cases (stage III) only 2 weeks. These results were similar to those of other studies conducted elsewhere but were at variance with our study made in 1985[256] in Japan in which 850 patients were divided

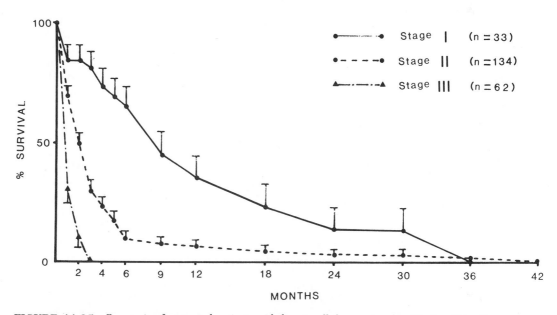

FIGURE 44-35 Prognosis of untreated patients with hepatocellular carcinoma. All stage III patients died within 3 months, whereas some stage I patients lived for more than 2 years. (Okuda K, et al. Natural history of hepatocellular carcinoma and prognosis in relation to treatment: study of 850 patients. Cancer 56:918, 1985)

into three stages and the median survival of untreated stage I patients was found to be 8.3 months (see Fig. 44-35). The staging scheme used in our study, which is now used by some European investigators,[30] is given in Table 44-10. In this scheme, only the size of the tumor and major cirrhosis-related factors (ascites and serum albumin and bilirubin) are considered. In the Primack scheme, in which weight loss, ascites, bilirubin, and portal hypertension signs were the basis of classification, speed of weight loss seemed to be a major prognostic determinant. No consideration of tumor size was made because all patients had a large mass at detection. The difficulty in staging the disease is the coexistent cirrhosis, which more often proves to be the major determinant of prognosis in Japan, whereas in African patients, cirrhosis is less common and less advanced and the tumor growth seems to determine the survival period.

Because of the low resectability rate in patients with HCC, various nonsurgical treatment modalities have been developed, as discussed below, but the efficacy is far from satisfactory and the prospect for the development of more effective treatments is dismal. The prevention of hepatitis virus infection and the treatment of chronic liver disease before it turns into cirrhosis seem to be the only solutions.

Surgical Treatment

Operative technique has been vastly improved over the years, and the early Lin's finger fracture method,[163] devised to shorten operating time and thereby reduce blood loss, is no longer used. Considerable progress has also been made, based on experience, in the preoperative assessment of hepatic functional reserve and prognosis, the type of operation to be used, and the extent of safe resection. The advances made in surgical management in the recent past are apparent if one compares the earlier and recent results compiled by the Liver Cancer Study Group of Japan. One of us (K.O.) analyzed 2411 histologically proven cases of HCC treated during the period from 1968 to 1977[252] and found that 831 of these cases had been treated surgically; simple laparotomy was done in 409 (49.2%) because the cancer was found untreatable on opening the abdomen, 98 had hepatic artery ligation, 24 portal vein ligation, and only 288 (11.9%) had hepatic resections, of which 40 (14%) were extended lobectomies. There were 27% operative deaths (death within 1 month), the 1-year survival was 33.3%, and 5-year survival 11.8%. Comparable figures obtained in the latest analysis for 2982 HCC cases treated in 1986 to 1987 showed that the overall resection rate was 20.9%, with practically no operative death,

and that 1012 of 1870 resections were curative. The increase in the resection rate was mainly due to the introduction of ultrasonography in diagnosis. In Spain, where there was no program for early detection, the resection rate among 289 HCC cases seen in 1983 to 1987 was only 5.6%.[30] In the survey in Japan, not a single case was treated by vascular ligation because the results had been poor and the same or even better arterial occlusion can be achieved by an angiographic embolization procedure; laparotomy alone occurred in only 1.2%. The 1-year survival rate was 78%, and the median survival of patients with HCC smaller than 2 cm was nearly 80 months[165] (Fig. 44-36). During these years, the strategy for early detection has been established, and the size of tumor at operation has been considerably reduced in this latest survey; 50% of resected HCCs were smaller than 5 cm. There have been more small resections (29%), segmentectomies (25%), and subsegmentectomies (22%) than lobectomies (16%) and extended lobectomies (4%). Intraoperative ultrasonography, introduced in Japan,[176,360] has been instrumental in the improvement of surgical results. Makuuchi developed an ultrasound-guided subsegmentectomy technique in which the target subsegment is colored by a dye injected into the feeding portal branch under ultrasound guidance.[177] Despite this progress, tumor recurrence is common and the major cause of postoperative death.[342] If a second operation is not possible, arterial embolization seems to be the only treatment.

Besides the size and location of the main mass and secondaries that determine the indication for surgery, hepatic functional reserve has to be carefully assessed. Some surgeons rely on the measurement of plasma clearance of an organic anion (indocyanine green), but the glucose tolerance test and other parameters are also used. Intraoperative measurement of the metabolic capacity of remnant liver has been advocated for determining the size limit for hepatic resection.[269] Obvious contraindicating factors are ascites and jaundice. It has not been determined whether esophageal varices that appear threatening endoscopically should be treated before surgery. The predictors for better postoperative survival include encapsulation of the mass and the absence of invasion in the resection margin or the capsule and of microsatellites.[153] The analysis of 2478 resected cases by the Liver Cancer Study Group of Japan similarly suggested better prognosis with the following parameters: presence of the fibrous capsule, absence of tumor invasion in the portal and hepatic veins, absence of capsular invasion, and a single mass.[166] In this analysis, there was no survivor after 44 months among 938

TABLE 44-10   *Staging Scheme for Prognosis and Efficacy of Treatment (Okuda)*

Stage	Tumor Size* >50% (+)	<50% (−)	Ascites (+)	(−)	Bilirubin >3 mg/dL (+)	<3 mg/dL (−)	Albumin <3 g/dL (+)	>3 g/dL (−)
I		(−)		(−)		(−)		(−)
II			1 or 2 (+)					
III			3 or 4 (+)					

(+), sign of advanced disease; (−), no sign of advanced disease.
*Sum of tumor areas in cross section of liver relative to the whole liver.

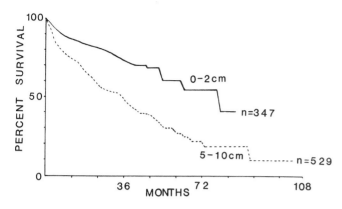

FIGURE 44-36 Relation between tumor size and survival after resection. The difference is significant (Liver Cancer Study Group of Japan, 1986 to 1987).

patients who had a noncurative resection. Fibrolamellar carcinoma is an exception, in that resectability is 50% to 75%[44,203] with an average survival of 32 to 68 months.[292] The value of cryosurgery for HCC not resectable because of cirrhosis remains to be evaluated.[393]

Nonsurgical Treatment

Systemic Chemotherapy. Many anticancer agents have been used singly or in combination through the intravenous or oral route, but the response rates have been low.[67] Some of the high response rates reported with doxorubicin have not been reproduced by others. A complete remission occasionally is obtained, but it is totally unpredictable. Kanematsu and coworkers[121] studied sensitivity of resected cancer tissues to various anticancer drugs in vitro and found that HCC was more sensitive than metastatic cancers. There is no in vitro system with which one can test drug sensitivity of HCC. Our study in stage III patients with HCC[256] showed that chemotherapy had a significant effect on their survival, suggesting that if other treatment modalities are not possible, chemotherapy ought to be given even to patients with advanced cancer.

Intraarterial Chemotherapy. The rationale for the intraarterial administration is to deliver drugs directly to cancer tissue in high concentrations. The drugs are injected in a single bolus into the hepatic artery after angiographic assessment[148] or by chronic infusion. In the original method for arterial infusion, the catheter was introduced operatively into the hepatic artery through the gastroduodenal artery, immobilized, and then connected to a chronic infusion pump.[331] Infusion could be continuous or intermittent. A number of modified techniques have since been introduced with the development of implantable pumps.[48] Nonoperative catheterization is preferred. A specially designed heparinized catheter has also been developed.[366] Such a catheter is passed into the hepatic artery and the other end connected to a reservoir or bellows, which is then implanted subcutaneously. We prefer the subclavian artery for passing the catheter because implantation of the reservoir is easy below the clavicle. The results have not been impressive in our hands[256] compared with other modes of chemotherapy. Gastroduodenal complications, such as ulcer, are not infrequent.

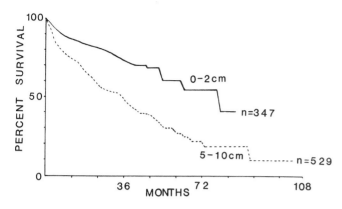

Arterial Embolization. Because HCC tissue, except for the capsule, depends on arterial supply,[208] cancer cells die when arterial blood flow is interrupted. Transcatheter arterial embolization (TAE), in which 1- to 2-mm Gelfoam particles are used, was first introduced in Japan in 1977[381] and is the most widely used modality of treatment in inoperable cases in the Far East[162,338] and perhaps elsewhere.[38] The effect is dramatic, as recognized from the sudden changes in tumor echo and formation of gas within the mass seen by CT.[74] The interior of the mass commonly liquefies. The effect is greater in a mass of the expanding gross type than in spreading-type HCC. This technique is contraindicated when there is tumor invasion in the portal trunk or its first-order branch because in such patients, occlusion of the hepatic artery induces extensive necrosis of the parenchyma.[343] Because occluding particles enter all the arterial branches, causing parenchymal damage, it is desirable to inject particles superselectively into the peripheral artery feeding the mass.

In our study on survival in relation to therapeutic modalities, the results with TAE were almost as good as those with hepatic resections in stage II patients[256] (Fig. 44-37). In a study at the National Cancer Hospital, Tokyo, all five patients with HCC smaller than 2 cm were living 3 years after TAE. In this study, Takayasu and associates[342] concluded that TAE was most effective in patients with multiple small (less than 2 cm) HCCs, provided there was no severe hepatic dysfunction or tumor thrombosis in the portal vein.

This technique is not without complications. In a study in London, early deaths occurred in some patients who had high serum ALP levels.[282] Dearterization by TAE usually is followed by rearterization, which lessens the therapeutic effect, requiring repeated embolizations; it may be achieved by using extrahepatic arteries for embolization.[321] Peripheral occlusion does not induce large rearterialization and is better in this respect. Injected particles may go into the cystic artery, causing aseptic cholecystitis,[150] or the splenic artery as a result of bouncing back of particles during the second arteriography for confirming the sites of embolization; splenic infarction results.[339] Because the fibrous capsule has dual blood supply, arterial embolization does not kill cancer cells that have invaded within the capsule. Attempts have been made with the technique of percutaneous transhepatic catheterization of the portal vein to embolize the portal branch going to the tumor for more complete killing of such cancer cells,[207] but the technique is not simple and the results have not been critically evaluated.

Chemoembolization and Targeting Chemotherapy. Along with TAE came the development of various techniques based on a similar rationale. Instead of occluding large-caliber arteries with Gelfoam particles, smaller arterial branches within the cancer may be occluded with smaller particles that contain an anticancer agent with the expectation of dual effects of embolization and chemotherapy. Microcapsules that are 0.2 mm in size and contain mitomycin C are just as effective as TAE.[223] In 1979, Konno and Maeda[147] synthesized a polystyrene–maleic acid conjugated with neocarzinostatin (SMANCS) and administered it mixed with Lipiodol into the hepatic artery. Under such conditions, Lipiodol is cleared from the parenchyma within 10 days or so, whereas it remains in the cancer tissue almost indefinitely (see section on Lipiodol CT), effecting slow release of the drug—targeting chemotherapy. Because SMANCS is not

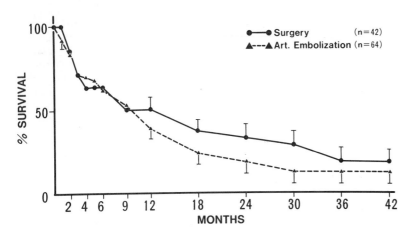

FIGURE 44-37 Comparison of survival curves for stage II patients treated by surgery and by arterial embolization. The difference is not significant. (Okuda K, et al. Natural history of hepatocellular carcinoma and prognosis in relation to treatment: study of 850 patients. Cancer 56:918, 1985)

commercially available, the practice is to prepare a mixture of the cytotoxic drug and Lipiodol with the aid of an angiographic agent having the same specific gravity as Lipiodol, a procedure called lipiodolization.[122] The drug in the aqueous phase would not remain with Lipiodol too long. In one study, cisplatin suspended in Lipiodol gave impressive results as assessed from the reduction of seromarkers.[307] Although Lipiodol itself causes microembolization within cancer tissue, it alone has no anticancer effect.[341] The trend in Japan and Taiwan is to treat inoperable cases with lipiodolization followed by TAE. One study in London comparing intravenous doxorubicin (Adriamycin) and lipiodolized doxorubicin in a small number of patients failed to show a difference.[118]

Radiation Therapy. It has generally been thought that external radiation alone is not effective unless combined with chemotherapy or immunotherapy. In our own experience with a linear accelerator in patients with HCC, a slow and progressive tumor regression frequently was observed. It was also learned that it induced a progressive atrophy of the liver parenchyma, leading to late hepatic failure in patients with Child C cirrhosis.[227] Large doses of irradiation over the upper abdomen commonly causes gastric ulcer, which does not heal readily, and therefore, an HCC located in the right lobe of a Child A liver may be a good candidate for external irradiation. A number of attempts have been made at internal radiation using radioactive substances bound to various antibodies, such as anti-AFP and antiferritin,[266,352] that have affinity to HCC tissue, but the results have not been exciting.

Intratumor Ethanol Injection. With the improved aiming using an ultrasound puncture transducer, it is now possible to inject a solution containing an anticancer agent directly into a small mass lesion. Drugs dissolved in an aqueous solution are quickly washed away, however, and do not remain long enough to exert cytotoxic effects. In 1983, we developed a technique in which absolute ethanol is repeatedly injected directly into a small mass until the mass is deemed to be totally coagulated. Several milliliters of ethanol is injected through a thin needle in each session, and at least five sessions are given; other options are to insert several needles simultaneously in one session[310] or to use a needle with several holes. The candidates for this treatment are inoperable patients who have one or two small HCCs in a cirrhotic liver. This technique is now widely adopted,[167,306] but long-term results have not been fully assessed. In our own

hands, the survival of patients treated by this modality was significantly prolonged compared with that of the control patients, who had had small HCCs but for various reasons did not receive treatment.[57] A group in Taiwan developed a special needle that permits injection of a small steel coil into the tumor as a landmark for subsequent follow-up.[306] Because a small inoperable HCC commonly is associated with advanced cirrhosis, tumor recurrence (new emergence of HCC elsewhere) is common after the treatment.[57] This technique has also been used by Livraghi and colleagues to disintegrate a portal tumor thrombus.[168]

Immunotherapy. A number of immunomodulators and immunostimulant agents have been used in animal and human HCC, but the results have not been satisfactory. The agents used include bacillus Calmette-Guérin vaccine; OK-432, a streptococcal preparation; interferon; interleukin-2; and lymphokine-activated killer cells (adoptive immunotherapy).[225,261] Occasional cases remit with regression of the tumor, but the overall results seem unsatisfactory.

Other Treatment Modalities. Hyperthemia has not been fully evaluated, although there have been preliminary studies combined with chemotherapy. Some mouse hepatoma cells are thyroid hormone–dependent in vitro, but attempts to exploit such characteristics of cancer cells in human cases have not been successful. It has also been shown that HCC cells have estrogen receptors, and attempts are being made to treat patients with HCC with antiestrogens, but the efficacy remains to be determined.

CHOLANGIOCARCINOMA

Definition

A cholangiocarcinoma is an intrahepatic malignant tumor composed of cells that resemble those of biliary epithelium. Synonyms include cholangiocellular carcinoma, peripheral cholangiocarcinoma, and intrahepatic bile duct carcinoma. Semantic confusion exists because some surgeons and pathologists call carcinoma of the extrahepatic bile duct cholangioma or cholangiocarcinoma, and the boundary between the intrahepatic and extrahepatic bile ducts has not been made clear. In the "General Rules for Surgical Studies on Cancer of the Bile Duct" issued by the Japanese Biliary Surgical Society, the point where the second-order bile ducts join to become the first-order (right and left hepatic) bile duct is considered the boundary between the intrahepatic and extrahepatic bile ducts.[117] A problem occurs in a carcinoma that arises in the hepatic hilum, the so-called Klatskin tumor, when it involves both sides of the boundary. For this reason, some authors include hilar carcinoma in the primary liver cancer.[58,249] One suggestion is that carcinoma of the extrahepatic bile duct be called bile duct carcinoma or carcinoma of the bile duct. Okuda and colleagues[249] proposed that hilar carcinoma and peripheral CCC be treated separately for analysis because the former behaves like extrahepatic bile duct carcinoma. Histologically, papillary growth occurs only in large bile ducts.

Epidemiology and Etiology

The incidence of CCC seems to vary less with the global region than does HCC, except for several areas in which liver fluke infestation is endemic, such as Thailand and Hong Kong. CCC constituted 0.49% of 136,475 autopsies during the period of 1958 to 1967 and 0.44% of 39,399 autopsies in 1987 in the Japan Autopsy Registries. In the Liverpool region, primary liver cancer was seen in 0.145% of 60,600 necropsies in 1947 to 1959, and CCC accounted for about one fifth of them.[46] In the Edmondson-Steiner series[58] of 48,900 necropsies in the United States, CCC occurred in only 0.05%. Thus, it seems that CCC is nearly 10 times as common in Japan as in the United States and the United Kingdom. The average age of patients is considerably older compared with HCC,[174,249,272,324] and the degree of male predominance is much less, ranging from 1 to 2.2.[6,58,172,174,249] The relative frequency of CCC among all primary liver cancers varies from 2.6% in Africa[324] to 25% in the United States,[58] as shown in Table 44-11. In western countries, it has been around 20% in most studies, whereas it is less than 10% in the areas where HCC is prevalent, such as South Africa and Singapore.[249,329] In other words, this ratio indirectly reflects the prevalence of HCC. In Japan, where HCC has been increasing at a rapid pace, this ratio has been reduced from 9.5% in 1968 to 1977[252] to 5.4% in 1982 to 1985 in the same setting as for the national survey.[166] For the same reason, the ratio of CCC to HCC is an indicator, albeit indirect, of the prevalence of CCC in the areas where the incidence of HCC is about the same. Both in Hong Kong and in South China,[159] it is about 1:5; both

areas are known for liver fluke endemicity. By contrast, it is 1:56 in Java, Indonesia,[70] and 1:38[324] to 1:20[94] in Africa, where liver fluke is uncommon but HCC is prevalent. These statistics seem to strongly suggest that prevalence of liver fluke infection is associated with the increased incidence of CCC. *Opisthorchis sinensis* infection commonly is seen in autopsies for CCC in Hong Kong. The northeastern part of Thailand is known for high prevalence of *Opisthorchis viverrini* infection. In one study in Thailand, 11 of 14 autopsy cases of CCC had *O viverrini* worms, whereas this fluke was found in none of 33 cases of HCC,[17] and in an another hospital-based case-controlled study, patients with *O viverrini* infection had a significantly higher incidence of CCC. According to Sonakul and coworkers,[320] the incidence of primary liver cancer among 154 patients with opisthorchiasis was 56.6%, and 77% of them were CCC. In a Hong Kong study by Belamaric,[14] 18 of 19 autopsy cases of CCC had severe infection of *O sinensis*, but none had cirrhosis. The tumor was located in proximity to parasitized ducts deep in liver parenchyma. AH typically was seen in the ductal wall around the flukes.

A number of recent studies in Japan suggest a causative relation between intrahepatic gallstones and CCC—5.7% to 11.7% of CCC cases had associated hepatolithiasis.[329] In the presence of intrahepatic stones, adenomatous, sometimes atypical hyperplasia of the bile duct epithelium commonly is seen in the vicinity of stones.[63,206] Repeated bouts of inflammation of the bile duct epithelium caused by stones may be a contributory factor. For the same reason, extrahepatic gallstones could have a similar role. In our study of 57 cases of CCC, 17.5% of them had stone disease,[249] and in a series of 102 autopsy cases in Japan, stones were found in 21%.[204] A group of pathologists at Kanazawa University recently described glandular tissues in large intrahepatic bile ducts and found atypical hyperplasia in 0.1% of 799 livers not bearing cancer, suggesting that some CCCs could arise from these peribiliary glands.[355]

The association of bile duct carcinoma with ulcerative colitis and primary sclerosing cholangitis is now well established. According to Ritchie and associates,[289] the incidence of bile duct carcinoma in ulcerative colitis patients is 1 in 256, and one third of these tumors occur within the liver. The entire colon usually is affected, and the average duration

TABLE 44-11 *Relative Frequency of Cholangiocarcinoma Among Primary Liver Cancers, Histologically Confirmed*

Author	Country	Year	Primary Liver Cancer, Total	Cholangiocarcinoma
Edmondson[58]	United States	1954	100	25 (25%)
MacDonald[172]	United States	1956	108	24 (22.2%)
Steiner[325]	Africa*	1960	860	22[†] (2.6%)
Cruckshank[46]	United Kingdom	1961	108	21 (20%)
Patton[272]	United States	1964	60	13 (21.7%)
Lopez-Corella[170]	Mexico	1968	37	7 (18.9%)
Miyaji[189]	Japan	1960	410	29 (7.1%)
Okuda[252]	Japan	1980	2829	268 (9.5%)
Liver Cancer Study Group of Japan[166]	Japan	1990	4765	256 (5.4%)

*African blacks only.
[†]Including cholangiolocellular carcinoma.
All but the last two studies are based on autopsies.

of colitis before cancer evolves is 5 (0 to 30) years. In the case of primary sclerosing cholangitis, cancer occurs at a relatively young age.[376] Chronic inflammation and glandular regeneration may predispose to carcinogenesis.[45] There are a number of reports on the association of cystic liver diseases and CCC. They include Meyenburg's complexes, congenital hepatic fibrosis, hepatic cysts, Caroli's diseases, and choledochal cysts. They are biliary system diseases and perhaps share a similar causative mechanism with stones and cholangitis. Cystic diseases complicated by CCC sometimes are mistaken for cystadenocarcinoma.[190]

Of the other known causative factors, Thorotrast is the best documented (see section on Thorotrast). In one study in Japan, hepatic cancers accounted for two thirds of the deaths caused by hepatic thorotrastosis, and CCC was the most frequent among them. According to Sugihara and Kojiro,[329] most Thorotrast-associated CCC was in the liver parenchyma, not associated with large bile ducts, and showed small to medium-size papillary growths of the bile duct epithelium with proliferating bile ductules around the portal tract. Similar changes have also been described by Rubel and associates[293] and termed duct dysplasia, cancer in situ.

Pathology

Cholangiocarcinoma is grossly gray-white, firm, and solid. According to its location, CCC is divided into the hilar and the peripheral type[249] (Fig. 44-38). Distinguishing CCC from extrahepatic bile duct carcinoma often is difficult when a massive tumor is located in the hilar portion, particularly in autopsy cases. Tumor invasion into the portal vein is relatively uncommon, but lymphatic invasion is frequent.

The growth patterns of CCC may be classified into nodular, infiltrative, diffuse, and periductal types.[329] In the nodular type, the tumor is relatively well demarcated but not encapsulated, as in HCC. Budding and multiple metastases typically are seen around the tumor. In the infiltrative type, a massive or relatively small tumor is growing in an infiltrative manner with an irregular boundary and multiple intrahepatic metastatic foci. In the diffuse type, numerous small and ill-defined tumor nodules are seen scattered throughout the liver. This type of CCC is relatively infrequent. In the periductal type, the tumor proliferates along the intrahepatic bile duct with infiltration into the adjacent liver parenchyma. Affected bile ducts typically are dilated.

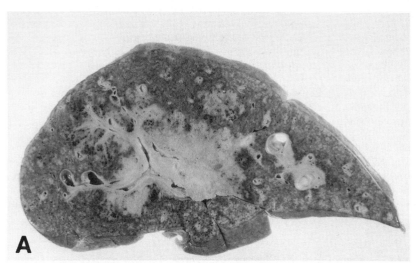

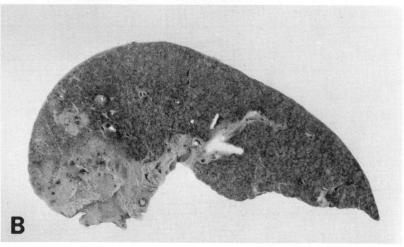

FIGURE 44-38 Gross appearance of cholangiocarcinoma. (**A**) Hilar type. The tumor is mostly located around the major bile ducts in the hilar region. (**B**) Peripheral type. The tumor is situated in the periphery of the right lobe.

Histologically, most CCCs are well to moderately differentiated tubular or papillotubular adenocarcinomas with abundant fibrous stroma (Fig. 44-39). Poorly differentiated adenocarcinoma and mucinous carcinoma also occur. Adenosquamous carcinoma and squamous cell carcinoma seldom are encountered.

Cholangiolocellular Carcinoma

Steiner and Higginson[325] first introduced the concept of cholangiolocellular carcinoma based on a study of 11 cases. They defined cholangiolocellular carcinoma as a specific type of primary liver cancer derived from the cholangioles or the canals of Hering. Grossly, this tumor is not different from the usual form of CCC. Histologically, however, cholangiolocellular carcinoma is characterized by the tubular structure consisting of cuboidal neoplastic cells showing an anastomosing cord-like pattern with abundant fibrous stroma (Fig. 44-40). Interestingly, the tumor cells are contiguous with liver cell cords with the replacing growth pattern at the tumor-nontumor boundary, unlike CCC.

Extrahepatic Metastasis

Lymphatic metastasis is much more common than hematogenous spread. Metastasis through the lymphatics to the hilar and peripancreatic lymph nodes occurs in about one half of CCC cases. Tokunaga[361] analyzed 45 autopsy cases of CCC and found extrahepatic metastasis in 77.8%. In his series, metastases were deemed to have been hematogenous in 51.1% and lymphatic in 64.4%; some showed both features.

Clinical Features

In the past, differential diagnosis between HCC and CCC was almost infeasible clinically because both present with a large hepatic mass and a rapidly downhill course. Early symptoms and complaints are not much different from those in HCC, except that signs of biliary obstruction are more common, as shown in Table 44-12. Because cirrhosis is not the underlying disease, signs attributable to cirrhosis and portal hypertension are absent, and exclusion of an extrahepatic primary by radiologic procedures makes a diagnosis of CCC more likely. Well-executed imaging can differentiate HCC and CCC in most instances with certain accuracy. When a hilar carcinoma is diagnosed, it cannot be made clear whether it is extrahepatic or intrahepatic, and therefore, in discussing clinical characteristics, one has to separate hilar carcinoma from the peripheral type of intrahepatic bile duct carcinoma,[249] which is CCC in a narrow sense of the term. The major difference is early jaundice and more frequent infections in hilar carcinoma. The prognosis of CCC was just as poor as that of advanced HCC in the past, but with early detection and surgical treatment, the prognosis of CCC has been considerably improved.

Diagnosis

Although no specific tumor markers are known, CEA and CA 19-9 are of diagnostic value. In a recent national study in Japan, CEA was positive in 53 (42.7%) of 124 cases of CCC, and it proved diagnostic in 30.3%.[165] Other reports cite higher positivity rates. CA 19-9 is more frequently positive in CCC,[190] and the combination of CEA and CA 19-9 is thought to be diagnostic in distinguishing CCC from HCC; this combination does not help in differential diagnosis of CCC and metastatic liver cancers, however. AFP, which is highly specific in HCC, may also be increased in some cases of CCC; in a national study in Japan, it was elevated in 39 (19.0%) of 205 cases.[165] The degree of elevation is much less compared with HCC.[190,249] Biochemical tests are not specific, except that ALP levels are elevated considerably in most patients. Hepatic function reserve is kept relatively well, despite the large size of mass in the absence of severe jaundice. Hypercalcemia occurs in some patients,[262] as is the case with sclerosing hepatic carcinoma.[263]

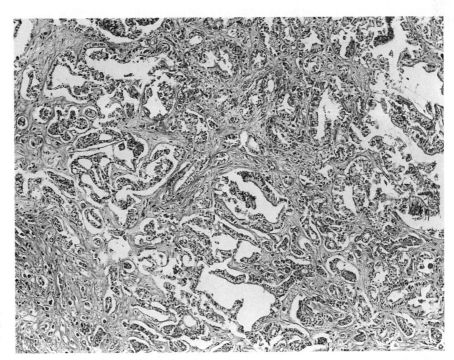

FIGURE 44-39 Histologically, this cancer consists of irregular glands of varying size formed by columnar tumor cells and abundant fibrous stroma ($\times$ 50).

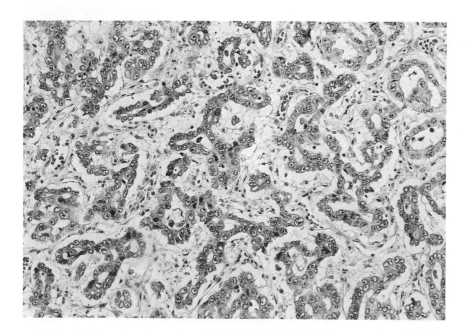

FIGURE 44-40   Cholangiolocellular carcinoma. Small, columnar tumor cells with eosinophilic cytoplasm form irregular tubules that are anastomosing among themselves (× 200).

Imaging diagnosis of CCC requires several modalities. On plain CT, CCC is seen as a low-density lesion, often with dilated bile ducts peripheral to it.[36] Because CCC is more often hypovascular, there is only mild enhancement on dynamic CT, unlike with HCC.[36] If a CCC near the hilum is compressing on a major portal vein branch, the lobe of the affected side is atrophied and readily recognized by CT.[340] CCC in the hilar area is hypodense or isodense in plain CT and may not be recognized but is seen enhanced on late-phase enhanced CT.[344] Calcification is not rare. On MRI, well-differentiated CCC has a high signal intensity, whereas scirrhous CCC demonstrates only a slightly higher signal intensity than the normal liver on T2-weighted spin-echo sequences. Bile duct dilatations within the liver and hilar lymph node metastases may be recognized by MRI.[54] On angiography, CCC is more often hypovascular or avascular, but there is a slight increase in vascularity with thin neoplastic vessels; the angiogram was interpreted as hypervascular in 41% (74 out of 180 cases) in a recent national survey in Japan.[165] Other angiographic features include irregular encasements, venous obstruction, arterio-arterial collaterals, and bile duct dilatation discerned on the arterial portogram. On ultrasonographic examination, CCC may be either hypoechoic or hyperechoic. If CCC has arisen in Thorotrast liver disease, the tumor is seen on CT as an area without Thorotrast within a liver parenchyma with diffuse high-density deposits. Direct cholangiography proves diagnostic in hilar carcinoma but not so much for peripheral-type CCC. In our own imaging study of 20 patients with CCC, including 3 with intraductal growths, the detection rate was 85% by ultrasonography, 67% by CT, and 79% by angiography, and there was intrahepatic biliary dilatation in 14 seen by ultrasonography; CT surpassed ultrasonography in the detection of intrahepatic bile duct dilatation.

Treatment and Prognosis

Cholangiocarcinoma responds poorly to chemotherapy. Early diagnosis and resection are the only reliable therapy.[126] Radiation therapy may be indicated postoperatively. In the Mizumoto and Kawarada[190] series in Japan, 11 of 15 CCC cases underwent hepatic resections—3 trisegmentectomies, 3 extended lobectomies, 3 lobectomies, and 2 lateral segmentectomies—and the longest survival was 6 years and 10 months (still living). There have been several case reports on

TABLE 44-12   *Early Symptoms and Laboratory Data on Admission in Patients with CCC (57 Cases)*

Symptom	Number	Percentage	Test	Average Value
Jaundice	33	57.9	Red blood cells (10^6/μL)	3.63
Abdominal pain	22	38.6	White blood cells (μL)	9261
Fever	10	17.5	Total protein (g/dL)	7.0
General malaise	9	15.8	γ-Globulin (g/dL)	1.5
Abdominal distention and fullness	7	12.3	Total cholesterol (mg/dL)	219
Anorexia	5	8.8	Total bilirubin (mg/dL)	10.3
Pruritus	3	5.3	AST (IU/L)	78
Weight loss	2	3.5	ALT (IU/L)	63

CCC, cholangiocarcinoma; AST, aspartate aminotransferase; ALT, alanine aminotransferase.

successful surgery for CCC, although they may be anecdotal. In a national study in Japan, 211 patients with CCC underwent hepatic resection during the period from 1978 to 1987. Among 86 patients in whom the resection was curative, the median survival period was 32 months and the 7-year survival rate was 42%[165] (Fig. 44-41). Without surgical treatment, the average survival period is about 6 months.[249,329]

COMBINED HEPATOCELLULAR AND CHOLANGIOCARCINOMA

Combined HCC and CCC (HCC-CCC) is composed of elements of both HCC and CCC in the same liver. Allen and coworkers[4] classified HCC-CCC into three categories: (1) tumors in which the areas of HCC and CCC are present separately (double cancer); (2) tumors in which both components are present adjacent to each other and mixed together as one mass (combined type); and (3) tumors in which both components are intimately mixed (mixed type). In another classification by Goodman and colleagues,[82] collision, transitional, and fibrolamellar types are separated.

We have found 10 cases (2.5%) of HCC-CCC among 393 consecutive autopsy cases of primary liver cancer. The average age, clinical symptoms, and biochemical data were not much different from those of HCC. Grossly, association of liver cirrhosis was seen in about 50% of cases. Each area of HCC and CCC was distinguished in some cases (Fig. 44-42), but more often, HCC-CCC showed a CCC-like appearance. Although the histogenesis of HCC-CCC is obscure, the following three concepts are possible: (1) double cancer, (2) HCC differentiating to CCC in part, and (3) the cancer arising in an intermediate (transitional) cell that differentiates into both HCC and CCC. Yano and coworkers[384] established a cell line from HCC that transformed to adenocarcinoma after culturing. Extrahepatic metastases are found in about 40% of the cases; HCC elements tend to metastasize to the

lung, but CCC elements metastasize to lymph nodes with preference.

Clinically, HCC-CCC is similar to HCC. In our experience, however, AFP levels were relatively low (within 10,000 ng/mL) with a positivity rate of 60%, and CEA, which seldom is positive in HCC, was positive in 88% of the cases, with a mean value of 7.5 ng/mL.

BILE DUCT CYSTADENOCARCINOMA

Bile duct cystadenocarcinoma is a rare, malignant cystic tumor lined by mucus-secreting columnar epithelium with papillary infoldings.[105] Its basic histologic features are similar to those of cystadenocarcinoma of the ovary and pancreas. Grossly, cysts are multilocular, and the cyst wall is irregularly thickened with or without tumor infiltration into the adjacent parenchyma. Histologically, the cysts are lined by mucin-secreting epithelium with varying degrees of stratification, budding, and papillary infolding (Fig. 44-43). It is common to see the transitional feature from benign single-layered columnar epithelium to malignant epithelial growth, but the differential diagnosis of benign cystadenoma and carcinoma often is difficult in the tumors without distinct invasion into the adjacent parenchyma. Transition from benign cystadenoma to cystadenocarcinoma has been observed.[105] CCC or adenocarcinoma arising in a liver with a cystic disease often is mistaken for cystadenocarcinoma.[190] Mizumoto and associates[191] proposed a histopathologic classification of cystic adenocarcinomas encompassing all such carcinomas based on 65 cases presented at a recent meeting in Japan, as shown in Figure 44-44. On ultrasonographic examination, the tumor is a globular or ovoid, thick-walled mass that often contains multiple septations or papillary infoldings; on CT, it appears as a low-density mass that contains mural nodules or internal septations[190] (Fig. 44-45). Kawarada and Mizumoto[126] described five cases treated surgically with a survival period longer than 3 years in four.

HEPATOBLASTOMA

A malignant tumor that arises in embryonic or fetal hepatocytes, hepatoblastoma is the most common liver tumor of childhood. Sometimes it occurs in adults. In a national survey in Japan (1968 to 1977), 56 of 61 cases of primary liver cancer under age 5 were hepatoblastomas, and there were 5 hepatoblastomas among 2698 adult primary liver cancers.[252] It is more frequent in boys (male/female ratio of 1.75:1).[327]

Pathology

Hepatoblastoma usually is found as a large mass lesion in the liver, and its gross appearance depends on the presence or absence of mesenchymal components. The association of liver cirrhosis is uncommon. Histologically, hepatoblastomas can be classified into epithelial and mixed epithelial and mesenchymal types.[327] In the epithelial components, there are two kinds of cells—fetal and embryonal. The fetal-type cells resemble the hepatocytes of the fetus and are arranged in twin cell–thick plates with an irregular trabecular pattern. Varying degrees of extramedullary hematopoiesis are observed in most fetal-type hepatoblastomas. The embryonic-type cells have a basophilic cytoplasm with a higher nucleus/cytoplasm ratio and grow in a trabecular or compact pattern. Tubular or rosette-like patterns typically are present. Extramedullary hematopoiesis is not found in this type. A transi-

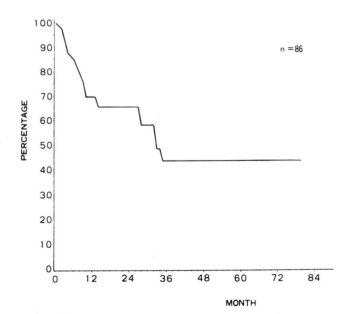

FIGURE 44-41 Survival curve for 86 cases of cholangiocarcinoma after resection (Liver Cancer Study Group of Japan, 1986 to 1987).

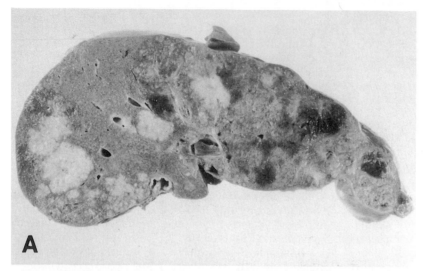

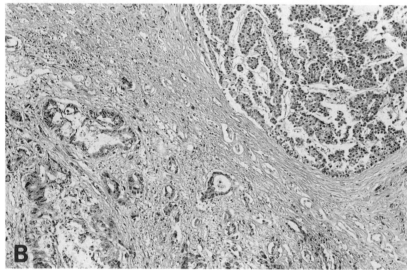

FIGURE 44-42 Combined hepatocellular carcinoma and cholangiocarcinoma. (**A**) Lesions of cholangiocarcinoma are seen as whitish gray areas, and hepatocellular carcinoma, as dark yellowish lesions occupying mainly the left lobe. (**B**) Histologic feature. Cholangiocarcinoma in the lower left and hepatocellular carcinoma in the upper right are not intermingled in this case.

tion between the fetal and the embryonal component often is present. Kasai and coworkers[123] proposed a separate anaplastic type of hepatoblastoma in which the tumor cells are small with scanty cytoplasm and lack mutual cohesiveness. This subtype of hepatoblastoma has a poorer prognosis. In the mixed epithelial and mesenchymal type of hepatoblastoma, various mesenchymal components, such as osteoid, chondroid, or spindle-shaped cells, are present in epithelial tumor tissues (Fig. 44-46).

Clinical Features

The presenting symptoms are enlarging abdomen accompanied by anorexia, weight loss, nausea, vomiting, and, sometimes, abdominal pain. Because cirrhosis is not the underlying condition, ascites, jaundice, and varices are uncommon objective signs. Associated paraneoplastic syndromes, such as precocious puberty with increased chorionic gonadotropin derived from cancer cells and thrombocytosis, have been reported. Urinary excretion of cystathionine produced by the tumor is increased in nearly 50% of patients.[77] Familial occurrence of hepatoblastoma among siblings and identical

twins has been described, and an association between hepatoblastoma and polyposis of the colon has been found in five families.[327] Congenital anomalies occurred in about 5.5% of the reported cases, according to Stocker and colleagues[327]; they included cleft palate, macroglossia, earlobe dysplasia, absence of one adrenal, umbilical hernia, and various cardiovascular and renal abnormalities. Serum AFP levels are elevated in most patients. In a recent national study in Japan, 18 of 19 patients with hepatoblastoma had increased AFP levels and 7 (36.8%) showed levels above 100,000 ng/mL.[165] HBsAg was negative in all 15 cases studied in this survey, but in an earlier survey, 2 of 16 cases were positive.[252]

Radiologically, about half the patients show calcification related to osteoid tissue formation on radiographs.[47] Angiography usually demonstrates tumor vascularity,[103] sometimes with a spoke-wheel pattern.[47] On ultrasonography, the tumor is basically echogenic, and calcification may be seen; hypoechoic areas represent necrosis or hemorrhage. On CT, the tumor is hypodense with minimal enhancement, and besides frequent calcification, nodularity or lobulation of the large mass may be seen.

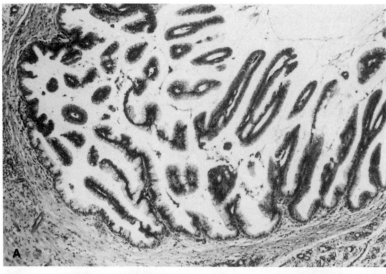

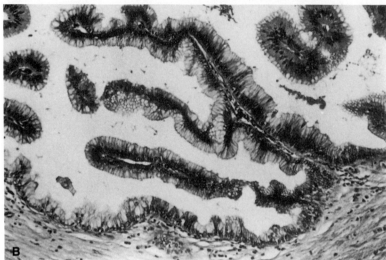

FIGURE 44-43 Histologic findings of resected cystadenocarcinoma of the liver (same case as in Fig. 44-45). The loculi are lined by columnar mucus-secreting epithelia with an obvious proliferative papillary growth (**A** × 15; **B** × 70). (Courtesy of Dr. Ryuji Mizumoto)

Treatment

At the time of diagnosis, 39% to 70% of tumors are considered unresectable. Preoperative chemotherapy or radiation may reduce the tumor size to permit resection. Because of the large size of the mass, operative mortality is high.[283] Long-term survival varies from 15% to 37%, largely depending on resectability and histologic type. The pure fetal cell type, if successfully resected, shows the best prognosis.

Malignant Mesenchymal Tumors

Malignant mesenchymal tumor of the liver is rare. According to the Registry of Autopsies in Japan, there were only 95 mesenchymal tumors among 17,417 autopsy cases of primary malignant tumors of the liver in 5 years from 1985 to 1989. It accounted for only 0.5% in the United States; Edmondson and Peters[61] found sarcomas in 1.2% of the 405 primary malignant tumors of the liver.

ANGIOSARCOMA

Angiosarcoma, which is derived from the endothelial cells, is the most common among malignant mesenchymal tumors of the liver, with a peak age incidence in the sixth and seventh decades and a male/female ratio of 3:1.[169] Synonyms are malignant hemangioendothelioma and hemangiosarcoma. Of the 17,417 autopsy cases of primary malignant tumors of the liver from 1985 to 1989 in Japan, only 40 were angiosarcoma. In the United States, about 25 cases occur each year.[65] Many hepatic angiosarcomas are causatively related to Thorotrast,[65,101,278,367] polyvinylchloride,[50,65] and arsenic.[66] According to Locker and associates,[169] 40% of 103 angiosarcomas were related to one of the following factors: Thorotrast (15 cases), polyvinylchloride (22 cases), arsenical ingestion (2 cases), radium implant (1 case), and hemochromatosis (3 cases). Other implicated factors include external radiation, copper,[275] hemochromatosis, steroids,[64] and phenelzine.[49]

A : Cystic adenocarcinoma

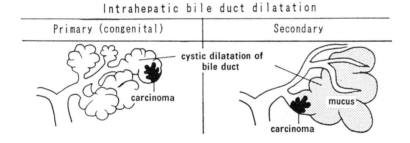

B : Bile duct carcinoma with intrahepatic bile duct dilatation

C : Degeneration cyst in malignant liver tumor

FIGURE 44-44 Classification of cystic adenocarcinoma of the liver based on 65 Japanese cases. (Mizumoto R, et al. Proposal of a new classification of cystic malignant tumours of the liver: classification of 65 cases reported at the 26th Annual Meeting of the Liver Cancer Society of Japan. J Gastroenterol Hepatol 6, 1991; courtesy of Dr. Ryuji Mizumoto)

Gross Appearance

Grossly, a various-size hemorrhagic tumor, angiosarcoma can be classified into four types: diffuse micronodular, multinodular, massive, and mixed multinodular and massive[141] (Fig. 44-47A). Extrahepatic metastasis is frequent. Of the 29 autopsy cases of Thorotrast-induced angiosarcoma in Japan, extrahepatic metastasis was found in 11 cases (37.9%), and metastasis to the lung was the most frequent (45.4%).

Histologic Features

Angiosarcoma is characterized by two cell types: spindle-shaped cells and polyhedral cells (see Fig. 44-47B). The spindle-shaped cells, which resemble fibroblasts, have elongated nuclei with one to two nucleoli and an extended cytoplasm. Polyhedral cells have round to ovoid nuclei with one to two distinct nucleoli and an abundant cytoplasm. They frequently are multinucleated and pleomorphic. Marked phagocytic activities, including erythrophagocytosis and cannibalism, commonly are observed in tumor cells, particularly in the polyhedral cells. Structurally, angiosarcoma consists of

combinations of sinusoidal, cavernous, and solid growth patterns. In the sinusoidal growth pattern, single or multilayered tumor cells proliferate along the sinusoids with varying degrees of sinusoidal dilatation and atrophy of liver cell cords. Occasionally, it is difficult to differentiate nontumorous sinusoidal dilatation with hypertrophic sinusoidal lining cells. Relatively thick fibrous stalks lined by tumor cells show papillary and cavernous patterns, which are common in angiosarcoma of soft tissue parts. Various-size solid tumor nests that consist mostly of spindle-shaped cells resembling fibrosarcoma occasionally are observed.

Clinical Features

The presenting symptoms include hepatomegaly, ascites, abdominal pain, anorexia, nausea, weight loss, fever, symptoms caused by tumor rupture, and splenomegaly. Hematologic abnormalities include anemia (sometimes caused by microangiopathic hemolysis), leukocytosis, and thrombocytopenia. In the presence of splenomegaly, there may be leukopenia. Serum bilirubin levels are elevated in about 60% of

118. Kalayci C, et al. Intraarterial Adriamycin and lipiodol for inoperable hepatocellular carcinoma: comparison with intravenous Adriamycin. J Hepatol 11:349, 1990

119. Kanai T, et al. Pathology of small hepatocellular carcinoma: a proposal for a new gross classification. Cancer 60:810, 1987

120. Kanematsu T, et al. The value of ultrasound in the diagnosis and treatment of small hepatocellular carcinoma. Br J Surg 72:23, 1985

121. Kanematsu T, et al. Sensitivity to six antitumor drugs differs between primary and metastatic liver cancers. Eur J Cancer Clin Oncol 24:1511, 1988

122. Kanematsu T, et al. A 5-year experience of lipiodolization: selective regional chemotherapy for 200 patients with hepatocellular carcinoma. Hepatology 10:98, 1989

123. Kasai M, et al. Histologic classification of liver cell carcinoma in infancy and childhood and its clinical evaluation. Cancer 25:551, 1970

124. Kashala LO, et al. Histopathologic feature of hepatocellular carcinoma in Zaire. Cancer 65:130, 1990

125. Kato N, et al. Detection of hepatitis C virus ribonucleic acid in the serum by amplification with polymerase chain reaction. J Clin Invest 86:1764, 1990

126. Kawarada Y, Mizumoto R. Cystic bile duct carcinoma of the liver: a report of 5 cases and proposal of a new classification. Gastroenterol Jpn 26:1991

127. Keen P, Martin P. Is aflatoxin carcinogenic in man? The evidence in Swaziland. Trop Geogr Med 23:44, 1971

128. Kenmochi K, et al. Relationship of histologic grade of hepatocellular carcinoma (HCC) to tumor size and demonstration of tumor cells of multiple different grades in single small HCC. Liver 7:18, 1987

129. Kew MC. Clinical, pathologic, and etiologic heterogeneity in hepatocellular carcinoma: evidence from South Africa. Hepatology 1:366, 1981

130. Kew MC, Geddes EW. Hepatocellular carcinoma in rural Southern African blacks. Medicine 61:98, 1982

131. Kew MC, Newburne PM. Tumor markers in hepatocellular carcinoma. In: Okuda K, Mackay IR, eds. Hepatocellular carcinoma. Geneva, Unione Internationale Contre le Cancer, 1982, p 123

132. Kew MC, et al. Tumor-associated isoenzymes of γ-glutamyl transferase in the serum of patients with hepatocellular carcinoma. Br J Cancer 50:451, 1984

133. Kew MC, et al. The role of membranous obstruction of the inferior vena cava in the etiology of hepatocellular carcinoma in southern African blacks. Hepatology 9:121, 1989

134. Kew MC, et al. Hepatitis C virus antibodies in southern African blacks with hepatocellular carcinoma. Lancet 335:873, 1990

135. King MA, et al. A comparison between des-γ-carboxy prothrombin and α-fetoprotein as markers of hepatocellular carcinoma in southern African blacks. J Gastroenterol Hepatol 4:17, 1989

136. Kingston JE, et al. Association between hepatoblastoma and polyposis coli. Arch Dis Child 58:959, 1983

137. Kiyosawa K, et al. Interrelationship of blood transfusion, non-A, non-B hepatitis and hepatocellular carcinoma: analysis by detection of antibody to hepatitis C. Hepatology 12:671, 1990

138. Klatskin G. Hepatic tumors: possible relationship to use of oral contraceptives. Gastroenterology 73:386, 1977

139. Kojiro M, et al. Hepatocellular carcinoma presenting as intrabile duct tumor growth: a clinicopathologic study of 24 cases. Cancer 49:2144, 1982

140. Kojiro M, et al. Hepatocellular carcinoma with intraatrial tumor growth: a clinicopathologic study of 18 autopsy cases. Arch Pathol Lab Med 108:989, 1984

141. Kojiro M, et al. Thorium dioxide–related angiosarcoma of the liver: pathomorphologic study of 29 autopsy cases. Arch Pathol Lab Med 109:853, 1985

142. Kojiro M, et al. Hepatocellular carcinoma with sarcomatous change: a special reference to the relationship with anticancer therapy. Cancer Chemother Pharmacol 23(Suppl):4, 1989

143. Kojiro M, et al. Comparative study of HCC between Japan and Spain. In: Sung JL, Chen DS, eds. Viral hepatitis and hepatocellular carcinoma. Amsterdam, Excerpta Med, 1990, p 545

144. Kojiro M, et al. Pathomorphologic characteristics of minute HCC. In: Sung JL, Chen DS, eds. Viral hepatitis and hepatocellular carcinoma. Amsterdam, Excerpta Med, 1990, p 535

145. Kondo F, et al. Biopsy diagnosis of well-differentiated hepatocellular carcinoma based on new morphologic criteria. Hepatology 9:751, 1989

146. Kondo F, Maeda H. Histological features and clinical course of large regenerative nodules: evaluation of their precancerous potentiality. Hepatology 12:592, 1990

147. Konno T, et al. Targeting chemotherapy of hepatocellular carcinoma: arterial administration of SMANCS/Lipiodol. In: Okuda K, Ishak KG, eds. Neoplasms of the liver. Tokyo, Springer, 1987, p 343

148. Kubo Y, Shimokawa Y. Arterial injection chemotherapy. In: Okuda K, Peters RL, eds. Hepatocellular carcinoma. New York, John Wiley & Sons, 1976, p 477

149. Kubo Y, et al. Detection of hepatocellular carcinoma during a clinical follow-up of chronic liver disease: observations in 31 patients. Gastroenterology 74:578, 1978

150. Kuroda C, et al. Gallbladder infarction following hepatic transcatheter arterial embolization. Radiology 149:85, 1983

151. Kwaan H, et al. Antifibrinolytic activity in primary carcinoma of the liver. Clin Sci 18:241, 1959

152. Lai CL, et al. Clinical features of hepatocellular carcinoma: review of 211 patients in Hong Kong. Cancer 47:27, 1981

153. Lai E C-S, et al. Long-term results of resection for large hepatocellular carcinoma: a multivariate analysis of clinicopathological features. Hepatology 11:815, 1990

154. Lam KC, et al. Hepatitis B virus and cigarette smoking: risk factors for hepatocellular carcinoma in Hong Kong. Cancer Res 42:5246, 1982

155. Larouze NB, et al. Host response to hepatitis-B infection in patients with primary hepatic carcinoma and their families: a case-control study in Senegal, West Africa. Lancet 2:534, 1976

156. Lee FI. Cirrhosis and hepatoma in alcoholics. Gut 7:77, 1966

156a. Lee FL, et al. Primary liver cell cancer occurring in association with Crohn's disease treated with prednisolone and azathioprine. Hepatogastroenterology 30:188, 1983

157. Leevy CM, et al. Diseases of the liver and biliary tract: standardization of nomenclature, diagnostic criteria, and diagnostic methodology. Washington, DC, Fogarty International Center Proceedings, 1976, no. 22, p 77

158. Levrero M, et al. Antibodies to hepatitis C virus in patients with hepatocellular carcinoma. J Hepatol 12:60, 1991

159. Liang PC, Tung C. Morphologic study and etiology of primary liver carcinoma and its incidence in China. Chin Med J [Engl] 79:336, 1959

160. Liaw YF, et al. Early detection of hepatocellular carcinoma in patients with chronic type B hepatitis: a prospective study. Gastroenterology 90:263, 1986

161. Liebman HA, et al. Des-γ-carboxy (abnormal) prothrombin as a serum marker of primary hepatocellular carcinoma. N Engl J Med 310:1427, 1984

162. Lin DY, et al. Hepatic arterial embolization in patients with unresectable hepatocellular carcinoma: a randomized controlled trial. Gastroenterology 94:453, 1988

163. Lin TY. Surgical treatment of primary liver cell carcinoma. In: Okuda K, Peters RL, eds. Hepatocellular carcinoma. New York, John Wiley & Sons, 1976, p 449

164. Liver Cancer Study Group of Japan. The general rules for the clinical and pathological study of primary liver cancer. Jpn J Surg 19:98, 1989

165. Liver Cancer Study Group of Japan. Follow-up of primary

liver cancer patients: report 9 (1986–1987). Kyoto, Department of Surgery II, Kyoto University, 1990

166. Liver Cancer Study Group of Japan. Primary liver cancer in Japan. Clinicopathologic features and results of surgical treatment. Ann Surg 211:277, 1990

167. Livraghi T, et al. US-guided percutaneous alcohol injection of small hepatic and abdominal tumors. Radiology 161:309, 1986

168. Livraghi T, et al. Percutaneous alcohol injection of portal thrombosis in hepatocellular carcinoma: a new possible treatment. Tumori 76:394, 1990

169. Locker GY, et al. The clinical features of hepatic angiosarcoma: a report of four cases and a review of the English literature. Medicine 58:48, 1979

170. Lopez-Corella E, et al. Primary carcinoma of the liver in Mexican adults. Cancer 22:678, 1969

171. Lubin E, Lewitus Z. Blood pool scanning in investigating hepatic mass lesions. Semin Nucl Med 2:128, 1972

172. MacDonald RA. Cirrhosis and primary carcinoma of the liver: changes in their occurrence at the Boston City Hospital 1897–1954. N Engl J Med 255:1179, 1956

173. MacDonald RA. Primary carcinoma of the liver. Arch Intern Med 99:266, 1957

174. MacSween RNM. A clinicopathological review of 100 cases of primary malignant tumors of the liver. J Clin Pathol 27:669, 1974

175. Madanagopalan N, et al. Clinical spectrum of chronic Budd-Chiari syndrome and surgical relief for "coarctation" of the inferior vena cava. J Gastroenterol Hepatol 1:359, 1986

176. Makuuchi M, et al. Intraoperative ultrasound examination for hepatectomy. Jpn J Clin Oncol 11:367, 1981

177. Makuuchi M, et al. Ultrasonically guided subsegmentectomy. Surg Gynecol Obstet 161:346, 1985

178. Margulis AR, et al. Nuclear magnetic resonance in the diagnosis of tumors of the liver. Semin Roentgenol 17:123, 1983

179. Mariani AF, et al. Regressive enlargement of a hepatic cell adenoma. Gastroenterology 77:1319, 1979

180. Marion P, et al. A virus of Beechy ground squirrels that is related to hepatitis B virus of humans. Proc Natl Acad Sci USA 77:2941, 1980

181. Mason WS, et al. Virus of Pekin ducks with structural and biological relatedness to human hepatitis B virus. J Virol 36:829, 1980

182. Matsui O, et al. Work in progress: dynamic sequential computed tomography during arterial portography in the detection of hepatic neoplasms. Radiology 146:721, 1983

183. Matsui O, et al. Adenomatous hyperplastic nodules in the cirrhotic liver: differentiation from hepatocellular carcinoma with MR imaging. Radiology 173:123, 1989

184. McFadzean AJS, Yeung RTT. Further observation on hypoglycemia in hepatocellular carcinoma. Am J Med 47:230, 1969

185. McMahon G, et al. Identification of an activated c-Ki-ras oncogene in rat liver tumors induced by aflatoxin Bl. Proc Natl Acad Sci USA 83:9418, 1986

186. Melato M, et al. Relationship between cirrhosis, liver cancer, and hepatic metastases: an autopsy study. Cancer 64:455, 1989

187. Melia WM, et al. Hepatocellular carcinoma in primary biliary cirrhosis: detection by α-fetoprotein estimation. Gastroenterology 87:660, 1985

188. Messing A, et al. Peripheral neuropathies, hepatocellular carcinoma and islet cell adenoma in transgenic mice. Nature 316:461, 1985

189. Miyaji T, Imai S. Pathological studies on 639 cases of hepatoma autopsied in Japan during the 10 years from 1946 to 1955 inclusive. Acta Hepatol Jpn 1:100, 1960

190. Mizumoto R, Kawarada Y. Diagnosis and treatment of cholangiocarcinoma of the liver. In: Okuda K, Ishak KG, eds. Neoplasms of the liver. Tokyo, Springer, 1987, p 381

191. Mizumoto R, et al. Proposal of a new classification of cystic malignant tumours of the liver: classification of 65 cases reported at the 26th Annual Meeting of the Liver Cancer Society of Japan. J Gastroenterol Hepatol 6:1991

192. Morgan AG, et al. A new syndrome associated with hepatocellular carcinoma. Gastroenterology 63:340, 1972

193. Mori T, et al. Statistical analysis of Japanese Thorotrast-administered autopsy cases. Environ Res 18:2313, 1975

194. Mori W. Cirrhosis and primary cancer of the liver: comparative study in Tokyo and Cincinnati. Cancer 20:627, 1967

195. Moroy T, et al. Two different mechanisms for hepatitis B virus–induced hepatocellular carcinoma. In: Zuckerman AJ, ed. Viral hepatitis and liver disease. New York, Alan R Liss, 1988, p 737

196. Moss AA, Stark DD. Magnetic resonance imaging of liver tumors. In: Okuda K, Ishak KG, eds. Neoplasms of the liver. Tokyo, Springer, 1987, p 301

197. Motohara K, et al. Detection of vitamin K deficiency by use of an enzyme-linked immunosorbent assay for circulating abnormal prothrombin. Pediatr Res 19:354, 1985

198. Munoz N, Bosch X. Epidemiology of hepatocellular carcinoma. In: Okuda K, Ishak KG, eds. Neoplasms of the liver. Tokyo, Springer, 1987, p 3

199. Munoz N, Linsell A. Epidemiology of primary liver cancer. In: Correa P, Haenszel W, eds. Epidemiology of cancer of the digestive tract. Hague, Martinus Nijhoff, 1982, p 161

200. Muramatsu Y, et al. Peripheral low-density area of hepatic tumors: CT pathologic correlation. Radiology 160:49, 1986

201. Nagasue N, Inokuchi K. Spontaneous and traumatic rupture of hepatoma. Br J Surg 66:248, 1979

202. Nagata Y, et al. Radiofrequency thermotherapy for malignant liver tumors. Cancer 65:1730, 1990

203. Nagorney DM, et al. Fibrolamellar carcinoma. Am J Surg 149:113, 1985

204. Nakajima T, et al. Histopathological study of 102 cases of intrahepatic cholangiocarcinoma: histologic classification and modes of spreading. Hum Pathol 19:1228, 1988

205. Nakamura T, et al. Obstruction of the inferior vena cava in the hepatic portion and the hepatic veins. Angiology 19:479, 1968

206. Nakanuma Y, et al. Are hepatolithiasis and cholangioma aetiologically related? A morphological study of 12 cases of hepatolithiasis associated with cholangiocarcinoma. Virchow Arch [A] 406:45, 1985

207. Nakao N, et al. Hepatocellular carcinoma: combined hepatic, arterial, and portal vein embolization. Radiology 161:303, 1986

208. Nakashima T. Vascular changes and hemodynamics in hepatocellular carcinoma. In: Okuda K, Peter RL, eds. Hepatocellular carcinoma. New York, John Wiley & Sons, 1976, p 169

209. Nakashima T, Kojiro M. Hepatocellular carcinoma: its pathology atlas. Tokyo, Springer, 1987, p 3

210. Nakashima T, et al. Primary hepatocellular carcinoma coincident with schistosomiasis japonica: a study of 24 necropsies. Cancer 36:1483, 1975

211. Nakashima T, et al. Histological growth pattern of hepatocellular carcinoma: relationship to orcein (hepatitis B surface antigen)–positive cells in cancer tissue. Hum Pathol 13:563, 1982

212. Nakashima T, et al. Pathology of hepatocellular carcinoma in Japan. 232 consecutive cases autopsied in ten years. Cancer 51:863, 1983

213. Nakayama T, et al. Arterioportal shunts on dynamic computed tomography. AJR 140:9532, 1983

214. Nayak NC, et al. Location of hepatitis B surface antigen in conventional paraffin sections of the liver. Am J Pathol 81:479, 1975

215. Neuberger J, et al. Oral contraceptive–associated liver tumours: occurrence of malignancy and difficulties in diagnosis. Lancet 1:273, 1980

216. Niederau CC, et al. Survival and causes of death in cirrhotic and in noncirrhotic patients with primary hemochromatosis. N Engl J Med 313:1256, 1985

217. Nishikawa J, et al. Lobar attenuation difference of the liver on computed tomography. Radiology 141:725, 1981

218. Obata H, et al. A prospective study on the development of hepatocellular carcinoma from liver cirrhosis with persistent hepatitis B virus infection. Int J Cancer 25:741, 1980

219. Ochiya N, et al. Molecular cloning of an oncogene from a human hepatocellular carcinoma. Proc Natl Acad Sci USA 83:4993, 1986

220. Ogata N, et al. Point mutation, allelic loss and increased methylation of c-Ha-ras gene in human hepatocellular carcinoma. Hepatology 13:31, 1991

221. O'Grady JG, et al. Liver transplantation for malignant disease. Results in 93 consecutive patients. Ann Surg 207:373, 1988

222. Ohnishi K, et al. The effect of chronic habitual alcohol intake on the development of liver cirrhosis and hepatocellular carcinoma: relation to hepatitis B surface antigen carriage. Cancer 49:672, 1982

223. Ohnishi K, et al. Arterial chemoembolization of hepatocellular carcinoma with mitomycin C microcapsules. Radiology 152:51, 1984

224. Ohnishi K, et al. Formation of hilar collaterals or cavernous transformation after portal vein obstruction by hepatocellular carcinoma: observation in ten patients. Gastroenterology 87:1150, 1984

225. Ohnishi S, et al. Adoptive immunotherapy with lymphokine-activated killer cells plus recombinant interleukin 2 in patients with unresectable hepatocellular carcinoma. Hepatology 10:349, 1989

226. Ohta T, et al. Paraneoplastic syndrome in hepatocellular carcinoma. Naika Mook 18:180, 1988

227. Ohto M, et al. Radiation therapy and percutaneous ethanol injection for the treatment of hepatocellular carcinoma. In: Okuda K, Ishak KG, eds. Neoplasms of the liver. Tokyo, Springer, 1987, p 335

228. Ohtomo K, et al. Hepatic tumors: dynamic MR imaging. Radiology 167:27, 1987

229. Ohtomo K, et al. Hepatocellular carcinoma and cavernous hemangioma: differentiation with MR imaging—efficacy of T2 values at 0.35 and 1.5 T. Radiology 168:621, 1988

230. Oka H, et al. Prospective study of early detection of hepatocellular carcinoma in patients with cirrhosis. Hepatology 12:680, 1990

231. Okazaki N, et al. Screening of patients with chronic liver disease for hepatocellular carcinomas by ultrasonography. Clin Oncol 10:241, 1976

232. Okazaki N, et al. Evaluation of the prognosis for small hepatocellular carcinoma based on tumor volume doubling time. A preliminary report. Cancer 63:2207, 1989

233. Okuda H, et al. Hepatocellular carcinoma (HCC) presumably associated with non-B hepatitis virus infection: clinical and pathological observations. Hepatology 2:113, 1982

234. Okuda H, et al. Clinicopathological features of hepatocellular carcinoma: comparison of seropositive and seronegative patients. Hepatogastroenterology 31:64, 1984

235. Okuda H, et al. Production of abnormal prothrombin (des-γ-carboxy prothrombin) by hepatocellular carcinoma: a clinical and experimental study. J Hepatol 4:357, 1987

236. Okuda H, et al. Production of des-γ-carboxy prothrombin by human hepatoma cells in culture. Hepatology 7:1128, 1987

237. Okuda H, et al. Production of abnormal vitamin K–dependent proteins by hepatocellular carcinoma. Hepatology 10:673, 1989

238. Okuda K. Clinical aspects of hepatocellular carcinoma: analysis of 134 cases. In: Okuda K, Peters RL, eds. Hepatocellular carcinoma. New York, John Wiley & Sons, 1976, p 387

239. Okuda K. Advances in hepatobiliary ultrasonography. Hepatology 1:662, 1981

240. Okuda K. Membranous obstruction of the inferior vena cava: etiology and relation to hepatocellular carcinoma. Gastroenterology 82:376, 1982

241. Okuda K. Early recognition of hepatocellular carcinoma. Hepatology 6:729, 1986

242. Okuda K. Hepatitis C virus and hepatocellular carcinoma. In: Tabor E, DiBisceglie A, Purcell RH, eds. Etiology, pathology, and treatment of hepatocellular carcinoma in North America. Woodlands, TX, Portfolio Publishing, 1991, p 119

243. Okuda K, Iio M. Radiological aspects of the liver and biliary tract. X-ray and radioisotope diagnosis. Chicago, Yearbook, 1976, p 267

244. Okuda K, Nakashima T. Primary carcinoma of the liver. In: Berk JE, et al, eds. Bockus' gastroenterology, vol 5. Philadelphia, WB Saunders, 1984, p 3315

245. Okuda K, et al. Demonstration of growing casts of hepatocellular carcinoma in the portal vein by celiac angiography: the thread and streaks sign. Radiology 117:303, 1975

246. Okuda K, et al. Clinical observations during a relatively early stage of hepatocellular carcinoma, with special reference to serum α-fetoprotein levels. Gastroenterology 69:226, 1975

247. Okuda K, et al. Angiographic demonstration of intrahepatic arterioportal anastomoses in hepatocellular carcinoma. Radiology 122:53, 1977

248. Okuda K, et al. Angiographic assessment of gross anatomy of hepatocellular carcinoma: comparison of celiac angiograms and liver pathology in 100 cases. Radiology 123:21, 1977

249. Okuda K, et al. Clinical aspects of intrahepatic bile duct carcinoma including hilar carcinoma: a study of 57 autopsy-proven cases. Cancer 39:232, 1977

250. Okuda K, et al. Clinicopathological features of encapsulated hepatocellular carcinoma. Cancer 40:1240, 1977

251. Okuda K, et al. Clinicopathological studies of minute hepatocellular carcinoma: analysis of 20 cases, including 4 with hepatic resection. Gastroenterology 73:109, 1977

252. Okuda K, et al. Primary liver cancers in Japan. Cancer 45:2663, 1980

253. Okuda K, et al. A clinical and pathological study of diffuse type hepatocellular carcinoma. Liver 1:280, 1981

254. Okuda K, et al. Hepatocellular carcinoma arising in noncirrhotic and highly cirrhotic livers: a comparative study of histopathology and frequency of hepatitis B markers. Cancer 49:450, 1982

255. Okuda K, et al. Gross anatomical features of hepatocellular carcinoma from three disparate geographic areas: proposal of new classification. Cancer 54:2165, 1984

256. Okuda K, et al. Natural history of hepatocellular carcinoma and prognosis in relation to treatment: study of 850 patients. Cancer 56:918, 1985

257. Okuda K, et al. Changing incidence of hepatocellular carcinoma in Japan. Cancer Res 47:4967, 1987

258. Okuda K, et al. Angiography in the diagnosis of liver disease. Semin Liver Dis 9:50, 1989

259. Okuda K, et al. Hepatocellular carcinoma without cirrhosis in Japanese patients. Gastroenterology 97:140, 1989

260. Okuda K, et al. Hepatocellular carcinoma presenting with pyrexia and leukocytosis: report of five cases. Hepatology 13:1991

261. Okuno K. Treatment of unresectable hepatoma via selective hepatic arterial infusion of lymphokine-activated killer cells generated from autologous spleen cells. Cancer 58:1001, 1986

262. Oldenburg WA, et al. Hypercalcemia and primary hepatic tumors. Arch Surg 117:1363, 1982

263. Omata M, et al. Sclerosing hepatic carcinoma: relationship to hypercalcemia. Liver 1:33, 1981

264. Omata M, et al. Duck hepatitis B virus and liver disease. Gastroenterology 85:260, 1983

265. Ong GB, Taw JL. Spontaneous rupture of hepatocellular carcinoma. Br Med J [Clin Res] 4:146, 1972

266. Order SE, et al. Radidolabelled antibodies in the treatment of non-resectable hepatocellular carcinoma: Johns Hopkins and Radiation Oncology Group experience. In: Bannasch P, et al, eds. Liver cell carcinoma. Dordrecht, Kluwer Academic Publishing, 1989, p 475

267. Orian JM, et al. New murine model for hepatocellular carcinoma: transgenic mice expressing metallothionein-ovine growth hormone fusion gene. J Natl Cancer Inst 82:393, 1990

268. Osborne BN, et al. Primary lymphoma of the liver: ten cases and a review of the literature. Cancer 56:2902, 1985

269. Ozawa K, et al. Clinical application of cytochrome a (+a3) of mitochondria from liver specimens: an aid in determining metabolic tolerance of liver remnant for hepatic resection. Ann Surg 180:868, 1974

270. Paradinas FJ, et al. High serum vitamin B_{12} binding capacity as a marker of the fibrolamellar variant of hepatocellular carcinoma. Br Med J [Clin Res] 285:840, 1982

271. Paterlini P, et al. Polymerase chain reaction to detect hepatitis B virus DNA and RNA sequences in primary liver cancer from patients negative for hepatitis B surface antigen. N Engl J Med 3233:80, 1990

272. Patton RB, Horn RC Jr. Primary liver carcinoma: autopsy study of 60 cases. Cancer 17:757, 1964

273. Peters RL. Pathology of hepatocellular carcinoma. In: Okuda K, Peters RL, eds. Hepatocellular carcinoma. New York, John Wiley & Sons, 1976, p 107

274. Petrelli NJ, et al. Hepatic resection for isolated metastasis from colorectal carcinoma. Am J Surg 149:205, 1985

275. Pimentel JC, Menezes AF. Liver disease in vineyard sprayers. Gastroenterology 72:275, 1977

276. Plengvanit U, et al. Intraperitoneal hemorrhage due to spontaneous rupture of primary liver cancer with particular reference to hepatic artery ligation. Ann Acad Med 9:264, 1980

277. Polio J, et al. Hepatocellular carcinoma in Wilson's disease: case report and review of the literature. J Clin Gastroenterol 11:220, 1989

278. Popper H, et al. Development of hepatic angiosarcoma induced by vinyl chloride, Thorotrast and arsenic: comparison with cases of unknown etiology. Am J Pathol 92:349, 1978

279. Popper H. Virus versus chemical hepatocarcinogenesis. J Hepatol 6:229, 1988

280. Popper H, et al. Woodchuck hepatitis and hepatocellular carcinoma: correlation of histologic with virologic observations. Hepatology 1:91, 1981

281. Popper H, et al. Hepatocarcinogenicity of woodchuck hepatitis virus. Proc Natl Acad Sci USA 84:866, 1987

282. Powell-Tuck J, et al. Prediction of early death after therapeutic hepatic arterial embolization. Br Med J [Clin Res] 288:1257, 1984

283. Price JB, et al. Major hepatic resections for neoplasia in children. Arch Surg 117:1139, 1982

284. Primack A, et al. A staging system for hepatocellular carcinoma: prognostic factors in Ugandan patients. Cancer 35:357, 1975

285. Prince AM, et al. A case-control study of the association between primary liver cancer and hepatitis B infection in Senegal. Int J Cancer 16:376, 1975

286. Purtilo DT, Gottlieb LS. Cirrhosis and hepatoma occurring at Boston City Hospital (1917–1968). Cancer 322:458, 1973

287. Registry of Hepatic Metastases. Resection of the liver for colorectal resection. Surgery 103:278, 1988

288. Reynolds SH, et al. Detection and identification of activated oncogenes in spontaneously occurring benign and malignant hepatocellular tumors of the BEC 3F1 mouse. Proc Natl Acad Sci USA 83:33, 1986

289. Ritchie J, et al. Biliary tract carcinoma with ulcerative colitis. Q J Med 43:263, 1974

290. Robinson WS, et al. The hepadna virus group. Hepatitis B and related viruses. In: Szmuness W, et al, eds. Viral hepatitis. Philadelphia, Franklin Institute Press, 1982, p 57

291. Rogler CE, et al. Deletion in chromosome 11p associated with a hepatitis B integration site in hepatocellular carcinoma. Science 230:319, 1985

292. Roles DB. Fibrolamellar carcinoma of the liver. In: Okuda K, Ishak KG, eds. Neoplasms of the liver. Tokyo, Springer, 1987, p 137

293. Rubel LR, et al. Thorotrast-associated cholangiocarcinoma: an epidemiologic and clinicopathologic study. Cancer 50:1408, 1982

294. Saito A, et al. Angio-echography in the diagnosis of hepatic tumors. Kan-Tan-Sui 15:1129, 1987

295. Sakuma K, et al. Relative risks of death due to liver disease among Japanese male adults having various statuses for hepatitis B s and e antigen/antibody in serum: a prospective study. Hepatology 8:1642, 1988

296. Sakurai M. A histopathologic study on the effect of alcohol on cirrhosis and hepatoma of autopsy cases in Japan. Acta Pathol Jpn 19:283, 1969

297. Salata H, et al. Porphyria cutanea tarda and hepatocellular carcinoma: frequency of occurrence and related factors. J Hepatol 1:477, 1985

298. Saracci R, Repetto F. Time trends of primary liver cancer: indication of increased incidence in selected cancer registry populations. J Natl Cancer Inst 65:241, 1980

299. Savitch I, et al. Uptake of Tc-99m-di-isopropylimino-diacetic acid by hepatocellular carcinoma: concise communication. J Nucl Med 24:1119, 1983

300. Sawabu N, et al. Clinical evaluation of specific γ-GTP isoenzyme in patients with hepatocellular carcinoma. Cancer 51:327, 1983

301. Shafritz DA, et al. Integration of hepatitis B virus DNA into the genome of liver cells in chronic liver disease and hepatocellular carcinoma: studies in percutaneous liver biopsies and post-mortem tissue specimens. N Engl J Med 305:1067, 1981

302. Shafritz DA, et al. Molecular biology of hepatocellular carcinoma: HBV DNA molecular forms and viral gene products in human liver tissue. In: Zuckerman AJ, ed. Viral hepatitis and liver disease. New York, Alan R Liss, 1988, p 731

303. Shaul Y, et al. A human hepatitis B viral enhancer element. EMBO J 4:427, 1985

304. Sheu JC, et al. Early detection of hepatocellular carcinoma by real-time ultrasonography: a prospective study. Cancer 56:660, 1985

305. Sheu JC, et al. Hepatocellular carcinoma: US evolution in the early stage. Radiology 155:463, 1985

306. Sheu JC, et al. Small hepatocellular carcinoma: intratumor ethanol treatment using new needle and guidance system. Radiology 163:43, 1987

307. Shibata J, et al. Hepatic arterial injection chemotherapy with cisplatin suspended in an oily lymphographic agent for hepatocellular carcinoma. Cancer 64:1586, 1989

308. Shikata T. Primary liver carcinoma and liver cirrhosis. In: Okuda K, Peters RL, eds. Hepatocellular carcinoma. New York, John Wiley & Sons, 1976, p 53

309. Shimokawa Y, et al. Serum glutamic oxalacetic transaminase/glutamic pyruvic transaminase ratios in hepatocellular carcinoma. Cancer 40:319, 1977

310. Shina S, et al. Multiple-needle insertion in percutaneous ethanol injection therapy for liver neoplasms. Gastroenterol Jpn 26:47, 1991

311. Shinagawa T, et al. Real-time ultrasonographic diagnosis of hepatocellular carcinoma: correlation of echograms and histopathological findings. Jpn J Gastroenterol 78:2404, 1981

312. Shinagawa T, et al. Diagnosis and clinical features of small hepatocellular carcinoma with emphasis of the utility of real-time ultrasonography: a study in 51 patients. Gastroenterology 86:495, 1984

313. Shirai F. Pathological study on hepatocellular carcinoma: ultrastructure of tumor-nontumor boundary. Acta Hepatol Jpn 23:1034, 1982

314. Simonetti RG, et al. Prevalence of antibodies to hepatitis C virus in hepatocellular carcinoma. Lancet 2:1338, 1989

315. Simson IW. Membranous obstruction of the inferior vena cava: etiology and relation to hepatocellular carcinoma. Gastroenterology 83:171, 1982

316. Small JA, et al. Early regions of JC virus and BL virus induce distinct and tissue-specific tumors in transgenic mice. Proc Natl Acad Sci USA 83:8288, 1986

317. Smalley SR, et al. Hepatoma in the noncirrhotic liver. Cancer 62:1414, 1988

318. Smoron GL, Battifora HA. Thorotrast-induced hepatoma. Cancer 20:1252, 1972

319. Solis JA, et al. Association of porphyria cutanea tarda and primary liver cancer: report of ten cases. J Dermatol (Tokyo) 9:131, 1982

320. Sonakul D, et al. Hepatic carcinoma with opisthorchiasis. Southeast Asian J Trop Med Public Health 9:215, 1978

321. Soo CDS, et al. Treatment of hepatic neoplasm through extrahepatic collaterals. Radiology 147:45, 1983

322. Soulier J-P, et al. A new method to assay des-γ-carboxy prothrombin. Results obtained in 75 cases of hepatocellular carcinoma. Gastroenterology 91:1258, 1986

323. Stadelnik RC, et al. Critical evaluation of hepatic scintiangiography for neoplasms of the liver. J Nucl Med 16:595, 1975

324. Steiner PE. Cancer of the liver and cirrhosis in trans-Saharan Africa and the United States of America. Cancer 13:1085, 1960

325. Steiner PE, Higginson J. Cholangiolocellular carcinoma of the liver. Cancer 12:753, 1959

326. Sternlieb I. Copper and the liver. Gastroenterology 78:1615, 1980

327. Stocker JT, et al. Undifferentiated embryonal sarcoma. Cancer 42:365, 1978

328. Su DL. Drinking water and liver cancer: an epidemiological approach to the etiology of this disease in China. Chin Med J [Engl] 92:748, 1979

329. Sugihara S, Kojiro M. Pathology of cholangiocarcinoma. In: Okuda K, Ishak KG, eds. Neoplasms of the liver. Tokyo, Springer, 1987, p 143

330. Sugihara S, et al. Pathomorphologic study on hyperplastic nodule of the liver: a special reference to the containment of cancerous foci. Acta Hepatol Jpn 31:324, 1990

331. Sullivan RD, et al. Chemotherapy of metastatic liver cancer by prolonged hepatic-artery infusion. N Engl J Med 270:321, 1964

332. Sumida M, et al. Accuracy of angiography in the diagnosis of small hepatocellular carcinoma. AJR 147:531, 1986

333. Summers J, et al. A virus similar to hepatitis B virus associated with hepatitis and hepatoma in woodchucks. Proc Natl Acad Sci USA 75:4533, 1978

334. Szmuness W. Hepatocellular carcinoma and the hepatitis B virus: evidence for a causal association. Prog Med Virol 24:40, 1978

335. Tada M, et al. Analysis of *ras* gene mutation in human hepatic malignant tumors by polymerase chain reaction and direct sequencing. Cancer Res 50:1121, 1990

336. Takayama T, et al. Malignant transformation of adenomatous hyperplasia to hepatocellular carcinoma. Lancet 336:1150, 1990

337. Takayasu K, Okuda K. Celiac angiography in the diagnosis of small hepatocellular carcinoma. In: Okuda K, Ishak KG, eds. Neoplasms of the liver. Tokyo, Springer, 1987, p 271

338. Takayasu K, et al. Hepatic arterial embolization for hepatocellular carcinoma. Radiology 150:661, 1984

339. Takayasu K, et al. Splenic infarction, a complication of transcatheter hepatic arterial embolization for liver malignancies. Radiology 151:371, 1984

340. Takayasu K, et al. Hepatic lobe atrophy following obstruction of the ipsilateral portal vein from hilar cholangiocarcinoma. Radiology 160:389, 1986

341. Takayasu K, et al. Hepatocellular carcinoma: treatment with intraarterial iodized oil with and without chemotherapeutic agents. Radiology 162:345, 1987

342. Takayasu K, et al. Clinical and radiological assessment of the results of hepatectomy for small hepatocellular carcinoma and therapeutic arterial embolization for postoperative recurrence. Cancer 64:1848, 1989

343. Takayasu K, et al. Hepatic artery embolization for inoperable hepatocellular carcinoma: progress and risk factors. Cancer Chemother Pharmacol 23:S123, 1989

344. Takayasu K, et al. CT of hilar cholangiocarcinoma: late contrast enhancement in six patients. AJR 154:1203, 1990

345. Takayasu K, et al. The diagnosis of small hepatocellular carcinoma: efficacy of various imaging procedures in 100 patients. AJR 155:49, 1990

346. Taketa K. α-Fetoprotein: reevaluation in hepatology. Hepatology 12:1420, 1990

347. Taketa K, et al. Lectin-reactive profiles of alpha-fetoprotein characterizing hepatocellular carcinoma and related conditions. Gastroenterology 99:508, 1990

348. Tanaka S, et al. Early diagnosis of hepatocellular carcinoma: usefulness of ultrasonically guided fine-needle aspiration biopsy. J Clin Ultrasound 14:11, 1986

349. Tanaka S, et al. Recent advances in ultrasonographic diagnosis of hepatocellular carcinoma. Cancer 63:1313, 1989

350. Tandon BN, et al. Study of an epidemic of jaundice, presumably due to toxic hepatitis, in northwest India. Gastroenterology 72:488, 1977

351. Tang ZY. Subclinical hepatocellular carcinoma: historical aspects and general consideration. In: Tang ZY, ed. Subclinical hepatocellular carcinoma. Beijing, China Academic Publishers, 1985, p 1

352. Tang ZY, et al. Radioimmunotherapy in the multimodality treatment of hepatocellular carcinoma with reference to second-look resection. Cancer 65:211, 1990

353. Tao LC, et al. Cytologic diagnosis of hepatocellular carcinoma by fine needle aspiration biopsy. Cancer 53:547, 1984

354. Taylor I. Colorectal liver metastasis: to treat or not to treat? Br J Surg 722:511, 1985

355. Terada T, Nakanuma Y. Pathological observations of intrahepatic peribiliary glands in 1000 consecutive autopsy livers. II. A possible source of cholangiocarcinoma. Hepatology 12:92, 1990

356. Terada T, et al. Iron-accumulating adenomatous hyperplastic nodule with malignant foci in the cirrhotic liver: histopathologic, quantitative iron, and magnetic resonance imaging in in vitro studies. Cancer 65:1994, 1990

357. Thompson RPH, et al. Cutaneous porphyria due to a malignant primary hepatoma. Gastroenterology 59:779, 1970

358. Tiollais P, et al. The hepatitis B virus. Nature 317:489, 1985

359. Tiribelli C, et al. Prevalence of hepatocellular carcinoma and relation to cirrhosis: comparison of two different cities of the world—Trieste, Italy, and Chiba, Japan. Hepatology 10:998, 1989

360. Tobe T. Hepatectomy in patients with cirrhotic livers: clinical and basic considerations. In: Nyhus LM, ed. Surgery annual, vol 16. E Norwalk, CT, Appleton-Century-Crofts, 1984, p 177

361. Tokunaga N. Pathomorphological study on primary liver cancer: a clinicopathologic study of cholangiocarcinoma. Acta Hepatol Jpn 25:549, 1984

362. Tomiya T, Fujiwara K. Plasma thrombin–antithrombin III complexes in diagnosis of primary hepatocellular carcinoma complicating liver cirrhosis. Cancer 67:481, 1991

363. Trichopoulos D, et al. Smoking and hepatitis B–negative primary hepatocellular carcinoma. J Natl Cancer Inst 65:111, 1980

364. Tsuchida S, et al. Purification of γ-glutamyltransferases from rat hepatomas and hyperplastic hepatic nodules, and comparison with the enzyme from rat kidney. Cancer Res 39:4200, 1979

365. Tsunetomi S, et al. Diagnosis of small hepatocellular carcinoma by computed tomography: correlation of CT findings and histopathology. J Gastroenterol Hepatol 4:395, 1989

366. Tylen U, et al. Heparinized catheter for long-term intraarterial infusion of 5-fluorouracil in liver metastases. Cardiovasc Radiol 2:111, 1979

367. Van Kaick G, et al. Der Beitrag der Computertomographie zur Quantifizierung der Thorotrast und zur thorotrastinduzierter Lebertumoren. Radiologe 26:123, 1986

368. Van Rensburg SJ, et al. Hepatocellular carcinoma and dietary aflatoxin in Mozambique and Transkei. Br J Cancer 51:713, 1985

369. Van Thiel DH, et al. Liver transplantation for hepatocellular carcinoma. In: Bannasch P, et al, eds. Liver cell carcinoma. Dordrecht, Kluwer Academic Publishing, 1989, p 499

370. Verhaeghe R, et al. Dysfibrinogenemia associated with primary hepatoma. Scand J Haematol 9:451, 1972

371. Vogelstein B, et al. Genetic alterations during colorectal tumor development. N Engl J Med 319:525, 1988

372. Wang HP, Rogler CE. Deletion in human chromosome arms 11p and 13q in primary hepatocellular carcinoma. Cytogenet Cell Genet 48:72, 1988

373. Wanless IR, et al. On the pathogenesis of focal nodular hyperplasia of the liver. Hepatology 5:1194, 1985

374. Waterhouse JAH, et al. Cancer incidence in five continents, vol 3. Lyon, International Agency for Research on Cancer, 1976

375. Waxman S, Gilbert HS. A tumor-related vitamin B_{12} binding protein in adolescent hepatoma. N Engl J Med 282:1053, 1973

376. Wee A, et al. Hepatobiliary carcinoma associated with primary sclerosing cholangitis and chronic ulcerative colitis. Hum Pathol 16:719, 1985

377. Wilkinson ML, et al. Wilson's disease and hepatocellular carcinoma: possible protective role of copper. Gut 24:767, 1983

378. Wogan GN. Aflatoxins and their relationship to hepatocellular carcinoma. In: Okuda K, Peters RL, eds. Hepatocellular carcinoma. New York, John Wiley & Sons, 1976, p 25

379. Wogen GN. The incidence of liver cell cancer by chemicals. In: Cameron HM, et al, eds. Liver cell cancer. Amsterdam, Elsevier, 1976, p 121

380. World Health Organization. World health statistics annual, 1978–1982. Vital statistics and causes of death. Geneva, WHO, 1982

381. Yamada R, et al. Hepatic arterial embolization in 120 patients with unresectable hepatoma. Radiology 148:397, 1983

382. Yamagiwa K. Kenntnis des primaren parenchymatosen Leberkarzinoms ("Hepatoma"). Virchow Arch [A] 206:437, 1911

383. Yamashita K, et al. Sugar chain of α-fetoprotein produced in human yolk sac tumor. Cancer Res 42:4691, 1983

384. Yano H, et al. A new human hepatocellular carcinoma cell line (KYN-1) with a transformation to adenocarcinoma. In Vitro 22:637, 1986

385. Yee JK. A liver-specific enhancer in the core promoter region of human hepatitis B virus. Science 246:658, 1989

386. Yokosuka O, et al. Duck hepatitis B virus DNA in liver and serum of Chinese duck: integration of viral DNA in a hepatocellular carcinoma. Proc Natl Acad Sci USA 82:5180, 1985

387. Yokosuka O, et al. Detection and direct sequencing of hepatitis B virus genome by DNA amplification method. Gastroenterology 100:175, 1991

388. Yoshida MD, et al. A rat strain that spontaneously develop severe hepatic necrosis and later hepatocellular carcinoma. J Hered 78:361, 1987

388a. Yoshida T. Über die experimentelle Erzeugung von Hepatoma durch die Fütterung mit o-Aminoazotoluolo Proc Imp Acad (Tokyo) 8:464, 1932

389. Yu MC, et al. Hepatitis, alcohol consumption, cigarette smoking, and hepatocellular carcinoma in Los Angeles. Cancer Res 43:6077, 1983

390. Yu SZ. Epidemiology of primary liver cancer. In: Tang ZY, ed. Subclinical hepatocellular carcinoma. Beijing, China Academic Publishing, 1985, p 189

391. Yumoto Y, et al. Hepatocellular carcinoma detected by iodized oil. Radiology 154:19, 1985

392. Zarbl H, et al. Direct mutagenesis of Ha-ras-l oncogenes by N-nitroso-N-methylurea during initiation of mammary carcinogenesis in rats. Nature 315:382, 1985

393. Zhou XD, et al. Clinical evaluation of cryosurgery in the treatment of primary cancer: report of 60 cases. Cancer 61:1889, 1988

394. Zhou XD, et al. Long-term survivors after resection for primary liver cancer: clinical analysis of 9 patients surviving more than ten years. Cancer 63:201, 1989

Diseases of the Liver, Seventh Edition, edited by
Leon Schiff and Eugene R. Schiff. J.B. Lippincott Company, Philadelphia © 1993.

45

Surgical Management of Primary and Metastatic Cancer of the Liver

Paul H. Sugarbaker

Most gastrointestinal cancers present in an advanced stage. To improve survival, one may attempt to prevent the disease or to bring about its early detection. Although these strategies should be more widely used, for various political and economic reasons, they have not been effective. Another strategy by which to improve the survival with intraabdominal cancer is to optimize therapy for advanced disease. For both hepatoma and primary colorectal cancer, early disease is curable in most patients with a simple surgical procedure. More effective treatment for advanced disease presents a major challenge for laboratory and clinical research efforts.

Natural History of Hepatocellular Carcinoma and Colorectal Metastases to the Liver

Despite a potentially curative resection of large bowel cancer, at least half of patients die of their disease, and liver metastases are involved in about half of these surgical treatment failures. Despite a complete surgical removal of primary liver cancer, over 70% of patients die of this disease. Rational decisions for the surgical management of these patients depend on the grade or biologic aggressiveness of the cancer and the anatomic location of the cancer. For hepatocellular cancer, both the grade of the cancer and its anatomic location present grave prognostic implications (Fig. 45-1). The primary tumor has a rapid doubling time, invades aggressively into surrounding tissues, and is early to disseminate into venules and lymphatic channels.[5,72] Because of its anatomic location, the tumor does not cause symptoms early in its natural history. Rather, an immense size of the primary tumor usually is observed at the time of diagnosis. Table 45-1 reviews some clinical features recognized in the natural history of hepatoma and other liver tumors.

Primary colorectal cancer differs greatly from hepatocellular cancer in its pattern of dissemination. Rather than synchronously embolizing diffusely to the systemic vasculature, colorectal cancer disseminates first local-regionally to sites within the abdominal cavity. Cancer dissemination usually is contained within the first lymphatic bed and the first capillary bed (liver) and to peritoneal surfaces. Disease dissemination limited to these anatomic sites can be surgically treated with curative intent.[38,41,78,87,92–94] Figures 45-1 and 45-2 contrast the patterns of dissemination of these two cancers. For hepatoma, there are only two phases in the dissemination of the disease. First, the primary tumor invades locally into

the liver. Next, it seeds distant (surgically unresectable) sites. As these metastases progress, they result in the cascade phenomenon and an overwhelming cancerous process. In contrast, for colorectal disease, there are, for some patients, three phases in the dissemination of the tumor. First, the primary tumor locally invades. Second, regional dissemination occurs: (1) lymphatic metastases to adjacent lymph nodes, (2) hematogenous metastases to liver and lungs, and (3) intraperitoneal spread to peritoneal surfaces. A window of time exists in which dissemination to any of these anatomic sites can be treated with curative intent. Colorectal cancer qualifies as a tumor with a metachronous (stepwise) pattern of dissemination. As cancer nodules in adjacent lymph nodes, liver, or peritoneal spaces increase in size, metastases from metastases occur. Only then does the cascade phenomenon begin and the host succumb to systemic cancer progression (see Table 45-1).

This concept of metachronous dissemination provides the biologic rationale for the surgical removal of hepatic metastases. There are vascular and lymphatic networks that temporarily interrupt cancer dissemination as a systemic process. The filtration systems that develop metastatic cancer and yet can be made surgically disease-free with curative intent are the adjacent lymphatics,[74,113] liver parenchyma,[87,92,93] and lung parenchyma.[78] Also, a curative approach to peritoneal implantation has been described.[93,94] A theoretical model in which a proportion of colorectal cancers show *isolated* sites of disease dissemination away from the primary tumor is shown in Figure 45-3.[100] In patients who are treated relatively early in the natural history of large bowel cancer, recurrent cancer is more likely to show first recurrence at a single anatomic site. Therefore, reoperative surgery is more likely to be successful. For example, in patients with Dukes' stage B, as opposed to Dukes' stage C, primary cancer, Hughes and coworkers[41] reported a 35% 5-year survival rate in liver resection for Dukes' stage B cancer and a 28% survival rate for Dukes' stage C cancer. This phenomenon of isolated sites of local-regional disease progression can only be appreciated if all malignant tissues are removed with negative margins of excision (surgical complete response). This concept of cancer dissemination necessitates a redefinition of the reasonable surgical limits of resection for advanced primary and recurrent large bowel cancer.

A principle of tumor biology that helps to explain this phenomenon of metachronous cancer spread is called *metastatic inefficiency*.[110,112] This theory seeks to interpret the dissemination of cancer through lymphatic and vascular channels by two powerful biologic principals. They are evolution and the

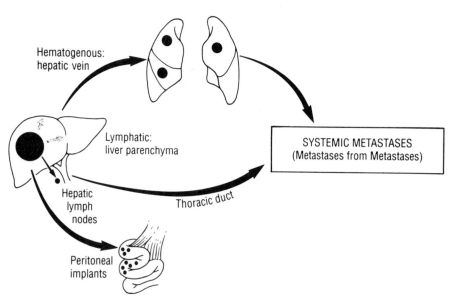

FIGURE 45-1   Primary liver cancer (hepatoma) dissemination.

laws of physics. In an evolutionary perspective, vascular and lymphatic channels have been precisely modified to distribute red blood cells, white blood cells, and platelets. Tumor cells enter at their own risk and are apparently destroyed in tremendous numbers in virtually all patients with cancer. Only as the number of tumor cells overwhelms the natural resistance of relevant capillary or lymphatic beds or as tumor cells gain through a process of selection unique cell surface properties do cancer cells implant and grow. Theoretically, billions of tumor cells are destroyed intravascularly on a daily basis for months and even years before implantation succeeds within an endothelial-lined and basement membrane–intact lymphatic or vascular channel.

Strict physical restrictions control the survival of cells within endothelial-lined spaces. Cancer cells may be too large to survive passage through capillary beds. Weiss (personal communication, June 1990) has suggested that their cell walls are too brittle, and they cannot survive the turbulence of the intravascular environment. Consequently, billions of tumor cells may be destroyed on a regular basis by a capillary bed. This assumes that the walls of blood vessels and lymphatic channels remain intact. Injured tissues have greatly increased propensity to tumor cell implantation and progression.[23] It is possible for one or a few metastases to have occurred within the liver and all the rest of the host's vascular and lymphatic system to remain free of disease. Metastatic disease within the liver must be isolated to that organ if the surgical removal of liver tumors is to result in cure. Because the clinician is better able to eliminate from liver resection, patients with extrahepatic disease, results with hepatic resec-

TABLE 45-1   *Comparative Oncology*

Clinical Feature	*Primary Liver Cancer*	*Primary Colorectal Cancer*	*Colorectal Liver Metastases*
Early symptoms or signs	Unusual	Pain, lower gastrointestinal bleeding, large bowel obstruction	Unusual
Tumor antigen	α-Fetoprotein	Carcinoembryonic antigen	Carcinoembrygonic antigen
Etiology	Hepatitis B implicated	Carcinogens in diet; high-fat, low-fiber diet, genetic predisposition	Portal vein tumor emboli
Size tumor	Increased size decreases survival	Increased bowel wall penetration but not size decreases survival	Size does not affect survival
Lymph node metastases	Signifies grave prognosis	Indicates 50% survival	Signifies grave prognosis
Tumor multiplicity	Signifies grave prognosis	NA	1–4 tumors carry same prognosis
Overall survival	<10%	40%	<10%
Survival operable patients	30%	50%	40%
Dissemination	Systemic	Local-regional	Systemic

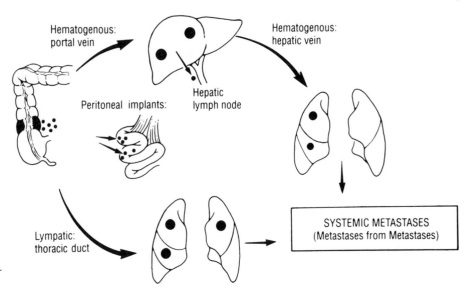

FIGURE 45-2 Colorectal cancer dissemination.

tion of colorectal metastases will continue to improve.[95] The presence or absence of occult extrahepatic disease must be the major prognostic factor determining the failure or success of hepatic resection.

A second important feature of colorectal cancer combines with metachronous dissemination to allow the resection of metastatic disease with curative intent. It involves the surgeon's ability to definitively locally control the primary cancer in a large proportion of patients. This feature distinguishes large bowel cancer from the other gastrointestinal cancers, such as gastric cancer, pancreatic cancer, and visceral sarcomas. Only with local control can the surgical benefits of the removal of metastatic disease show long-term survival.

An important concept in the biology of intraabdominal cancer suggests two general types of cancer dissemination. To understand the natural history of large bowel cancer, one must appreciate the difference between cancer spread and cancer metastases. Spread of cancer implies preoperative or

intraoperative dissemination of tumor emboli around the abdominal cavity. Spread results in local (resection site) recurrence or peritoneal carcinomatosis. The efficiency with which cells implant and grow within the abdominal cavity is extremely high. Even the lowest-grade mucinous colorectal tumors implant and grow with regularity within body cavities. In contrast, dissemination of tumor emboli by way of hematogenous or lymphatic routes is a complex biologic phenomena and qualifies as an inefficient process in most patients. This implantation inefficiency results from strict biologic and physical requirements of all implants that develop within a vascular channel.

Few, if any, physical or biologic restrictions prevent tumor implantation on the lining of a body cavity. Not only does surgical trauma encourage tumor entrapment and tumor growth as a result of fibrin deposition, but tumor progression is facilitated by the local production of growth factors.[16,98] The capability of a cancer embolus to implant and grow within a body cavity is not related to its ability to metastasize by way of blood vessels and lymphatic channels. Only high-grade invasive tumors metastasize. Both high- and low-grade tumors implant and grow within a body cavity. Consequently, the surgeon's success with the removal of hepatic metastases may be expected to increase sharply as resection site recurrence and peritoneal surface spread are eliminated as part of the natural history of this disease process. Great care should be taken in the surgical removal of the primary colorectal tumor so as not to allow for even a few tumor emboli to be lost into the free peritoneal cavity.

Colorectal cancer may be unique among intraabdominal neoplasms for several reasons. First, there is a stepwise progression of disease. This is because it is a relatively metastatically inefficient cancer, so that it is not uncommon for the liver to be the only site of distant cancer deposits. Second, it has a relatively low incidence of disease spread within the abdominal cavity, so that local control of the primary tumor and other sites of intraabdominal disease persistence is accomplished surgically. These clinical features remain important requirements of patients who are to have potentially curative liver resections.

Although the metastatic process from primary colorectal cancers to liver occurs by way of the portal vein, the blood

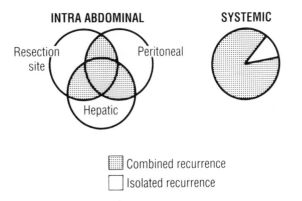

FIGURE 45-3 Surgical treatment failures of primary colorectal cancer. Isolated recurrences are observed in a proportion of patients, and when they occur, they should be resected with curative intent. (Modified from Sugarbaker PH, et al. Prospective randomized trial of intravenous versus intraperitoneal 5-fluorouracil in patients with advanced primary colon or rectal cancer. Surgery 98:414–421, 1985)

supply to hepatic tumors is arterial.[1,2,10,24,32,55,56,105] The transition from portal venous to hepatic arterial supply occurs early in the progression of the metastases. Even tumors 1 cm or less in diameter are nourished by hepatic arterial blood. For this reason, if one wants to infuse cytotoxic agents into liver tumors, the hepatic artery has been the most frequently used route of drug delivery.[18,47]

Noncolorectal Liver Metastases

Hepatic metastases commonly accompany malignant tumors at anatomic sites throughout the body.[111] Surgical treatment of these tumors is not indicated unless the metastatic process is isolated to the liver. A single exception to this concerns limited disease in the lungs plus liver or the abdominal cavity plus liver when surgery is able to achieve a disease-free status at both sites. From a tumor biology perspective, the only cancers that can be resected for cure are those whose primary site is anatomically located within the hepatic portal system. These cancers invade host tissues, gain access to venules (venous invasion), and then implant and grow within the hepatic portal system. As the tumors in the liver progress, they use almost exclusively hepatic arterial blood for expansion. The metastases that gain access to the hepatic parenchyma through the portal system are theoretically treatable for cure, if they can be detected and eradicated completely.

All the constraints that apply to colorectal cancers apply to the other intraabdominal tumors as one considers a patient for liver resection. The cancer must be metastatically inefficient, so that only one to four foci of metastatic disease exist within the liver. Also, no tumor deposits may exist at systemic sites as a result of seeding the systemic circulation. Disseminated cancer is a result of transhepatic migration of cancer cells[22] or of metastases from metastases.[8] The anatomic site of the primary cancer must also be rendered disease-free.

Rarely should one attempt the resection of liver metastases that result from primary tumors outside the portal system. The selective nature of the metastatic process does, however, support resection of hepatic metastases from extraabdominal sites in a few carefully selected patients.[3] Some laboratory tumors, when injected hematogenously, only produce liver

implants. The integrin system that exists on tumor cell surfaces may exhibit organ specificity. From a theoretical perspective, a melanoma, for example, occasionally may metastasize exclusively to the liver. The homing of melanoma cells to the liver may result in isolated liver metastases. Although long-term survival of these patients after liver resection has seldom been reported, anecdotal successes do exist. Meticulous work-up of these patients and careful intraoperative evaluation are indicated. Systemic chemotherapy may, in some patients, assist in preserving a state of metastatic inefficiency. Before proceeding with a liver resection with the primary tumor outside the portal system, one usually wants to observe a patient for several months. This delay helps the clinician to determine that other sites of metastatic disease are not present. A trial of induction chemotherapy often is recommended. An objective response observed in the macroscopic disease present within the liver may suggest that microscopic systemic sites of disease are eliminated.

Surgical Anatomy of the Liver

The liver is a large parenchymal structure secured by the evolutionary process beneath the right rib cage, so that it is not injured by vigorous exercise or extensive abdominal or chest trauma. This makes it surgically difficult to approach. Through large abdominal or abdominothoracic incisions and the use of self-retaining retractors, however, the surfaces of the liver can be inspected in their totality and the parenchyma bimanually palpated. The external markings on the liver are helpful in attempting to define its internal anatomy and the position of tumors. The falciform ligament defines the left hepatic plane. An imaginary line between the inferior vena cava and the gallbladder (Cantlie's line) defines the middle plane. A deep fissure on the posterior surface of the liver defines the caudate body on the left; the caudate process on the right (segment 1) is less clearly defined. Figure 45-4 shows the external surfaces of the liver. The organs adjacent to the visceral surface of the liver are identified by their respective impressions.

The lack of innervation of the liver allows tumors to grow to large size without symptoms. The parenchyma itself is de-

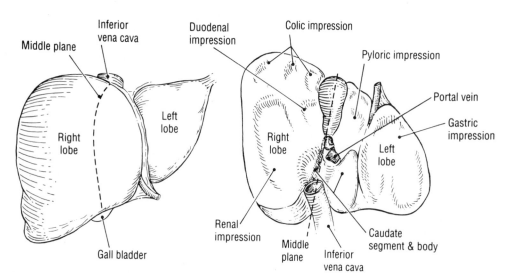

FIGURE 45-4 External surfaces of the liver. (Sugarbaker PH, Keminy N. Management of metastatic cancer to the liver. Adv Surg 22:1–56, 1989)

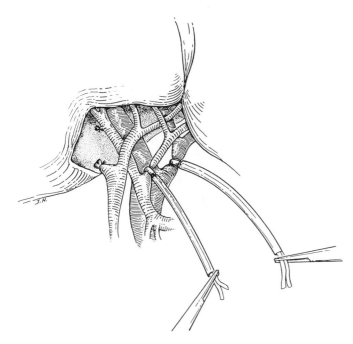

FIGURE 45-16 Preliminary control of left portal vein and left hepatic artery in a left lobe resection. (Modified from Sugarbaker PH. Left hepatectomy. In: Daly JM, Cady B, eds. Atlas of surgical oncology. St Louis, CV Mosby, 1993, pp 361–368)

the mobility of the portion of the liver to be resected. If one places the tissue being transected on strong traction, identification of vascular structures within the liver is greatly facilitated and the time required for parenchymal transection is greatly reduced.

SEGMENTAL RESECTIONS

Rarely, if ever, are deep transections of liver parenchyma performed that cross intersegmental planes (see Fig. 45-8). Although small tumors near the liver surface are removed by metastasectomy procedures (local resections), a tumor more than 3 cm in diameter is removed as a segmentectomy procedure. As many different segmentectomies have been performed as there are conceivable combinations. Segmental resections on the caudal liver segments (4b, 5, or 6) are easily performed and associated with minimal blood loss (see Fig. 45-8). Resections of cranial liver segments (4a, 7, or 8) are considerably more difficult and require amputation of the relevant hepatic vein close to the vena cava. In performing these segmental resections, one does not transect any portal structures until most of the parenchymal transection has been completed. This surgery can be conceptualized as hepatic vein surgery. As one appreciates by direct vision the relevant portal segmental structures as they arise from the major right or left portal pedicles, the segmental vein, artery, and bile duct are ligated, sutured, ligated, and then transected.

ing parenchymal transection. Small, stiff vascular clamps are placed across the hepatic veins outside the liver. The vessels are secured proximally and distally with a running suture (Fig. 45-17). If the hepatic veins are approached from beneath the liver after division of the caudate lobe veins, one can safely skeletonize about 1 cm of hepatic vein in nearly all patients. In addition to preventing intravascular tumor dissemination with manipulation of the cancer during resection, preliminary division of the hepatic veins adds greatly to

Cytoreductive Approach to Liver Tumors

One of the most powerful modern strategies in the treatment of cancer uses the concept of dose intensity. Improvements in survival have been seen in numerous cancers when chemotherapy was used in an aggressive manner over a short time period.[20,36] Combining intraarterial chemotherapy with

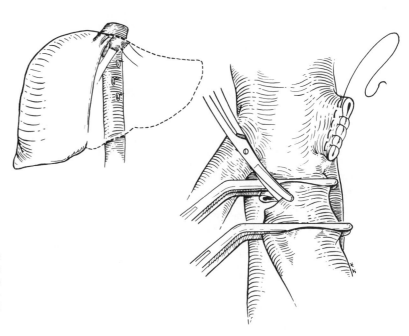

FIGURE 45-17 Preliminary division of the hepatic veins minimizes cancer cell embolization to the lungs and increases the mobility of the portion of the liver to be resected. (Modified from Sugarbaker PH. Left hepatectomy. In: Daly JM, Cady B, eds. Atlas of surgical oncology. St Louis, CV Mosby, 1993, pp 361–368)

surgical or radiotherapeutic cytoreduction is a new approach to regional dose intensity for hepatoma or colorectal metastases to the liver. New strategies for control of liver tumors have recently been described whereby numerous tumor nodules within the liver are resected or in some other way devitalized.[21,49,57,63,70,76,79,84] Methods for hepatic cytoreduction are itemized in Table 45-9. Cytoreduction implies complete devitalization of all visible tumor from the liver. It does not imply debulking because this implies that visible quantities of viable cancer remain after the surgical event. To achieve complete liver cytoreduction, one often may use several cytoreductive techniques. For example, electroevaporation may be used for peripheral tumors and then a grid of radioactive iodine 125 seeds positioned to control larger tumor nodules intimately related to the hepatic veins or portal vein bifurcation. Surgical and radiation cytoreduction techniques are not competitive but complementary, in that together they may devitalize all tumor nodules within the liver.

Either before or after complete cytoreduction of liver tumor, intraarterial chemotherapy is initiated. This treatment is an attempt to prevent the outgrowth of micrometastatic foci that usually are present in the liver in patients with multiple liver metastases.[40] Also, systemic chemotherapy is given because it may be of some benefit in suppressing the progression of disseminated disease.

TABLE 45-9 *Techniques for Hepatic Cytoreduction*

Technique	Comment
Ultrasonic dissection	Tiny rim of normal liver tissue is left on the tumor nodule; exposure may be greatly compromised on the underside of moderate to large tumor nodules; not appropriate for deep masses[49,63]
Cryosurgery	Time-consuming, may spare viable tumor along major vessels by the heat sink effect; not appropriate for deep masses[76]
Electrosurgical excision	Inadequate margins may result; exposure not compromised at deep margin; not appropriate for deep masses[70]
Microwave	Technology limited in its availability and in clinical testing[104]
Alcohol injection	Appropriate for small hepatomas in cirrhotic livers; uniformity of cell kill not established[57,84]
Grid of radioactive implants [125]I	Excellent to achieve local control around major vessels or deep within the liver; may result in tumor spill
Afterloading catheters	Excellent to achieve local control around major vessels or deep within the liver; may result in tumor spill[21]
Chemotherapy injection	Needs further clinical testing[79]

Intraarterial Chemotherapy

Because the liver has a solitary arterial blood supply, and because the hepatocyte has such marked resistance to chemotherapy toxicities, direct intraarterial administration of chemotherapy frequently has been used.[47] The high response rates seen with regional drug delivery come about because of two pharmacologic principles. First, there is a first-pass effect on concentration. The concentration of chemotherapy in arterial blood going to the tumor on the first pass is increased many times over that achieved for the same dose of drug given systemically. The actual concentration advantage for the first intraarterial pass of chemotherapy is proportional to the reduction in blood flow through the artery that has been cannulated. Second, many drugs have a first-pass effect on metabolism. These chemotherapeutic agents are metabolized at least in part by a single pass through the liver (such as FUdR or 5FU). Systemic toxicities are greatly reduced, so that a markedly increased total dose of regional drug instillation is possible. If adverse effects occur, the toxicities may be first expressed within the liver itself and usually by the biliary tree. The ductal structures do not have the capability to metabolize drug or to replicate as do hepatocytes. Little, if any, drug goes systemically to produce hematologic or other complications and warn the clinician to reduce or suspend drug administration. Therefore, without special monitoring, the biliary tree may be severely damaged by the intraarterial administration of drugs such as FUdR.[13,86]

One must be aware that the goals of intraarterial chemotherapy are limited. The anatomic site at which increased responses are expected include only the tissues that are infused. For most agents, greater responses systemically are not likely to be seen over and above those demonstrated for systemic chemotherapy. For drugs metabolized on a first pass, one expects reduced or absent systemic drug levels, and a greater incidence of systemic metastases is likely to be recorded.

The goal in intraarterial infusion chemotherapy is to change the natural history of hepatoma or colorectal hepatic metastases by helping to control intrahepatic disease. There have been four major problems with intraarterial chemotherapy treatments in the past. First, agents such as FUdR that were metabolized by a single pass through the liver were used. These agents manifested little or no systemic toxicities. This approach resulted in extensive complications within the biliary tree. Second, the absence of effective systemic treatment resulted in a higher likelihood for development of disseminated disease. Third, clinicians often failed to meticulously rule out extrahepatic disease, especially within anatomic sites difficult to image by radiologic tests. With both hepatocellular cancer and colorectal metastases to the liver, hepatic lymph nodes and peritoneal surfaces are involved in a significant proportion of patients. Only surgical exploration with careful inspection of the entire abdominal cavity and biopsy of suspicious lesions can rule out the presence of extrahepatic disease. Fourth, substantial regressions of intrahepatic tumors were not consolidated through the use of other multidisciplinary treatments that could be added onto the chemotherapy. Dose-intensive treatments used to augment intraarterial chemotherapy include cytoreduction by surgery or by radiation therapy (see Table 45-9). If consolidation treatments are not used, drug resistance occurs within several months. Because of the Gompertzian nature

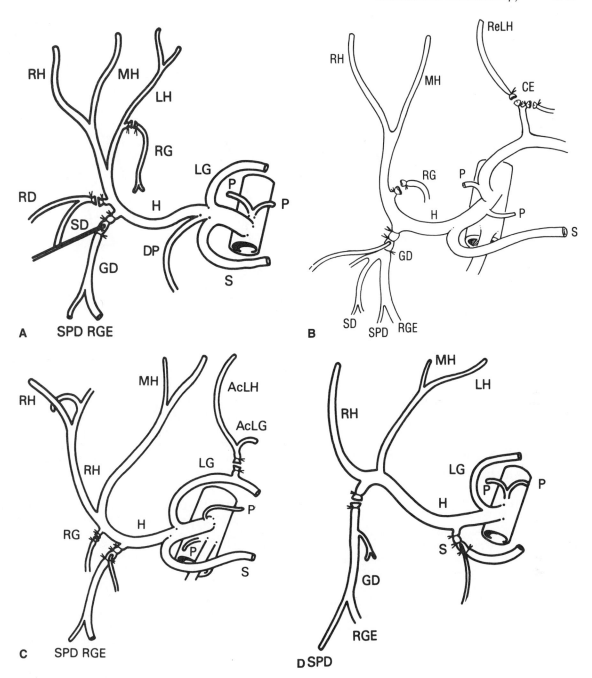

FIGURE 45-18 Technical aspects of hepatic artery cannulation. (**A**) Entire hepatic artery from celiac artery. (**B**) Replaced left hepatic artery from left gastric artery. (**C**) Accessory left hepatic artery from left gastric artery. (**D**) Early branching of left hepatic artery. (**E**) Replaced right hepatic artery from superior mesenteric artery. (**F**) Entire hepatic artery from superior mesenteric artery. RH, right hepatic; MH, middle hepatic; LH, left hepatic; RG, right gastric; LG, left gastric; H, hepatic; RD, right duodenal; SD, superior duodenal; GD, gastroduodenal; SPD, superior pancreatic duodenal; RGE, right gastroepiploic; P, phrenic; S, splenic; CE, celiac, ReLH, replaced left hepatic; CE, cardioesophageal; AcLH, accessory left hepatic; AcLG, accessory left gastric. (Modified from Sugarbaker PH, Schneider PD. Technique of hepatic infusion chemotherapy. In: van de Velde C, Sugarbaker PH, ed. Liver metastases. Boston, Martinus Nijhoff, 1984, pp 339–345)

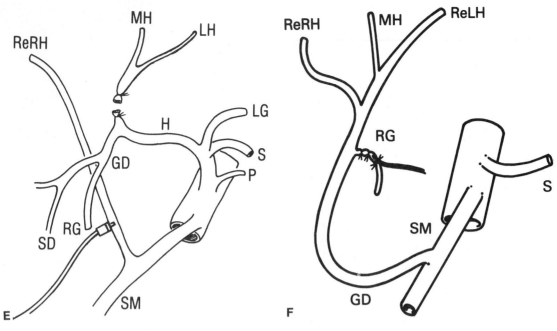

FIGURE 45-18   *(continued)*

of tumor growth, little benefit, in terms of prolonged survival, resulted.

Technical Aspects of Hepatic Artery Catheterization

Figure 45-18 shows the technical aspects of hepatic artery cannulation.[103] If only three to four monthly cycles of intraarterial chemotherapy are contemplated, then a port catheter system is adequate. If multiple cycles over many months are planned, then a continuous infusion pump may be preferable. The Infusaid pump maintains patency of the hepatic artery in a great many patients for years. The continuous administration of heparin at the tip of the catheter prevents platelet thrombi and the eventual arterial thrombosis observed with other catheter systems.[11]

Treatment Results

SURGICAL TREATMENT OF HEPATOMA

As indicated earlier, only about 20% of patients with hepatomas are candidates for surgery. Metastatic disease, large cancers involving both right and left lobes of the liver, multifocal disease in the liver, concomitant cirrhosis, lymph node involvement, and intraabdominal tumor found at the time of exploratory laparotomy all prevent a potentially curative resection. In those minority of patients who are resected for cure, about one third are alive and disease-free at 5 years. Patients with cirrhosis do less well, and few patients with hepatomas in cirrhosis survive 5 years. Figure 45-19 summarizes the results with resection of hepatocellular carcinoma.[37]

Patients with hepatoma have recently been treated with liver transplantation (see Chap. 43). Surgical resection in patients with large hepatomas has been unrewarding, with almost no patients surviving long term. Also, in those patients with smaller cancers in cirrhotic livers, the 5-year survival rate is low. Several groups have recently treated selected hepatoma patients with liver transplantation with favorable results being reported.

SURGICAL RESECTION OF COLORECTAL METASTASES ISOLATED TO THE LIVER

The results of surgery for colorectal metastases isolated to the liver are shown in Figure 45-20. Overall survival at 5 years approaches 30%.[39] These results continue to improve with time as clinicians gain expertise in eliminating occult distant metastases in this group of patients. The persistent 10% difference between survival and disease-free survival indicated that additional surgical procedures can be of benefit in these patients. Lung metastases and additional liver metastases are resectable with curative intent.[31,78] Although liver transplantation has been attempted in liver metastases patients, no favorable long-term results have been reported.

NONCOLORECTAL LIVER METASTASES

Long-term survival after surgical treatment is limited to patients whose primary tumors occur within the hepatic portal system.

TREATMENT WITH INTRAARTERIAL CHEMOTHERAPY

Summaries of the protocols using intraarterial chemotherapy in patients with colorectal metastases to the liver or primary liver cancer are shown in Tables 45-10 and 45-11.[9,13,14,34,46,48,51,52,65,75,82,83,109] In the two colorectal protocols in which survival was an endpoint, both showed significant

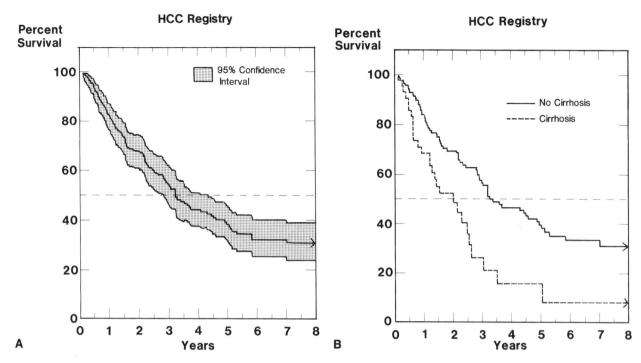

FIGURE 45-19 Survival of patients with hepatocellular cancer, HCC registry. (Tsao JI, Ashbun HJ, Hughes KS, et al. Hepatoma registry of the western world. In: Sugarbaker PH. Hepatobiliary cancer. Norwell, MA, Kluwer, 1993 [in press])

prolongation in survival in the patients with no extrahepatic disease. As the cytoreductive approach is tested in clinical trials, it is possible that the median survival of these patients will show additional improvement.

Failure Analysis for Patients Treated With Surgery

Hepatoma is a metastatically efficient tumor. With the primary cancer in the liver, the patterns of systemic metastases are throughout the entire intravascular bed. Lungs, brain,

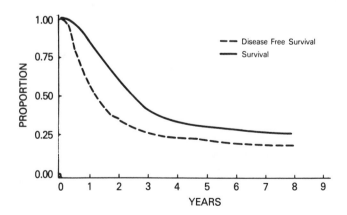

FIGURE 45-20 Survival and disease-free survival of patients with resected hepatic metastases. (Modified from Hughes KS, et al. Surgery for metastatic colorectal cancer to the liver: optimizing the results of treatment. Surg Clin North Am 69:339–359, 1989)

and adrenal metastases are frequent as well as deposits in the remaining liver parenchyma.

Steel and colleagues[88] and Hughes and coworkers[40] have studied the recurrence patterns after the resection of liver metastases from colorectal cancers. As expected, the sites of treatment failure are systemic. The hepatic resection effectively controlled disease within the liver in about two thirds of the patients. Both liver and lungs together were the most common sites at which recurrent disease was detected. Several groups recently called attention to a subgroup of patients in whom disease recurs in the liver only.[4,6,12,17,25,42,48,53,62,64,68,77,91,107] These patients probably have progression of occult disease in the liver that was metastatic from the primary tumor. These patients do not represent the cascade phenomenon. If the isolated repeat recurrence is detected in the liver, these patients represent a favorable group for long-term control. Presumably, they are a relatively metastatically inefficient group of patients selected from the group as a whole.

It is clear that metastatic disease is not a uniformly fatal process with large bowel cancer. Furthermore, recurrence of liver metastases after the resection is not necessarily a lethal process (see Fig. 45-20). Careful follow-up may select patients for curative repeat resection in the liver or curative resection of metastases from the lungs.

Follow-Up After Liver Resection

Recommendations for follow-up of these patients is shown in Table 45-12. We recommend frequent radiologic assessments of the patient for metastatic disease in addition to liver imaging. Frequent carcinoembryonic antigen assays should be

TABLE 45-10   Results of Intraarterial Chemotherapy for Colorectal Metastases Isolated to the Liver: Hepatic Artery FUdR Infusion With Internal Pump

Investigator	Patients	Prior Chemotherapy (%)	Partial Response	↓ CEA (%)	Median Survival (mo)	>50 Liver Involvement (%)
Niederhuber[65]	70	45	83	91	25	—
Balch[9]	50	40	—	83	26	—
Kemeny[51]	41	43	42	51	12	53
Shepard[83]	53	42	32	—	17	—
Cohen[14]	50	36	51	—	—	18
Weiss[109]	17	85	29	—	13	—
Schwartz[82]	23	—	15	75	18	—
Johnson[46]	40	—	47	—	12	34
Kemeny[48]	31	50	52	—	22	—
Ramming[75]	55	—	8	88	11	—

(Sugarbaker PH, Kemeny N. Metastatic cancer to the liver. In: DeVita V, Hellman S, Rosenberg SA, eds. Principles and practice of oncology. Philadelphia, JB Lippincott, 1988)

TABLE 45-11   Results of Chemotherapy for Colorectal Metastases Isolated to the Liver: Intrahepatic Versus Systemic Chemotherapy

Group	Patients	Intrahepatic		Systemic		P Value
		Drug	Percentage Response	Drug	Percentage Response	
MSKCC	163	FUdR	50	FUdR	20	.001
NCOG	143	FUdR	37	FUdR	10	.002
NCI	64	FUdR	62	FUdR	17	—
Consortium	43	FUdR	56	5FU	38	—
City of Hope	41	FUdR	56	5FU	0	—
Rogier		FUdR		5FU		

TABLE 45-12   Recommendations for 5-Year Follow-up After Resection of Colorectal Metastases Isolated to Liver: Use of 2,4,6 Plan

Year	Symptom Review and Physical Examination	CEA Assay	Chest Radiograph	CT Abdomen	Colonscopy or Barium Enema
1	2 monthly	2 monthly	6 monthly	6 monthly	Yearly*
2 and 3	4 monthly	4 monthly	Yearly	Yearly	Yearly*
4 and 5	6 monthly	6 monthly	Yearly	Yearly	3 yearly

*If two consecutive colon examinations are negative, the colonoscopy or barium enema can be repeated every 3 years.

performed. This is the most useful follow-up test in most patients.

Follow-up of patients with potentially curative resections of hepatoma are not as important. Further surgery or chemotherapy is not effective in prolonging survival or in bringing about a disease-free state. α-Fetoprotein assays and chest x-rays have been recommended.

References

1. Ackerman NB. The blood supply of experimental liver metastases. IV. Changes in vascularity with increasing tumor growth. Surgery 75:589–596, 1974
2. Ackerman NB, Hechmer PA. The blood supply of experimental liver metastases. V. Increased tumor perfusion with epinephrine. Am J Surg 140:625–631, 1980
3. Albelda SM, Buck CA. Integrins and other cell adhesion molecules. FASEB J 4:2868–2880, 1990
4. Anderson R, Tranberg KG, Bengmark S. Reresection of colorectal liver secondaries: a preliminary report. Hepat Pancreat Bil Surg 2:69–72, 1990
5. Anthony PP. Primary carcinoma of the liver: a study of 282 cases in Ugandan Africans. J Pathol 110:37–48, 1973
6. Augelli NV, Lucas RJ, Howells GA. Hepatic resections: an eight year experience at a community hospital. Am Surg 54:373–375, 1988
7. August DA, Ottow RT, Sugarbaker PH. Clinical perspective of human colorectal cancer metastasis. Cancer Metas Rev 3:303–324, 1984
8. August DA, Sugarbaker PH, Schneider PD. Lymphatic dissemination of hepatic metastases. Cancer 55:1490–1494, 1985
9. Balch CM, Urist MM. Intraarterial chemotherapy for colorectal liver metastases and hepatomas using a totally implantable drug infusion pump. Recent Results Cancer Res 100:123–147, 1986
10. Breedis C, Young G. The blood supply of neoplasms in the liver. Am J Pathol 30:969–985, 1954
11. Buch H, Grage TB, Vassilopoulos PP, et al. Intra-arterial infusion chemotherapy for hepatic carcinoma using a totally implantable infusion pump. Cancer 45:866–869, 1980
12. Butler J, Attiyeh FF, Daly JM. Hepatic resection for metastases of the colon and rectum. Surg Gynecol Obstet 162:109–113, 1986
13. Chang AE, et al. A prospective randomized trial of regional versus systemic continuous 5-fluorodeoxyuridine chemotherapy in treatment of colorectal liver metastases. Ann Surg 206:685–693, 1987
14. Cohen AM, Kaufman SD, Wood WC, et al. Regional hepatic chemotherapy using an implantable drug infusion pump. Am J Surg 145:529–533, 1983
15. Couinaud C. Principes directeurs des hepatectomies reglees. Chirurgie 106:8–10, 1980
16. Cunliffe WJ, Sugarbaker PH. Gastrointestinal malignancy: rationale for adjuvant therapy using early postoperative intraperitoneal chemotherapy (EPIC). Br J Surg 76:1082–1090, 1989
17. Dagradi AD, Mangiante GL, Marchiori LAM, Nicoli NM. Repeated hepatic resection. Int Surg 72:87–92, 1987
18. Daley JM, Butler J, Kemeny N, Yeh SDJ, Ridge JA, Botet J, Bading JR, DeCosse JJ, Benua RS. Predicting tumor response in patients with colorectal hepatic metastases. Ann Surg 202:384–393, 1985
19. Daly JM, Kemeny N, Oderman P, Botet J. Long-term hepatic arterial infusion chemotherapy. Arch Surg 119:936–941, 1984
20. DeVita VT, Hubbard SM, Longo DL. The chemotherapy of lymphomas: looking back, moving forward: the Richard and Hinda Rosenthal Foundation Award Lecture. Cancer Res 47:5810–5824, 1987
21. Dritschilo A, Grant EG, Harter KW, et al. Interstitial radiation therapy for hepatic metastases: sonographic guidance for applicator placement. AJR 147:275–278, 1986
22. Edwards JM, Kinmonth JB. Lymphovenous shunts in man. Br Med J [Clin Res] 4:579–581, 1969
23. Eggermont AMM, Steller EP, Marquet RL, Jeekel J, Sugarbaker PH. Local promotion of tumor growth after abdominal surgery is dominant over immunotherapy with interleukin-2 and lymphokine activated killer cells. Cancer Detect Prev 12:421–429, 1988
24. Ensminger WD, Gyves JW. Clinical pharmacology of hepatic arterial chemotherapy. Semin Oncol 10:176–182, 1983
25. Fortner JG. Recurrence of colorectal cancer after hepatic resection. Am J Surg 155:378–382, 1988
26. Fortner JG, Maclean BJ, Kim DK, Howland WS, Turnbull AD, Goldiner P, Carlon G, Beattie EJ Jr. The seventies evolution in liver surgery for cancer. Cancer 47:2162, 1981
27. Foster JH, Berman MM. Solid liver tumors. Philadelphia, WB Saunders, 1977
28. Francis DMA, Judson RT. Blood transfusion and recurrence of cancer of the colon and rectum. Br J Surg 74:26–30, 1987
29. Gennari L, Doci R, Bozzetti F, Veronesi U. Proposal for a clinical classification of liver metastases. Tumori 68:443, 1982
30. Gozzetti G, Mazziotti A, Bolondi L, Cavallari A, Grigioni W, Cassanova P, Bellusci R, Villanacci V, Labo G. Intraoperative ultrasonography in surgery for liver tumors. Surgery 99:523–530, 1986
31. Griffith KD, Sugarbaker PH, Chang AE. Repeat hepatic resections in recurrent colorectal metastases. Surgery 107:101–104, 1990
32. Healey JE. Vascular patterns in human metastatic liver tumors. Surgery 120:1187–1193, 1965
33. Hodgson WJB, DelGuercio LRM. Preliminary experience in liver surgery using the ultrasonic scalpel. Surgery 95:230–234, 1984
34. Hohn D, Stagg R, Friedman M, et al. The NCOG randomized trial of intravenous (IV) vs hepatic arterial (IA) FUdR for colorectal cancer metastatic to the liver. Proc Am Soc Clin Oncol 6:85, 1987
35. Hollinshead WH. The thorax, abdomen, and pelvis. Anatomy for surgeons, vol 2. New York, Harper & Row, 1971, p 330
36. Hryniuk WM. Average relative dose intensity and the impact on design on clinical trial. Semin Oncol 14:65–74, 1987
38. Hughes KS, Sugarbaker PH. Treatment of metastatic liver tumors. In: Rosenberg SA, ed. Surgical treatment of metastatic cancer. Philadelphia, JB Lippincott, 1987, pp 125–164
39. Hughes KS, Scheele J, Sugarbaker PH. Surgery for metastatic colorectal cancer to the liver: optimizing the results of treatment. Surg Clin North Am 69:339–359, 1989
40. Hughes KS, Simon R, Sugarbaker PH, et al. Resection of the liver for colorectal carcinoma metastases: a multi-institutional study of patterns of recurrence. Surgery 100:278–284, 1986
41. Hughes KS, Simon RM, Songhorabodi S, Sugarbaker PH, et al. Resection of the liver for colorectal carcinoma metastases: a multi-institutional study of indications for resection. Surgery 103:278–288, 1987
42. Huguet C, Bona S, Nordlinger B, Lagrange L, Parc R, Harb J, Benard F. Repeat hepatic resection for primary and metastatic carcinoma of the liver. Surg Gynecol Obstet 171:398–402, 1990
43. Huguet C, Nordlinger B, Galopin JJ, Bloch P, Gallot D. Normothermic hepatic vascular exclusion for extensive hepatectomy. Surg Gynecol Obstet 147:689–693, 1978
44. Jaffe BM, Donegan WL, Watson F, Spratt JS Jr. Factors influencing survival in patients with untreated hepatic metastases. Surg Gynecol Obstet 127:1–11, 1986
45. Joffe SN, Brackett KA, Sankar MY, Daikuzono N. Resection

of the liver with the ND laser. Surg Gynecol Obstet 163:437–442, 1986

46. Johnson LP, Wasserman PB, Rivkin SE. FUdR hepatic arterial infusion via an implantable pump for treatment of hepatic tumor. Proc Am Soc Clin Oncol 2:119, 1983

47. Kemeny MM, Sugarbaker PH. Treatment of metastatic cancer to liver. In: DeVita VT, Hellman S, Rosenberg SA, eds. Cancer: principles and practices of oncology, ed 3. Philadelphia, JB Lippincott, 1989, pp 2275–2298

48. Kemeny MM, Goldberg D, Beatty JD, et al. Results of a prospective randomized trial of continuous regional chemotherapy and hepatic resection as treatment of hepatic metastases from colorectal primaries. Cancer 57:492, 1986

49. Kemeny MM, Goldberg DA, Browning S, Metter GE, Miner P, Terz JJ. Experience with continuous regional chemotherapy and hepatic resection as treatment of hepatic metastases from colorectal primaries. Cancer 55:1265–1270, 1985

50. Kemeny N, Braun DW. Prognostic factors in advanced colorectal carcinoma: the importance of lactic dehydrogenase, performance status, and white blood cell count. Am J Med 74:786–794, 1983

51. Kemeny N, Daly J, Oderman P, et al. Hepatic artery pump infusion toxicity and results in patients with metastatic colorectal carcinoma. J Clin Oncol 2:595–600, 1984

52. Kemeny N, Daly J, Reichman B, et al. Intrahepatic or systemic infusion of fluorodeoxyuridine in patients with liver metastases from colorectal carcinoma. Ann Intern Med 107:459–465, 1987

53. Lange JF, Leese T, Bismuth H. Repeat hepatectomy for recurrent malignant tumors of the liver. Surg Gynecol Obstet 169:119–126, 1989

54. Lefor AT, Hughes KS, Shiloni E, Steinberg SM, Vetto JT, Papa MZ, Sugarbaker PH, Chang AE. Intraabdominal extrahepatic disease in patients with colorectal hepatic metastases. Dis Colon Rectum 31:100–103, 1988

55. Lin G, et al. Portal blood supply of liver metastases. AJR 143:53–55, 1984

56. Lin G, et al. Postmortem examination of the blood supply and vascular pattern of small liver metastases in man. Surgery 96:517–526, 1984

57. Livraghi T, Festi D, Monti F, Salmi A, Vettori C. US-guided percutaneous alcohol injection of small hepatic and abdominal tumors. Radiology 161:309–312, 1986

58. Lortat-Jacov JL, Robert HG. Hepatectomie droite reglee. Presse Med 60:549, 1952

59. Machi J, Isomoto H, Kurohiji T, Shirouzu K, Yamashita Y, Kakegawa T, Sigel B. Detection of unrecognized liver metastases from colorectal cancers by routine use of operative ultrasonography. Dis Colon Rectum 29:405–409, 1986

60. Makuuchi M. Abdominal intraoperative ultrasonography. Tokyo, Igaku-Shoin, 1987

61. Manual of cancer staging. Philadelphia, JB Lippincott, 1987

62. Minton JP, Chevinski AH, Hamilton WB. Repeated hepatic resection for colorectal metastases: EORTC Symposium on Advances in Gastrointestinal Tract Cancer. Research and Treatment Proceedings, Strasburg, France, November 15–17, 1989, p 188

63. Minton JP, Hamilton WB, Sardi A, et al. Results of surgical excision of one to 13 hepatic metastases in 98 consecutive patients. Arch Surg 124:46–48, 1989

64. Niederhuber JE. Arterial chemotherapy for metastatic colorectal cancer in the liver: Conference on Advantages in Regional Cancer Therapy. Giessen, West Germany, 1985

65. Niederhuber JE, Ensminger W, et al. Regional chemotherapy of colorectal cancer metastatic to the liver. Cancer 53:1336, 1984

66. Nelson RC, Chezmar JL, Sugarbaker PH, Bernardino ME. Comparison of angiography, CTP-portography, delayed CT and MRI for the preoperative evaluation of hepatic tumors. Radiology 172:27–34, 1989

67. Nelson RC, Chezmar JL, Sugarbaker PH, Murray DR, Bernardino ME. The ability of CT during arterial portography to preoperatively localize focal liver lesions to specific liver segments. Radiology 176:89–94, 1990

68. Nordlinger B, Parc R, Delva E, Quilichini MA, Hannoun L, Huguet C. Hepatic resection for colorectal liver metastases. Ann Surg 205:256–263, 1986

69. Okuda K, Ryu M, Tobe T. Surgical management of hepatoma. The Japanese experience. In: Wanebo HJ, ed. Hepatic and biliary cancer. New York, Marcel Dekker, 1987, pp 219–238

70. Ottow RT, Sugarbaker PH. Surgical therapy of liver cancer. In: Bottino JC, ed. Therapy of neoplasms confined to the liver and biliary tract. Boston, Martinus Nijhoff, 1984, pp 99–142

71. Ottow RT, Barbieri SA, Sugarbaker PH, Wesley RA. Liver transection: a controlled study of four different techniques in pigs. Surgery 97:596–601, 1985

72. Peters RL. Pathology of hepatocellular carcinoma. In: Okuda K, Peters RL, eds. Hepatocellular carcinoma. New York, John Wiley & Sons, 1976, pp 107–108

73. Pettavel J, Morgenthaler F. Traitement chimiotherapique des metastases hepatiques en fonction de leur evolution spontanee. Schweiz Med Wochenschr 99:588, 1969

74. Phillips RKS, Hittinger R, Blesovsky L, et al. Large bowel cancer: surgical pathology and its relationship to survival. Br J Surg 71:604–610, 1984

75. Ramming KP, O'Toole K. The use of the implantable chemoinfusion pump in the treatment of hepatic metastases of colorectal cancer. Arch Surg 121:1440–1444, 1986

76. Ravikumar TS, Steele GD. Hepatic cryosurgery. Surg Clin North Am 69:433–440, 1989

77. Rogier PH, et al. Efficacy and indications of intraarterial hepatic chemotherapy in liver metastases from colorectal cancer. UICC abstract, August 1990

78. Roth JA. Treatment of metastatic cancer to lung. In: Devita VT Jr, Hellman S, Rosenberg SA, eds. Cancer principles and practices of oncology, ed 3. Philadelphia, JB Lippincott, 1989, p 2273

79. Sarashina H, Todoroki T, Orii K, Ohara K, Otsu H, Iwasaki Y. Effects of preoperative radiotherapy on rectal cancer: preliminary report on combining radiation with intratumor injections of peplomycin and bromodeoxyuridine. Dis Colon Rectum 33:1017–1025, 1990

80. Schelle J. Segment oriented resection of the liver: rationale and technique. In: Lygidakis NG, Tytgat GNJ, eds. Hepatobiliary and pancreatic malignancies: diagnosis, medical and surgical therapy. New York, Thieme Medical Publishers, 1990

81. Schelle J. Report on liver anatomy to the Fourth International Congress on Hepato-Pancreatic Biliary Surgery, Hong Kong, 1992

82. Schwartz SI, Jones LS, McCune CS. Assessment of treatment of intrahepatic malignancies using chemotherapy via an implantable pump. Ann Surg 201:560–567, 1985

83. Shepard KV, Levin B, Karl RC, et al. Therapy for metastatic colorectal cancer with hepatic artery infusion chemotherapy using a subcutaneous implanted pump. J Clin Oncol 3:161–165, 1985

84. Sheu JC, Huang GT, Chen DS, Sung JL, Yang PM, Wei TC, Lai MY, Su CT, Tsang YM, Hsu HC, Su IH, Wu TH, Lin JT, Chuang CN. Small hepatocellular carcinoma: intratumor ethanol treatment using new needle and guidance systems. Radiology 163:43–48, 1987

85. Sigel B, Coelho JCU, Machi J, Flanigan DP, Donahue PE, Schuler JJ, Bietler JC. The application of real-time ultrasound imaging during surgical procedures. Surg Gynecol Obstet 157:33–37, 1983

86. Stagg RJ, Venook AP, Chase JL, Lewis BJ, Warren RS, Roh M, Mulvihill SJ, Grobman BJ, Rayner AA, Hohn DA. Alternating hepatic intra-arterial FUdR and 5-FU: a less toxic regimen for treatment of liver metastases from colorectal cancer. J Natl Cancer Inst 83:423–428, 1991

87. Steele G Jr, Bleday R, Mayer RJ, Lindblad AN, Petrelli N,

Weaver D, Herrera L, Leichman LP. A prospective evaluation of hepatic resection for colorectal carcinoma metastases to the liver: gastrointestinal tumor study group protocol 6584. J Clin Oncol 9:1105–1112, 1991

88. Steele G Jr, Osteen RT, Wilson RE, Brooks DC, Mayer RJ, Zamcheck N, Ravikumar TS. Patterns of failure after surgical cure of liver tumors: a change in the proximate cause of death and a need for effective systemic adjuvant therapy. Am J Surg 147:554–559, 1984

89. Stephenson KR, Steinberg SM, Hughes KS, Vetto JT, Sugarbaker PH, Chang AE. Preoperative blood transfusions are associated with decreased time to recurrence and survival after resection of colorectal liver metastases. Ann Surg 208:679–687, 1988

90. Steves MA, Vidal-Jove J, Sugarbaker PH, Gray R, Dolmatch B, Buck D, Maxwell D. Preoperative radiology evaluation of the liver by CT portography in patients with hepatic tumors. Am Surg 58:608–612, 1992

91. Stone MD, Cady B, Jenkins RL, McDermott WV, Steele GD. Surgical therapy for recurrent liver metastases from colorectal cancer. Arch Surg 125:718–722, 1990

92. Sugarbaker PH. Hepatic neoplasia. In: Bayless TM, ed. Current therapy in gastroenterology and liver disease. Philadelphia, BC Decker, 1986, pp 412–417

93. Sugarbaker PH. Surgical management of peritoneal carcinosis: diagnosis, prevention, and treatment. Langenbecks Arch Chir 373:189–196, 1988

94. Sugarbaker PH. Surgical treatment of peritoneal carcinomatosis. Can J Surg 32:164–170, 1989

95. Sugarbaker PH. Surgical decision-making for large bowel cancer metastatic to the liver. Radiology 174:621–626, 1990

96. Sugarbaker PH. Left hepatectomy. In: Daly JM, Cady B, eds. Atlas of surgical oncology. St Louis, CV Mosby, 1993, pp 361–368

97. Sugarbaker PH, Leighton SB. Hepatic parenchymal suction dissector. Surg Gynecol Obstet 163:267–269, 1986

98. Sugarbaker PH, Cunliffe W, Belliveau JF, DeBruijn EA, Graves T, Mullins R, Schlag P, Gianola F. Rationale for perioperative intraperitoneal chemotherapy as a surgical adjuvant for gastrointestinal malignancy. Regional Cancer Treat 1:66–79, 1988

99. Sugarbaker PH, Gianola FJ, Barofsky I, Hancock SL, Wesley R. 5-Fluorouracil chemotherapy and pelvic radiation in the treatment of large bowel cancer. Decreased toxicity in combined treatment with 5-fluorouracil administration through the intraperitoneal route. Cancer 58:826–831, 1986

100. Sugarbaker PH, Gianola FJ, Speyer JL, Wesley R, Barofsky I, Meyers CE. Prospective randomized trial of intravenous versus intraperitoneal 5-fluorouracil in patients with advanced primary colon or rectal cancer. Surgery 98:414–421, 1985

101. Sugarbaker PH, Nelson RC, Murray DR, Chezmar JL, Bernadino M. Liver computerized tomography for hepatic resection: a segmental approach. Surg Gynecol Obstet 171:189–195, 1990

102. Sugarbaker PH, Reining JW, Hughes KS. Diagnosis of hepatic metastases. In: Rosenberg SA, ed. Surgical treatment of metastatic disease. Philadelphia, JB Lippincott, 1987

103. Sugarbaker PH, van de Velde CJH, Veenhof CHN. A matrix for controlled clinical trials for the study of hepatic metastases: proceedings of a workshop. J Surg Oncol 31:94–99, 1986

104. Tabuse K, Katsumi M, Kobayashi Y, et al. Microwave surgery: hepatectomy using a microwave tissue coagulator. World J Surg 9:136–143, 1985

105. Taylor I. Cytotoxic perfusion for colorectal liver metastases. Br J Surg 65:109–114, 1978

106. Taylor I, et al. The blood supply of colorectal liver metastases. Br J Cancer 39:749, 1979

107. Tomas-de la Vega JE, Donahue EJ, Doolas A, Roseman DL, Straus A, Bonomi PD, Economou SG. A ten year experience with hepatic resection. Surg Gynecol Obstet 159:223–228, 1984

108. Tranberg KG, Rigotti P, Brackett KA, Bjornson HS, Fischer JE, Joffe SN. A comparison using the Nd-YAG laser, an ultrasonic surgical aspirator, or blunt dissection. Am J Surg 151:368–373, 1986

108a. Tsao JI, Ashbun HJ, Hughes KS, et al. Hepatoma registry of the western world. In: Sugarbaker PH, ed. Hepatobiliary cancer. Norwall, MA, 1993

109. Weiss GR, Garnick MB, Osteen R, et al. Long-term hepatic arterial infusion of 5-fluorodeoxyuridine for liver metastases using an implantable infusion pump. J Clin Oncol 1:337–344, 1983

110. Weiss JL. Metastatic inefficiency and regional therapy for liver metastases from colorectal carcinoma. Regional Cancer Treat 2:77–81, 1989

111. Weiss L. Liver metastases, ed 5. Boston, GK Hall, 1982

112. Weiss L. Metastatic inefficiency: causes and consequences. Cancer Rev 3:1–24, 1986

113. Wilson SM, Beahrs OH. The curative treatment of carcinoma of the sigmoid, rectosigmoid, and rectum. Ann Surg 183:556–563, 1976

Diseases of the Liver, Seventh Edition, edited by Leon Schiff and Eugene R. Schiff. J.B. Lippincott Company, Philadelphia © 1993.

Amebic and Pyogenic Liver Abscess

Kevin M. DeCock

Telfer B. Reynolds

Delay in diagnosis remains a major determinant of the severity of illness and outcome in amebic and pyogenic liver abscess. Lack of familiarity with the clinical features of these conditions on the part of clinicians and failure to consider the diagnosis are among the most important factors contributing to the continued morbidity and mortality.

The management of hepatic abscesses has been greatly influenced by advances in diagnostic imaging and interventional radiology. In amebic liver abscess, medical therapy alone is most often effective. A change has occurred in the therapeutic approach to pyogenic liver abscess, for which surgical drainage had until recently been considered mandatory. In recent times, antibiotic therapy alone, or in combination with percutaneous drainage, often has been shown to be curative, although surgery remains essential in some cases.

Amebic and pyogenic liver abscess share many common features. Clinically, the first diagnostic requirement is demonstration of the presence of an abscess, followed by determination of its nature. We have, for these reasons, elected to discuss amebic and pyogenic abscess together in the same chapter in an integrated manner.

Amebic Liver Abscess

HISTORICAL ASPECTS

Dysentery and hepatic abscesses were described by British physicians in India in the early 19th century.[84] Ipecacuanha was used for treatment, the active ingredient later being shown to be emetine. Losch,[110] in 1875, was the first author to give a detailed description of amebiasis in his report of a Russian woodcutter who died of the disease. In the same decade, Koch and Gaffky[99] and Kartulis[90] in Egypt reported original observations on amebic dysentery and liver abscess. The first recognized cases of amebic liver abscess in the United States were reported from Johns Hopkins Hospital in 1890 by Osler[141] and Simon.[184] A classic monograph on amebiasis was published from the same institution the next year.[37]

Confusion existed in the early 20th century concerning nomenclature and pathogenicity of different species of amebae. In the Philippines, experimental infections in prisoners made possible the distinction between *Entamoeba histolytica* (pathogenic) and *Escherichia coli* (nonpathogenic), showed that cysts were the infective stage, and demonstrated that not all people infected with *E histolytica* became ill.[204]

Important milestones in the history of chemotherapy for amebiasis have been the introduction of emetine for amebic dysentery and liver abscess by Rogers[162] in India in 1912;

the demonstration of the efficacy of chloroquine in hepatic amebiasis in 1948[33,34]; the introduction in 1959 of dehydroemetine,[26] a synthetic compound closely related to but less toxic than emetine; and the demonstration by Powell and colleagues,[152] in 1966, of cure in all forms of invasive amebiasis using metronidazole. These latter workers form part of a group of medical scientists from Durban, South Africa, whose collective work over more than 20 years has profoundly influenced the modern approach to amebiasis.

PARASITOLOGY

The term *amebiasis* signifies infection with the protozoan parasite *E histolytica* (Fig. 46-1). In most cases, infection is noninvasive and parasites are restricted to the intestinal lumen. Trophozoites, the active ameboid forms of the parasite, live in the lower bowel, where they browse on bacteria and other material in the host's feces, dividing by binary fission two or three times daily (Fig. 46-2). Noninvasive trophozoites are 10 to 20 μm in diameter and contain a nucleus and a number of vesicles in the granular cytoplasm. Their movement is sluggish and involves the formation of blunt pseudopodia limited by the ectoplasmic gel, into which streams the endoplasmic sol. The organisms are actively phagocytic for their food. Although metabolism is essentially anaerobic, the trophozoites can survive under conditions of low oxygen tension.

Under certain circumstances, the trophozoites expel their vacuoles and secrete a chitinous wall around themselves to form cysts. Cell division results in each cyst being quadrinucleate when mature. The cysts of *E histolytica* measure 10 to 14 μm in diameter and are distinguishable on the basis of their size and number of nuclei from those of the commensals *E coli* (14 to 20 μm; eight nuclei) and *Entamoeba hartmanni* (6 to 10 μm; four nuclei). These cysts are the infective stage; trophozoites die outside the human host and are destroyed by gastric acid when swallowed. Cysts in feces are viable for several days.

When ingested cysts reach the host's small intestine, their walls disintegrate and trophozoites are released that mature as they travel down to the large bowel. Any cause of diarrhea or intestinal hurry, including noninfectious conditions, can prevent encystment and result in the passage of active trophozoites in stool.

Undefined factors stimulate trophozoites of *E histolytica* to become invasive. Invasive organisms are more active and larger than their nonpathogenic predecessors, measuring up

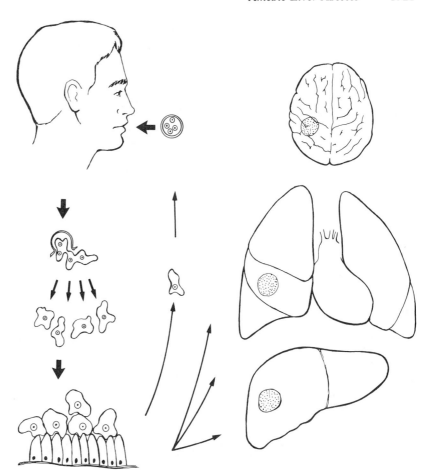

FIGURE 46-1   Life cycle of *Entamoeba histolytica*.

to 50 μm in diameter. The hallmark of invasive intestinal amebiasis is the demonstration in stool, rectal mucosal scrapings, or biopsy specimens of trophozoites that contain ingested red blood cells. Amebic cysts or trophozoites in stool are not diagnostic of invasive disease.

It is unclear what factors render certain strains of *E histolytica* invasive. Association with bacteria may enhance the pathogenicity of some strains.[207] A number of differences exist in the surface characteristics of trophozoites from different strains when cultured in vitro.[177] The injection of amebae

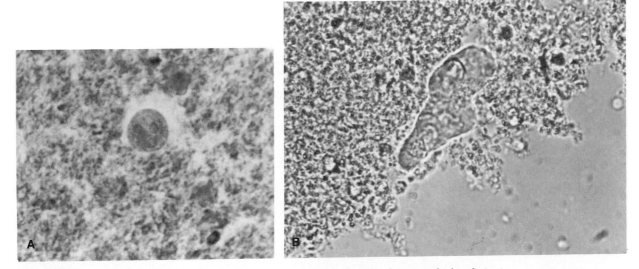

FIGURE 46-2   (**A**) Cyst of *Entamoeba histolytica* in stool. (**B**) Trophozoite of *Entamoeba histolytica* in aspirate from amebic liver abscess.

from pathogenic human infections into laboratory animals resulted in pathology in the new hosts, whereas noninvasive human infections were of low virulence in the animals.[193] Invasive strains do not always cause disease, as has been demonstrated in experimental human infections.[204] Resistance to complement-mediated lysis has been demonstrated in some pathogenic strains.[160] Biochemical examination of the isoenzyme characteristics of strains of different geographic origin and of varying pathogenicity recently associated certain enzyme markers with invasiveness.[173] The association between biochemically distinguishable zymodemes of *E histolytica* and pathogenicity has been the most promising advance in understanding the wide variations in disease. An immunofluorescent technique using monoclonal antibodies has been reported as capable of distinguishing pathogenic from nonpathogenic strains.[191] No other distinguishing features between pathogenic and nonpathogenic organisms are evident on light or electron microscopy or by examination using other methods.

HOST RESPONSE

Antigenic determinants capable of eliciting an antibody response have been detected in subcellular fractions of trophozoites that contain ribosomal, lysosomal, and soluble cytoplasmic matter as well as in material derived from the trophozoite surface.[178] *E histolytica* antigen has been detected in serum, feces, and material from liver abscesses in infected patients.[177]

The complex humoral response to amebic infection results primarily in the production of immunoglobulin G antibody. Immunoglobulin M class antibody also appears, although immunoglobulin E is lacking.

Immune serum and antiamebic globulin have been shown experimentally to have a lytic effect on amebae.[177] Complement may be required to mediate this effect; in experimental infections in animals, prior depletion of complement with cobra venom produced more extensive infections.[27]

In humans, the humoral response serves as a marker of prior invasive disease. A review[167] emphasizes the importance of cell-mediated immunity in protecting against invasive amebiasis. Exposure to amebic antigen leads to T-lymphocyte sensitization and proliferation, lymphokine production, and macrophage activation.[167] In vitro tests of cell-mediated immunity and skin reactivity to amebic antigen may be suppressed early in the course of infection but recover with successful therapy. Immunosuppressive drugs in animals promote the development of experimental amebic liver abscesses,[21] and clinical observations in humans suggest that these drugs enhance invasiveness. In vitro studies of the interaction between human white blood cells and virulent amebae suggest that monocyte-derived activated macrophages may be important effector cells in the immune response against *E histolytica*.[168]

Alcoholism and malnutrition frequently have been quoted as host factors that promote invasive amebiasis, although definite evidence for this is lacking.[44] The sex of the host is an important factor, with hepatic amebiasis being about 3 to 10 times more common in males than in females after puberty. Reinfection after successful treatment of invasive amebiasis is possible, although relatively uncommon.

PATHOGENESIS AND PATHOLOGY

Amebae reach the liver through portal blood. It is unlikely that lymphatic spread can occur, since amebae have never been reported in abdominal lymph glands and they do not appear to enter the bloodstream through the thoracic duct.[35,48]

Most amebic abscesses develop in the right lobe of the liver near the dome. The right lobe is probably more often affected than the left lobe because it has a larger volume. In addition, it receives a major part of the venous drainage from the cecum and ascending colon, parts of the bowel frequently affected by amebiasis.[8]

Amebic liver abscesses are well-demarcated lesions (Fig. 46-3) that initially contain yellow-brown fluid that later attains its classic orange-brown "anchovy sauce" appearance (Fig. 46-4). The fluid represents necrotic liver tissue mixed with blood. It is odorless, unless secondarily infected, and usually contains few or no neutrophils. For this reason, the term *abscess*, although traditional, is not strictly accurate.

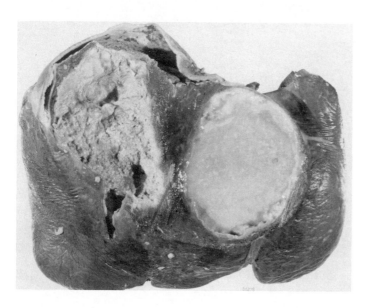

FIGURE 46-3 Autopsy specimen of hepatic amebiasis. Two discrete abscesses occupy almost the entire liver.

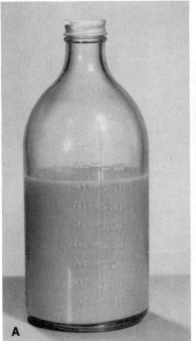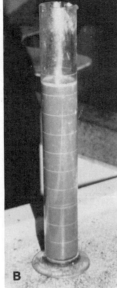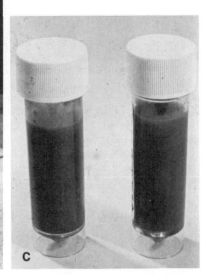

FIGURE 46-4   Amebic liver abscess contents ("anchovy sauce"). The color may vary from light brown (**A**) to orange (**B**) or dark brown (**C**).

The edge of the amebic lesion has a shaggy, fibrinous wall that consists of necrotic material, compressed hepatocytes, and a mixture of inflammatory cells. Amebae most often are found at the periphery of an abscess, although frequently no parasites can be identified in abscess aspirate. Lysis of hepatic cells occurs in periportal regions. The surrounding unaffected liver is hyperemic and edematous, explaining the clinical finding of hepatomegaly that often seems disproportionate to the size of the abscess cavity. A mixed inflammatory cell infiltrate may be seen in adjacent hepatic parenchyma.

Bile is probably lethal to amebae, and infection of the gallbladder and bile ducts does not occur. Healing of amebic abscesses progresses without scarring, although the defect in the parenchyma may persist for a long time.

Amebic hepatitis, a term used by some earlier workers,[45] is no longer considered a specific entity. Reports of a diffuse hepatitis with amebae throughout the liver have never been substantiated. There are, however, descriptions by experienced physicians of tender hepatomegaly without overt abscess formation in patients with amebiasis, with improvement after specific chemotherapy.[36,159] Such cases may represent an early stage of hepatic amebiasis, in which microscopic lesions are presumed to coalesce to form a discrete abscess. In addition, in endemic tropical regions, nonspecific changes in the liver, including Kupffer cell hyperplasia and portal tract inflammation, are frequent in patients with different intestinal infections.[80]

EPIDEMIOLOGY

Infection with *E histolytica* affects one tenth of the world's population and is considered responsible for at least 40,000 deaths annually, most infections occurring in the developing countries of the tropics and subtropics.[95,96,115,205] Infection prevalence varies greatly and in some regions exceeds 50%. One study from the Gambia, West Africa, documented infection rates approaching 100% annually.[24]

The association between amebiasis and warm climates results from the poor sanitation and lack of hygiene that accompany underprivileged living conditions. Infection occurs mainly by the fecal–oral route, with transmission resulting from contamination of food by flies, unhygienic handling of food, and spread within the family. Raw sewage contaminating water supplies occasionally causes infection, as may the use of human feces as fertilizer and of unclean water for freshening food.

Disease incidence is difficult to assess because of the unreliable nature of case reporting. Conclusions from several reviews are that invasive amebiasis, including liver abscess, is especially common in sub-Saharan Africa, Asia, Mexico, and parts of South America.[53,54] Real but ill-defined geographic variations exist in the prevalence of liver abscess among infected people. Such regional differences may be partially explained by showing variation in virulence and distribution among parasite strains of differing isoenzyme patterns (zymodemes).[49]

Transmission of amebiasis can also occur in the developed world.[106] Although amebic liver abscess was described some years ago in an unfortunate German worker 14 weeks after he fell into a sewage tank,[98] infection is now rarely waterborne.[106] Person-to-person spread, as may occur in institutions or in slum areas with large immigrant populations, accounts for most cases.[180,187,188] An unusual mode of transmission in an outbreak of amebiasis was the paramedical practice of colonic irrigation.[28] In occasional patients, no source of infection is evident.[154,170]

In recent years, an increased incidence of amebiasis has been noted in urban male homosexual populations.[47,93,113,150] Recognition of the association between homosexuality and amebiasis is attributed to Most,[130] who, in a lecture titled "Manhattan: 'A Tropical Isle'?" reported a minor outbreak in New York City. Although amebic liver abscess has been documented in male homosexuals,[124,197,208] no increase in frequency has been reported in the acquired immunodeficiency syndrome.[9] Homosexual modes of transmission are probably oroanal or genitoanal with orogenital contact. Examination of the isoenzyme characteristics of amebae isolated from homosexual subjects has shown a high prevalence of nonpathogenic zymodemes.[10,66,122,172] This may help to explain the relative rarity of amebic liver abscess in homosexual men compared with the epidemic prevalence of intestinal infection.

Heterosexual venereal transmission with infection of the male and female genitalia has been described, although the reported cases were not associated with liver abscess.[131,195]

CLINICAL FEATURES

Amebic liver abscess is 3 to 10 times as common in men as in women. Most patients are young adults, although all age groups can be affected. With care, a relevant epidemiologic history usually can be elicited. Most patients are emigrants from or residents of endemic areas and poor. In the more affluent, a history of international travel by the patient or his or her close contacts may be relevant. In a patient with compatible symptoms, any history, no matter how remote, of travel to or residence in a developing country should raise the differential diagnosis of amebiasis. Specific questions about homosexual activity should be asked. A history of previous dysentery is infrequent and generally unhelpful unless accompanied by dependable laboratory reports.

Symptoms of amebic liver abscess are slow in onset and usually are present for several days or weeks before medical attention is sought.[3,6,40,91,108,196,198] Initial complaints are vague and include malaise, fever, anorexia, and abdominal discomfort. In established cases, pain is most often the dominant symptom and is maximal in the right hypochondrium. About three fourths of patients complain of fever, often with chills and sweats, particularly at night. Anorexia, nausea, and vomiting are common, and many patients lose weight. Chest symptoms are present in about one fourth of patients and include right-sided pleuritic pain and cough. Diaphragmatic irritation may result in right shoulder pain and hiccoughs. Occasional patients recognize abdominal swelling. Concurrent intestinal disease, such as dysentery or diarrhea, is rare.

Infrequently, the onset of disease is abrupt and the symptoms mimic those of an abdominal surgical emergency.[105] Sometimes patients complain of ill health for many months, with constitutional symptoms such as weight loss and anemia predominating. In a small minority, the only manifestation is fever.

On examination, most patients are ill, sallow, and sweaty, and they may appear anemic and toxic. They tend to remain ambulant until close to hospitalization, by which time movement is clearly painful, and they may seek a certain position on lying down for maximum comfort. Fever and tenderness over the liver are almost invariable, with the tenderness sometimes being most impressive over the right lower inter-costal area. Sometimes the liver is visibly enlarged or expands the lower rib cage to give the abdomen an asymmetric appearance. Most often the liver is palpable, and in rare cases, it is huge and extends down to the pelvis. The physical signs may be subtler when the abscess is in the left lobe of the liver. Epigastric and left hypochondrial tenderness and enlargement of the left lobe could raise this possibility.[8]

Careful examination of the chest reveals abnormalities in up to half of patients. Movement of the right side may be limited by pain. Dullness to percussion over the right lower lung field is common and implies a raised right hemidiaphragm or pleural effusion. Occasionally there are fine crepitations on auscultation or a pleural or pericardial friction rub.

Jaundice is rare and, when present, usually of a minor degree. It indicates severer illness. Deeper jaundice usually results from multiple or large amebic abscesses or from lesions situated near the inferior surface of the liver with compression of the larger intrahepatic ducts.[138,143]

Wherever amebiasis occurs in adults, children also may be infected.[75,117,123,161,175] Most reported cases of liver abscess in childhood have been in children under age 3, with some affected at only 1 month of life. The sex ratio of cases in children is almost equal. Fever and tender hepatomegaly are the usual physical signs, with the latter sometimes difficult to elicit in a crying child. Associated intestinal amebiasis and multiple hepatic abscesses seem more frequent in children than adults, and malnutrition is an important accompaniment. Amebic liver abscess often seems a severer disease in childhood.

Treatment with corticosteroids enhances the invasiveness of *E histolytica*, and cases exist in which administration of such drugs to patients with benign infections apparently resulted in hepatic amebiasis.[13,51,52,86,176,192] Sometimes liver abscess occurs in pregnancy,[33,38,43,127,134,203] and such cases frequently are misdiagnosed. A Nigerian autopsy study demonstrated a higher prevalence and mortality from amebiasis in pregnant compared with nonpregnant women.[2] It has been suggested that the immunologic and hormonal alterations of pregnancy predispose to invasive disease. Finally, there is a widespread clinical impression that amebic liver abscess is rare in patients with chronic liver disease, although isolated cases have been documented.[15,57]

DIAGNOSIS

Conventional Laboratory Tests

Anemia is common in amebic liver abscess, with about half the patients having hemoglobin values below 12 g/dL. Although usually normochromic and normocytic, a hypochromic blood picture may occur despite adequate iron stores.[116] A neutrophilic leukocytosis is usual, and a high proportion of bands may be seen. Although the white blood cell count is between 10,000 and 20,000/μL, isolated cases with leukemoid reactions are described. Eosinophilia is not a feature of amebiasis. The erythrocyte sedimentation rate is raised.

Results of liver tests often are abnormal and of value in focusing attention on the liver, although derangements may be minor and nonspecific. Slight elevation of alkaline phosphatase levels and reduction of serum albumin levels are the most frequent abnormalities. Normal liver tests do not exclude the diagnosis of hepatic abscess. Significant elevation of the bilirubin level in hepatic amebiasis is unusual.

Diagnostic Imaging

About half of patients show elevation of the right hemidiaphragm on the chest roentgenogram (Fig. 46-5), the changes in contour being typically most marked anteriorly and medially.[31] Fluoroscopy may demonstrate reduced or absent diaphragmatic movement. Blunting of the right costophrenic angle from a sympathetic pleural effusion is common, as are minor right lower lobe parenchymal abnormalities from atelectasis. Abdominal films may show hepatomegaly but are not helpful. Barium studies and infusion tomography are now outdated techniques for diagnosing amebic abscess.[5,156]

Technetium sulfur colloid scanning (Fig. 46-6), the first modality that allows direct assessment of space-occupying liver lesions, is sensitive but lacks specificity.[94,156] Other hepatic masses, such as tumors and cysts, may produce similar "cold" areas. Gallium scans often are used to complement sulfur colloid examinations.[156] Unlike pyogenic abscesses and primary hepatocellular cancers, amebic abscesses concentrate gallium only at the periphery of the abscess. The disadvantages of these tests include their low specificity, the time required for their completion, and the difficulty of working with isotopes.

Ultrasonography (Fig. 46-7) is quick, safe, economical, and easily repeatable.[4,23,41,156,157,201] Ultrasound scanning readily distinguishes solid from fluid-filled lesions, and if necessary, the apparatus can be brought to the patient's bedside. The technique is applicable even in areas with limited facilities.[41] A disadvantage of ultrasonography is its dependence on the interest and skill of the investigator.

Ultrasonic signs quoted as typical of hepatic amebic abscess are (1) a round or oval shape; (2) a lack of significant wall echoes, so that there is abrupt transition from normal liver to the lesion; (3) a hypoechoic appearance compared with normal liver, with diffuse echoes throughout the abscess; (4) a peripheral location, usually close to the liver capsule;

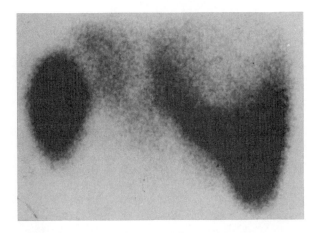

FIGURE 46-6 Isotope liver–spleen scan in a patient with amebic liver abscess. Right posterior oblique view. A large defect is seen in the superior aspect of the right lobe of the liver.

and (5) a distal sonic enhancement.[156,157] Atypical features that have been documented include an irregular shape and a hyperechoic appearance.[39]

Computed tomographic (CT) scanning (Fig. 46-8) shows amebic abscesses as well-defined, round, low-density lesions, which may have a nonhomogeneous internal structure.[156] CT scanning is particularly useful in precise localization and definition of extent of disease (eg, in cases complicated by rupture). Both CT scanning and ultrasonography may be used for guidance in cases in which aspiration is indicated. Disadvantages of CT scanning are its cumbersome nature and expense and the ionizing radiation inherent to the investigation.

Parasitology and Serodiagnosis

Concurrent hepatic abscess and amebic dysentery are unusual; stool examinations in large series of patients with amebic abscesses have been negative in three fourths of cases or more. Parasitologic examination of a stool specimen can neither prove nor exclude hepatic amebiasis, although it may be

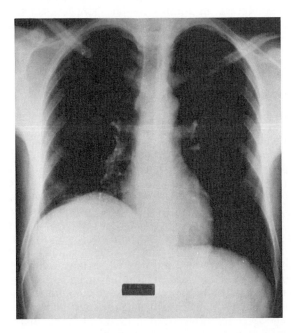

FIGURE 46-5 Chest radiograph in a young Mexican American man with amebic liver abscess. Note the elevated right hemidiaphragm.

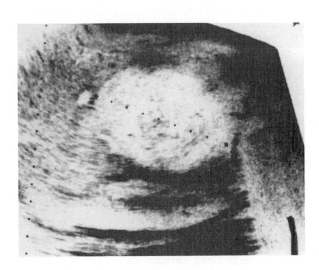

FIGURE 46-7 Ultrasound of liver in a young Mexican American with amebic liver abscess. Sagittal view through right lobe of liver.

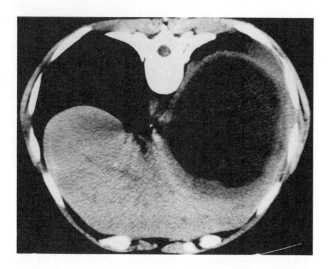

FIGURE 46-8 CT scan in a patient with amebic liver abscess. The scan was performed with the patient lying prone. A large right lobe liver abscess is shown. The lesion was subsequently aspirated.

relevant for subsequent management. The quality of practical parasitology in hospital laboratories varies widely. Overdiagnosis is especially common, with stool leukocytes frequently reported as trophozoites of *E histolytica*.[29,186]

Serodiagnostic tests used include complement fixation, immunodiffusion, indirect fluorescent antibody tests, indirect hemagglutination (IHA), counterimmunoelectrophoresis, and enzyme-linked immunosorbent assay (ELISA).[85,98,145,177] Commercially produced diagnostic kits for use at the bedside, such as those using latex agglutination, are also available. Clinicians should familiarize themselves with local facilities and the accepted sensitivity and specificity of the tests in question.

Positive tests are expected in virtually all cases of extraintestinal amebiasis as well as in most cases of amebic dysentery. Serology can only prove that a patient has suffered invasive infection with *E histolytica*, not that a particular illness is the result of that infection.

The IHA test is highly sensitive and widely available. A serologic titer of 1:512 is usual, although not invariable, in acute invasive disease. Titers may continue to rise after presentation, and on occasion, the test is negative when the patient is first seen but positive a few days later. The IHA test may remain positive for months or years after invasive infection.

ELISA is a cheap and sensitive technique that has been widely applied to the serodiagnosis and seroepidemiologic study of many parasitic diseases.[12] Its use for the diagnosis of amebiasis is likely to increase.

Agreement between the various test systems is not absolute, and it is possible that different antibodies are being detected. Serodiagnostic tests are crucial in diagnosis, but their results must be interpreted in their clinical and epidemiologic context.

COMPLICATIONS

The most frequent complication of amebic liver abscess is rupture, the direction and consequences of which depend on the site of the primary lesion. Rupture can occur into the chest, pericardium, peritoneal cavity, and intraabdominal organs and through the skin. In one study of fatal amebiasis, 41 of 90 cases with liver abscess had ruptured.[92]

Rupture into the chest may result in hepatobronchial fistula, lung abscess, or amebic empyema, although most pleural effusions in patients with amebic abscess are clear, sterile, "sympathetic" exudates.[7,81,82,200,202] Transdiaphragmatic rupture and pleural effusions are most common on the right side. Symptoms of rupture through the diaphragm include pain (which may be constant, pleuritic, or referred to the shoulder), dyspnea, and shock. Cough is frequent, and when rupture is into the bronchial tree, it may be associated with hemoptysis and expectoration of abscess contents. Rare patients suffer silent rupture and present simply with amebic empyema. Reported long-term complications of transdiaphragmatic rupture include pulmonary fibrosis, bronchiectasis, pleural thickening, and chronic empyema.

Left lobe abscesses are especially prone to rupture into the pericardium.[83,111] Sometimes this dangerous complication is preceded by the development of a serous pericardial effusion. Patients present with obscure heart failure, pericarditis, or cardiac tamponade. Constrictive pericarditis may develop later in patients who survive.

Like hepatobronchial fistula, rupture into the bowel may achieve spontaneous drainage.[14] Intraperitoneal rupture is more common and presents as signs of peritonitis, local pain, and tenderness or simply with ascites.[50,68,128,185] Although such patients may be gravely ill, intraperitoneal rupture of an amebic liver abscess is a less serious event than amebic peritonitis from perforation of the large bowel in amebic dysentery. Rare cases have ruptured into the kidneys or pancreas.

Secondary infection of an amebic liver abscess is unusual and most often iatrogenic, the result of aspiration.[64] Other documented complications, all exceptionally rare, include fulminant hepatic failure,[169] hemobilia,[101,153] reversible portal hypertension,[133] and inferior vena caval obstruction,[79,174] associated in one case with nephrotic syndrome.[79] Amebic cerebral abscess, an unusual complication, results from hematogenous spread. This must be distinguished from primary amebic meningoencephalitis resulting from infection with certain free-living species of amebae.

Pyogenic Liver Abscess

HISTORICAL ASPECTS

Liver abscess was recognized by ancient physicians,[70] but modern study of the condition dates back to the late 19th century. In the preantibiotic era, appendicitis was the most frequent underlying cause, accounting for one third of cases reported in the world literature.[140] The first documentation of pyogenic liver abscess secondary to appendicitis is ascribed to Waller in 1846.[140] French physicians referred to the condition as *le foie appendiculaire*, and this complication was observed in up to 4% of patients with appendicitis.[61] The early literature was reviewed by Ochsner and colleagues,[140] who extensively discussed surgical management of pyogenic liver abscess. The first successful use of an antibiotic, sulfanilamide, in conjunction with surgical drainage for multiple hepatic abscesses was reported in 1938.[142] In 1947, anaerobic organisms were cultured from pyogenic liver abscesses and successfully treated with penicillin.[125] Although surgical treatment has remained the most widely accepted form of therapy, McFadzean and colleagues,[121] in 1953, effectively treated pyogenic liver abscesses with antibiotics and closed percutaneous drainage. A report from the University of Southern California in 1979 documented successful treatment of pyogenic liver abscess in selected cases using antibiotics alone.[112]

EPIDEMIOLOGY

Worldwide, pyogenic liver abscess is much less common than amebic abscess, but in Western communities without significant immigrant populations, pyogenic abscess is more frequent. Accurate incidence figures are lacking, but 8 to 16 cases per 100,000 hospital admissions is an accepted estimate.[70,120,136] The prevalence at autopsy has been quoted as 0.3% to 1.5%.[70,183] Pyogenic liver abscess, therefore, is a rare condition, making prospective controlled studies difficult.

This is a disease of middle-aged and older people, and the sexes are affected about equally. Geographic variations in disease frequency are not obvious, and there is no racial susceptibility.

PATHOGENESIS AND PATHOLOGY

Pyogenic infection may be carried to the liver in hepatic arterial or portal venous blood and in bile.[16,136,140] Arterial spread results from generalized septicemia or from distant localized infections, whereas portal venous spread more often complicates intraabdominal sepsis, such as diverticulitis or peritonitis, from other causes. The classic changes of pylephlebitis, with the portal vein and its branches containing blood clot and pus, are now seldom seen.

A frequent cause of liver abscess is cholangitis, complicating benign or malignant biliary obstruction and endoscopic or operative intervention. Parasitic invasion of the biliary tree by roundworms or flukes also may lead to biliary infection.[36] The important subject of recurrent pyogenic cholangitis (oriental cholangiohepatitis) is outside the scope of the present discussion.

Abscess formation may complicate blunt or penetrating trauma, including liver biopsy and surgery. Foreign bodies have long been recognized as potential sources of infection,[140] and penetration or perforation of bowel by diverse objects such as toothpicks and pins is well described.[22,140] Direct extension of infection to the liver may occur secondary to such conditions as empyema of the gallbladder and subphrenic abscess. Umbilical sepsis is an important cause of liver abscess in infants.

Sometimes secondary infection complicates congenital or acquired hepatic abnormalities such as hydatid or nonparasitic cysts, amebic abscesses, and choledochal cysts. Necrosis and infection of primary or secondary hepatic cancers are recognized. A significant proportion of cases have no obvious cause. Spread to the liver by way of the portal vein is probable in such instances. Lymphatic spread does not seem to occur.

Abscesses may be multiple or single, with those originating from blood-borne spread of infection usually being multiple. The gross lesions give overlying liver tissue a pale appearance. The abscess cavities are variable in size and frequently coalesce, and advanced cases have a honeycombed appearance. A fibrous capsule may surround the lesions, which contain a polymorphonuclear cell infiltrate and necrotic liver tissue. Most abscesses are in the right lobe of the liver.[16,140]

MICROBIOLOGY

In the preantibiotic era, the most common organisms incriminated as causing liver abscess were *E coli*, streptococci, and staphylococci.[140] About half of abscesses and all blood cultures were bacteriologically sterile. Today, with awareness of the exacting growth requirements of many organisms, cultures of blood or abscess contents are positive in most cases.

E coli remains the single bacterium most frequently isolated in most reported series.[16,109,120,126,139,148] Other important aerobic organisms are various gram-negative bacilli, including species of *Klebsiella*, *Proteus*, and *Pseudomonas*, and gram-positive enteric organisms, such as *Streptococcus faecalis* and *Streptococcus faecium*. The latter two agents are referred to as enterococci. Other gram-positive aerobic infections are less common. *Staphylococcus aureus* and *Streptococcus pyogenes* may complicate penetrating trauma, and the former occasionally is associated with unusual immunologic deficiency states, such as Job's syndrome[77] and chronic granulomatous disease.[147]

The importance of anaerobic and microaerophilic organisms in liver abscess is a recent recognition.[165,166] Attention to detail concerning the collection of specimens, their transportation to the laboratory, and their subsequent processing increases the recovery of these bacteria. As many as one third to one half of patients may be infected with such organisms. Anaerobic organisms incriminated include *Bacteroides* sp, *Fusobacterium* sp, anaerobic streptococci (*Peptostreptococcus* and *Peptococcus* spp), and, rarely, *Clostridium* sp. Microaerophilic streptococci are considered by some authors as the most common of all organisms that cause liver abscess.[129] These fastidious organisms require an environment rich in carbon dioxide for successful culture. *Streptococcus milleri* is the most important member of the group. The confusing classification of these organisms has recently been discussed.[25,56] Many lesions are polymicrobial infections.

Unusual organisms documented as causing liver abscess on occasion include species of *Salmonella*, *Haemophilus*, and *Yersinia*. Actinomycosis, tuberculosis, and melioidosis also may be associated with liver abscess.

CLINICAL FEATURES

Clinical presentation is variable, with some patients complaining of acute symptoms referable to the right upper quadrant and others having no localizing features.[16,17,70,78,87,109,119,120,136,139,140,146,148,163,189] The sex ratio is virtually equal, and most Western patients are middle aged or older. A history of previous abdominal pathology should be carefully sought. Most of the clinical findings in patients with amebic liver abscess may also be associated with pyogenic abscesses. Sometimes conditions that predispose to impaired immunity, such as diabetes, are present.

Most patients complain of constitutional symptoms, such as malaise, anorexia, nausea, vomiting, and weight loss, and many notice fever, rigors, and sweats. Abdominal pain is frequent, most often localized to the right hypochondrium. Some patients present with generalized abdominal pain, mimicking a surgical emergency, whereas others present simply with fever. The history most often is of short duration but occasionally extends over weeks or months. Rarely, pyogenic liver abscess is virtually asymptomatic[144] or presents as a space-occupying lesion of the liver.

On examination, most patients are ill and febrile. Anemia and finger clubbing may be present in long-standing cases. Jaundice occurs in about one third of patients. Tachycardia, tender hepatomegaly, and right hypochondrial tenderness are frequent. Respiratory signs indicative of a small right pleural effusion, atelectasis, or raised hemidiaphragm are regularly found.

The complications of pyogenic liver abscess are essentially the same as those of hepatic amebiasis (see above) but, in addition, include the consequences of severe sepsis. Associated diseases such as diverticulitis with peritonitis, Crohn's disease, biliary tract obstruction, and cancer may all influence the clinical picture. Whether abscesses are solitary or multiple also determines the clinical course, with multiple abscesses carrying a more unfavorable prognosis. Septic complications of pyogenic abscess include septicemia and metastatic abscess, direct extension, hypotension and shock, adult respiratory distress syndrome, mental obtundation, and renal failure.

DIAGNOSIS

Conventional Laboratory Tests

Routine laboratory tests are incapable of distinguishing pyogenic from amebic abscesses. At least half of patients have hemoglobin levels below 12 g/dL, an elevated white blood cell count with a left shift is detected in up to three fourths of cases, and the erythrocyte sedimentation rate is invariably raised. Bilirubin and alkaline phosphatase levels often are elevated. Hyperbilirubinemia may result from sepsis but also may reflect biliary tract disease. The latter can also cause alkaline phosphatase elevations, although this may result from the abscess per se or from associated cancer. Aminotransferase levels often are raised to a minor degree. Albumin levels reflect disease severity, and levels below 2 g/dL carry a poor prognosis.[109] Most patients have a prolonged prothrombin time. Although liver tests may be deranged in sepsis of any origin, elevated vitamin B_{12} levels reflect intrahepatic pathology.[135]

Diagnostic Imaging

About half the patients with pyogenic liver abscess have some abnormality on the chest roentgenogram, and the range of abnormal features is similar to that seen in hepatic amebiasis. If infection is with gas-forming organisms, air–fluid levels may be seen below the diaphragm on chest or abdominal films.

Scintigraphy with technetium sulfur colloid is sensitive for detecting lesions more than 2 cm in diameter, although smaller lesions may be missed.[164] Gallium scanning has to be performed in addition if scintigraphy is to be diagnostic. Pyogenic liver abscesses avidly take up gallium, despite occasional false-negatives.[67]

Ultrasonography (Fig. 46-9) shows pyogenic abscesses as round, ovoid, or elliptic lesions within the liver parenchyma, most often not contiguous with the liver capsule.[137] The margin of each lesion is irregular and echo-poor. Abscesses are mostly hypoechoic compared with normal liver parenchyma, and they contain a variable number of internal echoes. A hyperechoic appearance occasionally is seen, particularly when gas-forming organisms are present.[107]

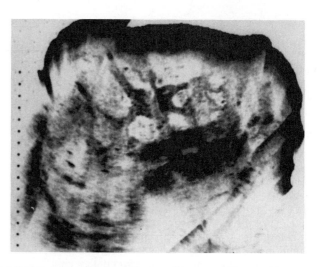

FIGURE 46-9   Ultrasound scan of liver in a 38-year-old woman with multiple pyogenic liver abscesses (Transverse view).

CT scanning (Fig. 46-10) is highly sensitive for diagnosis of intraabdominal abscesses.[100,164] The lesions show in the liver as areas of decreased attenuation. An advantage of CT scanning over ultrasonography is that the quality of the scan is not affected by bowel gas or foreign objects such as tubes and dressings.

Selective hepatic angiography has been used for diagnosis of hepatic abscesses but is no longer a necessary investigation.[16,62]

Microbiology

Multiple blood cultures should be taken before the initiation of therapy. Although many authors quote 50% as the expected rate of positive cultures,[120,136] in some reports, the success rate has been almost 100%.[77] The role of diagnostic aspiration of abscess contents is discussed below. If aspiration is performed, pus, not swabs, should be submitted to the laboratory, as promptly as possible.[55,129] Aspirated pus is variably colored, usually not dark brown or red-brown as is amebic abscess content, and frequently is foul smelling. It should be

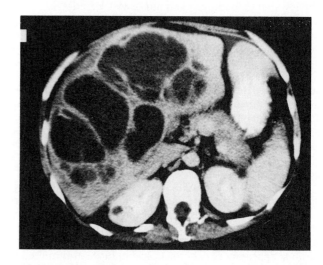

FIGURE 46-10   CT scan of liver in the same patient as in Figure 46-9. Aspiration confirmed the lesions to be pyogenic abscesses.

transported to the laboratory in the syringe used for aspiration, to avoid exposure to air. The physician should be in close communication with the microbiologist about the handling of specimens. Gram stain usually shows organisms unless there has been substantial preceding antibiotic treatment. The submitted material should be cultured for aerobic, anaerobic, and microaerophilic organisms.

Diagnostic Approach to Liver Abscess

The presence of a liver abscess may be suggested by the patient's history, physical examination, and results of laboratory tests but is confirmed by imaging techniques. It is unnecessary to subject patients to every type of scan available, and the choice of initial investigation should be governed by local facilities and expertise. Ultrasonography is our preferred initial investigation, although it is the most operator dependent of the various imaging modalities. If high-quality ultrasonography cannot be guaranteed or if the clinician suspects the presence of an abscess despite negative ultrasound, CT scanning is indicated. We find scintigraphy the least helpful of the scanning modalities.

The features of amebic and pyogenic liver abscess are compared in Table 46-1.[17,69] In our own experience, the features most predictive of the diagnosis have been the patient's age, sex, and ethnicity (young immigrant males favor amebiasis); symptoms and signs (severe constitutional illness and underlying pathology favor pyogenic abscess); degree of derangement of liver tests (usually more abnormal in pyogenic illness); and response to chloroquine (specific for amebic abscess). The diagnosis of the cause of the abscess should not be made on the results of scans alone, although sometimes the latter are highly predictive.[155] In most cases, a confident diagnosis is reached combining epidemiologic, clinical, and radiologic features with the results of blood cultures and amebic serology. If amebic liver abscess is suspected on clinical or epidemiologic grounds, we begin treatment with chloroquine; this treatment is specific for hepatic amebiasis but not for pyogenic abscess. The response to chloroquine, or the lack of it, is in itself a useful diagnostic test. Metronidazole may successfully treat anaerobic pyogenic infections, and therapeutic response is, therefore, not specific for amebiasis.[88] Negative amebic serology virtually excludes the diagnosis of hepatic amebiasis, despite rare cases in which serologic tests become positive after the patient's initial presentation. If invasive amebiasis seems likely despite an initial negative result, the test should be repeated.

Aspiration of abscesses may be performed for either diagnostic or therapeutic purposes. Diagnostic aspiration usually is performed under ultrasound or CT guidance and involves the removal of a small quantity of abscess material through a fine needle for diagnostic studies. In regions of the world in which sophisticated imaging techniques are not available, aspiration has to be performed blind. In such an event, unless an obvious swelling is present, the needle should be cautiously inserted in the area of maximal hepatic tenderness.

TABLE 46-1 *Comparison of Amebic and Pyogenic Liver Abscess*

Criteria	Amebic	Pyogenic
Age	Any; mostly younger	Any, mostly older
Sex	Males more than females	Equal
Epidemiologic features	Residence or travel in endemic area; poverty; poor hygiene; homosexuality	None; occasional association with roundworm or fluke infection
Associated medical conditions	Rare	Common (eg, surgery; biliary tract disease; diverticulitis; tumors)
Significant jaundice	Rare	Common
Multiple abscesses	Infrequent	Common
Complications	Rupture	Rupture; extension; sepsis
Liver tests	Mildly deranged; alkaline phosphatase elevated, albumin reduced	More markedly abnormal; direct bilirubin, LDH, AST, globulins elevated; albumin reduced
Amebic serology	Positive	Negative (unless previously exposed)
Blood cultures	Negative; if positive, it indicates superinfection	Frequently positive
Response to chloroquine	Yes	No
Response to metronidazole	Yes	Sometimes
Abscess contents	Thick fluid; variable color, yellow-brown, nonodorous	Pus; creamy yellow, mostly foul-smelling
Medical therapy effective	Almost always	Often
Percutaneous drainage required	Very rarely	Sometimes
Surgery required	Almost never	Sometimes
Mortality with prompt diagnosis	Very low	Appreciable

The frequency with which diagnostic aspiration need be undertaken varies with local patterns of disease. Aspiration seldom is indicated in patients with amebic liver abscess, in whom there usually is time to safely await the results of amebic serology and response to therapy with chloroquine. When it is obtained, the aspirate from an amebic abscess usually is orange-brown, odorless, and bacteriologically sterile. In pyogenic abscess, however, diagnostic aspiration may be critically important for microbiologic diagnosis when this has not already been obtained from blood cultures. The detection of malodorous pus and the identification of organisms on Gram's stain may provide immediate assistance in the choice of antibiotic therapy or may modify the choice of antibiotic used. We now recommend diagnostic aspiration in all cases of suspected or proven pyogenic abscess unless there has already been demonstrated an excellent response to antibiotic therapy.

Diagnostic aspiration is indicated in the critically ill, in whom there is no time to wait for results of blood cultures and serodiagnostic tests; in patients with negative blood cultures and amebic serology; and in those with either type of abscess not responding to medical therapy. In pyogenic abscess, the latter raises the possibility of infection with an organism not covered by administered antibiotics; in hepatic amebiasis, bacterial superinfection needs to be excluded.

Figure 46-11 shows our algorithm for diagnosis and treatment of hepatic abscess.

Treatment

AMEBIC LIVER ABSCESS

The management of amebiasis has been usefully reviewed by Knight.[95,96]

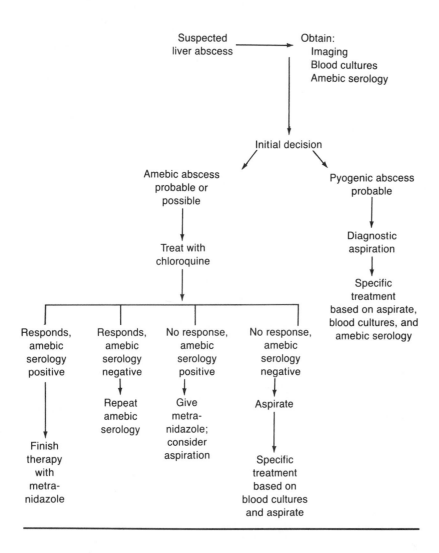

Indications for diagnostic aspiration
   Diagnosis of pyogenic abscess
   Critically ill patient requiring diagnosis
Indications for therapeutic aspiration
   Failure to respond to treatment
   Imminent rupture

FIGURE 46-11 Diagnostic and therapeutic approach to suspected liver abscess.

Chemotherapeutic Agents
Table 46-2 lists chemotherapeutic agents.

Metronidazole. Metronidazole is the treatment of choice for all forms of invasive amebiasis.[59] It is a nitroimidazole that is well absorbed after oral administration, and it is excreted mainly by way of the kidneys. Reduction of the drug's nitro group by *E histolytica* produces toxic metabolites that interfere with nucleic acid synthesis. Adverse effects include nausea, anorexia, metallic taste, urethral and vaginal burning, dark urine, and a disulfiram-like reaction with alcohol. Central nervous system effects such as vertigo, ataxia, and peripheral neuropathy have also been reported. A transient leukopenia occasionally is observed. Reports of possible carcinogenicity, mutagenicity, and teratogenicity under experimental conditions have not been matched by adverse effects in humans, and the advantages of metronidazole for severe disease, including in pregnancy, outweigh its theoretic dangers. In practice, the gastrointestinal adverse effects cause the most trouble.

The usual dosage of metronidazole is 750 mg three times daily for 5 to 10 days. In actual fact, a choice of regimens is available, and large single doses (2.4 g) given for shorter periods, such as 3 days, may be equally effective.[151] The usual pediatric dose is 35 to 50 mg/kg/d in three divided doses. In very ill patients, some clinicians extend treatment to 15 days or even beyond. As with many infectious diseases, the duration of treatment prescribed often is somewhat arbitrary. Patients who cannot take oral metronidazole may be treated with the parenteral preparation.[30,63,103] Metronidazole is effective treatment for invasive intestinal disease but is not completely reliable as a luminal amebicide.

Occasional treatment failures have been reported in addition to cases of hepatic amebiasis developing after metronidazole therapy for intestinal disease.[1,60,72,73,75,102,149,190,206] Other nitroimidazoles offer no advantage over metronidazole. The best known is tinidazole, which is perhaps associated with less nausea. The usual adult dosage is 2 g/d.

Chloroquine. The antimalarial drug chloroquine, a 4-aminoquinoline, acts by binding to parasite deoxyribonucleic acid.[96,95] High concentrations in liver tissue are obtained after oral administration. It has a half-life up to 1 week and is excreted predominantly through the kidneys.

Adverse effects are nausea, abdominal discomfort, and pruritus. Retinopathy is only a potential problem in patients taking long-term chloroquine, as for malaria prophylaxis or rheumatoid arthritis. The usual dose is 1 g/d for 2 days followed by 500 mg/d for 20 days. The only controlled trial of chloroquine versus metronidazole for amebic liver abscess showed no difference in efficacy, other than slightly quicker response with metronidazole.[32] Chloroquine has no action against intestinal infection.

Emetine and Dehydroemetine. Emetine is the oldest as well as the most potent amebicidal drug available. It is given by intramuscular or subcutaneous injection and slowly excreted through the kidneys. The drug acts by interfering with protein synthesis. The usual dosage is 1 mg/kg/d to a maximum of 60 mg/d for 10 days. Duration of treatment

TABLE 46-2 *Drugs Used in Treatment of Amebic Liver Abscess*

Drug	Conventional Dosage	Adverse Effects
Metronidazole	Adult: 750 mg tid for 5–10 d (alternative schedule 2.4 g once daily for 3–5 d)	Anorexia, nausea, metallic taste, dark urine, disulfiram-like reaction, central nervous system effects, leukopenia
	Pediatric: 35–50 mg/kg/d in three divided doses for 5–10 d	Carcinogenicity in animals; mutagenicity in bacteria
	Also effective for intestinal amebiasis	
Chloroquine	Adult: Loading dose 1 g daily for 1–2 d, then 500 mg/d for 20 d	Nausea, vomiting, pruritus; cardiotoxicity in overdose; retinopathy with long-term ingestion
	Pediatric: 10 mg base/kg	
	Ineffective for intestinal amebiasis	
Emetine	1 mg/kg by intramuscular or subcutaneous injection (maximum 60 mg/d) for up to 10 d, not to be repeated within 1 mo	Cardiotoxicity, nausea, vomiting, diarrhea, renal impairment, pain or necrosis at injection site
	Ineffective as a luminal amebicide	
Dehydroemetine	1.25 mg/kg intramuscular or subcutaneous injection (maximum 90 mg/d) for up to 10 d	As for emetine, although less cardiotoxic
	Ineffective as a luminal amebicide	
Luminal amebicides Diloxanide furoate*	Adult: 500 mg for 10 d Pediatric: 20 mg/kg/d in three divided doses	Few adverse effects: mild gastrointestinal disturbance, flatulence
Diiodohydroxyquin	Adult: 650 mg tid for 20 d Pediatric: 30–40 mg/kg/d in three divided doses; maximum 2 g/d	Furunculosis, dermatitis, chills, fever, and abdominal discomfort; neuropathy, myelopathy, and optic atrophy with longer use; subacute myelooptic neuropathy associated particularly with related compound iodochlorhydroxyquin

*Available in the United States from Parasitic Diseases Division, Centers for Disease Control, Atlanta, GA 30333.

should be kept to a minimum, preferably less than 6 days. Adverse effects have rendered this drug obsolete except in the severest of cases. Adverse effects include vomiting, diarrhea, renal impairment, and pain or necrosis at the site of injection. The most serious adverse effect is cardiotoxicity, any sign of which is an indication for stopping the drug. Emetine has no luminal amebicidal activity.

Dehydroemetine is a synthetic preparation with a similar action to emetine but associated with less cardiotoxicity. It is equally effective therapeutically but excreted more rapidly. The daily dose is 1.25 mg/kg, given by intramuscular or subcutaneous injection, to a maximum of 90 mg/d. It should be given in preference to emetine, if available. Cardiotoxicity may be more likely with concurrent administration of chloroquine.[179]

Management of the Patient

Therapy with chloroquine is begun while awaiting amebic serology in cases of suspected amebic liver abscess. Metronidazole is substituted once there is firm laboratory support for the diagnosis. Five days of metronidazole is curative in most patients, although in the very ill, treatment is continued for 10 to 14 days. Chloroquine is continued as well in such cases. Emetine, or preferably dehydroemetine, is reserved for patients who do not respond to treatment and used in conjunction with metronidazole.

Critically ill patients and those who do not respond to medical therapy within 48 to 72 hours should undergo diagnostic aspiration to confirm the diagnosis and exclude bacterial superinfection. Therapeutic percutaneous aspiration is indicated for cases not responding to treatment and for patients in whom rupture seems imminent. Therapeutic aspiration is performed with a large-bore needle, preferably under ultrasound or CT guidance, to evacuate as much abscess material as possible. Abscess size should not in itself be a deciding factor about aspiration, although large abscesses are perhaps especially likely to respond slowly to medical treatment. Left lobe lesions must be carefully assessed, in view of their propensity to rupture into the pericardium. Provided diagnosis is not excessively delayed, most patients can be managed medically without aspiration. Resolution of amebic abscesses as assessed by diagnostic imaging techniques is slower than for pyogenic abscesses.[181] After successful therapy of an amebic abscess, defects may remain evident on ultrasonography for months or even years[154,158] (Fig. 46-12). Such lesions contain thin, serous fluid.[154] They should not be aspirated and need no specific treatment.

Medical therapy is also the cornerstone of treatment of amebic liver abscess with complications. The role of surgery in such cases is controversial. Amebic empyema should probably be drained, usually by a needle or chest tube and more rarely by open thoracotomy. Untreated, chronic empyema and pleural thickening may result.[81] Amebic empyema occasionally is erroneously diagnosed on thoracentesis that yields typical amebic pus, when the aspirating needle in such cases has actually traversed the high right diaphragm into the liver abscess cavity. Hepatobronchial fistula may be self-limiting. If secondary lung abscess develops, this can be treated medically, but bacterial contamination must be searched for.

Rupture into the pericardium is an emergency that require immediate pericardiocentesis. If aspiration through a needle is unsuccessful, then drainage through a pericardial window is indicated. Constrictive pericarditis may develop at a later stage despite appropriate acute management and may require pericardiectomy.[111]

Rupture of an amebic abscess into the peritoneal cavity is frequently only discovered at laparotomy for an undiagnosed acute abdomen. If the diagnosis at operation is clear, the peritoneal cavity should be lavaged, the abscess drained, and medical therapy promptly instituted. Secondary bacterial contamination is a major complication, and efforts should be made to avoid it by limiting surgical maneuvers to a minimum. Unless there is failure to respond to therapy, operation is not indicated for peritoneal rupture diagnosed by paracentesis.[68]

It is reasonable to assume that intestinal infection preceded a liver abscess and to treat all patients with a luminal amebicide. Metronidazole is not wholly effective in this regard and does not always eradicate cyst passage. Diloxanide furoate and diiodohydroxyquin are the preferred agents. The

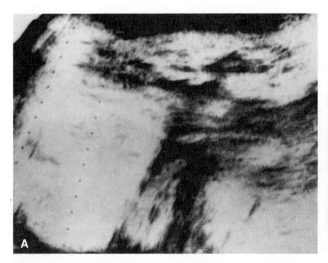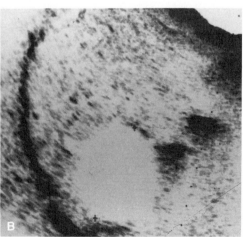

FIGURE 46-12 (A) Ultrasound of liver showing a large amebic abscess. Transverse view. (B) A cystic residual defect is seen 5 years later and was followed unchanged for another 2 years. Sagittal view.

respective adult dosages are 500 mg three times daily for 10 days and 650 mg three times daily for 20 days, conventionally given after completion of treatment of hepatic disease.

Prognosis

Amebiasis is an eminently treatable disease, and probably the major factor that determines outcome is the rapidity with which the diagnosis is reached. Paradoxically, lack of familiarity with amebic liver abscess in areas well served medically may result in higher mortality than in countries with limited facilities.[46] In uncomplicated disease, the case-fatality rate should be less than 1%.[6] The highest death rate is associated with rupture into the pericardium, 32% to 100% in different series.[7,83,111] In general, rupture into the peritoneal cavity or the chest has a mortality up to 20%. The prognosis of rupture need not be as dire as suggested by autopsy studies,[92] provided diagnosis and treatment are instituted without delay.

PYOGENIC LIVER ABSCESS

The traditional treatment for pyogenic liver abscess has been open surgical drainage, combined with broad-spectrum antibiotics.[11] In recent times, percutaneous drainage of intraabdominal abscesses has become widely accepted practice,[58,65,74,89,199] and this technique has also been applied to hepatic abscesses.[19,71,104,114,146,182] This approach is not new; McFadzean and coworkers[121] reported a successful outcome in 13 of 14 patients with pyogenic liver abscess treated by percutaneous needle drainage and antibiotics in 1953. The procedure is now preferably performed under ultrasound or CT guidance, and if aspiration is considered inadequate, a pigtailed catheter with side holes may be left in situ until drainage stops. The complications of this procedure include bleeding, perforation of intraabdominal structures, infection, and catheter displacement.

It has been shown that a significant proportion of patients can be managed medically without therapeutic aspiration or surgery,[16,20,42,77,112,194] despite some reports to the contrary.[118,126] We recommend diagnostic aspiration in all cases prior to commencing antibiotics if pyogenic abscess is a likely diagnosis. When diagnostic aspiration is being performed, as much pus as possible should be removed with the one intervention. In general, antibiotics effective against gram-negative bacilli as well as against microaerophilic and anaerobic organisms should be prescribed until a microbiologic diagnosis has been established. Duration of antibiotic treatment is empirical, and should be guided by clinical response. A total of at least 3 or 4 weeks of therapy is usual, with 1 to 2 weeks of treatment after resolution of fever and leukocytosis.

Management of the Patient

We consider patients with negative amebic serology who do not respond to chloroquine to be suffering from pyogenic abscess. The results of blood and aspirate cultures determine our selection of antibiotics, although we always include an agent effective against anaerobes in the regimen while culture results are pending. *S milleri* is sensitive to penicillin-like drugs but not to metronidazole. Frequently used combinations to initiate therapy are ampicillin, an aminoglycoside or a third-generation cephalosporin, and clindamycin or metronidazole. Exact microbiologic diagnosis subsequently allows administration of specific antimicrobial therapy. Failure to show some improvement within 48 to 72 hours of begin-

ning appropriate antibiotic therapy leads us to undertake drainage, usually by way of a catheter. Diagnostic aspiration is performed by the radiologist, under ultrasound or CT guidance, with the internist in attendance to assist in the appropriate handling of specimens. We have used our approach successfully in several dozen patients. In most cases, parenteral antibiotics can be replaced by oral medication after 10 to 14 days, with treatment being continued for an additional 2 weeks.

The belief that many patients can be managed medically is tempered by recognition that some patients urgently require drainage. Clinical judgment must be used to carry out swift therapeutic aspiration in those cases in need of it. In addition, surgery remains indicated in a proportion of patients, such as those with biliary tract disease or associated intraabdominal infection and cases not responding to the management outlined previously. Surgery also usually is required for abscesses complicated by rupture or extension. Close supervision of the patient, flexibility in approach, and cooperation between internist, radiologist, microbiologist, and surgeon are essential.

Prognosis

Traditionally, mortality rates approaching 100% have been quoted for undrained liver abscess.[110,126,148] Reports of successful medical management, with or without aspiration, describe case-fatality rates as low as 10%.[77,112] As in amebic abscess, delay in diagnosis and treatment have a major effect on outcome.[171] The prognosis is also related to underlying disease, and an overall mortality of 30% is probably realistic. Mortality seems greater in patients with multiple abscesses. The rarity of pyogenic liver abscess and the wide variation in associated disease make controlled studies of different methods of treatment difficult.

References

1. Abioye AA. Drug and immunodiagnostic resistant amoebic liver abscess in Ibadan: an elucidation of a possible mechanism. J Trop Med Hyg 79:252, 1976
2. Abioye AA, Edington GM. Prevalence of amoebiasis at autopsy in Ibadan. Trans R Soc Trop Med Hyg 66:754, 1972
3. Abuabara SF, Barrett JA, Hau T, Jonasson O. Amebic liver abscess. Arch Surg 117:239, 1982
4. Abul-Khair MH, Kenawi MM, Korashy EE, Arafa NM. Ultrasonography and amoebic liver abscesses. Ann Surg 93:221, 1981
5. Adamali N, Wankya BM, Maneno J. Infusion tomography of the liver in the diagnosis of amoebic liver abscess: a preliminary report. East Afr Med J 55:414, 1979
6. Adams EB, MacLeod IN. Invasive amebiasis. II. Amebic liver abscess and its complications. Medicine 56:325, 1977
7. Adeyemo AO, Aderounmu A. Intrathoracic complications of amoebic liver abscess. J R Soc Med 77:17, 1984
8. Alkan WJ, Kalmi B, Kalderon M. The clinical syndrome of amebic abscess of the left lobe of the liver. Ann Intern Med 55:800, 1961
9. Allason-Jones E, Mindel A, Sargeaunt P, Katz D. Outcome of untreated infection with *Entamoeba histolytica* in homosexual men with and without HIV antibody. Br Med J [Clin Res] 297:654, 1988
10. Allason-Jones E, Mindel A, Sargeaunt P, Williams P. *Entamoeba histolytica* as a commensal intestinal parasite in homosexual men. N Engl J Med 315:353, 1986

11. Altemeier WA. Pyogenic liver abscess. In: Schiff L, Schiff ER, eds. Diseases of the liver, ed 5. Philadelphia, JB Lippincott, 1982, pp 1221–1238

12. Ambroise-Thomas P, Desgeorges PT, Monget D. Diagnostic immuno-enzymologique (ELISA) des maladies parasitaires par une micromethode modifiée. Bull WHO 56:797, 1978

13. Amin N. Amoebiasis and corticosteroids. Br Med J [Clin Res] 2:1084, 1978

14. Armen RC, Fry M, Heseltine PNR. Spontaneous colonic drainage: a rare complication of an amebic liver abscess. West J Med 142:253, 1985

15. Atoba MA, Otulana BA, Adebajo AO. Primary liver carcinoma associated with infective liver disease. Trop Geogr Med 40:244, 1988

16. Balasegaram M. Management of hepatic abscess. Curr Probl Surg 18:285, 1981

17. Barbour GL, Juniper K. A clinical comparison of amebic and pyogenic abscess of the liver in sixty-six patients. Am J Med 53:323, 1972

18. Barnes PF, De Cock KM, Reynolds TB, Ralls PW. A comparison of amebic and pyogenic abscess of the liver. Medicine 66:472, 1987

19. Berger LA, Osborne DR. Treatment of pyogenic liver abscesses by percutaneous needle aspiration. Lancet 1:132, 1982

20. Bertoli D, Del Poggio P, Mazzolari M, Randone G. Management of liver abscesses. Lancet 1:743, 1982

21. Biagi FF, Robledo E, Servin H, Marvan G. Influence of some steroids in the experimental production of amebic hepatic abscess. Am J Trop Med Hyg 12:318, 1963

22. Bloch DB. Venturesome toothpick: a continuing source of pyogenic hepatic abscess. JAMA 252:797, 1984

23. Boultbee JE, Simjee AE, Rooknoodeen F, Engelbrecht HE. Experiences with grey scale ultrasonography in hepatic amoebiasis. Clin Radiol 30:683, 1979

24. Bray RS, Harris WG. The epidemiology of infection with *Entamoeba histolytica* in the Gambia, West Africa. Trans R Soc Trop Med Hyg 71:401, 1977

25. Brennan RO, Durack DT. The viridans streptococci in perspective. In: Remington JS, Swartz MN, eds. Current clinical topics in infectious diseases, vol 5. New York, McGraw-Hill, 1984, p 253

26. Brossi A, Baumann N, Chopard-dit-Jean LH, et al. Syntheseversuche in der Emetine-Reihe. 4. Mitteilung Racemisches 2-Dehydroemetine. Helv Chir Acta 42:772, 1959

27. Capin R, Capin NR, Carmona M, Ortiz-Ortiz L. Effect of complement depletion on the induction of amebic liver abscess in the hamster. Arch Invest Med (Mex) 11:173, 1980

28. Centers for Disease Control. Amebiasis associated with colonic irrigation—Colorado. MMWR 30:101, 1981

29. Centers for Disease Control. Pseudo-outbreaks of intestinal amoebiasis: California. MMWR 34:125, 1985

30. Chowcat NL, Wyllie JH. Intravenous metronidazole in amoebic enterocolitis. Lancet 2:1143, 1976

31. Cockshott P, Middlemiss H. Amoebiasis. In: Clinical radiology in the tropics. Edinburgh, Churchill Livingstone, 1979, pp 130–132

32. Cohen HG, Reynolds TB. Comparison of metronidazole and chloroquine for the treatment of amoebic liver abscess. Gastroenterology 69:35, 1975

33. Conan NJ. The treatment of amebic hepatitis with chloroquine. Bull NY Acad Med 24:545, 1948

34. Conona NJ. Chloroquine in amebiasis. Am J Trop Med 28:107, 1948

35. Connor DH, Neafie RC, Meyers WM. Amebiasis. In: Binford CH, Connor DH, eds. Pathology of tropical and extraordinary diseases, vol 1. Washington, DC, Armed Forces Institute of Pathology, 1976, pp 308–316

36. Cook GC. Tropical gastroenterology. Oxford, Oxford University Press, 1980

37. Councilman WT, La Fleur HA. Amoebic dysentery. Bull Johns Hopkins Hosp 2:395, 1891

38. Cowan DB, Houlton MCC. Rupture of an amoebic liver abscess in pregnancy. S Afr Med J 53:460, 1978

39. Dalrymple RB, Fataar S, Goodman A, et al. Hyperechoic amoebic liver abscesses: an unusual ultrasonic appearance. Clin Radiol 33:541, 1982

40. De Bakey ME, Ochsner A. Hepatic amoebiasis: a 20 year experience and analysis of 263 cases. Int Abstr Surg 92:209, 1951

41. De Cock KM, Calder JF. Ultrasonic diagnosis of abdominal disease in Kenya. Trans R Soc Trop Med Hyg 75:632, 1981

42. De Cock KM, Bhatt KM, Bhatt SM, et al. Management of liver abscesses. Lancet 1:743, 1982

43. De Silva K. Intraperitoneal rupture of an amoebic liver abscess in a pregnant woman at term. Ceylon Med J 15:51, 1970

44. Diamond LS. Amebiasis: nutritional implications. Rev Infect Dis 4:843, 1982

45. Diaz CA. Amebic hepatic abscess. In: Padilla y Padilla CA, Padilla GM, eds. Amebiasis in man. Springfield, IL, Charles C Thomas, 1974, pp 92–109

46. Dorrough RL. Amebic liver abscess. South Med J 60:305, 1967

47. Dritz SK, Ainsworth TE, Garrard WF, et al. Patterns of sexually transmitted enteric diseases in a city. Lancet 2:3, 1977

48. Edington GM, Gilles HM. Amoebiasis and the liver. In: Pathology in the tropics, vol 2, ed 2. London, Edward Arnold, 1976, pp 71–73

49. Editorial. Is that amoeba harmful or not? Lancet 1:732, 1985

50. Eggleston FC, Handa AK, Verghese M. Amebic peritonitis secondary to amebic liver abscess. Surgery 91:46, 1982

51. Eisert J, Hannibal JE, Sanders SL. Fatal amebiasis complicating corticosteroid management of pemphigus vulgaris. N Engl J Med 261:843, 1959

52. El-Hennawy M, Abd-Rabbo H. Hazards of cortisone therapy in hepatic amoebiasis. J Trop Med Hyg 81:71, 1978

53. Elsdon-Dew R. The epidemiology of amoebiasis. In: Dawes B, ed. Advances in parasitology. New York, Academic Press, 1968, pp 1–62

54. Elsdon-Dew R. Amebiasis as a world problem. Bull NY Acad Med 47:438, 1971

55. Eykyn S, Phillips I. Pyogenic liver abscess. Br Med J [Clin Res] 280:1617, 1980

56. Facklam RR. The major differences in the American and British streptococcus taxonomy schemes with reference to *Streptococcus milleri*. Eur J Clin Microbiol 3:91, 1984

57. Falaiye JM, Okeke GCE, Fregene AO. Amoebic abscess in the cirrhotic liver. Gut 21:161, 1980

58. Ferrucci JT, Van Sonnenberg E. Intra-abdominal abscess: radiological diagnosis and treatment. JAMA 246:2728, 1981

59. Finegold SM. Metronidazole. Ann Intern Med 93:585, 1980

60. Fisher LS, Chow AW, Lindquist L, Guze LB. Failure of metronidazole in amebic liver abscess. Am J Med Sci 271:65, 1976

61. Fitz RH. Perforating inflammation of the vermiform appendix: with special reference to its early diagnosis and treatment. Am J Med Sci 92:321, 1886

62. Freeny PC. Acute pyogenic hepatitis: sonographic and angiographic findings. AJR 135:388, 1980

63. Gall SA, Edmisten C, Vernon RP. Intravenous metronidazole in the treatment of ruptured amebic liver abscess. South Med J 73:1274, 1980

64. Gathiram V, Simjee AE, Bhamjee A, et al. Concomitant and secondary bacterial infection of the pus in hepatic amoebiasis. S Afr Med J 65:951, 1984

65. Gerzof SG, Robbins AH, Johnson WC, et al. Percutaneous catheter drainage of abdominal abscesses. N Engl J Med 305:653, 1981

66. Goldmeier D, Sargeaunt P, Price AB, et al. Is *Entamoeba histolytica* in homosexual men a pathogen? Lancet 1:641, 1986.

67. Gooneratne NS, Imarisio JJ. Decreased uptake of 67 gallium

citrate (67 Ga) by a bacterial hepatic abscess. Gastroenterology 73:1147, 1977

68. Greaney GC, Reynolds TB, Donnovan AJ. Ruptured amebic liver abscess. Arch Surg 120:555, 1985

69. Greenstein AJ, Barth J, Dicker A, et al. Amebic liver abscess: a study of 11 cases compared with a series of 38 patients with pyogenic liver abscess. Am J Gastroenterol 80:472, 1985

70. Greenstein AJ, Lowenthal D, Hammer GS, et al. Continuing changing patterns of disease in pyogenic liver abscess: a study of 38 patients. Am J Gastroenterol 79:217, 1984

71. Greenwood LH, Collins TL, Yrizarry JM. Percutaneous management of multiple liver abscesses. AJR 139:390, 1982

72. Gregory PB. A refractory case of hepatic amoebiasis. Gastroenterology 70:585, 1976

73. Griffin FM. Failure of metronidazole to cure hepatic amebic abscess. N Engl J Med 288:1397, 1973

74. Haaga JR, Weinstein AJ. CT-guided percutaneous aspiration and drainage of abscesses. AJR 135:1187, 1980

75. Harrison HR, Crowe CP, Fulginiti VA. Amebic liver abscess in children: clinical and epidemiologic features. Pediatrics 64:923, 1979

76. Henn RM, Collin DB. Amebic abscess of the liver: treatment failure with metronidazole. JAMA 224:1394, 1973

77. Herbert DA, Fogel DA, Rothman J, et al. Pyogenic liver abscesses: successful non-surgical therapy. Lancet 1:134, 1982

78. Heymann AD. Clinical aspects of grave pyogenic abscess of the liver. Surg Gynecol Obstet 149:209, 1979

79. Huddle KR. Amoebic liver abscess, inferior vena-caval compression and the nephrotic syndrome. S Afr Med J 61:758, 1982

80. Hutt MSR. Some aspects of liver disease in Ugandan Africans. Trans R Soc Trop Med Hyg 65:273, 1971

81. Ibarra-Perez C. Thoracic complications of amebic abscess of the liver: report of 501 cases. Chest 79:672, 1981

82. Ibarra-Perez C, Selman-Lama M. Diagnosis and treatment of amebic "empyema." Am J Surg 134:283, 1977

83. Ibarra-Perez C, Green L, Calvillo-Juarez M, de la Cruz JV. Diagnosis and treatment of rupture of amebic abscess of the liver into the pericardium. J Thorac Cardiovasc Surg 64:11, 1972

84. Imperato PJ. A historical overview of amebiasis. Bull NY Acad Med 57:175, 1981

85. Juniper KS, Worrell CL, Minshew MC, et al. Serologic diagnosis of amebiasis. Am J Trop Med Hyg 21:157, 1972

86. Kanani SR, Knight R. Relapsing amoebic colitis of 12 years' standing exacerbated by corticosteroids. Br Med J [Clin Res] 2:613, 1969

87. Kandel G, Marcon NE. Pyogenic liver abscess: new concepts of an old disease. Am J Gastroenterol 79:65, 1984

88. Kane JG, Parker RH. Metronidazole and hepatic abscess: a false-positive response. JAMA 236:2653, 1976

89. Karlson KB, Martin EC, Frankuchen EI, et al. Percutaneous abscess drainage. Surg Gynecol Obstet 154:44, 1982

90. Kartulis S. Zur Aetiologie der Dysenterie in Aegypten. Arch Pathol Anat 105:521, 1886

91. Katzenstein D, Rickerson V, Braude A. New concepts of amebic liver abscess derived from hepatic imaging, serodiagnosis, and hepatic enzymes in 67 consecutive cases in San Diego. Medicine (Baltimore) 61:237, 1982

92. Kean BH, Gilmore HR, Van Stone WW. Fatal amebiasis: report of 148 fatal cases from the Armed Forces Institute of Pathology. Ann Intern Med 44:831, 1956

93. Kean BH, William DC, Luminais SK. Epidemic of amoebiasis and giardiasis in a biased population. Br J Vener Dis 55:375, 1979

94. Kew MC, Osler HI, McCann WG, et al. Radiocolloid imaging in primary liver cancer and amoebic liver abscess. S Afr Med J 56:127, 1979

95. Knight R. The chemotherapy of amoebiasis. J Antimicrob Chemother 6:577, 1980

96. Knight R. Hepatic amoebiasis. Semin Liver Dis 4:277, 1984

97. Knobloch J, Mannweiler E. Development and persistence of antibodies to *Entamoeba histolytica* in patients with amebic liver abscess: analysis of 216 cases. Am J Trop Med Hyg 32:727, 1983

98. Knobloch J, Funke M, Bienzle U. Autochthonous amoebic liver abscess in Germany. Trop Med Parasitol 31:414, 1980

99. Koch R, Gaffky G. Bericht uber die Thatigkeit der zur Erforschung der cholera in jahre 1883 nach Egypten und Indien Enstandten Kommission. Arb Kaisere Ges 3:1, 1887

100. Koehler PR, Moss AA. Diagnosis of intra-abdominal and pelvic abscesses by computerized tomography. JAMA 244:49, 1980

101. Koshy A, Khuroo MS, Suri S, et al. Amebic liver abscess with hemobilia. Am J Surg 138:453, 1979

102. Koutsaimanis KG, Timms PW, Ree GH. Failure of metronidazole in a patient with hepatic amebic abscess. Am J Trop Med Hyg 28:768, 1979

103. Kovaleski T, Malangoni MA, Wheat LJ. Treatment of an amebic liver abscess with intravenous metronidazole. Arch Intern Med 141:132, 1981

104. Kraulis JE, Bird BL, Colapinto ND. Percutaneous catheter drainage of liver abscess: an alternative to open drainage? Br J Surg 67:400, 1980

105. Krettek JE, Goldstein LI, Busuttil RW. The symptoms of an amebic abscess of the liver stimulating an acute surgical abdomen. Surg Gynecol Obstet 148:552, 1979

106. Krogstad DJ, Spencer HC, Healy GR, et al. Amebiasis: epidemiologic studies in the United States, 1971–1974. Ann Intern Med 88:89, 1978

107. Kuligowska E, Connors SK, Shapiro JH. Liver abscess: sonography in diagnosis and treatment. AJR 138:253, 1982

108. Lamont AC, Wicks ACB. Amoebic liver abscess in Rhodesian Africans. Trans R Soc Trop Med Hyg 70:302, 1976

109. Lazarchick J, de Souza E, Silva NA, et al. Pyogenic liver abscess. Mayo Clin Proc 48:349, 1973

110. Losch FA. Massive development of amebas in the large intestine (translated from the original). Am J Trop Med Hyg 24:383, 1975

111. Macleod IN, Wilmot AJ, Powell SJ. Amoebic pericarditis. QJ Med 35:293, 1966

112. Maher JA, Reynolds TB, Yellin AE. Successful medical treatment of pyogenic liver abscess. Gastroenterology 77:618, 1979

113. Marr JS. Amebiasis in New York City: a changing pattern of transmission. Bull NY Acad Med 57:188, 1981

114. Martin EC, Karlson KB, Frankuchen E, et al. Percutaneous drainage in the management of hepatic abscesses. Surg Clin North Am 61:157, 1981

115. Martinez-Palomo A, Martinez-Baez M. Selective primary health care: strategies for control of disease in the developing world. X. Amebiasis. Rev Infect Dis 5:1093, 1983

116. Mayet FGH, Powell SJ. Anemia associated with amebic liver abscess. Am J Trop Med Hyg 13:790, 1964

117. McCarty E, Pathmanand C, Sunakorn P, Scherz RG. Amebic liver abscess in childhood. Am J Dis Child 126:67, 1973

118. McCorkell SJ, Niles NL. Pyogenic liver abscesses: another look at medical management. Lancet 1:803, 1985

119. McDonald MI. Pyogenic liver abscess: diagnosis, bacteriology and treatment. Eur J Clin Microbiol 3:506, 1984

120. McDonald MI, Corey GR, Gallis HA, Durack DT. Single and multiple pyogenic liver abscesses: natural history, diagnosis and treatment, with emphasis on percutaneous drainage. Medicine (Baltimore) 63:291, 1984

121. McFadzean AJS, Chang KPS, Wong CC. Solitary pyogenic abscess of the liver treated by closed aspiration and antibiotics: a report of 14 consecutive cases of recovery. Br J Surg 41:141, 1953

122. McMillan A, Gilmour HM, McNeillage G, Scott GR. Amoebiasis in homosexual men. Gut 25:356, 1984

123. Merritt RJ, Coughlin E, Thomas DW, et al. Spectrum of amebiasis in children. Am J Dis Child 136:785, 1982

124. Meyers JD, Kuharic HA, Holmes KK. *Giardia lamblia* infection in homosexual men. Br J Vener Dis 53:54, 1977
125. Michel ML, Wirth RW. Multiple pyogenic abscesses of the liver: cure by penicillin in case due to anaerobic streptococci. JAMA 133:395, 1947
126. Miedema BW, Dineen P. The diagnosis and treatment of pyogenic liver abscesses. Ann Surg 200:328, 1984
127. Mitchell RW, Teare AJ. Amoebic liver abscess in pregnancy. Br J Obstet Gynaecol 91:393, 1984
128. Monga NK, Wig JD, Sood KC, et al. Amebic peritonitis. Int Surg 62:431, 1977
129. Moore-Gillon JC, Eykyn SJ, Phillips I. Microbiology of pyogenic liver abscess. Br Med J [Clin Res] 283:819, 1981
130. Most H. Manhattan: "a tropical isle"? Am J Trop Med Hyg 17:333, 1968
131. Mylius RE, Tenseldam REJ. Venereal infection by *Entamoeba histolytica* in a New Guinea native couple. Trop Geogr Med 14:20, 1962
132. Naidoo PM, Keeton G, Stein L, et al. Hepatic amoebiasis. S Afr Med J 48:1159, 1974
133. Naik SR, Achar BG, Mehta SK. Reversible portal hypertension in amoebic liver abscess: a case report. J Trop Med Hyg 81:116, 1978
134. Navaratne RA. Postpartum intraperitoneal rupture of an amoebic liver abscess. Ceylon Med J 17:160, 1972
135. Neale G, Caughey DE, Mollin DL, Booth CC. Effects of intrahepatic and extrahepatic infection on liver function. Br Med J [Clin Res] 1:382, 1966
136. Neoptolemos JP, Macpherson DS. Pyogenic liver abscess. Br J Hosp Med 26:48, 1981
137. Newlin N, Silver TM, Stuck KJ, Sandler MA. Ultrasonic features of pyogenic liver abscesses. Radiology 139:155, 1981
138. Nigam P, Gupta AK, Kapoor KK, et al. Cholestasis in amoebic liver abscess. Gut 26:140, 1985
139. Northover JMA, Jones BJM, Dawson JL, Williams R. Difficulties in the diagnosis and management of pyogenic liver abscess. Br J Surg 69:48, 1982
140. Ochsner A, DeBakey M, Murray S. Pyogenic abscess of the liver. II. An analysis of forty-seven cases with review of the literature. Am J Surg 40:292, 1938
141. Osler W. On the *Amoeba coli* in dysentery and in dysenteric liver abscess. Bull Johns Hopkins Hosp 1:53, 1890
142. Ottenberg R, Berck M. Sulfanilamide therapy for suppurative pylephlebitis and liver abscesses. JAMA 111:1374, 1938
143. Ou Tim L, Segal I, Hodkinson HJ. Amoebic liver abscess in patients presenting with jaundice. S Afr Med J 55:179, 1979
144. Palmer ED. The changing manifestations of pyogenic liver abscess. JAMA 231:192, 1975
145. Patterson M, Healy GR, Shabot JM. Serologic testing for amoebiasis. Gastroenterology 78:136, 1980
146. Perera MR, Kirk A, Noone P. Presentation, diagnosis and management of liver abscess. Lancet 2:629, 1980
147. Perry HB, Boulanger M, Pennoyer D. Chronic granulomatous disease in an adult with recurrent abscesses. Arch Surg 115:200, 1980
148. Pitt HA, Zuidema GD. Factors influencing mortality in the treatment of pyogenic hepatic abscess. Surg Gynecol Obstet 140:228, 1975
149. Pittman FE, Pittman JC. Amebic liver abscess following metronidazole therapy for amebic colitis. Am J Trop Med Hyg 23:146, 1974
150. Pomerantz BM, Marr JS, Goldman WD. Amebiasis in New York City 1958–1978: identification of the male homosexual high risk population. Bull NY Acad Med 56:232, 1980
151. Powell SJ. Therapy of amebiasis. Bull NY Acad Med 47:469, 1971
152. Powell SJ, MacLeod I, Wilmot AJ, Elsdon-Dew R. Metronidazole in amoebic dysentery and amoebic liver abscess. Lancet 2:1329, 1966
153. Powell SJ, Sutton JB, Lautre G. Haemobilia in amoebic liver abscess. S Afr Med J 47:1555, 1973
154. Price ME. Amoebic liver abscess in a Norfolk factory worker. Br Med J [Clin Res] 283:1175, 1981
155. Ralls PW, Barnes PF, Radin DR, Colletti P, Halls J. Sonographic features of amebic and pyogenic liver abscess: a blinded comparison. AJR 149:499, 1987.
156. Ralls PW, Colletti PM, Halls JM. Imaging in hepatic amebic abscess. In: Ravdin JI, ed. Amebiasis: human infection by *Entamoeba histolytica*. New York, John Wiley & Sons, 1988, pp 664–719
157. Ralls PW, Colletti PM, Quinn MF, Halls J. Sonographic findings in hepatic amebic abscess. Radiology 145:123, 1982
158. Ralls PW, Quinn MF, Boswell WD, et al. Patterns of resolution in successfully treated hepatic amebic abscess: sonographic evaluation. Radiology 149:541, 1983
159. Ramachandran S, De Saram R, Rajapakse CNA, Sivalingam S. Hepatic manifestations during amoebic dysentery. Postgrad Med J 49:261, 1973
160. Reed SL, Sargeaunt PG, Braude AI. Resistance to lysis by human serum of pathogenic *Entamoeba histolytica*. Trans R Soc Trop Med Hyg 77:248, 1983
161. Rode H, Davies MRQ, Cywes S. Amoebic liver abscesses in infancy and childhood. S Afr J Surg 16:131, 1978
162. Rogers L. The rapid cure of amoebic dysentery and hepatitis by hypodermic injections of soluble salts of emetine. Br Med J [Clin Res] 1:14, 1912
163. Rubin RH, Swartz MN, Malt R. Hepatic abscess: changes in clinical, bacteriologic and therapeutic aspects. Am J Med 57:602, 1974
164. Rubinson HA, Isikoff MB, Hill MC. Diagnostic imaging of hepatic abscesses: a retrospective analysis. AJR 135:735, 1980
165. Sabbaj J. Anaerobes in liver abscess. Rev Infect Dis 6:S152, 1984
166. Sabbaj J, Sutter V, Finegold SM. Anaerobic pyogenic liver abscesses. Ann Intern Med 77:629, 1972
167. Salata RA, Radvin JI. Review of the human immune mechanisms directed against *Entamoeba histolytica*. Rev Infect Dis 8:261, 1986
168. Salata RA, Pearson RD, Ravdin JI. Interaction of human leukocytes and *Entamoeba histolytica*: killing of virulent amebae by the activated macrophage. J Clin Invest 76:491, 1985
169. Saltzman DA, Smithline N, Davis JR. Fulminant hepatic failure secondary to amebic abscesses. Dig Dis 23:561, 1978
170. Sanderson IR, Walker-Smith JA. Indigenous amoebiasis: an important differential diagnosis of chronic inflammatory bowel disease. Br Med J [Clin Res] 289:823, 1984
171. Sandford NL, Bradbear RA, Powell LW. Pyogenic liver abscess: a neglected diagnosis. Aust NZ J Med 14:597, 1984
172. Sargeaunt PG, Oates JK, MacLennan I, et al. *Entamoeba histolytica* in male homosexuals. Br J Vener Dis 59:193, 1983
173. Sargeaunt PG, Williams JE, Grene JD. The differentiation of invasive and non-invasive *Entamoeba histolytica* by isoenzyme electrophoresis. Trans R Soc Trop Med Hyg 72:519, 1978
174. Schmid BD, Lalyre Y, Sigel B, et al. Inferior vena cava obstruction complicating amebic liver abscess. Dig Dis Sci 27:565, 1982
175. Scragg J. Amoebic liver abscess in African children. Arch Dis Child 35:171, 1960
176. Seale JP, Lee JH. An unusual complication of corticosteroid therapy for sarcoidosis. Med J Aust 1:252, 1977
177. Sepulveda B, Martinez-Palomo A. Immunology of amoebiasis by *Entamoeba histolytica*. In: Cohen S, Warren KS, eds. Immunology of parasitic infections, ed 2. Oxford, Blackwell, 1982, pp 170–191
178. Sepulveda B, Martinez-Palomo A. Amebiasis. In: Warren KS, Mahmoud AAF, eds. Tropical and geographical medicine. New York, McGraw-Hill, 1984, pp 305–318
179. Seshadri MS, John L, Varkey K, Koshy TS. Ventricular tachycardia in a patient on dehydroemetine and chloroquine for amoebic liver abscess. Med J Aust 1:406, 1979
180. Sexton DJ, Krogstad DJ, Spencer HC Jr, et al. Amebiasis in

a mental institution: serologic and epidemiologic studies. Am J Epidemiol 100:414, 1974

181. Sheen IS, Chien CS, Lin DY, Liaw YF. Resolution of liver abscesses: comparison of pyogenic and amebic liver abscesses. Am J Trop Med Hyg 40:384, 1989

182. Sheinfeld AM, Steiner AE, Rivkin LB, et al. Transcutaneous drainage of abscesses of the liver guided by computed tomography scan. Surg Gynecol Obstet 155:662, 1982

183. Sherman JD, Robbins SL. Changing trends in the casuistics of hepatic abscess. Am J Med 28:943, 1960

184. Simon CE. Abscess of the liver: perforation into the lung; *Amoeba coli* in sputum. Bull Johns Hopkins Hosp 1:97, 1890

185. Singh KP, Sreemannarayana MB, Mehdiratta KS. Intraperitoneal rupture of amebic liver abscess. Int Surg 62:432, 1977

186. Smith JW. Identification of fecal parasites in the Special Parasitology Survey of the College of American Pathologists. Am J Clin Pathol 72:371, 1979

187. Spencer HC, Hermos JA, Healey GR, et al. Epidemic amebiasis in an Arkansas community. Am J Epidemiol 104:93, 1976

188. Spencer HC, Muchnick C, Sexton DJ, et al. Endemic amebiasis in an extended family. Am J Trop Med Hyg 26:628, 1977

189. Stenson WF, Eckert T, Avioli LA. Pyogenic liver abscess. Arch Intern Med 143:126, 1983

190. Stillman AE, Alvarez V, Grube D. Hepatic amebic abscess: unresponsiveness to combination of metronidazole and surgical drainage. JAMA 229:71, 1974

191. Strachan WD, Chiodini PL, Spice WM, Moody AH, Ackers JP. Immunological differentiation of pathogenic and nonpathogenic isolates of *Entamoeba histolytica*. Lancet 1:561, 1988

192. Stuiver PC, Goud THJLM. Corticosteroids and liver amoebiasis. Br Med J [Clin Res] 2:394, 1978

193. Tanimoto-Weki M, Vazquez-Saavedra JA, Calderon P, Aguirre-Garcia J. Resultados de la inoculacion al hamster de trofozoitos obtenidos de portadores asintomaticos de *E. histolytica*. Arch Invest Med (Mex) 4(Suppl 1):105, 1973

194. Thomas CT, Berk SL, Thomas E. Management of liver abscesses. Lancet 1:742, 1982

195. Thomas JA, Antony AJ. Amoebiasis of the penis. Br J Urol 48:269, 1976

196. Thompson JE, Forlenza S, Verma R. Amebic liver abscess: a therapeutic approach. Rev Infect Dis 7:171, 1985

197. Thompson JE, Freischlag J, Thomas DS. Amebic liver abscess in a homosexual man. Sex Transm Dis 10:153, 1983

198. Triger DR. Amoebic liver abscess in Wessex: a retrospective survey of 24 cases. J Trop Med Hyg 81:54, 1978

199. Van Sonnenberg E, Ferruci JT, Mueller PR. Percutaneous radiographically guided catheter drainage of abdominal abscesses. JAMA 247:190, 1982

200. Verghese M, Eggleston FC, Handa AK, Singh CM. Management of thoracic amebiasis. J Thorac Cardiovasc Surg 78:757, 1979

201. Vickary FR, Cusick G, Shirley IM, Blackwell RJ. Ultrasound and amoebic liver abscess. Br J Surg 64:113, 1977

202. Vickers PJ, Bohra RC, Sharma GC. Hepatopulmonary amebiasis: a review of 40 cases. Int Surg 67:427, 1982

203. Wagner VP, Smale LE, Lischke JH. Amebic abscess of the liver and spleen in pregnancy and the puerperium. Obstet Gynecol 45:562, 1975

204. Walker EL, Sellards AW. Experimental entamoebic dysentery. Philippine J Sci 8:253, 1913

205. Walsh JA. Estimating the burden of illness in the tropics. In: Warren KS, Mahmoud AAF, eds. Tropical and geographical medicine. pp 185–196

206. Weber DM. Amebic abscess of liver following metronidazole therapy. JAMA 216:1339, 1971

207. Wittner M, Rosenbaum RM. Role of bacteria in modifying virulence of *Entamoeba histolytica*: studies of amebae from axenic cultures. Am J Trop Med Hyg 19:755, 1970

208. Ylvisaker JT, McDonald GB. Sexually acquired amebic colitis and liver abscess. West J Med 132:153, 1980

Diseases of the Liver, Seventh Edition, edited by
Leon Schiff and Eugene R. Schiff. J.B. Lippincott Company, Philadelphia © 1993.

Parasitic Diseases of the Liver

Zoheir Farid

Michael E. Kilpatrick

Peter L. Chiodini

This chapter covers the diagnosis, clinical presentation, and treatment of the major protozoal and helminthic infections that may affect the liver. Emphasis is placed on early diagnosis and current effective chemotherapy. Table 47-1 summarizes the clinically relevant human parasitic diseases that can involve the liver and biliary tracts.[12,14,21,54,64,105,111,118,125,127]

PROTOZOAL INFECTIONS

Amebiasis

Amebic abscess of the liver is discussed in detail in Chapter 46. This chapter presents only a brief summary to emphasize the importance of this protozoal infection and involvement of the liver.

Amebiasis is an infection of the colon caused by the protozoan *Entamoeba histolytica.* Clinical features may vary from no symptoms to mild to severe diarrhea. Extraintestinal *E histolytica* infection involving the liver is the third most important human parasitic infection following malaria and schistosomiasis. The hepatic amebic abscess does not contain pus but rather proteinaceous debris with trophozoites at the periphery of the cavity. The abscess may rupture into the peritoneum, pleura, lung, or pericardium. The differential diagnosis of amebic liver abscess includes pyogenic liver abscess, hydatid cyst, and hepatoma. The introduction of immunoserology (counterimmunoelectrophoresis [CIEP]), ultrasound, and computed tomography (CT) has greatly facilitated diagnosis; metronidazole has revolutionized treatment (Figs. 47-1 and 47-2).[4,36,37,48,91,94,97]

Malaria

The liver is involved during two stages of the life cycle, first in the preerythrocytic phase and then in the erythrocytic phase, the stage responsible for the development of clinical illness in human malaria. A detailed and authoritative account of the malaria life cycle is to be found in Garnham.[49]

PATHOLOGY

The Preerythrocytic Stage

Sporozoites injected by a mosquito bite circulate through the bloodstream to the liver, where they enter hepatocytes. Some sporozoites may enter Kupffer cells but they develop no further and die within a day.[49] Development in the hepatocyte to a mature schizont (30 to 70 μm diameter) occurs.

Rupture of the schizont releases merozoites into the bloodstream, where they invade erythrocytes. The number of merozoites varies according to the species of parasite, with some 10,000 in *Plasmodium vivax* and 30,000 in *P falciparum.* The time course for maturation also varies by species, the minimum being 5.5 days for *P falciparum* and 15 days for *P malariae.*

P falciparum and *P malariae* have no residual liver stages, but *P vivax* and *P ovale* have persistent exoerythrocytic stages. The hypnozoite is a unicellular stage that remains constant in size and appearance until activated by an as yet unidentified trigger. They then undergo division and develop into mature schizonts.

The duration and latency of the hypnozoite varies between strains of *P vivax;* for example, in *P vivax hibernans* all sporozoites develop to hypnozoites with a latency of 8 to 9 months, whereas in the Chesson strain of *P vivax,* more than half the sporozoites proceed to immediate development, with the rest becoming hypnozoites that are then activated at various intervals[49] (Fig. 47-3).

Erythrocytic Stages

Effects on the Hepatic Sinusoids. The degree of hepatic damage depends on the species of malaria parasite and the severity of the infection; the most serious effects result from infection with *P falciparum.*

In most patients, unconjugated bilirubin predominates as a result of hemolysis, but where the bilirubin is high, conjugated bilirubin predominates, as a result of hepatocyte dysfunction. Cholestasis may occur in, for example, some patients with black-water fever. The serum albumin may be low and the prothrombin time moderately prolonged. There may be moderate elevation of aminotransferases and 5′ nucleotidase.[123] In severe falciparum malaria, hypoglycemia, probably due to decreased hepatic gluconeogenesis,[83] and lactic acidosis, secondary to reduced hepatic clearance, are serious complications. Changes occur in triglycerides, phospholipids, free fatty acids, cholesterol, esterified cholesterol, and nonesterified fatty acids.[123] Hills[56] has reported abnormal sulfobromophthalein sodium (Bromsulphalein) retention in jaundiced cases of malaria.

Molyneux and colleagues,[83] using the indocyanine green method, showed that hepatic blood flow was reduced during

TABLE 47-1 *Parasitic Diseases of the Liver*

Protozoal Infections
Amebiasis	Babesiosis
Malaria	Leishmaniasis

Helminthic Infections

Nematodes
  Ascariasis
  Toxocariasis
  Strongyloidiasis
  Capillariasis
  Trichiniasis
Cestodes
  Echinococcosis

Trematodes
  Blood flukes
    Schistosomiasis
  Liver flukes
    Fascioliasis
    Clonorchiasis
    Opisthorchiasis
    Dicrocoeliasis
  Lung flukes
    Paragonimiasis

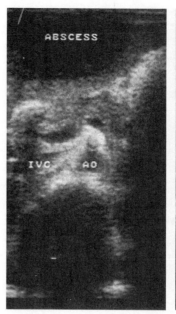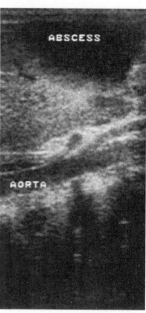

FIGURE 47-2 Transverse (**right**) and longitudinal (**left**) scans showing an anterior left lobe abscess.

the acute phase of severe noncerebral *P falciparum* malaria but returned to normal during convalescence. This is possibly explained by sequestration or microcirculatory obstruction by parasitized erythrocytes in the portal circulation, leading to reduced portal venous blood flow.

Effects on Kupffer Cells and Sinusoidal and Portal Macrophages.

In an acute attack of malaria in a nonimmune person, including young children in endemic areas, there is hypertrophy of hepatic macrophages, and large amounts of hemozoin pigment are present in the Kupffer cells. Pigment appears in the Kupffer cells and the sinusoidal macrophages within 6 days of an acute attack of malaria. It persists for a long period but usually disappears within 6 months. Kupffer cells and sinusoidal macrophages also phagocytose nonparasitized as well as parasitized erythrocytes.

Necropsy and Histopathologic Findings.

Most information has come from cases of *P falciparum* malaria; the other species infecting humans rarely cause death during the acute attack. The findings in cases of infection with other species of human malaria are similar to but less severe than those due to *P falciparum*.

Macroscopically, the liver is chocolate or slate-gray colored, congested, and tense. There may be loss of the lobular pattern but no gross necrosis or hemorrhage.

Liver biopsy specimens from jaundiced malaria patients usually show Kupffer cell hyperplasia and mononuclear cell infiltration. There are prominent pigment deposits in Kupffer cells. Other series showed no structural changes, or slight hepatocyte swelling, whereas some series reported centrizonal necrosis. After successful treatment, the changes resolve, and Cook[23] thought it extremely unlikely that long-term hepatic sequelae ever result from human malaria.

Electron microscopy of liver tissue from severe *P falciparum* malaria showed hypertrophy of Kupffer cells and sinusoidal macrophages. Hepatocyte swelling, changes in the endoplasmic reticulum and mitochondria, and loss of microvilli at the sinusoidal pole were reported.[26]

Animal Models.

In rhesus monkeys experimentally infected with *P knowlesi*, the liver shows sinusoidal dilatation around the central veins, with necrosis of hepatocytes in the centrilobular region.[100]

Also in rhesus monkeys infected with *P knowlesi*, portal angiography showed constriction in all branches of the portal vein and diminished sinusoidal perfusion. The changes were mediated by sympathetic activity and reversed by adrenergic blockade.[74]

The Liver in Hyperreactive Malarial Splenomegaly (Formerly Tropical Splenomegaly Syndrome).

In endemic areas, as malarial antibody concentration increases and immunity increases, Kupffer cell hypertrophy partially

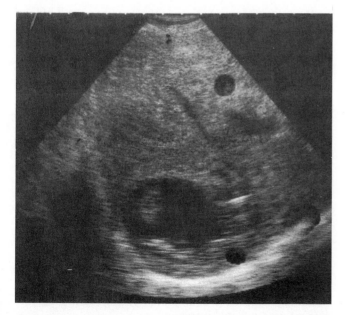

FIGURE 47-1 Sector scan of a liver with a posterosuperior right lobe liver abscess seen near the diaphragm.

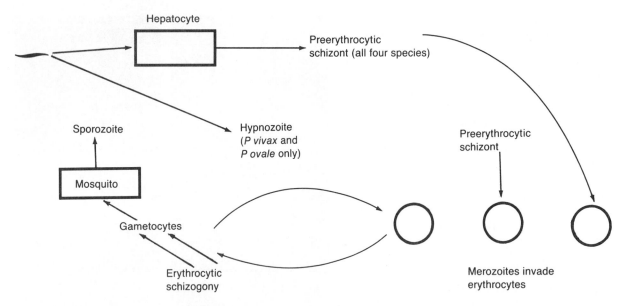

FIGURE 47-3   Schematized life cycle of the human malaria parasite.

resolves and hepatic sinusoidal lymphocytes and plasma cells proliferate. In a few cases, particularly dense hepatic sinusoidal lymphocytosis develops. Associated with this is massive splenomegaly, markedly elevated malarial antibody concentration, and raised serum IgM.

Hyperreactive malarial splenomegaly (HMS) is thought to result from an aberrant immunologic response to all four species of *Plasmodium* that infect humans, leading to overproduction of B lymphocytes and immunocomplexes.

Bates and colleagues[11] examined the hypothesis that HMS may evolve into a malignant lymphoproliferative disorder. It was already known that in about 10% of African HMS patients, the disease resembled chronic lymphatic leukemia (CLL), with a marked lymphocytosis in blood and bone marrow. In addition, some patients with HMS become resistant to treatment with antimalarial drugs such that splenic regression fails to occur on proguanil therapy. These facts led to a suggestion that HMS might be a premalignant condition.

Bates and associates[11] studied 22 Ghanaian patients with HMS or lymphocytosis whom they categorized by degree of response to proguanil therapy. DNA extracted from their peripheral blood cells was screened by DNA probe for rearrangements of the Jh region of the immunoglobulin gene. Clonal rearrangements of the Jh region were found in all 3 patients with no response to proguanil, in none of 13 patients with a sustained response, and in 2 of 6 patients with moderate response or relapse on proguanil therapy. The authors claim that detection of these rearrangements and thus clonal lymphoproliferation in patients whose clinical features lay between HMS and CLL supports the hypothesis that HMS might be a premalignant condition.

CLINICAL FEATURES OF MALARIA, WITH REFERENCE TO THE LIVER

Neither the preerythrocytic schizont nor the hypnozoite give rise to symptoms or signs in human malaria.

The asexual erythrocytic stages are responsible for production of clinical illness in malaria. Jaundice is common in adults, especially if they have severe *P falciparum* infection, but is uncommon in African children. It has been suggested that the immune status of the patient helps determine the extent of hepatocellular dysfunction. Clinical liver failure is not seen in human malaria unless the patient has concomitant viral hepatitis.[123] Tender hepatomegaly, with some splenomegaly, is common, especially in young children and nonimmune adults.

DIAGNOSIS OF MALARIA WITH SPECIAL REFERENCE TO THE LIVER

As with any condition, diagnosis of malaria rests on the triad of history, examination, and investigation.

History
Patients may complain of headache, fever, rigors, and muscle aches. The features are nonspecific and nondiagnostic. A major pitfall in history taking is failure to take a travel history or elicit a history of blood transfusion, residence near an international airport, or self-injection.

Examination
Results of examination can vary considerably from the absence of any physical signs to the presence of multisystem disease in an unconscious, jaundiced patient with pulmonary edema and bleeding mucous membranes secondary to disseminated intravascular coagulation. None of the physical signs present in human malaria is diagnostic.

Misdiagnosis
The nonspecific clinical features of malaria have led to serious errors of diagnosis. The most common misdiagnosis is influenza, but where the disease has a significant effect on the liver, it can be misdiagnosed as acute viral hepatitis, a potentially lethal error if the patient actually is suffering from *P falciparum* malarial infection.

The differential diagnosis of malaria with hepatic changes

includes viral hepatitis, amebic infection of the liver, typhoid fever, cytomegalovirus infection, Epstein-Barr virus hepatitis, Q fever, and jaundice secondary to pneumococcal pneumonia or pyomyositis.[23]

Diagnosis of acute malaria rests on the examination of thick and thin blood films by an experienced microscopist. Thrombocytopenia is a useful clue that should encourage the microscopist to look again at "negative" films and to request repeat samples. Sequestration of parasites in the capillaries and postcapillary venules in synchronous infections with *P falciparum*, recent antimalarial chemoprophylaxis, or partial antimalarial therapy may be responsible for a truly negative blood film when the patient actually has malaria, but an important and potentially remediable cause of false-negative blood film reports in the presence of malaria is observer error.

Serologic investigation (eg, by the indirect fluorescent antibody test [IFAT] or by enzyme-linked immunosorbent assay [ELISA]) is useful for retrospective diagnosis, and is fundamental to the diagnosis of HMS.

Treatment

A detailed description of the treatment of malaria is beyond the scope of this chapter. *P malariae* is treated with chloroquine alone; there is no hypnozoite stage. *P vivax* and *P ovale* are treated with chloroquine, which deals with the erythrocytic stages, followed by primaquine (provided the patient's glucose-6-phosphate dehydrogenase status is normal) to deal with hypnozoites in the liver.

The treatment of *P falciparum* malaria infection is becoming more complicated due to the ever-increasing spread of chloroquine resistance. The reader is referred to the WHO publication on severe and complicated malaria[123] for a detailed review of the topic. Expert advice on the diagnosis and treatment of malaria is available in the United States from the Centers for Disease Control (Atlanta), and in the United Kingdom from the Hospital for Tropical Diseases (London).

The elimination of quinine proceeds mainly by hepatic biotransformation (80%), with 20% eliminated by the kidneys. The total systemic clearance of quinine is reduced in malaria, especially if severe, with parallel reduction of renal and hepatic clearance.[123]

After successful therapy of acute malaria, the liver changes resolve.

Babesiosis

Babesiosis is a protozoan disease with a zoonotic transmission. An infected tick transmits the *Babesia* sp to humans through a bite. The merozoites invade the erythrocytes in the vertebrate host. Infection in humans varies from asymptomatic to severe disease. In animals, the liver becomes involved when sequestration of parasitized red blood cells (RBCs) occurs in the capillary beds.

LIFE CYCLE

This parasite multiplies within RBCs by budding, not by schizogony, as seen with malaria. The vertebrate reservoirs in nature are primarily mice, but deer, foxes, raccoons, cattle, horses, and dogs are other vertebrates that may be infected. The larvae, nymphs, and adults of various ticks play the major role in transmission. *Ixodes dammini*, *I ricinus*, and *I per-*

suleatus all are identified as vectors of babesiosis. *B microti* has been identified in the New England area of the United States, whereas *B bovis* and *B divergens* are present in Europe. Transmission as a result of blood transfusion has been documented.[108]

PATHOGENESIS AND CLINICAL FEATURES

The *Babesia* merozoite requires complement factors to invade the erythrocyte, and then multiplies within the cell by budding. There are no schizonts or gametocytes, as with malaria, and there is no exoerythrocytic cycle. In animals, sequestration of RBCs in capillaries causes an acute respiratory distress syndrome when the lungs are involved and organ damage when the liver, kidneys, or muscles are involved.

Most cases of *B microti* infection in humans are asymptomatic. Mildly symptomatic infections generally resolve with supportive care. Treatment is required for patients with high rates of parasitism or with significant clinical illness. In Europe, babesiosis has been described only in asplenic patients (*B bovis*), whereas in the United States, it is described in splenic, immunocompetent patients (*B microti*); symptomatic patients present with fever, headache, and fatigue 1 to 4 weeks after exposure. In *B bovis* or *B divergens* infection, severe anemia, icterus, and hemoglobinuria occur with protracted infection. Hepatosplenomegaly may occur.[61,126]

DIAGNOSIS

Diagnosis is confirmed by observation of the organism within the RBCs in Giemsa-stained blood smears. IFAT has proved reliable in humans and animals. ELISA promises to be a good test for rapid field diagnosis.[99]

TREATMENT

The use of clindamycin, 1.2 g parenterally twice daily or 600 mg orally three times a day for 7 days, and quinine, 650 mg orally three times a day for 7 days, quickly relieves clinical symptoms and reduces parasitemia in *B microti* infection. Therapy of human infection with bovine species has proved more difficult, especially because these patients usually have been splenectomized previously. Pentamidine in combination with trimethoprim sulfamethoxazole may be helpful. Concurrent exchange blood transfusion may be required.

Leishmaniasis

Visceral leishmaniasis is caused by infection with protozoan parasites of the *Leishmania donovani* complex. The parasites exist in mammalian hosts as amastigotes within cells of the reticuloendothelial system, within which they multiply by binary fission. They are ingested by sandfly vectors of the genus *Phlebotomus* (old world) or *Lutzomyia* (new world), in which they develop to flagellated promastigotes. After inoculation into a new mammalian host, the promastigotes are opsonized and phagocytosed by macrophages, within which they lie in parasitophorous vacuoles and develop to amastigotes. In India, humans act as reservoir for visceral leishmaniasis, but elsewhere the mechanism is zoonosis, with a variety of small mammals or dogs as reservoir hosts.

Visceral leishmaniasis is endemic in the Mediterranean

littoral of southern Europe, North Africa, and the Middle East; and in Central Asia, the former Soviet Union, Pakistan, India, Bangladesh, and China. In Africa, visceral leishmaniasis is endemic in Sudan, Kenya, Ethiopia, and Somalia, and occurs sporadically in a number of other countries south of the Sahara.[106] It is important to remember that many areas endemic for visceral leishmaniasis receive a substantial number of tourists and other overseas visitors each year; the physician in the temperate zone must be alert to the possibility of visceral leishmaniasis presenting after the traveller has returned home.

LIFE CYCLE

There is some variation between endemic areas in the age at which visceral leishmaniasis occurs. In Mediterranean areas there is a high attack rate in infants, especially those aged less than 2 years. In the Indian subcontinent, older children and young adults mainly are affected, and in Africa, young men account for most of the sporadic cases. In epidemics of visceral leishmaniasis, however, all ages, especially young children, can be affected.[106]

PATHOLOGY

The usual host cells for *Leishmania* are cells of the mononuclear phagocyte system. Amastigotes are found in much smaller numbers in cells of low phagocytic potential in which they multiply less well,[101] but have been reported in hepatic parenchymal cells. Neutrophils do not harbor large numbers of amastigotes. *Leishmania* can remain dormant in the liver in cryptic infections.[92,93]

Visceral leishmaniasis usually affects the spleen and liver, but bone marrow and lymph nodes often are involved.[76] Parasites may be found in normal skin in some cases.

There may be considerable proliferation of Kupffer cells, containing numerous parasites,[103] although this is not an invariable feature and on occasion few or even none may be found. Parasite-laden cells may be both diffusely distributed and aggregated in granulomata, and associated with some cellular infiltrate in which plasma cells usually predominate.[101]

Moreno and associates[85] reported hepatic fibrin-ring granulomas in three patents with visceral leishmaniasis. Small intralobular granulomata were haphazardly distributed throughout the liver parenchyma. They were formed by histiocytes mixed with lymphocytes, neutrophils, and eosinophils. All showed characteristic eosinophilic fibrinoid material, usually within the granulomas, sometimes with a ring arrangement around a central empty vacuole. The liver biopsy specimen contained occasional *Leishmania* amastigotes, but they were found only rarely along with fibrinoid necrosis in the same granuloma. Ridley,[101] who with Jopling described the leprosy spectrum, has addressed the question of a spectrum in the histologic processes taking place in visceral leishmaniasis. He noted that although amastigotes often multiply freely in intact macrophages, sometimes the organisms are scarce and the host cells take on a histiocytic form. These cells may evolve toward epithelioid cells, although fully developed epithelioid cells have not been shown in human visceral leishmaniasis. Pampiglione and colleagues[92,93] recorded epithelioid granulomata in cases of cryptic visceral leishmaniasis but not in symptomatic cases.

Ridley[101] concluded that there may be a spectrum but that it probably was not important, because parasites of the *L donovani* complex were organisms of low virulence usually present in large numbers, rarely inducing strong delayed hypersensitivity.

Ridley[101] thought that the high parasite load that was usual in active visceral leishmaniasis was relevant to the low incidence of necrosis compared to cutaneous leishmaniasis. Necrosis has been recorded in the liver in visceral leishmaniasis when the parasite load was low.

Extracellular deposition of a periodic acid–Schiff-positive substance that gives the same staining reaction as collagen often occurs in the liver, as well as in the spleen and lymph nodes. Amyloidosis is rare.[101] When healing occurs, fibrous scars are formed and the liver may take on a pseudocirrhotic appearance.[6]

CLINICAL FEATURES

A papular lesion (leishmanioma) can occur at the site of primary inoculation[76] but may not necessarily be followed by visceral dissemination. There is a wide range of clinical disease, from rapidly progressive fulminant infection through mild cases and subclinical infection.[106]

The incubation period is 2 to 6 months, but there is wide variation, with figures between 10 days and 9 years on record.[98]

Acute presentations with sudden high fever and rigors or with progressively rising fever over 1 week are well described. Such cases may progress rapidly to death within 1 week; subside without the diagnosis being suspected; recur after 2 or 3 weeks; or persist for several weeks, subside at first, and then present again after some months with clinical features suggesting insidious onset.[98]

The classic description of visceral leishmaniasis includes progressive splenomegaly, hepatomegaly, anemia, wasting, and fever.[103]

The major symptoms at presentation are as follows:

- Fever, which is more noticeable in acute cases. There is little to be gained by analysis of fever pattern because the classic pattern of double diurnal peaks is uncommon.[98]
- Abdominal swelling and abdominal pain, both due to splenomegaly. Diarrhea and dysentery of bacillary or amebic origin can occur, although a leishmanial etiology has been postulated, since parasitized macrophages may be found in the lamina propria.
- Cough, epistaxis, bleeding gums, hemorrhage into skin, menorrhagia, or amenorrhea have been reported. Eventually, weight loss, lassitude, and weakness occur.[98]

In patients with acquired immunodeficiency syndrome (AIDS) and visceral leishmaniasis, the classic features may be absent; for example, there may be absence of hepatic or splenic enlargement, absence of hyperglobulinemia, and infection of unusual sites (eg, lungs).[52]

PHYSICAL SIGNS

In full-blown visceral leishmaniasis, the patient has a protuberant abdomen, muscle wasting of thorax and limbs, anemia, and dry, rough hair. Cutaneous pigmentation of the face, feet, and hands occurs, although there is geographic variation in the extent to which it occurs. In India the disease is known as *black sickness*, hence the term *kala azar*. Depigmentation of the skin has also been recorded (eg, in Kenya).[98] Splenomegaly, although not invariable, is usually massive when present, especially in well established disease.

Hepatomegaly often occurs. Cole,[20] in a classic description of visceral leishmaniasis in East Africa, noted that in comparison to splenomegaly, hepatomegaly was slower to develop and to recede, was less marked, and occurred less often. On occasion, however, hepatomegaly may predominate over splenomegaly.

Hepatocellular jaundice may occur in severe disease. Ascites is a late sign that may be associated with generalized edema.[98] Generalized lymphadenopathy occurs commonly, particularly in Mediterranean and African foci, and may be the presenting feature; this is a potential cause of diagnostic confusion.[106]

Complications include secondary bacterial infections, and respiratory tract infections (pneumonia, pulmonary tuberculosis) are important causes of death in visceral leishmaniasis. Pneumococcal meningitis also is recorded. Diarrhea is common, as mentioned. Hemorrhage may occur, usually as epistaxis, but occasionally from the gastrointestinal tract.[106]

Recovery from visceral leishmaniasis may be followed by development of post–kala azar dermal leishmaniasis (PKDL). This may present as hypopigmented macules, erythema, or nodules in the Indian form or as a punctate, measles-like rash in the African form. The skin in PKDL contains *Leishmania* amastigotes, which are numerous in the nodular form.[98] Patients with PKDL may be important epidemiologically, especially in areas where humans act as the reservoir for visceral leishmaniasis.

LABORATORY FINDINGS

Nonspecific features include anemia, usually normochromic, normocytic, sometimes with a hemoglobin as low as 4 g/100 mL, and leukopenia, especially neutropenia, with total white cell counts of 1 to 2 × 10⁹/L. The platelet count also is reduced. The pancytopenia is largely the result of hypersplenism. Proliferative glomerulonephritis and interstitial nephritis may occur. The prothrombin time often is slightly increased, and the albumin low.

There is a massive polyclonal increase in IgG, much of which is not specific to *Leishmania*.

DIFFERENTIAL DIAGNOSIS

The clinical features of visceral leishmaniasis are largely nonspecific and, in the early stages of clinical assessment, the range of possible diagnosis is relatively wide. Based on extensive personal experience, Manson-Bahr[77] has given the following differential diagnosis:

In cases presenting as fever of unknown origin, visceral leishmaniasis must be distinguished from malaria, relapsing fever, trypanosomiasis, brucellosis, liver abscess, and tuberculosis.
In cases of chronic onset with splenomegaly and anemia, consider malaria, hyperreactive malarial splenomegaly, myeloid leukemia, lymphoma, hepatic cirrhosis, hepatosplenic schistosomiasis, thalassemic hemoglobinopathies, and systemic histoplasmosis.
Where dysproteinemia predominates, consider macroglobulinemia, multiple myelomatosis, and lymphoma.

Occasionally, visceral leishmaniasis may give rise to nasopharyngeal granulomas that must be distinguished from tuberculosis, systemic mycoses, or carcinoma.

The differential diagnosis of PKDL includes leprosy, syphilis, yaws, or superficial mycoses.

DEFINITIVE DIAGNOSIS

As with any disease, diagnosis of visceral leishmaniasis is founded on the triad of history, examination, and investigation. The first two, although important, yield only nonspecific information, and definitive diagnosis rests on microscopic demonstration of amastigotes in tissue samples.

The best yield is obtained from splenic aspiration, with parasites demonstrable in 90% of active cases of visceral leishmaniasis. Splenic aspiration is contraindicated in patients with a small, soft spleen, in children under 5 years of age, and in patients with an abnormal prothrombin, clotting, or bleeding time.[77] The procedure must be undertaken with care and should be performed by a clinician experienced in the technique.

Liver biopsy is almost as sensitive as splenic aspiration, whereas bone marrow aspiration yields positive results in 80% of active cases. Amastigotes have been plentiful in bone marrow samples obtained from AIDS patients with visceral leishmaniasis.[52]

Examination of lymph gland juice obtained by aspiration of enlarged nodes yields positive results in about 60% of cases.

Examination of peripheral blood or slit skin smears is not helpful for routine diagnosis. In cases of *Leishmania* infection in patients with AIDS, however, amastigotes have been readily demonstrated in clinically unaffected skin.

Smears or tissue dabs for microscopy should be stained with Giemsa stain at pH 6.8. Aliquots of the samples should be cultured on NNN medium or on Schneider's insect tissue culture medium. Positive samples yield a growth of promastigote organisms.

Indirect Methods of Diagnosis

The formol gel test is nonspecific and relies on the high IgG levels present in visceral leishmaniasis. It is positive in a number of other diseases, including malaria, macroglobulinemia, and leprosy.

Serodiagnosis

A variety of serodiagnostic methods are available. Those in common use include IFAT, ELISA, and the direct agglutination test. Expert advice on serodiagnosis is available in the United States from the Parasitic Disease Section, Centers for Disease Control, and in the United Kingdom from the Department of Parasitology, Hospital for Tropical Diseases.

The leishmanin skin test (or Montenegro test) is negative in acute visceral leishmaniasis, becoming positive after successful treatment.

DNA probes are under evaluation for the diagnosis of visceral leishmaniasis. Isoenzyme analysis using cultured promastigotes is of value in speciation, and monoclonal antibody typing also is available.

TREATMENT

No specific measures are required to deal with hepatic involvement. The principles of therapy include supportive treatment, which may include blood transfusion in severe anemia, prompt diagnosis, and therapy of secondary bacterial infections, and specific antileishmanial chemotherapy. The agents available include the following:

1. Pentavalent antimonials (sodium stibogluconate and meglumine antimonate) are the agents of choice. γ-Interferon is synergistic with sodium stibogluconate, and the combination has proved effective in refractory cases.
2. Allopurinol plus pentavalent antimonials can be used in cases unresponsive to antimonials alone.[15]
3. Alternative agents to antimonials are pentamidine, paromomycin, or amphotericin B.
4. Liposomal amphotericin B has given good results in a single case report,[24] and deserves further evaluation in visceral leishmaniasis.

Patients with AIDS and visceral leishmaniasis often prove refractory to therapy or relapse after cessation of treatment.[52]

HELMINTHIC INFECTIONS

Nematodes

Most nematodes are free-living, nonsegmented roundworms with separate sexes. All nematodes are structurally similar, with a thick cuticle covering their body. In some species, the life cycle is simple; the eggs leave the host in feces, embryonate in soil, and reenter the host by the oral route to develop directly to adult worms in the intestine. In other species, the cycle is more complex, involving intermediate invertebrate or vertebrate hosts with a complex migration route once inside the host. Some species are capable of penetrating directly into the host through the unbroken skin.[28]

ASCARIASIS

The adult female *Ascaris lumbricoides* measures 20 to 40 cm in length, whereas the male measures 15 to 30 cm. Humans are infected by ingesting the embryonated eggs, often by eating raw, contaminated vegetables.

Ascaris Life Cycle
Ascaris eggs hatch in the small intestine, and larvae penetrate the intestinal wall, enter the portal circulation and reach the liver, pass through to the heart, and thence to the pulmonary artery and lungs. In the lungs, further growth and development takes place; then the larvae leave the alveolar spaces and migrate up the respiratory tract to the pharynx, are swallowed, and grow to sexually mature adults in the intestine 2 to 3 months from the time of egg ingestion. The shedding of eggs in feces, which contaminates the soil, allows the cycle to continue. *A lumbricoides* has a worldwide distribution.

Pathogenesis and Clinical Features
The second- and third-stage ascaris larvae are large and antigenic. Their passage through the liver parenchyma and entry into the lung alveoli causes damage, and if the infection is heavy, symptoms may be severe. When many larvae are migrating simultaneously, patients may experience enlargement of the liver, intense pneumonitis, and generalized tox-

icity that may last more than 2 weeks. This is similar to the acute phase of schistosomiasis and fascioliasis.

The clinical features of acute ascariasis are often cough, fever, wheezing, and dyspnea. Chest radiography reveals opacification and the white blood cell count shows eosinophilia. As the worms mature in the intestine, symptoms will depend on the worm burden. In light infections, the patient may have no symptoms. In heavy infections, the main problem is mechanical, with small bowel obstruction. If the worms migrate up the biliary ducts into the liver, obstructive jaundice, intrahepatic abscesses, or cholangitis may occur. Heavy infections in children may contribute to malnutrition.[12,13,66]

Diagnosis
Diagnosis is confirmed by finding the characteristic eggs in the feces. Diagnosis can be suspected in patients presenting with abdominal colic, enlarged, tender liver, fever, and eosinophilia. Ultrasonography may show the worms in the biliary ducts.

Treatment
Infected people may be cured with a single dose of mebendazole, 500 mg, or, alternatively, with mebendazole, 100 mg twice daily for 3 days; pyrantel pamoate, 10 mg/kg, to a maximum of 1 g; or levamisol, 2.5 mg/kg.[22,124]

TOXOCARIASIS

The adult nematodes *Toxocara canis* and *T cati* live in the lumen of the small intestine of dogs and cats, respectively. Humans are infected by ingestion of the embryonated eggs containing second-stage larvae. These hatch in the small intestine, penetrate the intestinal wall, and enter the portal circulation to wander aimlessly from organ to organ, maturing to the third larval stage. The liver, brain, and eye are the organs most frequently affected.

Toxocariasis is a cosmopolitan infection of dogs and cats, and infection of humans with the larvae is worldwide. It is mainly a disease of children. *T canis* infection is one of the most common causes of the visceral larva migrans syndrome.

Pathogenesis and Clinical Features
Two disease syndromes are recognized—generalized visceral larva migrans and an acute phase similar to those caused by the other invasive helminths, with patients presenting with fever, eosinophilia, hepatomegaly, and even asthma. As the larvae burrow into the tissues of either the liver, lungs, brain, or eye, they cause hemorrhage, necrosis, and secondary inflammation.

When larvae become trapped in the tissues, they incite a granuloma formation with a preponderance of eosinophils; later, fibrosis and calcification may result. Larvae trapped in the retina with granuloma formation may impair vision and often are mistaken for a retinal tumor (ocular larva migrans). Larvae trapped in the liver will result in granuloma formation with eosinophils, leading to an enlarged, tender liver. The pathologic changes in the liver are mostly in the form of small eosinophilic abscesses with central necrosis showing Charcot-Leyden crystals. Lesions in the brain may lead to encephalitis and convulsions.[12,90,118]

Diagnosis

The definitive diagnosis of toxocariasis is made by identification of the larvae in tissues. A strongly positive ELISA test to detect antibodies helps to indicate a presumptive diagnosis of toxocariasis. Liver biopsy may be necessary to differentiate hepatic involvement from hepatic capillariasis.[51]

Treatment

Diethylcarbamazine administered orally in a dose of 3 mg/kg three times daily for 21 days is standard therapy.

Alternatively, thiabendazole may be given in a dose of 50 mg/kg/d for 5 days. Both drugs kill the larvae, preventing migration and additional damage. Albendazole in a dose of 10 mg/kg/d for 5 days has been reported to be effective in the treatment of visceral, ocular, and cutaneous larva migrans. Prednisone should be used in the acute toxemic phase of the infection, particularly in severe ophthalmic cases.[102,113,124]

STRONGYLOIDIASIS

Infection with *Strongyloides stercoralis* usually is asymptomatic. In patients with heavy infections and in immunosuppressed patients, symptoms are present. The infection is widespread in the tropics, the subtropics, and in southern and eastern Europe and the United States. Adult worms live in the human intestine.

Life Cycle

The slender female adult worm measures 2 mm in length. They burrow in the mucosa of the intestine and lay the noninfective rhabditiform larvae, which are shed in the feces. The adult male worms are then expelled. The shed larvae develop in moist soil into free-living, male and female worms within about 1 week. Humans are infected by the infective filariform larvae, which penetrate the intact skin, are carried to the lungs, migrate through the alveoli to reach the bronchial tree, and are swallowed to reach the intestine where they mature. The whole cycle takes about a month. Autoinfection occasionally occurs if the rhabditiform larvae change into the infective filariform stage in the intestines, and reinfection then occurs by penetration of either the bowel wall or the perianal skin.

Pathogenesis and Clinical Features

As with the other invasive helminths, acute infection may lead to an itchy eruption followed by a low-grade fever accompanied by cough, wheeze, abdominal pain, diarrhea, and eosinophilia.

The liver is affected in immunosuppressed people when the hyperinfection syndrome develops as enormous numbers of filariform larvae are reinvading the body through the bowel wall. The filariform larvae may invade any organ, including the liver, lung, or even brain. Symptoms depend on the affected organ. If the larvae migrate to the liver, a severe granulomatous reaction with clinical evidence of jaundice and deranged liver functions may occur.[12,13,118]

Diagnosis

Serologic tests for diagnosis include CIEP and ELISA, but definitive diagnosis is made through the finding of rhabditiform larvae or infective larvae in the feces or bowel aspiration and bowel biopsy specimens.[53]

Treatment

Longer courses are required in the hyperinfestation syndrome. The drug of choice is albendazole; it is given in a dose of 400 mg/d for 3 consecutive days for adults and children over 2 years of age. A second course of treatment may be necessary.[22,124]

CAPILLARIASIS

Capillaria (Hepaticola) hepatica is a common nematode parasite of the rat and less frequently of mice, hares, dogs, beavers, and monkeys. Human infection is rare. The thin adult female worm measures about 20 mm; the male is half that length. They live in the liver tissues and eggs are laid in the parenchyma. Humans become infected by eating food containing the embryonated eggs passed in the feces by the infected scavenger animal. The larvae hatch from the infected eggs in the intestine, enter the portal venous system, and reach the liver, where they mature to adults in about 1 month.

The clinical presentation in confirmed infection with this parasite in humans involves acute or subacute hepatitis, with hepatomegaly and hypereosinophilia. The granuloma formation around the eggs in the liver may have to be differentiated from hepatic amebiasis or even a liver mass. Signs of *C hepatica* are those of any invasive helminth infection. The differential diagnosis includes Loffler's syndrome, acute trichiniasis, schistosomiasis, fascioliasis, and visceral larva migrans. Diagnosis is made by liver biopsy. There are no reports of successful treatment.[12,89]

TRICHINIASIS

Trichiniasis has a cosmopolitan distribution.

Humans usually are infected with *Trichinella spiralis* by eating raw or undercooked pork containing the infectious larvae. These are freed in the stomach or duodenum, enter the small intestine, and penetrate the mucosal epithelium, where they live and rapidly mature into adult male and female worms. The male measures about 1.5 mm and the female 3 mm in length. By the sixth day of infection, the first-stage larvae are liberated. These penetrate the intestinal mucosa to enter the general circulation and become distributed throughout the body; they may become localized in various locations, including the myocardium, cerebrospinal fluid, brain, and rarely the liver and gallbladder. They later reenter the bloodstream, finally to reach the striated muscle, where they become encapsulated. Clinical signs and symptoms usually are associated with heavy infections and include diarrhea, fever, myalgia, periorbital edema, and leukocytosis with marked eosinophilia. Rarely, hepatic histologic study may show invasion of the hepatic sinusoid by *Trichinella* larvae, and if biliary tract obstruction results, jaundice may develop. Diagnosis is made by a combination of history of eating raw pork and the clinical manifestation of fever with marked eosinophilia (again, the clinical manifestation of invasive helminths). ELISA or IFAT for specific anti-*Trichinella* antibody may be helpful, but both give negative results in the first few weeks after infection. Muscle biopsy may confirm the diagnosis. Steroids may be needed in the acute phase to relieve allergic and inflammatory symptoms before starting treatment with either mebendazole 200 mg/d for 5 days or albendazole 400 mg/d for 3 days.[12,17,21,87,105,124] Thiabendazole is an alternative. Anthelmintic therapy of trichinosis may be unsatisfactory in established infections, however.

Trematodes

All trematodes (flukes) are parasitic. Some live within the lumen of organs, some live in blood vessels, whereas others infect solid organs such as the liver and lung. The adult worms vary in morphology. The sexes are separate in the blood flukes, whereas in the intestinal and tissue flukes, both male and female reproductive organs exist in the same parasite. All flukes are surrounded by a tegument with spines. Embryonated or nonembryonated eggs may be produced. Fertilized eggs pass from the human host into water where snails are infected, and then cercariae leave the snail and either encyst or penetrate the human to complete the life cycle. The larvae that encyst on plants or various aquatic animals must be eaten by humans to complete their life cycle.

THE BLOOD FLUKES

Schistosomiasis

Schistosomiasis (bilharziasis) is a disease caused by trematodes of the genus *Schistosoma*, affecting mainly the genitourinary and gastrointestinal systems. Three species cause most of the infections in humans. *S haematobium* in Africa and the Middle East causes urinary schistosomiasis. *S mansoni* in Africa, South America, and the Caribbean and *S japonicum* in the Far East cause intestinal and hepatosplenic schistosomiasis. In southeast Asia, infection with *S mekongi* may be a cause of liver disease, and in central Africa, *S intercalatum* may cause colonic disease.[1,7,25,63,64]

Life Cycle.   The life cycles of the three main human-infecting species are similar. Humans are infected by contact with fresh water containing cercariae. The cercariae penetrate the skin and within 24 hours reach the peripheral venules and lymphatics, and are carried to the pulmonary vessels. They travel to the lungs, probably through the bloodstream, and reach the liver, where they develop in the portal venous system. After 6 to 12 weeks, the adult male and female worms, measuring 10 to 20 mm long, migrate to their final habitat. Adult *S haematobium* worms live in the plexus of veins of the urinary bladder, prostate, and the uterus, where they lay eggs and produce the clinical features of urinary schistosomiasis. *S mansoni* worms inhabit tributaries of the inferior mesenteric veins and produce intestinal schistosomiasis. *S japonicum* worms inhabit venules of the superior mesenteric veins and present the clinical manifestation of intestinal schistosomiasis.

Each female worm, depending on species, lays 300 to 3000 eggs daily, and may live for 10 to 30 years. The eggs are laid in the terminal venules and enter the lumen of the organ. *S haematobium* eggs enter the urinary bladder and are passed in the urine, whereas *S mansoni* and *S japonicum* eggs enter the intestine and are passed in the feces. The eggs hatch immediately in fresh water, liberating free-swimming miracidia that survive up to 24 hours. If the miracidia penetrate a specific snail host (genus *Bulinus* for *S haematobium*, *Biomphalaria* for *S mansoni*, and *Oncomelania* for *S japonicum*), daughter sporocysts produce cercariae within 4 to 6 weeks. The cercariae pass into water when the sporocyst ruptures. They remain infective for 2 to 3 days and the life cycle is completed when they come into contact with humans.[7,29,50]

Pathology.   The schistosome eggs that pass through the blood vessel and organ walls cause necrotizing and inflammatory changes. Eggs that stay in the tissues result in the formation of bilharzial granulomas. The inflammatory reaction, which may be diffuse or localized in a pseudotuberculoid pattern, is rich in eosinophils in the early phases, along with macrophages, lymphocytes, plasma cells, and scattered foreign body giant cells surrounding the egg. Over time, the lesions progress to marked fibrosis with less cellularity and degenerated, calcified eggs. The pathologic process of schistosomiasis is a result of the host's reaction to the eggs in various tissues. The severity of the disease is related to the delayed hypersensitivity reaction to the deposited egg. Rarely, there is a severe reaction in the tissue forming eosinophilic abscesses around dead worms. The fibrosis following the schistosomal reaction is the cause of serious complications, specifically periportal hepatic fibrosis and obstructive uropathy (Fig. 47-4).[31,78,88,116,117,120–122]

Clinical Features.   Three disease syndromes are recognized in schistosomiasis—dermatitis, acute toxemic schistosomiasis (Katayama's syndrome), and chronic schistosomiasis.

DERMATITIS.   Itching with erythema and a papular rash may develop within minutes of exposure to cercaria-infested water (swimmer's itch). Symptoms usually last 2 to 3 days and usually are seen in the primary infection. This hypersensitivity reaction to cercarial penetration often is diagnosed in young children exposed to infected waters for the first time.[12]

ACUTE TOXEMIC SCHISTOSOMIASIS (KATAYAMA'S SYNDROME).   The clinical presentation of acute toxemic schistosomiasis usually occurs 4 to 6 weeks after initial exposure and coincides with early egg-laying. This acute phase of the infection, essentially a form of serum sickness, is mainly seen in city dwellers or young patients exposed for the first time. They present with fever, diarrhea, hepatomegaly, and hypereosinophilia. The fever may, in some cases, last for 4 to 6 weeks and patients often are referred to hospital for investigation of fever of unknown origin. Children often deny any history of water exposure and the first indication of acute schistosomiasis is the marked eosinophilia and tender hepatomegaly. In this acute phase, eggs usually are not present in the feces; diagnosis can be inferred by ELISA or rapid CIEP detection of a markedly elevated specific IgM. Acute toxemic schistosomiasis and acute fascioliasis have similar clinical presentations, but serology can be used to differentiate them.[16,18,19,40,55,62,112]

CHRONIC SCHISTOSOMIASIS.   Untreated acute schistosomiasis progresses to the third stage of chronic schistosomiasis. The granulation reaction of the host to the eggs and the subsequent fibrosis are responsible for the clinical picture of chronic schistosomiasis. *S mansoni* and *S japonicum* worms live in the portal and mesenteric vessels, and pathologic processes mainly affect the intestinal tract and liver. *S haematobium* is found in the vesical plexus, and affects mainly the urinary tract. Rarely, the lungs and central nervous system are affected when eggs or worms passing through collateral circulation lodge in these organs.

In *S mansoni* infection, eggs begin to appear in the feces about 8 to 10 weeks after exposure. This early egg passage usually is asymptomatic, but patients may complain of intermittent diarrhea. Later, blood, pus, and mucus generally accompany the diarrhea until frank attacks of dysentery develop. The attacks may become severe, leading to loss of weight, dehydration, and serious malnutrition.

In African intestinal schistosomiasis, pseudopolyps develop in the colon of patients. These may be single or multiple. They generally involve the rectosigmoid colon or the lower third of the descending colon; rarely, they are extensive, involving the whole descending and transverse colon. Severe hypoproteinemia caused by the protein-losing enteropathy usually develops in these patients, and they present with dependent edema and ascites. Clubbing and hypertrophic osteoarthropathy develops in some patients. Early diagnosis of these patients is important because therapy can resolve the inflammatory pseudopolyps and reverse the hypoproteinemia and other symptoms. Occasionally, a large mass will develop in the descending colon as a result of the inflammatory response to egg deposition.

Eggs carried back to the liver by collateral circulation cause a severe granulomatous reaction. This delayed hypersensitivity reaction to the schistosome eggs produces marked periportal fibrosis, leading to presinusoidal portal hypertension and congestive splenomegaly. With severe schistosomal infection, portal hypertension increases and ascites develops, and occasionally hypersplenism with refractory anemia occurs. Gastroesophageal varices and hematemesis are the most serious developments. In pure hepatosplenic schistosomiasis, although periportal fibrosis exists, the liver parenchyma is spared, and the liver functions remain normal.

A serious disease combination is schistosomiasis and hepatitis B infection. Unfortunately, hepatitis B is frequent in populations at risk for schistosomiasis. Patients with advanced bilharzial hepatosplenomegaly often are hepatitis B carriers in whom chronic active hepatitis with cirrhosis develops. Liver carcinoma is common in these patients. Response to antischistosomal therapy is poor and eventually hepatocellular failure, jaundice, and hepatic coma develop. A few patients have endocrine dysfunction and present with gynecomastia, scanty body hair, and stunted growth.

In *S japonicum* and *S mekongi* infection, eggs are laid mainly in the venules of the superior mesenteric veins, and severe lesions results in the small intestine. Eggs carried to the liver lead to fibrosis, portal hypertension, and splenomegaly, and patients present with dysenteric symptoms, hepatic fibrosis, splenomegaly, and ascites. Ectopic lesions in the lungs and central nervous system are more common in *S japonicum*.[9,25,28,42,63,65,67,71–73,75]

Diagnosis. A history of exposure to schistosome-infested water, however briefly, combined with abdominal pain, diarrhea, or dysentery, and peripheral eosinophilia should arouse suspicion. Feces should be examined repeatedly for eggs. Immunodiagnosis, using CIEP or ELISA, has proved useful in the identification of specific antibodies, permitting early diagnosis of the acute toxemic phase of the infection (the Katayama syndrome) before eggs are detected in the feces in patients exposed for the first time. Sigmoidoscopy and colonoscopy may reveal involvement of the rectum and sigmoid and transverse colon (schistosomal tubercles and polyps), and rectal biopsy may be necessary to find eggs. In chronic disease, barium enema air-contrast radiographs usually are necessary to show the extent of colonic involvement, and liver biopsy and abdominal ultrasonography will demonstrate schistosomal periportal fibrosis[2,3,8,30,57,81] (Figs. 47-5 and 47-6).

Treatment. The two effective oral drugs available for the treatment of all stages of *S mansoni* infection are praziquantel and oxamniquine. Oxamniquine is given orally in a dose of 20 to 30 mg/kg/d for 3 days, whereas praziquantel is given either as a single dose of 30 to 45 mg/kg or, in heavy infections, in a total dose of 60 mg/kg divided into three equal portions and given in 1 day. Both cause minor side effects, usually epigastric pain with some nausea. Both drugs can be given to patients with schistosomal hepatosplenomegaly. Both result in over a 90% egg reduction and a cure rate of 70% to 90%.

Acute toxemic schistosomiasis is best treated with praziquantel, 75 mg/kg divided in three doses given 4 hours apart in 1 day. Steroids (prednisone, 5 mg three times daily) are used to control the fever and toxemia for 2 to 3 days before starting specific therapy. This acute phase of the infection is seen mainly in *S mansoni* and *S japonicum* infections, and rarely in *S haematobium* infection.

In *S japonicum* and *S mekongi* infections, praziquantel is the drug of choice and should be given in a dose of 25 mg/kg body weight three times a day for 3 consecutive days.

In advanced complicated hepatosplenic schistosomiasis, surgical intervention may include injection sclerotherapy for severe variceal bleeding, splenectomy in serious hypersplenism, or shunt operation in uncontrolled portal hypertension. These procedures should be done only in facilities specializing in such techniques. Since the introduction of single-dose oral praziquantel therapy for schistosomiasis, such advanced, complicated cases rarely are seen.[22,25,27,33–35,38,39,45,68,95,110,119,124]

THE LIVER FLUKES

This section deals with the hermaphroditic liver flukes—*Fasciola hepatica*, *Clonorchis sinensis*, *Opisthorchis felineus*, *O viverrini*, and *Dicrocoelium dendriticum*. All have similar life cycles. The metacercaria (encysted larva) is the infective stage; infection is acquired by ingestion of the metacercaria, which contaminate plants, fish, crabs, or ants. The metacercaria excyst within the lumen of the small intestine and the immature flukes migrate to the biliary tract of the host. Eggs are passed in the feces into water, and hatch into miracidia that enter the intermediate snail host and asexually divide into sporocysts, rediae, and cercariae. The cercariae emerge and encyst on vegetables or in tissues of fish or crustaceans.[29]

Fascioliasis

Life Cycle. Infection with the cosmopolitan, large (30 mm in length) *F hepatica* results from eating watercress or other plants infected with metacercaria. The metacercaria excyst in the small intestine and the immature flukes burrow through the wall of the intestine, pass through the peritoneal cavity, and penetrate into the liver, reaching the bile ducts where they mature in about 2 months. Eggs reach the duodenum through the bile ducts and those passed out in the

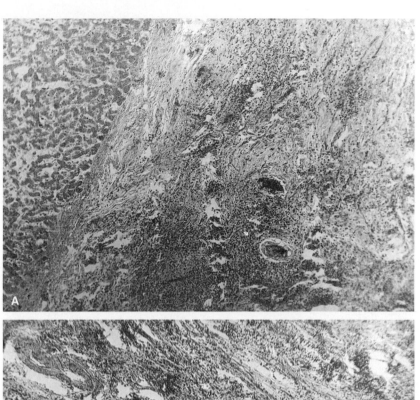

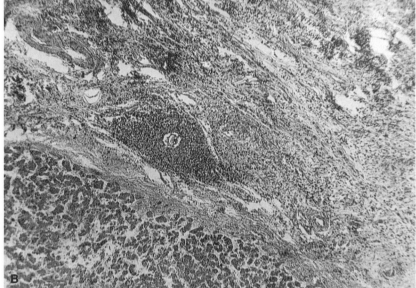

FIGURE 47-4 (**A**) Schistosomal liver showing respected limiting plate, marked portal fibrosis, scattered *Schistosoma* ova, and dense inflammatory reaction (H&E, × 100). (**B**) Schistosomal liver showing intact limiting plate, marked portal fibrosis, and granulomatous reaction surrounding *Schistosoma* ova (H&E, × 100). (**C**) Schistosomal liver showing respected limiting plate, dense portal fibrosis, proliferating bile ducts, and scattered calcified *Schistosoma* ova (H&E, × 100). (**D**) Schistosomal rectal polyp with fibrotic core entangling numerous calcified ova surrounded by hyperplastic rectal mucosa (H&E, × 100). (Courtesy of Professor Elia A. Ishak, Department of Pathology, Cairo University, Cairo, Egypt)

feces into fresh water continue the cycle. *F hepatica* is the sheep liver fluke.

Pathogenesis and Clinical Picture. *F hepatica* is a large liver fluke and heavy infection can cause severe illness. The worms live in the bile ducts and biliary system of the liver where their eggs cause inflammation and fibrosis. They often stray into the gallbladder. During the acute phase of the infection, patients will present with fever, eosinophilia, and anemia. Children in particular may become acutely ill and often are referred to hospital as cases of prolonged undiagnosed fever. Examination usually reveals an enlarged, tender liver; occasionally, ascites develops in children. If bile duct obstruction occurs, jaundice results, and when bacterial cholangitis develops, patients may present with a complicated clinical picture of vague upper abdominal pain and polymorphonuclear neutrophil leukocytosis. In light chronic in-

fections, patients may complain only of abdominal pain and diarrhea.[41,43,44]

Diagnosis. Prolonged fever, abdominal pain, diarrhea, and an enlarged, tender liver plus eosinophilia should alert the physician to an occult helminthic infection. The geographic history should suggest the possible helminth, and immunoserologic investigation with fecal examination for eggs confirms the diagnosis. In fascioliasis, using a purified *Fasciola* antigen, CIEP and ELISA usually give strongly positive results. Ultrasonography may show the worms in the liver, biliary system, or in the gallbladder.[10,81,104]

Treatment. Although praziquantel is the drug of choice for the other liver flukes, it is not effective in the treatment of *F hepatica* infection. Bithionol in a dose of 50 mg/kg/d for 10 doses is an effective drug. Intramuscular

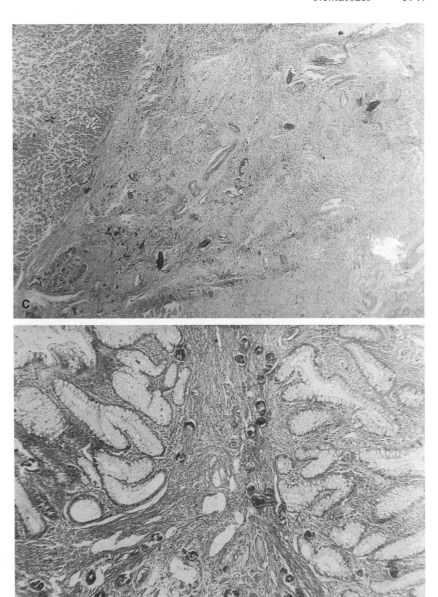

dehydroemetine, 1 mg/kg/d for 14 doses, is an alternative drug.[46,123]

Clonorchiasis, Opisthorchiasis, and Dicrocoeliasis

The morphology, life cycle, and pathogenic effects of the remaining species of liver flukes that commonly infect humans are similar and are discussed briefly together.

C sinensis is widespread in China, Japan, Korea, and Vietnam. The cercariae of *C sinensis* infect more than 80 species of fresh-water fish, and humans are infected by eating raw or slightly pickled fish infected with the metacercaria.

O felineus occurs in many wild and domestic animals in eastern Europe, and human infection is common in Poland and Russia. *O viverrini* is the most common liver fluke infection in north Thailand, and dogs and cats act as reservoirs of infection. Similar to clonorchiasis, humans are infected with both of these flukes by eating various infected fresh-water fish, uncooked, contaminated with the metacercariae.

D dendriticum is a small liver fluke; humans are accidentally infected by swallowing ants containing the metacercariae. Human infection has been reported from Nigeria, Sweden, Russia, and Saudi Arabia. Sheep, cattle, and camels act as reservoirs of infection.

The adult worms of these flukes live and lay eggs in the biliary system of the liver, leading to inflammation and fibrosis of the biliary ducts. Heavily infected patients may present with fever, eosinophilia, jaundice, and an enlarged, tender liver. Again, if bacterial cholangitis develops, patients may present with an enlarged, tender gallbladder and a polymorphonuclear neutrophil leukocytosis. Cancer of the bile ducts has been linked to *C sinensis* and *O viverrini* infections.

Diagnosis is established by repeated fecal examinations and finding the eggs characteristic of the species appropriate for a specific geographic area. As purer antigens become avail-

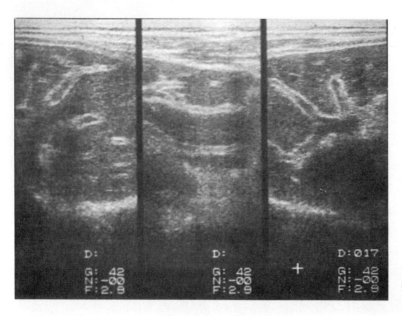

FIGURE 47-5   Three scans in a schistosomal liver are shown. The characteristic bilharzial pattern is seen as portal tract thickening with portal venous radicles within.

able, ELISA may confirm the specific helminthic infection. *C sinensis, O felineus, O viverrini,* and *D dendriticum* infections are successfully treated with praziquantel. The dose is 20 mg/kg three times daily for 2 days.[32,47,59,69,70,79,82,84,96,109,114,115,124]

THE LUNG FLUKES

The adult trematode genus *Paragonimus* measures 7 to 12 mm in length and typically lives encapsulated in pockets of the lungs. Rarely, it may involve the liver. Humans are infected by eating raw freshwater crabs, shrimp, or crayfish

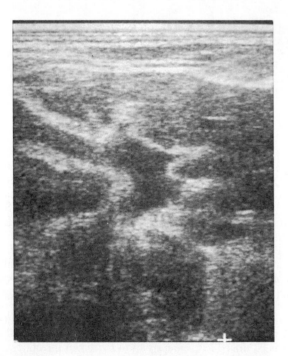

FIGURE 47-6   Typical bilharzial liver pattern showing echolucent left portal vein with portal tract thickening around its radicles.

containing the metacercariae. These excyst in the intestine and the larvae then penetrate the intestinal wall, pass into the peritoneal cavity, and enter and remain in the abdominal muscles for several days. They then penetrate the diaphragm, enter the pleural cavity, and burrow into the lungs where they develop into adult worms. The life cycle is completed when the infected person either coughs the eggs out or swallows them and then passes them in the feces. The eggs complete embryonating after discharge from the body into fresh water, and a free-swimming miracidium finds its typical freshwater snail host. The cercariae subsequently emerge to infect the crustaceans, mainly crayfish, and encyst into metacercariae.

Paragonimiasis

Infection with *Paragonimus* sp occurs mainly in southeast Asia and has been reported from Japan, Korea, China, Taiwan, Thailand, Malaysia, and the Philippines. Infection also occurs in west Africa. It is primarily a lung infection.

Pathogenesis and Clinical Picture.   The worms in tissues typically produce a granulomatous reaction that gradually becomes encapsulated. In the abdominal cavity, abscesses may develop and in the muscular tissues the worms may provoke the formation of cysts. Because of their tortuous migration route, the worms may develop in ectopic foci, including the liver. In the liver, these flukes will induce a leukocytic infiltration with eosinophils and finally multiple small cystic abscesses containing thick, purulent fluid. Patients usually complain of fever and dull abdominal pain with tender hepatomegaly. Eosinophilia is present.[12,21,80,105]

Diagnosis.   Specific diagnosis is made by finding the characteristic eggs in the sputum, aspirated pleural effusion, feces, or from biopsy of cutaneous lesions.

Treatment.   Praziquantel is the drug of choice for adults and children over 4 years of age; the dose is 25 mg/kg three times a day for 2 consecutive days.[105,124]

Cestodes

The cestodes (tapeworms) live in the intestinal tract of their host. They vary in size, some exceeding 10 m in length with others only a few millimeters long. The adult worms have a head (scolex) and a segmented body (strobila). Each segment is known as a proglottid. The scolex has suckers, hooks, or grooves with which the adult worms attach themselves to the intestinal wall. The last segments of the body contain the fertilized eggs, and usually detach from the body and release the eggs into the intestine for subsequent passage in the feces. The eggs either are eaten by the intermediate host to undergo further development, or hatch and then infect the intermediate host to undergo further morphogenesis to the next stage. Ultimately, the definitive host must eat the infective larval tapeworms to become infected. Each segment of the body of the adult worm contains a set of male and female reproductive organs, so that each proglottid has sperm and ova, and self-fertilization results. Embryonation of the eggs occurs and the gravid proglottid may contain many infectious eggs. The larval stage of the tapeworm *Echinococcus granulosus* is the main tapeworm affecting the human liver.[29]

ECHINOCOCCOSIS (HYDATID DISEASE)

Infection of humans with the cestode *E granulosis* occurs through eating food, usually lettuce or green salads, contaminated with dog feces containing the embryonated infectious eggs. Humans, sheep, and cattle are intermediate hosts of the infection. The domestic dog is the main definitive host, with the adult worms living in the intestine.

The minute adult tapeworm measures 3 to 6 mm in length and is composed of a scolex, neck, and usually three proglottids. Human infection occurs mainly in sheep-raising areas of South America, Algeria, Egypt, South Africa, Asia Minor, central Asia, and northern China. The infection also occurs in certain areas of New Zealand, Australia, Canada, and the United States.

Life Cycle

Eggs hatch in the human intestine and the emerging larvae (oncospheres) pass through the wall of the intestinal tract to enter the portal system and penetrate into the liver parenchyma, where they transform into hydatid cysts. The right lobe of the liver usually is more affected than the left. Rarely, other organs, including the lung, brain, and bone, may be affected. The hydatid cyst takes several months to mature and several years to reach a large size, which may be as great as 30 cm diameter in the liver tissue. The cyst is a fluid-filled structure consisting of a thick, noncellular, laminated membrane surrounding a thin, cellular, germinal membrane. The whole cyst is surrounded by a fibrous host tissue capsule. Protoscoleces grow by budding from the inner germinal membrane of the cysts. Small brood capsules may contain as many as 12 protoscoleces, and each single protoscolex, if eaten, can develop into an adult worm in the domestic dog or other canidae. Dogs acquire the infection by eating organs of slaughtered sheep, cattle, or other animals containing the hydatid cyst. A single hydatid cyst can lead to thousands of adult worms infecting the intestine of the dog, which then passes the ova in feces, transmitting the infection to the intermediate hosts of human and sheep.

Pathogenesis and Clinical Picture

About 70% of hydatid cysts develop in the liver, 20% in the lungs, and the rest in rarer sites, including the brain and bones. As the cysts grow, they cause pressure symptoms. Patients usually present with a low-grade fever, an enlarged, tender liver with predominantly right lobe involvement, and eosinophilia. As the cysts grow, the liver may compress the base of the lungs or the cysts may rupture into the lungs, leading to breathlessness and cough with bloody sputum.

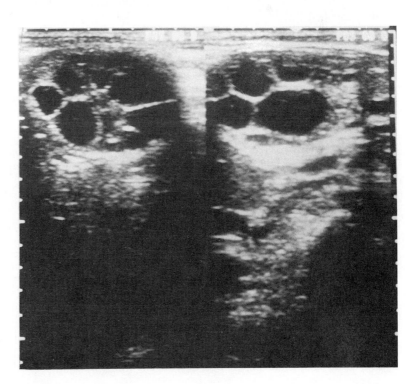

FIGURE 47-7 Two scans showing multilocular hepatic cyst with internal echoes in some of the locules, in a case of hydatid cyst.

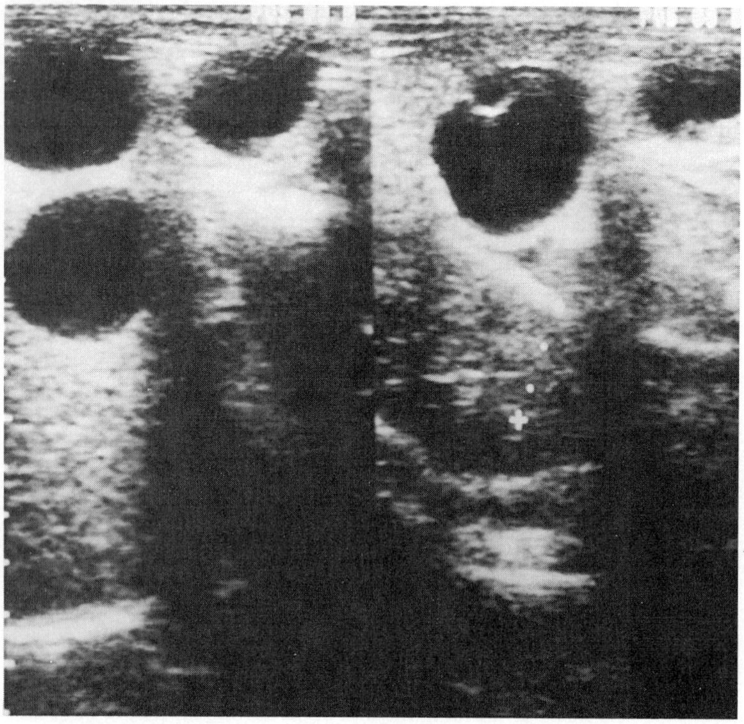

FIGURE 47-8 Multiple hydatid cysts of the liver. One cyst shows a smaller "daughter" cyst inside.

Rupture of the cysts into the lungs or abdomen, either from a blow or spontaneously, may lead to severe anaphylactic shock and sudden death. Rupture into the biliary tree results in cholangitis and duct obstruction. If the cyst becomes infected, the signs and symptoms are those of an abscess of the liver or of the involved organ. If the cysts invade the brain or bone, patients may present with symptoms of intracerebral space-occupying lesion or of bone fracture, respectively. Eventually the cysts die, the fluid is absorbed, and the walls become calcified.[12,13,107]

Diagnosis

Diagnosis is made indirectly. Aspiration of the cyst or biopsy should not be attempted because leakage may cause spread of the infection or anaphylaxis. Immunoserology and radiology have greatly facilitated diagnosis. ELISA and the complement fixation test are helpful. ELISA gives positive results in about 90% of hepatic hydatid cysts. Serology combined with ultrasonography and CT of the liver, lungs, and abdomen to outline the presence of cysts have superseded other forms of diagnosis. In certain centers, detection of circulating antigens to hydatid infection has now become possible. Differential diagnosis must include hepatic abscess (bacterial or amebic) or hepatic neoplasm[58] (Figs. 47-7 and 47-8).

Treatment

Albendazole in an adult dose of 400 mg twice daily in 28-day blocks with 14 days off between blocks of therapy has proved effective.[5,60,86] The optimal duration of therapy is not yet defined. In those cysts that are operable, albendazole therapy usually is followed by surgical removal of the cyst.

Accessible cysts should be removed surgically. In multiple cysts of the liver or lungs, hemihepatectomy or lobectomy may be necessary. If cysts cannot be removed surgically, they can be sterilized by removing the hydatid fluid and introducing a scolicidal agent such as 0.5% silver nitrate, but only specialized centers should deal with these complicated cases.

Two other species of echinococcus rarely infect humans, *E multilocularis* and *E vogeli*. Both may cause widespread hydatid disease of the liver and both can be fatal. The adult stage of *E multilocularis* usually infects sylvatic canine mammals such as the fox. Human infection has been reported from North America, Canada, and Russia. *E vogeli* infection has been reported from Colombia.

Both infections develop in the liver into an alveolar type of cyst and spread like a neoplasm. Albendazole has been shown to be of some value in arresting progress of the infection when surgery is ineffective.

References

1. Abdel Wahab MF. Schistosomiasis in Egypt. Boca Raton, FL, CRC Press, 1982
2. Abdel Wahab MF, et al. Characteristic sonographic pattern of schistosomal hepatic fibrosis. Am J Trop Med Hyg 40:72, 1989
3. Abdel Wahab MF, et al. Sonographic studies of schoolchildren in a village endemic for S. *mansoni*. Trans R Soc Trop Med Hyg 84:69, 1990
4. Ahmed L, et al. Ultrasonography in the diagnosis and management of 52 patients with amebic liver abscess in Cairo. Rev Infect Dis 12:330, 1990
5. Ammann WR, et al. Recurrence rate after discontinuation of long-term mebendazole therapy in alveolar echinococcosis (preliminary results). Am J Trop Med Hyg 43:506, 1990
6. Andrion JA, Comino A. Visceral leishmaniasis (kala azar): hepatic involvement. Pathology 18:485, 1986
7. Ansari N, ed. Epidemiology and control of schistosomiasis (bilharziasis). Baltimore, University Park Press, 1973
8. Araki T, et al. Hepatic *Schistosomiasis japonica* identified by CTI. Radiology 157:757, 1985

9. Bassily S, et al. Chronic hepatitis B in patients with *Schistosoma mansoni.* J Trop Med Hyg 86:67, 1983

10. Bassily S, et al. Sonography in diagnosis of fascioliasis. Lancet 1:1270, 1989

11. Bates I, et al. Use of immunoglobulin gene rearrangements to show clonal lymphoproliferation in hyper-reactive malarial splenomegaly. Lancet 331:505, 1991

12. Beaver PC, Jung RC, Cupp EW, eds. Clinical parasitology, ed 9. Philadelphia, Lea & Febiger, 1984

13. Bell DR. Lecture notes on tropical medicine, ed 3. London, Blackwell Scientific Publications, 1990

14. Brownwold E, et al, eds. Harrison's principles of internal medicine, ed 11. New York, McGraw-Hill, 1987

15. Bryceson A. Therapy in man. In: Peters W, Killick-Kendrick R, eds. The leishmaniases in biology and medicine. New York, Academic Press, 1987, pp 847–907

16. Centers for Disease Control. Acute schistosomiasis with transverse myelitis in American students returning from Kenya. MMWR 33:445, 1984

17. Chan SW, et al. Serodiagnosis of human trichinosis using a gel filtration antigen and indirect IgG–ELISA. Trans R Soc Trop Med Hyg 84:721, 1990

18. Chapman PJC, et al. Acute schistosomiasis (Katayama fever) among British air crew. Br Med J 297:1101, 1988

19. Cohen J, et al. Schistosomal myelopathy. Br Med J 1:1258, 1977

20. Cole ACE. Kala-azar in East Africa. Trans R Soc Trop Med Hyg 37:409, 1944

21. Cook GC. Tropical gastroenterology. New York, Oxford University Press, 1980

22. Cook GC. Chemotherapy of parasitic infections. Curr Opin Infect Dis 1:423, 1988

23. Cook GC. Hepatic structure and function in experimental and human malaria: In Bianchi L, Gerok W, Maier KP, Deinhardt F, eds. Infectious diseases of the liver. Falk Symposium 54. Boston, Kluwer Academic Publishers, 1989, pp 191–213

24. Davidson RN, et al. Liposomal amphotericin B in drug-resistant visceral leishmaniasis. Lancet 337:1061, 1991

25. Davis A. Recent advances in schistosomiasis. Q J Med 58:95, 1986

26. De Brito T, et al. Human liver biopsy in *P. falciparum* and *P. vivax* malaria: a light and electron microscopy study. Virchows Arch [A] 348:220, 1989

27. De Cock KM. Human schistosomiasis and its management. J Infect 8:5, 1984

28. De Cock KM. Hepatosplenic schistosomiasis: a clinical review. Gut 27:734, 1986

29. Despommier DD, Karapelou JW, eds. Parasite life cycles. New York, Springer-Verlag, 1987

30. Doehring-Schwerdtfeger E, et al. Ultrasonographical investigation of periportal fibrosis in children with *S. mansoni* infection: evaluation of morbidity. Am J Trop Med Hyg 42:581, 1990

31. Dunn MA, Kamel R. Hepatic schistosomiasis. Hepatology 1:653, 1981

32. Elkins DB, et al. A high frequency of hepatobiliary disease and suspected cholangiocarcinoma associated with heavy O. *viverrini* infection in a small community in north-east Thailand. Trans R Soc Trop Med Hyg 84:715, 1990

33. El Masry NA, et al. Treatment of bilharzial colonic polyposis with praziquantel. J Infect Dis 52:1360, 1985

34. El Masry NA, et al. A comparison of the efficacy and side effects of various regimens of praziquantel for the treatment of schistosomiasis. Trans R Soc Trop Med Hyg 82:719, 1988

35. El Rooby AS. Management of hepatic schistosomiasis. Semin Liver Dis 5:263, 1985

36. Farid Z, et al. Hepatic amebiasis: diagnostic counterimmunoelectrophoresis and metronidazole (Flagyl) therapy. Am J Trop Med Hyg 26:822, 1977

37. Farid Z, et al. Amebic liver abscess presenting as fever of unknown origin (FUO): serology, isotope scanning and metronidazole therapy in diagnosis and treatment. J Trop Med Hyg 85:255, 1982

38. Farid Z, Wallace CK. Schistosomiasis and praziquantel. Ann Intern Med 99:883, 1983

39. Farid Z, et al. Schistosomiasis and praziquantel. Ann Intern Med 101:882, 1984

40. Farid Z, et al. Acute schistosomiasis mansoni (Katayama syndrome). Ann Trop Med Parasitol 80:563, 1986

41. Farid Z, et al. Unsuccessful use of praziquantel to treat acute fasciola in children. J Infect Dis 154:920, 1986

42. Farid Z. Schistosoma mansoni infection: intestinal schistosomiasis. Med Interne 55:2281, 1988

43. Farid Z, et al. Treatment of acute toxaemic fascioliasis. Trans R Soc Trop Med Hyg 82:299, 1988

44. Farid Z, et al. Praziquantel and fasciola hepatica infection. Trans R Soc Trop Med Hyg 83:813, 1989

45. Farid Z, et al. Praziquantel and acute urban schistosomiasis. Trop Geogr Med 41:172, 1989

46. Farid Z, et al. The treatment of acute *F. hepatica* infection in children. Trop Geogr Med 42:95, 1990

47. Flavell DJ. Liver fluke infection as an etiological factor in bile-duct carcinoma in man. Trans R Soc Trop Med Hyg 75:814, 1981

48. Freeman O, et al. Amebic liver abscess: the effect of aspiration on the resolution or healing time. Ann Trop Med Parasitol 84:281, 1990

49. Garnham PCC. Malaria parasites of man: life-cycles and morphology (excluding ultrastructure). In: Wernsdorfer WH, McGregor I, eds. Malaria: principles and practice of malariology. Edinburgh, Churchill Livingstone, 1988, pp 61–96

50. Gilles HM. Schistosomiasis: an overview. Med Interne 55:2280, 1988

51. Glickman LT. Toxocariasis. In: Warren KS, Mahmoud AAF, eds. Tropical and geographical medicine. New York, McGraw-Hill, 1990, pp 431–437

52. Godfrey-Faussett P, et al. Parasites in the immuno-compromised host. In: Warren KS, ed. Immunology and molecular biology of parasitic infections. London, Blackwell Scientific Publications 1993

53. Goka AKJ, et al. Diagnosis of strongyloides and hookworm infections: comparison of faecal and duodenal fluid microscopy. Trans R Soc Trop Med Hyg 84:829, 1990

54. Goldsmith R, Heyneman D, eds. Tropical medicine and parasitology. Norwalk, CT, Appleton & Lange, 1989

55. Hassib F. Schistosomal myelopathy. Br Med J 189, 1977

56. Hills AG. Malarial jaundice. Am J Med Sci 212:45, 1971

57. Hillyer GV, et al. Immunodiagnosis of infection with S. *haematobium* and S. *mansoni* in man. Am J Trop Med Hyg 29:1254, 1980

58. Hira PR, et al. An enzyme-linked immunosorbent assay using an arc 5 antigen for the diagnosis of cystic hydatid disease. Ann Trop Med Parasitol 84:157, 1990

59. Horstmann RD, et al. High efficacy of praziquantel in the treatment of 22 patients with clonorchis/opisthorchis infections. Tropenmed Parasit 32:157, 1981

60. Horton RJ. Chemotherapy of *Echinococcus* infection in man with albendazole. Trans R Soc Trop Med Hyg 83:97, 1989

61. Imes GD Jr, Neafie RC. Babesiosis. In: Binford CH, Connor DH, eds. Pathology of tropical and extraordinary diseases. Washington, DC, Armed Forces Institute of Pathology, 1976, pp 301–302

62. Istre GR, et al. Acute schistosomiasis among Americans rafting the Omo River, Ethiopia. JAMA 251:508, 1984

63. Jordan P, Webbe G, eds. Human schistosomiasis. Springfield, IL, Charles C Thomas, 1969

64. Katz M, Despommier DD, Gwadz R, eds. Parasitic diseases, ed 2. New York, Springer-Verlag, 1989

65. Kaplan MM, Compton CC. A 25-year-old Cambodian native with hematemesis. N Engl J Med 319:37, 1988

66. Khuroo MS, Zargar SA. Biliary ascariasis: a common cause of biliary and pancreatic disease in an endemic area. Gastroenterology 88:418, 1985

67. Kilpatrick ME, et al. Presymptomatic schistosomal colonic polyposis. Ann Trop Med Parasitol 76:109, 1982

68. King CH, Mahmoud AA. Drugs 5 years later: praziquantel. Ann Intern Med 110:290, 1989

69. Kurathong S, et al. *Opistorchis viverrini* infection and cholangiocarcinoma. Gastroenterology 89:151, 1985

70. Kurathong S, et al. *Opisthorchis viverrini* infection in rural and urban communities in northeast Thailand. Trans R Soc Trop Med Hyg 81:411, 1987

71. Latent schistosomiasis. (Editorial) Br Med J 835, 1976

72. Lehman JS, et al. Intestinal protein loss in schistosomal polyposis of the colon. Gastroenterology 59:433, 1970

73. Madwar MA, et al. The relationship between uncomplicated schistosomiasis and hepatitis B infection. Trans R Soc Trop Med Hyg 83:233, 1989

74. Maegraith B, Fletcher A. The pathogenesis of mammalian malaria. Adv Parasitol 10:49, 1972

75. Mahmoud AAF. Schistosomiasis. N Engl J Med 297:1329, 1977

76. Manson-Bahr PEC. East African kala-azar with special reference to the pathology, prophylaxis and treatment. Trans R Soc Trop Med Hyg 53:123, 1959

77. Manson-Bahr PEC. Diagnosis. In: Peters W, Killick-Kendrick E, eds. The leishmaniasis in biology and medicine. New York, Academic Press, 1987, pp 703–729

78. McCully RM, Barron CN, Cheever AW. Schistosomiasis (bilharziasis). In: Binford CH, Connor DH, eds. Pathology of tropical and extraordinary diseases. Washington, DC, Armed Forces Institute of Pathology, 1976, pp 482–508

79. McFadzean AJS, Yeung RTT. Acute pancreatitis due to *Clonorchis sinensis*. Trans R Soc Trop Med Hyg 60:466, 1966

80. Meyers WN, Neafie RC. Paragonimiasis. In: Binford CH, Connor DH, eds. Pathology of tropical and extraordinary diseases. Washington, DC, Armed Forces Institute of Pathology, 1976, pp 517–523

81. Mikhail EM, et al. Counterimmunoelectrophoresis for the rapid and specific diagnosis of acute fascioliasis and schistosomiasis. Trans R Soc Trop Med Hyg 84:400, 1990

82. Mohamed AR, Mummery V. Human dicrocoeliasis: report on 208 cases from Saudi Arabia. Trop Geogr Med 42:1, 1990

83. Molyneux ME, et al. Reduced hepatic blood flow and intestinal malabsorption in severe falciparum malaria. Am J Trop Med Hyg 40:470, 1989

84. Monroe LS. Gastrointestinal parasites. In: Berk JE, ed. Bockus' gastroenterology. Philadelphia, WB Saunders, 1985, p 4250

85. Moreno A, et al. Hepatic fibrin-ring granulomas in visceral leishmaniasis. Gastroenterology 95:1123, 1988

86. Morris DL, et al. Albendazole in hydatid disease. Br Med J 286:103, 1983

87. Most H. Trichinosis: preventable yet still with us. N Engl J Med 298:1178, 1978

88. Nash TE, et al. Schistosome infections in humans: perspectives and recent findings. Ann Intern Med 97:740, 1982

89. Neafie RC, Conner DH, Cross JH. Capillariasis (intestinal and hepatic). In: Binford CH, Connor DH, eds. Pathology of tropical and extraordinary diseases. Washington, DC, Armed Forces Institute of Pathology, 1976, pp 402–408

90. Neafie RC, Conner DH. Visceral larva migrans. In: Binford CH, Connor DH, eds. Pathology of tropical and extraordinary diseases. Washington, DC, Armed Forces Institute of Pathology, 1976, pp 433–436

91. Nishoka NS, Donnelly SS. A 72-year-old Chinese woman with recent abdominal pain and a right-sided abdominal mass. N Engl J Med 323:467, 1990

92. Pampiglione S, et al. Studies on Mediterranean leishmaniasis: 1. An outbreak of visceral leishmaniasis in northern Italy. Trans R Soc Trop Med Hyg 68:349, 1974

93. Pampiglione S, et al. Studies on Mediterranean leishmaniasis: 2. Asymptomatic cases of visceral leishmaniasis. Trans R Soc Trop Med Hyg 68:447, 1974

94. Patterson M, et al. Serologic testing for amebiasis. Gastroenterology 78:136, 1980

95. Pearson R, Guerrant R. Praziquantel: a major advance in antihelminthic therapy. Ann Intern Med 99:195, 1983

96. Purtillo DT. Clonorchiasis and hepatic neoplasms. Trop Geogr Med 28:21, 1976

97. Ralls PW, et al. Patterns of resolution in successfully treated hepatic amebic abscess: sonographic evaluation. Radiology 149:541, 1983

98. Rees PH, Kager PA. Visceral leishmaniasis and post-kala-azar dermal leishmaniasis. In: Petters W, Killick-Kendrick R, eds. The leishmaniasis in biology and medicine. New York, Academic Press, 1987, pp 583–615

99. Reiter I, Weiland G. Recently developed methods for the detection of babesial infections. Trans R Soc Trop Med Hyg 83:21, 1989

100. Ridgon RH, Thomas WKS. A study of the pathological lesions in *P. knowlesi* infection in *M. rhesus* monkeys. Am J Trop Med Hyg 22:329, 1942

101. Ridley DS. Pathology. In: Peters W, Killick-Kendrick R, eds. The leishmaniases in biology and medicine. New York, Academic Press, 1987, pp 665–701

102. Sanguini S, et al. Albendazole in the therapy of cutaneous larva migrans. Trans R Soc Trop Med Hyg 84:831, 1990

103. Sen Gupta PC, et al. The liver in kala-azar. Ann Trop Med Parasitol 50:252, 1956

104. Shaheen HI, et al. Dot enzyme-linked immunosorbent assay (dot-ELISA) for the rapid diagnosis of human fascioliasis. J Parasitol 75:549, 1989

105. Sherlock S. Diseases of the liver and biliary system, ed 7. Philadelphia, FA Davis, 1985

106. Smith DH. Visceral leishmaniasis: human aspects. In: Gilles HM, ed. Recent advances in tropical medicine. Edinburgh, Churchill Livingstone, 1984, pp 79–87

107. Sparks AK, Connor DH, Neafie RC. Echinococcosis. In: Binford CH, Connor DH, eds. Pathology of tropical and extraordinary diseases. Washington, DC, Armed Forces Institute of Pathology, 1976, pp 530–533

108. Spielman A, et al. Ecology of *Ixodes dammini*-borne human babesiosis and Lyme disease. Annu Rev Entomol 30:439, 1985

109. Strauss WG. Clinical manifestations of clonorchiasis: a controlled study of 105 cases. Am J Trop Med Hyg 11:625, 1962

110. Strickland GT, et al. Clinical characteristics and response to therapy in Egyptian children heavily infected with *S. mansoni*. J Infect Dis 146:20, 1982

111. Strickland GT, ed. Hunter's tropical medicine, ed 6. Philadelphia, WB Saunders, 1984

112. Stuiver C. Acute schistosomiasis (Katayama fever). Br Med J 288:221, 1984

113. Sturchler D. Thiabendazole vs. albendazole in treatment of toxocariasis: a clinical trial. Ann Trop Med Parasitol 83:473, 1989

114. Sun T. Pathology and immunology of *C. sinensis* infection of the liver. Ann Clin Lab Sci 14:208, 1984

115. Uflacker R, et al. Parasitic and mycotic causes of biliary obstruction. Gastrointest Radiol 7:173, 1982

116. Warren KS. Schistosomiasis: host–pathogen biology. Rev Infect Dis 4:771, 1982

117. Warren KS, et al. Morbidity in schistosomiasis japonica in relation to intensity of infection: a study of 2 rural brigades in Anhui Province, China. N Engl J Med 309:1533, 1983

118. Warren KS, Mahmoud AAF, eds. Tropical and geographic medicine, ed 2. New York, McGraw-Hill, 1990

119. Watt G, et al. Praziquantel in treatment of cerebral schistosomiasis. Lancet 1:529, 1986
120. Watt G. Hepatosplenic schistosomiasis. N Engl J Med 319:1286, 1988
121. Watt G. Schistosoma japonicum infection: Asiatic intestinal schistosomiasis. Med Interne 55:2284, 1988
122. Webbe G. Schistosomiasis: some advances. Br Med J 283:1104, 1981
123. World Health Organization. Severe and complicated malaria: second edition. Trans R Soc Trop Med Hyg 2:1, 1990
124. World Health Organization. WHO model prescription information: drugs used in parasitic diseases. Geneva, World Health Organization, 1990
125. Wright R, et al. Liver and biliary disease, ed 2. Philadelphia, WB Saunders 1985
126. Wright IG, et al. Immunopathophysiology of babesial infections. Trans R Soc Trop Med Hyg 83:11, 1989
127. Wyngaarden JB, Smith LH, eds. Cecil's textbook of medicine, ed 18. Philadelphia, WB Saunders, 1988

Diseases of the Liver, Seventh Edition, edited by
Leon Schiff and Eugene R. Schiff. J.B. Lippincott Company, Philadelphia © 1993.

48

Leptospirosis

Jay P. Sanford

Definition

Leptospirosis is the name applied to disease caused by all leptospires, regardless of specific serotype. Previously, a number
of names were used to describe various clinical syndromes,
such as Weil's disease for icteric leptospirosis caused by the
icterohaemorrhagiae serogroup, swineherds' disease for that
caused by the pomona serogroup, canicola fever for leptospirosis due to the canicola serogroup, mud fever, autumn fever,
field fever, 7-day fever, and Fort Bragg fever. The recognition
of considerable overlap between clinical syndromes and specific serogroups of leptospira has led to the discontinuation
of such terminology.

History

The separation of leptospiral jaundice from other infectious
diseases of the liver occurred in two stages, the first, clinical,
and the second, nearly 30 years later, bacteriologic.[1] The
term *Weil's disease* was used first by Goldschmidt in 1887 to
designate the form of infectious jaundice that Professor Weil
of Heidelberg had established as a separate entity in 1886
from a study of four patients.[10,32] Two of the cases had occurred in 1870 and the other two in 1882, but they each
presented such similar features that Weil considered them to
be the same disease. The four patients were men, and each
had a febrile illness with neurologic symptoms, hepatomegaly, splenomegaly, jaundice, and renal involvement. After a
relatively short course, the patients recovered; however, three
had a recurrence of fever after an afebrile period of 1 to 7
days. Although he could not demonstrate either its anatomic
basis or the infective agent, Weil suggested that the cases represented a new entity. Actually, Landouzy had described the
disease in 1883 and had associated it with work in sewers.[16]
Subsequently, there developed skepticism as to whether
Weil's disease was a separate entity. Inada and associates[12]
were convinced of the existence of Weil's disease as an illness
characterized by conjunctival congestion, muscular pain,
fever, jaundice, hemorrhagic diathesis, albuminuria, and a
fairly high death rate. They stated that splenic enlargement
was uncommon, occurring in about 10% of patients. In
November, 1914, in Kyushu, Inada and coworkers first saw
spirochetes in the liver tissue of a guinea pig that had been
inoculated with blood from a patient with Weil's disease.
They obtained similar results with blood from 13 of 17 other
cases of Weil's disease and failed to find spirochetes in guinea
pigs inoculated with blood from patients with other infec-

tions, including catarrhal jaundice. They named the organism *Spirochaeta icterohaemorrhagiae*. They cultured the organism and showed that it could gain entry into guinea pigs
through abraded and even apparently intact skin, that spirochetes could be seen in patients' urine, and that antibodies
appeared in patients' serum and persisted for a number of
years.[12] Noguchi[19] carefully studied the *S icterohaemorrhagiae* of Inada and colleagues, strains from British cases in
Flanders during World War I, and strains from wild rats in
the United States. He considered the morphology to be sufficiently characteristic to justify the creation of a new genus,
which he named *Leptospira*.[19] Stimson[25] described a spiro-
chete in sections of the kidney of a patient in New Orleans
who died of presumed yellow fever. He named the organism
(?*Spirochaeta*) *interrogans*. His description of the organism
and photographs taken in 1940 by Sellards[21] from Stimson's
original sections show that the organism was a leptospire.

Etiology

Leptospires are finely coiled, motile aerobic spirochetes approximately 0.1 μm wide and 6 to 20 μm long. They have
bent or hooked ends often resembling question marks; hence
the name *interrogans*. The cell wall has a three-layered structure similar to that of gram-negative bacteria.[14] Leptospira are
resistant to metronidazole.

The genus *Leptospira* contains only one species, *L interrogans*, so named because of the priority established by Stimson,[25] which is subdivided into two complexes, interrogans
and biflexa. The interrogans complex includes the pathogenic strains, whereas the biflexa complex includes sapro-
phytic strains. Within each complex, the organisms show antigenic variations that are stable and allow them to be classed
as serotypes (serovars). Serotypes with common antigens are
arranged into serogroups (vars). Despite common usage to the
contrary, an example of the correct designation of *Leptospira*
is as follows: canicola serogroup of *L interrogans* or *L interrogans* serovar canicola. The interrogans complex now contains about 240 serotypes of pathogenic leptospires arranged
in 23 serogroups (the numbers in the following parentheses
refer to the numbers of serotypes within the serogroups): icterohaemorrhagiae (18), hebdomidis (30), autumnalis (17),
canicola (12), australis (12), tarassovi (17), pyrogenes (12),
bataviae (10), javanica (8), pomona (8), ballum (3), cynoptei
(3), celledoni (3), grippotyphosa (5), panama (2), shermani
(1), ranarum (2), and bufonis (1). At least 27 serotypes of
leptospira occur naturally in the United States.

Epidemiology

Leptospirosis is thought to be the most widespread zoonosis in the world.[27] It occurs throughout the world, except for Antarctica, and is most prevalent in the tropics. In southeast Asia, the Marquesas Islands, and Trinidad, 15% to 28% of people are seropositive. Leptospirosis is still endemic in the Po valley of Italy.[5] Although leptospirosis is not common in the United States, it has been reported from all regions, including arid areas such as Arizona. Between 1980 and 1992, 40 to 100 cases were reported.[4] Infection in humans is an incidental occurrence and is not essential in the maintenance of leptospirosis. The disease occurs in a wide range of domestic and wild animal hosts. In many species, such as opossum, skunk, raccoon, and fox, infectivity ratios in the range of 10% to 50% are not unusual. Interspecies spread of specific serotypes of leptospires among animal hosts is frequent; for example, pomona, a serotype principally associated with livestock, has been demonstrated in dogs. Infection in animals may vary from inapparent illness to fatal disease. Asymptomatic host animals may carry high numbers of leptospires in their kidneys (more than 10^{10} organisms per gram). The carrier state, in which the host may shed leptospires in its urine for months or years, develops in many animals. Immunization of dogs may not prevent the carrier or shedder state.[9]

Survival of pathogenic leptospires in nature is governed by factors including pH of the urine of the host, pH of the soil or water into which they are shed, and ambient temperature. Leptospires shed in a carrier's urine have been found in the soil to a depth of 1 cm with a radius 1 to 2 cm beyond the urine spot. Most spots retain infective capacity for 6 to 48 hours. Acid urine permits only limited survival; however, if the urine is neutral or alkaline, is shed into a similar moist environment that has low salinity, is not badly polluted with microorganisms or detergents, and has a temperature above 22°C (71.6°F), leptospires may survive for several weeks. Human infection can occur either by direct contact with urine or tissue of an infected animal or indirectly through contaminated water, soil, or vegetation. The usual portals of entry in humans are abraded skin, particularly about the feet, and exposed conjunctival, nasal, and oral mucous membranes. Swallowing contaminated water during immersion has been associated with high attack rates.[6] Transmission of a serovar, hardjo, which infected cows and was shed in their milk, from an infected mother to her nursing infant has been reported.[3] The previously held concept that organisms can penetrate intact skin has been questioned. Although leptospires have been isolated from ticks, these arthropods are unimportant in transmission.

With the ubiquitous infection of animals, leptospirosis in human beings can occur in all age groups, at all seasons, and in both sexes. It is primarily a disease of teenaged children and young adults (about one half of all patients are between the ages of 10 and 39 years), however, occurs predominantly in men (80%), and develops most frequently in hot weather (in the United States, one half of infections occur from July to October).[11,34] The wide spectrum of animal hosts results in both urban and rural human disease. Leptospirosis has been considered an occupational disease; however, improved methods of rat control and better standards of hygiene have reduced the incidence among occupational groups such as coal miners and sewer workers. The epidemiologic pattern has changed; in the United States, United Kingdom, Europe, and Israel water-associated and cattle-associated leptospirosis has become most common. Fewer than 20% of patients have direct contact with animals, and those who have such contact are usually farmers, trappers, or abattoir workers. In the United States in the majority of patients, exposure is incidental; two thirds of cases occur in children, students, or housewives. Swimming or partial immersion in contaminated water, such as by riding a motorcycle through contaminated pools of water, has been implicated in one fifth of patients and has accounted for most of the recognized common-source outbreaks. In Hawaii, one fourth of cases have been associated with aquaculture industries. In the United Kingdom, fish farm workers show a moderately increased risk. Several soldiers assigned to the British Army on the Rhine have contracted leptospirosis after falling into rivers.

Pathology

Postmortem examinations of patients who died of leptospirosis have been confined almost exclusively to people with icteric leptospirosis (Weil's disease). Gross examination has revealed bile staining of the tissues. Hemorrhages, petechial or ecchymotic, occur in almost all organs but are most prominent in striated muscle, kidneys, adrenals, liver, stomach, spleen, and lungs.[1] The liver and kidneys are of normal size or slightly enlarged. Lungs are edematous with varying degrees of focal or diffuse hemorrhage.

Histologic alterations in the liver are neither specific nor diagnostic. Proliferation of liver cells as evidenced by mitotic figures and cells with two nuclei, cloudy swelling, dissociation of hepatic cords, enlargement of Kupffer cells, and varying degrees of necrosis (usually slight and focal) occur. Biliary stasis involving the central, but not the peripheral, portion of the lobule is frequent. The degree of functional damage to the liver in fatal cases often is poorly correlated with the degree of histopathologic changes. Leptospires rarely are demonstrated in the liver.

Microscopic changes of the kidneys often are striking. In the acute phase, lesions predominantly involve the tubules and vary from simple dilatation of distal convoluted tubules to degeneration, necrosis, and basement membrane rupture. Interstitial edema and cellular infiltrates consisting of lymphocytes, neutrophilic leukocytes, histiocytes, and plasma cells are uniformly present. Glomerular lesions either are absent or consist of mesangial hyperplasia and focal foot process fusion, which are interpreted as nonspecific changes associated with acute inflammation and protein filtration. Special staining techniques using silver impregnation methods have demonstrated organisms in the lumina of renal tubules but rarely in other organs.

In skeletal muscle, focal necrotic and necrobiotic changes thought to be typical of leptospirosis occur. Biopsies early in the illness demonstrate swelling, vacuolization, and, subsequently, hyalinization. Leptospiral antigen has been demonstrated in these lesions by the fluorescent antibody technique. Healing ensues with minimum fibrosis through the formation of new myofibrils. Microscopic evidence of myocarditis, including focal hemorrhages, interstitial edema, and focal infiltration with lymphocytes and plasma cells can be seen. Pulmonary findings consist of a patchy, localized hemorrhagic pneumonitis. Bile staining of leptomeninges and choroid plexus may be seen. Microscopic changes in the brain and meninges are minimal and are not diagnostic.

Clinical Manifestations

GENERAL FEATURES

The incubation period after immersion or accidental laboratory exposure has shown extremes of 2 and 26 days; the usual range is 7 to 13 days and the average is 10 days.[1,9]

Leptospirosis is a typically biphasic illness. During the first, or leptospiremic, phase, leptospires are present in the blood and cerebrospinal fluid.[8] The onset is typically abrupt, and initial symptoms include headache, which is usually frontal, less often retroorbital, and occasionally bitemporal or occipital.[2] Severe muscle aching occurs in most patients, involving the muscles of the thighs and lumbar areas most prominently, and is often accompanied by severe pain on palpation. Patients often complain of leg pain with walking.[20] The myalgia may be accompanied by extreme cutaneous hyperesthesia (causalgia). Chills followed by a rapidly rising temperature are prominent. After the abrupt onset, the leptospiremic phase typically lasts 4 to 9 days. Features during this interval include recurrent chills, high spiking temperatures (usually 38.9°C [102°F] or greater), headache, and continued severe myalgia. Anorexia, nausea, and vomiting are encountered in one half or more of the patients. Occasionally, patients have diarrhea. Pulmonary manifestations, usually either a cough or chest pain, have varied in frequency of occurrence from less than 25% to 86%. Hemoptysis occurs but is uncommon in the United States and Europe, although it is a common feature, noted in 40% of patients, in Korea and China.[20] Examination during this phase reveals an acutely ill, febrile patient, with a relative bradycardia and normal blood pressure, although European authors comment on early hypotension. Disturbances in sensorium may be encountered in up to 25% of all patients and in half of patients with icteric (Weil's) disease.[17] The most characteristic physical sign is conjunctival suffusion, which usually first appears on the third or fourth day. It may be lacking in some patients but more often is overlooked. This may be associated with photophobia, but serous or purulent secretion is unusual. Less common findings include pharyngeal injection, cutaneous hemorrhages, and skin rashes that usually are macular, maculopapular, or urticarial and usually occur on the trunk. Uncommon findings are splenomegaly, hepatomegaly, lymphadenopathy, and jaundice. The first phase terminates after 4 to 9 days, usually with defervescence and improvement in symptoms. This coincides with the disappearance of leptospires from the blood and cerebrospinal fluid.

The second phase, which has been characterized as the immune phase, correlates with the appearance of circulating IgM antibodies.[8] The concentration of C3 in serum remains within normal range. Clinical manifestations show greater variability than those of the first phase. After a relatively asymptomatic period of 1 to 3 days, the fever and earlier symptoms recur, and meningismus may develop. The fever rarely exceeds 38.9°C (102°F) and usually is of 1 to 3 days' duration. It is not uncommon for fever to be absent or transient. Even when symptoms or signs of meningeal irritation are absent, routine examination of cerebrospinal fluid after the seventh day has revealed pleocytosis in 50% to 90% of patients.[8] Less common features include iridocyclitis, optic neuritis, and other nervous system manifestations, including encephalitis, myelitis, and peripheral neuropathy. Transient ischemic attacks in childhood and adolescence caused by cerebral leptospiral arteritis have been reported by Chinese clinicians.

Some clinicians recognize a third, or convalescent, phase, usually between the second and fourth weeks, when both fever and aching may recur. The pathogenesis of this stage is not understood.

Leptospirosis during pregnancy may be associated with an increased risk of fetal loss.

SPECIFIC FEATURES

Weil's disease accounts for 1% to 6% of cases of leptospirosis, although the proportion is as high as 62% in a series from Portugal.[17] Serovar *L icterohaemorrhagiae* accounts for 40% of those with Weil's disease, and the remainder are caused by multiple serovars. Weil's disease is defined as severe leptospirosis with jaundice, usually accompanied by azotemia, hemorrhages, anemia, disturbances in consciousness, and continued fever. There is uncertainty as to the pathogenesis of the syndrome, that is, whether it represents direct toxic damage due to leptospires or whether it is the consequence of immune response to leptospiral antigens. The consensus favors toxic damage.

The onset and first stage are identical with those of the less severe forms of leptospirosis. The distinctive features of Weil's disease appear from the third to the sixth day but do not reach their peak until well into the second stage. As in milder forms of leptospirosis, there is a tendency for defervescence on about the seventh day; however, with recurrence, fever is marked and may persist for several weeks. Either renal or hepatic manifestations may predominate. Hepatic disturbances include tenderness in the right upper quadrant and hepatic enlargement, both of which are common when jaundice is present. Serum glutamic-oxaloacetic transaminase (SGOT) values are rarely increased more than five-fold regardless of the degree of hyperbilirubinemia, which predominantly is conjugated (direct); as an example, serum bilirubin is 40 mg/dL, whereas SGOT is 170 IU/dL. The predominant mechanism appears to be an intracellular block to bilirubin excretion.

Renal manifestations consist primarily of proteinuria, pyuria, hematuria, and azotemia. Dysuria is rare. Serious renal damage usually occurs in the form of acute tubular necrosis associated with oliguria. The peak elevation of blood urea nitrogen usually is seen on the fifth to seventh day. Hemorrhagic manifestations, which are most prevalent in this group of patients, include epistaxis, hemoptysis, gastrointestinal bleeding, hemorrhage into the adrenal glands, hemorrhagic pneumonitis, and subarachnoid hemorrhage. Fatal subarachnoid hemorrhage without thrombocytopenia and thrombotic thrombocytopenic purpura have been reported.[15] These manifestations have been explained on the basis of diffuse vasculitis with capillary injury. In addition, hypoprothrombinemia and thrombocytopenia have been observed in some patients.

Laboratory Features

In anicteric patients, leukocyte counts vary from leukopenic levels to mild elevations. In patients with jaundice, leukocytosis as high as 70,000 cells/µL may be present. Regardless of the total leukocyte count, however, neutrophilia of over 70% is encountered very frequently during the first stage.

Hemolytic substances have been demonstrated in cultures of pathogenic leptospires. In contrast to many hemolysins of bacterial origin that are not hemolytic in vivo, leptospiral hemolysins appear to be active in vivo. In patients with jaundice, anemia may be severe and most characteristically is due to intravascular hemolysis. Other mechanisms of anemia include that secondary to azotemia and blood loss secondary to hemorrhage. Anemia due to leptospirosis is unusual in anicteric patients.

Thrombocytopenia sufficient to be associated with bleeding may be encountered. Additional hematologic abnormalities include elevation of the erythrocyte sedimentation rate in more than half of patients, although this rate usually remains below 50 mm/h.

Urinalysis during the leptospiremic phase reveals mild proteinuria, casts, and an increase in cellular elements. In anicteric infections, these abnormalities rapidly disappear after the first week. Proteinuria and abnormalities in the urine sediment usually are not associated with elevations in blood urea nitrogen. Because the anicteric form of the disease often has gone undiagnosed, estimates of the frequency of azotemia and jaundice probably are high. Azotemia has been reported in approximately one fourth of patients. In three fourths of these patients, the blood urea nitrogen is less than 100 mg/dL. Azotemia usually is associated with jaundice. Serum bilirubin levels may reach 65 mg/dL; however, in two thirds of patients, the levels are less than 20 mg/dL. During the first phase, one half of the patients have increased serum creatine phosphokinase levels, with mean values of five times normal.[14] Such increases are not seen in viral hepatitis, and a slight increase in transaminase with a definite increase in creatine phosphokinase suggests leptospirosis rather than viral hepatitis.

Diagnosis

Diagnosis is based on culture of the organism or serologic proof of its existence. The most common initial diagnoses in patients with leptospirosis are meningitis, hepatitis, nephritis, fever of undetermined origin, and influenza.[2] Leptospires may be isolated quite readily during the first phase from blood and cerebrospinal fluid or during the second phase from the urine. Leptospires may be excreted in the urine for up to 11 months after the onset of illness and may persist despite antimicrobial therapy. Whole blood should be injected immediately into tubes containing semisolid medium such as Fletcher's or EMJH medium. If culture medium is not available, leptospires reportedly will remain viable up to 11 days in blood to which anticoagulants, preferably sodium oxalate, have been added. Citrate should not be used because it inhibits leptospires. Animal inoculation (preferably either suckling hamster or guinea pig) may be used and is of particular value if specimens are contaminated. Direct examination of blood or urine by the dark-field method has been used; however, this method so frequently results in failure or misdiagnosis that it should not be used.[24] Serologic methods are applicable during the second phase; antibodies appear from the 6th to the 12th days of illness. Five serologic tests are available: microscopic agglutination (MA), macroscopic agglutination (slide test, ST), hemolytic, indirect hemagglu-

tination (IHA), and complement fixation.[13] The MA test is the standard procedure used for serologic diagnosis, but it is complex, requiring the maintenance of cultures of live leptospires (23 being used). The test is partially serovar specific. Agglutinins elicited by leptospires of a particular serovar often agglutinate leptospires of other serovars in the same serogroup. Absorption studies on serum from an infected person indicate the infecting serovar with a high degree of probability. The ST is commonly used in hospitals to screen sera for infection. Antigens used include ballum, canicola, icterohaemorrhagiae, bataviae, grippotyphosa, pyrogenes, autumnalis, pomona, wolfii, australis, tarassovi, and georgia. The IHA test uses glutaraldehyde fixation of sheep erythrocytes coated with an alcohol-extracted antigen from a single leptospiral serovar (andaman). An enzyme-linked immunosorbent assay test for leptospirosis has been developed that shows a high degree of specificity and sensitivity compared with the MA test.[30] It is not yet commercially available. Diagnostic criteria are as follows: a case is confirmed by the isolation of leptospires on culture or seroconversion from a titer of below 1:50 to over 1:200 or by a four-fold or greater change in MA titer between acute and convalescent serum specimens studied at the same laboratory; a case is presumed if the finding is an MA titer of at least 1:200 or a positive ST reaction on a single serum specimen obtained after the onset of symptoms.

DIFFERENTIAL DIAGNOSIS

During the initial 48 to 96 hours of illness, leptospirosis is virtually indistinguishable from infection due to hantavirus (hemorrhagic fever with renal syndrome, Korean hemorrhagic fever) or scrub typhus (tsutsugamushi disease). Because of the initial similarity, I have used the term *lepthantagamushi* syndrome. With the recognition of hantavirus infections in Europe and the potential for specific but differing treatment regimens for each, this differential diagnosis is becoming increasingly important.[35]

Before consideration of specific infections that may be associated with jaundice, it should be noted that, in a patient with underlying liver disease, jaundice may appear or worsen from a variety of causes, including infections. Drugs being used to treat an infected patient also may cause jaundice. Table 48-1 provides a summary of major considerations. In young children, Kawasaki disease (mucocutaneous lymph node syndrome) shares many features with leptospirosis. In older children and young adults, the toxic shock syndrome, which has been associated with an exotoxin produced by some strains of *Staphylococcus aureus* related to phage group I, produces a syndrome that, clinically, is virtually indistinguishable from leptospirosis. Similarly, staphylococcal bacteremia may masquerade as leptospirosis. Through a mechanism that has not been defined, pyelonephritis is sometimes, albeit rarely, associated with jaundice. Consideration of leptospirosis requires a high index of suspicion and a careful epidemiologic history of potential contact with animal urine or water.

Prognosis

The prognosis depends on both the virulence of the organism and the general condition of the patient. Between 1974 and 1981, mortality in reported cases in the United States varied annually between 2.4% and 16.4%, averaging 7.1%.[4] A

TABLE 48-1 *Differential Diagnosis of Infectious Causes of Jaundice*

Mechanism of Jaundice	Disease Entity	Category of Patient		
		Neonate	Child	Adult
Hemolysitic	Infection in patients with abnormal red blood cells	×	×	×
	Malaria	×	×	×
	Babesiosis		×	×
	Bartonellosis		×	×
	Bacteroides bacteremia	×	×	×
	Clostridium perfringens toxemia	×	×	×
Obstructive	Cholangitis with infection	×	×	×
Hepatocellular	Viral hepatitis	×	×	×
	Infectious mononucleosis	×	×	×
	TORCH syndrome*	×		
	Coxsackievirus	×	×	×
	Yellow fever	×	×	×
	Lassa fever		×	×
	Ebola virus		×	×
	Marburg disease		×	×
	Psittacosis		×	×
	Q fever		×	×
	Gonococcal perihepatitis		×	×
	Kawasaki's disease	×	×	
	Toxic shock syndrome (phage group I staphylococci)		×	× (young)
	Granulomatous hepatitis		×	×
	Syphilis			
	Congenital	×		
	Secondary		×	×
	Leptospirosis		×	×
	Bacteremia	×		
	Hepatic abscess	×	×	×
	Pyelonephritis (rare)			×
	Parasites			
	Amebiasis		×	×
	Clonorchiasis			×
	Schistosomiasis			×

*Toxoplasmosis, rubella, cytomegalovirus, herpes simplex.

mortality as high as 48% in 1971 is reported from Barbados.[7] Age is the most significant host factor related to mortality. In a representative series, mortality rose from 10% in men under 50 years of age to 56% in those over 51 years of age. The virulence of the infecting leptospires correlates best with the development of jaundice. In anicteric patients, death is extremely rare, but with the development of jaundice, mortality in various series has ranged from 15% to 40%. Death usually is secondary to hemorrhage, especially gastrointestinal or renal failure. The long-term prognosis after the acute renal and hepatic lesions of leptospirosis is good. Glomerular filtration rates return to normal, usually within 2 months; however, a few patients show residual tubular dysfunction, such as a defect in renal concentrating capacity. In a small series of patients, ophthalmologic sequelae and headache persisted for 6 to 29 years.[23]

Treatment

A variety of antimicrobial drugs, including penicillin, streptomycin, the tetracycline congeners, chloramphenicol, erythromycin, and ciprofloxacin, have been effective in vitro and in experimental leptospiral infections.[22] Data concerning the efficacy of antibiotics in human beings have been conflicting. Studies have shown efficacy for both penicillin G and doxycycline in leptospirosis.[18,26,29] Although initiation of treatment within 4 days of onset of illness may be more effective, in severely ill patients, initiation of treatment with penicillin G even later has been beneficial.[29] Within 4 to 6 hours after initiation of penicillin G therapy, a Jarisch-Herxheimer type of reaction may occur, although none occurred in 24 patients with proven leptospirosis who were monitored for reactions after intravenous penicillin.[31] A prospective, double-blind study has demonstrated that doxycycline, 200 mg orally once a week, is highly effective prophylaxis.[26] In a companion prospective double-blind study, doxycycline, 100 mg orally twice daily for 7 days, reduced duration of illness and favorably affected fever, malaise, headache, and myalgias.[18] Treatment prevented leptospiruria. Both studies were based on disease acquired in Panama. The epidemiologic conditions and clinical illnesses were typical of leptospirosis generally. It is reasonable to assume that the conclusions are applicable to other areas and would probably apply to other tetracyclines provided appropriate dosage adjustments were made. In a prospective, randomized, placebo-controlled trial in the Philippines, administration of penicillin G, 1.5 million IU intravenously every 6 hours, significantly reduced the duration of fever, clinical illness, and duration of hospital stay, and prevented leptospiruria even when started late in the course of a patient's disease.[29]

The clinical impression is that early bed rest may minimize subsequent morbidity. Azotemia and jaundice require meticulous attention to fluid and electrolyte therapy. Because the renal damage is reversible, patients with azotemia should be considered for peritoneal dialysis or hemodialysis.[33] Case reports have suggested that exchange transfusion is beneficial in the management of patients with extreme hyperbilirubinemia.

References

1. Alston JM, Broom JC. Leptospirosis in man and animals. Edinburgh, E & S Livingstone, 1958
2. Berman SJ, et al. Sporadic anicteric leptospirosis in South Vietnam: a study of 150 patients. Ann Intern Med 79:167, 1973
3. Bolin CA, Koellner P. Human to human transmission of Leptospira interrogans by milk. J Infect Dis 158:246, 1988
4. Centers for Disease Control. Summary of notifiable diseases, United States 1991. MMWR 40:53, 1991; 41:940, 1992
5. Ciceroni L, Pinto A, Cacciapuoti B. Recent trends in human leptospirosis in Italy. Eur J Epidemiol 4:49, 1988
6. Corwin A, Ryan A, Bloys W, Thomas R, Deniega B, Watts D. Waterborne outbreak of leptospirosis among United States military personnel in Okinawa, Japan. Int J Epidemiol 19:743, 1990
7. Damude DF, et al. The problem of human leptospirosis in Barbados. Trans R Soc Trop Med Hyg 73:169, 1979
8. Edwards GA, Domm M. Human leptospirosis. Medicine 39:177, 1960
9. Feigin RD, Anderson DC. Human leptospirosis. CRC Crit Rev Clin Lab Sci 5:413, 1975
10. Goldschmidt F. Ein Leintrag zur neuen infections krankheit Weil's. Dtsch Arch Klin Med 40:238, 1877
11. Heath CW Jr, Alexander AD. Leptospirosis in the United States: analysis of 483 cases in man, 1949–1961. N Engl J Med 273:857, 915, 1965
12. Inada R, et al. The etiology, mode of infection, and specific therapy of Weil's disease (spirochaetosis icterohaemorrhagiae). J Exp Med 23:377, 1916
13. Johnson RC. The biology of parasite spirochetes. New York, Academic Press, 1976
14. Johnson WD Jr, et al. Serum creatine phosphokinase in leptospirosis. JAMA 233:981, 1975
15. Laing RW, Teh C, Toh CH. Thrombotic thrombocytopenic purpura (TTP) complicating leptospirosis: a previously undescribed association. J Clin Pathol 43:961, 1990
16. Landouzy LTJ. Fievre bilieuse en hepatique. Gaz Hop (Paris) 56:809, 1883
17. Lecour H, Miranda M, Magro C, Rocha A, Goncalves V. Human leptospirosis: a review of 50 cases. Infection 17:8, 1989
18. McClain JB, et al. Doxycycline therapy for leptospirosis. Ann Intern Med 100:696, 1984
19. Noguchi H. Spirochaeta icterohaemorrhagiae in American wild rats and its relation to Japanese and European strains. J Exp Med 25:755, 1917
20. Park SK, Lee SH, Rhee YK, et al. Leptospirosis in Chonbuk Province of Korea in 1987: a study of 93 patients. Am J Trop Med Hyg 41:345, 1989
21. Sellards AW. The interpretation of (? Spirochaeta) interrogans of Stimson (1907) in the light of subsequent developments. Trans R Soc Trop Med Hyg 33:545, 1940
22. Shalit I, Barnea A, Shakar A. Efficacy of ciprofloxacin against *Leptospira interrogans* serogroup licterohaemorrhagiae. Antimicrob Agents Chemother 35:788, 1989
23. Shpilberg O, Shaked Y, Maier MK, Samra D, Samra Y. Long-term follow-up after leptospirosis. South Med J 83:405, 1990
24. Smith TF, et al. Pseudospirochetes, a cause of erroneous diagnosis of leptospirosis. Am J Clin Pathol 72:459, 1979
25. Stimson AM. Note on an organism found in yellow fever tissue. Public Health Rep 22:541, 1907
26. Takafuji ET, et al. An efficacy trial of doxycycline chemoprophylaxis against leptospirosis. N Engl J Med 310:497, 1984
27. Turner LH. Leptospirosis. Br Med J 1:537, 1973
28. Turner LH. Classification of spirochetes in general and of the genus *Leptospira* in particular. In: Johnson RC, ed. The biology of parasitic spirochetes. New York, Academic Press, 1976, pp 95–106
29. Watt G, Padre LP, Tuazon ML, Calubaquib C, Santiago E, Ranoa CP, Laughlin LW. Placebo-controlled trial of intravenous penicillin for severe and late leptospirosis. Lancet 1:433, 1988
30. Watt G, Alquiza LM, Padre LP, Tuazon ML, Laughlin LW. The rapid diagnosis of leptospirosis: a prospective comparison of the dot enzyme-linked immunosorbent assay and the genus specific microscopic agglutination test at different stages of illness. J Infect Dis 157:840, 1988
31. Watt G, Padre LP, Tuazon ML, Calubaquib C. Limulus lysate positivity and Herxheimer-like reactions in leptospirosis: a placebo-controlled study. J Infect Dis 162:564, 1990
32. Weil A. Uber eine eigentumliche mit Milztumor, Icterus und Nephirtis einbergehende akute infektions krankheit. Dtsch Arch Klin Med 39:209, 1886
33. Winearls CG, et al. Acute renal failure due to leptospirosis: clinical features and outcome in six cases. Q J Med 53:487, 1984
34. Wong ML, et al. Leptospirosis: a childhood disease. J Pediatr 90:532, 1977
35. World Health Organization. Tick-borne encephalitis and hemorrhagic fever with renal syndrome in Europe. EURO Reports and Studies No. 104. Copenhagen, WHO, 1986.

Diseases of the Liver, Seventh Edition, edited by
Leon Schiff and Eugene R. Schiff. J.B. Lippincott Company, Philadelphia © 1993.

49

Acquired Immunodeficiency Syndrome and the Liver

K. Rajender Reddy

Lennox J. Jeffers

Acquired immunodeficiency syndrome (AIDS), a retroviral infection caused by the human immunodeficiency virus (HIV), has generated more interest than any other single disease over the past decade. Practically every solid and hollow organ system has been noted to be involved in this syndrome, mainly by opportunistic infections and by tumors such as Kaposi's sarcoma and non-Hodgkin's lymphoma. The spectrum of hepatobiliary abnormalities noted is vast, with some specific abnormalities related to the liver and the biliary tract; more frequently, however, abnormalities within the liver are part of a systemic illness[6a,11,23,25,30,32,40a,55,67,68,81,81b,85,86,96,102,111,131,133] (Table 49-1).

Unusual biliary tract diseases are now well recognized as part of the syndrome.[1,7,14,17,38,42,48,54,56,57,74,76,105,112,128] Multiple illnesses may be noted at one point in time rather than a single event being responsible for an entire clinical picture. Furthermore, the many infections and neoplasms to which these patients are susceptible makes AIDS one of the few conditions in which newer hepatobiliary diagnoses are frequently considered due to observations of newer clinical features. Because of atypical clinical manifestations that are regularly being reported in this condition and because of unknown manifestations that are yet to be appreciated, the physician may need to deviate from a systematic approach and resort to an invasive procedure, such as liver biopsy or a cholangiogram, much earlier than would be done during the care of other acute and chronic liver diseases.

This chapter attempts to review the wide range of hepatobiliary abnormalities noted in AIDS patients, with the goal of helping physicians to apply this knowledge during their day-to-day practices involving AIDS patients.

Acute Human Immunodeficiency Virus Infection Syndrome

An acute mononucleosis-like syndrome due to HIV has been described in all AIDS risk groups, including health care workers. The clinical presentation is similar to infectious mononucleosis and includes fever, sweats, malaise, myalgia, anorexia, nausea, diarrhea, and nonexudative pharyngitis.[125] Skin rash, diffuse lymphadenopathy, and hepatosplenomegaly may occur, along with an elevation in serum transaminases and alkaline phosphatase.[29]

Immunohistochemical evidence of HIV in various components of the liver has been observed. Three different stain-

ing patterns by anti-P24–antibody have been observed in Kupffer cells, granulomas, probably histiocytes, and sinusoidal endothelial cells.[43] Similarly, in situ hybridization technique has noted HIV DNA in sinusoidal endothelial cells in a small number of hepatocytes in addition to the expected finding in lymphocytes.[69] Both macrophages and endothelial cells in the liver have been demonstrated to express CD4 molecule, a receptor for HIV.[114] These observations are of interest and significance and may be a step toward a better understanding of pathophysiologic mechanisms involved in the several unusual hepatic manifestations of AIDS.

Viral Hepatitis

Viral hepatitis A, B, C, and D infections commonly occur in high-risk groups such as homosexuals, intravenous drug abusers, and sexually promiscuous heterosexuals.[15] These groups also are at risk for HIV infection, and it is not uncommon to encounter more than one viral infection in patients from these populations. Hemophiliacs and health care workers are particularly at risk for hepatitis B and C infections as well as for HIV infection. Coinfections may be asymptomatic or clinically evident as chronic liver disease. Immune mechanisms are invoked in the pathogenesis of hepatitis B virus (HBV) infection; therefore, its expression may be altered by HIV. Hepatitis C virus (HCV) and hepatitis D virus (HDV) are well-known parenterally transmitted infections, and their expression has been studied in HIV-positive individuals, although not much has been written on this subject.[34,61,75,79]

HEPATITIS A

Hepatitis A virus (HAV) is transmitted by a fecal–oral route and is caused by an RNA virus that results in acute, but not chronic, hepatitis. Although HAV infection has far greater significance in developing countries, where it can be seen in epidemic proportions, it has been observed among promiscuous homosexuals and intravenous drug abusers in the Western world. Anal–oral transmission most likely occurs among homosexuals, and parenteral exposure by contaminated needles, although infrequent, is most likely responsible for HAV infection among intravenous drug abusers.[15,19] A higher seroprevalence (30%) of antibody to HAV (anti-HAV) has been noted among homosexual men as compared with heterosexual controls.[19] Superimposed fulminant HAV in in-

TABLE 49-1　*Diseases Affecting the Hepatobiliary System and Histologic Changes in AIDS*

Viral Hepatitis	*AIDS Cholangiopathy*
Hepatitis A	Acalculous cholecystitis
Hepatitis B	Sclerosing cholangitis
Hepatitis C (non-A, non-B)	Papillary stenosis
Hepatitis D	Lymphoma of the biliary tree
Cytomegalovirus	
Epstein-Barr virus	*Neoplasms*
Herpes simplex virus	Kaposi's sarcoma
Human immunodeficiency	Non-Hodgkin's lymphoma
virus	Hodgkin's lymphoma
	(infrequent)
Opportunistic Infections	
Mycobacterium avium–	*Drug-Induced Hepatitis*
intracellulare	See Table 49-2
Cryptosporidium	
Pneumocystis carinii	*Histologic Findings*
Mycobacterium tuberculosis	Steatosis (fatty liver)
Coccidioides immitis	Granulomatous hepatitis
Candida albicans	Portal inflammation
Histoplasma capsulatum	Sinusoidal dilation
Cryptococcus neoformans	Bacillary peliosis hepatis

travenous drug abusers with chronic liver disease has been reported.[2] Acute HAV infection in homosexual men and intravenous drug abusers may have a more severe course, which is possibly related to the presence of underlying chronic liver disease.[2,65] Recently, an inactivated hepatitis A vaccine was licensed in the United Kingdom and in a few European countries that has been shown to be immunogenic in 99.8% of patients after two doses.[41] We hope that this vaccine will also be licensed in the United States, so that it can be targeted at high-risk groups for this infection.

HEPATITIS B AND D

A higher seroprevalence of HbsAg and delta antigen has been noted in patients with AIDS as compared with those without AIDS, perhaps secondary to a greater degree of immunosuppression, facilitating viral replication.[61] Antibodies to delta antigen, however, were noted more often in non-AIDS patients, a finding probably related to a relatively better immunogenic state.[61] Although there may be differences in prevalence of delta markers between AIDS and non-AIDS, in two studies an influence on HBV and HDV replication was not noted to be modified by HIV infection.[34,79] Clinical evidence of more severe liver disease, however, has been observed in HDV-HBV–coinfected patients in the presence of HIV infection.[82] Chronic viral hepatitis B is immunologically mediated; therefore, its clinical course and viral expression may be altered by HIV, a virus with significant influence on the host immune system. There is direct and circumstantial evidence to support the view that HBV infection is immunologically mediated, and an immunoincompetent host is more likely to have chronic hepatitis B.[23a] Transmission of HBV and HDV occurs parenterally and sexually, although HDV is less efficiently transmitted sexually and is relatively a greater problem in other geographic areas than in North America.[61,79] It is not uncommon to see HBV and HDV in HIV-infected patients since these infections share similar modes of transmission.[34,61,79]

In HIV–HBV coinfection, a higher degree of viral replication as represented by increased DNA polymerase has been observed.[31,90] In addition, a more significant immunohistochemical demonstration of hepatitis B core antigen (HBcAg) and hepatitis B e antigen (HBeAg) in the liver has been noted in HIV–HBV coinfection as compared with HBV infection alone.[31,78] Furthermore, serum aminotransferases in HIV-positive patients are significantly lower than those in HIV-negative patients, and this has been associated with a lower degree of hepatocellular necrosis (Color Fig. 29E and F), which again is thought to be due to immune tolerance for HBV facilitated by HIV-related immunosuppression.[63,77,90,106] Rustgi and coworkers[106] have suggested that HIV infection in chronic hepatitis B may lead to amelioration of hepatocyte necrosis and facilitate a high viremic state. Reactivation of both HBV and HDV infections related to subsequent infection with HIV have been reported, and this is analogous to HBV reactivation seen in cancer, chemotherapy, and other immunoincompetent states.[117] In HIV infection, reappearance of hepatitis B surface antigen (HBsAg) has been observed in previously HBsAg-negative patients, in patients positive for antibody to HBsAg, and in patients positive for antibody to HBcAg.[66,86a,126] Experience to the contrary, however, with no correlation between viral replication, immunohistochemical expression of viral markers, and disease activity, has also been reported.[91,100] Similarly, there has been lack of correlation between fulminant viral hepatitis and the presence or absence of antibody to HIV (anti-HIV).[3] One can gather from the various studies reported that a spectrum of changes is seen in patients with multiple infections (HBV, HDV, HIV). There is even a report of HIV infection facilitating progression of HBV-related liver disease on to liver failure and death.[43a]

Most patients with AIDS have serologic markers of HBV infection, although many have evidence of past infection rather than ongoing viral replication.[32,106] One can postulate that exposure to HBV infection occurred before exposure to HIV infection and that these patients were able to seroconvert because, if it occurred after HIV infection, HBV infection most likely would progress to chronic hepatitis B.[36] In HIV-infected individuals exposed to HBV, the likelihood of progression on to HBV carrier stage has been observed to be several times higher than that in HIV-negative individuals.[36,122]

Efforts to prevent HBV among high-risk groups through administration of hepatitis B vaccine have been ongoing for several years. HIV-infected patients had a suboptimal (less than 70%) response to HBV vaccine, as compared with a 90% response in the immunocompetent population.[13,18,35] This difference is independent of lymphocyte subsets, status of cutaneous delayed hypersensitivity, and presence or absence of cytomegalovirus (CMV) infection.[18] Furthermore, revaccination in HIV-positive nonresponders and suboptimal responders had poor results, as compared with the 50% response rate seen in HIV-negative patients after revaccination.[35,35a] HIV-infected homosexuals who did respond to the vaccine, however, demonstrated short- and long-term protection for up to 7 years, similar to the immunocompetent population.[35,35a]

α-Interferon (α-IFN) has been extensively evaluated in the treatment of chronic hepatitis B and has been shown to decrease the HBV replicative state.[90a] Several poor prognostic features for response have been observed, among which is HIV infection.[77] Additionally, homosexuality, independent of HIV status, has been a factor associated with suboptimal response, which is most likely related to the observed immunologic changes in this group.[21,92]

Despite conflicting and contradictory data, the opinion emerges that HIV-related immunosuppression does alter expression of HBV markers, severity of liver disease, and response to hepatitis B vaccination and α-interferon treatment. Furthermore, delta infection may adversely influence the severity of liver disease in HBV and HIV infections.

HEPATITIS C

Unlike HBV, which is efficiently transmitted parenterally and sexually, HCV is a predominantly parenterally transmitted infection and therefore is more prevalent in intravenous drug abusers than in homosexuals. Supporting evidence for a predominant parenteral transmission of HCV is the high seroprevalence of HCV markers in parenteral drug abusers,[26b] which parallels HBV markers, in contrast to the lower seroprevalence of HCV markers than HBV markers among homosexuals.[78a] HCV–HIV coinfection, however, appears to increase the sexual transmission of HCV, presumably through HIV-influenced increase in hepatitis C viremia.[26c]

The influence of HIV on the natural history of chronic hepatitis C has not been as well evaluated as its influence on chronic hepatitis B. One brief report[75] has implied that the clinical course of posttransfusion non-A, non-B (presumably C) chronic hepatitis may be adversely influenced by HIV infection. Characteristic features of this study included an elderly population, a 3% seroprevalence of anti-HIV, and transfusion as the mode of acquisition of HIV and non-A, non-B hepatitis infections.[75]

α-IFN is used in the treatment of chronic hepatitis C in anti-HIV–negative patients. Adverse immunologic effects of HIV, influencing the response to α-IFN, appear to have persuaded investigators to exclude HIV-infected patients in large studies. A report that evaluated α-IFN in HIV–HCV coinfections has noted similar responses to chronic hepatitis C without HIV infection.[9]

Other Viral Infections

Cytomegalovirus infection is common in AIDS patients, and the spectrum can range from mere evidence of past CMV infection, as noted in homosexuals,[64,80] to a fulminant and disseminated illness.[30,48,81,81b,102] Both a hepatitis-like illness and biliary tract disease may be seen as a consequence of this infection (see section on cholangiopathy), and a predominant elevation of alkaline phosphatase may be seen biochemically.[48,88] Intranuclear inclusion bodies, producing an owl's eye sign within the hepatocytes, vascular endothelial cells, and biliary endothelium, are well-recognized features in association with a granulomatous reaction.[7,14,30,38]

By in situ hybridization techniques, viral DNA of CMV, herpes simplex virus, Epstein-Barr virus, HBV, HIV, and human T-cell leukemia/lymphoma virus type I have been noted in nuclei and cytoplasm of hepatocytes, monocytes, and lymphocytes and in perisinusoidal lining cells. Some of these viruses also expressed DNA in the biliary epithelium.[69] These viruses have been noted as multiple infections in several patients and, furthermore, without clinical manifestations of these infections.[69]

Fulminant hepatitis due to herpes simplex virus type II[137] or adenovirus[62] is rare.

Drug-Induced Hepatitis

It is not uncommon for a patient with AIDS to be taking multiple hepatotoxic drugs.[6a,69a,113a] These drugs may be used to treat an opportunistic infection or may be primarily directed at HIV. Isoniazid, rifampin, and trimethoprim-sulfamethoxazole are the most common among the potentially hepatotoxic drugs responsible for hepatic dysfunction (Table 49-2). Most often, the drugs cause a hepatitis-like clinical and biochemical picture, but affected patients may have a cholestatic biochemical profile, particularly if they have hepatic involvement by an infection or neoplasm. Zidovudine can cause a mixed hepatitis–cholestasis profile,[24a] and 2'3'-deoxyinosine causes a predominant hepatitis-like illness. 2'3'-Deoxyinosine has rarely been implicated in fulminant hepatic failure.[58a] Underlying poor nutritional status or the concomitant use of cytochrome P-450 inducers may increase susceptibility to various drugs. The decision to continue or discontinue a drug should depend on the certainty of the diagnosis, severity of the illness, availability of alternative drugs, and likelihood of a particular drug causing hepatitis. It is prudent to stop the implicated drug if the patient develops jaundice and to switch to alternative, equally effective drugs if available.

Opportunistic Infections

A multitude of opportunistic bacterial and fungal infections have been found in the liver. Mycobacterial infections have been noted consistently in the liver both antemortem and at autopsy.[9a,30,32,40,55,58,67,70,81,85,94,97,102,111] Most often, *Mycobacterium avium-intracellulare* (MAI) organisms have been noted,[40,59,70] and occasionally, atypical mycobacteria have been responsible for infection, including *M xenopi*[26a] and *M kansasii*.[110] The incidence of *M tuberculosis* infection in the liver generally has trailed MAI, except in the Haitian subpopulation, where it has been more common than atypical mycobacteria.[32] Often, hepatic granulomas (Color Fig. 29A) are noted in association with these infections, and these usually are ill-formed granulomas[32,55,70] (see Color Fig. 29B). A poor granulomatous response in AIDS is not surprising because of suppressed T-lymphocyte activity, which is necessary for expression of granulomatous hypersensitivity. It is uncommon to see a well-formed granuloma, which, in the case of MAI, is composed of foamy blue histiocytes with abundant acid-fast bacilli on special stains (see Color Fig. 29C and D). Because the immunoincompetent state fails to elicit a granulomatous reaction, only acid-fast organisms have been noted on special stains.[32] Cultures of liver biopsy specimens do yield these organisms, but a diagnosis is often established on histopathologic evaluation with special stains.[32,85,111] A predominant elevation of alkaline phosphatase has been observed,[12,55] but this has not been a consistent feature.[32]

TABLE 49-2   *Drugs Used in the Treatment of Acquired Immunodeficiency Syndrome*

Drug Category	Hepatocellular	Cholestatic	Granulomatous	Mixed
Analgesics	Acetaminophen Ibuprofen Indomethacin Salicylates	Propoxyphene		Naproxen Piroxicam Sulindac
Anticonvulsants	Diphenylhydantoin Valproate*	Diphenylhydantoin	Diphenylhydantoin	Carbamazephine Phenobarbital

Antimicrobials	Amphotericin B
	Clindamycin
	Ethionamide
	Isoniazid
	Ketoconazole
	Metronidazole
	Oxacillin
	Aminosalicylic acid
	Pentamidine
	Pyrazinamide
	Quinacrine
	Rifampin†
	Sulfonamides
	Sulfones (dapsone)
	Tetracycline*
	Trimethoprim–
	  sulfamethoxazole
	Zidovudine
		Carbenicillin
		Erythromycin
		Ketoconazole
		Rifampin
		Thiabendazole
		Trimethoprim–
		  sulfamethoxazole
		Zidovudine
			Trimethoprim–
			  sulfamethoxazole
				Trimethoprim–
				  sulfamethoxazole

Miscellaneous	Disulfiram Vitamin A Prochlorperazine	Anabolic steroids Chlorpromazine Contraceptive steroids Prochlorperazine		Chlordiazepoxide Diazepam

*Microvesicular steatosis may occur.
†Cholestasis predominates, but hepatocellular damage may also occur.
(Adapted from Lewis JH, Zimmerman HJ. Drug-induced liver disease. Med Clinic North Am 73:775–792, 1989; Schwarz ED, Greene JB. Diagnostic considerations in the human immunodeficiency virus–infected patient with gastrointestinal or abdominal symptoms. Semin Liv Dis 12:142–153, 1992; and Bach N, Thelse ND, Schaffner F. Hepatic histopathology in the acquired immunodeficiency syndrome. Semin Liver Dis 12:205–212, 1992).

Opportunistic fungal infections that involve the liver usually are part of a disseminated disease.[16] Cryptococcal hepatitis[8,60,120] (see Color Fig. 29H) occurs along with cryptococcal meningoencephalitis, and this is associated with significantly elevated alkaline phosphatase.[30,32] Mucicarmine-positive cryptococcal organisms are noted histologically. *Histoplasma capsulatum*,[4,9a,16,44,109] *Candida albicans*,[27,37,51,87] *Sporothrix schenckii*,[71] and *Coccidioides immitis*[111] are other fungal infections that have occurred as part of a disseminated process, and nonspecific biochemical or radiologic characteristics can be attributed to these infections. Special stains and cultures are helpful in establishing these diagnoses when atypical clinical features are present.[16]

Protozoan infections of the liver are relatively infrequently encountered. *Pneumocystis carinii* infection often causes pneumonia, with occasional dissemination to various organs, including the liver.[28,72,98,99,107,134] *P carinii* hepatitis has occurred in patients on inhaled pentamidine, indicating that such prophylaxis only prevented pulmonary pneumocystosis.[93] An associated hypoalbuminemia may be related to underlying poor nutritional status.[93] Visceral leishmaniansis[26] with hepatic involvement has also been reported.[133]

Sinusoidal Abnormalities

A spectrum of sinusoidal abnormalities that includes sinusoidal dilation, perisinusoidal fibrosis, and peliosis hepatis has been observed in AIDS.[20,22,89,114,115] Often, the sinusoidal dilation is an incidental finding, has no zonal predilection, and is of no major clinical consequence. An ultrastructural study specifically examined sinusoidal dilation in HIV infection, and lesions of the sinusoidal barrier were noted mainly as a predominance of numerous hyperplastic sinusoidal macrophages.[114,115] In situ hybridization and immunohistochemical studies have noted HIV in the liver, and it has been postulated that endothelial cell injury and sinusoidal dilation may be directly or indirectly related to the presence of HIV.[43,114,115]

Peliosis hepatis represents a blood-filled cystic space in hepatic parenchyma that often does not have an endothelial lining; this is a common finding in AIDS (see Color Fig. 29G). Before its description in AIDS, peliosis hepatis was seen as a consequence of chronic infections, such as pulmonary tuberculosis; advanced malignancy; and use of anabolic steroids and other drugs, such as azathioprine.[129,135]

Clinically, patients may have abdominal pain associated with hepatomegaly, but it is most likely to be an incidental finding either antemortem or at autopsy.[20,22,29] Transaminases may be mildly or moderately elevated, with a relatively higher alkaline phosphatase, and computed tomography (CT) may show defects.[20,89] Microscopically, these are multiple, randomly distributed lesions; and laparoscopically, they are multiple, tiny, 2- to 4-mm blue-red areas on the liver surface.[20,50]

Convincing evidence indicates that peliosis hepatis associated with HIV infection is caused by a bacillus and therefore should be termed *bacillary peliosis hepatis*.[89] A histopathologic and ultrastructural study looked at HIV-associated peliosis hepatis in comparison with HIV-negative peliosis hepatis and noted clumpy, granular, purple material on Warthin-Starry stain that ultrastructurally proved to be bacilli. Furthermore, there was an associated cutaneous bacillary angiomatosis in HIV-positive patients that was not an accompaniment of HIV-negative peliosis. Additional associated conditions included Kaposi's sarcoma of the skin, abdominal lymphadenopathy, and infections such as MAI and *Cryptococcus neoformans*. A subsequent study led to the identification of the bacillus known to cause bacillary peliosis hepatis and cutaneous bacillary angiomatosis.[118] Using murine antiserum studies, electrophoretic patterns of outer membrane proteins, and restriction endonuclease digestion patterns of DNA, the bacillus has been designated *Rochalimaea henselae*, a fastidious, gram-negative bacillus distinct from *R quintana*, which is the etiologic agent of trench fever.

The pathogenetic mechanisms involved in the induction of peliosis hepatis are unclear, although one speculation is that the bacillus elaborates an angiogenic factor similar to one elaborated by *Bartonella bacilliformis*,[29a] and clinical response to erythromycin in bacillary peliosis hepatis has been noted.[89] Additional cofactors may be direct HIV infection of the liver, associated HIV-related cachexia syndrome, and granulomatous hepatitis related to one or more infections. Kaposi's sarcoma, a vascular neoplasm seen often in AIDS, may be considered at the extreme end of the spectrum of sinusoidal abnormalities, with sinusoidal dilation and angiosarcomatous changes merely representing transitional stages.[22]

Lipid-laden perisinusoidal cells, along with hypertrophy of Kupffer cells and endothelial cell inclusions, have been noted in AIDS.[24] This, conceivably, could be due to hypervitaminosis A, although this has not been proved, and it may represent a nonspecific finding, possibly induced by drugs or systemic or hepatic infections.

Fatty Infiltration

Fatty infiltration of the liver is perhaps the single most common abnormality in AIDS, both clinically and histologically.[32,111] It may be related to the underlying cachexia syndrome or may be due to hyperalimentation, or may be associated with drugs or infections, particularly hepatitis C. Clinically, significant hepatomegaly may be noted, associated with a predominantly elevated alkaline phosphatase. Symptoms such as fevers, jaundice, and pruritus are absent. Ultrasound examination may identify fatty infiltration, but CT scan should depict the decreased density of the liver and thus is more definitive. Microscopically, macrovesicular fat is noted, which is randomly distributed throughout the lobule without any zonal predilection. A rare case of Reye's syndrome, causing microvesicular fat, has been reported in an adult with AIDS.[52] Steatohepatitis is uncommon, and liver failure or portal hypertension due to these observations are not noted.[9a,32] Fat, however, can be a part of alcoholic hepatitis, in which case the clinical features may be similar to alcoholic hepatitis in the HIV-negative patient.

Cholangiopathy

Cholangiopathy is a well-recognized entity in AIDS, and patients present with one or more of the following symptoms, mimicking bacterial cholangitis: fever, right upper quadrant abdominal pain, nausea, vomiting, jaundice, and hepatomegaly.[14,38,74,105,112] AIDS cholangiopathy, however, is often a nonbacterial infection and is predominantly caused by CMV and *Cryptosporidium* sp. It can be of noninfectious cause, and it is rarely caused by Kaposi's sarcoma[14] or non–cleaved-cell lymphoma infiltrating the biliary tree.[56] Sometimes, despite extensive search, the cause remains unknown. Because HIV has been identified in small and large bowel mucosa,[82a] a direct HIV infection of the biliary mucosa has been suggested as a cause of AIDS cholangiopathy.[14] AIDS cholangiopathy has been reported predominantly in homosexuals.[14,38,74]

Hepatic biochemical tests may reveal a predominant elevation of alkaline phosphatase, and hyperbilirubinemia may be seen.[14,105] Ultrasonography often demonstrates a dilated intrahepatic and extrahepatic biliary tree; therefore, CT is seldom necessary.[14] The diagnosis is established by cholangiography, and endoscopic retrograde cholangiopancreatography (ERCP) has been the preferred route over transhepatic cholangiogram. Dilation of the extrahepatic bile ducts is often due to stenosis of the papilla of Vater. A radiologic picture mimicking sclerosing cholangitis is not unusual; a serrated intrahepatic and extrahepatic biliary tree with irregularities of the wall are noted. A focal, irregular beaded appearance of the intrahepatic biliary radicles is common. Irregularities of the bile duct may be pronounced, which may be due to connective tissue swelling and thickening. The observed cholangiographic abnormalities can be categorized into four groups: (1) sclerosing cholangitis and papillary stenosis, (2) papillary stenosis alone (Fig. 49-1), (3) sclerosing cholangitis alone, and (4) long, extrahepatic bile duct strictures.[14,76] ERCP facilitates therapeutic intervention through papillotomy and biliary tree stent placement and also provides an opportunity to establish the cause of cholangiopathy.[14,74,112] Endoscopic ampullary biopsies have revealed CMV intranuclear inclusions and associated chronic inflammatory changes.[14] Similarly, *Cryptosporidium* sp and MAI organisms have been recovered from periampullary and duodenal biopsy specimens. Biopsy of surgically removed gallbladders has revealed intranuclear inclusions of CMV along with numerous *Cryptosporidium* sp organisms attached to gland epithelium.[7] Ultrastructurally, trophozoite and mature schizont *Cryptosporidium* sp organisms have been noted. Oocysts of cryptosporidium have been identified in bile and stool specimens using a modified acid-fast stain. Hepatic histology either is normal or demonstrates mild, nonspecific portal or focal inflammation with associated mild cholestasis.[105] Hepatobiliary cryptosporidiosis and CMV infection may mimic metastatic cancer to the liver.[38,127] A simultaneous cryptosporidial involvement of the gastrointestinal tract

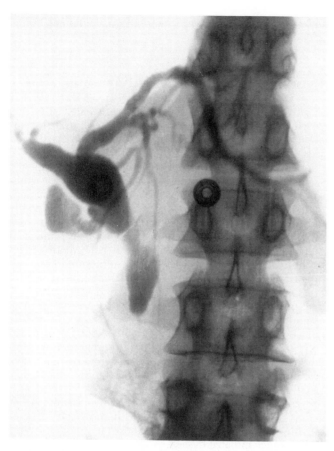

FIGURE 49-1   ERCP demonstration of papillary stenosis due to cryptosporidial infection in AIDS. (Courtesy of Nezam H. Afdhal, MD, Boston City Hospital)

has led to the postulation that the infection may reach the liver and gallbladder by a contiguous spread from the gastrointestinal tract.[14] Although logic dictates that endoscopic intervention with papillotomy and stent placement would relieve symptoms and biochemical abnormalities, observations that have not demonstrated a consistent benefit have been made. Pain relief has been observed, but alkaline phosphatase levels have been noted to progressively rise despite stents and decreases in ductal dilation; this phenomenon is most likely due to intrahepatic sclerosing cholangitis.[14,76,112]

CMV dissemination appears to precede the development of cholestatic liver enzymes and cholangiopathy.[48] About one third of patients with disseminated CMV infection were noted to develop, within 3 months, cholestatic liver enzymes, and in a third of these patients, there was radiologic evidence of cholangiopathy.[48] Ganciclovir treatment has not influenced the course of cholestatic abnormalities.[48]

AIDS-related cholangiopathy, unlike primary idiopathic sclerosing cholangitis, is sometimes associated with cholecystitis. An acute cholecystitis has been observed histologically, along with gangrenous change, hemorrhagic mucosal necrosis, acute and chronic inflammation, edema, and mucosal ulceration with fibrinous material. The cholecystitis may be of both calculous and acalculous variety. CMV and *Cryptosporidium* sp are often implicated in cholecystitis,[1,7,55,57,105] and *Candida albicans*,[17] and *Salmonella typhimurium*[105] are

infrequently responsible. Cholecystitis is often due to opportunistic infections. Rarely, gram-negative bacteria, *Klebsiella pneumoniae* and *Pseudomonas aeruginosa*, have been cultured from the gallbladder.[7]

AIDS-related cholangiopathy is one of the few conditions in AIDS patients for which therapeutic intervention most likely is of some help, particularly in improving the quality of life. An endoscopic sphincterotomy can be done and often provides relief in papillary stenosis. Similarly, biliary tract stenting provides relief of symptoms. No medical therapy directed at either *Cryptosporidium* sp or CMV has been shown to be of benefit. Surgical intervention is seldom carried out unless there is concern about gangrenous cholecystitis. The patient may be too ill to tolerate surgery, and transhepatic cholecystostomy is an alternative in patients with acute cholecystitis.

Laparoscopy

Limited experience has been reported with laparoscopy in AIDS partly because of the lack of widespread familiarity with this procedure. Several observations have been made, including ascites with high protein content ranging from 3.1 to 5.4 g/dL.[50,132] Laparoscopically, most often, these patients were noted to have non-Hodgkin's lymphoma involving the peritoneum and liver. Multiple white, raised plaques have been described on the peritoneum along with multiple 2- to 5-mm nodules on omentum in non-Hodgkin's lymphoma. Peritoneal and hepatic plaque-like lesions are not specific for lymphoma, however, and have been observed in disseminated cryptococcosis and *P carinii* infections. Likewise, tiny (smaller than 5 mm in diameter) nodular lesions have occurred as a consequence of mycobacterial infections. Histologically, caseating and noncaseating granulomas with acid-fast bacilli have been reported, and cultures have been positive for *M tuberculosis* and MAI; occasional cases of splenic abscesses due to *M tuberculosis* have been noted. Chylous ascites has been an infrequent observation. Massive intraabdominal adhesions, some with the appearance of violin strings, have been observed, and these were often due to *M tuberculosis*.

Unusual causes of peritonitis in AIDS include toxoplasmosis[47] and coccidioidomycosis.[10] A nonspecific chronic peritonitis has been described laparoscopically for which a clearcut cause has not been determined, even at autopsy.[132] HIV infection previously was noted to be associated with nonspecific pericarditis, meningitis, pneumonitis, and glomerulonephritis, and this leads to speculation about whether a nonspecific peritonitis may have been directly caused by HIV infection. CMV infection was excluded in cases of nonspecific peritonitis using polymerase chain reaction for viral DNA, but the possibility of other bizarre or unknown infections has not been ruled out because ultrastructural studies have not been done in these patients.[132]

Laparoscopically, cirrhosis has been noted in some AIDS patients,[50,101] which is not surprising given the likelihood that they may be alcoholic[49] or have either HBV[49] or HCV infection. Ascites in such cases, if present, has a low-protein content.[101] Identification of *Salmonella enteritidis* group B as the cause of spontaneous bacterial peritonitis in a cirrhotic patient with ascites has led to the diagnosis of AIDS in one patient. Spontaneous salmonella bacteremia has been well described in AIDS but is an uncommon cause of spontaneous bacterial peritonitis in cirrhotic patients with ascites. Laparoscopy has also been helpful in diagnosing Kaposi's sarcoma involving the liver; and in one case, the diagnosis of Kaposi's sarcoma in a patient with a markedly elevated alkaline phosphatase led to the diagnosis of AIDS.[39]

Liver Disease in Pediatric Patients With AIDS

The range of hepatobiliary abnormalities has not been well evaluated in pediatric AIDS patients as compared with adults with AIDS. A large retrospective autopsy study noted several histologic abnormalities either singly or in combination, and these included giant cell transformation, CMV inclusions, Kaposi's sarcoma, diffuse lymphoplasmacytic infiltrate, granulomatous hepatitis, mild portal inflammation, necrosis around central veins, steatosis, and cholestasis.[53] To a large extent, abnormalities noted within the liver were nonspecific and not reflective of pathology noted elsewhere. Diffuse parenchymal lymphoplasmacytic infiltrate was noted in two children, and they had associated lymphoid interstitial pneumonitis. Giant cell hepatitis had a higher frequency, with a lower frequency of granulomas in children as compared with adults. Otherwise, the abnormalities were comparable to findings in adult AIDS patients. Biliary tree abnormalities similar to those found in AIDS cholangiopathy were not noted in pediatric patients. This may be due to various factors: study of pediatric AIDS patients being an autopsy study[53]; cholangiographic studies are more difficult to perform in pediatric patients, particularly via endoscopic route; and finally, pediatric AIDS patients represent a minority of all patients with AIDS. Kaposi's sarcoma and lymphoma were noted in children under 2 years of age, indicating that tumors can occur early in life.[53] Chronic active hepatitis has been reported in children with HIV infection.[23b,124]

Ultrastructural Changes

Only a few ultrastructural studies of the liver, with the exception of one large study evaluating changes in peliosis hepatis and sinusoidal dilatation,[115] have been reported involving case reports. An earlier report described ultrastructural changes in the liver in immunocompromised humans that were similar to changes seen in chimpanzees inoculated with NANB hepatitis sera.[130] Cytoplasmic tubular structures and clusters of 23-nm double-shelled particles were seen that were distinct from several of the commonly noticed viral particles, such as Dane particles, Epstein-Barr virus, CMV, and herpes simplex virus. Further work in this arena remains to be done, and the significance of these findings is unknown. A more interesting observation has been the identification of a microsporidian protozoan of the genus *Encephalitozoon* in a patient with AIDS that caused a clinical hepatitis-like illness.[123] Light microscopy revealed focal granulomatous and suppurative necrosis, chiefly in the portal areas, and gram-positive, cocci-like organisms were noted on a hematoxylin–eosin stain. Ultrastructurally, several spores, sporoblasts, and a sporont of *E cuniculi* were noted, and this infection proved to be fatal. This was the first morphologic documentation of *E cuniculi* in humans.

Lymphoma and Kaposi's Sarcoma

It is well recognized that AIDS is associated with the development of lymphoma, chiefly non-Hodgkin's lymphoma.[45,46,84,103,113,136a] Lymphomas most often have been seen in male homosexuals and are of the B-cell and non-B, non-T–cell types.[46,136a] Hodgkin's lymphoma is infrequently seen.[46] Extranodal involvement of multiple organs is significantly higher than is seen in lymphomas in the general population, and these are highly aggressive and respond poorly to treatment, often resulting in early death.[46,136a] About 10% of patients with lymphomas appear to have liver involvement, and a common extranodal site is bone marrow. Hepatic involvement may be detected on ultrasound examination as small hypoechoic nodules.[73] CT scan is more helpful because it also evaluates the spleen and retroperitoneum.[84,113] Features noted on imaging studies are suggestive but not diagnostic, and a definitive diagnosis can be made by CT-guided biopsy or laparoscopy.[50,84,132] Since bone marrow involvement is more frequent, however, a bone marrow aspiration and biopsy should be considered before more invasive procedures (CT-guided or laparoscopic biopsy) are undertaken.

Kaposi's sarcoma is the most common neoplasm in AIDS and is seen predominantly in male homosexuals.[40a] Frequently, hepatic involvement is diagnosed postmortem and is part of a disseminated disease. Abdominal pain and hepatosplenomegaly with predominant elevation of alkaline phosphatase may be the clinical features in the occasional case diagnosed antemortem.[39] Ultrasonography[73] and CT may demonstrate defects within the liver and spleen that appear hypoattenuated with enhancement on delayed scans; these features, however, are not specific for Kaposi's sarcoma. Laparoscopically, they are seen as soft, purple, 2- to 3-mm nodules.[50]

The protean hepatobiliary manifestations reported in AIDS are in a unique category because they often are not seen in other hepatobiliary diseases. Hepatic biochemical test abnormalities are common with or without associated symptoms or signs of acute or chronic liver disease. The abnormalities may be due to medications, concomitant chronic viral hepatitis, and alcohol abuse. Significant fatty infiltration may be responsible in some cases, and there may be associated hepatomegaly with evidence of it better appreciated by CT than ultrasonography. Jaundice may be due to significant drug-related hepatotoxicity or AIDS cholangiopathy, but it is seldom due to opportunistic infections and tumors, unless the tumors were strategically located in the portal region, obstructing or directly involving the biliary tree. A spectrum of vascular lesions has been reported, and bacillary peliosis hepatis is unique to this condition. AIDS cholangiopathy represents one of the few conditions in which symptomatic relief can be provided with appropriate intervention. Therefore, evidence of a dilated biliary tree on ultrasound should be an indication for cholangiographic study with therapeutic intervention as necessary (ie, papillotomy with or without stent placement).

The decision to perform a percutaneous liver biopsy is important and should be made after carefully evaluating the potential risks and benefits. There has been an anecdotal report of significant bleeding after percutaneous biopsy in these patients, even in the absence of an overt coagulation disorder.[33] Liver biopsy may be performed to evaluate persistent abnormal hepatic biochemical tests in the absence of any symptoms that might be considered of hepatobiliary origin. More often, however, percutaneous biopsy should be considered in patients with abnormal hepatic biochemical tests associated with unexplained fevers or hepatomegaly with or without abdominal pain. Imaging studies such as ultrasonography and CT may help identify neoplastic involvement of the liver, spleen, and abdominal lymph nodes. In these patients, a guided liver biopsy, either laparoscopically or radiologically, is preferable to a blind percutaneous biopsy. Ascites is best evaluated laparoscopically, but the technical capability may not be available at all institutions. It is uncommon to see an opportunistic infection solely confined to the liver; it usually is part of a multisystem disease. Therefore, less invasive studies, such as bone marrow biopsy and even bronchoscopy, should be considered for diagnosing a multisystem disease before percutaneous liver biopsy. However, some data support doing a percutaneous liver biopsy first because this procedure had a higher yield than bone marrow aspiration biopsy in detecting mycobacterial infection.[95]

Although a great deal of knowledge has been accumulated on intrahepatic diseases in AIDS diagnosed by liver biopsy, the usefulness of the information regarding its influence on implementing proper therapy and thereby influencing survival has been questioned.[111] Among the several invasive diagnostic modalities available in hepatobiliary diseases, cholangiography, particularly ERCP, is the least controversial because of its therapeutic potential. Laparoscopy has been helpful in evaluating patients with ascites, particularly high-protein ascites, and this has helped establish several diagnoses, including lymphoma, mycobacterial disease, and other conditions, such as *P carinii* and *Cryptosporidium* sp infections.[50,132] The debate regarding the role of liver biopsy is likely to continue until definitive data are produced, particularly regarding its influence on management and survival. It is prudent, however, to continue to evaluate hepatic histology in carefully selected patients to gain new information with potentially diagnostic and therapeutic value on a condition that is in a state of rapid evolution.

References

1. Aaron JS, Wynter CD, Kirton OC, et al. Cytomegalovirus associated with acalculous cholecystitis in a patient with acquired immunodeficiency syndrome. Am J Gastroenterol 83:879–881, 1988
2. Akriviadis EA, Redeker AG. Fulminant hepatitis A in intravenous drug abusers with chronic liver disease. Ann Intern Med 110:838–839, 1989
3. Amoroso P, Lettieri G, Giorgio A, et al. Lack of correlation between fulminant form of viral hepatitis and retrovirus infection associated with the acquired immune deficiency virus (AIDS) in drug addicts. Br Med J 292:376–377, 1986
4. Ankobiah WA, Vaidya K, Powell S, et al. Disseminated histoplasmosis in AIDS: clinicopathologic features in seven patients from a non-endemic area. NY State J Med 90:234–238, 1990
6a. Bach N, Theise ND, Schaffner F. Hepatic histopathology in AIDS. Semin Liv Dis 12:205–212, 1992
7. Blumberg RS, Kelsey P, Perrone T, et al. Cytomegalovirus and cryptosporidium associated acalculous gangrenous cholecystitis. Am J Med 76:1118–1123, 1984
8. Bonacini M, Nussbaum J, Ahluwalia C. Gastrointestinal, hepatic, and pancreatic involvement with Cryptococcus neoformans in AIDS. J Clin Gastroenterol 12:295–297, 1990
9. Boyer N, Marcellin P, Degott C, et al. Recombinant interferon-α for chronic hepatitis C in patients positive for antibody to human immunodeficiency virus. J Infect Dis 165:723–726, 1992
9a. Boylston AW, Cook HT, Francis ND, et al. Biopsy pathology of AIDS. J Clin Pathol 40:1–8, 1982
10. Byrne WR, Dietrich RA. Disseminated coccidioidomycosis with peritonitis in a patient with the acquired immunodeficiency syndrome: prolonged survival associated with skin test reactivity to coccioidin. Arch Intern Med 149:947–948, 1989
11. Cappell MS. Hepatobiliary manifestations of the acquired immune deficiency syndrome. Am J Gastroenterol 86:1–15, 1991
12. Cappell MS, Schwartz MS, Biempica L. The clinical utility of biopsy in patients with serum antibodies to the human immunodeficiency virus. Am J Med 88:123–130, 1990
13. Carne CA, Weller IVD, Waite J, et al. Impaired responsiveness of homosexual men with HIV antibodies to plasma derived hepatitis B vaccine. Br Med J 294:866–868, 1987
14. Cello JP. Acquired immunodeficiency syndrome cholangiopathy: spectrum of disease. Am J Med 86:539–546, 1989
15. Centers for Disease Control. Hepatitis A among drug abusers. MMWR 37:297–300, 305, 1988
16. Chandler FW. Pathology of the mycoses in patients with the acquired immunodeficiency syndrome (AIDS). Curr Top Med Mycol 1:1–23, 1985
17. Cockerill FR, Hurley DV, Malagelada JR, et al. Polymicrobial cholangitis and Kaposi's sarcoma in blood product transfusion-related acquired immune deficiency syndrome. Am J Med 80:1237–1241, 1986
18. Collier AC, Corey L, Murphy VL, et al. Antibody to human immunodeficiency virus (HIV) and suboptimal response to hepatitis B vaccination. Ann Intern Med 109:101–105, 1988
19. Corey L, Holmes KK. Sexual transmission of hepatitis A in homosexual men: incidence and mechanism. N Engl J Med 302:435–438, 1980
20. Czapar CA, Weldon-Linne M, Moore DM, et al. Peliosis hepatis in the acquired immunodeficiency syndrome. Arch Pathol Lab Med 110:611–613, 1986
21. Dobozin BS, Judson FN, Cohn DL, et al. The relationship of abnormalities of cellular immunity to antibodies to HTLV III in homosexual men. Cell Immunol 98:156–171, 1986
22. du Mayne JFD. Hepatic vascular lesions in AIDS. JAMA 254:53–54, 1985
23. du Mayne JFD, Marche C, Penalba C, et al. Hepatic lesions in acquired immunodeficiency syndrome: a study of 20 cases. Presse Med 14:1177–1180, 1985
23a. Dierstag JL. Immunologic mechanisms in chronic viral hepatitis. In: Vyas GN, Dienstag JL, Hoofnagle JH, eds. Viral hepatitis and liver disease. Orlando, Grune & Stratton, 1984, pp 135–66
23b. Duffy LF, Daum F, Kahn E. Hepatitis in children with acquired immunodeficiency syndrome. Gastroenterology 90:173–81, 1986
24. Dupon M, Kosaifi T, Le Bail B, et al. Lipid-laden perisinusoidal cells in patients with acquired immunodeficiency syndrome. Liver 11:211–219, 1991
24a. Dubin G, Braffman MN. Zidovudine-induced hepatotoxicity. Ann Intern Med 110:85–86, 1989
25. Dworkin BM, Stahl RE, Giardina MA, et al. The liver in acquired immune deficiency syndrome: emphasis on patients with intravenous drug abuse. Am J Gastroenterol 82:231–236, 1987

26. Federico G, Cauda R, Piccigallo E, et al. Visceral leishmaniasis in patients with AIDS: description of 2 cases. Pathologica 81:591–600, 1989

26a. Eng RHK, Forrester C, Smith SM, et al. *Mycobacterium xenopi* infection in a patient with acquired immunodeficiency syndrome. Chest 86:145–147, 1984.

26b. Esteban JI, Esteban R, Viladomia, et al. Hepatitis C virus antibodies among risk groups in Spain. Lancet 2:294–297, 1989

26c. Eyster ME, Alter HJ, Aledort LM, et al. Heterosexual cotransmission of hepatitis C virus (HCV) and human immunodeficiency virus. Ann Intern Med 115:764–768, 1991

27. Finkelstein R, Wichtig C, Hashmonai M. Candida albicans liver abscesses. Infection 13:243–244, 1985

28. Fishman EK, Magid D, Kuhlman JE. Pneumocystis carinii involvement of the liver and spleen: CT demonstration. J Comput Assist Tomogr 14:146–148, 1990

29. Girard PM, et al. Acute hepatitis during HIV primary infection. Third International Conference on AIDS. Abstract THP 169. Washington, DC, June 1987

29a. Garcia FU, Wojta J, Broadley KN, et al. *Barrtonella bacilliformis* stimulates endothelial cells *in vitro* and is angiogenic *in vivo*. Am J Pathol 136:1125–1135, 1990

30. Glasgow BJ, Anders K, Layfield LJ, et al. Clinical and pathologic findings of the liver in the acquired immune deficiency syndrome (AIDS). Am J Clin Pathol 83:582–588, 1985

31. Goldin RD, Fish DE, Hay A, et al. Histological and immunohistochemical study of hepatitis B virus in human immunodeficiency virus. J Clin Pathol 43:203–205, 1990

32. Gordon SC, Reddy KR, Gould EE, et al. The spectrum of liver disease in the acquired immunodeficiency syndrome. J Hepatol 2:475–484, 1986

33. Gordon SC, Veneri RJ, McFadden RF, et al. Major hemorrhage after percutaneous liver biopsy in patients with AIDS. (Letter) Gastroenterology 100:1787, 1991

34. Govindarajan S, Edwards VM, Stuart ML, et al. Influence of human immunodeficiency virus infection on expression of chronic hepatitis B and D virus infections. In: Zuckerman AJ, ed. Viral hepatitis and liver disease. New York, Alan R Liss, 1988, pp 201–204

35. Hadler SC. Hepatitis B prevention and human immunodeficiency virus (HIV) infection. (Editorial) Ann Intern Med 109:92–94, 1988

35a. Hadler SC, Judson F, Echenberg D, et al. Effect of prior human immunodeficiency virus infection or the outcome of hepatitis B virus infection. (Abstract) J Med Virol 21:87A, 1987

36. Hadler SC, Judson F, O'Malley PM, et al. Outcome of hepatitis B virus in homosexual men and its relation to prior human immunodeficiency virus infection. J Infect Dis 163:454–459, 1991

37. Haron E, Feld R, Tuffnell P, et al. Hepatic candidiasis: an increasing problem in immunocompromised patients. Am J Med 83:17–26, 1987

38. Hasan F, Jeffers LJ, Dickinson G, et al. Hepatobiliary cryptosporidiosis and cytomegalovirus infection mimicking metastatic cancer to the liver. Gastroenterology 100:1743–1748, 1991

39. Hasan F, Jeffers LJ, Welsh S, et al. Hepatic involvement as the primary manifestations of Kaposi's sarcoma in AIDS. Am J Gastroenterol 84:1449–1451, 1989

40. Hawkins CC, Gold JW, Whimbey E, et al. *Mycobacterium avium* complex infections in patients with the acquired immunodeficiency syndrome. Ann Intern Med 105:184–188, 1986

40a. Herndier BG, Friedman SL. Neoplasms of the gastrointestinal tract and hepatobiliary system in AIDS. Semin Liver Dis 12:205–212, 1992

41. Hepatitis A: a vaccine at last. (Editorial) Lancet 339:1198–1192, 1992

42. Hinnant K, Schwartz A, Rotterdam H, et al. Cytomegaloviral cryptosporidial cholecystitis in two patients with AIDS. Am J Surg Pathol 13:57–60, 1989

43. Housset C, Boucher O, Girard PM, et al. Immunohistochemical evidence for human immunodeficiency virus-1 infection of liver Kupffer cells. Hum Pathol 21:404–408, 1990

43a. Housset C, Pol S, Carnot F. Interactions between HIV-1, hepatitis delta virus and hepatitis B virus infection in 260 chronic carriers of hepatitis B virus. 15:578–83, 1992

44. Huang CT, McGarry T, Cooper S, et al. Disseminated histoplasmosis in the acquired immunodeficiency syndrome: report of five cases from a nonendemic area. Arch Intern Med 147:1181–1184, 1987

45. Ioachim HL, Cooper MC, Hellman GC. Hodgkin's disease and the acquired immunodeficiency syndrome. (Letter) Ann Intern Med 101:876–877, 1984

46. Ioachim HL, Cooper MC, Hellman GC. Lymphomas in men at high risk for AIDS, a study of 21 cases. Cancer 56:2831–2842, 1985

47. Israelski DM, Skowron G, Leventhal, et al. Toxoplasma peritonitis in a patient with acquired immunodeficiency syndrome. Arch Intern Med 148:1655–1657, 1988

48. Jacobson MA, Cello JP, Sande MA. Cholestasis and disseminated cytomegalovirus disease in patients with the acquired immunodeficiency syndrome. Am J Med 84:218–224, 1988

49. Jacobson JM, Worner TM, Sacks HS, et al. Human immunodeficiency virus and hepatitis B infections in alcoholics. In: Alcohol, immunomodulation, and AIDS. New York, Alan R Liss, 1990, pp 67–73

50. Jeffers LJ, Cheinquer H, Alzate I, et al. Laparoscopic and histologic findings in patients with the human immunodeficiency virus. Gastrointest Endosc (submitted)

51. Johnson TL, Barnett JL, Appelman HD, et al. Candida hepatitis: histopathologic diagnosis. Am J Surg Pathol 12:716–720, 1988

52. Jolliet P, Widmann JJ. Reye's syndrome in adult with AIDS. Lancet 335:1457, 1990

53. Jonas MM, Roldan EO, Lyons HJ, et al. Histopathologic features of the liver in pediatric acquired immune deficiency syndrome. J Pediatr Gastroenterol Nutr 9:73–81, 1989

54. Kahn DG, Garfinkle JM, Klonoff DC, et al. Cryptosporidial and cytomegaloviral hepatitis and cholecystitis. Arch Pathol Lab Med 111:879–881, 1987

55. Kahn SA, Saltzman BR, Klein RS, et al. Hepatic disorders in the acquired immune deficiency syndrome: a clinical and pathological study. Am J Gastroenterol 81:1145–1148, 1986

56. Kaplan LD, Kahn J, Jacobson M, et al. Primary bile duct lymphoma presenting as Kaposi's sarcoma in a homosexual man with the acquired immunodeficiency syndrome (AIDS). Ann Intern Med 110:161–162, 1989

57. Kavin H, Jonas RB, Chowdhury L, et al. Acalculous cholecystitis and cytomegalovirus infection in the acquired immunodeficiency syndrome. Ann Intern Med 104:53–54, 1986

58. Kielhofner MA, Hamill RJ. Focal hepatic tuberculosis in a patient with acquired immunodeficiency syndrome. South Med J 84:401–404, 1991

58a. Kew Lai K, Yang DL, Zawaiki JK, Cooley TP. Fulminant hepatic failure associated with 2'3'-dideoxyinose (ddI). Ann Intern Med 115:283–284, 1991

59. Klatt EC, Jensen DF, Meyer PR. Pathology of *Mycobacterium avium-intracellulare* infection in acquired immunodeficiency syndrome. Hum Pathol 18:709–714, 1987

60. Kovacs JA, Kovacs AA, Polis M, et al. Cryptococcosis in the acquired immunodeficiency syndrome. Ann Intern Med 103:533–538, 1985

61. Kreek MJ, Des Jarlais DC, Trepo CL, et al. Contrasting prevalence of delta hepatitis markers in parenteral drug abusers with and without AIDS. J Infect Dis 162:538–541, 1990

62. Krilov LR, Rubin LG, Frogel M, et al. Disseminated adenovirus infection with hepatic necrosis in patients with human immunodeficiency virus infection and other immunodeficiency states. Rev Infect Dis 12:303–307, 1990

63. Krogsgaard K, Orskov B, Ole Nielson J, et al. The influence of HTLV-III infection on the natural history of hepatitis B virus infection in male homosexual HBsAg carriers. Hepatology 7:37–41, 1987

64. Lange M, Klein EB, Kornfield H, et al. Cytomegalovirus isolation from healthy homosexual men. JAMA 252:1908–1910, 1984

65. Laskin KJ, Black M. Fulminant hepatitis A in intravenous-drug abusers. (Letter) Ann Intern Med 110:845–846, 1989

66. Lazizi Y, Grangeot-Keros L, Delfraissy JF, et al. Reappearance of hepatitis B virus in patients infected with the human immunodeficiency virus type I. J Infect Dis 158:666–667, 1988

67. Lebovics E, Dworkin BM, Heier SK, et al. The hepatobiliary manifestations of human immunodeficiency virus infection. Am J Gastroenterol 83:1–7, 1988

68. Lebovics E, Thung SN, Schaffner F, et al. The liver in the acquired immunodeficiency syndrome: a clinical and histologic study. Hepatology 5:293–298, 1985

69. Li XM, Cheinquer H, Reddy KR, et al. Post-mortem detection, by in situ hybridization, of DNA of various viruses in the liver in acquired immunodeficiency syndrome. (submitted)

69a. Lewis JH, Zimmerman HJ. Drug-induced liver disease. Med Clinic North Am 73:775–792, 1989

70. Light RW. Hepatic mycobacterial disease and AIDS. Hepatology 11:506–507, 1990

71. Lipstein-Kresch E, Isenberg HD, Singer C, et al. Disseminated *Sporothrix schenckii* infection with arthritis in a patient with acquired immunodeficiency syndrome. J Rheumatol 12:805–808, 1985

72. Lubat E, Megibow AJ, Balthazar EJ, et al. Extrapulmonary *Pneumocystis carinii* infection in AIDS: CT findings. Radiology 174:157–160, 1991

73. Luburich P, Bru C, Ayuso MC, et al. Hepatic Kaposi sarcoma in AIDS: US and CT findings. Radiology 175:172–174, 1990

74. Margulis SJ, Honig CL, Soave A, et al. Biliary tract obstruction in the acquired immunodeficiency syndrome. Ann Intern Med 105:207–210, 1986

75. Martin P, Di Bisceglie AM, Kassianides C, et al. Rapidly progressive non-A, non-B hepatitis in patients with human immunodeficiency virus infection. Gastroenterology 97:1559–1561, 1989

76. McCarty M, Choudhri AH, Helbert M, et al. Radiological features of AIDS related cholangitis. Clin Radiol 40:582–585, 1989

77. McDonald JA, Caruso L, Karayiannis P, et al. Diminished responsiveness of male homosexual chronic hepatitis B virus carriers with HTLV-II antibodies to recombinant α-interferon. Hepatology 7:719–723, 1987

78. McDonald JA, Harris S, Waters JA, et al. Effect of human immunodeficiency virus (HIV) infection on chronic hepatitis B hepatic viral antigen display. J Hepatol 4:337–342, 1987

78a. Melbye M, Biggar RJ, Wantzin P, et al. Sexual transmission of hepatitis C virus: cohort study (1981–89) among European homosexual men. Br Med J 301:210–212, 1990

79. Monno L, Angarano G, Santantonio T, et al. Lack of HBV and HDV replicative activity in HBsAg-positive intravenous drug addicts with immune deficiency due to HIV. J Med Virol 34:199–205, 1991

80. Mintz L, Drew WL, Miner RC, et al. Cytomegalovirus infections in homosexual men: an epidemiological study. Ann Intern Med 99:326–329, 1983

81. Nakanuma Y, Liew CT, Peters RL, et al. Pathologic features of the liver in acquired immunodeficiency syndrome (AIDS). Liver 6:158–166, 1986

81b. Niedt GW, Schirella RA. Acquired immunodeficiency syndrome: clincopathologic study of 56 autopsies. Arch Pathol Lab Med 109:727–734, 1985

82. Novick DM, Farci P, Croxson TS, et al. Hepatitis D virus and human immunodeficiency virus antibodies in parenteral drug abusers who are hepatitis B surface antigen positive. J Infect Dis 158:795–802, 1988

82a. Nelson JA, Wiley CA, Reynolds-Kohler C, et al. Human immunodeficiency virus detected in bowel epithelium from patients with gastrointestinal symptoms. Lancet 1:259–262, 1988

83. Novick DM, Lok ASF, Thomas HC. Diminished responsiveness of homosexual men to antiviral therapy for HBsAg-positive chronic liver disease. J Hepatol 1:29–35, 1984

84. Nyberg D, Jeffrey R, Federle M, et al. AIDS-related lymphomas: evaluation by abdominal CT. Radiology 159:59–63, 1986

85. Orenstein MS, Tavitian A, Yonk B, et al. Granulomatous involvement of the liver in patients with AIDS. Gut 26:1220–1225, 1985

86. Palmer M, Braly L, Schaffner F. The liver in acquired immune deficiency disease. Semin Liver Dis 7:192–202, 1987

86a. Ortiz-Interian CJ, de Medina MD, Perez GO, et al. Recurrence and clearance of hepatitis B surface antigenemia in a dialysis patient infected with the human immunodeficiency virus. Am J Kidney Dis 16:154–156, 1990

87. Pastakia B, Shawker TH, Thaler M, et al. Hepatosplenic candidiasis: wheels within wheels. Radiology 166:417–421, 1988

88. Payne TH, Cohn DL, Davidson AJ, et al. Marked elevations of serum alkaline phosphatase in patients with AIDS. J AIDS 4:238–243, 1991

89. Perkocha LA, Geaghan SM, Benedict Yen TS, et al. Clinical and pathological features of bacillary peliosis hepatis in association with human immunodeficiency virus infection. N Engl J Med 232:1581–1586, 1990

90. Perrillo RP, Regenstein FG, Roodman ST. Chronic hepatitis B in asymptomatic homosexual men with antibody to the human immunodeficiency virus. Ann Intern Med 105:382–383, 1986

90a. Perrillo RP, Schiff ER, Davis GL. Hepatitis Interventional Therapy Group. A randomized, controlled trial of interferon alfa-2b alone and after prednisone withdrawal for the treatment of chronic hepatitis B. N Engl J Med 323:295–301, 1990

91. Piccigallo E, Jeffers LJ, Reddy KR, et al. Immunocytochemical detection of hepatitis B surface and core antigens in the liver of patients anti-HIV positive and anti-HIV negative with HBsAg-positive chronic liver disease. Third International Conference on Acquired Immunodeficiency Syndrome (AIDS), Washington, DC June 1–5, 1987

92. Pinching AJ, Jeffries DJ, Donaghy, et al. Studies of cellular immunity in male homosexuals in London. Lancet 2:126–130, 1983

93. Poblete RB, Rodriguez K, Foust RT, et al. *Pneumocystis carinii* hepatitis in the acquired immunodeficiency syndrome (AIDS). Ann Intern Med 110:737–738, 1989

94. Pottipati AR, Dave PB, Gumaste V, et al. Tuberculous abscess of the liver in acquired immunodeficiency syndrome. J Clin Gastroenterol 13:549–553, 1991

95. Prego V, Glatt AE, Roy V, et al. Comparative yield of blood culture for fungi and mycobacteria, liver biopsy, and bone marrow biopsy in the diagnosis of fever of undetermined origin in human immunodeficiency virus-infected patients. Arch Intern Med 150:333–336, 1990

96. Prufer-Kramer L, Kramer A, Weigel R, et al. Hepatic involvement in patients with human immunodeficiency virus infection: discrepancies between AIDS patients and those with earlier stages of infection. J Infect Dis 163:866–869, 1991

97. Radin DR. Intraabdominal *Mycobacterium tuberculosis* vs *Mycobacterium avium-intracellulare* infections in patients with AIDS: distinction based on CT findings. Am J Roentgenol 156:487–491, 1991

98. Radin DR, Baker EL, Klatt EC, et al. Visceral and nodal calcification in patients with AIDS-related Pneumocystis carinii infection. Am J Roentgenol 154:27–31, 1990

99. Raviglione MC. Extrapulmonary pneumocystis: the first 50 cases. Rev Infect Dis 12:1127–1138, 1990

100. Rector WG Jr, Govindarajan S, Horsburgh CR Jr, et al. Hepatic inflammation, hepatitis B replication, and cellular immune function in homosexual males with chronic hepatitis B and antibody to human immunodeficiency virus. Am J Gastroenterol 83:262–266, 1988

101. Reddy KR, Chan JC, Smiley D, et al. Spontaneous group B Salmonella enteritidis peritonitis in cirrhotic ascites and acquired immune deficiency syndrome. Am J Gastroenterol 83:882–884, 1988

102. Reichert CM, O'Leary TJ, Levens DL, et al. Autopsy pathology in the acquired immune deficiency syndrome. Am J Pathol 112:357–382, 1983

103. Robert NJ, Schneiderman H. Hodgkin's disease and the acquired immunodeficiency syndrome. (Letter) Ann Intern Med 101:142–143, 1984

105. Roulot D, Valla D, Brun-Vezinet F, et al. Cholangitis in the acquired immunodeficiency syndrome: report of two cases and review of the literature. Gut 28:1653–1660, 1987

106. Rustgi VK, Hoofnagle JH, Gerin JL, et al. Hepatitis B virus infection in the acquired immunodeficiency syndrome. Ann Intern Med 101:795–797, 1984

107. Sachs JR, Greenfield SM, Sohn M, et al. Disseminated Pneumocystis carinii infection with hepatic involvement in a patient with the acquired immune deficiency syndrome. Am J Gastroenterol 86:82–85, 1991

109. Salzman SH, Smith RL, Aranda CP. Histoplasmosis in patients at risk for the acquired immunodeficiency syndrome in a nonendemic setting. Chest 93:916–921, 1988

110. Scherer R, Sable R, Sonnenberg M, et al. Disseminated infection with *Mycobacterium kansasii* in the acquired immunodeficiency syndrome. Ann Intern Med 105:710–712, 1986

111. Schneiderman DJ, Arenson DM, Cello JP, et al. Hepatic disease in patients with the acquired immune deficiency syndrome (AIDS). Hepatology 7:925–930, 1987

112. Schneiderman DJ, Cello JP, Laing FC. Papillary stenosis and sclerosing cholangitis in the acquired immunodeficiency syndrome. Ann Intern Med 106:546–549, 1987

113. Scoazec JY, Degott C, Brousse N, et al. Non-Hodgkin's lymphoma presenting as a primary tumor of the liver presentation, diagnosis and outcome in eight patients. Hepatology 13:870–875, 1991

113a. Schwarz ED, Greene JB. Diagnostic consideration in the human immunodeficiency virus–infected patient with gastrointestinal or abdominal symptoms. Semin Liver Dis 12:142–153, 1992

114. Scoazec JY, Feldman G. Both macrophages and endothelial cells of the human hepatic sinusoid express the CD4 molecule, a receptor for the human immunodeficiency virus. Hepatology 12:505–510, 1990

115. Scoazec JY, Marche C, Girard PM, et al. Peliosis hepatis and sinusoidal dilation during infection by the human immunodeficiency virus (HIV): an ultrastructural study. Am J Pathol 131:38–47, 1988

117. Shattock AG, Finlay H, Hillary IB. Possible reactivation of hepatitis D with chronic δ antigenaemia by human immunodeficiency virus. Br Med J 294:1656–1657, 1987

118. Slater LN, Welch DF, Min KW. *Rochalimaea henselae* causes

bacillary angiomatosis and peliosis hepatis. Arch Intern Med 152:602–606, 1992

120. Staib F. Detection of *Cryptococcus neoformans* in biopsy specimens from the spleen and the liver of AIDS patients: critical comments. Mykosen 29:551–555, 1986

122. Taylor PE, Stevens CE, Rodriguez de Cordoba S, et al. Hepatitis B virus and human immunodeficiency virus: possible interactions. In: Zuckerman AJ, ed. Viral hepatitis and liver disease. New York, Alan R Liss, 1988, pp 198–200

123. Terada S, Reddy KR, Jeffers LJ, et al. Microsporidian hepatitis in the acquired immunodeficiency syndrome. Ann Intern Med 107:61–62, 1987

124. Thung SN, Gerber MA, Benkov KJ, et al. Chronic active hepatitis in a child with human immunodeficiency virus infection. Arch Pathol Lab Med 112:914–916, 1988

125. Tindall B, Barker S, Donovan B, et al. Characteristics of the acute clinical illness associated with human immunodeficiency virus infection. Arch Intern Med 143:945–949, 1988

126. Vento S, Di Perri G, Luzzati R, et al. Clinical reactivation of hepatitis B in anti-HBs-positive patients with AIDS. (Letter) Lancet 1:332–333, 1989

127. Vieco PT, Rochon L, Lisbona A. Multifocal cytomegalovirus-associated hepatic lesions simulating metastases in AIDS. Radiology 176:123–124, 1990

128. Viteri AI, Greene JF. Bile duct abnormalities in the acquired immune deficiency syndrome. Gastroenterology 92:2014–2018, 1987

129. Wakabayashi T, Onda H, Tada T, et al. High incidence of peliosis hepatis in autopsy cases of aplastic anemia with special reference to anabolic steroid therapy. Acta Pathol Jpn 34:1079–1086, 1984

130. Watanabe S, Reddy KR, Jeffers L, et al. Electron microscopic evidence of non-A, non-B hepatitis markers and virus-like particles in immunocompromised humans. Hepatology 4:628–632, 1984

131. Welch K, Finkbeiner W, Alpers CE, et al. Autopsy findings in the acquired immune deficiency syndrome. JAMA 252:1152–1159, 1984

132. Wilcox CM, Forsmark CE, Darragh T, et al. High-protein ascites in patients with the acquired immunodeficiency syndrome. Gastroenterology 100:745–748, 1991

133. Wilkins MJ, Lindley R, Dourakis SP, et al. Surgical pathology of the liver in HIV infection. Histopathology 18:459–464, 1991

134. Worner TM. Disseminated *Pneumocystis carinii* infection in AIDS. (Letter) Am J Gastroenterol 86:1857, 1991

135. Zafrani ES, Cazier A, Baudelot AM, et al. Ultrastructural lesions of the liver in human peliosis: a report of 12 cases. Am J Pathol 114:349–359, 1984

136. Zafrani ES, Pinaudeau Y, Dhumeaux D. Drug-induced vascular lesions of the liver. Arch Intern Med 143:495–502, 1983

136a. Ziegler JL, Beckstead JA, et al. Non-Hodgkin's lymphoma in 90 homosexual men: relation to generalized lymphadenopathy and the acquired immunodeficiency syndrome. N Engl J Med 311:565–570, 1984

137. Zimmerli W, Bianchi L, Gudat F, et al. Disseminated herpes simplex type 2 and systemic *Candida* infection in a patient with previous asymptomatic human immunodeficiency virus infection. J Infect Dis 157:597–598, 1988

Diseases of the Liver, Seventh Edition, edited by
Leon Schiff and Eugene R. Schiff. J.B. Lippincott Company, Philadelphia © 1993.

50

The Liver and Its Effect
on Endocrine Function
in Health and Disease

Elizabeth J. Smanik

Hope Barkoukis

Kevin D. Mullen

Arthur J. McCullough

The liver is primarily a metabolic organ that coordinates a
variety of hormonal, biochemical, and physiologic processes.
These processes fall into two major categories. Within the
first category are those functions that occur primarily within
the liver such as bile acid and urea synthesis, protein secretion, xenobiotic metabolism, signal transduction gene
expression, ligand binding, membrane transport, and cell–
matrix and cell–cell interaction. The second category comprises those functions that orchestrate simultaneous processes
and integrate the entire body into a well coordinated functioning unit. This latter category includes such functions as
the acute-phase response, interorgan nutrient trafficking,
growth processes, protein–energy balance, and modulation of
hormonal actions. Of course, such a classification is largely
artificial because both processes are intimately related to initiating and continually fine tuning each other's functional
goals.

Although both types of functions are significantly controlled by endocrinologic mechanisms, the hormonal influence on the latter integrative functions has more clearly defined areas of clinical interest. Consequently, this latter
category is emphasized here, but readers are referred to reviews that have focused on those processes occurring primarily within the liver.[327] Because all these hepatic functions are
controlled to a large extent by hormonal action,[294] it is not
surprising that liver disease should cause a wide spectrum of
endocrine alterations and, in turn, that endocrine diseases
may alter liver status; the most important of these include
insulin resistance with altered nutrient metabolism, hepatic
steatosis associated with obesity, thyroid disease, and abnormal sex steroid metabolism.

Hormonal aspects also are critical to hepatic differentiation and function. It is unclear, however, if the endocrine
response of the liver occurs independently of the primary hypothalamic–pituitary–gonadal axis or is sequentially linked in
response to imbalance. Steroid, thyroid, and peptide hormones without exception interact with hepatic protein syn-

thesis, glucose, fatty acid, cholesterol, drug and toxin metabolism, and bile secretion such that an understanding of the
molecular dynamics existing between the endocrine signaling system and the hepatic response is important. This review
also updates information about the molecular aspects of hormone action and summarize its functional implications. In
addition, the clinical consequences of the endocrine action
of the human liver as it pertains to the diseased state is described. Before specific conditions can be discussed, it is important to review the mechanism of peptide and steroid hormone action in the liver.

HORMONE ACTION

The liver regulates intermediary metabolism with both short-
and long-term control to modulate conditions of varying nutrient influx with constitutive needs. Fine tuning of this control in the liver, as well as in most other tissues, includes
hormonal pathways. The molecular steps have been extensively studied in the past three decades in target tissue and in
vitro systems. The mechanisms derived from these studies are
operative in all tissue and thus are relevant to endocrine liver
function (Fig. 50-1). Hormones bind to a protein receptor
with the following characteristic features:

- High affinity (Kd dissociation constant range of 10^{-9} to
  10^{-11} mol/L)
- Saturability (B_{max} within physiologic concentration ranges
  and low abundance relative to total cellular protein concentration; $1:10^4$ to 10^5)
- Specificity
- Reversability (measured association Ka and dissociation Kd
  constants)
- Correlation of the concentration of receptors required for
  binding with the ability to induce the biologic effect

Thus, the hormone–receptor interaction dictates the specific
physiologic effect that constitutes the major differences

This work was supported in part by National Institutes of Health grant
DK-39527 and a grant from the MetroHealth Hospital Foundation.

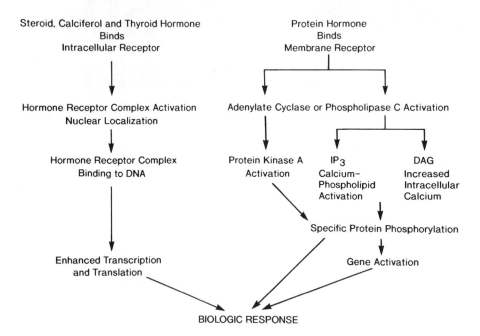

FIGURE 50-1   Schematic diagram indicating the major steps involved in the intracellular mechanism of action of steroid, calciferol, thyroid, and protein hormones. IP$_3$, inositol-1,4,5-triphosphate; DAG, diacyl glycerol. IP$_3$ and DAG are products of phosphodiesterase hydrolysis of phosphatidyl inositol-4,5-diphosphate.

among steroids, protein hormones, thyroid hormones, and catecholamines.

Steroid and Thyroid Hormones

Steroid hormones include androgens, estrogens, progestins, mineralocorticoids, glucocorticoids, 25-hydroxycholecalciferol, and 1,25 dihydroxycholecalciferol. These are synthesized in a common pathway from cholesterol, a universal constituent of cell membranes, and therefore appear to be ancient in an evolutionary sense. They share the four fused ring structure, cyclopentanophenanthrene. The liver shares responsibility with the kidney in the bioactivation of thyroid hormone. Both plasma-binding proteins, thyroxine-binding globulin (TBG) and thyroxine-binding prealbumin (TBPA), are synthesized in the liver and bind thyroxine (T$_4$), triiodothyronine (T$_3$), and their metabolites and affect hormone turnover. The liver accounts for 85% of the conversion of T$_4$ to T$_3$.[406,540] The only pathway to yield a bioactive metabolite is the conversion of T$_4$ to T$_3$ via deiodinase. A specific deiodinase that converts about 40% of circulating T$_4$ to reverse T$_3$ ($_r$T$_3$), a biologically inactive metabolite, is found in the brain, placenta, and skin and functions as a homeostatic mechanism. T$_3$ binds to its receptor 10 times more avidly than T$_4$ and is 10 times more biologically potent than T$_4$. As with the iodothyronines, steroid hormones are lipophilic. They associate with plasma proteins to maintain solubility and prolong their biologic half-life. They passively traverse cellular membranes along concentration gradients and bind intracellular soluble receptors to maintain high intracellular concentrations of hormone. Hormone receptor number varies in the cell with alterations in physiologic state as well as with disease. After binding to a receptor, the soluble hormone–receptor complex undergoes a number of changes, termed *transformation* or *activation*, including a conformational change and reduction in its overall size (Fig. 50-2). This is due to loss of one or two nonsteroid binding components (eg, the 90-kd heat shock protein, which enables the

complex to accumulate in the nucleus and bind DNA with high affinity[237]; see Fig. 50-1). Additionally, the receptor protein may undergo phosphorylation, which enhances nuclear binding or allows receptor recycling.

All steroids and thyroid receptors share a similar structural organization that includes nonoverlapping, linearly arranged functional domains. They possess a variable N-terminal region and a highly conserved C terminus. At least four functional domains have been identified in the glucocorticoid receptor as the prototype for other steroid and thyroid receptor systems: (1) the N-terminal site of antigenic recognition, (2) a DNA binding site in the central region, (3) a hormone binding region in the carboxy terminus, and (4) a small hinge region between the DNA and hormone binding sites that may be important for stereochemical interactions (see Fig. 50-2). Hormone–receptor complex binding to DNA acts to accelerate the rate of hormone–receptor association with DNA. DNA association with the activated hormone–receptor complex is specific for the DNA response element at the promoter site of a target gene. The specified DNA binding sites for several steroid and thyroid hormone receptors have been identified by nuclease footprint analysis. The binding site involves a hormone receptor dimer that binds a highly conserved region, the hormone responsive element (HRE), which is an enhancer region and is located upstream to the promotor region (see Fig. 50-2). An enhancer is a DNA sequence that is transcribed by RNA polymerase II and is required for full activity of a promoter region. Hormone–receptor complex binding to DNA is located in a half turn of the major groove of DNA and is organized as two zinc-containing, protein finger-like regions that are enriched with cysteine residues.[169,192] Other proteins that regulate gene expression bind DNA in a similar manner, suggesting that this organization is functionally important.[140] The glucocorticoid, mineralocorticoid, androgen, and thyroid hormone receptors have been purified and cDNA probes have been isolated. The nucleotide sequences for various cDNAs have been compared. Remarkable homology is found among the DNA binding sites for glucocorticord, progesterone, androgen, and

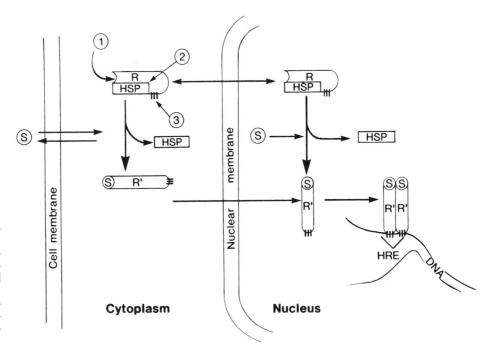

FIGURE 50-2 Intracellular mechanisms of steroid hormone action. S, steroid hormone; R, unbound hormone receptor; HSP, heat shock protein; R′, activated receptor bound to steroid; 1, steroid-binding site; 2, hinge region; 3, receptor DNA-binding site; HRE, hormone response element or specific DNA-binding domain.

mineralocorticoid receptors on the one hand and estrogen, thyroid, vitamin D, retinoic acid, the oncogene *erb* A, and ecdysterone, an insect hormone, in another related subgroup. These similarities in nucleotide sequences support the concept of a superfamily of multiple hydrophobic ligands that may be divided into subgroups that bind receptor dimer proteins and associate in turn with DNA.

Steroid hormone DNA binding leads to at least three responses: (1) a *direct* increase in the efficacy of transcription interaction by stabilizing the transcription complex at the steroid-specific enhancer region, the HRE; (2) an *indirect* increase that necessitates the synthesis of a protein that then activates gene expression; and 3) *gene repression*. In addition, negative regulation by glucocorticoids of α-fetoprotein transcription has been described in rat liver.[196] The mechanism whereby hormone receptor–DNA binding affects response is thought to involve transient structural alteration of the chromosome at the site of binding that relaxes its structure and enhances its nuclease sensitivity.[555] Further definition awaits cocrystallization of these ternary complexes. Estrogen[58] and glucocorticoids[115] additionally act on mRNA processing and degradation along with posttranslational processing.

Protein Hormones

Protein hormones are water soluble and bind to protein receptors that span the bilipid plasma membrane of a target cell (see Fig. 50-1). Hormone binding occurs in the extracellular portion of the receptor near the amino terminus in cysteine-rich regions. The protein hormone receptor traverses the membrane with functional domains near the carboxy terminus extending into the cytoplasm. Both epidermal growth factor (EGF) and insulin receptors have tyrosine kinase activity in the cytoplasmic regions. The receptor elicits its action according to one of several mechanisms, including stimulation or inhibition of cyclic adenosine monophosphate (cAMP) production, and stimulation of intracellular calcium

production with or without production of phosphatidylinositol (see Fig. 50-1). Several hormones such as insulin, growth hormone, prolactin, EGF, and insulin-like growth factors (IGF-I, IGF-II) act independently of any identified secondary messengers (Table 50-1). The production of cAMP by adenylate cyclase plays a critical role in the mechanism of action of a number of protein hormones (see Fig. 50-1). The quadrimeric enzyme complex has three subunits in the guanosine triphosphate (GTP)-dependent regulatory complex—α, β, and λ—and a catalytic subunit, and is located on the cytoplasmic side of the plasma membrane.[293] Hormone receptor binding may either activate or inhibit the magnesium-dependent production of cAMP from adenosine triphosphate. Multiple hormone receptor complexes may interact independently with one adenylate cyclase complex in a given target cell.[62] The stimulatory and inhibitory subunits as part of the GTP-dependent regulatory complex act separately on one catalytic subunit of adenylate cyclase.[171] In eukaryote cells, cAMP phosphorylates and binds to protein kinase A to initiate a phosphorylation–dephosphorylation cascade that mediates hormonal action. Although diverse functions regulated by hormones include steroidogenesis, protein secretion, ion transport, carbohydrate and fat metabolism, and gene regulation, the specific phosphoproteins involved in this step within the target cell remain under investigation.

The binding of certain hormones, such as gonadotropin-releasing hormone to pituitary cells to release luteinizing hormone (LH), and α-adrenergic catecholamines to liver cells to inhibit glycogen synthetase, involves an increase in intracellular calcium as the specific second messenger (see Table 50-1). Many enzymes, such as pyruvate carboxylase, glycogen synthetase, and pyruvate dehydrogenase, exhibit calcium-dependent activity. Inositol-1,4,5-triphosphate (IP3), a product of phosphodiesterase hydrolysis of phosphatidylinositol 4, 5-biphospate in plasma membrane, is closely related to intracellular calcium activity.[37] Ultimately, phosphorylation of proteins completes the response initiated by these hormone–receptor interactions. Several hormones, including

TABLE 50-1 *Hormones That Bind Cell Membrane Receptors*

cAMP Mediated
α_2,* β_2-adrenergic catecholamines
Corticotropin
Angiotensin II*
Antidiuretic hormone
Calcitonin
Chorionic gonadotropin
Corticotropin-releasing hormone
Follicle-stimulating hormone
Glucagon
Lipotropin
Luteinizing hormone
Melanocyte-stimulating hormone
Parathyroid hormone
Somatostatin*
Thyroid-stimulating hormone

Calcium or Phosphatidyl Inositol Mediated
α-Adrenergic catecholamine
Acetylcholine
Angiotensin II
Antidiuretic hormone
Gonadotropin-releasing hormone
Thyrotropin-releasing hormone
Thyroid-stimulating hormone
Vasoactive intestinal peptide

Unknown Intracellular Messenger
Chorionic somatomammotropin
Epidermal growth factor
Fibroblast growth factor
Growth hormone
Insulin
Insulin-like growth factors
Nerve growth factor
Oxytocin
Platelet-derived growth factor
Prolactin

cAMP, cyclic adenosine monophosphate.
*Hormones that inhibit adenylate cyclase.
(Modified in part from Granner D. Hormones of the gonads. In: Murray R, et al, eds. Harper's biochemistry, ed 21. Norwalk, CT, Appleton & Lange, 1988)

insulin, IGFs, growth hormone, and prolactin do not use any of the known second messengers already described. Both the IGF and EGF receptors have intrinsic tyrosine kinase activity that is closely linked to hormone binding.[557] Novel intracellular mechanisms of signaling for these hormones may be involved.[45]

Hormone Receptor Actions in the Liver

The earliest reports of estrogen, androgen, and glucocorticoid liver receptors were in rats.[156,291,442,539] Elegant work has shown the estrogen receptor (ER) in rat and human liver to share classic features seen in rat uterine studies.[123,413] Specific characteristics unique to ER in the liver are (1) an age-related induction in ER number in both males and females[131]; (2) gender-specific response to estrogen with increased receptor number in females and decreased in males[125]; (3) growth

hormone, prolactin, and glucocorticoid control of ER concentration[368] and induction of the female pattern of hepatic steroid metabolism[199]; and (4) tissue-specific opposite effects in the estrogenic bioactivity of antiestrogens.[261] The nonsteroidal triarylethylene antiestrogens such as tamoxifen and nafoxidine are potent growth inhibitors and thus serve as therapy in human hormone-dependent breast cancers with ER activity. Yet these synthetic drugs demonstrate a wide spectrum of tissue and species activity and vary from pure antagonist in chick oviduct with no estrogen response to pure agonist in rat liver with significant estrogen effect. As the use of these drugs increases, close watch for estrogen-like actions on the liver is needed.[241] These issues are relevant because human hepatic steroid and drug metabolism is sex dependent.[197,404]

ER activity is recognized in human normal liver,[121,411] hepatic adenomas,[22,162,412] focal nodular hyperplasia,[492] hepatocellular carcinoma,[151] hepatoblastoma,[223] and hepatitis B virus-infected male and female livers with low levels of progesterone receptors and HSP 27.[81] Clinical response seen in hepatic adenoma regression with cessation of oral contraceptives,[129,258] adenoma growth with pregnancy,[306] and partial regression of hepatomas in 40% of patients treated with a synthetic progestin, megestrol acetate,[151] lends credence to the functional relevance of estrogen action in the liver. Further studies are needed because growth promotion by estrogens is not universal[498] and ER–DNA association may be atypical in liver tissue.[131] The use of mycotoxins as growth-promotant substitutes for diethylstilbestrol in food-producing animals is another example of a potential association of clinical findings with liver ER. Zearalenone, an estrogen product of the mold, *Fusarium*, which grows in corn, wheat, and maize, is associated with human liver tumor induction.[462] Zearalenone derivatives avidly bind ER in both male and female rat liver.[414]

Androgen receptors (AR) have been found in human[151] and in rat liver.[15] AR in the liver requires a normally functioning pituitary because cytoplasmic and nuclear AR activity is lost with hypophysectomy.[126] Unlike ER, cimetidine has no effect on AR in the liver.[512] α_{2u}-Globulin is an androgen-dependent protein synthesized in male rat liver and is a major urinary protein component.[441] Females do not produce α_{2u}-globulin unless they undergo ovariectomy and androgen exposure. In such treated females, α_{2u}-globulin-producing hepatocytes appear in a specific pattern with immunolabeled cells first seen adjacent to the central vein. Next, a perivenular ring of cells acquire α_{2u}-globulin synthesis ability. Finally, hepatocytes along cords emanating from the central vein acquire competency. This perivenular to periportal path is opposite to the direction of blood flow and DNA labeling. Thus, hormonal expression in hepatocytes may involve cell-to-cell communication and polarity as critical elements in their mechanisms of action.[444] Although liver AR mRNA and α_{2u}-globulin levels decline in senescent animals, a 40% reduction in dietary caloric intakes retards this loss, suggesting nutritional interplay with endocrine action.[487] At least two actions of AR have been postulated in the liver: (1) to maintain androgen-regulated hepatic function and (2) to promote hepatic carcinogenesis. Liver AR populations were decreased in two animal models of liver damage, the alcohol-fed rat and carbon tetrachloride-induced cirrhosis.[124,391] Nagasue and colleagues[358] have reported a three-fold increase in AR content of hepatocellular carcinomas compared with adjacent normal liver tissue. At least two rat models of hepa-

sequently, there is some overlap in the receptor specificity for these peptides.[316] Insulin binds the IGF-I receptor with 1% of the affinity of IGF-I. Similarly, IGF-I and IGF-II bind to the insulin receptors with only 2% of insulin's affinity for its receptors,[87] but can cause hypoglycemia.[456] Both IGF-I and IGF-II and insulin receptors are heterotetrameric structures with two α subunits (molecular weight of about 135 kd) and two β subunits (molecular weight of about 95 kd).[513] The α subunits contain the ligand binding sites, which undergo structural change after ligand binding. This ligand receptor binding activates tyrosine kinase activity and phosphorylation of protein thought to be needed for specific IGF and insulin signaling.[87,244] The IGF-I and insulin receptors also interact with each other. Activation of one activates the other.[254] Consequently, IGF-I and insulin have overlapping binding and signal transduction characteristics, while individually maintaining specific effects of nutrients on growth and metabolism.[119] The IGF-II receptor closely resembles the mannose-6-phosphate receptor, which appears important to intracellular transport of proteins to the lysosomes.

An important concept is that IGF-I and IGF-II function as paracrine–autocrine hormones as well as classical endocrine hormones.[87,154] Many cell types, including fibroblasts, can secrete IGF[8,89,357] and fibroblast-like cells in connective tissue have been found to contain mRNA for both IGF-I and IGF-II.[201] Because the cells are found ubiquitously in tissues throughout the body, secretion of IGF has been hypothesized to stimulate growth locally (an effect that can be blocked in culture by antibodies to IGF-I or its receptor).[84,448] Consistent with this concept, IGF-I is synthesized in rapidly dividing cells involved in wound injury and repair.[440] Thus, IGF-I and IGF-II synthesis may play a role in both hepatic proliferative and regenerative response to injury, as has been suggested in regenerating and fetal rat liver.[70,467]

Turning to the more classic hormone mechanisms, growth hormone and nutrition appear to be the two major factors that control IGF synthesis and IGF plasma levels. Growth hormone interacts with two types of receptors in the hepatocyte membrane, a somatogenic receptor and a lactogenic receptor.[422] These receptors are influenced by gender,

with somatogenic receptors being present in both male and female livers, whereas lactogenic receptors are normally found only in female livers.[422] Although growth hormone stimulation of lactogenic receptors may play a physiologic role in somatomedin production,[85] growth hormone control of hepatic somatomedin production is mediated predominantly by somatogenic receptors.[12,149,218] Growth hormone-stimulated hepatic IGF-I secretion has been demonstrated in hypophysectomized rats,[86,106,537] isolated perfused rat livers,[262,325,455,466] cultured hepatocytes,[43,321,490] and hepatic explants.[458] This growth hormone-stimulated IGF-I secretion then participates in a negative feedback loop on growth hormone secretion. This negative feedback occurs through two mechanisms.[33,57] First, IGF-I stimulates the hypothalamus to secrete somatostatin (a potent inhibitor of growth hormone release). Second, IGF-I interferes with growth hormone-releasing factor stimulation of growth hormone gene expression in the pituitary. Both of these mechanisms may be involved in the growth hormone secretory patterns associated with fasting.[216]

In addition to growth hormone, nutritional status is another major factor influencing IGF-I synthesis and secretion. Malnutrition inhibits IGF-I secretion,[88] and serum IGF-I levels have been used as a nutritional marker during nutrient therapy.[319,344] Normal subjects who are fasted for 5 days have a 70% fall in plasma IGF-I levels, an abnormality that is reversed by refeeding[87] (Fig. 50-8) and is not responsive to growth hormone administration.[338] The mechanism by which malnutrition decreases serum IGF levels is multifactorial.[87] Fasting decreases growth hormone binding to hepatocytes,[301] an abnormality that is likely to occur at the level of transcription of growth hormone receptor.[491] Additionally, fasting decreases IGF-I mRNA,[133] again at the transcriptional level.[491] These abnormalities also occur in nonhepatic tissues such as muscle, intestine, brain, and kidney.[296] In contrast to fasting, protein restriction decreases serum IGF-I levels but has little or no effect on growth hormone binding.[302] Furthermore, growth hormone does not elicit an IGF-I response in the face of protein restriction. These data suggest a post–growth hormone receptor abnormality associated with pro-

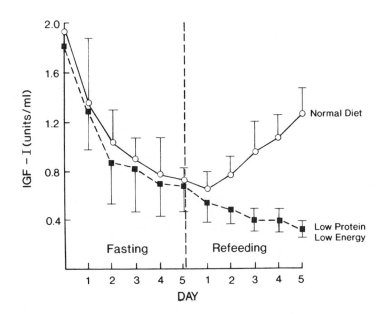

FIGURE 50-8 The response of serum IGF-I levels to periods of fasting and refeeding is provided. These results were obtained in five normal control patients placed on either a normal or low-protein, low-energy diet. (Modified from Clemmons DR, Underwood LE. Nutritional regulation of IGF-I and IGF binding proteins. Annu Rev Nutr 11:393–412, 1991)

tein restriction.[304] Not only does nutritional status influence growth hormone and serum–tissue levels of IGF-I, but IGF binding proteins also decrease with malnutrition. These binding proteins exist in at least three different molecular forms, have high affinity for IGF, and each seems to have a specific influence on IGF metabolism.[87] These binding proteins are important in controlling serum IGF levels, and also influence IGF binding to target tissues and the entry of IGF into tissue. They also potentiate IGF effects[16,23] by mechanisms that remain largely unknown.[87]

Because chronic liver disease is associated with malnutrition[329] and decreased IGF-I, which itself is influenced by dietary intake, the interaction of nutritional status and liver disease may have important metabolic and clinical sequelae in cirrhosis. Unfortunately, those studies that have investigated IGF levels in liver disease have not carefully controlled the nutritional status. Consequently, the effect of hepatic injury per se on serum IGF levels remains unclear. Because studies have demonstrated that exogenously administered growth hormone to humans[315,410,447,560] and IGF-I to animals[119,231] can be given safely, this form of therapy may prove useful in the future management of liver disease, once a greater understanding is gained of the pathophysiologic aspects of IGF metabolism in liver disease. Improved knowledge in this area should lead to improved strategies for nutritional and hormonal therapy in these patients.

Diabetes Mellitus and the Liver

Patients with diabetes mellitus have been reported to have a spectrum of histopathologic findings on examination of the liver[49,101,139,359,494,503]:

- Glycogen deposition
  - Intranuclear
  - Cytoplasmic
- Fatty liver
- Fatty liver with portal fibrosis
- Nonalcoholic steatohepatitis
- Increased iron deposition
  - Hemochromatosis
  - Hemosiderosis
- Portal tract or bile duct abnormality
  - Common bile duct stones
  - Large duct obstruction
- Cirrhosis

Whether these abnormalities are attributable to diabetes alone, concomitant obesity, or even to other causes of liver disease is not easy to discern from the literature. In addition, as described earlier, glucose intolerance secondary to liver disease (so-called hepatogenous diabetes) develops in many patients. Thus, it is probable that the incidence of liver disease in patients labeled as diabetics may be an overestimate because of the inclusion of some of these patients with hepatogenous diabetes.[333] Nonetheless, despite some limitations with the epidemiologic data, it appears that diabetic patients, particularly those with the adult onset type, have an increased incidence of significant liver disease, including cirrhosis, compared with the general population.[101,139,494,545]

Throughout this section, diabetes is classified into three main types: (1) type I, insulin-dependent diabetes or juvenile onset diabetes; (2) type II, which characteristically is associated with increased insulin levels and hyperglycemia and was formerly known as adult onset diabetes; and (3) secondary diabetes due primarily to pancreatic disease. Impaired glucose tolerance may represent either an early presymptomatic phase of type II diabetes or, as noted earlier, be indicative of hepatogenous diabetes.[333] Generally, hepatogenous diabetes is not associated with fasting hyperglycemia, which helps to distinguish it from type II diabetes.[361]

Diabetes-associated liver disease is primarily a pathologic diagnosis without specific clinical signs and liver test abnormalities to indicate the extent or severity of liver pathologic involvement found on biopsy. Thus, the topic generally is discussed under pathologic rather than clinical headings. Pathologic findings likely to be encountered in diabetic patients who have liver tissue examined were just listed. The initial diagnosis of liver disease in diabetics is being detected more frequently by radiologic procedures. Accordingly, the broadening spectrum of clinical presentations of diabetes-related liver disease is given in this list:

- Mildly abnormal liver tests with or without hepatomegaly
- Hepatomegaly, hepatic pain, abnormal liver tests
- Incidental discovery on imaging studies with or without abnormal liver tests
- Hepatomegaly with features of portal hypertension
- Decompensated cirrhosis
- Jaundice, cholangitis, raised alkaline phosphatase level
- Incidental discovery at laparotomy or autopsy

Clearly, diabetic patients are not immune to other causes of liver disease. Thus, before attributing liver abnormalities in diabetic patients to simple fatty liver, other diseases should be considered and excluded.

TYPES OF LIVER INJURY

Glycogen Deposition

Vacuolization of hepatocyte nuclei due to glycogen deposition may be present in 80% of diabetic patients subjected to liver biopsy.[101,137] The mechanism for this phenomenon is poorly understood. The combination of glycogenated nuclei and severe steatosis found in a liver biopsy often suggests the patient has diabetes.[494] Nuclear vacuolization is not specific to diabetic patients; it also is found in Wilson's disease, sepsis, tuberculosis, and other diseases.[101] Marked hepatomegaly due to extensive cytoplasmic glycogen deposition in poorly controlled type I diabetic patients has been reported. When accompanied by growth retardation, obesity, a florid facies, and hypercholesterolemia, this entity in children is known as Mauriac's syndrome.[320] Milder forms of the syndrome may be seen in diabetic patients commenced on insulin therapy for diabetic ketoacidosis.[59,137,214,307] Once adequate diabetic control is achieved, the hepatomegaly usually regresses.

Because fatty liver and nonalcoholic steatohepatitis are discussed in some detail in Chapter 31, only some of the salient features of those problems in diabetic patients are discussed here.

Fatty Liver

Excessive fat deposition in the liver is common in type II diabetic patients. An average incidence of 50% has been reported, which may be an overestimate because only diabetic patients with abnormal liver test results or hepatomegaly tend to have biopsies performed.[101,148,494] Type I diabetic patients rarely have fatty liver except in situations of poor control.[494] Although the true incidence of fatty liver in diabetic patients is unknown, one ultrasound study[148] suggested that 23% of a population of stable diabetic outpatients had evidence of fatty liver. As radiologists became more adept at identifying fatty liver on imaging studies (computed tomography [CT] and ultrasound), and further reports of validation of these techniques for detecting fatty liver appear,[453] it is becoming more feasible to determine the true extent of this problem in diabetic patients. Regardless of the accuracy of noninvasive techniques in detecting fat in the liver, the only way to distinguish fatty liver from the precirrhotic (albeit slowly progressive) condition of nonalcoholic steatohepatitis is by liver biopsy.[454]

Despite many investigators stressing that steatosis and the more advanced lesion of steatohepatitis in diabetic patients do not correlate with the severity of glucose intolerance,[49,101,359,454,533] a report suggests the opposite is true.[479] Rather than the extent of obesity being the main factor correlating with the severity of findings on liver biopsy in obese diabetic patients, Silverman and colleagues[479] found that the degree of abnormality of glucose intolerance was more predictive. Whether this was due to a more careful evaluation of diabetic status in their morbidly obese patients compared with other studies of patients with fatty liver, is not apparent.[388,494] This issue might best be resolved by comparing the degree of severity of fatty liver with the level of glycosylated hemoglobin, rather than simply depending on random fasting blood sugar level tests. Against this concept are reports of severe fatty liver preceding the onset of hyperglycemia in a number of patients with strong family histories of diabetes.[21] The mechanism for excess fat deposition in the liver of diabetic patients probably arises from one or more of the following processes: (1) increased lipolysis, (2) increased uptake of fatty acids by the liver, (3) increased production of hepatic triglycerides, and (4) limited capacity to export synthesized triglycerides. The relative roles of obesity and diabetes in mediating the deposition of excessive fat in the liver of diabetic patients through one or more of these mechanisms are difficult to ascertain because most type II diabetic patients are obese.[494]

Diagnosis of fatty liver is best achieved with liver biopsy; however, it is not practical to perform biopsies on all diabetic patients with abnormal liver test results or hepatomegaly. Typically, serum transaminase levels are either normal or only modestly raised (less than three-fold elevations) in fatty liver. Unlike in alcoholic liver disease, the alanine aminotransferase level frequently is greater than the aspartate aminotransferase level.[494] Many clinicians recommend hepatic ultrasound as the first test in evaluating liver abnormalities in diabetic patients.[148,453] Clearly, if the patient is massively obese, a CT scan may be preferable. Reliable reports of findings compatible with fatty liver are being received from radiologists. Coupled with improvement or normalization of liver test results with weight reduction, this suggests that the diagnosis is indeed fatty liver.[388,454] It remains to be seen if the reported[388] impressive improvement in liver abnormalities with weight reduction in overweight patients applies to obese diabetic patients as well (only 8% of the patients in that study were diabetic). The only treatment for fatty liver in type II diabetes that can be recommended is weight reduction. This not only may improve liver status but also should reduce insulin requirements or lower insulin levels.[388,454] Hyperinsulinemia has been suggested as a factor in diabetes-related liver disease.[545] One drawback of weight reduction as a treatment for liver abnormalities in obese diabetic patients is that it may

induce the formation of gallstones.[285] This problem potentially could be prevented by prophylactic use of ursodeoxycholic acid.

Fatty Liver With Portal Fibrosis

This entity appears to be a variant of fatty liver. As the term implies, fibrosis is seen in portal areas, typically in a stellate pattern.[1] Whether this pathologic finding progresses to cirrhosis with or without intervening nonalcoholic steatohepatitis remains to be determined.

Nonalcoholic Steatohepatitis

Various terms for this have been used over the years (fatty liver hepatitis, diabetic hepatitis, and so forth). The presentation for this condition is similar to that for simple fatty liver in diabetic patients (see section on diabetes mellitus and the liver). Liver test abnormalities do not distinguish between fatty liver and nonalcoholic steatohepatitis.[454] Thus, as more patients are noted to have fatty liver by radiologic imaging studies, the subgroup with nonalcoholic steatohepatitis may be missed unless liver biopsy is performed. Whether this is of any clinical consequence is debatable because recommendation for weight loss is the treatment of choice whatever the biopsy shows.[454] If a liver biopsy demonstrates nonalcoholic steatohepatitis, then the main issue to resolve is whether the lesion is truly nonalcoholic. Despite reports that nonalcoholic steatosis can be distinguished from alcoholic hepatitis based on histologic findings alone,[139] it is the experience of some groups that histologic distinction can be difficult.[116,274,277,297,359,454,468,479,494] (Further discussion of nonalcoholic steatohepatitis can be found in Chapter 31.) Whether this lesion is responsible for an increased incidence of cirrhosis in diabetic patients[101,494,503] is uncertain but remains a possibility because it has been documented that steatohepatitis has progressed to cirrhosis in a number of cases.[139,494]

Increased Iron Deposition

Clearly, if excessive iron is noted on liver biopsy in a diabetic patient, the first consideration is whether the patient has hemochromatosis.[145,324] Hemochromatosis, alcoholism with or without pancreatic insufficiency, and cirrhosis can be associated with excessive liver iron deposition.[183] The major difference between these processes is that the amount of iron deposited in liver in hemochromatosis is far higher and leads to cirrhosis.[324] Mild to moderate increases in hepatic iron content can be seen in chronic pancreatitis, in part due to failure of the pancreas to alkalinize the duodenum. This results in increased iron absorption, as does alcohol, which can lead to diagnostic confusion in some cases,[183] particularly in patients with alcoholic liver disease.

Portal Tract–Bile Ductular Abnormalities

Diabetes secondary to chronic pancreatitis can be associated with histologic features of extrahepatic biliary obstruction due to common bile duct strictures.[290] Occasionally, this can lead to biliary cirrhosis.[290,550] Generally, the diabetic aspect of these patients' medical problems is minor compared with the dominating symptoms of pain and malabsorption due to chronic pancreatitis.[550] Although this entity might come to light on liver biopsy, the best technique for detection of this problem is ultrasonography followed by cholangiography.[290] Because of the higher incidence of gallstones in diabetic patients,[31] liver biopsies displaying marked neutrophil infiltration in the portal tracts may signify ascending cholangitis even in the absence of classic symptoms. An analysis of the issue of cholecystectomy in diabetic patients with asymptomatic gallstones did not favor prophylactic gallbladder removal.[152]

Cirrhosis

In their exhaustive review of liver diseases and diabetes mellitus in 1970, Creutzfeldt and colleagues[101] concluded that "the frequent co-incidence of different liver diseases with diabetes mellitus is not the consequence of diabetes." In light of documentation since this report of the progression of steatohepatitis in diabetic patients to cirrhosis,[139] we must assume that there is some risk for the development of cirrhosis in diabetic patients. Because obesity without overt diabetes also has been documented occasionally to result in cirrhosis,[1] the relative roles of diabetes and obesity in contributing to the *possible* increase of cirrhosis in diabetic patients remain unclarified. Because of major uncertainties in the criteria for diagnosing diabetes in older autopsy studies, the real incidence of cirrhosis in patients with diabetes is unknown.[101] It is possible that study of a large cohort of diabetic patients using modern techniques of hepatic imaging and liver biopsy eventually could determine the risk of cirrhosis in patients with type II diabetes.

Other than the known potential for the progression of steatohepatitis to cirrhosis, no pathophysiologic mechanism for the possible increase in cirrhosis in diabetic patients has been proved.[49,101,503] Some cases of biliary cirrhosis due to pancreatitis-associated common bile duct obstruction may be occurring.[550] Hepatotoxicity due to oral hypoglycemic drug therapy conceivably may play some role.[48,178,360,461,519] As mentioned earlier, high insulin levels have been suggested potentially to be involved in inducing the lesion of steatohepatitis with fibrosis.[545] One of the more plausible suggestions over the years was that viral hepatitis was more common in diabetic patients.[101,494] There seems, however, little evidence supporting this with objective serologic markers of viral hepatitis. The role of chronic hepatitis C in liver disease in diabetic patients, however, has yet to be investigated. When insulin injection practices were not as hygienic as today, viral hepatitis may well have been a real risk for diabetic patients. The diabetic population at risk for liver disease does tend to have frequent contact with medical workers, blood transfusions during cardiac surgery, and other potentially risky situations for contracting viral hepatitis. Studies are awaited on the diabetic population to ascertain if they have an increased incidence of any form of viral hepatitis.

CLINICAL PRESENTATION OF LIVER DISEASE IN DIABETIC PATIENTS

Liver disease in diabetic patients can present in many different ways, as noted earlier. The most common is mildly abnormal liver test results. Assessment of these patients requires the same approach as it does in the nondiabetic population. In other words, not all liver problems are due to fatty liver in diabetic patients, and a diligent evaluation for other causes of liver disease should not be denied these patients. Occasionally, rarer entities with possible association with diabetes, such as nodular regenerative hyperplasia[509] or hepatic adenomas,[147] are discovered with investigations such as ultrasound and liver biopsy. More often, a diagnosis is made based

on the patient's lack of hepatotoxic (including alcohol) exposure, a compatible ultrasound examination, and negative test results for other causes of liver disease. If a trial of weight reduction reduces liver test abnormalities or hepatomegaly (if detected), then often the diagnosis of fatty liver is thought to be sound, without necessitating recourse to a confirmatory liver biopsy.[454] Occasionally, focal deposition of fat in the liver can lead to diagnostic confusion, particularly with metastatic liver disease.[82] Significantly elevated alkaline phosphatase levels in a diabetic patient always should be investigated, with the emphasis that the particular liver test abnormality rarely should be attributed to simple fatty liver alone. Although poorly documented in the literature, all clinicians are aware of the tendency of diabetic patients to present with severe extrahepatic biliary tract disease in the absence of florid symptoms and signs. Thus, even a hint of biliary tract disease in a diabetic patient should be investigated promptly. As in the nondiabetic patient, patients with diabetes can present with florid decompensated cirrhosis. Often, if they are scrutinized, evidence for portal hypertension can be ascertained from their prior medical records. Isolated thrombocytopenia, leukopenia, or raised globulin levels should suggest to physicians that their otherwise healthy-appearing diabetic patient may have more than just fatty liver. Because of obesity, however, hepatomegaly often is not detected in type II diabetic patients and liver disease is never suspected unless liver test abnormalities are present. Occasionally, fatty liver, nonalcoholic steatohepatitis, and even cirrhosis are discovered accidentally for the first time at laparotomy.

Hypoglycemia in Liver Disease

Symptomatic hypoglycemia is a common complication of fulminant hepatic failure.[452] Massive reduction in functioning hepatic mass has been known to be associated with hypoglycemia since the early 1920s.[308] In massive liver injury, the capacity of the liver to produce glucose from glycogenolysis and gluconeogenesis is reduced below a critical level. Loss of the normal metabolism of insulin by the liver with resulting hyperinsulinemia,[518] in addition to other hormonal alterations in fulminant hepatic failure, also contributes to hypoglycemia. Presumably, conditions like Reye's syndrome and fatty liver of pregnancy that are not associated with hepatic necrosis lead to hypoglycemia because of acquired mitochondrial enzyme abnormalities.[213] Mild hypoglycemia with less severe viral hepatitis has been reported to be common (about half of cases) in one series,[141] but was not confirmed in another study.[253]

Hypoglycemia in patients with fulminant hepatic failure can be severe and require massive glucose administration to correct.[452] This problem can occur abruptly, which is one of the many reasons why patients with fulminant hepatic failure should be managed in intensive care units.

In contrast to fulminant hepatic failure, hypoglycemia is rare in chronic liver disease, even in its most advanced states.[561] Insulin resistance,[72,226,333,401,447,500,535] preferential use of nonglucose substrates for energy in the fasted state,[353] and possibly preservation of gluconeogenesis by the kidney may protect patients with cirrhosis from hypoglycemia. Similar mechanisms may protect these patients from alcoholic hypoglycemia and insulin therapy-induced hypoglycemia, which appears to be rare in patients with cirrhosis. Septicemia, especially with septic shock,[370] and the development of hepatocellular carcinoma[331] are the two situations in which symptomatic hypoglycemia can develop in patients with chronic liver disease. Two types of hypoglycemia are recognized with hepatocellular carcinoma, which may be accompanied by other features of the paraneoplastic syndromes associated with this tumor (erythrocytosis, hypercalcemia, hypercholesterolemia).[92] Type A cases are the most common (87% of cases), and these patients typically have poorly differentiated, rapidly growing tumors.[331] Hypoglycemia appears only in the preterminal stage of the disease in those patients who suffer from severe muscle wasting. Severe malnutrition in cirrhosis may cause hypoglycemia due to a decreased muscle mass, which is the major carbon source for gluconeogenesis.[157,158] In type A cases, however, the hypoglycemia is thought to be due to glucose consumption of the tumor exceeding the capacity of the residual noncancerous liver to produce glucose.[331] The less common type B case is seen in patients with well differentiated tumors who can experience the abrupt onset of hypoglycemia, which may be extremely difficult to correct. The mechanism for hypoglycemia in these patients is obscure but appears to be due to an acquired defect in glycogenolysis[92] rather than the production of an insulin-like substance by the tumor, which was implicated and then refuted in earlier studies.[144,463] Reduced hepatic production of glucose has been demonstrated in patients with hepatocellular carcinoma[269] despite high glycogen content in the tumor and remaining liver.[92]

Thyroid Disorders and the Liver

HYPERTHYROIDISM

Disturbances in liver function have been reported in both hyperthyroidism and in hypothyroidism (Table 50-5). Mild, nonspecific increases in transaminase and serum alkaline phosphatase levels often are seen in thyrotoxicosis.[6,65,507] Apparently, both bone and liver contribute to the raised alkaline phosphatase levels that are a fairly consistent feature of hyperthyroidism.[98] Jaundice is rare in thyrotoxicosis; it seems to have been a feature of thyrotoxicosis in the era of less effective antithyroid therapy than is currently available.[24,65,546] When it is observed, jaundice has been attributed to congestive hepatopathy due to thyrotoxicosis-induced heart failure,[193] but it has been clearly observed in the absence of heart failure,[193] especially in thyroid storm patients.[221] As noted earlier, more recent reports of histologic changes in the livers of patients with hyperthyroidism do not demonstrate centrilobular necrosis,[6] which was present in earlier series.[24,65,546] The mechanism of liver injury in thyrotoxicosis is thought to be caused in part by relative centrilobular hypoxia due to increased hepatocyte demand for oxygen without a concomitant increase in hepatic blood flow.[533] A similar mechanism has been proposed for alcohol-induced liver injury.[379] Jaundice appearing in patients with milder cases of hyperthyroidism should raise the issue of an underlying liver disease or Gilbert's disease.[193]

HYPOTHYROIDISM

Hypothyroidism frequently is associated with increased serum levels of creatine kinase, aldolase, lactic dehydrogenase, and aspartate aminotransferase.[259] Alanine aminotransferase

TABLE 50-5 *Thyroid Disorders and the Liver*

Hyperthyroidism
  Mildly abnormal LFT results, especially alkaline phosphatase
  Jaundice in thyroid storm
Hypothyroidism
  Half of patients have mild LFT abnormalities
  Myxedematous ascites
Associated disease
  Primary biliary cirrhosis
  Primary cholangitis
  Chronic active hepatitis
Therapy-associated
  Liver toxicity with antithyroid drugs
  Interferon-induced thyroid dysfunction
Acute hepatitis
  Increased T_4 levels due to increased TBG
  Variable serum T_3 levels
Chronic liver disease
  Normal, low, or elevated T_4 levels
  Decreased conversion of T_4 to T_3
  Decreased serum T_3 levels
  Increased rT_3 concentration
  Normal or slight elevation of TSH

LFT, liver function test; T_4, thyroxine; TBG, thyroxine-binding globulin; T_3, triiodothyronine; rT_3, reverse triiodothyronine; TSH, thyroid-stimulating hormone.

levels also may be elevated on occasion. Because of routine multipanel biochemical testing, unless creatine kinase levels are measured, liver disease often is suspected in undiagnosed hypothyroid patients. Creatine kinase levels can be highly elevated, predominantly as the result of an increase in the muscle–isoenzyme fraction.[259] Thus, most if not all of the serum enzyme changes seen in hypothyroidism appear to result from muscle rather than liver. Hypothyroid myopathy may be an early manifestation of thyroid dysfunction and be associated with minimal thyroid test result abnormalities.[259] Some of its symptoms can be confused with nonspecific symptoms commonly seen in patients with liver disease (eg, myalgias, fatigue, cramps), which adds to diagnostic confusion in some cases.

Another less common manifestation of hypothyroidism that can raise the issue of liver disease is so-called myxedematous ascites.[83,259,450] Typically, this is a high-protein ascites unassociated in many cases with any signs of heart failure. Its mechanism is obscure, although one report described central congestive fibrosis of the liver in a number of patients.[10] Generally, no liver disease is evident as a cause for the syndrome. It can appear in mild hypothyroidism[259] and can be associated with massive and intractable ascites. Its frequent association with pleural and pericardial effusions can be helpful in leading to its consideration as a cause of ascites. Resolution of these effusions is seen with adequate thyroid replacement therapy, as is true of the serum enzyme abnormalities described earlier.

THYROID ABNORMALITIES IN LIVER DISEASE

Autoimmune chronic active hepatitis and primary biliary cirrhosis are associated with a high incidence of thyroid dysfunction.[102,506] In one study, nearly one quarter of patients with primary biliary cirrhosis were diagnosed as having hypothyroidism.[102] Because of frequently raised thyroid binding globulin levels in primary biliary cirrhosis and chronic active hepatitis, the diagnosis of hypothyroidism can be missed unless both free T_4 and thyroid-stimulating hormone (TSH) levels are measured.[465] As noted earlier, the appearance of significant liver test abnormalities in patients with thyroid diseases should raise the possibility of coincidental liver disease (eg, high alkaline phosphatase level in the hypothyroid patient could signify primary biliary cirrhosis). Sclerosing cholangitis also may be associated with a higher incidence of thyroid problems.[20,256]

Therapy-Associated Abnormalities

Occasionally, hepatotoxicity due to antithyroid drugs has been observed.[298,390] Concerns that propranolol therapy of portal hypertension would worsen thyroid test abnormalities in chronic liver disease by virtue of its inhibition of the conversion of T_4 to T_3[99] seem unfounded based on one study.[34] The use of propylthiouracil to treat alcoholic liver disease, although inconclusively efficacious,[200,247] does seem to have low toxicity. Reports on the impact of propylthiouracil on thyroid test result abnormalities in alcoholic liver disease are awaited.

One major issue in the thyroid is the potential toxicity of interferon therapy for chronic viral hepatitis. Although it is uncommon, one study reported an incidence of significant thyroid dysfunction in 5% of patients being treated for chronic hepatitis C.[38] Induction of autoimmunity to the thyroid is thought to be the basis of these abnormalities. Either thyrotoxicosis due to acute thyroiditis or hypothyroidism has been observed.[38] Weight loss in excess of the usual 5% to 10% range seen in chronic α-interferon therapy[425] may be an indication of hyperthyroidism in some patients. As mentioned earlier, the myopathy of hypothyroidism may be missed in a patient on interferon therapy because of the similarity between the symptoms of the myopathy and those induced by interferon therapy itself (muscle aching, and the like). Thus, monitoring of thyroid status in interferon-treated patients might be advisable, particularly if side effects from interferon treatment seem to be more severe than those normally observed.

THYROID TEST ABNORMALITIES IN LIVER DISEASE

Most clinicians confronted with the literature on acquired abnormalities of thyroid tests in patients with liver disease assume one needs to be an endocrinologist to interpret all the reported findings. In general, however, it can be assumed that most patients are euthyroid if they have a normal high-sensitivity TSH level and a normal free T_4 level. The latter test is routinely performed and obviates the need to take into account the variation in thyroid-binding globulin levels seen in patients with liver disease. Much of the confusion in the published literature dealing with thyroid test result abnormalities in liver disease, which at times appears contradictory, can be attributed to patients being studied at different stages of their disease.

Acute Liver Disease

Patients with acute liver disease tend to have elevated serum levels of total T_4 without signs of hyperthyroidism. The mechanism for this appears to be due primarily to increased thyroid-binding globulin levels.[159,438] Patients with more severe liver injury may have low thyroid-binding globulin and T_4 levels, but the data on this issue are mixed.[211] Because thyroid-binding globulin apparently is synthesized by the liver, it has been proposed that its production is reduced in more advanced disease.[27] Serum T_3 levels in acute liver disease are extremely variable,[533] but the ratio of T_3 to T_4 seems to correlate with the severity of liver damage and to have some prognostic significance.[211] The relationship of the varying reports of thyroid test result abnormalities in acute liver disease to the report of an incidence of thyroid enlargement in slightly over one quarter of patients with acute viral hepatitis remains to be confirmed and clarified.[207] Resolution of thyroid test abnormalities and goiter have been reported with recovery from acute hepatic diseases.[159,207]

Chronic Liver Disease

As mentioned earlier, primary biliary cirrhosis and autoimmune chronic active hepatitis alter thyroid test results in a fashion similar to that seen in acute liver disease (increased T_4 levels). Male patients with prominent feminization due to portosystemic shunting of blood can have high total T_4 levels, which seems to be due primarily to high thyroid-binding globulin levels.[53] Estrogen-induced induction of thyroid-binding globulin sialylation may be the mechanism for this phenomenon, allowing decreased hepatic uptake and clearance of the molecule. Free T_4 levels in these patients are normal.

More commonly, the following constellation of thyroid test result abnormalities is seen in patients with cirrhosis:

- Slightly elevated, normal, or lower levels of total serum T_4[220] due to increased, normal, or decreased synthesis of thyroid-binding globulins, respectively
- Normal to slightly elevated free T_4 levels
- Reduction in serum levels of T_3
- Increased levels of rT_3
- Normal or mild elevations of serum TSH levels

Decreased serum T_3 levels are found most consistently and reflect the severity of liver disease.[27,211,367] This perhaps is not surprising because peripheral conversion of T_4 to T_3 predominantly occurs in the liver.[211] rT_3, on the other hand, appears to be produced at extrahepatic sites.[27] Despite all of these changes, most patients generally are considered to be euthyroid. Subsets of patients with alcoholic cirrhosis have a submaximal TSH response to thyrotropin-releasing hormone (TRH), however, indicating hypothalamic–pituitary dysfunction.[531,533] Reports of thyroid gland volume reduction in alcoholic patients with cirrhosis, however, have not been attributable to this defect.[206,533] As stressed earlier, if in doubt about the thyroid status of a patient with liver disease, the advent of high-sensitivity TSH and free T_4 testing makes it easy to determine if an individual patient is euthyroid. Hepatocellular carcinoma has been reported to be associated with increased serum levels of thyroid-binding globulin.[245,373] The mechanism for this phenomenon, which can be found in 18% to 69% of patients, may be due to synthesis of the globulin by the tumor.[168,245,502] When it occurs, it can be a useful marker for assessment of treatment response (surgical resection or chemotherapy).[502] Despite impressively increased levels of total T_4, these patients generally are euthyroid.[373]

Sex Steroids and the Liver

SEXUAL DIMORPHISM OF HEPATIC FUNCTION

As early as 1937, Holck and colleagues[217] noted that female rats were anesthetized with half the dose of amobarbital required in males. Other barbiturates such as pentobarbital have prolonged duration of anesthetic effect in female compared with male rats.[217] No sex differences were found with hexobarbital or chloral hydrate, so that not all hepatic metabolic enzymes similarly respond. These sex-related alterations in enzyme activity have been defined as dimorphism. Hepatic enzymes such as lidocaine-N-deethylase have gender-dependent levels of activity (Table 50-6). These enzymes also may be induced by phenobarbital, which reduces these

TABLE 50-6 *Sex Differences in Hepatic Proteins*

Male	Female
Microsomal Oxidative Enzymes	
Estrogen-2α-hydroxylase	Steroid 5α-reductase
Estrogen-4-hydroxylase	
2α-, 2β-, 6β-, 15β-, 16α, 18 testosterone hydroxylase	
Hexobarbitol hydroxylase	
Benzo(a)pyrene hydroxylase	
Enzymes	
Ethylmorphine demethylase	Bile acid sulfotransferase
Lidocaine-N-deethylase	7α-Testosterone hydroxylase
Imipramine-N-demethylase	Phosphorylase a
Imipramine-N-oxidase	Carbonic anhydrase
Diazepam-3-hydroxylase	Monoamine oxidase
Diazepam-N-demethylase	Glutathione peroxidase
Aminopyrine demethylase	Cholinesterase
Acetominophen sulfotransferase	Glucose-6-phosphate dehydrogenase
Carbonic anhydrase	6-Phosphogluconate dehydrogenase
Histidase	HMG-CoA reductase
Aldehyde oxidase	
Glutathione-5-transferase (ligandin)	
UDP-glucuronyl transferase	
Receptors	
Androgen	Estrogen
LDL	Prolactin
	β-Adrenergic catecholamines
Hepatic Proteins	
β₂-Microglobulin	
Male-specific estrogen binder	
Bond's protein	
Serum Proteins	
α₂ᵤ-Globulin	Ceruloplasmin
α₁-Antitrypsin	Sex hormone-binding globulin
	Transcortin
	Thyroxine-binding globulin
	Vitellogenin
	Thiamine and riboflavin binding proteins

UDP, uridine diphosphate; LDL, low-density lipoprotein; HMG-CoA, 3-hydroxy-3-methylglutaryl coenzyme A.

sex differences.[114] Hepatic enzymes that metabolize drugs or steroids, levels of androgen, estrogen, low-density lipoprotein and prolactin receptors, several serum proteins that are synthesized and secreted by the liver, induction of fatty liver,[477] and diet-induced cirrhosis[426] are sex-dependent in mammals and in humans, to a somewhat lesser extent. Males are more capable of hepatic microsomal oxidation, females of reductive activity.[404] In general terms, this translates into a variety of drugs acting two to five times longer or more potently in females than in males. This is due to differences in enzymatic rates of metabolism. Sexual dimorphism makes teleologic sense because it provides the liver in the oviparous female with the capability transiently to produce most of the lipids and yoke proteins needed in egg formation.[442] Vitamin-binding proteins and detoxification enzymes produced by the female liver protect the embryo from circulating waste products and control steroid metabolism. Continued sex hormone–specific regulation of hepatic function postpartum is maintained through hepatic hormones and their respective receptors. Hepatic proteins that vary in amount due to gender in humans and rats are listed in Table 50-6 in relation to their function. Sex steroid alteration of hepatic protein levels or activity may differ from gender-directed hepatic dimorphism. Normal male hepatic function requires androgens both as a surge early in life, for male imprinting of the hypothalamus and pituitary to ensure full enzyme activity in adulthood, and in some instances postpuberty, to maintain maximal activity. Castration abolishes the activity of these male hepatic proteins and testosterone administration restores it. Pregnant rats, when given high doses of cimetidine, an H₂ antagonist with antiandrogenic activity, showed a 40% decrease in estrogen 2-hydroxylase (a male-specific liver enzyme) activity in adult male offspring.[125] Although the molecular process of hepatocarcinogenesis is complex and multifactorial, males are at increased risk. An association has been made with increased male hepatic sulfotransferase activity and the production of N-2-fluorenylacetamide, a carcinogen.[305] Sex steroids alter hepatic enzymes involved in glucose metabolism in a gender-dependent manner as well. Studies have shown that the lipogenic enzymes glucose-6-phosphate dehydrogenase, 6-phosphogluconate dehydrogenase, hexokinase, phosphofructokinase, and fumarase have more activity in females than males.[276] This parallels a general trend in females of more activity in androgen inactivation with higher levels of 5α-reductase and conversion to estrogens than in males.[110] Female animals have at least twice as much liver alcohol dehydrogenase activity than males.[419] Liver alcohol dehydrogenase turnover is stimulated by androgen levels rather than estrogen-related alterations, because only male gonadectomy affects enzyme activity. Female gonadectomy has no effect.[342] Estrogen treatment of males reverses neonatal imprinting and feminizes hepatic function. Androgen exposure in female brains masculinizes hepatic metabolism.[197] Sex steroid control of steroid metabolism in the liver also involves the hypothalamic–pituitary axis, because hypophysectomy eliminates sex differences.[197]

HYPOTHALAMIC–PITUITARY CONTROL

Both the hypothalamus and anterior pituitary regulate the sexual dimorphism of hepatic function.[264] Electrical ablation of the anterior periventricular hypothalamic area and amygdala in males feminizes hepatic metabolism. Somatostatin was identified as the essential neurohormone in this process. Somatostatin treatment of castrated male rats feminizes liver function, whereas it has no effect on intact males. Somatostatin and androgen administration to castrated males decreased in part the feminization process.[531] Thus, the hypothalamic input in the hypothalamic–pituitary–liver axis can be modified by sex steroids. Estradiol implantation in the paraventricular or anterior pituitary region in male rats feminizes hepatic function. The female pulsatile pattern of growth hormone secretion feminizes hepatic steroid metabolism in the rat.[345]

Decreased pituitary sensitivity in the male alcoholic involves more than gonadotropin cells because chlorpromazine, TRH, and sleep-induced prolactin secretion is inappropriately normal in patients with cirrhosis, TRH-induced growth hormone release is enhanced, and TRH-induced TSH secretion was significantly decreased compared with controls.[528,531]

MALE IMPRINTING

The liver is inherently female in its metabolic pattern.[114] The term *imprinting* has been applied to brain, gonad, and hepatic postnatal differentiation due to hormonal exposure that results in the irreversible establishment of a male pattern of response.[198] Both androgens and growth hormone are required before puberty to induce a male pattern of hepatic proteins. In rats, the pattern of growth hormone secretion is sex specific: a male pulsatile periodicity with peaks every 3 to 4 hours and low baseline levels, and a female random peak pattern and high baseline levels. In male rats treated with portacaval anastomosis with evidence of portal hypertension, growth retardation occurs despite an intact male pattern of growth hormone secretion (McCullough AJ, unpublished observation, June 1991), so that growth hormone action in the liver is multifaceted. Exposure of a hypophysectomized rat neonate to the continuous administration of growth hormone results in feminized liver function.[346] Hepatic metabolism in the male is partially decreased after puberty by castration and thus requires androgen exposure throughout life to maintain maximal male-specific enzyme and protein activities.[107,130] Female hepatic metabolic patterns require normal growth hormone secretion. Testosterone exposure to female neonatal rats was without effect in adult hepatic metabolic enzyme acativity. Androgen exposure in the 35- to 50-day-old postpubertal female increased arylhydrocarbon hydroxylase levels to male values, suggesting a window period of hormonal sensitivity in female hepatic metabolic patterns.[387]

Liver Disease and Alterations in the Reproductive Endocrine Axis

ALCOHOLIC LIVER DISEASE

Of the many liver diseases, alcohol-related injury is the most destructive of reproductive function. Both androgen deficiency and feminization clinically occur in alcoholic men, and oligoamenorrhea occurs in alcoholic women. Classic studies first demonstrated the occurrence of feminization with alcohol-related cirrhosis and postulated that severe liver disease decreased metabolism and clearance of steroids and resulted in endocrine dysfunction. It has since been shown

in human and animal studies that alcohol-related sex steroid imbalance and feminization are found throughout the range of liver pathology, from normal to cirrhosis.[9] Thus, alcohol toxicity, liver disease, and reproductive perturbation are interrelated, multifaceted processes. Much of our understanding of the effects of alcohol on the reproductive endocrine status is due to the critical studies done by Van Thiel, Gavaler, and colleagues. Thorough and timely reviews that include this effort have been published.[516,518,533] This review focuses on human data in this area with reference as needed to information derived from animal studies.

Men

Alcohol interferes with normal function in male testes, pituitary, hypothalamus, and adrenal gland. Alcohol ingestion alters testosterone synthesis and metabolism differently in the absence or presence of cirrhosis. In the absence of liver disease, alcohol levels above 100 mg/dL decrease the amplitude of episodic plasma testosterone secretion within 24 hours and by 5 days reduce significantly the mean plasma testosterone level.[179] Studies in animals suggest no acute effect of ethanol on testicular 3α-hydroxysteroid dehydrogenase activity; however, chronic exposure decreases this enzyme activity by 30%.[77] Ethanol also decreases the intracellular concentration of a cofactor required in testosterone synthesis, NAD^+. This effect is reversible in vitro. In vivo, NAD^+ depletion favors androstenedione production over that of testosterone. Thus, ethanol exposure can inhibit testosterone synthesis in several steps. An increase in serum LH is seen in men at the onset of peak blood ethanol levels.[335] LH and follicle stimulating hormone (FSH) are normal after the first 24-hour period of alcohol ingestion when measured both in secretory patterns and amplitudes in the normal man. These data taken together suggest that a primary effect of acute alcohol exposure is gonadotoxic in the man. After a 72-hour period of alcohol exposure, serum testosterone levels decreased and LH levels increased in normal men.[530] Chronic alcohol exposure (5 to 22 days) decreases plasma LH levels. A diminished response of LH release due to stimulation using luteinizing-releasing factor (LRF) was found in normal men exposed to alcohol and in alcoholic persons with a range of liver disease. This response is unlike the exaggerated one seen in patients with primary gonadal dysfunction and the increase seen with repeated LRF stimulation in hypothalamic hypogonadotropic hypogonadism. Thus, the dual effects of ethanol, as proposed by Van Thiel, involve gonadal toxicity and pituitary hyperresponsiveness.[529] In men with cirrhosis, normal, low, and elevated LH and FSH levels have been measured (Table 50-7).[11,118] Pituitary gonadotropin reserve has been measured in response to clomiphene and LRF stimulation infusion. In men with cirrhosis, a normal, diminished, and rarely a stimulated pattern of LH and FSH secretion was found,[179,548] suggesting that the hypothalamic–pituitary axis alterations are not uniformly predictable. Relative or absolute pituitary gonadotropin deficiency in general is seen in end-stage alcoholic cirrhosis and includes basal and stimulatable gonadotropin activity. It appears to be irreversible in men and may correlate with encephalopathy.[11] A significant negative association between gonadotropin-stimulated testosterone secretion and LRH-stimulated gonadotropin release has been reported in men with cirrhosis.[118] One interpretation of these findings may be enhanced feedback by testosterone at low concentrations on anterior pituitary function.

TABLE 50-7   *Basal Hormone Values in Patients With Alcohol-Related Cirrhosis Compared to Normal Men and Women* *

Hormone	Men		Women	
	Cirrhotic	Normal	Cirrhotic	Normal
T_{free} (nmol/L)	6.6 ± 4.8[14]	10–35[551]	< 3.5	0.59 ± 0.06[79]
T_{total} (ng/mL)	$5.57 \pm .50$[286]	4.24 ± 1.67	1.45 ± 0.22[68]	1.36 ± 0.14
MCR_T (L/d/m²)	338 ± 121[11]	543 ± 142	—	321 ± 12[180]
Androstenedione (nmol/L)	8.12 ± 2.8[14]	3.83 ± 1.7	6.65 ± 1.33[68]	5.90 ± 0.44
$Estradiol_{free}$ (nmol/L)	$0.64 \pm .44$[11]	0.47 ± 0.32	—	0.07–0.22[551]
$Estradiol_{total}$ (pg/mL)	29.3 ± 2.2[396]	23.3 ± 2.0	—	101 ± 23.9[79]
$MCR_{Estradiol}$ (L/d/m²)	722 ± 311[11]	878 ± 295	—	—
$Estrone_{total}$ (pg/mL)	74.2 ± 8.0[396]	26.0 ± 1.7	1.15 ± 0.07[68]	1.29 ± 0.21
$Estriol_{total}$ (pg/mL)	11.5 ± 1.9[396]	6.5 ± 0.7	—	—
SHBG (mg/dL)	4.32 ± 3.2[529]	0.52 ± 0.29	0.394 ± 0.26[68]	0.340 ± 0.23
Luteinizing hormone (U/L)	20.5 ± 2.9[528]	9.2 ± 1.1	—	5–25[551]
FSH (U/L)	23.9 ± 3.8[528]	7.4 ± 0.6	—	5–20[551]

MCR, metabolic clearance rate; SHBG, sex hormone-binding globulin; FSH, follicle-stimulating hormone; T, testosterone.
*Values are means ± standard deviation. The units for data from reference 68 are nmol/L.

Chronic alcohol ingestion (24 days) decreases by 40% testosterone binding to sex hormone–binding globulin (SHBG), the major androgen carrier protein in plasma.[182] One study has demonstrated an inverse relationship between the severity of liver disease and basal testosterone levels. In addition, basal serum testosterone does not correlate with outcome in alcoholic men with cirrhosis.[504] Ample data support a four- to eight-fold elevation in SHBG serum concentration in chronic alcoholic men,[525,529] (see Table 50-7). The metabolic clearance rate (MCR) for testosterone increases after 4 weeks of drinking alcohol, although data are confusing in other studies. $MCR_{testosterone}$ is the product of hepatic testosterone extraction and hepatic blood flow. Hepatic blood flow increases 50% with alcohol intake.[78] Alcohol also enhances steroid metabolism in the man by increasing hepatic steroid A-ring reductase activity from 0.82 ± 0.35 to 2.87 ± 2.38 nmol/L/min/mg protein.[179] There were no differences in the conversion rate of testosterone to estradiol, estrone, and androstenedione after 28 days of alcohol intake.[179] No changes in the production rates of androstenedione and estradiol were found in normal men after alcohol intake.[179] In addition to the gonadotoxic effects of alcohol, alcohol intake without liver disease enhances hepatic metabolism of testosterone without increases in estrogen or pituitary gonadotropins. In contrast, alcohol intake in the presence of cirrhosis (1) decreased testosterone binding affinity to SHBG, (2) increased conversion of androstenedione to estrone, and (3) decreased MCR for testosterone.[180] These alterations attempt to maintain testosterone levels and shift metabolism toward estrogens. In humans with cirrhosis, plasma estrone and estradiol levels are elevated.[378] In rats, partial portal vein ligation further increased ethanol-induced estradiol and estrone levels, suggesting portosystemic shunting may enhance systemic estrogen levels.[527] Estrogen elevation appears to involve multiple factors, such as adrenal stimulation with production of estrogenic precursors, altered estrogen metabolism, protein binding and clearance, and less effective enterocirculation due to portosystemic shunting. Although alcohol increases aromatase activity in rat liver,[181] and aromatase is found in human liver,[485] there is no evidence for alcohol effects on human hepatic aromatase. The hepatic extraction ratio of steroids was measured in alcoholic men with cirrhosis and found to be 20% to 50% of total body clearance compared with normal men; hence, peripheral handling of steroids may play a critical regulatory role in steroid balance.[191] Although the hepatic extraction of androstenedione, testosterone, estradiol, progesterone, and 17-hydroxyprogesterone varies to a high degree of correlation with the degree of hepatic elimination impairment as measured by indocyanine green extraction, these ratios failed to predict plasma steroid concentrations, and thus other factors also must be important.

Hypogonadism—Testicular Atrophy.   Early descriptions of testicular atrophy in association with Laennec's cirrhosis in 1909 and 1910[14,524] emphasized the importance of chronic alcoholism and not cirrhosis in the genesis of testicular changes. Clinically, the normal measured testis diameter in an adult averages 4.6 cm, with a range of 3.5 to 5.5 cm, which corresponds to a volume of 12 to 25 mL.[194] Hypogonadism or a testicular diameter of less than 2.5 cm occurs in 30% to 75% of men with cirrhosis. In comparing data, it must be recognized that orchidometer measurements of testicular volumes less than 20 mL may be overestimates.[194] Impotence is reported in alcoholic men with cirrhosis in up to 80% to 90% of patients, with either abnormal seminal fluid or no ability to produce an ejaculate. Additional signs of hypogonadism include decreased beard growth, decreased axillary and torso hair, and delayed prostate hypertrophy. Two types of prostate hypertrophy exist, an early, stromal type that is dependent on estrogenic stimulation of fibromuscular tissue, and a later, epithelial hyperplasia variant that is androgen dependent.[521] Men with cirrhosis have a 41% incidence of epithelial hyperplasia compared with age-matched noncirrhotic men (71%), whereas there were no differences in the stromal type of prostate hypertrophy.[150] The association of hypogonadism with advanced liver disease is not an absolute one. In alcohol-fed and liver-injured animal models, testicular atrophy, decreased testosterone, and a decreased ability to produce progeny were found without significant liver disease. Normal testes have been noted in cases of severe cirrhosis in humans.[517] Conflicting data exist in comparison of alcoholic and nonalcoholic men with cirrhosis, because testicular atrophy was significantly more common in alcohol-related disease. No correlation of testicular abnormalities and liver histologic results was found in the study of 30 alcoholic persons,[288] yet the extent of testicular damage did increase with increasing amounts of alcohol consumed.[40,248] Several studies have explored the cellular mechanisms of alcohol toxicity in the testis. Alcohol reduces LH receptor binding and cAMP production in the testis.[177] Low ethanol concentrations (25 mg/dL) blocked 44% of testosterone synthesis and secretion in tissue culture.[132] Acetaldehyde in the same system achieved equal inhibition at a 1000-fold lower concentration.[90] An additional study in rats suggests acetaldehyde may mediate the gonadal toxicity of ethanol.[80] In perfused rat testes, acetaldehyde blocks testosterone production.[520] This inhibition is reversed by coincubation with 4-methylpyrazole, an alcohol dehydrogenase inhibitor, or penicillamine, which inactivates acetaldehyde.[164] There is an inducible alcohol dehydrogenase enzyme unique to the testes that may generate acetaldehyde, a more potent toxin than alcohol. Leydig cell microsomal enzymes have lower activity and an inhibitory redox state due to alcohol exposure. In the absence of the trophic influence of testosterone, atrophy of germ cell epithelium and seminiferous tubules occurs with subsequent testicular fibrosis.[529] Testicular interstitial or Leydig cells appear normal or even hyperplastic, yet have numerous derangements of mitochondria and microsomes.[534] Testicular atrophy is increased in men with cirrhosis under the age of 40 years,[349] although it is independent of age in another study.[30] Alcohol noncompetitively blocks testicular retinol (vitamin A) bioactivation, an essential factor in normal spermatogenesis.

Hypogonadism in the alcoholic man involves toxicity of alcohol and acetaldehyde within the testis, the suppression by alcohol of gonadotropic (LH, FSH) secretory patterns and gonadotropic content of the anterior pituitary, and alcohol effects on the central nervous system input to the hypothalamus. In patients with portosystemic shunting, further diversion of adrenal and testicular androgens to peripheral tissue such as fat and muscle, which contain aromatase, may perpetuate a relative androgen deficit and estrogen surplus that contributes to the cessation of spermatogenesis. Although this mechanism is tenable, further studies need to be done. Those protective mechanisms that prevail in alcoholic men with cirrhosis without hypogonadism remain unidentified. The nature of alcohol alteration of germ epithelium and Leydig cell testosterone production is unclear. The mechanisms of decreased pituitary sensitivity and hypothalamic alterations by alcohol remain to be defined. In addition, reversible features of these alterations need to be identified so that specific therapy may be possible.

Feminization—Gynecomastia. Hypogonadism and feminization are different abnormalities,[522] with testicular atrophy usually preceding feminization. Men with chronic liver disease frequently are feminized. The frequency of such characteristics appears to be increased in alcoholic liver disease. The incidence of characteristics of feminization has been reported to be 64% for female escutcheon, 36% for palmar erythema, 34% for cutaneous spiders, and 14% for gynecomastia.[282] Gynecomastia may be seen at birth and puberty in normal male development. Its incidence increases with age, adrenocorticoid and testicular tumors, thyrotoxicosis, malnutrition, paraplegia, and hospitalization. Obesity as measured by body mass index (BMI) may occur with gynecomastia in up to 85% of patients without liver disease, if the BMI is greater than 25 kg/m^2.[365] Prevalence of gynecomastia in men with cirrhosis usually is 67% and is unrelated to BMI. In an aged-matched comparison of alcoholic men with cirrhosis with nonalcoholic, nonobese hospitalized men, no differences in the number of patients with gynecomastia were found (50% versus 44%).[74] The patients with cirrhosis had decreased serum testosterone and increased estradiol, whereas the control group with gynecomastia had normal sex steroid values. No correlations were found between medications, extent of malnutrition, sex steroid hormone levels, the ratio of either total or free fraction of steroid hormones, and gynecomastia.[74,79] Other studies of gynecomastia in alcoholic men with cirrhosis have shown an association with increased plasma estrone and estriol despite normal total and unbound estradiol.[191] Thus, multiple factors and variable breast tissue sensitivity to hormonal change must be implicated in the etiology of gynecomastia associated with alcoholic cirrhosis.[79] At least one speculation has been put forth that a heightened sense of awareness rather than true association exists between alcoholic cirrhosis and gynecomastia. Serum prolactin levels are increased four-fold in alcoholic men with cirrhosis with gynecomastia compared with control subjects,[532] yet mild and reversible liver disease appears to reduce basal prolactin and enhance TRH-stimulatable hormone secretion in alcoholic men compared with control subjects.[531] Other studies have failed to show an association between hyperprolactinemia and gynecomastia.[511] Although prolactin synthesis is estrogen responsive, estrogen levels in liver disease do not correlate with prolactin, further complicating issues.[9] Prolactin levels are thought to be increased in association with, but not causative in, the development of gynecomastia.[55]

Biochemical features of estrogenization seen in alcoholic men include increases in serum levels of neurophysin (3-fold), SHBG (8-fold), prolactin (4.5-fold), and growth hormone (3-fold) compared with basal levels in normal men. When compared with estrogen levels, the appearance and degree of increase of these serum proteins do not correlate. Thus, evidence is inconclusive in men that biochemical feminization is due to high circulating levels of the estrogens. It is fairly consistent that estrone levels are increased 2- to 4-fold in men with alcoholic liver disease[260] due to increased peripheral aromatization of androstenedione and adrenal synthesis of estrone. Estrone is one twelfth as potent an estrogen as estradiol.[215]

A hypothesis that deserves further study suggests that part of the estrogenization may be due to excessive ingestion and retention of nonsteroidal estrogen-like substances in our food chain and in alcoholic beverages that have biologic activity (ie, phytoestrogens).[282,283] It has been demonstrated in quail and sheep that estrogenization can occur due to excessive ingestion of nonsteroidal estrogen-like plant substance in clover.[281] Ether extracts of male alcoholic plasma demonstrated estrogen-like binding affinity in 20% of samples not accountable by known hormones present in the serum.[282] Thus, tissue sensitivity to endogenous and exogenous estrogen may be increased in the presence of alcohol such that subcellular studies are needed to define such mechanisms in target tissues such as the breast, testes, prostate, uterus, ovary, pituitary, adipose tissue, and hair follicle.

Sex Differences in Alcohol-Induced Liver Disease

An autopsy study from 1936 to 1942[489] was the first to note sex differences in mortality among alcoholic patients with cirrhosis, with a mean age of death from any cause of 56.3 years for men and 48.6 years for women. Death from cirrhosis occurred at 45.7 years in women and 55.1 years in men.[489] Cirrhosis occurred in 250 cases, with 190 men and 60 women. This study and another[436] also demonstrated that 20% of men versus 85% of women died of liver failure. Carcinoma was coincident with cirrhosis in 9 of the 250 autopsies. A study of 14 men and 12 women who presented with acute alcoholic hepatitis and were followed nearly 2 years also indicated more toxicity in women, with 7 of 12 women and 2 of 14 men progressing to cirrhosis. It is noteworthy that four of seven of the female patients with cirrhosis had the disease despite documented alcohol abstinence.[389] Several reports identified that women have more severe liver disease at the initial hospital admission, with shorter-interval histories of alcohol intake at lower amounts.[389,548] Peguignot and colleagues[392] studied 227 hospitalized alcoholic patients with cirrhosis and found women to have a three times higher risk for cirrhosis than men. The study determined that risk for developing cirrhosis was significant at a daily dose of alcohol of 60 g in men and 20 g in women.[165,392]

Women

One of three alcoholic persons in the United States is a woman,[526] and a significant proportion (15%) of women deny alcoholism. The incidence of alcoholic hepatitis in Denmark as measured as a female/male ratio is rising from 0.11 in 1970 to 0.35 in 1984,[343] and in England it has risen from 0.2 in 1967 to 1971 to 0.47 in 1972 to 1975.[265] Referrals for treatment of women in alcoholic clinics have increased nearly sixfold in this same period. In gender-comparative studies, women presented with alcoholic hepatitis after 10.2 ± 4.4 years of drinking and a total of 633 ± 260 kg of alcohol, compared with 18.6 ± 6.7 years and 1389 ± 703 kg of alcohol in men.[389] A shorter duration of alcohol intake is seen in women in whom gastrointestinal hemorrhage, gastritis, hypertension, anemia, malnutrition, and obesity develop.[7] On the basis of study of 1000 patients with cirrhosis, cirrhosis occurred twice as often in women than men.[547] Alcoholic hepatitis develops in more black women than men in the United States,[289] although a reverse ratio was noted in another study.[163] Before 1970, the greatest rate increase of mortality due to cirrhosis in the United States was in black women.[55] Certainly, ample data support the idea that women are at more risk for liver injury than men. Alcoholic women with liver disease have increased serum immunoglobin (IgG and IgM) and smooth muscle antibody levels compared with men, suggesting that alcohol may elicit a greater immunologic response in women.[265] The risk for cirrhosis increases with dose of alcohol in men and women.[392] Interestingly, 5-year survival with cirrhosis in alcoholic women is similar to that in men with cirrhosis—45%—and is significantly improved by abstinence from alcohol,[343] challenging the British and European hypotheses that women are more susceptible to alcohol's toxicity than men.[265,347,389] The female gender is

a positive prognostic factor in cirrhosis in studies by the Copenhagen group.[172,459]

Female alcoholics are defeminized and have severe hypogonadism. Unlike men, steroid production in the woman is not acutely altered by alcohol. Early necropsy studies in chronic alcoholic premenopausal women showed evidence of hypogonadism: ovarian atrophy, the absence of corpora lutea, cystic dilatation of Graafian follicles, stromal hyperplasia in the ovary, adenofibrosis in the breast, narrowed adrenocortices, and estrogenized epithelium in the cervix.[19,523,558] Conflicting data exist on the uterine status in women with cirrhosis. Both atrophic and hyperplastic endometrium with amenorrhea and menometrorrhagia have been reported.[292] Clinically, hypogonadism is seen in chronic alcoholic women with a decrease in developing follicles and corpora lutea, oligoamenorrhea, a loss in breast and pelvic fat accumulation, and infertility. Biochemically, serum estradiol and progesterone are below normal, with increased FSH and a small increase in LH. Reports of sex steroid production and clearance rates in women with cirrhosis are minimal. There is altered hypothalamic response with decreased GRH release as a result of clomiphene exposure; however, normal gonadotropin response to clomiphene was seen in six postmenopausal and three premenopausal alcoholic women with chronic liver disease.[219] There is a report of two women admitted for detoxification during alcoholic hepatitis with a history 3.5 to 4 years of amenorrhea while heavily drinking alcohol. Both women noted menses within 2 to 12 weeks of abstinence from alcohol, suggesting gonadal impairment in premenopausal alcoholic women may be reversible.[449] Cirrhosis and pregnancy rarely concur, and occur more often in non–alcohol-related cirrhosis.[52] In a series of nine pregnancies from Iran involving postnecrotic cirrhosis in six women, chronic active hepatitis in one, and posthepatitic cirrhosis in two, hepatic decompensation was no more apparent than in control patients. Increased fetal risk as seen in stillbirths and premature deliveries was found in four cases.[52]

Acute alcohol administration does not alter the pituitary–gonadal axis in nonalcoholic women. When measured in the late follicular phase of young women with blood alcohol levels of 88 mg/dL, serum LH and estradiol were unchanged, whereas prolactin was increased compared with control subjects.[334] In luteal phase studies, no alcohol impairment of ovarian function was measured in terms of estradiol, progesterone, and testosterone serum levels. In addition, pituitary function as measured by secretion of LH, FSH, prolactin, and growth hormone was minimally altered.[514] In chronic alcoholic women, 2- to 4-fold elevations of prolactin were seen throughout the menstrual cycle in another study.[515] Most (85%) women with cirrhosis have evidence of enhanced estrogen response.[19] Chronic alcoholic women admitted for detoxification have 2- to 3-fold increased serum androstenedione and dehydroepiandrosterone throughout the entire menstrual cycle,[128] suggesting increased adrenal activity. Increased estrone production was the primary estrogen change found in six women with cirrhosis, with nearly a 10-fold increase in plasma conversion of androstenediol to estriol.[128] Studies measuring serum testosterone and SHBG in alcoholic women with and without cirrhosis found no differences from control levels[68] and yet another gender difference—elevated serum androstenedione in alcoholic women negatively correlated with liver histologic results (see Table 50-7).[68] Thus, much evidence exists for hypogonadism in the alcoholic woman. Peak levels of serum alcohol vary with the menstrual cycle and increase during the follicular phase.[165] Sex-dependent differences in SHBG and pituitary hormones are apparent.

Hormone Replacement

The effect of alcohol abstinence on impotence and loss of libido has been studied in 60 alcoholic men, and 25% of these had spontaneous recovery of sexual function.[526] No spontaneous recoveries occurred in men with testicular atrophy or who had inadequate LRF-stimulated secretion of LH and FSH. Liver histologic study did not predict this recovery. Neither clomiphene (20 mg/d) nor human chorionic gonadotropin administration (5000 IU twice weekly) brought return of sexual function in the 45 men who remained impotent for the 2 years of alcohol abstinence in this study. Fluoxymesterone, a nonaromatizable androgen, has been given up to 80 mg/d to those patients without spontaneous recovery of sexual function, and 25% of these men had return of sexual function. Azoospermia was the expected and only adverse side effect. Oxandrolone treatment of men with alcoholic hepatitis increased dietary intake and may improve long-term survival compared with placebo-treated control subjects.[336] Bromocriptine therapy in alcoholic persons has been unsuccessful.[348] Single-dose oral testosterone increases testosterone, dihydrotestosterone, androstenedione, and estrone levels in the serum for 2 to 24 hours in nonalcoholic men and to a greater extent in alcoholic men with cirrhosis. In addition, serum estradiol was increased in men with cirrhosis and not in normal men after testosterone administration.[174] Several blinded, controlled trials using oral testosterone for up to 4 years failed to show improvement of libido, erection, and ejaculatory function compared with placebo.[173,175,504] No benefits in liver function, complications of cirrhosis, and prognosis were reported. Serum hormone levels in alcoholic men who received oral testosterone for 1 year showed increased testosterone, estrone, and nonprotein-bound estradiol, decreased LH and FSH, and no change in prolactin.[166] It is unclear if this increase in estrogen and suppression of gonadotropins offsets androgen repletion benefits. More therapeutic trials for sexual dysfunction due to alcoholic liver disease must be conducted. These should include patients before the development of testicular atrophy and involve alcoholic abstinence, nonaromatizable androgen repletion with fluoxymesterone, mesterone, or 4-chlorotestosterone, and nontoxic inhibition of acetaldehyde production.[166]

Adrenal Cortical Function

Necropsy studies in patients with cirrhosis have demonstrated macroscopically normal-size adrenal glands with decreased lipid content in most.[292] Alcohol-related cirrhosis may impair the circadian patterns in glucocorticoid secretion, and evidence exists for enhanced aldosterone secretion.[318] Yet, a normal response to corticotropin (ACTH) stimulation of adrenal secretion in patients with cirrhosis also has been reported.[260] Urinary excretion of 17-hydroxycorticosteroids and 17-ketosteroids is increased in normal and alcoholic men given oral alcohol.[19] Reduction of hydrocortisone is decreased in the cirrhotic liver. Conjugation of corticosteroid metabolites is preserved in liver disease.[135] Acute alcohol intoxication has been reported in four men and two women associated with clinical findings suggestive of Cushing's syndrome. These patients have decreased peripheral muscle mass, truncal obesity, hypertension, and facial erythema. Biochemical assessment showed a mean elevated baseline morning cortisol level of 44.5 ± 21.2 mg/dL, and inadequate response to dexamethasone suppression was demonstrated in three patients. These abnormalities resolved after hospitalization and alcohol abstinence. A second group of patients with nonalcoholic liver disease had normal morning serum cortisol levels.[481] Cobb and colleagues[91] have shown in perfused rat adrenal glands that acetaldehyde increases corticosterone secretion 54%, suggesting a direct effect of this substance on the adrenal glands. ACTH stimulation test results in 31 adult men with hemochromatosis were found to be normal.[480] There is normal plasma cortisol and a normal response to ACTH stimulation of adrenal secretion in patients with hemochromatosis.[135]

NONALCOHOLIC LIVER DISEASE

A limited amount of information suggests that hypogonadism exists in association with nonalcoholic chronic liver disease. In general, hypogonadism is less prevalent and less severe in these cases. Testicular atrophy has been reported in hepatoma and in pancreatic carcinoma that is metastatic to liver.[349] In a comparative study, 21 nonalcoholic patients with liver disease were divided into three groups—11 with chronic active hepatitis, 5 with primary biliary cirrhosis, and 5 with cryptogenic cirrhosis—and were compared with alcoholic patients with liver disease and a control group. Nearly half of the patients with nonalcoholic liver disease admitted to decreased sexual function and impotence. Ten to 20% higher proportions of sexual dysfunction were noted in a comparable group with alcohol-related liver disease. Men with either chronic active hepatitis or cryptogenic cirrhosis reported only 13% and 7% loss in libido, respectively.[415] Testicular atrophy and gynecomastia were nearly nonexistent in chronic active hepatitis.[495] Men with non–alcohol-related liver disease have moderately decreased testosterone and dehydroepiandrosterone and normal estradiol levels compared with normal men. Despite similar Child-Pugh scores, more alcoholic men had decreased body hair and gynecomastia to a greater extent than the nonalcoholic liver disease group.[14] Less gynecomastia was noted in men with chronic active hepatitis, postnecrotic cirrhosis, and noncirrhotic portal hypertension compared with alcoholic persons with cirrhosis, although patient numbers were small.[155]

Hemochromatosis

Hypogonadism is found in most patients with hemochromatosis, with features of testicular atrophy, reduced body hair, altered fat distribution, decreased libido, and gynecomastia frequently reported. Testicular atrophy was found in 27 of 31 male patients with hemochromatosis who were studied, and was associated with female fat distribution in 1 case and gynecomastia in 4.[480] Basal serum testosterone and SHBG levels were normal in men with testicular atrophy and hemochromatosis despite a high proportion of patients with decreased libido or impotence.[543] Growth hormone levels were evenly divided into decreased, normal, and elevated levels. Serum FSH and LH levels were at the upper limit of normal.[480] In another study, basal LH and testosterone levels were below normal in 8 of 10 men and 2 of 2 women with hemochromatosis.[39] These patients also were not responsive to LRF or clomiphene administration. Basal and stimulated FSH levels were normal in this study. Markedly decreased pituitary response was measured by clomiphene and LRF challenge in all 10 men studied with hemochromatosis.[510] Iron deposition is recognized in gonadotropic and lactotropic cells in the anterior pituitary,[393] whereas hemosiderin deposition in the testes is predominantly in vessel wall and connective tissue.[510] Loss of spermatozoa, atrophy of the seminiferous tubules, and tubular wall thickening are seen on histologic examination of tissue from patients with hemochromatosis.[495] It is unresolved if hypogonadism in hemochromatosis is due to testicular or pituitary dysfunction, or a combination of both. Chronic administration of human chorionic gonadotropin increases testosterone in patients with hypogonadism and hemochromatosis.[170] The pituitary defect involves only the gonadotropic cells of the anterior pituitary, because ACTH, TSH, growth hormone, and prolactin levels were normal in most male patients with hemochromatosis who were studied.[76,332] As in alcohol-related hypogonadism, this clinical entity in patients with hemochromatosis often occurs before advanced liver disease.[11] Gynecomastia and spider nevi are less commonly seen in patients with hemochromatosis than in alcoholic persons with cirrhosis.[415] Serum estrogen levels in hemochromatosis have been reported to be normal.[544] Phlebotomy does not improve impotence in hemochromatosis, although symptomatic improvement has been shown with testosterone administration.[145,364] Gonadal effects of hemochromatosis in female patients have not been reported in detail.

Wilson's Disease, Biliary Cirrhosis, and Infiltrative Processes

Unlike hemochromatosis, Wilson's disease is not associated with gonadal or pituitary dysfunction because copper accumulation does not occur in these specific tissues. Copper association with amino acids has been shown to stimulate secretion of LRF, which may enhance gonadal function.[18] Sarcoidosis, amyloidosis, histiocytosis X, and tuberculosis may infiltrate hypothalamic and pituitary tissues as well as the liver. Alteration of the hypothalamic–pituitary–gonadal axis in these processes occurs due to infiltration of the neuroendocrine tissue, and not as a consequence of isolated liver disease. In a study of 25 patients with primary biliary cirrhosis, no differences in age of onset or duration of menopause were found compared with an age-matched control group.[26] Patients with primary biliary cirrhosis had increased estrone, androstenedione, and SHBG and similar testosterone and decreased dihydrotestosterone levels compared with control subjects. Amenorrhea is associated with nonalcoholic chronic liver disease in women. No correlation was found in duration of amenorrhea and duration of cirrhosis in 12 women of whom 7 had chronic active hepatitis.[105] Pituitary and gonadal hormone levels in these patients were divided into hypogonadotrophic and normogonadotrophic patterns, so that no singular pattern of endocrine dysfunction was apparent. A significant inverse correlation was found between duration of amenorrhea and metacarpal bone density, suggesting increased risk for bone complications.

SUMMARY

There is no consensus on the value of specific therapy directed against hormonal abnormalities in chronic liver disease. The factors controlling the interaction between hormonal status and survival in chronic liver disease are complex, and many of the pathophysiologic factors involved in altered hormonal metabolism remain to be defined in these patients. Sufficient evidence is emerging, however, to prohibit the clinician from considering these hormonal abnormalities merely a curious side effect of liver damage. Interventional hormonal therapies need to be considered in the overall management plans for these patients.

Acknowledgments

We thank Ms. Judy Gainer and Mrs. Molly O'Connell-Pasquale for their expert work in preparing the manuscript.

References

1. Adler M, Schaffner F. Fatty liver hepatitis and cirrhosis in obese patients. Am J Med 67:811–816, 1979
2. Adlercreutz H, Tenhunen R. Some aspects of the interaction between natural and synthetic female sex hormones and the liver. Am J Med 49:630–648, 1970
3. Alberti KGMM, Reord CO, Williamson DH, Wright R. Metabolic changes in active chronic hepatitis. Clin Sci 42:596–605, 1982
4. Alford FP, Dudley FJ, Chisholm DJ, Findlay DM. Glucagon metabolism in normal subjects and in cirrhotic patients before and after portosystemic venous shunt surgery. Clin Endocrinol 11:413–424, 1979
5. Arroyo V, Planas R, Gaya J, Deulofeu R, Rimola A, Perez-Ayuso RM, Rivera F, Rodes J. Sympathetic nervous activity, renin-angiotensin system and renal extraction of prostaglandin E_2 in cirrhosis: relationship to functional renal failure and sodium and water excretion. Eur J Clin Invest 13:271–278, 1983
6. Ashkar FS, Miller R, Smoak WM, Gilson AJ. Liver disease in hyperthyroidism. South Med J 64:462–465, 1971
7. Ashley MJ, Olen JS, LeRiche WH, Kornaczewski A, Schmidt W, Rankin JG. Morbidity in alcoholics: evidence for accelerated development of physical disease in women. Arch Intern Med 137:883–887, 1977
8. Atkinson PR, Weidman ER, Bhaumick KB, Bala RM. Release of somatomedin-like activity by cultured WF-38 human fibroblasts. Endocrinology 106:2006–2012, 1980
9. Bahnsen M, Gluud C, Johnsen SG, Bennett P, Svenstrup S, Micic S, Dietrickson O, Svendsen LB, Brodthagen UA. Pituitary-testicular function in patients with alcoholic cirrhosis of the liver. Eur J Clin Invest 11:473–479, 1981
10. Baker A, Kaplan M, Wolfe H. Central congestive fibrosis of the liver in myxedematous ascites. Ann Intern Med 77:927–929, 1972
11. Baker HWG, Burger HG, deKretser DM, Dulmanes A, Hudson B, O'Connor S, Paulsen CA, Purcell N, Rennie GC, Seah CS, Taft HP, Wang C. A study of the endocrine manifestations of hepatic cirrhosis. Q J Med 15:145–178, 1976
12. Bala RM, Bohnet HG, Carter JN, Friesen HG. Effect of ovine prolactin on serum somatomedin bioactivity in hypophysectomized female rats. Can J Physiol Pharmacol 56:984–992, 1978
13. Ballman M, Hartmann H, Deacon CF. Hypersecretion of proinsulin does not explain the hyperinsulinemia of patients with liver cirrhosis. Clin Endocrinol 25:351–361, 1986
14. Bannister P, Oakes J, Sheridan P, Losowsky MS. Sex hormone changes in chronic liver disease: a matched study of alcoholic versus non-alcoholic liver disease. Q J Med 63:305–313, 1987
15. Bannister P, Sheridan P, Losowsky MS. Identification and characterization of the human androgen receptor. Clin Endocrinol 23:495–502, 1985
16. Bar RS, Clemmons DR, Boes M, Busby WH, Booth BA,

Dake BL, Sandra A. Transcapillary permeability and sub-endothelial distribution of endothelial and amniotic fluid IGF-binding proteins in rat heart. Endocrinology 127:1078–1086, 1990

17. Bareca T, Franceschini R, Cataldi A, Rolandi E. Plasma somatostatin response to an oral mixed test meal in cirrhotic patients. J Hepatol 12:40–44, 1991

18. Barnea A, Cho G. Evidence that copper-amino acid complexes are potent stimulators of the release of luteinizing hormone-releasing hormone from isolated hypothalamic granules. Endocrinology 115:936–943, 1984

19. Barr RW, Sommers SC. Endocrine abnormalities accompanying hepatic cirrhosis and hepatoma. J Clin Endocrinol Metab 17:1017–1029, 1957

20. Bartholomew LG, Cain JC, Woolner LB, Utz DC, Ferris DO. Sclerosing cholangitis: its possible association with Reidel's struma and fibrous retroperitonitis. N Engl J Med 269:8–12, 1963

21. Batman PA, Scheur PJ. Diabetic hepatitis preceding the onset of glucose intolerance. Histopathology 9:237–243, 1985

22. Baum JK, Holtz F, Bookstein JJ, Klein EW. Possible association between benign hepatomas and oral contraceptives. Lancet 2:926–929, 1973

23. Baxter RC, Martin JL, Beniac VA. High molecular weight insulin-like growth factor binding protein complex: purification and properties of the acid labile sub-unit from human serum. J Biol Chem 264:11843–11848, 1989

24. Beaver DC, Pemberton J. The pathologic anatomy of the liver in exophthalmic goiter. Ann Intern Med 7:687–708, 1933

25. Becker MD, Cook GC, Wright AD. Paradoxical elevation of growth hormone in chronic active hepatitis. Lancet 2:1035–1039, 1969

26. Becker U, Almdal T, Christensen E, Gluud C, Farholt S, Bennett P, Svenstrup B, Hardt F. Sex hormones in postmenopausal women with primary biliary cirrhosis. Hepatology 13:865–869, 1991

27. Becker U, Gluud C, Bennett P. Thyroid hormones and thyroxine-binding globulin in relation to liver function and serum testosterone in men with alcoholic cirrhosis. Acta Med Scand 324:367–373, 1988

28. Bendtsen F, Henriksen JH, Sorensen TIA, Christensen NJ. Effect of oral propranolol on circulating catecholamines in cirrhosis: relationship to severity of liver disease and splanchnic haemodynamics. J Hepatol 10:198–204, 1990

29. Bendtsen F, Christensen NJ, Sorensen TIA, Henriksen JH. Effect of oral propranolol administration on azygos, renal and hepatic uptake and output of catecholamines in cirrhosis. Hepatology 14:237–243, 1991

30. Bennett HS, Baggenstoss AH, Butt HR. The testes, breast and prostate of men who die of cirrhosis of the liver. Am J Clin Pathol 20:814–828, 1950

31. Bennion LJ, Grundy SM. Risk factors for the development of cholelithiasis in man. N Engl J Med 1161–1167, 1978

32. Benoit JN, Barrowman JA, Harper SL, Kvietys PR, Granger DN. Role of humoral factors in the intestinal hyperemia associated with chronic portal hypertension. Am J Physiol 247:G486–G493, 1984

33. Berelowitz M, Szabo M, Frohman LA, Firestone S, Chu L, Hintz RL. Somatomedin C mediates growth hormone negative feedback by effects on both the hypothalamus and the pituitary. Science 212:1279–1285, 1981

34. Bernardi M, DePalma R, Trevisani F, et al. "Low T₃ syndrome" in cirrhosis: effect of β-blockade. Am J Gastroenterol 84:727–731, 1989

35. Bernardi M, Trevisani F, Santini C, Zoli G, Baraldini M, Ligabue A, Gasbarrini G. Plasma norepinephrine, weak neurotransmitters, and renin activity during active tilting in liver cirrhosis: relationship with cardiovascular homeostasis and renal function. Hepatology 3:56–64, 1983

36. Berne C, Fagius J, Niklason F. Sympathetic response to oral carbohydrate administration: evidence from microelectrode nerve recordings. J Clin Invest 84:1403–1409, 1989

37. Berridge MJ. Inositol trisphosphate and diacylglycerol: two interacting second messengers. Ann Rev Biochem 56:159–193, 1987

38. Berris, B, Feinman SV. Thyroid dysfunction and liver injury following alpha-interferon treatment of chronic viral hepatitis. Dig Dis Sci 36:1657–1660, 1991

39. Bezwoda WR, Bothwell TH, VanderWalt LA, Kronheim S, Pimstone BL. An investigation into gonadal dysfunction in patients with idiopathic haemochromatosis. Clin Endocrinol 6:377–385, 1977

40. Bhalla VK, Chen CJH, Gnanaprakasam MS. Effects of in vivo administration of human gonadotropin and ethanol on the processes of testicular receptor depletion and replenishment. Life Sci 24:1315–1324, 1979

41. Bhathena SJ, Voyles NR, Smith S, Recant L. Decreased glucagon receptors in diabetic rat hepatocytes. J Clin Invest 61:1488–1497, 1978

42. Bichet DG, Van Putten VJ, Schrier RW. Potential role of increased sympathetic activity in impaired sodium and water excretion in cirrhosis. N Engl J Med 307:1552–1557, 1982

43. Binoux M, Hossenlopp P, Lassarre C, Seurin D. Somatomedin production by rat liver in organ culture. I. Validity of the technique. Influence of the released material on cartilage sulphation: effects of growth hormone and insulin. Acta Endocrinol 93:73–82, 1980

44. Bjorntop P, Sjostrom L. Carbohydrate storage in man: speculations and some quantitative considerations. Metabolism 27(Suppl):1853–1865, 1978

45. Blackshear PJ. Insulin-stimulated protein biosynthesis as a paradigm of protein kinase C-independent growth factor. Clin Res 37:15–25, 1989

46. Blanchet L, Lebrec D. Changes in splanchnic blood flow in portal hypertensive rats. Eur J Clin Invest 12:327–330, 1982

47. Blei AT, Robbins DC, Drobny E, Baumann G, Rubenstein AH. Insulin resistance and insulin receptors in hepatic cirrhosis. Gastroenterology 83:1191–1199, 1982

48. Bloodworth JMB, Hamwi GJ. Histopathologic lesions associated with sulfonylurea administration. Diabetes 10:90–98, 1959

49. Bloodworth JMB. Diabetes mellitus and cirrhosis of the liver. Arch Intern Med 108:95–101, 1961

50. Blundell TL, Humbel RE. Hormone families: pancreatic hormones and homologous growth factors. Nature 287:781–783, 1980

51. Bonnadonna RC, Groop LC, Zych K, Shank M, DeFronzo RA. Dose dependent effect of insulin on plasma free fatty acid turnover and oxidation in humans. Am J Physiol 259:E736–E750, 1990

52. Borhanmanesh F, Haghighi P. Pregnancy in patients with cirrhosis of the liver. Obstet Gynecol 36:315–324, 1970

53. Borst GC, Eil C, Burman KD. Euthyroid hyperthyroxinemia. Ann Intern Med 98:366–378, 1983

54. Bosch J, Gomis R, Kravetz D. Role of spontaneous portal-systemic shunting in hyperinsulinism of cirrhosis. Am J Physiol 247:G206–212, 1984

55. Bowen OR. Alcohol and health. United States Department of Health and Human Services, National Institute on Alcohol Abuse and Alcoholism, publication no. 87–1519. Washington, DC, p 18

56. Bratusch-Marrain P, Smith D, DeFronzo RA. The effect of growth hormone on glucose metabolism and insulin secretion in man. J Clin Endocrinol Metab 55:973–982, 1982

57. Brazeau P, Guillemen R, Ling N, Van Wyk JJ, Humbel R. Inhibition by somatomedin of growth hormone secretion stimulated by hypothalamic growth hormone-releasing factors (somatocrinin, GRF) or the synthetic peptide hpGRF. CR Acad Sci Paris 295:651–666, 1982

58. Brock ML, Shapiro DJ. Estrogen stabilizes vitellogenin

mRNA against cytoplasmic degradation. Cell 34:207–214, 1983

59. Bronstein HD, Kantrowitz PA, Schaffner F. Marked enlargement of the liver and transient ascites associated with the treatment of diabetic acidosis. N Engl J Med 261:1314–1318, 1959

60. Brown AL, Graham DE, Nissley SP, Hill DJ, Strains AS, Rechler MM. Developmental regulation of insulin-like growth factor II mRNA in different rat tissues. J Biol Chem 261:13144–13150, 1986

61. Bruno JF, Olchovsky D, White JD, Leidy JW, Song Jinfen, Berelowitz M. Influence of food deprivation in the rat on hypothalamic expression of growth hormone releasing factor and somatostatin. Endocrinology 127:2111–2116, 1990

62. Butcher RW, Baird CE. Effects of prostaglandins on adenosine 3′, 5′-monophosphate levels in fat and other tissues. J Biol Chem 243:1713–1717, 1968

63. Cabre E, Periago JL, Abad-LaCruz A, Gil A, Gonzalez-Huix F, Sanchez de Medina F, Gassull MA. Polyunsaturated fatty acid deficiency in liver cirrhosis: its relation to associated protein-energy malnutrition. Am J Gastroenterol 83:712–727, 1988

64. Cahill GR Jr, Herrera MC, Morgan AO, Soeldner JS, Steinke J, Levy PL. Hormone-fuel interrelationships during fasting. J Clin Invest 45:1751–1769, 1966

65. Cameron GR, Karunaratne W. Liver changes in exophthalmic goiter. J Pathol 41:267–282, 1935

66. Campillo B, Chapelain C, Bonnet JC, Frisdal E, Devanlay M, Bouissou P, Fouet P, Wirquin E, Atlan G. Hormonal and metabolic changes during exercise in cirrhotic patients. Metabolism 39:18–24, 1990

67. Campillo B, Fouet P, Bonnet JC, Atlan G. Sub-maximal oxygen consumption in liver cirrhosis. J Hepatol 10:163–167, 1990

68. Carlstrom K, Eriksson S, Rannevik G. Sex steroids and steroid binding proteins in female alcoholic liver disease. Acta Endocrinol 111:75–79, 1986

69. Carnelro deMoura M, Curz AG. Carbohydrate metabolism studies in cirrhosis of the liver. Am J Dig Dis 13:891–906, 1968

70. Caro JF, Poulos J, Ittoop O, Pories WJ, Flickinger EG, Sinha MK. Insulin-like growth factor I binding in hepatocytes from human liver: human hepatoma and normal, regenerating, and fetal liver. J Clin Invest 81:976–981, 1988

71. Castellano TJ, Schiffman RL, Jacob MC, Loeb JN. Suppression of liver cell proliferation by glucocorticoid hormone: a comparison of normally growing and regenerating tissue in the immature rat. Endocrinology 102:1107–1112, 1978

72. Cavallo-Perin P, Bruno A, Nuccio P, Dall'Omo AM, Fronda GR, Avagnina P, Molino G, Rozzo C, Pagano G. Insulin resistance in human liver cirrhosis is not modified by portosystemic surgical shunt. Acta Endocrinol 112:377–382, 1986

73. Cavallo-Perin P, Cassader M, Bozzo C, Bruno A, Nuccio P, Dall'Omo AM, Marucci M, Pagano G. Mechanism of insulin resistance in human liver cirrhosis: evidence of a combined receptor and post receptor defect. J Clin Invest 75:1659–1665, 1985

74. Cavanaugh J, Niewoehner CB, Nuttall FQ. Gynecomastia and cirrhosis of the liver. Arch Intern Med 150:563–565, 1990

75. Ceci F, Muscaritoli M, Cangiano C, et al. Effect of exogenous triglyceride infusion on the plasma amino acid profile in liver cirrhosis. Clin Nutr 7:151–156, 1988

76. Charbonnel B, Chupen M, LeGrand A, Guillon J. Pituitary function in idiopathic haemochromatosis: hormonal study in 36 male patients. Acta Endocrinol 98:178–183, 1981

77. Chiao Y-B, Johnston DE, Gavaler JS, Van Thiel DH. Effect of chronic ethanol feeding on testicular content of enzymes required for testosteronogenesis. Alcoholism 5:230–236, 1981

78. Childs AW, Kivel RM, Lieberman A. Effect of ethyl alcohol on hepatic circulation, sulfo-bromophthalein clearance and hepatic glutamic-oxalacetic transaminase production in man. Gastroenterology 45:176–181, 1963

79. Chopra IJ, Tulchinsky D, Greenway FL. Estrogen–androgen imbalance in hepatic cirrhosis. Ann Intern Med 79:198–203, 1973

80. Cicero TJ, Bell RD. Effects of ethanol and acetaldehyde on the biosynthesis of testosterone in the rodent testes. Biochem Biophys Res Commun 94:814–819, 1980

81. Civica DR, Jorge AD, Jorge O, Milutin C, Hosokawa R, Lestren MD, Muzzio E, Schulkin S, Schirbur R. Estrogen receptors, progesterone receptors and heat shock 27-kD protein in liver biopsy specimens from patients with hepatitis B virus infection. Hepatology 13:838–844, 1991

82. Clain JE, Stephens DH, Charboneau JW. Ultrasonography and computed tomography in focal fatty liver. Gastroenterology 87:948–952, 1984

83. Clancy RL, Mackay IR. Myxoedematous ascites. Med J Aust 2:415–416, 1979

84. Clemmons DR, Elgin RG, Han VKM, Casella SJ, D'Ercole AJ, Van Wyk JJ. Cultured fibroblast monocytes secrete a protein that alters the cellular binding of somatomedin C/insulin-like growth factor I. J Clin Invest 77:1548–1556, 1986

85. Clemmons DR, Underwood LE, Ridgway EC, Kliman B, Van Wyk JJ. Hyperprolactinemia is associated with increased immunoreactive somatomedin C in hypopituitarism. J Clin Endocrinol Metab 52:731–735, 1981

86. Clemmons DR, Thissen JP, Maes M, Ketelslegers JM, Underwood LE. Insulin-like growth factor I (IGF-I) infusion into hypophysectomized or protein-deprived rats induced specific IGF binding proteins in serum. Endocrinology 125:2967–2972, 1985

87. Clemmons, DR, Underwood LE. Nutritional regulation of IGF-I and IGF binding proteins. Annu Rev Nutr 11:393–412, 1991

88. Clemmons DR, Klibanski A, Underwood LE, McArthur JW, Ridgway EC, Van Wyk JJ. Reduction of plasma immunoreactive somatomedin-C during fasting in humans. J Clin Endocrinol Metab 53:1247–1250, 1981

89. Clemmons DR, Underwood LE, Van Wyk JJ. Hormonal control of immunoreactive somatomedin production by cultured human fibroblasts. Clin Invest 67:10–19, 1981

90. Cobb CF, Ennis MF, Van Thiel DH, Gavaler JS, Lester R. Acetaldehyde and ethanol are direct testicular toxins. Forum 29:641–644, 1978

91. Cobb CF, Van Thiel DH, Ennis MF, Gavaler JS, Lester R. Is acetaldehyde an adrenal stimulant? Curr Surg 36:431–434, 1979

92. Cochrane M, William R. Humoral effects of hepatocellular carcinoma. In: Okuda K, Peters RL, eds. Hepatocellular carcinoma. New York, John Wiley & Sons, 1976, pp 369–384

93. Collins JR, Lacy WW, Stiel JM. Glucose intolerance and insulin resistance in patients with liver disease. Arch Intern Med 126:608–614, 1970

94. Collins JR, Crofford OB. Glucose intolerance and insulin resistance in patients with liver disease. Arch Intern Med 124:142–148, 1969

95. Conn, HO, Schreiber W, Elkington SG. Cirrhosis and diabetes II. Dig Dis Sci 16:227–239, 1971

96. Conn HO, Daughaday WH. Cirrhosis and diabetes. V. Serum growth hormone levels in Laennec's cirrhosis. J Lab Clin Med 76:678–688, 1970

97. Conn HO, Schreiber W, Elkington SG, Elkington SG. Cirrhosis and diabetes I. Am J Dig Dis 14:837–852, 1969

98. Cooper DS, Kaplan MM, Ridgway EC, et al. Alkaline phosphatase isoenzyme patterns in hyperthyroidism. Ann Intern Med 90:164–168, 1979

99. Cooper DS, Daniels GH, Landenson PW, Ridgway EC. Hyperthyroxinemia in patients treated with high-dose propranolol. Am J Med 73:867–871, 1982

100. Courtney-Moore M, Cherrington AD, Cline G, Pagliassotti

MJ, Jones EM, Neal DW, Badet C, Shulman GI. Sources of carbon for hepatic glycogen synthesis in the conscious dog. J Clin Invest 88:578–587, 1991

101. Creutzfeldt W, Frerich SH, Sickinger K. Liver disease and diabetes mellitus. In: Popper H, Schaffner F. Progress in liver disease, vol 3. New York, Grune & Stratton, 1970, pp 371–407

102. Crowe JP, Christensen E, Butler J, Wheeler P, Doniach D, Keenan J, Williams R. Primary biliary cirrhosis: the prevalence of hypothyroidism and its relationship to thyroid antibodies and sicca syndrome. Gastroenterology 78:1437–1441, 1980

103. Cruise JL, Cotecchia S, Michalapoulos G. Norepinephrine decreases EGF binding in primary rat hepatocyte cultures. J Cell Physiol 127:39–44, 1986

104. Cruise JL, Knechtle SJ, Bollinger RR, Kuhn C, Michalopoulos G. α_1-Adrenergic effects and liver regeneration. Hepatology 7:1189–1194, 1987

105. Cundy TF, Butler J, Pope RM, Saggai-Malek AK, Wheeler MJ, Williams R. Amenorrhea in women with non-alcoholic chronic liver disease. Gut 31:202–206, 1990

106. D'Ercole AJ, Stiles AD, Underwood LE. Tissue concentrations of somatomedin C: further evidence for multiple sites of synthesis and paracrine mechanisms of action. Proc Natl Acad Sci USA 81:935–941, 1984

107. Dannon GA, Porubek DJ, Nelson SD, Waxman DJ, Guengerich FP. 17β-Estradiol 2- and 4-hydroxylation catalyzed by rat hepatic cytochrome P-450: role of individual forms, inductive effects, developmental pattern and alteration by gonadectomy and hormone replacement. Endocrinology 118:1952–1960, 1986

108. Danowski TS, Gillespie HK, Fergus EB, Puntereri AJ. Significance of blood sugar and serum electrolyte changes in cirrhosis following glucose, insulin, glucagon or epinephrine. Yale J Biol Med 29:361–375, 1956

109. DeFronzo RA, Jacot E, Jequier E, Maeder E, Wahren J, Felber JP. The effect of insulin on the disposal of intravenous glucose: results from indirect calorimetry and hepatic and femoral venous catheterization. Diabetes 30:1000–1007, 1981

110. DeFronzo RA, Ferrannini E, Hendler R, Felig P, Wahren J. Regulation of splanchnic peripheral glucose uptake by insulin and hyperglycemia in man. Diabetes 32:35–45, 1983

111. DeFronzo RA, Ferrannini E. Regulation of hepatic glucose metabolism in humans. Diab Metab Rev 3:415–459, 1987

112. DeFronzo RA, Gunnarson R, Bjorkman O, Olsson M, Wahren J. Effects of insulin on peripheral and splanchnic glucose metabolism in non-insulin-dependent (type II) diabetes mellitus. J Clin Invest 76:149–155, 1985

113. DelPrato S, Castellino P, Siminson DC, DeFronzo RA. Hyperglucagonemia and insulin-mediated glucose metabolism. J Clin Invest 79:547–556, 1987

114. Denlinger CL, Vesell ES. Hormonal regulation of the developmental pattern of epoxide hydrolases: studies in rat liver. Biochem Pharmacol 38:603–610, 1989

115. Diamond DJ, Goodman HM. Regulation of growth hormone mRNA synthesis by dexamethasone and triiodothyronine. J Mol Biol 181:41–62, 1985

116. Diehl AM, Goodman Z, Ishak KG. Alcohol-like liver disease in nonalcoholics: a clinical and histological comparison with alcohol-induced liver injury. Gastroenterology 95:1056–1062, 1988

117. Dietrich R, Bachmann C, Lauterburg BH. Exercise-induced hyperammonemia in patients with compensated chronic liver disease. Scand J Gastroenterol 25:329–334, 1990

118. Distiller LA, Sagel J, Dubowitz B, Kay G, Carr PJ, Katz M, Kew MC. Pituitary-gonadal function in men with alcoholic cirrhosis of the liver. Horm Metab Res 8:461–465, 1976

119. Douglas RG, Gluckman PD, Ball K, Breier B, Shaw JHF. Effects of infusion of insulin-like growth factors (IGF) I, IGF (II), and insulin on glucose and protein metabolism in fasted lambs. J Clin Invest 88:614–622, 1991

120. Dudley FJ, Alford FP, Chisholm DJ, Findlay DM. Effect of portasystemic venous shunt surgery on hyperglucagonemia in cirrhosis: paired studies of pre and post shunted subjects. Gut 20:817–824, 1979

121. Duffy MJ, Duffy GJ. Estradiol receptors in human liver. J Steroid Biochem 9:233–235, 1978

122. Dzurikoka V, Niederland TR, Brixova E, Dzurik R, Hupkoua V, Holoman J. Abnormal carbohydrate metabolism in patients with liver cirrhosis: in vitro study. Diabetologia 8:202–205, 1972

123. Eagon PK, Fisher SE, Imhoff AF, Porter LE, Stewart RR, Van Thiel DH, Lester R. Estrogen-binding proteins of male rat liver: influences of hormonal changes. Arch Biochem Biophys 201:486–499, 1980

124. Eagon PK, Willett JE, Seguiti SM, Appler ML, Gavaler JS, Van Thiel DH. Androgen-responsive functions of male rat liver: effect of chronic alcohol ingestion. Gastroenterology 93:1162–1169, 1987

125. Eagon PK, Porter LE, Francavilla A, DiLeo A, Van Thiel DH. Estrogen and androgen receptors in liver: their role in liver disease and regeneration. Semin Liver Dis 5:59–69, 1985

126. Eagon PK, Seguiti SM, Rogerson BJ, McGuire TF, Porter LE, Seeley DH. Androgen receptor in rat liver: characterization and separation from a male-specific estrogen-binding protein. Arch Biochem Biophys 268:161–175, 1989

127. Eden S. Age and sex related differences in episodic growth hormone secretion in the rat. Endocrinology 105:555–560, 1979

128. Edman CD, MacDonald PC, Combes B. Extraglandular production of estrogen in subjects with liver disease. Gastroenterology 69:819A, 1975

129. Edmondson HA, Reynolds TB, Henderson B, Benton B. Regression of liver cell adenomas associated with oral contraceptives. Ann Intern Med 86:180–182, 1977

130. Einarsson K, Gustafsson J-A, Stenberg A. Neonatal imprinting of liver microsomal hydroxylation and reduction of steroids. J Biol Chem 248:4987–4997, 1973

131. Eisenfeld AJ, Aten R, Weinberger M, Haselbacher G, Halpern K, Krakoff L. Estrogen receptor in the mammalian liver. Science 191:862–864, 1976

132. Ellengboe J, Varanelli CC. Ethanol inhibits testosterone biosynthesis by direct action on leydig cells. Res Commun Chem Pathol Pharmacol 24:87–102, 1979

133. Emler T, Maiter D, Gerard G, Underwood LE, Maes M, Ketelslegers JM. Reduction in insulin-like growth factor I by dietary protein restriction is age dependent. Pediatr Res 26:415–419, 1989

134. Erdstein J, Wisebord S, Mishken SY, Mishken S. The effect of several sex steroid hormones on the growth rate of three Morris hepatoma tumor lines. Hepatology 9:621–624, 1989

135. Evans A, Spring S, Nelson RS. Adrenal hormone therapy in viral hepatitis I. The effect of ACTH in the acute disease. Ann Intern Med 38:1115–1133, 1953

136. Evans WS, Faria ACS, Christiansen E, Ho KY, Weiss J, Rogol AD, Johnson ML, Blizzard RM, Veldhuis JK, Thorner MD. Impact of intensive venous sampling on characterization of pulsatile GH release. Am J Physiol 252:E549–E556, 1987

137. Evans RW, Littler TR, Pemberton HS. Glycogen storage in the liver in diabetes mellitus. J Clin Pathol 8:110–113, 1955

138. Fain JN, Garcia-Sainz JA. Adrenergic regulation of adipocyte metabolism. J Lipid Res 24:945–966, 1983

139. Falchuk KR, Fiske SC, Haggitt RC, Felderman M, Trey C. Pericentral hepatic fibrosis and intracellular hyalin in diabetes mellitus. Gastroenterology 78:535–541, 1980

140. Farrall L, Rhodes D, Klug A. Mapping of the sites of protection on a 5s RNA gene by the xenopus transcription factor IIIA: a model for the interaction. J Mol Biol 192:577–591, 1986

141. Felig P, Brown N, Levine RA, Klatskin G. Glucose homeostasis in viral hepatitis. N Engl J Med 283:1436–1440, 1970

142. Felig P, Wahren J, Hendler R. Influence of oral glucose inges-

tion on splanchnic glucose and gluconeogenic substrate metabolism in man. Diabetes 24:468–475, 1975

143. Ferrannini E, Bjorkman O, Reichard GA, Pilo A, Olsson M, Wahren J, DeFronzo RA. The disposal of an oral glucose load in healthy subjects. Diabetes 34:580–588, 1985

144. Field JB, Keen H, Johnson P, Herrint B. Insulin-like activity of non-pancreatic tumors associated with hypoglycemia. J Clin Endocrinol 23:1229–1236, 1963

145. Finch SC, Finch CA. Idiopathic hemochromatosis, an iron storage disease. Medicine 34:381–430, 1955

146. Floras JS, Legault L, Morali GA, Hara K, Blendis LM. Increased sympathetic outflow in cirrhosis and ascites: direct evidence from intraneural recordings. Ann Intern Med 114:373–380, 1991

147. Foster JH, Donohue TA, Berman MM. Familial liver cell adenomas and diabetes mellitus. N Engl J Med 299:239–241, 1978

148. Foster KJ, Dewbury K, Griffith AH, Price CP, Wright R. Liver disease in patients with diabetes mellitus. Postgrad Med J 56:767–772, 1980

149. Francis MJO, Hill DJ. Prolactin-stimulated production of somatomedin by rat liver. Nature 255:167–169, 1975

150. Frea B, Annoscia S, Stanta G, Lozzi C, Carmignani G. Correlation between liver cirrhosis and benign prostatic hyperplasia: a morphological study. Urol Res 15:311–314, 1987

151. Friedman MA, Demanes DJ, Hoffman PG. Hepatomas: hormone receptors and therapy. Am J Med 73:362–366, 1982

152. Friedman LS, Roberts MS, Brett AS, Marton KI. Management of asymptomatic gallstones in the diabetic patient: a decision analysis. Ann Intern Med 109:913–919, 1988

153. Fujita S, Takimoto T, Kobayashi M, Shigeta Y, Hoshi M. Erythrocyte insulin receptors in patients with chronic liver diseases. Horm Metab Res 14:51–52, 1982

154. Furlanetto RW, Underwood LE, Van Wyk JJ, D'Ercole AJ. Estimation of somatomedin-C levels in normals and patients with pituitary disease. J Clin Invest 60:648–657, 1977

155. Galvao-Teles A, Burke CW, Anderson DC, Marshall JC, Corker CS, Bown RL, Clark ML. Biologically active androgens and estradiol in men with chronic liver disease. Lancet 1:173–177, 1973

156. Gametchu B, Harrison RW. Characterization of a monoclonal antibody to the rat liver glucocorticoid receptor. Endocrinology 114:274–279, 1984

157. Garber AJ, Bier DM, Cryer PE, et al. Hyperglycemia in compensated chronic renal insufficiency: substrate limitation of gluconeogenesis. Diabetes 23:982–986, 1974

158. Garber AJ, Karl IE, Kipnis DM. Alanine and glutamine synthesis and release from skeletal muscle. II. The precursor role of amino acids in alanine and glutamine synthesis. J Biol Chem 251:836–843, 1976

159. Gardner, DF, Carithers RL Jr, Utiger RD. Thyroid function in patients with acute and resolved hepatitis B infection. Ann Intern Med 96:450–452, 1982

160. Garvey WT, Olefsky JM, Marshall S. Insulin induces progressive insulin resistance in cultured rat adipocytes. Diabetes 35:258–267, 1986

161. Garvey WT, Olefsky JM, Marshall S. Insulin receptor down regulation is linked to an insulin induced post receptor defect in the glucose transport system in rat adipocytes. J Clin Invest 76:22–30, 1985

162. Gastard J, Gosselen M, Brelagne JF, Hannouche N, Samperez S, Jouan P, Launos B. Dosage des recepteurs de l'oestradiol dans un adenome hepatique observe apres prise d'oestroprogestatifs. Nouv Presse Med 9:43, 1980

163. Gaudin C, Braillon A, Selz F, Cuche JL, Lebrec D. Free and conjugated catecholamines in patients with cirrhosis. J Lab Clin Med 115:589–592, 1990

164. Gavaler JS, Gay V, Egler K, Van Thiel DH. Evaluation of the differential in vivo toxic effects of ethanol and acetaldehyde on the hypothalamic-pituitary gonadal axis using 4-methylpyrazole. Alcoholism 7:332–336, 1983

165. Gavaler JS. Sex related differences in ethanol-induced liver disease: artifactual or real? Alcoholism (NY) 6:186–196, 1982

166. Gavaler JS, Van Thiel DH. Gonadal dysfunction and inadequate sexual performance in alcoholic cirrhotic men. Gastroenterology 95:1680–1683, 1988

167. Gavin JR, Roth J, Neville DM, DeMeyts P, Buell DN. Insulin-dependent regulation of insulin receptor concentrations: a direct demonstration in cell culture. Proc Natl Acad Sci USA 71:84–88, 1974

168. Gershengorn GC, Larsen PR, Robbin J. Radioimmunoassay for serum thyroxine-binding globulin: results in normal subjects and in patients with hepatocellular carcinoma. J Clin Endocrinol Metab 42:907–911, 1976

169. Giguere V, Hollenberg SM, Rosenfeld MG, Evans RM. Functional domains of the human glucocorticoid receptor. Cell 46:645–652, 1986

170. Gilbert-Dreyfus M. La fonction testiculaire dans l'hemochromatoses-idiopatheque. Rev Franc Endocrinol Clin Nutr Metab 10:191–203, 1969

171. Gilman AG. G proteins and dual control of adenylate cyclase. Cell 36:577–579, 1984

172. Gines P, Quintero E, Arroyo V, Teres J, Bruguera M, Rimola A, Caballera J, Rodes J, Rozman C. Compensated cirrhosis: natural history and prognostic factors. Hepatology 7:122–128, 1987

173. Gluud C, Bennett P, Svenstrup B, Micic S, the Copenhagen Study Group for Liver Diseases. Effect of oral testosterone treatment on serum concentrations of sex steroids, gonadotrophins and prolactin in alcoholic cirrhotic men. Aliment Pharmacol Ther 2:119–128, 1988

174. Gluud C, Dejgaard A, Bennett P, Svenstrup B. Androgens and oestrogens before and following oral testosterone administration in male patients with and without alcoholic cirrhosis. Acta Endocrinol 115:385–391, 1987

175. Gluud C, Wantzen P, Eriksen J, the Copenhagen Study Group for Liver Diseases. No effect of oral testosterone treatment in sexual dysfunction in alcoholic cirrhotic men. Gastroenterology 95:1582–1587, 1988

176. Glynn MJ, Powell-Tuck J, Reaveley DA, Murray-Lyon IM. High lipid parenteral nutrition improves portal systemic encephalopathy. JPEN 12:457–461, 1988

177. Gnanaprakasam MS, Chen CJH, Sutherland JC, Bhalla VK. Receptor depletion and replenishment processes: in vivo regulation of gonadotropin receptors by luteinizing hormone, follicle stimulating hormone, and ethanol in rat testes. Biol Reprod 20:991–1000, 1979

178. Goodman RC, Dean PJ, Radparvar A, Kitabchi AE. Glyburide-induced hepatitis. Ann Intern Med 106:837–839, 1987

179. Gordon GG, Southern AL. Metabolic effects of alcohol on the endocrine system. In: Leiber DS, ed. Metabolic aspects of alcoholism. Baltimore, University Park Press, 1977, p 277

180. Gordon GG, Olivo J, Rafii F, Southern AL. Conversion of androgens to estrogens in cirrhosis of the liver. J Clin Endocrinol Metab 40:1018–1026, 1975

181. Gordon GG, Southern AL, Vitlek J, Lieber CS. The effect of alcohol ingestion on hepatic aromatase activity and plasma steroid hormones in the rat. Metabolism 28:20–24, 1979

182. Gordon GG, Altman K, Southern AL, Rubin E, Lieber CS. The effect of alcohol (ethanol) administration on sex hormone metabolism in normal men. N Engl J Med 295:793–797, 1976

183. Grace ND, Powell LW. Iron storage disorders of the liver. Gastroenterology 64:1257–1283, 1974

184. Granich S. The induction in vitro of the synthesis of δ-amino levulinic acid synthetase in chemical porphyria: a response to certain drugs, sex hormones, and foreign chemicals. J Biol Chem 241:1359–1375, 1966

185. Greco AV, Altomonto L, Ghirlanda G, Rebuzzi AG, Manna R, Bertoli A. Somatostatin infusion in liver cirrhosis: glucagon control of glucose homeostasis. Diabetologia 18:187–191, 1980

186. Greco AV, Rebuzzi AG, Altomonte L, Manna R, Bertoli A, Ghirlanda G. Glucose, insulin and somatostatin infusion for the determination of insulin resistance in liver cirrhosis. Horm Metab Res 11:547–549, 1979

187. Greco AV, Bertoli A, Ghirlanda G, Manna R, Altomonte L, Rebuzzi AG. Insulin resistance in liver cirrhosis: decreased insulin binding to circulating monocytes. Horm Metab Res 12:577–581, 1980

188. Greco AV, Bertoli A, Caputo S, Altomonte L, Manna R, Ghirlanda G. Decreased insulin binding to red blood cells in liver cirrhosis. Acta Diabetol Lat 20:251–256, 1983

189. Greco AV, Altomonte L, Ghirlanda G, D'Anna LM, Manna R, Caputo S, Uccuoli L. Glucagon and glucose intolerance in liver cirrhosis. Acta Endocrinol 118:337–345, 1988

190. Greco AV, Crucitti F, Chirlanda G, Manna R, Altomonte L, Rebuzzi AG, Bertoli A. Insulin and glucagon concentrations in portal and peripheral veins in patients with hepatic cirrhosis. Diabetologia 17:23–28, 1979

191. Green JRB, Mowat AG, Fisher RA, Anderson DC. Plasma oestrogens in men with chronic liver disease. Gut 17:426–430, 1976

192. Green S, Chambon P. Oestradiol induction of a glucocorticoid-responsive gene by a chimaeric receptor. Nature 325:75–77, 1987

193. Greenberger WJ, Milligan FD, DeGroot LJ, Isslebacher KJ. Jaundice and thyrotoxicosis in the absence of congestive heart failure. Am J Med 36:840–846, 1964

194. Griffin JE, Wilson JD. Disorders of the testes and the male reproductive tract. In: Wilson JD, Foster DW, eds. Williams' textbook of endocrinology. Philadelphia, WB Saunders, 1992, pp 799–852

195. Groop LC, Bonadonna RC, DelPrato S, Ratheiser K, Zych K, Ferrannini E, DeFronzo RA. Glucose and free fatty acid metabolism in non-insulin dependent diabetes mellitus. J Clin Invest 84:205–213, 1989

196. Guertin M, Barel P, Barlkowiak J, Anderson A, Belanger L. Rapid suppression of α₁-fetoprotein gene transcription by dexamethasone in developing rat liver. Biochemistry 22:4296–4302, 1983

197. Gustafsson, J-A, Mode A, Norstedt G, Skett P. Sex steroid induced changes in hepatic enzymes. Annu Rev Physiol 45:51–60, 1983

198. Gustafsson J-A, Stenberg A. Irreversible androgenic programming at birth of microsomal and soluble rat liver enzymes active on 4-androstene-3, 17-dione and 5α-androstane-3α, 17β-diol. J Biol Chem 249:711–718, 1974

199. Gustafsson J-A, Stenberg A. On the obligatory role of the hypophysis in sexual differentiation of hepatic metabolism in rats. Proc Natl Acad Sci USA 73:1462–1465, 1976

200. Halle P, Pare P, Kaptein E, Kanel G, Redeker AG, Reynolds TB. Double-blind controlled trial of propylthiouracil in patients with severe acute alcoholic hepatitis. Gastroenterology 82:925–931, 1982

201. Han VKM, D'Ercole AJ, Lund PK. Cellular location of somatomedlin (insulin-like growth factor) messenger RNA in the human fetus. Science 236:193–197, 1987

202. Hansel W, Concannon PW, McEntee K. Plasma hormone profiles and pathological observations in medroxy-progesterone acetate-treated beagle bitches. In: Garattini S, Berendes HW, eds. Pharmacology of steroid contraceptive drugs. New York, Raven Press, 1977, pp 145–191

203. Harewood MS, Proietto J, Dudley F, Alford FP. Insulin action and cirrhosis: insulin binding and lipogenesis in isolated adipocytes. Metabolism 31:1241–1246, 1982

204. Haug A, Spydevold O, Hostmark AT. Effect of orchidectomy and testosterone substitution on enzyme activity and DNA content in rat liver and epididymal fat. Int J Biochem 17:31–36, 1985

205. Hayakawa T, Dondo T, Shibata T, Kitagawa M, Ono H, Sakai Y, Takeichi M, Yamamoto R, Kodaira R. Serum insulin-like growth factor II in chronic liver disease. Dig Dis Sci 34:338–342, 1989

206. Hegedus L. Decreased thyroid gland volume in alcoholic cirrhosis of the liver. J Clin Endocrinol Metab 58:930–933, 1984

207. Hegedus L. Thyroid gland volume and thyroid function during and after acute hepatitis infection. Metabolism 35:495–498, 1986

208. Henriksen JH, Ring-Larsen H, Christensen NJ. Sympathetic nervous activity in cirrhosis: a survey of plasma catecholamine studies. J Hepatol 1:55–65, 1984

209. Henriksen JH, Christensen NJ, Ring-Larsen H. Noradrenalin and adrenalin in various vascular beds in patients with cirrhosis: relation to hemodynamics. Hepatology 1:293–304, 1981

210. Henrikson JH, Ring-Larsen H, Kanstrup IL, Christensen NJ. Splanchnic and renal elimination of catecholamines in cirrhosis: evidence of enhanced sympathetic activity in patients with decompensated cirrhosis. Gut 25:1134–1143, 1984

211. Hepner GW, Chopra IJ. Serum thyroid hormone levels in patients with liver disease. Arch Intern Med 139:1117, 1979

212. Hernandez A, Zorilla E, Gershberg H. Decreased insulin production, elevated growth hormone levels and glucose intolerance in liver disease. J Lab Clin Med 73:25–33, 1969

213. Heubi JE, Partin JC, Partin JS, Schubert WK. Reye's syndrome: current concepts. Hepatology 7:155–164, 1987

214. Hildes JA, Sherlock S, Welsh V. Liver and muscle glycogen in normal subjects, in diabetes mellitus and in acute hepatitis. Clin Sci 7:287–295, 1949

215. Hisaw FL. Comparative effectiveness of estrogens on fluid imbibition and growth of the rats' uterus. Endocrinology 64:276–289, 1959

216. Ho KY, Veldhuis JD, Johnson ML, Furianetto R, Evans WS, Alberti KGMM, Thorner MO. Fasting enhances growth hormone secretion and amplifies the complex rhythms of growth hormone secretion in man. J Clin Invest 81:968–975, 1988

217. Holck HGO, Kanan MA, Mills LM, Smith EL. Studies upon sex-difference in rats in tolerance to certain barbituates and nicotine. J Pharmacol Exp Ther 60:323–346, 1937

218. Holder AT, Wallis M. Actions of growth hormone, prolactin, and thyroxine on serum somatomedin-like activity and growth in hypopituitary dwarf mice. J Endocrinol 74:223–228, 1977

219. Hugues JN, Perret G, Adessi G, Coste T, Modigliani E. Effect of chronic alcoholism on the pituitary-gonadal function of women during menopausal transition and in the post-menopausal period. Biomedicine 29:279–283, 1978

220. Inada M, Sterling K. Thyroxine turnover and transport in Laennec's cirrhosis of the liver. J Clin Invest 46:1275–1282, 1967

221. Ingbar IH. Thyroid storm or crisis. In: Werner SC, Ingber SH, eds. The thyroid: a fundamental and clinical text. New York, Harper & Row, 1978, pp 800–804

222. Insel JR, Kolterman OG, Saekow, Olefsky JM. Short term regulation of insulin receptor affinity in man. Diabetes 29:132–139, 1980

223. Iqbal MJ, Wilkinson ML, Johnson PJ, Williams R. Sex steroid receptor proteins in foetal, adult and malignant liver tissue. Br J Cancer 48:791–796, 1983

224. Issekutz B, Issekutz TB, Elahi D. Glucose kinetics during oral glucose tolerance test in normal, methyl prednisolone treated and alloxan diabetic dogs. Diabetes 23:645–650, 1974

225. Iversen J, Vilstrup H, Tygstrup N. Insulin sensitivity in alcoholic cirrhosis. Scand J Clin Lab Invest 43:565–573, 1983

226. Iversen J, Vilstrup H, Tygstrup N. Kinetics of glucose metabolism in relation to insulin concentrations in patients with alcoholic cirrhosis and in healthy persons. Gastroenterology 87:1136–1143, 1984

227. Iversen J. Adrenergic receptors and the secretion of glucagon and insulin from the isolated, perfused canine pancreas. J Clin Invest 52:2102–2116, 1973

228. Iwasaki Y, Sato H, Ohkubo A, Sanjo T, Futagawa S, Subiura M, Tsuji S. Effect of spontaneous portal-systemic shunting on

plasma insulin and amino acid concentrations. Gastroenterology 78:677–683, 1980

229. Iwasaki Y, Ohkubo A, Kajinuma H, Akanuma Y, Kosaka K. Degradation and secretion of insulin in hepatic cirrhosis. J Clin Endocrinal Metab 47:774–779, 1978

230. Jackson RA, Peters N, Advani V. Forearm glucose uptake during the oral glucose tolerance test in normal subjects. Diabetes 22:442–458, 1973

231. Jacob R, Barrett E, Plewe G, Fagin KD, Sherwin RS. Acute effects of insulin-like growth factors on glucose and amino acid metabolism in the awake fasted rat. J Clin Invest 83:1717–1723, 1989

232. Jansson JO, Eden S, Isaksson O. Sexual dimorphism in the control of growth hormone secretion. Endocrinol Rev 6:128–150, 1985

233. Jansson JO, Frohman LA. Differential effects of neonatal and adult androgen exposure on the growth hormone secretory pattern in male rats. Endocrinology 120:1551–1557, 1987

234. Jenkins DJA, Thorne MJ, Taylor RH, Bloom SR, Sarson DL, Jenkins AL, Blendis LM. Slowly digested carbohydrate food improves impaired carbohydrate tolerance in patients with cirrhosis. Clin Sci 66:649–657, 1984

235. Jenkins DJA, Shapira N, Greenberg G, Jenkins AL, Collier GR, Poduh C, Wolever TMS, Anderson GH, Blendis LM. Low glycemic index foods and reduced glucose, amino acid and endocrine responses in cirrhosis. Am J Gastroenterol 84:732–739, 1989

236. Jenkins DJA, Thorne MJ, Taylor RH, Bloom SR, Sarson DL, Jenkins AL, Anderson GH, Blendis LM. Effect of modifying the rate of digestion of a food on the blood glucose, amino acid, and endocrine responses in patients with cirrhosis. Am J Gastroenterol 82:223–230, 1987

237. Joab I, Radanyi C, Renoir M, Buchow T, Catelli M-G, Binart N, Mester J, Baulieu EE. Common non-hormone binding component in nontransformed chick oviduct receptors of four steroid hormones. Nature 308:850–853, 1984

238. John WJ, Phillips R, Ott L, Adams LJ, McClain CJ. Resting energy expenditure in patients with alcoholic hepatitis. JPEN 13:124–127, 1989

239. Johnston DG, Alberti KGMM, Wright R, Smith-Laing G, Stewart AM, Sherlock S, Faber O, Binder C. C-peptide and insulin in liver disease. Diabetes 27(Suppl):201–206, 1978

240. Jones AL, Marver HS, Kroe EM. An electron microscopic and biochemical study of the effects of progesterone on the rat hepatocyte. Anat Rec 166:326, 1970

241. Jordan VC. Effect of tamoxifen (ICI 46, 474) on initiation and growth of DMBA-induced rat mammary carcinomata. Eur J Cancer 12:419–424, 1975

242. Kabadi UM, Eisenstein AB, Konda J. Elevated plasma ammonia level in hepatic cirrhosis: Role of glucagon. Gastroenterology 88:750–756, 1985

243. Kabadi UM, Eisenstein AB, Tucci J, Pellicone J. Hyperglucagonemia in hepatic cirrhosis: its relation to hepatocellular dysfunction and normalization on recovery. Am J Gastroenterol 79:143–149, 1984

244. Kadowaki T, Koyasu S, Nishida E, Tobe K, Izumi T, Takahu F, Sakai H, Yahara I, Kasuga M. Tyrosine phosphorylation of common and specific sets of cellular proteins rapidly induced by insulin, insulin-like growth factor I and epidermal growth factor in an intact cell. J Biol Chem 262:7342–7350, 1987

245. Kalk WJ, Kew MC, Danilewitz MD, Jacks F, Van Der Waltla, Levin J. Thyroxine binding globulin and thyroid function tests in patients with hepatocellular carcinoma. Hepatology 2:72–76, 1982

246. Kaneto A, Kosada K. Stimulation of glucagon and insulin secretion by acetyl-choline infused intrapancreatically. Endocrinology 95:676–681, 1974

247. Kaplowitz N. Propylthiouracil treatment for alcoholic hepatitis: should it and does it work? Gastroenterology 82:1468–1471, 1982

248. Karhrinen PJ, Penttila A, Liesto K, Mannikko A, Valimaki M, Mottonen M, Ylikahri R. Changes in germinal tissue and leydig cells correlated with ethanol consumption in males with and without liver disease. In: Chambers PL, Prazrosi P, Chambers M, eds. Disease metabolism and reproduction in the toxic response to drugs and other chemicals, vol 7. Berlin, Springer-Verlag, 1984, pp 155–158

249. Kashimata M, Hiramatsu M, Minami N. Differential secretory pattern of growth hormone controls the number of hepatic epidermal growth factor receptors in the rat. J Endocrinol 123:75–81, 1989

250. Kasperska-Czyzy Kowa T, Heding LG, Czyayka. Serum levels of true insulin, C-peptide and pro-insulin in peripheral blood of patients with cirrhosis. Diabetologia 25:506–509, 1983

251. Keller U, Gerber PPG, Buhler FR, Stauffacher W. Role of the splanchnic bed in extracting circulating adrenaline and noradrenaline in normal subjects and in patients with cirrhosis of the liver. Clin Sci 67:45–49, 1984

252. Keller U, Sonnenberg GE, Burckhardt D, Perruchoud A. Evidence for an augmented glucagon dependence of hepatic glucose production in cirrhosis of the liver. J Clin Endocrinol Metab 54:961–968, 1982

253. Kelly M, Walsh H, Doyle C, O'Sullivan DJ, O'Regan J, Whelton M. Glucose homeostasis in viral hepatitis. Digestion 6:286, 1973

254. Khan CR, White MF. The insulin receptor and molecular mechanisms of insulin action. J Clin Invest 82:1151–1156, 1988

255. Khan CR, Goldfine ID, Neville DM Jr, DeMeyts P. Alterations in insulin binding induced by changes in vivo in the levels of glucocorticoids and growth hormone. Endocrinology 103:1054–1066, 1978

256. Kittredge RD, Nash AD. The many facets of sclerosing fibrosis. AJR 122:288–298, 1974

257. Klapper DG, Svoboda ME, Van Wyk JJ. Sequence analysis of somatomedin C: confirmation of identity with insulin-like growth factor I. Endocrinology 112:2215–2220, 1983

258. Klatskin G. Hepatic tumors: possible relationship to use of oral contraceptives. Gastroenterology 73:386–394, 1977

259. Klein I, Levey GS. Unusual manifestation of hypothyroidism. Arch Intern Med 144:123–128, 1984

260. Kley HK, Keck E, Kruskenyser HL. Estrone and estradiol in patients with cirrhosis of the liver: effects of ACTH and dexamethasone. J Clin Endocrinol Metab 43:557–560, 1976

261. Kneifel MA, Katzenellenbogen BS. Comparative effects of estrogen and antiestrogen on plasma renin substrate levels and hepatic estrogen receptors in the rat. Endocrinology 108:545–552, 1981

262. Kogawa M, Takano K, Hizuka N, Asakawa K, Shizume K. Effect of GH and insulin on the regeneration of somatomedin by perfused rat liver. Endocrinol Jpn 29:141–147, 1982

263. Krahenbul S, Weber FL, Brass EP. Decreased hepatic glycogen content and accelerated response to starvation in rats with carbon tetrachloride-induced cirrhosis. Hepatology 14:1189–1195, 1991

264. Kramer RE, Greiner JW, Rumbaugh RC, Sweeney TD, Colby HD. Requirement of the pituitary gland for gonadal hormone effects on hepatic drug metabolism in rats. J Pharmacol Exp Ther 208:19–23, 1979

265. Krasner N, Davis M, Portmann B, Williams R. Changing pattern of alcoholic liver disease in Great Britain: relation to sex and signs of autoimmunity. Br Med J 1:1497–1500, 1977

266. Krusynska Y, Williams N, Perry M, Home P. The relationship between insulin sensitivity and skeletal muscle enzyme activities in hepatic cirrhosis. Hepatology 8:1615–1619, 1988

267. Kurland KJ, Pilkis SJ. Indirect versus direct routes of hepatic glycogen synthesis. FASEB J 3:2277–2281, 1989

268. Lamas E, Zindy F, Seurin D, Guguen-Guillouzo C, Brechot C. Expression of insulin-like growth factor II and receptors for insulin-like growth factor II, insulin-like growth factor I and

insulin in isolated and cultured rat hepatocytes. Hepatology 13:936–940, 1991

269. Landau BR, Wills N, Craig JW, Leonards JR, Moriwaki T. The mechanism of hepatoma-induced hypoglycemia. Cancer 15:1088–1096, 1962

270. Landau BR, Wahren J. Quantification of the pathways followed in hepatic glycogen formation from glucose. FASEB J 2:2368–2375, 1988

271. Landreneau RJ, Horton JW, McClelland RN. Mesenteric venous hypertension: importance after portal systemic shunting? Surgery 106:11–20, 1989

272. Lautt WW, Legare DJ, D'Almeida MS. Adenosine as putative regulator of hepatic arterial flow (the buffer response). Am J Physiol 248:H331–H338, 1985

273. Leatherdale BA, Chase RA, Rogers J, Alberti KGMM, Davies P, Record CD. Forearm glucose uptake in cirrhosis and its relationship to glucose tolerance. Clin Sci 59:191–198, 1980

274. Lee RG. Non-alcoholic steatohepatitis: a study of 49 patients. Hum Pathol 20:594–598, 1989

275. Lee SS, Johansen K, Lebrec D. Circulatory changes induced by portal venous diversion and mesenteric hypertension in rats. Hepatology 15:117–121, 1992

276. Lee VM, Szepesi B, Hansen RJ. Gender linked differences in dietary induction of hepatic glucose-6-phosphate dehydrogenase, 6 phosphogluconate dehydrogenase and malic enzyme in the rat. J Nutr 116:1547–1554, 1986

277. Leevy CM. Fatty liver: a study of 270 patients with biopsy proven fatty liver and a review of the literature. Medicine 4:249–276, 1962

278. Leffert HL. Growth control of differentiated fetal rat hepatocytes in primary monolayer culture. VII Hormonal control of DNA synthesis and its possible significance to the problem of liver regeneration. J Cell Biol 62:792–801, 1974

279. Leffert HL, Koch KS. Proliferation of hepatocytes. In: Porter R, Whelan J, eds. Hepatotrophic factors. CIBA Foundation Symposium No. 55. Amsterdam, Elsevier, 1978, pp 61–94

280. Leffert HL, Koch KS, Moran T, Rubalcava B. Hormonal control of rat liver regeneration. Gastroenterology 76:1470–1482, 1979

281. Leiukkainen T. The effect of testosterone, progesterone and estrogen on the acetylating activity in rat liver and kidney preparations. Acta Physiol Scand 51:254, 1961

282. Leopold SA, Erwin M, Oh J, Browning B. Phytoestrogens: adverse effects on reproduction in California quail. Science 191:98–100, 1976

283. Lester R, Van Thiel DH, Eagon PK, Imhoff AF, Fisher SE. Hypothesis concerning the effects of dietary non-steroidal estrogen on the feminization of male alcoholics. In: Research Monograph 2, Alcohol and Nutrition, DHEW Publication. Washington, DC, United States Department of Health and Human Services, 1979, pp 383–388

284. Levey S, Robinson A. Introduction to the general principles of hormone–receptor interactions. Metabolism 31:639–644, 1982

285. Liddle RA, Goldstein RB, Saxton J. Gallstone formation during weight reduction dieting. Arch Intern Med 149:1750–1753, 1989

286. Liegel J, Fabre LF, Howard PY, Farmer RW. Plasma testosterone binding globulin (SGB) in alcoholic subjects. Physiologist 15:198, 1972

287. Lillioja S, Mott DM, Zawadzki JK, Young AA, Abbott WG, Bogardus C. Glucose storage is a major determinant of in vivo "insulin resistance" in subjects with normal glucose tolerance. J Clin Endocrinal Metab 62:922–927, 1986

288. Lindholm J, Fabricius-Bjerre N, Bahnsen M, Boresen P, Hagen C, Christensen T. Sex steroids and sex-hormone binding globulin in males with chronic alcoholism. Eur J Clin Invest 8:273–276, 1978

289. Lischner MW, Alexander JF, Galambos JT. Natural history of alcoholic hepatitis. I. The acute disease. Am J Dig Dis 16:481–494, 1971

290. Littenberg G, Afroudakis A, Kaplowitz N. Common bile duct stenosis from chronic pancreatitis: a clinical and pathologic specimen. Medicine 58:385–412, 1979

291. Litwack G, Morey T. In: Freedman PF, Rabin BR, eds. The effects of drugs on cellular control mechanisms. London, Macmillan, 1972, pp 95–105

292. Lloyd CW, Williams RH. Endocrine changes associated with Laennec's cirrhosis of the liver. Am J Med 4:315–330, 1948

293. Lochrie MA, Simon MI. G protein multiplicity in eukaryotic signal transduction systems. Biochemistry 27:4957–4965, 1988

294. Long CL, Lowry SF. Hormonal regulation of protein metabolism. JPEN 14:555–562, 1990

295. Lopez S. Insulin dependent changes in subcellular distribution of liver insulin receptors in obese Zucker rats. Diabetologia 31:922–927, 1988

296. Lowe WJ, Adamo M, Werner H, Roberts CT, LeRoith D. Regulation by fasting of insulin-like factor I and its receptor: effects on gene expression and binding. J Clin Invest 84:619–626, 1989

297. Ludwig J, Viggiano TR, McGill DB, Ott BJ. Non-alcoholic steatohepatitis: Mayo Clinic experiences with a hitherto unnamed disease. Mayo Clin Proc 55:434–438, 1980

298. Lunzer M, Huang SN, Ginsberg J, Ahmed M, Sherlock S. Jaundice due to carbimizole. Gut 16:913–917, 1975

299. Luyck AS, Lefebvre PJ. Mechanisms involved in the exercise induced increase in glucagon secretion in rats. Diabetes 23:81–92, 1974

300. MacGorman LR, Rizza RA, Gerich JE. Physiologic concentrations of growth hormone exert insulin-like and insulin antagonistic effects on both hepatic and extrahepatic tissues in man. J Clin Endocrinol Metab 53:556–559, 1981

301. Maes M, Underwood LE, Ketelslegers JM. Plasma somatomedin-C in fasted and refed rats: close relationship with changes in liver somatogenic (GH) but not lactogenic (PRL) binding sites. J Endocrinol 97:243–252, 1983

302. Maes M, Underwood LE, Ketelslegers JM. Low somatomedin C in protein deficiency: relationship with changes in liver somatogenic and lactogenic binding sites. Mol Cell Endocrinol 37:301–309, 1984

303. Magnusson I, Chandramouli V, Schumann WC, Kumaran K, Wahren J, Landau BR. Quantification of the pathways of hepatic glycogen formation on ingesting a glucose load. J Clin Invest 80:1748–1754, 1987

304. Maiter DM, Maes M, Underwood LE, Fliessen T, Gerard G, Ketelslegers JM. Early changes in serum concentrations of somatomedin-C induced by dietary protein deprivation: contributions of growth hormone receptor and post receptor defects. J Endocrinol 118:113–120, 1988

305. Malejka-Gigante D, Magat WJ, Decker RW. Sex hormone-mediated effects on the phase I and phase II metabolism of N-2-fluorenylacetamide: modulation of 9-hydroxylation. Biochem Pharmacol 38:1075–1082, 1989

306. Malt RA, Hershberg RA, Miller WL. Experience with benign tumors of the liver. Surg Gynecol Obstet 130:285–291, 1970

307. Manderson WG, McKiddie MT, Manners DJ, Stark JR. Liver glycogen accumulation in unstable diabetes. Diabetes 17:13–16, 1968

308. Mann FC, Magath TB. Studies on the physiology of the liver. II. The effect of removal of the liver on the blood sugar. Arch Intern Med 30:73–84, 1922

309. Marchesini G, Bianchi G, Zoli M, Dondi C, Forlani G, Melli A, Bua V, Vannini P, Pisi E. Plasma amino acid response to protein ingestion on patients with liver cirrhosis. Gastroenterology 85:283–290, 1983

310. Marchesini G, Forlani G, Zoli M, Dondi C, Bianchi G, Bua V, Vannini P, Pisi E. Effect of euglycemic insulin infusion on plasma levels of branched-chain amino acids in cirrhotics. Hepatology 3:184–187, 1983

311. Marchesini G, Zoli M, Dondi C, Angiolini A, Melli A, Pisi E. Ammonia induced changes in pancreatic hormones and

plasma amino acids in patients with liver cirrhosis. Dig Dis Sci 27:406–412, 1982

312. Marchesini G, Bianchi GP, Vilstrup H, Checchia GA, Patrono D, Zoli M. Plasma clearances of branched-chain amino acids in control subjects and in patients with cirrhosis. J Hepatol 4:108–117, 1987

313. Marchesini G, Pacini G, Bianchi G, Patrono D, Cobelli C. Glucose disposal β-cell secretion and hepatic insulin extraction in cirrhosis: a minimal model assessment. Gastroenterology 99:1715–1722, 1990

314. Marco J, Diego J, Villanueva ML, Diaz-Ficrros M, Valverde I, Segovia J. Elevated plasma glucagon levels in cirrhosis of the liver. N Engl J Med 289:1107–1111, 1973

315. Marcus R, Butterfield G, Holloway L, Gilliland L, Baylink DJ, Hintz RL, Sherman BM. Effects of short term administration of recombinant human growth hormone to elderly people. J Clin Endocrinol Metab 70:519–527, 1990

316. Marshall RN, Underwood LE, Voina SJ, Foushee DB, Van Wyk JJ. Characterization of insulin and somatomedin receptors in human placental membranes. J Clin Endocrinol Metab 39:283–292, 1974

317. Marti V, Burwen SJ, Wells A, Barker ME, Huling S, Feren AM, Jones AL. Localization of epidermal growth factor receptor in hepatocyte nuclei. Hepatology 13:15–20, 1991

318. Martini GA. Extrahepatic manifestations of cirrhosis. Clin Gastroenterol 4:439–460, 1975

319. Mattox TW, Brown RO, Boucher BA, Buonpane EA, Fabian TC, Luther RW. Use of fibronectin and somatomedin-C as markers of enteral nutrition support in traumatized patients using a modified amino acid formula. JPEN 12:592–596, 1988

320. Mauriac P. Hepatomegalie, nanisme, obesite dans le diabete infantile, pathogenie du syndrome. Presse Med 54:826–827, 1946

321. Mayer PW, Schalch DS. Somatomedin synthesis by a subclone of Buffalo rat liver cells: characterization and evidence for immediate secretion of de novo synthesized hormone. Endocrinology 113:588–594, 1983

322. Mayer-Alber A, Hartmann H, Stumpe F, Creutzfeldt W. Mechanism of insulin resistance in CCL₄-induced cirrhosis of rats. Gastroenterology 102:223–229, 1992

323. McCaleb ML, Izzo MS, Lockwood DH. Characterization and partial purification of a factor from human uremic serum that induces insulin resistance. J Clin Invest 75:391–396, 1985

324. McClain CJ, Marsano L, Burk RF, Bacon B. Trace metals in liver disease. Semin Liver Dis 11:321–339, 1991

325. McConaghey P, Sledge CB. Production of "sulphation factors" by the perfused liver. Nature 225:1249–1251, 1970

326. McCullough AJ, Mullen KD, Smanik EJ, Tabbaa M, Szauter K. Nutritional therapy and liver disease. Gastroenterol Clin North Am 18:619–643, 1989

327. McCullough, AJ, Tavill AS. Hepatic protein metabolism: basic and applied biochemical and clinical aspects. In: Arias IM, Frenkel M, Wilson JHP, eds. The liver annual. New York, Elsevier, 1987, pp 48–90

328. McCullough AJ, Mullen KD, Kalhan SC. Measurement of total body and extracellular water in cirrhotic patients with and without ascites. Hepatology 14:1102–1111, 1991

329. McCullough AJ, Tavill AS. Disordered energy and protein metabolism in liver disease. Semin Liver Dis 11:265–277, 1991

330. McDonald TJ, Dupre J, Caussignac Y, Radziuk J, ManVliet S. Hyperglucagonemia in liver cirrhosis with portal systemic venous anastomoses: responses of plasma glucagon and gastric inhibitory polypeptide to oral or intravenous glucose in cirrhotics with normal or elevated fasting plasma glucose levels. Metabolism 28:300–307, 1979

331. McFadzean AJS, Yeung RTT. Further observations on hypoglycemia in hepatocellular carcinoma. Am J Med 47:220–225, 1969

332. McNeil LW, McKee LC, Lorber D, Rabin D. The endocrine manifestations of hemochromatosis. Am J Med Sci 285:7–13, 1983

333. Megyesi C, Samols E, Marks V. Glucose tolerance and diabetes in chronic liver disease. Lancet 2:1051–1055, 1967

334. Mendelson JH, Mello NK, Ellengboe J. Acute alcohol intake and pituitary gonadal hormones in normal human females. J Pharmacol Exp Ther 218:23–26, 1981

335. Mendelson JH, Mello NK, Ellengboe J. Effects of acute alcohol intake on pituitary-gonadal hormones in normal human males. J Pharmacol Exp Ther 202:676–682, 1977

336. Mendenhall CL, Anderson S, Garcia-Pont P, Goldberg S, Kiernan T, Seeff B, Sorrell M, Tamburro S, Wiesner R, Tellerman R, Chedid A, Chen T, Rabin L. Veterans administration cooperative study on alcoholic hepatitis: short-term and long-term survival in patients with alcoholic hepatitis treated with oxandrolone and prednisolone. N Engl J Med 311:1464–1470, 1984

337. Mendenhall CL, Anderson S, Weesner RE, Goldberg SJ, Crolic KA. Protein-calorie malnutrition associated with alcoholic hepatitis. Am J Clin Nutr 38:849–859, 1983

338. Merimee TJ, Zapf J, Froesch ER. Insulin-like growth factors in fed and fasted states. J Clin Endocrinol Metab 55:999–1002, 1982

339. Merli M, Riggio O, Romiti A, Ariosto F, Mango L, Pinto G, Savioli M, Capocaccia L. Basal energy production rate and substrate use in stable cirrhotic patients. Hepatology 12:106–112, 1990

340. Merli M, Iapechino S, Bolognese A, Bruni A, Cantafora A, Riggio O, Capocaccia L. Fatty acid composition of adipose tissue in patients with chronic liver disease. J Hepatol 3:104–110, 1986

341. Merli M, Eriksson LS, Hagenfeldt L, Wahren J. Splanchnic and leg exchange of free fatty acids in patients with liver cirrhosis. J Hepatol 3:348–355, 1986

342. Mezey E, Potter JJ. Effect of castration on the turnover of rat liver alcohol dehydrogenase. Biochem Pharmacol 34:369–372, 1985

343. Milman N, Graudal N, Strom P, Franzman M-B. Alcoholic hepatitis in females. Acta Med Scand 223:119–124, 1988

344. Minuto F, Barreca A, Adami GF, Fortini P, Del Monte P, Cella F, Scopinaro N, Girodano G. Insulin-like growth factor-I in human malnutrition: relationship with some body composition and nutritional parameters. JPEN 13:392–396, 1989

345. Mode A, Gustafsson J-A, Jansson J-O, Eden S, Isaksson O. Association between plasma levels of growth hormone and sex differentiation of hepatic steroid metabolism in the rat. Endocrinology 111:1692–1699, 1982

346. Mode A, Norstedt G, Simic B. Continuous infusion of growth hormone feminizes hepatic steroid metabolism in the rat. Endocrinology 108:2103–2108, 1981

347. Morgan MY, Sherlock S. Sex-related differences among 100 patients with alcoholic liver disease. Br Med J 1:939–941, 1977

348. Morgan MY. The effect of bromocriptine on sexual function and hormonal profiles in chronic alcoholic men with liver disease. In: Langer M, Chiandussi L, Chopra IJ, Martini L, eds. The endocrines and the liver. New York, Academic Press, 1982, pp 165–171

349. Morrione TG. Effect of estrogens on the testes in hepatic insufficiency. Arch Pathol 37:39–48, 1944

350. Morrison WL, Bouchier IAD, Gibson JNA, Rennie MJ. Skeletal muscle and whole body protein turnover in cirrhosis. Clin Sci 78:613–619, 1990

351. Mortiaux A, Dawson A. Plasma free fatty acids in liver disease. Gut 2:304–309, 1961

352. Muggeo M, Tiengo A, Fedele D, Crepaldi G. Altered control of growth hormone secretion in patients with cirrhosis of the liver. Arch Intern Med 139:1157–1160, 1979

353. Mullen, KD, Denne S, McCullough AJ, Savin JM, Bruno

D, Tavill AS, Kalhan SC. Leucine metabolism in stable cirrhosis. Hepatology 6:622–630, 1986

354. Muller WA, Paloona GR, Auilar-Parada E, Unger RH. Abnormal alpha-cell function in diabetes. N Engl J Med 283:109–115, 1970

355. Muscaritoli M, Cangiano C, Cascino A, Ceci F, Caputo V, Martino P, Serra P, Rossi Fanelli F. Exogenous lipid clearance in compensated liver cirrhosis. JPEN 10:599–603, 1986

356. Myers SR, McGuinness OP, Neal DW, Cherrington AD. Intraportal glucose delivery alters the relationship between net hepatic glucose uptake and the insulin concentration. J Clin Invest 87:930–939, 1991

357. Nagaoka I, Trapnell BC, Crystal RG. Regulation of insulin-like growth factor I gene expression in the human macrophage-like cell line U 937. J Clin Invest 85:448–455, 1990

358. Nagasue N, Ito A, Yukaya H, Ogawa Y. Androgen receptors in hepatocellular carcinoma and surrounding parenchyma. Gastroenterology 89:643–647, 1985

359. Nagore N, Scheuer PJ. The pathology of diabetic hepatitis. J Pathol 156:155–160, 1988

360. Nakao NL, Gelb AM, Stenger RJ, Siegel JH. A case of chronic liver disease due to tolazamide. Gastroenterology 89:192–195, 1985

361. National Diabetes Data Group. Classification and diagnosis of diabetes mellitus and other categories of glucose intolerance. Diabetes 28:1039–1057, 1979

362. Naylor CD, O'Rourke K, Desky AS, Baker JP. Parenteral nutrition with branched-chain amino acids in hepatic encephalopathy: a meta-analysis. Gastroenterology 97:1033–1042, 1989

363. Nicholls KM, Shapiro MD, VanPutten VJ, Kluge R, Chung HM, Bichet DG, Schrier RW. Elevated plasma norepinephrine concentrations in decompensated cirrhosis: association with increased secretion rates, normal clearance rates and suppressibility by central blood volume expansion. Circ Res 56:457–461, 1985

364. Niederau C, Stremmel W, Strohmeyer G. Eisenuberladung und Haemochromatose. Internist (Berlin) 22:546–554, 1981

365. Niewoehner CB, Nuttall FQ. Gynecomastia in a hospitalized male population. Am J Med 77:633–638, 1984

366. Nissley SP, Rechler MM. Insulin-like growth factors: biosynthesis receptors and IGF-carrier proteins. In: Li CH, ed. Hormonal proteins and peptides. New York, Academic Press, 1985, pp 127–203

367. Nomura S, Pittman CS, Chambers JB, Buck MW, Shimizu T. Reduced peripheral conversion of thyroxine to triiodothyroxine in patients with hepatic cirrhosis. J Clin Invest 56:643–652, 1975

368. Norstedt G, Wrange O, Gustafsson J-A. Multihormonal regulation of the estrogen receptor in rat liver. Endocrinology 108:1190–1196, 1981

369. Nosadini R, Avogaro A, Mollo F, Maresco HC, Tieng A, Duner E, Merkel C, Gatta A, Zuin R, deKreutzenberg S, Trevisan R, Crepaldi G. Carbohydrate and lipid metabolism in cirrhosis: evidence that hepatic uptake of gluconeogenic precursors and of free fatty acids depends on effective hepatic flow. J Clin Endocrinol Metab 58:1125–1132, 1984

370. Novel O, Bernuau J, Rueff B, Benhamou JP. Hypoglycemia: a common complication of septicemia in cirrhosis. Arch Intern Med 141:1477–1478, 1981

371. Novin D, Robinson K, Culbreth LA, Tordoff MG. Is there a role for the liver in the control of food intake? Am J Clin Nutr 42:1050–1062, 1985

372. Nygren A, Adner N, Sundblad L, Wiechel KL. Insulin uptake by the human alcoholic cirrhotic liver. Metabolism 34:48–52, 1985

373. Ober KP, Lowder SC. Massive hyperthyroxinemia in a euthyroid patient with hepatocellular carcinoma. Am J Med 86:621–623,1989

374. Ohnishi K, Mishima A, Takashi M, Tsuchiya S, Iida S, Iwama S, Groto N, Kono K, Nakajima Y, Suzuki N, Musha

375. H, Okuda K. Effects of intra- and extrahepatic portal systemic shunts on insulin metabolism. Dig Dis Sci 28:201–206, 1983

375. Okuno M, Nagayama M, Takai T, Rai A, Nakao S, Kamino K, Umeyama K. Postoperative total parenteral nutrition in patients with liver disorders. J Surg Res 39:93–102, 1985

376. Olefsky JM, Sperling MA, Reaven GM. Does glucagon play a role in the insulin resistance of patients with adult nonketotic diabetes? Diabetologia 13:327–330, 1977

377. Olefsky JM, Reaven GM. Effects of sulfonylurea therapy on insulin binding to mononuclear leukocytes of diabetic patients. Am J Med 60:89–95, 1976

378. Olivo J, Gordon GG, Rafii F. Estrogen metabolism in hyperthyroidism and cirrhosis of the liver. Steroids 26:47–56, 1975

379. Orrego H, Kalant K, Israel Y, et al. Effect of short term therapy with propylthiouracil in patients with alcoholic liver disease. Gastroenterology 76:105–115, 1979

380. Ostrowski JL, Ingleton PM, Underwood JCE, Parsons MA. Increased hepatic androgen receptor expression in female rats during diethylnitrosamine liver carcinogenesis: a possible correlation with liver tumor development. Gastroenterology 94:1193–1200, 1988

381. Owen LN, Buggs MH. Contraceptive steroid toxicology in the beagle dog and its relevance to human carcinogenicity. Curr Med Res Opin 4:309–329, 1976

382. Owen OE, Felig P, Morgan AP, Wahren J, Cahill GF Jr. Liver and kidney metabolism during prolonged starvation. J Clin Invest 48:574–583, 1969

383. Owen OE, Trapp VE, Reichard GA, Mozzoli MA, Moctezuma J, Paul P, Skutches CL, Boden G. Nature and quantity of fuels consumed in patients with alcoholic cirrhosis. J Clin Invest 72:1821–1832, 1983

384. Owen OE, Mozzoli MA, Reichle FA, Kreulen TH, Owen RS, Boden G, Polansky M. Hepatic and renal metabolism before and after portasystemic shunts in patients with cirrhosis. J Clin Invest 76:1209–1217, 1985

385. Owen OE, Reichle FA, Mozzoli MA, Kreulen T, Patel MS, Elfenbein IB, Golsorkhi M, Chang KH, Rao NS, Sue HS, Boden G. Hepatic, gut and renal substrate flux rates in patients with hepatic cirrhosis. J Clin Invest 68:240–252, 1981

386. Painson JC, Tannenbaum GS. Sexual dimorphism of somatostatin and growth hormone factor signaling in the control of pulsatile growth hormone secretion in the rat. Endocrinology 128:2858–2866, 1991

387. Pak RCK, Tsim KWK, Cheng CHK. Pubertal gonadal hormones in modulating the testosterone dependency of hepatic aryl hydrocarbon hydroxylase in female rats. Pharmacology 29:121–127, 1984

388. Palmer M, Shaffner F. Effect of weight reduction or hepatic abnormalities in overweight patients. Gastroenterology 99:1408–1413, 1990

389. Pares A, Caballeria J, Bruguera M, Torres M, Rodes J. Histological course of alcoholic hepatitis: influence of abstinence, sex and extent of hepatic damage. J Hepatol 2:33–42, 1986

390. Parker WA. Propylthiouracil-induced hepatotoxicity. Clin Pharm 1:471–472, 1982

391. Parsons MA, Bannister P, Ingleton PM, Underwood JCE, Losowsky MS. Hepatic androgen receptors in evolving cirrhosis of the rat. J Endocrinol 108:119, 1986

392. Peguignot G, Chabet C, Eydoux H, Courcoul MA. Augmentation du risque de cirrhosis en function de la ration d'alcool. Rev Alcoholism 20:191–202, 1974

393. Peillon F, Racadot J. Modifications histopathologiques de l'hypophyse dans six cas d'hemochromatose. Ann Endocrinol (Paris) 31:259–270, 1970

394. Pelkonen R, Kallio H, Suoranta H, Karonen SL. Plasma insulin, C-peptide and blood glucose in portal, hepatic and peripheral veins in liver cirrhosis: effect of intravenous tolbutamide. Acta Endocrinol 97:496–502, 1981

395. P'eng FK, Lui WY, Chang TJ, Kao HL, Wu LH, Liu TY, Chi CW. Glucocorticoid receptors in hepatocellular carcinoma and adjacent liver tissue. Cancer 62:2134–2138, 1988

396. Pentihainen PJ, Pentihainen LA, Azarnoff DL, Dujovne LA. Plasma levels and excretion of estrogens in urine in chronic liver disease. Gastroenterology 69:20–27, 1975

397. Perez G, Trimarco B, Undaro B. Glucoregulatory response to insulin-induced hypoglycemia in Laennec's cirrhosis. J Clin Endocrinol Metab 46:778–783, 1978

398. Perley MJ, Kipnsis DM. Plasma insulin responses to oral and intravenous glucose: studies in normal and diabetic subjects. J Clin Invest 46:1954–1971, 1967

399. Peterson RE. Adrenocorticol steroid metabolism and adrenal cortical function in liver disease. J Clin Invest 39:320–321, 1960

400. Petrides AS, DeFronze RA. Glucose metabolism in cirrhosis: a review with some perspectives for the future. Diabetes Metab Rev 5:691–709, 1989

401. Petrides AS, Luzi L, Reuben A, Riely C, DeFronzo RA. Effect of insulin and plasma amino acid concentration on leucine metabolism in cirrhosis. Hepatology 14:432–441, 1991

402. Petrides AS, Groop LC, Riely CA, DeFronzo RA. Effect of physiologic hyperinsulinemia on glucose and lipid metabolism in cirrhosis. J Clin Invest 88:561–570, 1991

403. Petrides AS, Passlack W, Reinhauer H, Stremmel W, Strohmeyer G. Insulin binding to erythrocytes in hyperinsulinemic patients with pre-cirrhotic hemochromatosis and cirrhosis. Klin Wochenschr 65:877–878, 1987

404. Pfaffenberger CD, Horning EC. Sex differences in human urinary steroid metabolic profiles determined by gas chromatography. Anal Biochem 80:329–343, 1977

405. Pilo A, Navalesi R, Ferrannini E. Insulin kinetics after portal and peripheral injection of ^{25}I-insulin: data analysis and modeling. Am J Physiol 230:1626–1629, 1976

406. Pittman CS. Hormone metabolism. In: DeGroat LJ, Cahill CF, O'Dell JWD, et al, eds. Endocrinology, vol 1. New York, Grune & Stratton, 1979, p 365

407. Polonsky KS, Pugh W, Jaspan JB. C-peptide and insulin secretion. J Clin Invest 74:1821–1829, 1984

408. Polonsky KS, Rubenstein AH. C-peptide as a measure of the secretion and hepatic extraction of insulin. Diabetes 33:468–494, 1984

409. Pomposelli JJ, Moldawer LL, Palombo JD, Babayan VK, Bistrian BR, Blackburn GL. Short-term administration of parenteral glucose–lipid mixtures improves protein kinetics in portacaval shunted rats. Gastroenterology 91:305–312, 1986

410. Ponting GA, Ward HC, Halliday D, Sim AJW. Protein and energy metabolism with biosynthetic human growth hormone in patients on full intravenous nutritional support. JPEN J Parenter Enteral Nutr 14:437–441, 1990

411. Porter LE, Elm MS, Dugas MC, Van Thiel DH, Eagon PK. Characterization and quantitation of human hepatic estrogen receptor. Gastroenterology 81:704–712, 1983

412. Porter LE, Elm MS, Van Thiel DH, Eagon PK. Estrogen receptor in human liver nuclei. Hepatology 4:1085, 1984

413. Porter LE, Elm MS, Van Thiel DH, Eagon PK. Hepatic estrogen receptor in human liver disease. Gastroenterology 92:35–45, 1987

414. Powell-Jones W, Raeford S, Lucier GW. Binding properties of zearalenone mycotoxins to hepatic estrogen receptors. Mol Pharmacol 20:35–42, 1981

415. Powell LW, Mortimer R, Harris OD. Cirrhosis of the liver: a comparative study of the 4 major etiological groups. Med J Aust 1:941–950, 1971

416. Proietto J, Dudley FJ, Aitken P. Hyperinsulinemia and insulin resistance of cirrhosis: the importance of hypersecretion. Clin Endocrinol 21:657–665, 1984

417. Proietto J, Nankervis A, Aitken P, Dudley FJ, Caruso G, Alford FP. Insulin resistance in cirrhosis: evidence for a postreceptor defect. Clin Endocrinol 21:677–688, 1984

418. Pugh RNH, Murray-Lyon IM, Dawson JL, Pietroni MC, Williams R. Transection of the oesophagus for bleeding oesophageal varices. Br J Surg 60:646–649, 1973

419. Rachamin G, MacDonald JA, Walid S, Clapp JJ, Khann JM, Israel Y. Modulation of alcohol dehydrogenase and ethanol metabolism by sex hormones in the spontaneously hypertensive rat. Biochem J 186:484–490, 1980

420. Radzuik J, McDonald TJ, Rubenstein D. Initial splanchnic extraction of ingested glucose in normal man. Metabolism 27:657–669, 1978

421. Randle PJ, Garland PB, Hales CN, Newsholme EA. The glucose fatty-acid cycle: its role in insulin sensitivity and the metabolic disturbances of diabetes mellitus. Lancet 1:785–789, 1963

422. Ranke MB, Stanley CA, Tenore A, Rodbard D, Bongiovanni AM, Parks JS. Characterization of somatogenic and lactogenic binding sites in isolated rat hepatocytes. Endocrinology 99:1033–1039, 1976

423. Re RN, Vizard DL, Brown J, Bryan SE. Angiotensin II receptors in chromatin fragments generated by micrococcal nuclease. Biochem Biophys Res Commun 119:220–227, 1984

424. Reaven GM. Role of insulin resistance in human disease. Diabetes 37:1595–1607, 1988

425. Renault PF, Hoofnagle JH. Side effects of alpha interferon. Semin Liver Dis 9:273–277, 1989

426. Reuben M. Influence of age and sex on dietary-induced cirrhosis. Arch Environ Health 18:792–797, 1969

427. Riggio O, Merli M, Cantafora A, DiBiase A, Lalloni L, Leonetti F, Miazzo P, Rinaldi V, Rossi-Fanelli F, Tamburrano G, Capocaccia L. Total and free fatty acid concentrations in liver cirrhosis. Metabolism 33:646–651, 1984

428. Riggio O, Merli M, Cangiano C, Capocaccia R, Cascino A, Lala A, Leonetti F, Mauceri M, Pepe M, Rossi-Fanelli F, Savioli M, Tamburrano G, Capocaccia L. Glucose intolerance in liver cirrhosis. Metabolism 31:627–634, 1982

429. Riley WJ, McCaan VJ. Impaired glucose tolerance and growth hormone in chronic liver disease. Gut 22:301–305, 1981

430. Rinderknecht E, Humbel RE. Primary structure of human insulin-like growth factor II. FEBS Lett 89:283–288, 1978

431. Rinderknecht E, Humbel RE. The amino acid sequence of human insulin-like growth factor I and its structural homology with pro-insulin. J Biol Chem 253:769–778, 1978

432. Ring-Larsen H, Hesse B, Henriksen JH, Christensen NJ. Sympathetic nervous activity and renal and systemic hemodynamics in cirrhosis: plasma norepinephrine concentration, hepatic extraction and renal disease. Hepatology 2:304–310, 1982

433. Rizza RA, Mandarino LJ, Gerich JE. Effect of growth hormone on insulin action in man: mechanisms of insulin resistance, impaired suppression of glucose production, and impaired stimulation of glucose utilization. Diabetes 31:663–669, 1982

434. Rizza RA, Mandarino LJ, Genest J, Genest J, Baker BA, Gerich JE. Production of insulin resistance by hyperinsulinemia in man. Diabetologia 28:70–75, 1985

435. Roginsky MS, Zansi I, Cohn SH. Skeletal and lean body mass in alcoholics with and without cirrhosis. Calcif Tissue Res Suppl 21:381–391, 1976

436. Rolleston H, McNee JW. Diseases of the liver, gallbladder and bile ducts. New York, MacMillan, 1929, p 256

437. Romijn, JA, Endert E, Sauerwein HP. Glucose and fat metabolism during short-term starvation in cirrhosis. Gastroenterology 100:731–737, 1991

438. Ross DS, Daniels GH, Dienstag JL, Ridgway EC. Elevated thyroxine levels due to increased thyroxine binding globulin in acute hepatitis. Am J Med 74:564–569, 1983

439. Rossner S, Johansson C, Wallius G, Aly A. Intralipid clearance and lipoprotein pattern in men with advanced alcoholic liver cirrhosis. Am J Clin Nutr 32:2022–2026, 1979

440. Rotwein P, Folz RH, Gordon JI. Biosynthesis of human insulin-like growth factor I (IGF-I). J Biol Chem 262:11807–11812, 1987

441. Roy AK, Chatterjee B. Sexual dimorphism in the liver. Annu Rev Physiol 45:37–50, 1983

442. Roy AK, Melen BS, McMinn DM. Androgen receptor in rat liver: hormonal and developmental regulation of the cytoplasmic receptor and its correlation with the androgen-dependent synthesis of α_2U-globulin. Biochem Biophys Acta 354:213–232, 1974

443. Roy AK, Neuhaus OW, Harmeson CR. Preparation and characterization of a sex-dependent rat urinary protein. Biochem Biophys Acta 127:72–81, 1966

444. Roy AK, Sarkar FH, Nag AC, Mancini MA. Role of cytodifferentiation and cell-cell communication in the androgen dependent expression of α_2U globulin gene in rat liver. In: Serrero G, Hayaski J, eds. Cellular endocrinology: hormonal control of embryonic and cellular differentiation. New York, Alan R Liss, 1986, pp 401–415

445. Rubenstein AH, Clark JL, Melani F, Steiner DF. Secretion of pro-insulin, C-peptide by pancreatic β cells and its circulation in blood. Nature 224:697–699, 1969

446. Rubenstein AH, Potenger LA, Mako M, Gets GS, Steiner DF. The metabolism of pro-insulin and insulin by the liver. J Clin Invest 51:112–121, 1972

447. Rudman D, Feller AG, Nagraj HS, Gergans GA, Lalitha PY, Goldberg AF, Schlenker RA, Cohn L, Rudman IW, Mattson DE. Effects of human growth hormone in men over 60 years old. N Engl J Med 323:1–6, 1990

448. Russell WE, Van Wyk JJ, Pledger WJ. Inhibition of the mitogenic effects of plasma by a monoclonal antibody to somatomedin-C. Proc Natl Acad Sci USA 81:2389–2392, 1984

449. Ryback RS. Chronic alcohol consumption and menstruation. JAMA 238:2143, 1977

450. Sachdev Y, Hall R. Effusions into body cavities in hypothyroidism. Lancet 1:564–566, 1977

451. Samaan NA, Stone DB, Eckhardt RD. Serum glucose, insulin and growth hormone in chronic hepatic cirrhosis. Arch Intern Med 124:149–152, 1969

452. Samson RI, Trey C, Timme AH, Saunders SJ. Fulminating hepatitis with recurrent hypoglycemia and hemorrhage. Gastroenterology 53:291–300, 1967

453. Scatarige JC, Scott WW, Donovan PJ, Siegelmann SS, Sanders RC. Fatty infiltration of the liver: ultrasonographic and computed tomography correlation. J Ultrasound Med 3:9–14, 1984

454. Schaffner F, Thaler H. Non-alcoholic fatty liver disease. In: Popper H, Schaffner F, eds. Progress in liver diseases, vol 8. Philadelphia, Grune & Stratton, 1986, pp 283–297

455. Schalch DS, Heinrich UE, Draznin B, Johnson CJ, Miller LL. Role of the liver in regulating somatomedin activity: hormonal effects on the synthesis and release of insulin-like growth factor and its carrier protein by the isolated perfused rat liver. Endocrinology 104:1143–1151, 1979

456. Scheiwiller E, Guler HP, Merryweather J, Scandella C, Maerki W, Zapf J, Froesch ER. Growth restoration of insulin-deficient diabetic rats by recombinant human insulin-like growth factor I. Nature 323:169–171, 1986

457. Schimpff, Lebrec D, Donnadiu M. Serum somatomedin activity measured as sulphation factors in peripheral, hepatic and renal veins of patients with alcoholic cirrhosis. Acta Endocrinol 88:729–734, 1978

458. Schimpff RM, Donnadieu M, Gautier M. Somatomedin activity measured as sulphation factor in culture media from normal human liver and connective tissue explants: effects of human growth hormone. Acta Endocrinol 98:24–29, 1981

459. Schlichting P, Christensen E, Andersen PK, Fauerholdt L, Juhl E, Poulsen H, Tygstrup N, the Copenhagen Study Group for Liver Diseases. Prognostic factors in cirrhosis identified by Cox's regression model. Hepatology 3:889–895, 1983

460. Schneeweiss B, Graninger W, Ferenci P, Eichinger S, Grimm G, Schneider B, Laggner AN, Lenz K, Kleinberger G. Energy metabolism in patients with acute and chronic liver disease. Hepatology 11:387–393, 1990

461. Schneider HL, Hornback, KD, Kninz JL, Efrusy ME. Chlor-

propamide hepatotoxicity: report of a case and review of the literature. Am J Gastroenterol 79:721–724, 1984

462. Schoental R. The role of nicotinamide and of certain other modifying factors in diethylnitrosamine carcinogenesis. Cancer 40:1833–1840, 1977

463. Schonfeld A, Babbott D, Gundersen K. Hypoglycemia and polycythemia associated with primary hepatoma. N Engl J Med 265:231–233, 1961

464. Schulman GI, Cline G, Schumann WC, Chandramouli V, Kumaran K, Landau BR. Quantitative comparison of the pathways of hepatic glycogen repletion in fed and fasted humans. Am J Physiol 259:E335–E341, 1990

465. Schussler GC, Schaffner F, Korn F. Increased serum thyroid hormone binding and decreased free hormone in chronic active liver disease. N Engl J Med 297:510–515, 1978

466. Schwander JC, Hauri C, Zapf J, Froesch ER. Synthesis and secretion of insulin-like growth factor and its binding protein by the perfused rat liver: dependence on growth hormone status. Endocrinology 113:297–305, 1983

467. Scott CD, Ballesteros M, Baxter RC. Increased expression of insulin-like growth factor-II/mannose-6-phosphate receptor in regenerating rat liver. Endocrinology 127:2210–2216, 1990

468. Seki K, Minami Y, Nishikawa M, Kawata S, Miyoshi S, Imai Y, Tarvi S. "Non-alcoholic steatohepatitis," induced by massive doses of synthetic estrogen. Gastroenterol Jpn 18:197–203, 1983

469. Shanbhogue RLK, Bistrian BR, Jenkins RL, Jones C, Benotti P, Blackburn GL. Resting energy expenditure in patients with end stage liver disease and in normal population. JPEN 11:305–308, 1987

470. Shankar TP, Fredi JL, Himmelstein S, Solomon SS, Duckworth WC. Elevated growth hormone levels and insulin resistance in patients with cirrhosis of the liver. Am J Med Sci 291:248–254, 1986

471. Shankar TP, Solomon SS, Duckworth WC, Jerkins T, Iyer RS, Bobal MA. Growth hormone and carbohydrate intolerance in cirrhosis. Horm Metab Res 20:579–583, 1988

472. Shankar TP, Solomon SS, Duckworth WC, Himmelstein S, Gray S, Jerkins T, Bobal MA. Studies on glucose intolerance in cirrhosis of the liver. J Lab Clin Med 102:459–469, 1983

473. Sherwin RS, Joshi P, Hendler R, Felig P, Conn HO. Hyperglucagonemia in Laennec's cirrhosis: the role of portal-systemic shunting. N Engl J Med 290:239–242, 1974

474. Sherwin RS, Fisher M, Bessoff J, Snyder N, Hendler R, Conn HO, Felig P. Hyperglucagonemia in cirrhosis: altered secretion and sensitivity to glucagon. Gastroenterology 74:1224–1228, 1978

475. Shikita M, Sato F. 20α-Hydroxysteroid dehydrogenase and reductive metabolism of progesterone in mammalian cell cultures. Arch Biochem 133:336–344, 1969

476. Shurberg JL, Resnick RH, Koff RS, Ros E, Baum RA, Pallotta JA. Serum lipid, insulin and glucagon after portocaval shunt in cirrhosis. Gastroenterology 72:301–304, 1977

477. Sidranskey H, Farber E. Sex differences in induction of periportal fatty liver by methionine deficiency in the rat. Proc Soc Exp Biol Med 98:293–297, 1958

478. Silva G, Gomis R, Bosch J, Casamitjana R, Mastai R, Nauasa M, Rivera F, Rodes J. Hyperglucagonism and glucagon resistance in cirrhosis: paradoxical effect of propranolol on plasma glucagon levels. J Hepatol 6:325–331, 1988

479. Silverman JF, O'Brien KF, Long S, Leggett N, Khazanie PG, Pories WJ, Norris HT, Caro JF. Liver pathology in morbidly obese patients with and without diabetes. Am J Gastroenterol 85:1349–1355, 1990

480. Simon M, Franckemont P, Murie N, Ferrand B, van Cauwenberge H, Bourel M. Study of somatotropic and gonadotropic pituitary function in idopathic haemochromatosis (31 cases). Eur J Clin Invest 2:384–389, 1972

481. Smals AGH, Njo KT, Knoben JM, Ruland CM, Kloppenborg PWC. Alcohol-induced cushinoid syndrome. J R Coll Physicians 12:36–41, 1977

482. Smanik EJ, Mullen DK, Giroski W, McCullough AJ. The influence of portacaval anastomosis on gonadal and anterior pituitary hormones in a rat model standardized for gender, food intake and time after surgery. Steroids 56:237–241, 1991

483. Smith-Laing G, Sherlock S, Faber OK. Effects of spontaneous portal-systemic shunting on insulin metabolism. Gastroenterology 76:685–690, 1979

484. Smith-Laing G, Orskov H, Gore MBR, Sherlock S. Hyperglucagonemia in cirrhosis: relationship to hepatocellular damage. Diabetologia 19:103–108, 1980

485. Smuk M, Schwers J. Aromatization of androstenedione by human adult liver in vitro. J Clin Endocrinol Metab 45:1001–1012, 1977

486. Soeters P, Weir G, Ebeid AM, James JH, Fischer JE. Insulin and glucagon following portocaval shunt. Gastroenterology 69:867–871, 1975

487. Song CS, Rao TR, Demyan WF, Mancini MA, Chatterjee B, Roy AK. Androgen receptor messenger ribonucleic acid (mRNA) in the rat liver: changes in mRNA levels during maturation, aging and caloric restriction. Endocrinology 128:349–356, 1991

488. Sonnenberg GE, Keller V, Burckhardt D. Ursachen der Hyperinsulinemia bei Patienten mit Leber Cirrhose: Portocavale Shunts oder Verminderate Degradations-Faenigkeit der Eber. Verh Dtsch Ges Inn Med 86:771–775, 1980

489. Spain DM. Portal cirrhosis of the liver: a review of 250 necropsies with references to sex differences. Am J Clin Pathol 15:215–218, 1945

490. Spencer EM. Synthesis by cultured hepatocytes of somatomedin and its binding protein. FEBS Lett 99:157–161, 1979

491. Starus DS, Takemoto CD. Effect of fasting on insulin-like growth factor (IGF-I) and growth hormone receptor mRNA levels on IGF-I transcription in rat liver. Mol Endocrinol 4:91–100, 1990

492. Stauffer JQ, Lapinski MW, Harold DJ, Myers JK. Focal nodular hyperplasia of the liver and intrahepatic hemorrhage in young women on oral contraceptives. Ann Intern Med 83:301–306, 1975

493. Stewart A, Johnston DG, Alberti KGMM, Nattrass M, Wright R. Hormone and metabolite profiles in alcoholic liver disease. Eur J Clin Invest 13:397–403, 1983

494. Stone BG, Van Thiel DH. Diabetes mellitus and the liver. Semin Liver Dis 5:8–28, 1985

495. Stremml W, Kley HK, Kruskemper HL, Strohmeyer G. Differing abnormalities in estrogen and androgen and insulin metabolism in idiopathic hemochromatosis versus alcoholic liver disease. Semin Liver Dis 5:84–93, 1985

496. Swart GR, Zillikens MC, VanVuure JK, van den Berg JW. Effect of a late evening meal on nitrogen balance in patients with cirrhosis of the liver. Br Med J 299:1202–1203, 1989

497. Takano K, Hizuka N, Shizume K, Hayashi N, Motoike Y, Obata H. Serum somatomedin peptides measured by somatomedin A radioreceptor assay in chronic liver disease. J Clin Endocrinol Metab 45:828–832, 1977

498. Tam SP, Archer TK, Deeley RA. Effects of estrogen on apolipoprotein secretion by the human hepatocarcinoma cell line, Hep G2. J Biol Chem 260:1670–1675, 1985

499. Tannenbaum GS, Martin JB. Evidence for an endogenous ultradian rhythm governing growth hormone secretion in the rat. Endocrinology 98:562–570, 1976

500. Taylor R, Heine RJ, Collins J, James OWF, Alberti KGMM. Insulin action in cirrhosis. Hepatology 5:64–71, 1985

501. Teng CS, Ho PWM, Yeung RTT. Down-regulation of insulin receptors in post necrotic cirrhosis of the liver. J Clin Endocrinol Metab 55:524–530, 1982

502. Terui S, Morihn Y, Yamamoto H, Koyama Y. Thyroxine-binding globulin as a marker of liver tumors. Cancer Detect Prev 10:371–378, 1987

503. Thaler H. Relation of steatosis to cirrhosis. Clin Gastroenterol 4:273–280, 1975

504. The Copenhagen Study Group for Liver Diseases. Testosterone treatment of men with alcoholic cirrhosis: a double-blind study. Hepatology 6:807–813, 1986

505. Thiebaud D, DeFronzo RA, Jacot E, Golay A, Acheson K, Maeder E, Jequier E, Felber JP. Effect of long chain triglyceride infusion on glucose metabolism in man. Metabolism 31:1128–1136, 1982

506. Thompson WJ, Hart IR. Chronic active hepatitis and Graves disease. Am J Dig Dis 18:111–119, 1973

507. Thompson P, Strum D, Boehm T, Wartofsky L. Abnormalities of liver function tests in thyrotoxicosis. Milit Med 143:548–551, 1978

508. Thornburn AW, Gumbiner B, Bulacan F, Brechtel G, Henry RR. Multiple defects in muscle glycogen synthase activity contribute to reduced glycogen synthesis in non-insulin dependent diabetes mellitus. J Clin Invest 87:489–495, 1991

509. Thung SN, Gerber MA, Bodenheimer HC. Nodular regenerative hyperplasia of the liver in a patient with diabetes mellitus. Cancer 49:543–546, 1982

510. Tourniaire J, Fevre M, Mazenod B, Ponsen G. Effect of clomiphene citrate and synthetic LHRH on serum luteinizing hormone (LH) in men with idiopathic hemochromatosis. J Clin Endocrinol Metab 38:1122–1124, 1974

511. Turkington RW. Serum prolactin levels in patients with gynecomastia. J Clin Endocrinol Metab 34:62–66, 1972

512. Turocy JF, Chiang AN, Seeley DH, Eagon PK. Effects of H$_2$-antagonists on androgen imprinting of male hepatic functions. Endocrinology 117:1953–1961, 1985

513. Ullrich A, Gray A, Tam AW, Yang-Feng T, Tsubokawa M. Insulin-like growth factor I receptor primary structure: comparison with insulin receptor suggests structural determinants that define functional specificity. EMBO J 5:2503–2512, 1986

514. Valimaki M, Harkonen M, Ylikahri R. Acute effects of alcohol on female sex hormones. Alcoholism 7:289–293, 1983

515. Valimaki M, Pelkonen R, Harkonen M, Tiomala P, Koestenen P, Rorne R, Ylikahri R. Pituitary-gonadal hormones and adrenal androgens in non-cirrhotic female alcoholics after cessation of alcohol intake. Eur J Clin Invest 20:177–181, 1990

516. Van Thiel DH. Disorders of the hypothalamic–pituitary–gonadal and thyroidal axes in patients with liver disease. In: Zakim D, Boyer TD, eds. Hepatology: a textbook of liver disease. Philadelphia, WB Saunders, 1990, pp 513–530

517. Van Thiel DH. Feminization of chronic alcoholic men: a formulation. Yale J Biol Med 52:219–225, 1979

518. Van Thiel DH. The liver and the endocrine system. In: Arias IM, Jakoby WB, Popper H, Schachter D, Shafritz DA, eds. The liver: biology and pathobiology. New York, Raven Press, 1988, pp 1007–1031

519. Van Thiel DH, de Belle R, Mellow M, Widerlite L, Philips E. Tolazamide hepatotoxicity. Gastroenterology 67:506–510, 1974

520. Van Thiel DH, Cobb CF, Herman GB, Perez HA, Estes L, Gavaler JS. An examination of various mechanisms for ethanol induced testicular injury: studies utilizing the isolated perfused rat testes. Endocrinology 109:2009–2015, 1981

521. Van Thiel DH, Gavaler JS. Prostate hypertrophy in the elderly cirrhotic patient: an estrogenic or androgenic response? Hepatology 9:167–168, 1989

522. Van Thiel DH, Gavaler JS, Eagon PK. Feminization in alcoholic liver disease: the role of ethanol and alcoholic liver disease. MIDA Research Monograph 55:32–41, 1984

523. Van Thiel DH, Gavaler JS, Lester R. Ethanol: a gonadal toxin in the female. Drug Alcohol Depend 2:373–380, 1977

524. Van Thiel DH, Gavaler JS, Lester R, Goodman MD. Alcohol-induced testicular atrophy: an experimental model for hypogonadism occurring in chronic alcoholic men. Gastroenterology 69:326–332, 1975

525. Van Thiel DH, Gavaler JS, Lester R, Loriaux DL, Braunstein GD. Plasma estrone, prolactin, neurophysin and sex steroid-binding globulin in chronic alcoholic men. Metabolism 24:1015–1019, 1975

526. Van Thiel DH, Gavaler JS, Sanghoi A. Recovery of sexual

function in abstinent alcoholic men. Gastroenterology 84:677–682, 1982

527. Van Thiel DH, Gavaler JS, Slone FL, Cobb CF, Smith WI, Bron KM, Lester R. Is feminization in alcoholic men due in part to portal hypertension: a rat model. Gastroenterology 78:81–91, 1980

528. Van Thiel DH, Lester R. Further evidence for hypothalamic–pituitary dysfunction in alcoholic men. Alcoholism 2:265–270, 1978

529. Van Thiel DH, Lester R, Sherins RJ. Hypogonadism in alcoholic liver disease: evidence for a double defect. Gastroenterology 67:1188–1199, 1974

530. Van Thiel DH, Lester R, Vaitukaitis J. Evidence for a defect in pituitary secretion of luteinizing hormone in chronic alcoholic men. J Clin Endocrinol Metab 47:499–507, 1978

531. Van Thiel DH, McClain CJ, Elson MK, McMillen MJ. Hyperprolactinemia and thyrotropin-releasing factor (TRH) responses in men with alcoholic liver disease. Alcoholism 2:344–348, 1978

532. Van Thiel DH, Smith WI, McClain CJ, Lester R. Abnormal prolactin and growth hormone responses to thyrotropin releasing hormone in chronic alcoholic men. Med Curr Alcohol 5:71–79, 1979

533. Van Thiel DH, Stone BG, Schade RR. The liver and its effect on endocrine function in health and diseases. In: Schiff L, Schiff ER, eds. Diseases of the liver, ed 6. Philadelphia, JB Lippincott, 1987, pp 129–162

534. Van Thiel DH, Tarter RE, Rosenblum E, Gavaler JS. Ethanol, its metabolism and gonadal effects: does sex make a difference? In: Alcohol research from bench to bedside. Haworth Press, 1989, pp 131–169

535. Vannini P, Forbani G, Marchesini G. The euglycemic clamp technique in patients with liver cirrhosis. Horm Metab Res 16:341–343, 1984

536. Van Wyk JJ. The somatomedins: Biologic actions and physiologic control mechanisms. In: Li CH, ed. Hormonal proteins and peptides. Orlando, FL, Academic Press, 1984, pp 81–125

537. Vassilopoulou-Selin R, Phillips LS. Extraction of somatomedin activity from rat liver. Endocrinoloogy 110:582–589, 1982

538. Vigneri R, Goldfine ID, Wong KY, Smith GJ, Pezzino V. The nuclear envelope: the major site of insulin binding in rat liver nuclei. J Biol Chem 253:2098–2103, 1978

539. Viladiu P, Delgado C, Pensky J, Pearson OH. Estrogen binding protein of rat liver. Endocr Res Commun 2:273–280, 1985

540. Visser TJ. Tentative review of recent in vitro observations of the enzymatic deiodination of iodothyronines and its possible physiologic implications. Mol Cell Endocrinol 10:241–247, 1978

541. Wahrenberg HP, Engfelt P, Bolinder J. Acute adaptation in adrenergic control of lipolysis during exercise in humans. Am J Physiol 253:E383–390, 1987

542. Walker C, Peterson W, Unger R. Blood ammonia levels in advanced cirrhosis during therapeutic elevation of the insulin:glucagon ratio. N Engl J Med 291:168–171, 1974

543. Walsh CH, Wright AD, Williams JW, Holden G. A study of pituitary function in patients with idiopathic hemochromatosis. J Clin Endocrinol Metab 43:866–872, 1976

544. Walton C, Kelly WF, Laing I, Bullock DE. Endocrine abnormalities in idiopathic haemochromatosis. Q J Med 52:99–110, 1983

545. Wanless IR, Bargman JM, Oreopoulos DB, Vas SI. Subcapsular steatonecrosis in response to peritoneal insulin delivery: a clue to the pathogenesis of steatonecrosis in obesity. Modern Pathol 2:69–74, 1989

546. Weller CV. Hepatic lesions associated with exophthalmic goiter. Trans Assoc Am Physicians 45:71–85, 1930

547. Wilkinson P, Kornaczewski A, Rankin JG, Santamaria JN. Physical disease in alcoholism: initial survery of 1000 patients. Med J Aust 1:1217–1225, 1971

548. Wilkinson P, Santamaria JN, Rankin JG. Epidemiology of alcoholic cirrhosis. Austral Ann Med 18:222–226, 1969

549. Willet I, Esler M, Burke E, Leonard P, Dudley F. Total and renal sympathetic nervous system activity in alcoholic cirrhosis. J Hepatol 1:639–648, 1985

550. Wilson C, Auld CP, Schlinkert R, Hasan AH, Imrie CW, MacSween RNM, Carter DC. Hepatobiliary complications of chronic pancreatitis. Gut 30:520–527, 1989

551. Wilson JD, Foster DW. Williams' textbook of endocrinology. Philadelphia, WB Saunders, 1992

552. Wu JC, Daughaday WH, Lee SD, Hsiao TS, Chou CK, Lin HD, Tsai YT, Chiang BN. Radioimmunoassay of serum IGF-I and IGF-II in patients with chronic liver diseases and hepatocellular carcinoma with or without hypoglycemia. J Lab Clin Med 112:589–594, 1988

553. Wu A, Grant DB, Hambley J, Levi AJ. Reduced serum somatomedin activity in patients with chronic liver disease. Clin Sci 47:359–365, 1974

554. Yalow RS, Berson SA. Insulin resistance. In: Ellenberg M, Pifkin H, eds. Diabetes mellitus: theory and practice. New York, McGraw-Hill, 1970, pp 389–402

555. Yamamoto KR. Steroid receptor regulated transcription of specific genes and gene network. Annu Rev Genet 19:209–252, 1985

556. Yeung RTT, Wang CCL. A study of carbohydrate metabolism in post necrotic cirrhosis of liver. Gut 15:907–912, 1974

557. Yu KT, Czech MP. Tyrosine phosphorylation of the insulin receptor β subunit activates the receptor-associated tyrosine kinase activity. J Biol Chem 259:5277–5286, 1984

558. Yung Y, Russfield AB. Prolactin cells in the hypophysis of cirrhotic patients. Arch Pathol 94:265–269, 1972

559. Zapf J, Morell B, Walter H, Laron Z, Froesch ER. Serum levels of insulin-like growth factor (IGF) and its carrier protein in various metabolic disorders. Acta Endocrinol 95:505–509, 1980

560. Ziegler TR, Young LS, Ferrari-Baliviera E, Demling RH, Wilmore DW. Use of human growth hormone combined with nutritional support in a critical care unit. JPEN 14:574–581, 1990

561. Zimmerman HJ, Thomas LJ, Scherr EH. Fasting blood sugar in hepatic disease with reference to infrequency of hypoglycemia. Arch Intern Med 91:577–584, 1953

Diseases of the Liver, Seventh Edition, edited by
Leon Schiff and Eugene R. Schiff. J.B. Lippincott Company, Philadelphia © 1993.

51

The Liver in Pregnancy

Caroline A. Riely

For a variety of reasons, liver disease in pregnancy is poorly understood by many practitioners of internal medicine. First, medical problems arising during the course of gestation usually are cared for by the obstetrician. Many of the reports of liver diseases in pregnancy have appeared in the obstetric literature. As a consequence, most medical specialists have little familiarity with medicine in pregnancy. In addition, the pregnant state is accompanied by striking alterations in physiology, most of which are unfamiliar to the specialist in internal medicine. Finally, pregnancy presents some special medical problems, diseases that are either unique to pregnancy (most notably the toxemias—preeclampsia and eclampsia), or that are exacerbated by pregnancy and present in an unusual guise. As a consequence, these disorders often are overlooked or misunderstood by the medical specialist.

Similarly, pregnancy is not commonplace in clinics specializing in liver disease. It does occur, however, and is not rare among women who are reformed alcoholics or who have adequately treated, steroid-responsive chronic active hepatitis. Good, prospectively collected data on the incidence of pregnancy in patients with liver disease are not available. The incidence of liver disease occurring in pregnancy has been estimated, usually from collation of reported cases, but the figures are only rough estimates, at best. The reported incidence of jaundice (implying fairly severe liver disease) in pregnancy ranges from 1 in 1500 or 1600[104,177] to 1 in 2500.[125] The incidence of subicteric hepatic dysfunction must be higher. For example, cholestasis of pregnancy may occur in as many as 10% of pregnancies.[182]

Nevertheless, the study of liver diseases in pregnancy is a rewarding one, as is reflected by the many excellent reviews available on this topic.[79,91,104,120,128,158,163,242,248,249,256,262,269,283] Of particular interest to the hepatologist are the diseases unique to pregnancy (eg, cholestasis of pregnancy or acute fatty liver of pregnancy) that have interesting parallels with or contrasts to liver disorders occurring in the nonpregnant population. Complete elucidation of the pathogenesis of these diseases is unavailable but will be based on a thorough understanding of the normal physiologic changes in pregnancy.

Alterations Associated With the Pregnant State

PHYSIOLOGY

Normal pregnancy is associated with a series of dramatic hemodynamic changes (Table 51-1). There is a marked peripheral arterial vasodilatation, somewhat akin to the marked decrease in peripheral vascular resistance seen in cirrhosis.[258] The blood volume increases by an average of 48%, with a wide range but with an increase consistent over consecutive gestations for each person.[222] This change, consisting ultimately of an average increase of 1500 mL of plasma and 500 mL of red blood cells, begins in the first trimester, is more marked in the second trimester, and increases only slightly more in the third trimester. There is an associated increase in cardiac output and in heart rate.[311] The stroke volume increases gradually to reach a peak at 32 weeks of gestation then decreases back to the prepregnancy norm. Renal blood flow and glomerular filtration rate increase during gestation. Hepatic blood flow does not change compared with prepregnancy levels, but the fractional blood flow to the liver drops from 35% in nonpregnant state to 29% during pregnancy.[203] The gravid uterus presents an increasing obstruction to blood return through the inferior vena cava as term approaches.[150] There is increased return to the heart through the azygos system and esophageal varices may occur in normal pregnant women near term. Also as term approaches, there is an increasingly hypercoagulable state.[126] The hemodynamic changes are magnified by Valsalva maneuvers during labor and a peak in cardiac output is reached during the second stage. In the days to weeks after delivery, these hemodynamic alterations revert to normal, aided by the blood loss at delivery.

Normal pregnancy also is associated with changes in gastrointestinal physiology. There is a decrease in lower esophageal sphincter tone, which may be the cause of the heartburn that so frequently affects pregnant women.[54] There is an overall decrease in gastrointestinal motility, with a resulting prolongation in transit time.[305] The gallbladder in both men and women has progesterone receptors, but most men lack the estrogen receptors found in the gallbladder in women.[227] There is an increase in fasting gallbladder volume and an increase in residual volume after contraction, the so-called sluggish gallbladder of pregnancy.[31,77] Nevertheless, the gallbladder in pregnancy still contracts appropriately, emptying 40% of its contents, as it does in the nonpregnant state.[224] These changes in smooth muscle motility correlate with increases in serum progesterone values and may be related etiologically to this putative smooth muscle relaxant. Indeed, progesterone levels fall precipitously within 4 days after delivery, correlating well with the prompt return to baseline in gallbladder and gastrointestinal tract motility.[34] Studies of biliary lipids and bile acid kinetics during pregnancy have shown an increase in the lithogenic index of bile, associated with an increase in biliary cholesterol secretion and a decrease in both the synthesis of chenodeoxycholic acid relative

TABLE 51-1   *Changes Associated With Normal Pregnancy*

Physiology

  ↑ Blood volume, cardiac output

  ↓ Mean peripheral vascular resistance

  ↑ Renal blood flow

  ↑ Azygous vein flow

Hypercoagulable state

  ↓ Lower esophageal sphincter tone

  ↑ Gallbladder volume

  ↓ Cheno/cholate synthesis

  ↑ Cholesterol secretion in bile

  ↑ Lithogenicity of bile

  ↓ Rate of enterohepatic cycling of bile acid pool

Physical examination

  Blood pressure: ↓ in second trimester, returns to prepregnancy norm at term

  ↑ Pulse

  Spider angiomas

  Palmar erythema

  Impalpable liver

TABLE 51-2   *Changes in Laboratory Values During Normal Pregnancy*

Decreased	Increased	Unchanged
Hemoglobin	White blood cell	Transaminases
Albumin	count	Serum bile acids
BUN	Fibrinogen	5′Nucleotidase, GGTP
Uric acid	Ceruloplasmin	
	α_2-Globulins	
	Cholesterol	
	Triglycerides	
	BSP retention	
	Alkaline phosphatase	
	Urinary porphyrins	

BUN, blood urea nitrogen; BSP, bromsulfophthalein; GGTP, γ-glutamyl transpeptidase.

to cholic acid and the rate of enterohepatic cycling of the bile acid pool.[149,324] These changes may reflect sequestration of the bile acid pool in the distended gallbladder, as well as changes in bile acid synthesis modulated by gestational hormones.

PHYSICAL EXAMINATION

During pregnancy, the physical examination changes (see Table 51-1). Serial measurements of blood pressure show a decrease in the second trimester that is followed by an increase back toward the values of early pregnancy as term approaches. The pulse rate increases. Typical spider angiomata that fade after delivery often develop in pregnant women.[21] Palmar erythema also is commonly found. The expanding uterus makes physical examination of the liver difficult and hepatomegaly rarely can be detected.

LABORATORY VALUES

The normal range for many laboratory values changes during pregnancy[75] (Table 51-2). The increase in blood volume and resulting hemodilution are reflected in a decrease in hemoglobin concentration and serum albumin. This hemodilution, together with an increase in fractional renal blood flow, results in a decrease in blood urea nitrogen and in uric acid levels, which normalize as term approaches. During normal pregnancy, there is a decrease in serum levels of carnitine, perhaps implying relative carnitine deficiency.[10] Increases are found in the normal levels of white blood cells and of various proteins such as fibrinogen, ceruloplasmin, and α_2-globulins. Serum lipids change strikingly, with a 50% increase in serum cholesterol and a three-fold increase in serum triglyc-

erides.[220] Urinary excretion of the porphyrin precursors δ-aminolevulinic acid and porphobilinogen increases slightly during pregnancy.[39,64] Urinary orotic acid excretion appears to be unchanged.[94]

The question of the existence of a physiologic cholestasis of pregnancy has long been debated. Studies of serum bile acid levels during gestation show either normal values[253] or small but significant increases, usually within the range of normal.[87,109,182] The metabolism of another organic anion, bromsulfophthalein (BSP), has been investigated extensively. Estrogenic steroids are known to increase the retention of BSP after a simple bolus intravenous injection.[161,233] More sophisticated studies using infusion techniques have shown a decrease in the transport maximum for BSP and an increase in hepatic storage capacity as gestation advances.[55,84] Other studies, however, have shown unexpected changes in the albumin binding of BSP during pregnancy.[57] This compound is no longer available commercially in the United States, although the agent still is useful for research purposes.[233]

Standard liver function test results are normal during the entire course of pregnancy with a single exception: the alkaline phosphatase level rises as term approaches. This is due to the presence of a heat-stable fraction of placental origin. Test results of so-called hepatic alkaline phosphatase, such as 5′-nucleotidase or γ-glutamyl transpeptidase (GGTP), remain normal throughout pregnancy or rise only minimally toward term.[75,306] Any consistent elevation in transaminase or bilirubin should warn the clinician of possible liver disease in the pregnant woman.

HEPATIC HISTOLOGY

Hepatic histologic status is not altered by pregnancy.[11,130] Ultrastructure of the liver reveals no significant abnormalities, with proliferation of the smooth endoplasmic reticulum and other nonspecific and nonpathologic changes.[217]

SYNDROME OF PREECLAMPSIA–ECLAMPSIA

Any clinician who cares for pregnant women should be conversant with the syndrome of toxemia of pregnancy, now designated preeclampsia–eclampsia.[49,240,250,323] This syndrome usually is foreign to internists and gastroenterologists, because it is unique to the pregnant state in humans or, rarely, concurrent with hydatidiform mole. It occurs in the second half of pregnancy, usually in the third trimester, although it also can present in the puerperium, after delivery. It is more common in, although not limited to, the primiparous woman and more common in multiple gestations (eg, twins). It is not rare, occurring in 3% to 11% of all pregnancies. Once it has occurred, it is not more likely to complicate subsequent pregnancies. It is a multisystem disease associated with a variety of epiphenomena, most typically edema, proteinuria, and hypertension.[229] There may be involvement of the central nervous system with hyperreflexia and, defining eclampsia, seizures. There is no direct correlation between the severity of the various manifestations; for example, seizures are not limited to cases with severe hypertension. Hypertension should be judged relative to the individual patient's previous blood pressure determinations. An elevation of 30 mmHg systolic or 15 mmHg diastolic over mid-trimester levels should be considered pathologic. Any blood pressure of greater than 140/90 mmHg in a pregnant woman is pathologic. The serum uric acid level often is elevated relative to pregnancy norms, and any value over 6 mg/dL should suggest this syndrome.[259] Treatment is delivery, after which the process abates. The infants of affected pregnancies have an increased incidence of being small for gestational age or stillborn.

The pathogenesis of this disorder is unknown, although it is known to be associated with a failure of the normal expansion of intravascular volume[222] and with an exaggeration of the activated state of coagulation and fibrinolysis normally seen in pregnancy.[126] Affected patients fail to demonstrate the decrease in vascular resistance appropriate to advancing pregnancy.[99] A study has shown that platelet responsiveness to vasopressin is exaggerated early in the gestation of women who go on to manifest preeclampsia.[327] These results imply that platelet dysfunction is pivotal in the pathogenesis of preeclampsia, a disorder presumed to originate in the trophoblast. The prevalence of this condition among family members has suggested genetic factors, possibly with inheritance as an autosomal recessive. Many possible etiologies have been proposed,[7] but none proven. Most obstetricians favor the postulate of vasospasm with enhanced vasoconstrictor tone, associated with vascular injury and microangiopathy, possibly due to alterations in eicosanoid (prostaglandin, prostacyclin, thromboxane) homeostasis.

Pregnancy Occurring in Women With Preexisting Liver Disease

In the usual practice of hepatology, pregnancy rarely is encountered. Most patients with liver disease are not women of childbearing age. In addition, most women with serious liver disease are infertile because of the associated anovulatory state. Nevertheless, pregnancy can occur in women with preexisting liver disease, and when it does, it presents some special problems.[301] Among them is the question of the effect of the liver disease, or its treatment, on the fetus. Alcoholic liver disease, as an example, often is associated with infertility. Most alcoholics do not have liver disease, however, and pregnancy in a fertile alcoholic woman can result in fetal alcohol syndrome in the infant, including typical facies, malformations, and developmental delay. Several such infants have been reported to have liver disease, with fatty liver and

portal and perisinusoidal fibrosis, suggestive of alcoholic liver disease.[174] For the most part, however, liver disease or its treatment is not teratogenic and, if they can succeed in getting pregnant, women with liver disease do not have an increased risk for bearing children with congenital anomalies. On the other hand, they do have more maternal problems with pregnancy, and a greater risk for prematurity or stillbirth.

CIRRHOSIS AND PORTAL HYPERTENSION

Worsening jaundice with progressive liver failure, ascites, and hepatic coma have been reported during the course of pregnancy in women with cirrhosis.[30,260] Whether this exacerbation of hepatic dysfunction is caused by the gestation or merely coincident with it is unclear. It is clear, however, that women with cirrhosis can sustain pregnancy without any worsening of hepatic function.[30,319] Published reports document an increase in the incidence of stillbirths and premature delivery in women with cirrhosis.[30,48,257]

Women with noncirrhotic portal hypertension, such as that seen in congenital hepatic fibrosis or portal vein thrombosis, do not have diminished fertility and pregnancy may be encountered in this setting with some frequency. Worsening of preexisting portal hypertension might be anticipated in the setting of the marked increase in blood volume and in azygos flow seen in normal pregnancy. Prospective surveys of the course of pregnancy in patients with portal hypertension, either cirrhotic or noncirrhotic in origin, are not available. Published reports probably are biased toward complications occurring in this setting. Variceal hemorrhage during pregnancy or labor has been reported with some frequency.[48,257,277] Spontaneous rupture of a splenic artery aneurysm has been reported as a complication of pregnancy in women with portal hypertension[17] but is also a known complication of pregnancy in normal women. Patients with a past history of variceal hemorrhage who have had shunt surgery before the beginning of pregnancy have a lower incidence of hemorrhage during the pregnancy than do comparable women who have not had surgery. It is not clear, however, that the incidence of variceal hemorrhage is increased during pregnancy compared with the incidence in nonpregnant patients with known varices. Nor does the history of hemorrhage in one gestation predict the outcome of subsequent pregnancies.[38] There are many reports of successful shunt surgery without fetal wastage during gestation in women who have bled from varices. Elective ablation of varices by sclerotherapy in the pregnant woman has been proposed, but, given the uncertainty about its effectiveness and about the significance of the problem during pregnancy, such a suggestion seems premature.

SPECIFIC LIVER DISEASES

Chronic Hepatitis B and D

In general, pregnancy is well tolerated by women who are chronic carriers of hepatitis B, with reactivation of the virus and exacerbation of the disease during or after gestation being the exception rather than the rule.[228,260] The placenta forms an excellent barrier against transmission of the large virus, and intrauterine infection with hepatitis B is rare. It does occur, however, probably as a result of transplacental leakage, as can occur in threatened abortion.[179,216] The major problem for women who are chronic carriers of hepatitis B is the risk of maternal-to-infant (vertical) transmission of the infection at delivery. Transmission at birth is more likely (90%) if the mother is HBeAg-positive[12,284] or has high circulating levels of hepatitis B virus (HBV) DNA.[132] The rate of transmission may be lower if the delivery is done by cesarean section.[173] This is not indicated, however, as appropriate immunoprophylaxis of the newborn with both hepatitis B hyperimmune globulin and vaccine interrupts transmission in over 90%.[50,285] Several studies have demonstrated that prenatal testing limited only to high-risk group mothers fails to detect many carriers,[137,165] and routine prenatal screening of all pregnant women for HBsAg is the standard of care.[29,5,98,142,226] Infants born to carriers of the hepatitis B precore mutant, women who are positive for anti-HBe along with high levels of HBV DNA in the serum are at particular risk for fulminant hepatitis B in the first 2 to 4 months after birth.[47,271,289] Therefore, immunoprophylaxis should be given to infants from all mothers who are HBsAg-positive, regardless of HBe status. Hepatitis D (delta) also can be transmitted from mother to infant at birth.[63]

Chronic Hepatitis C
Uneventful pregnancy without worsening disease or fetal complications in women with presumed hepatitis C has been reported.[129] Transmission from chronic carrier mothers to their offspring has been documented but appears to be much less efficient than is vertical transmission of hepatitis B.[316] Rates of transmission are much increased in human immunodeficiency virus (HIV)–infected women who transmit HIV, as well as hepatitis C virus, to their infants.[93,290]

Steroid-Responsive Chronic Active Hepatitis
This distinct clinical syndrome is known by a variety of names, including autoimmune or lupoid chronic active hepatitis, but is perhaps best qualified by its most distinctive clinical characteristic, the rapid and complete (or close to complete) remission obtained in response to immunosuppression with corticosteroids, either alone or in combination with azathioprine. This disorder presents frequently in young women, many of whom become anovulatory in response to the active and severe hepatitis, which has often progressed to cirrhosis by the time of diagnosis. Women appropriately treated for this disease with immunosuppression regain their fertility, and have been reported to have successful pregnancies, without any increase in fatality.[69,172,282] Flare-up of the underlying disease has been reported during pregnancy, but it is unclear that this is related to the pregnant state.[319] Cessation of therapy during pregnancy in such patients has been associated with relapse of the disease. Azathioprine has not been reported to be teratogenic in this setting of low-dose therapy. Such women are at increased risk, however, for obstetric complications such as preeclampsia and stillbirth or prematurity.[282]

Primary Biliary Cirrhosis
Pregnancy in women affected with this diseases has been reported and may be associated with an increase in cholestasis that resolves after delivery.[319] Another report documented improvement in cholestasis during gestation.[211]

Wilson's Disease
Women with ovulatory failure due to Wilson's disease regain fertility when treated, often promptly. Either they, or their physicians, may be tempted to decrease or stop therapy during gestation.[310] But, as is the case in the nonpregnant patient

with Wilson's disease, cessation of therapy can have devastating effects and should not be attempted.[254,266] Penicillamine has been reported to be associated with cutis laxa in the newborn, an effect of its ability to decopper the body.[244] Although similar birth defects have not yet been reported in women using trientene, they are to be anticipated.[310] Clearly, the major risk to the mother in stopping therapy much outweighs the potential risk to the fetus and therapy should be continued; successful pregnancy in treated women is the rule.[51,72,309,310] Like other women with cirrhosis, patients with Wilson's disease may be at increased risk for intrauterine growth retardation and preeclampsia, and should be followed by an expert in maternal–fetal medicine.

Hepatic Neoplasia
Hepatic adenomas or tumors of focal nodular hyperplasia associated with previous therapy with oral contraceptive agents have been reported to enlarge and present[187] or to rupture during subsequent pregnancy.[148,261] Surgical removal before conception or during pregnancy has been successful, although it may put the pregnancy at risk.[187] Similarly, hepatocellular carcinoma also may rupture into the peritoneum during pregnancy.[210]

Familial Hyperbilirubinemia
The unconjugated hyperbilirubinemia of Gilbert's syndrome is not exacerbated by the pregnant state.[85] In Dubin-Johnson syndrome, however, the conjugated hyperbilirubinemia worsens during gestation but returns to prepregnancy levels after delivery.[53,68]

Familial Intrahepatic Cholestatic Syndromes
Reported experience with pregnancy in these rare syndromes is meager. In Alagille's syndrome[243] and in Byler's syndrome, the underlying cholestasis is said to worsen during pregnancy.

Porphyria
These genetic disorders of heme metabolism, which may be exacerbated by estrogenic hormones, may provide problems for affected women and their offspring during pregnancy. Porphyria cutanea tarda rarely has been reported to have its initial presentation during pregnancy.[225] Acute porphyric attacks often complicate the course of pregnancy in patients with acute intermittent porphyria, variegate porphyria, or hereditary coproporphyria,[39,140] and may result in intrauterine growth retardation or, rarely, maternal death. On the other hand, many women with acute porphyria, particularly those with little clinical expression of the defect, weather pregnancy with no problems. The nausea and vomiting of hyperemesis gravidarum, coupled with antiemetic therapy, has been reported to precipitate an initial attack of acute intermittent porphyria.[197]

After Liver Transplantation
Women with chronic liver disease often regain their fertility after liver transplantation. Pregnancy occurring in transplanted women is no longer unusual, and is well tolerated for the most part, with no increased risk to the graft.[170,196] There is an increased incidence of preeclampsia in transplanted women and they should be observed carefully during gestation by an expert in maternal–fetal medicine. If pregnancy is not desired, contraceptive methods (preferably barrier) should be instituted rapidly after transplantation, be-

cause conception has been reported as early as 3 weeks after grafting.

Given this rather incomplete picture of the outcome of pregnancy in women with liver disease, what advice should the clinician give to the patient with chronic liver disease who is, or desires to be, pregnant? First, such women should expect to have difficulty conceiving. They should be informed that if they have cirrhosis they may be at increased risk for variceal hemorrhage that could be life-threatening during gestation, particularly if they are known to have esophageal varices or have had a past history of variceal bleeding. There is no increased incidence of congenital malformations in the offspring of women with cirrhosis, but there is a greater likelihood of stillbirth or prematurity. There is little evidence that pregnancy worsens the underlying liver disease. Should such women desire to have children despite these risks and succeed in getting pregnant, they should be referred to obstetricians specializing in maternal–fetal medicine who are well versed in the anticipated complications.

Usual Liver Diseases Complicating Pregnancy

Common liver diseases, unrelated etiologically to the pregnant state, may occur concurrently with it. In some special disorders, pregnancy exacerbates the condition, leading to altered prevalence and morbidity in the pregnant woman.

DISORDERS NOT EXACERBATED BY PREGNANCY

Hepatitis B
In general, viral diseases are neither more common nor more severe in pregnancy.[123] In patients with documented acute infection with hepatitis B, pregnancy is not associated with an increased mortality[52,117,144,177] or teratogenicity.[299] Infection during gestation should not prompt termination of the pregnancy. Women exposed to hepatitis B during gestation may be vaccinated without any reported increase in congenital anomalies,[176] and the vaccine is immunogenic in this setting.[14]

Drug Hepatitis
Because of concern about teratogenicity in the fetus, pregnant women in general take fewer medications than the nonpregnant population. When they do take medications, however, they run the same risk for adverse drug reactions as others. Typical hepatitic reactions have been reported to anesthetic agents (halothane[119] and methoxyflurane[247]). Adverse reactions to erythromycin estolate[193] and to propylthiouracil[202] have been documented in pregnancy. On the other hand, there is no documented increased incidence of such adverse reactions during pregnancy. For example, 1300 pregnant women took isoniazid for tuberculosis without ill effect.[273]

Liver Transplantation
Transplantation of the liver has been accomplished during pregnancy with[202] or without fetal wastage.[86,89,170,195] Such heroic surgery must be considered with extreme care in this setting. If the condition prompting transplantation is caused by pregnancy (eg, acute fatty liver of pregnancy), prompt di-

agnosis, followed by interruption of the pregnancy with maximal support of the mother, is the treatment of choice.

Metastasis to Liver
The liver is not palpable in normal pregnant women, and the detection of hepatomegaly on physical examination should signal a pathologic condition needing immediate evaluation. Patients with extensive tumor invasion of the liver may present with abdominal or back pain, with rupture of the liver, or with hepatic failure. The usual source is a common tumor, such as carcinoma of the colon[204,208,303,326] or the pancreas.[89] Breast cancer may also present with hepatomegaly during pregnancy. It is possible that the modest immunosuppressive state associated with pregnancy is permissive in allowing extensive spread and growth in this setting.

Other Complicating Illnesses
Severe systemic infections with sepsis, particularly urinary tract infections, may be associated with jaundice in the pregnant woman,[177] as also occurs in the nonpregnant state. Amebic abscess or echinococcal cysts of the liver also have been reported to occur in pregnancy.[58,304]

DISORDERS EXACERBATED BY PREGNANCY

Hepatitis E
For decades it was unclear why hepatitis is more frequent and more severe in pregnant women, particularly in developing countries. During epidemics of infectious hepatitis, the illness is reported to occur more frequently in pregnant women than in nonpregnant women or in men[92,152] and, particularly during the third trimester, is associated with increased morbidity and mortality compared with nonpregnant patients.[4,151,152] Within the course of gestation, clinical hepatitis occurs most commonly in the third trimester as contrasted with the first two trimesters.[3,22,29,117,144,177,189] In developing countries, hepatitis is more likely to follow a fulminant, fatal course in pregnant women than in nonpregnant women or in men, particularly during the third trimester.[29,52,92,144,152,189,322] This predisposition to increased fatality has not been reported from the United States or France.[117,177,275] Most of these studies were done without serologic testing for hepatitis A or B. Where testing for hepatitis B was available, pregnant women with "hepatitis" had a lower than expected incidence of hepatitis B positivity.[52,144,177]

It now becomes evident that the hepatitis characterized in these reports is hepatitis E, a newly discovered, single-stranded RNA virus of the calciviridae family.[328] This is a common infection in all of the developing world where contamination of water with sewerage occurs. It occurs both sporadically and in epidemics, particularly after flooding. It is both more often clinically detectable and more likely to be severe in pregnant women during the third trimester, when the case fatality rate is 20%.[101] This virus has been isolated from the stool of infected people[141] and it has been cloned.[231] Serologic testing will be available soon. Pregnant women should consider carefully travel to endemic areas, which include parts of Asia (India, southern Russia), Africa and the Middle East, and Mexico.

Herpes Simplex Hepatitis
When it occurs in the third trimester of pregnancy, hepatitis due to systemic infection with herpes simplex virus is likely to be severe, and half of the reported cases of fulminant her-

petic hepatitis have occurred in pregnant women.[97,159,318] Affected patients have a viral prodrome, including fever and upper respiratory tract symptoms. Despite marked abnormalities in aminotransferase levels and prothrombin time, they usually are anicteric at presentation. A vesicular eruption is diagnostically useful but may not present visibly. Cultures and histology on liver biopsy are helpful in the differential diagnosis, which should include severe liver disorders due to pregnancy, such as acute fatty liver of pregnancy and preeclamptic liver disease. Therapy with acyclovir is successful, and affected women need not be delivered.

Why these two viral infections should be so much more severe, and cause such increased hepatic injury, in the third trimester of pregnancy is unclear. Alterations in T-cell function have been reported in pregnancy and may relate to this enhanced susceptibility.[279] Herpes simplex hepatitis is known to be more severe in certain immunocompromised states, such as in patients on chronic immunosuppression after transplantation.

Biliary Tract Disease and Pancreatitis

As mentioned earlier, pregnancy decreases gallbladder motility and increases the lithogenicity of bile. Pregnancy has long been considered to be a risk factor in the development of gallstones, and epidemiologic studies confirm that pregnancy is associated with an increased risk for gallstones but only for a 5-year period after the pregnancy. Thereafter, the risk drops back to that of the never-pregnant population.[291] In teenagers with gallstones, a past history of pregnancy is common.[41] Gallstones and biliary sludge may (or may not[251]) be observed by ultrasonography to accumulate over gestation. Sludge in the gallbladder usually resolves within a year after delivery with return to nonpregnant physiology, whereas gallstones are less likely to disappear.[191]

Acute cholecystitis may occur in pregnancy and operative cholecystectomy may be accomplished during gestation, although there may be an increase in either maternal or fetal morbidity, particularly if surgery is performed in the first trimester.[67,115] In large studies of cholecystectomy in women, this procedure was performed only rarely during pregnancy,[80,221] suggesting that acute cholecystitis unresponsive to conservative medical management is not a common occurrence in pregnancy. Less invasive approaches to the problem of biliary lithiasis in pregnancy have been successful. Choledocholithiasis can be managed by endoscopic retrograde cholangiopancreatography with sphincterotomy.[16,25] Laparoscopic cholecystectomy also has been reported to be successful in pregnancy.[223] As in the nonpregnant state, cholecystitis due to *Salmonella* infection may occur during pregnancy.[270]

Acute pancreatitis may complicate pregnancy. Usually, this occurs in the setting of cholelithiasis,[139,194] and gallstones should be sought in any affected patient. Gallstone pancreatitis should be treated aggressively, either operatively[27] or endoscopically.[16] Pancreatitis complicating pregnancy may be associated etiologically with acute fatty liver of pregnancy[198,236] or with preeclampsia.[320] Mild pancreatitis may occur in association with severe hyperemesis gravidarum, presumably as so-called refeeding pancreatitis. Familial hypertriglyceridemia, exacerbated by the physiologic hypertriglyceridemia of pregnancy, may present in pregnancy with pancreatitis.[62]

Choledochal cyst may present during pregnancy with abdominal pain, a mass, and jaundice.[287] Such patients may represent cases of congenital choledochal cyst that was exacerbated by the effects of pregnancy on biliary motility. Spontaneous rupture of a choledochal cyst[134] and of an apparently normal common hepatic duct have been reported in pregnancy.[218]

Budd-Chiari Syndrome

Both pregnancy and therapy with oral contraceptive agents are associated with a hypercoagulable state.[126,181] The Budd-Chiari syndrome (venoocclusive disease of the major hepatic veins) occurs with increased frequency in women on oral contraceptives.[178,294] Reports from India suggest that it also is more common in pregnant women, occurring usually immediately after delivery.[56,153] Similar cases have been reported from Spain[90] and Israel.[246] Closer evaluation of affected women demonstrates an underlying myeloproliferative disorder (eg, polycythemia rubra vera) in many in whom this syndrome develops during pregnancy.[296,297] The prognosis for this syndrome when it occurs in the setting of pregnancy is ominous, as it is for idiopathic venoocclusive disease. Nevertheless, successful, uncomplicated pregnancy has been reported in several patients who had Budd-Chiari syndrome associated with oral contraceptives or underlying myeloproliferative syndrome.[294,302]

Liver Disease Associated Etiologically With Pregnancy

Within this category are diseases unique to the pregnant state in humans. The most important distinction among them is whether they are associated with preeclampsia or not. Those disorders associated with preeclampsia require the appropriate treatment for preeclampsia, namely, termination of the pregnancy. Those not associated with preeclampsia resolve with cessation of pregnancy but do not require this therapy to protect the life of the mother. Crucial in arriving at the correct diagnosis for these disorders of pregnancy is knowledge of the gestational age of the pregnancy, because conditions associated with preeclampsia occur only in the second half of pregnancy.

DISORDERS NOT ASSOCIATED WITH PREECLAMPSIA

Hyperemesis Gravidarum

Nausea and vomiting are so common in the first trimester of pregnancy that morning sickness is thought of as being one of the first signs to the woman that she is pregnant. When this condition becomes protracted and severe, requiring hospitalization for treatment of dehydration with ketosis, the diagnosis of hyperemesis gravidarum is made. Abnormalities in liver function have been reported in this setting[2,171] and, in the era before intravenous hydration, this disorder was a cause of death with jaundice in the pregnant woman.

The cause of the nausea and vomiting typical of early pregnancy has yet to be identified. Early reports stressed the psychopathologic dimension of this symptom,[78] and this theory persists in the medical community.[111,127] But epidemiologic studies in large groups of pregnant women have demonstrated an association of vomiting early in pregnancy with primiparity, young age, nonsmoking, and obesity.[157] There also is a clear association of vomiting early in pregnancy with

34. Braverman DZ, et al. Postpartum restoration of pregnancy-induced cholecystoparesis and prolonged intestinal transit time. J Clin Gastroenterol 10:642, 1988

35. Breen KJ, et al. Idiopathic acute fatty liver of pregnancy. Gut 11:822, 1970

36. Breen KJ, et al. Uncomplicated subsequent pregnancy after idiopathic fatty liver of pregnancy. Obstet Gynecol 40:813, 1972

37. Brenard R, et al. Benign recurrent intrahepatic cholestasis: a report of 26 cases. J Clin Gastroenterol 11:546, 1989

38. Britton RC. Pregnancy and esophageal varices. Am J Surg 143:421, 1982

39. Brodie MJ, et al. Pregnancy and the acute porphyrias. Br J Obstet Gynecol 84:726, 1977

40. Brown MS, et al. The initial presentation of fatty liver of pregnancy mimicking acute viral hepatitis. Am J Gastroenterol 82:554, 1987

41. Buiumsohn A, et al. Cholelithiasis and teenage mothers. J Adolesc Health Care 11:339, 1990

42. Burk RF Jr. Selenium deficiency in search of a disease. Hepatology 8:421, 1988

43. Burroughs AK, et al. Idiopathic acute fatty liver of pregnancy in 12 patients. Q J Med 204:481, 1982

44. Cammu H, et al. Idiopathic acute fatty liver of pregnancy associated with transient diabetes insipidus: case report. Br J Obstet Gynecol 94:173, 1987

45. Cano RI, et al. Acute fatty liver of pregnancy: complication by disseminated intravascular coagulation. JAMA 231:159, 1975

46. Carrel T, et al. Rupture of a subcapsular liver hematoma in the post-partum associated syndrome of HELLP. Helv Chir Acta 57:29, 1990

47. Chang MH, et al. Fulminant hepatitis in children in Taiwan: the important role of hepatitis B virus. J Pediatr 111:34, 1987

48. Cheng Y-S. Pregnancy in liver cirrhosis and/or portal hypertension. Am J Obstet Gynecol 128:812, 1977

49. Chesley LC. History and epidemiology of preeclampsia–eclampsia. Clin Obstet Gynecol 27:801, 1984

50. Chin J. Prevention of chronic hepatitis B virus infection from mothers to infants in the United States. Pediatrics 71:289, 1983

51. Chin RKH. Pregnancy and Wilson's disease. (Letter) Am J Obstet Gynecol 165:488, 1991

52. Christie AB, et al. Pregnancy hepatitis in Libya. Lancet 2:1976, 1976

53. Cohen L, et al. Pregnancy, oral contraceptives, and chronic familial jaundice with predominantly conjugated hyperbilirubinemia. Gastroenterology 62:1182, 1972

54. Cohen S. The sluggish gallbladder of pregnancy. N Engl J Med 302:397, 1980

55. Combes B, et al. Alterations in sulfobromophthalein sodium removal mechanisms from blood during normal pregnancy. J Clin Invest 42:1431, 1963

56. Covillo FV, et al. Budd-Chiari syndrome following pregnancy. Missouri Medicine 81:356, 1984

57. Crawford JS, et al. Binding of bromosulfophthalein by serum albumin from pregnant women, neonates and subjects on oral contraceptives. Br J Anaesth 40:723, 1968

58. Crow JP, et al. Echinococcal disease of the liver in pregnancy. HPB Surgery 2:115, 1990

59. Dammann HG, et al. In vivo diagnosis of massive hepatic infarction by computed tomography. Dig Dis Sci 27:73, 1982

60. Davies MH, et al. Acute liver disease with encephalopathy and renal failure in late pregnancy and the early puerperium: a study of fourteen patients. Br J Obstet 87:1005, 1980

61. Davis JS, et al. Tetracycline toxicity: a clinicopathologic study with special reference to liver damage and its relationship to pregnancy. Am J Obstet Gynecol 95:523, 1966

62. DeChalain TMB, et al. Hyperlipidemia, pregnancy and pancreatitis. Surg Gynecol Obstet 167:469, 1988

63. Deinhardt F, et al. Viral hepatitis. Bull WHO 60:661, 1982

64. DeKlerk M, et al. Urinary porphyrins and porphyrin precursors in normal pregnancy. S Afr Med J 49:581, 1975

65. dePagter AGF, et al. Familial benign recurrent intrahepatic cholestasis: interrelation with intrahepatic cholestasis of pregnancy and from oral contraceptives. Gastroenterology 71:202, 1976

66. Depue RH, et al. Hyperemesis gravidarum in relation to estradiol levels, pregnancy outcome, and other maternal factors: a seroepidemiologic study. Am J Obstet Gynecol 156:1137, 1987

67. Dixon NP, et al. Aggressive management of cholecystitis during pregnancy. Am J Surg 154:292, 1987

68. DiZoglio J, et al. The Dubin-Johnson syndrome and pregnancy. Obstet Gynecol 42:560, 1973

69. Dubois RS, et al. Chronic active hepatitis and pregnancy: a report of two cases in adolescence. Am J Gastroenterol 77:649, 1982

70. Ducroz B, et al. The HELLP syndrome: is this a clinical form of thrombotic angiopathy? J Gynecol Obstet Biol Reprod 19:729, 1990

71. Duma RJ, et al. Acute fatty liver of pregnancy. Ann Intern Med 63:851, 1965

72. Dupont P, et al. Pregnancy in a patient with treated Wilson's disease: a case report. Am J Obstet Gynecol 163:1527, 1990

73. Durr JA, et al. Diabetes insipidus in pregnancy associated with abnormally high circulating vasopressinase activity. N Engl J Med 316:1070, 1987

74. Ebert EC, et al. Does early diagnosis and delivery in acute fatty liver of pregnancy lead to improvement in maternal and infant survival? Dig Dis Sci 29:453, 1984

75. Elliott JR, et al. Normal clinical chemical values for pregnant women at term. Clin Chem 17:156, 1971

76. Espinosa J, et al. The effect of phenobarbital on intrahepatic cholestasis of pregnancy. Am J Obstet Gynecol 119:234, 1974

77. Everson GT, et al. Gallbladder function in the human female: effect of the ovulatory cycle, pregnancy, and contraceptive steroids. Gastroenterology 82:711, 1982

78. Fairweather DVI. Nausea and vomiting in pregnancy. Am J Obstet Gynecol 102:135, 1968

79. Fallon HJ. Liver diseases. In: Burrow GN, Ferris TF, eds. Medical complications during pregnancy, ed 2. Philadelphia, WB Saunders, 1982, p 278

80. Feller A, et al. Acute fatty liver of pregnancy: a possible disorder of carnitine metabolism. Gastroenterology 84:1150, 1983

81. Ford SM, et al. Case report: transient vasopressin-resistant diabetes insipidus of pregnancy. Obstet Gynecol 68:726, 1986

82. Frezza M, et al. Reversal of intrahepatic cholestasis of pregnancy in women after high dose S-adenosyl-L-methionine administration. Hepatology 4:274, 1984

83. Frezza M, et al. S-adenosylmethionine for the treatment of intrahepatic cholestasis of pregnancy: results of a controlled clinical trial. Hepatogastroenterology 37:122, 1990

84. Frezza M, et al. Alteration in sulfobromphthalein hepatic storage capacity (S) in non-pregnant women previously affected with intrahepatic cholestasis of pregnancy (ICP). Acta Obstet Gynecol Scand 65:577, 1986

85. Friedlaender P, et al. Icterus and pregnancy. Am J Obstet Gynecol 97:894, 1967

86. Friedman E, et al. Malignant insulinoma with hepatic failure complicating pregnancy. South Med J 81:86, 1988

87. Fulton IC, et al. Is normal pregnancy cholestatic? Clin Chim Acta 130:171, 1983

88. Furhoff AK, et al. Jaundice in pregnancy: a follow-up study of women originally reported by L. Thorling: present health of the women. Acta Med Scand 196:181, 1974

89. Gamberdella FR. Pancreatic carcinoma in pregnancy: a case report. Am J Obstet Gynecol 149:15, 1984

90. Gatell-Artigas JM, et al. Pregnancy and the Budd-Chiari syndrome. (Letter) Dig Dis Sci 27:89, 1982
91. Geall MG, et al. Liver disease in pregnancy. Med Clin North Am 58:817, 1974
92. Gelpi AP. Viral hepatitis complicating pregnancy: mortality trends in Saudi Arabia. Int J Gynaecol Obstet 17:73, 1979
93. Giovannini M, et al. Maternal–infant transmission of hepatitis C virus and HIV infections: a possible interaction. (Letter) Lancet 1:1166, 1990
94. Glasgow AM, et al. Urinary orotic acid in pregnancy. Am J Obstet Gynecol 149:464, 1984
95. Goodlin RC. Severe pre-eclampsia: another great imitator. Am J Obstet Gynecol 125:747, 1976
96. Goodlin RC. Preeclampsia as the great imposter. J Obstet Gynecol 164:1577, 1991
97. Goyert GL, et al. Anicteric presentation of fatal herpetic hepatitis in pregnancy. Obstet Gynecol 65:585, 1985
98. Greenspoon JS, et al. Necessity for routine obstetric screening for hepatitis B surface antigen. J Reprod Med 34:655, 1989
99. Groenendijk R, et al. Hemodynamic measurements in preeclampsia: preliminary observations. Am J Obstet Gynecol 150:232, 1984
100. Gross S, et al. Maternal weight loss associated with hyperemesis gravidarum: a predictor of fetal outcome. Am J Obstet Gynecol 160:906, 1989
101. Gust ID, et al. Report of a workshop: waterborne non-A, non-B hepatitis. J Infect Dis 156:630, 1987
102. Gwee MCT. Can tetracycline-induced fatty liver in pregnancy be attributed to choline deficiency? Med Hypotheses 9:157, 1982
103. Hackenberg R, et al. Symptomatik eines rupturierten Leberhamatoms als schwere Komplikation des HELLP-syndroms. Geburtshilfe Frauenheilkd 51:313, 1991
104. Haemmerli UP. Jaundice during pregnancy. Acta Med Scand [Suppl] 444:1, 1966
105. Harada A, et al. Comparison of thyroid stimulators and thyroid hormone concentrations in the sera of pregnant women. J Clin Endocrinol Metab 48:793, 1979
106. Harper M, et al. Vasopressin-resistant diabetes insipidus, liver dysfunction, hyperuricemia and decreased renal function: a case report. J Reprod Med 32:862, 1987
107. Harpey JP, et al. Multiple acyl-cCoA dehydrogenase deficiency occurring in pregnancy and caused by a defect in riboflavin metabolism in the mother. J Pediatr 103:394, 1983
108. Hatfield AK, et al. Idiopathic acute fatty liver of pregnancy: death from extrahepatic manifestations. Dig Dis 17:167, 1977
109. Heikkinen J, et al. Changes in serum bile acid concentrations during normal pregnancy, in patients with intrahepatic cholestasis of pregnancy and in pregnant women with itching. Br J Obstet Gynaecol 88:240, 1981
110. Heikkinen J. Serum bile acids in the early diagnosis of intrahepatic cholestasis of pregnancy. Obstet Gynecol 61:581, 1983
111. Henker FO III. Psychotherapy as adjunct in treatment of vomiting during pregnancy. South Med J 69:1585, 1976
112. Henny CP, et al. Review of the importance of acute multidisciplinary treatment following spontaneous rupture of the liver capsule during pregnancy. Surg Gynecol Obstet 156:593, 1983
113. Herbert WNP, et al. Improving survival with liver rupture complicating pregnancy. Am J Obstet Gynecol 142:530, 1982
114. Heyborne KD, et al. Prolongation of premature gestation in women with hemolysis, elevated liver enzymes and low platelets: a report of five cases. J Reprod Med 35:53, 1990
115. Hiatt JR, et al. Biliary disease in pregnancy: strategy for surgical management. Am J Surg 151:263, 1986
116. Hibbard LT. Spontaneous rupture of the liver in pregnancy: a report of eight cases. Am J Obstet Gynecol 126:334, 1976
117. Hieber JP, et al. Hepatitis and pregnancy. J Pediatr 91:545, 1977
118. Hirsch EH, et al. Hepatic infarction in ulcerative colitis during pregnancy. Gastroenterology 78:571, 1980
119. Holden TE, et al. Hepatic infarction in ulcerative colitis during pregnancy. Obstet Gynecol 40:586, 1972
120. Holzbach RT. Jaundice in pregnancy. Am J Med 61:367, 1976
121. Holzbach RT, et al. Familial recurrent intrahepatic cholestasis of pregnancy: a genetic study providing evidence for transmission of a sex-limited, dominant trait. Gastroenterology 85:175, 1983
122. Holzbach RT, et al. Recurrent intrahepatic cholestasis of pregnancy. JAMA 193:542, 1965
123. Horstmann DM. Viral infections. In: Burrow GN, Ferris TF, eds. Medical complications during pregnancy, ed 2. Philadelphia, WB Saunders, 1982, p 333
124. Hou SH, et al. Acute fatty liver of pregnancy: survival with early cesarean section. Dig Dis Sci 29:449, 1984
125. Hurwitz MB. Jaundice in pregnancy: a 10 year study and review. S Afr Med J 44:219, 1970
126. Hyde E, et al. Intravascular coagulation during pregnancy and the puerperium. J Obstet Gynaecol Br CommonW 80:1059, 1973
127. Iatrakis GM, et al. Vomiting and nausea in the first 12 weeks of pregnancy. Psychother Psychosom 49:22, 1988
128. Iber FL. Jaundice in pregnancy: a review. Am J Obstet Gynecol 91:721, 1965
129. Infeld DS, et al. Chronic persistent hepatitis and pregnancy. Gastroenterology 77:524, 1979
130. Ingerslev M, et al. Biopsy studies on the liver in pregnancy: I. normal histological features of the liver as seen on aspiration biopsy. Acta Obset Gynecol Scand 25:352, 1945
131. Ingerslev M, et al. Biopsy studies on the liver in pregnancy: III. liver biopsy in albuminuria of pregnancy, eclampsism, and eclampsia. Acta Obstet Gynecol Scand 25:361, 1945
132. Ip HMH, et al. Prevention of hepatitis B virus carrier state in infants according to maternal serum levels of HBV DNA. Lancet 1:406, 1989
133. Israel EJ, et al. Maximal response to oxytocin of the isolated myometrium from pregnant patients with intrahepatic cholestasis. Acta Obstet Gynecol Scand 65:581, 1986
134. Jackson BT, et al. Perforated choledochus cyst. Br J Surg 58:38, 1971
135. Jacobs MB. Hepatic infarction related to oral contraceptive use. Arch Intern Med 144:642, 1984
136. Jewett JF. Eclampsia and rupture of the liver. N Engl J Med 297:1009, 1977
137. Jonas MM, et al. Failure of centers for disease control criteria to identify hepatitis B infection in a large municipal obstetrical population. Ann Intern Med 107:335, 1987
138. Joske RA. Acute fatty liver of pregnancy. Gut 9:489, 1968
139. Jouppila P, et al. Acute pancreatitis in pregnancy. Surg Gynecol Obstet 139:879, 1974
140. Kanaan C, et al. Pregnancy and acute intermittent porphyria. Obstet Gynecol Surv 44:244, 1989
141. Kane MA, et al. Epidemic non-A, non-B hepatitis in Nepal. JAMA 252:3140, 1984
142. Kane MA, et al. Routine prenatal screening for hepatitis B surface antigen. (Editorial) JAMA 259:408, 1988
143. Kaplan MM. Current concepts: acute fatty liver of pregnancy. N Engl J Med 313:367, 1985
144. Karouf M, et al. Hepatite et grossesse a Tunis: a propos de 103 cas compares a 100 cas en dehors de la grossesse. J Gynecol Biol Reprod 9:887, 1980
145. Kauppila A, et al. Raised serum human chorionic gonadotropin concentrations in hyperemesis gravidarum. Br Med J 1:1670, 1979
146. Kauppila A, et al. Low serum selenium concentration and glutathione peroxidase activity in intrahepatic cholestasis of pregnancy. Br Med J 294:150, 1987
147. Kelton JG. Management of the pregnant patient with idio-

pathic thrombocytopenic purpura. Ann Intern Med 99:796, 1983

148. Kent DR, et al. Effect of pregnancy on liver tumor associated with oral contraceptives. Obstet Gynecol 51:148, 1978

149. Kern FJ, et al. Biliary lipids, bile acids, and gallbladder function in the human female. J Clin Invest 68:1229, 1981

150. Kerr MG, et al. Studies of the inferior vena cava in late pregnancy. Br Med J 1:532, 1964

151. Khuroo MS. Study of an epidemic of non-A, non-B hepatitis: possibility of another human hepatitis virus distinct from posttransfusion non-A, non-B type. Am J Med 68:818, 1980

152. Khuroo MS, et al. Incidence and severity of viral hepatitis in pregnancy. Am J Med 70:252, 1981

153. Khuroo MS, et al. Budd-Chiari syndrome following pregnancy: report of 16 cases, with roentgenologic, hemodynamic and histologic studies of the hepatic outflow tract. Am J Med 68:113, 1980

154. Kiilholma P. Serum copper and zinc concentrations in intrahepatic cholestasis of pregnancy: a controlled study. Eur J Obstet Gynecol Reprod Biol 21:207, 1986

155. Killam AP, et al. Pregnancy-induced hypertension complicated by acute liver disease and disseminated intravascular coagulation: five case reports. Am J Obstet Gynecol 123:823, 1975

156. Kirby NG. Primary hepatic pregnancy. Br Med J 1:296, 1969

157. Klebanoff MA, et al. Epidemiology of vomiting in early pregnancy. Obstet Gynecol 66:612, 1985

158. Klein N, et al. Liver disease. In: Lee RV, ed. Current obstetric medicine, vol 1. St Louis, Mosby–Year Book, 1991, p 99

159. Klein NA, et al. Herpes simplex virus hepatitis in pregnancy. Gastroenterology 100:239, 1991

160. Koch KL, et al. Gastric dysrhythmias and nausea of pregnancy. Dig Dis Sci 35:961, 1990

161. Kreek MJ, et al. The response to challenge with the synthetic estrogen, ethinyl estradiol. N Engl J Med 277:1391, 1967

162. Kreek MJ. Female sex steroids and cholestasis. Semin Liver Dis 7:8, 1987

163. Krejs GJ. Jaundice during pregnancy. Semin Liver Dis 3:73, 1983

164. Krueger KJ, et al. Hepatic infarction associated with eclampsia. Am J Gastroenterol 85:588, 1990

165. Kumar ML, et al. Should all pregnant women be screened for hepatitis B. Ann Intern Med 107:273, 1987

166. Kunelis CT, et al. Fatty liver of pregnancy and its relationship to tetracycline therapy. Am J Med 38:359, 1965

167. Kuoppala T, et al. Vitamin D and mineral metabolism in intrahepatic cholestasis of pregnancy. Eur J Obstet Gynecol Reprod Biol 23:45, 1986

168. Laatikainen K. The effect of cholestyramine and phenobarbital on pruritus and serum bile acid levels in cholestasis of pregnancy. Am J Obstet Gynecol 132:501, 1978

169. LaBrecque DR, et al. Four generations of arteriohepatic dysplasia. Hepatology 2:467, 1982

170. Laifer SA, et al. Pregnancy and liver transplantation. Obstet Gynecol 76:1083, 1990

171. Larrey D, et al. Recurrent jaundice caused by recurrent hyperemesis gravidarum. Gut 25:1414, 1984

172. Lee MG, et al. Pregnancy in chronic active hepatitis with cirrhosis. J Trop Med Hyg 90:245, 1987

173. Lee SD, et al. Role of caesarean section in prevention of mother–infant transmission of hepatitis B virus. Lancet 2:833, 1988

174. Lefkowich JH, et al. Hepatic fibrosis in fetal alcohol syndrome: pathologic similarities to adult alcoholic liver disease. Gastroenterology 85:951, 1983

175. Levine MG, et al. Total parenteral nutrition for the treatment of severe hyperemesis gravidarum: maternal nutritional effects and fetal outcome. Obstet Gynecol 72:102, 1988

176. Levy M, et al. Hepatitis B vaccine in pregnancy: maternal and fetal safety. Am J Perinatol 8:227, 1991

177. Levy VG, et al. Les icteres au cours de la grossesse. Med Chir Dig 6:111, 1977

178. Lewis JH, et al. Budd-Chiari syndrome associated with oral contraceptive steroids. Dig Dis Sci 28:673, 1983

179. Lin H-H, et al. Transplacental leakage of HBeAg-positive maternal blood as the most likely route in causing intrauterine infection with hepatitis B virus. J Pediatr 111:877, 1987

180. Long RG, et al. Pre-eclampsia presenting with deep jaundice. J Clin Pathol 30:212, 1977

181. Lowe GDO, et al. Increased blood viscosity in young women using oral contraceptives. Am J Obstet Gynecol 137:840, 1980

182. Lunzer M, et al. Serum bile acid concentrations during pregnancy and their relationship to obstetric cholestasis. Gastroenterology 91:825, 1986

183. Luwuliza-Kirunda JMM. Primary hepatic pregnancy: case Report. Br J Obstet Gynaecol 85:311, 1978

184. Mabie WC, et al. Computed tomography in acute fatty liver of pregnancy. Am J Obstet Gynecol 158:142, 1988

185. MacKenna J, et al. Acute fatty metamorphosis of the liver: a report of two patients who survived. Am J Obstet Gynecol 127:400, 1977

186. MacKenna J, et al. Preeclampsia associated with hemolysis, elevated liver enzymes, and low platelets: an obstetric emergency? Obstet Gynecol 62:751, 1983

187. Maged DA, et al. Noncystic liver mass in the pregnant patient. South Med J 83:51, 1990

188. Malatjalian DA, et al. Acute fatty liver of pregnancy: light and electron microscopic studies. Gastroenterology 84:1384, 1983

189. Mallia CP, et al. Fulminant virus hepatitis in late pregnancy. Ann Trop Med Parasitol 76:143, 1982

190. Manas KJ, et al. Hepatic hemorrhage without rupture in preeclampsia. N Engl J Med 312:424, 1985

191. Maringhini A, et al. Sludge and stones in gallbladder after pregnancy: prevalence and risk factors. J Hepatol 5:218, 1987

192. McClements BM, et al. Idiopathic acute fatty liver of pregnancy: three cases including a subsequent normal pregnancy. Ulster Med J 59:217, 1990

193. McCormack WM, et al. Hepatotoxicity of erythromycin estolate during pregnancy. Antimicrob Agents Chemother 12:630, 1977

194. McKay AJ, et al. Pancreatitis, pregnancy, and gallstones. Br J Obstet Gynaecol 87:47, 1980

195. Merritt WT, et al. Liver transplantation during pregnancy: anesthesia for two procedures in the same patient with successful outcome of pregnancy. Transplant Proc 23:1996, 1991

196. Meyers RL, et al. Childbirth after liver transplantation. Transplantation 29:432, 1980

197. Milo R, et al. Acute intermittent porphyria in pregnancy. Obstet Gynecol 43:450, 1989

198. Minakami H, et al. Recurrent pancreatitis in the third trimester in 2 consecutive pregnancies: its relationship to liver histology—a case report. Asia Oceania J Obstet Gynaecol 15:147, 1989

199. Minakami H, et al. Preeclampsia: a microvesicular fat disease of the liver. Am J Obstet Gynecol 159:1043, 1988

200. Moldin P, et al. Acute fatty liver of pregnancy with disseminated intravascular coagulation. Acta Obstet Gynecol Scand 57:179, 1978

201. Mori M, et al. Morning sickness and thyroid function in normal pregnancy. Obstet Gynecol 72:355, 1988

202. Morris CV, et al. An unusual presentation of fulminant hepatic failure secondary to propylthiouracil therapy. Clin Transplant 311, 1989

203. Munnell EW, et al. Liver blood flow in pregnancy: hepatic vein catheterization. J Clin Invest 26:952, 1947

204. Natkunam R, et al. Peripartum haemoperitoneum. Aust NZ J Surg 61:323, 1991

205. Neerhof MG, et al. Hepatic rupture in pregnancy. Obstet Gynecol Surv 44:407, 1989

206. Neirynck C, et al. Spontaneous rupture of the liver with hemoperiton. J Chir 128:231, 1991
207. Nelson EW, et al. Spontaneous hepatic rupture in pregnancy. Am J Surg 134:817, 1977
208. Nesbitt JC, et al. Colorectal carcinoma in pregnancy. Arch Surg 120:636, 1985
209. Neuman M, et al. Maternal death caused by HELLP syndrome (with hypoglycemia) complicating mild pregnancy-induced hypertension in a twin gestation. Am J Obstet Gynecol 162:372, 1990
210. Nganwuchu AM, et al. Rupture of a nodule of hepatocellular carcinoma simulating uterine rupture in late pregnancy. Trop Doct 21:45, 1991
211. Nir A, et al. Pregnancy and primary biliary cirrhosis. Int J Gynaecol Obstet 28:279, 1989
212. Nixon WCW, et al. Icterus in pregnancy: a clinico-pathological study including liver biopsy. J Obstet Gynaecol Br Empire 54:642, 1947
213. O'Grady JP, et al. Splenic artery aneurysm rupture in pregnancy: a review and case report. Obstet Gynecol 50:627, 1977
214. Ober WB, et al. Acute fatty metamorphosis of the liver associated with pregnancy. Am J Med 19:743, 1955
215. Ockner SA, et al. Fulminant hepatic failure caused by acute fatty liver of pregnancy treated by orthotopic liver transplantation. Hepatology 11:59, 1990
216. Ohto H, et al. Intrauterine transmission of hepatitis B virus is closely related to placental leakage. J Med Virol 21:1, 1987
217. Perez VS, et al. Ultrastructure of human liver at the end of normal pregnancy. Am J Obstet Gynecol 110:428, 1971
218. Piotrowski JJ, et al. Case reports: spontaneous bile duct rupture in pregnancy. HPB Surg 2:205, 1990
219. Pockros PJ, et al. Idiopathic fatty liver of pregnancy: findings in ten cases. Medicine 68:1, 1984
220. Potter JM, et al. The hyperlipidemia of pregnancy in normal and complicated pregnancies. Am J Obstet Gynecol 153:165, 1979
221. Printen KJ, et al. Cholecystectomy during pregnancy. Am Surg 44:432, 1978
222. Pritchard JA. Changes in blood volume during pregnancy and delivery. Anesthesiology 26:393, 1965
223. Pucci RO, et al. Case report of laparoscopic cholecystectomy in the third trimester of pregnancy. Am J Obstet Gynecol 165:401, 1991
224. Radberg G, et al. Gastric and gallbladder emptying in relation to the secretion of cholecystokinin after a meal in late pregnancy. Digestion 42:174, 1989
225. Rajka G. Pregnancy and porphyria cutanea tarda. Acta Derm Venereol (Stockh) 64:444, 1984
226. Ramia S, et al. Perinatal transmission of hepatitis B virus infection: a recommended strategy for prevention and control. Br J Obstet Gynecol 89:141, 1991
227. Ranelletti FO, et al. Estrogen and progesterone receptors in the gallbladders from patients with gallstones. Hepatology 14:608, 1991
228. Rawal BK, et al. Symptomatic reactivation of hepatitis B in pregnancy. Lancet 337:364, 1991
229. Redman CWG. Platelets and the beginnings of preeclampsia. N Engl J Med 323:478, 1990
230. Reid R, et al. Fetal complications of obstetric cholestasis. Br Med J 1:870, 1976
231. Reyes GR, et al. Isolation of a cDNA from the virus responsible for enterically transmitted non-A, non-B hepatitis. Science 247:1335, 1990
232. Reyes H, et al. Prevalence of intrahepatic cholestasis of pregnancy in Chile. Ann Intern Med 88:487, 1978
233. Reyes H, et al. Sulfobromophthalein clearance tests before and after ethinyl estradiol administration, in women and men with familial history of intrahepatic cholestasis of pregnancy. Gastroenterology 81:226, 1981
234. Reyes H. The enigma of intrahepatic cholestasis of pregnancy: lessons from Chile. Hepatology 2:86, 1982
235. Ribalta J, et al. S-adenosyl-L-methionine in the treatment of patients with intrahepatic cholestasis of pregnancy: a randomized, double-blind, placebo-controlled study with negative results. Hepatology 13:1084, 1991
236. Riely CA. Acute fatty liver of pregnancy. Semin Liver Dis 7:47, 1987
237. Riely CA. Case studies in jaundice of pregnancy. Semin Liver Dis 8:191, 1988
238. Riely CA, et al. Histology of HELLP syndrome in preeclampsia: laboratory abnormalities fail to predict severity. Hepatology 14:101, 1991
239. Riely CA, et al. Acute fatty liver of pregnancy: a reassessment based on observations in nine patients. Ann Intern Med 106:703, 1987
240. Roberts JM. Pregnancy-related hypertension. In: Creasy RK, Resnik R, eds. Maternal–fetal medicine. Philadelphia, WB Saunders, 1984, p 703
241. Rolfes DB, et al. Acute fatty liver of pregnancy: a clinico-pathologic study of 35 cases. Hepatology 5:1149, 1985
242. Rolfes DB, et al. Liver disease in pregnancy. Histopathology 10:555, 1986
243. Romero R, et al. Arteriohepatic dysplasia in pregnancy. Am J Obstet Gynecol 147:108, 1983
244. Rosa FW. Teratogen update: penicillamine. Teratology 33:127, 1986
245. Rosenbloom AA, et al. The circulating vasopressinase of pregnancy: species comparison with radioimmunoassay. Am J Obstet Gynecol 121:316, 1975
246. Rosenthal T, et al. The Budd-Chiari syndrome after pregnancy: report of two cases and review of the literature. Am J Obstet Gynecol 113:789, 1972
247. Rubinger D, et al. Hepatitis following the use of methoxyflurane in obstetric analgesia. Anesthesiology 43:593, 1975
248. Rustgi VK. Liver disease in pregnancy. Med Clin North Am 73:1041, 1989
249. Rustgi VK, et al. Gastrointestinal and hepatic complications in pregnancy. New York, John Wiley & Sons, 1986
250. Saftlas AF, et al. Epidemiology of preeclampsia and eclampsia in the United States, 1979–1986. Am J Obstet Gynecol 162:460, 1990
251. Sali A, et al. Effect on pregnancy on gallstone formation. Aust N Z J Obstet Gynaecol 29:386, 1989
252. Samsioe G, et al. Studies in cholestasis of pregnancy. V. Gallbladder disease, liver function tests, serum lipids and fatty acid composition of serum lecithin in the non-pregnant state. Acta Obstet Gynecol Scand 54:417, 1975
253. Samuelson K, et al. Radioimmunoassay of serum bile acids in normal pregnancy. Acta Obstet Gynecol Scand 59:417, 1980
254. Scheinberg IH, et al. Wilson's disease. Philadelphia, WB Saunders, 1984
255. Schoeman MN, et al. Recurrent acute fatty liver of pregnancy associated with a fatty-acid oxidation defect in the offspring. Gastroenterology 100:544, 1991
256. Schorr-Lesnick B, et al. Liver diseases unique to pregnancy. Am J Gastroenterol 86:659, 1991
257. Schreyer P, et al. Cirrhosis: pregnancy and delivery—a review. Obstet Gynecol Surv 37:304, 1982
258. Schrier RW. Body fluid volume regulation in health and disease: a unifying hypothesis. Ann Intern Med 113:155, 1990
259. Schuster E, et al. Plasma urate measurements and fetal outcome in preeclampsia. Gynecol Obstet Invest 12:162, 1981
260. Schweitzer IL, et al. Pregnancy in hepatitis B antigen positive cirrhosis. Obstet Gynecol 48:535, 1976
261. Scott LD, et al. Oral contraceptives, pregnancy, and focal nodular hyperplasia of the liver. JAMA 251:1461, 1984
262. Seymour CA, et al. Liver and gastrointestinal function in pregnancy. Postgrad Med J 55:343, 1979
263. Shaw D, et al. A prospective study of 18 patients with cholestasis of pregnancy. Am J Obstet Gynecol 142:621, 1982
264. Sheehan HL. The pathology of acute yellow atrophy and de-

layed chloroform poisoning. J Obstet Gynaecol Br Empire 47: 49, 1940

265. Sherlock S. Acute fatty liver of pregnancy and the microvesicular fat diseases. Gut 24:265, 1983

266. Shimono N, et al. Fulminant hepatic failure during perinatal period in a pregnant women with Wilson's disease. Gastroenterol Jpn 26:69, 1991

267. Sibai BM. The HELLP syndrome (hemolysis, elevated liver enzymes, and low platelets): much ado about nothing? Am J Obstet Gynecol 162:311, 1990

268. Sibai BM, et al. Maternal–perinatal outcome associated with the syndrome of hemolysis, elevated liver enzymes, and low platelets in severe preeclampsia–eclampsia. Am J Obstet Gynecol 155:501, 1986

269. Simon JA. Biliary tract disease and related surgical disorders during pregnancy. Clin Obstet Gynecol 26:810, 1983

270. Sinapolice RX, et al. Hemoglobin SD disease associated with cholecystitis and cholelithiasis in pregnancy. Obstet Gynecol 60:388, 1982

271. Sinatra FR, et al. Perinatal transmitted acute icteric hepatitis B in infants born to hepatitis B surface antigen-positive and anti-hepatitis Be-positive carrier mothers. Pediatrics 70:557, 1982

272. Sjovall K, et al. Serum bile acid levels in pregnancy with pruritus. Clin Chim Acta 13:20, 1966

273. Snider DE, et al. Treatment of tuberculosis during pregnancy. Am Rev Respir Dis 122:65, 1980

274. Snyder RR, et al. Etiology and management of acute fatty liver of pregnancy. Clin Perinatol 13:813, 1986

275. Snydman DR. Current concepts: hepatitis in pregnancy. N Engl J Med 313:1398, 1985

276. Somner DG, et al. Hepatic rupture with toxemia of pregnancy: angiographic diagnosis. Am J Radiol 132:455, 1979

277. Soto-Albors CE, et al. Portal hypertension and hypersplenism in pregnancy secondary to chronic schistosomiasis. J Reprod Med 29:345, 1984

278. Soules MR, et al. Nausea and vomiting of pregnancy: role of human chorionic gonadotropin and 17-hydroxyprogesterone. Obstet Gynecol 55:966, 1980

279. Sridama V, et al. Decreased levels of helper T cells: a possible cause of immunodeficiency in pregnancy. N Engl J Med 307:352, 1982

280. Stander HJ, et al. Acute yellow atrophy of the liver in pregnancy. Am J Obstet Gynecol 28:61, 1934

281. Stellato TA, et al. Fetal salvage with maternal total parenteral nutrition: the pregnant mother as her own control. JPEN J Parenter Enteral Nutr 12:412, 1988

282. Steven MM, et al. Pregnancy in chronic active hepatitis. Q J Med 48:519, 1979

283. Steven MM. Pregnancy and liver disease. Gut 22:592, 1981

284. Stevens CE, et al. HBeAg and anti-HBe detection by radioimmunoassay: correlation with vertical transmission of hepatitis B virus in Taiwan. J Med Virol 3:237, 1979

285. Stevens CE, et al. Yeast-recombinant hepatitis B vaccine: efficacy with hepatitis B immune globulin in prevention of perinatal hepatitis B virus transmission. JAMA 257:2612, 1987

286. Swaminathan R, et al. Thyroid function in hyperemesis gravidarum. Acta Endocrinol 120:155, 1989

287. Taylor TV, et al. Choledochal cyst of pregnancy. J R Coll Surg 22:424, 1977

288. Tchobroutsky C, et al. The HELLP syndrome: a special form of hypertension in pregnancy. J Gynecol Obstet Biol Reprod 18:325, 1989

289. Terazawa S, et al. Hepatitis B virus mutants with precore-region defects in two babies with fulminant hepatitis and their mothers positive for antibody to hepatitis B E antigen. Pediatr Res 29:5, 1991

290. Thaler MM, et al. Vertical transmission of hepatitis C virus. Lancet 338:17, 1991

291. Thijs C, et al. Pregnancy and gallstone disease: an empiric demonstration of the importance of specification of risk periods. Am J Epidemiol 134:186, 1991

292. Thorling L. Jaundice in pregnancy. Acta Med Scand 302:1, 1955

293. Tiitinen A, et al. Placental protein 10 (PP10) in normal pregnancy and cholestasis of pregnancy. Br J Obstet Gynaecol 92: 1137, 1985

294. Tsung SH, et al. Budd-Chiari syndrome in women taking oral contraceptives. Clin Lab Sci 10:528, 1980

295. United States Department of Health and Human Services. Prevention of perinatal transmission of hepatitis B virus: prenatal screening of all pregnant women for hepatitis B surface antigen. MMWR 37:341, 1988

296. Valla D. Obstruction of the hepatic veins. Dig Dis 8:226, 1990

297. Valla D, et al. Primary myeloproliferative disorder and hepatic vein-thrombosis: a prospective study of erythroid colony formation in vitro in 20 patients with Budd-Chiari syndrome. Ann Intern Med 103:329, 1985

298. van der Weiden RMF, et al. Transient diabetes insipidus of pregnancy. Eur J Obstet Gynecol Reprod Biol 25:331, 1987

299. van Os HC, et al. The influence of contamination of culture medium with hepatitis B virus on the outcome of in vitro fertilization pregnancies. Am J Obstet Gynecol 165:152, 1991

300. Vanjak D, et al. Intrahepatic cholestasis of pregnancy and acute fatty liver of pregnancy. Gastroenterology 100:1123, 1991

301. Varma RR. Course and prognosis of pregnancy in women with liver disease. Semin Liver Dis 7:59, 1987

302. Vons C, et al. Successful pregnancy after Budd-Chiari syndrome. (Letter) Lancet 2:975, 1984

303. Voorhis BV, et al. Colon carcinoma complicating pregnancy: a report of two cases. J Reprod Med 34:923, 1989

304. Wagner VP, et al. Amoebic abscess of the liver and spleen in pregnancy and the puerperium. Obstet Gynecol 45:562, 1975

305. Wald A, et al. Effect of pregnancy on gastrointestinal transit. Dig Dis Sci 27:1015, 1982

306. Walker FB, et al. Gamma glutamyl transpeptidase in normal pregnancy. Obstet Gynecol 43:745, 1974

307. Wallstedt A, et al. A controlled study of autonomic function and electrogastrography in hyperemesis gravidarum. Gastroenterology 100:A847, 1991

308. Wallstedt A, et al. Prevalence and characteristics of liver dysfunction in hyperemesis gravidarum. Clin Res 38:970, 1991

309. Walshe JM. Pregnancy in Wilson's disease. Q J Med 46:73, 1977

310. Walshe JM. The management of pregnancy in Wilson's disease treated with trientine. Q J Med 58:81, 1986

311. Walters WAW, et al. Changes in the maternal cardio-vascular system during human pregnancy. Surg Gynecol Obstet 131:765, 1970

312. Weber FL, et al. Abnormalities of hepatic mitochondrial urea-cycle enzyme activities and hepatic ultrastructure in acute fatty liver of pregnancy. J Lab Clin Med 94:27, 1979

313. Weigel MM, et al. Nausea and vomiting of early pregnancy and pregnancy outcome: an epidemiological study. Br J Obstet Gynaecol 96:1304, 1989

314. Weigel RM, et al. Nausea and vomiting of early pregnancy and pregnancy outcome: a meta-analytical review. Br J Obstet Gynaecol 96:1312, 1989

315. Weinstein L. Syndrome of hemolysis, elevated liver enzymes, and low platelet count: a severe consequence of hypertension in pregnancy. Am J Obstet Gynecol 142:159, 1982

316. Wejstal R, et al. Mother to infant transmission of hepatitis C virus infection. J Med Virol 30:178, 1990

317. Wenk RE, et al. Tetracycline-associated fatty liver of pregnancy, including possible pregnancy risk after chronic dermatologic use of tetracycline. J Reprod Med 26:135, 1981

318. Wertheim RA, et al. Fatal herpetic hepatitis in pregnancy. Obstet Gynecol 62:38, 1983

319. Whelton MJ, et al. Pregnancy in patients with hepatic cirrhosis: management and outcome. Lancet 2:995, 1968
320. Wilkinson EJ. Acute pancreatitis in pregnancy: a review of 98 cases and a report of 8 new cases. Obstet Gynecol Surv 28:281, 1973
321. Wilson JAP. Intrahepatic cholestasis of pregnancy with marked elevation of transaminases in a black American. Dig Dis Sci 32:665, 1987
322. Wong DC, et al. Epidemic and endemic hepatitis in India: evidence for a non-A, non-B hepatitis virus etiology. Lancet 2:876, 1980
323. Worley RJ. Pathophysiology of pregnancy-induced hypertension. Clin Obstet Gynecol 27:821, 1984
324. Ylostalo P, et al. Gallbladder volume and serum bile acids in cholestasis of pregnancy. Br J Obstet Gynaecol 89:59, 1982
325. Young N, et al. Antibody to cardiolipin causing hepatic infarction in a post partum patient with systemic lupus erythematosus. Australas Radiol 35:83, 1991
326. Zakut H, et al. Colon carcinoma in pregnancy: case report and review of the literature. Clin Exp Obstet Gynecol 11:27, 1984
327. Zemel MB, et al. Altered platelet calcium metabolism as an early predictor of increased peripheral vascular resistance and preeclampsia in urban black women. N Engl J Med 323:434, 1990
328. Zuckerman AJ. Hepatitis E virus. Br Med J 300:1475, 1990

Diseases of the Liver, Seventh Edition, edited by Leon Schiff and Eugene R. Schiff. J.B. Lippincott Company, Philadelphia © 1993.

52

The Liver in Circulatory Failure

Sheila Sherlock

A rise in pressure in the right atrium is readily transmitted to the hepatic veins. Liver cells are particularly vulnerable to diminished oxygen supply so a failing heart, lowered blood pressure, or reduced hepatic blood flow are reflected in impaired hepatic function. The left lobe of the liver may suffer more than the right.

Hepatic Changes in Acute Heart Failure and Shock

Hepatic changes are common in acute heart failure and in shock due to trauma, burns, hemorrhage, sepsis, peritonitis, or black water fever. Light microscopy shows a congested zone 3 with local hemorrhage (Fig. 52-1). Focal necrosis with eosinophilic hepatocytes, hydropic change, and polymorphonuclear infiltration usually is centrizonal. Midzonal necrosis may be due to tangential section cutting, but in some instances is unexplained.[6] The reticulin framework is preserved within the necrotic zone. With recovery, particularly after trauma, mitoses may be prominent.

Hepatic calcification can develop in zone 3 after shock.[30] This might be related to the disturbance of intracellular calcium homeostasis as a result of ischemic liver injury.

Changes can be related to the duration of the shock: if longer than 24 hours, hepatic necrosis is almost constant; if less than 10 hours, it is unusual.

The fall in blood pressure leads to a reduction in hepatic blood flow, and the oxygen content of the blood is reduced. Hepatic arterial vasoconstriction follows the fall in systemic blood pressure. The centrizonal (zone 3) cells receive blood at a lower oxygen tension than the peripheral (zone 1) cells[12] and therefore more readily become anoxic and necrotic (Fig. 52-2).

The hepatocyte injury is largely due to oxygen lack. Insufficient substrates and accumulation of metabolites contribute; the mechanisms are multiple. The absence of available oxygen results in loss of mitochondrial oxidative phosphorylation. Impaired membrane function and reduced protein synthesis contribute,[12] and there are alterations in hepatocellular ion homeostasis.[3] Much of the tissue damage develops during reperfusion, when there is a large flux of oxygen-derived free radicals.[33] These initiate lipid peroxidation with disruption of membrane integrity. Lysosomal membranes may be peroxidased with the release of enzymes into the cytoplasm.

Treatment is unsatisfactory. Free radical trapping agents such as vitamin E, glutathione, and ascorbic acid are being evaluated. Allopurinol, a specific inhibitor of xanthine oxidase, the enzyme that generates free radicals from oxygen, may be useful.[22]

Some patients show mild icterus, and jaundice has been recorded in severely traumatized patients. Serum transaminase levels increase markedly and the prothrombin time rises.

Ischemic Hepatitis

This condition is defined as marked and rapid elevation of serum transaminase levels in the setting of an acute fall in cardiac output.[10] Acute hepatic infarction is an alternative definition. The picture simulates acute virus hepatitis.

The patient usually suffers from cardiac disease, often ischemic, or a cardiomyopathy. He or she has an acute fall in cardiac output, often due to an arrhythmia or myocardial infarction. Zone 3 necrosis without inflammation results. Clinical evidence of hepatic failure is absent; in particular, congestive cardiac failure is inconspicuous.

Serum bilirubin and alkaline phosphatase values increase slightly, but serum transaminase levels rise rapidly and strikingly to more than 1000 IU/L.[18] Values return speedily toward recovery in less than 1 week. Mortality is high (58.6%) and depends on the underlying cause and not the liver injury.[14] Tests for hepatitis A, B, and C are negative, and hepatotoxic drugs cannot be incriminated. If the liver has been previously damaged by chronic congestive heart failure, acute circulatory failure may lead to the picture of fulminant hepatic failure.[25]

Postoperative Jaundice

Jaundice developing soon after surgery may have multiple causes.[16] Increased serum bilirubin follows blood transfusion, particularly of stored blood. The hemoglobin in 500 mL of blood contains about 250 mg of bilirubin, the normal daily production. Extravasated blood in the tissues gives an additional bilirubin load.

Impaired hepatocellular function follows surgery, anesthetics, and shock. Severe jaundice develops in approximately 2% of patients, with shock resulting from major trauma.[26] Hepatic perfusion is reduced. This will be particularly evident if the patient is in incipient circulatory failure and the cardiac output is already reduced. Renal blood flow also falls.

Halothane anesthetics, especially if multiple, may be followed by a hepatitis-like picture. This is rare less than 7 days after a first operation. Other drugs used in the operative pe-

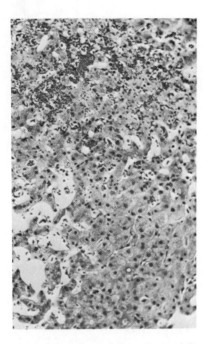

FIGURE 52-1 Ischemic heart failure. Serum bilirubin 2.1 mg/dL. Liver cells have disappeared from the center of the lobule and are replaced by frank hemorrhage (H&E, × 120). (Sherlock S. The liver in heart failure: relation of anatomical, functional and circulatory changes. Br Heart J 13:273, 1951)

riod, such as the promazines, must also be considered. Sepsis, per se, can produce deep jaundice, which may be cholestatic.

In the United States, glucose-6-phosphatase dehydrogenase deficiency affects about 10% of African Americans. In such patients, the administration of the many drugs at the time of surgery may precipitate hemolysis and jaundice.

Rarely, a cholestatic jaundice may be noted on the first or second postoperative day. It reaches its height between 4 and 10 days and disappears by 14 to 18 days. Serum biochemical changes are variable. Sometimes, but not always, the alkaline phosphatase and transaminase levels are increased.[28] The se-

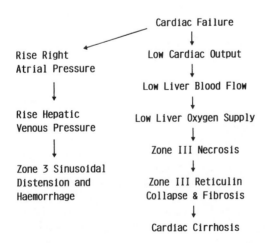

FIGURE 52-2 Factors leading to cardiac cirrhosis and zone 3 hemorrhage in patients with cardiac failure.

rum bilirubin value can rise to levels of 23 to 39 mg/dL. The picture simulates extrahepatic biliary obstruction.[11] Patients have all had an episode of shock and been transfused. Zone 3 hepatic necrosis, however, is not conspicuous and hepatic histologic specimens show only minor abnormalities. The mechanism of the cholestasis is uncertain. This picture must be recognized[12] and, if necessary, needle biopsy of the liver performed.

Jaundice may develop in severely ill patients in intensive care after severe trauma or postoperative intraabdominal sepsis; this reflects severe multiple organ failure and a poor prognosis.[32] The jaundice usually is of the cholestatic type, with raised conjugated serum bilirubin and alkaline phosphatase levels and only slightly increased transaminases.

Experimentally, bile flow falls after hemorrhagic shock. Endotoxemia and sepsis may activate inflammatory mediators, leading to vascular damage, increased permeability, edema, and impaired oxygen transport.[4] With better intensive care, the number of patients with multiple organ failure is falling.

Jaundice After Cardiac Surgery

Jaundice is frequent and develops in 20% of patients having cardiopulmonary bypass surgery.[5] It carries a poor prognosis. The jaundice is detected by the second postoperative day. Serum bilirubin is conjugated, suggesting failure of canalicular biliary excretion. The serum alkaline phosphatase value may be normal or only slightly increased, and transaminase levels are raised, often becoming very high.[16] Older patients are particularly at risk. Jaundice is significantly associated with multiple valve replacement, high blood transfusion requirements, and a longer bypass time.

Many factors contribute. The patient may have a liver that has already suffered from prolonged heart failure. Operative hypotension, shock, and hypothermia may have occurred. Infections, drugs (including anticoagulants), and anesthetics must be considered. Liver blood flow drops by about 20%,[13] and the serum bilirubin load is increased by blood transfusion. The pump may contribute by decreasing erythrocyte survival and by adding gaseous microemboli, platelet aggregates, and debris to the circulation.

Hepatitis C is now the most common cause of posttransfusion hepatitis. The acute attack may be virtually asymptomatic, and the patient may present months or years later with chronic hepatitis or cirrhosis. Hepatitis B is rare since blood has been screened routinely. Cytomegalohepatitis may develop after cardiac surgery.

The Liver in Congestive Heart Failure
PATHOLOGY

Hepatic autolysis is particularly rapid in the patient dying of heart failure.[29] Autopsy material is therefore unreliable for the assessment of the effects of cardiac failure on the liver in life.

The liver usually is enlarged and purplish with rounded edges. As cardiac cirrhosis develops, the liver shrinks. Nodularity is never as great as with other types of cirrhosis. The cut surface shows prominent hepatic veins, which may be thickened. The liver drips blood. Central zones are promi-

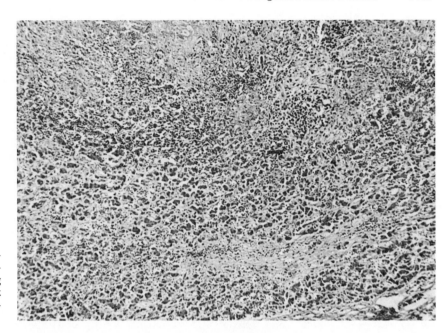

FIGURE 52-3   Cut surface of liver from patient dying of congestive heart failure. Note dilated hepatic veins. Light areas corresponding to peripheral fatty zones alternate with dark areas corresponding to central zonal congestion and hemorrhage.

nent with alteration of yellow (fatty change) and red areas (centrizonal hemorrhage), giving a nutmeg-like appearance (Fig. 52-3).

The hepatic venule always is dilated, and the sinusoids entering it are engorged for a variable distance toward the periphery. In severe cases, there is frank hemorrhage with focal necrosis of liver cells. The liver cells show a variety of degenerative (zone 1) changes, but each portal tract (zone 3) is surrounded by relatively normal cells to a depth that varies inversely with the extent of the atrophy. Surviving cells usually retain their glycogen. Biopsy sections show significant fatty change in about one third. This contrasts with the usual postmortem material. Cellular infiltration is inconspicuous.

The zone 3 degenerating cells often are packed with brown lipochrome pigment. As they disintegrate, pigment lies free among cellular debris. Bile thrombi, particularly in zone 1, may be seen in deeply jaundiced patients. Zone 3 periodic acid–Schiff-positive, diastase-resistant hyaline globules also may be seen.[17]

Zone 3 reticulin condensation follows loss of liver cells (Fig. 52-4). Next, reticulin and collagen increase and the central vein shows phlebosclerosis. If the heart failure continues or relapses, bridges develop between central veins so that the unaffected portal zone is surrounded by a ring of fibrous tissue (reversed lobulation; Fig. 52-5). Later, the portal zones are involved and a complex cirrhosis results. A true cardiac cirrhosis is rare.

Electron microscopy shows atrophy of zone 3 cells, probably related to new fibers in the space of Disse, which interfere with blood–hepatocyte transfer. Canaliculi may dilate and rupture.

MECHANISM

Zone 3 hepatocytes receive blood at a lower oxygen tension than those in zone 1. Hypoxia causes degeneration of zone 3 liver cells, dilatation of sinusoids, and slowing of bile secretion. The liver attempts to compensate by increasing the oxygen extracted as the blood flows across the sinusoidal bed.

Collagenosis of the space of Disse may play a minor role in impairing oxygen diffusion.

Necrosis correlates with a reduced systemic blood pressure and hence with a low cardiac output. The hepatic venous pressure increases in proportion to the rise in central venous pressure, and this correlates with zone 3 congestion.[1]

CLINICAL FEATURES

Mild jaundice is common, but deeper icterus is particularly associated with chronic congestive failure, due, for example, to coronary artery disease or mitral stenosis.[24] In hospitalized patients, cardiorespiratory disease is the most common cause of a raised serum bilirubin level. Jaundice increases with prolonged and repeated bouts of congestive heart failure.[8] Edematous areas escape, because bilirubin is protein bound and does not enter edema fluid with a low protein content.

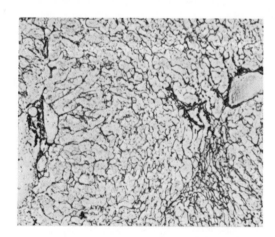

FIGURE 52-4   The liver in congestive heart failure. Reticulin stains show condensation at the lobular center (H&E, × 120). (Sherlock S. The liver in heart failure: relation of anatomical, functional and circulatory changes. Br Heart J 13:273, 1951)

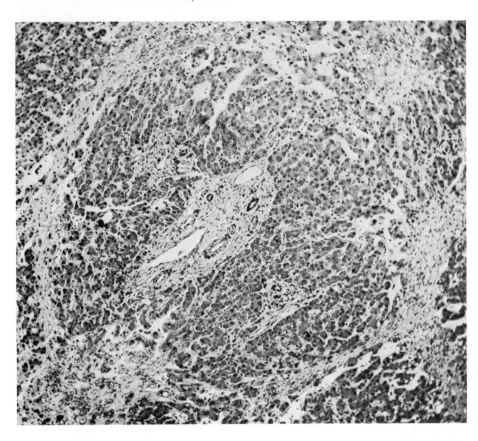

FIGURE 52-5 Fibrous tissue bands pass from central vein to central vein. There is reversed lobulation and a fully developed cardiac cirrhosis. Portal tracts show only slight fibrosis (H&E, × 90).

Jaundice is partly hepatic because the greater extent of zone 3 necrosis, the deeper is the icterus[29] (Figs. 52-6 and 52-7).

Cholestasis due to bile thrombi or to pressure on bile ducts by distended veins is unlikely.

Bilirubin released from infarcts, whether pulmonary, splenic, or renal, or simply from pulmonary congestion, overloads the anoxic liver. Patients in cardiac failure who become jaundiced with minimal hepatocellular damage usually have clear evidence of pulmonary infarction.[29] In keeping with bilirubin overload, the serum shows unconjugated bilirubinemia.

The patient may complain of right abdominal pain, probably due to stretching of the nerve endings in the capsule of the enlarged liver. The firm, smooth, and tender lower edge may reach the umbilicus.

A rise in right atrial pressure is transmitted readily to the hepatic veins. This is particularly so in tricuspid incompetence when the hepatic vein pressure tracing resembles that obtained from the right atrium. Palpable systolic pulsation of the liver can be related to this transmission of pressure. Presystolic hepatic pulsation occurs in tricuspid stenosis. The expansion may be felt bimanually with one hand over the liver anteriorly and the other over the right lower ribs posteriorly. This expansibility distinguishes it from the palpable epigastric pulsation due to the aorta or a hypertrophied right ventricle. Correct timing of the pulsation is important.

In heart failure, pressure applied over the liver increases the venous return and the jugular venous pressure rises due to the inability of the failing right heart to handle the increased blood flow.

The hepatojugular reflux is of value for the identification of the jugular venous pulse and to establish that venous channels between the hepatic and jugular veins are patent.

The reflux is absent if the hepatic veins are occluded or if the main mediastinal or jugular veins are blocked. It is useful in diagnosing tricuspid regurgitation.[21]

DOPPLER SONOGRAPHY

Arterial pressure is reflected all the way to the portal system. Pulsed duplex Doppler sonography shows increased pulsatility in the portal vein, depending on the severity of the heart failure.[15] Patients with high arterial pressures do not always have pulsatile flow, however.[7]

Ascites is associated with a particularly high venous pressure, a low cardiac output, and severe, zone 3 necrosis. This description applies to patients with mitral stenosis and tricuspid incompetence or constrictive pericarditis. In such pa-

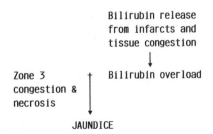

FIGURE 52-6 Factors leading to jaundice in patients with cardiac failure.

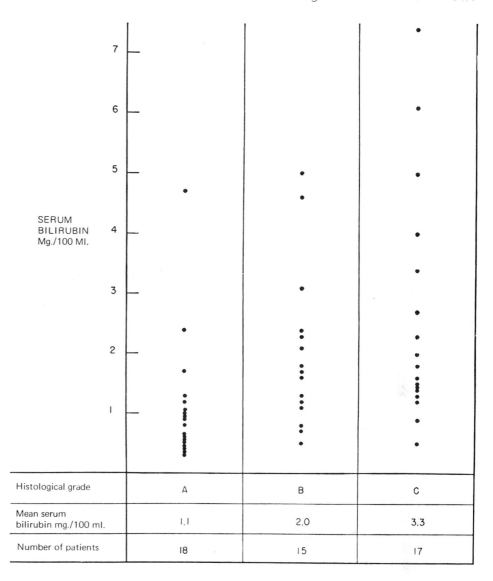

Histological grade	A	B	C
Mean serum bilirubin mg./100 ml.	1.1	2.0	3.3
Number of patients	18	15	17

FIGURE 52-7 Relation of extent of hepatic necrosis to serum bilirubin concentration. (Sherlock S. The liver in heart failure: relation of anatomical, functional and circulatory changes. Br Heart J 13:273, 1951)

tients, the ascites may be out of proportion to the edema and to the symptoms of congestive heart failure. The ascitic fluid protein content is raised to 2.5 g/dL or more, similar to that observed in Budd-Chiari syndrome.[27]

Confusion, lethargy, and coma are occasional accompaniments of heart failure and are related to cerebral anoxia. Occasionally, the whole picture of impending hepatic coma may be seen.[24]

Splenomegaly is frequent. Other features of portal hypertension usually are absent except in very severe cardiac cirrhosis associated with constrictive pericarditis. At autopsy, however, 6.7% of 74 patients with congestive heart failure showed esophageal varices, although only in 1 was there evidence of bleeding.

Cardiac cirrhosis should be suspected in patients with prolonged, decompensated mitral valve disease with tricuspid incompetence or in patients with constrictive pericarditis. The prevalence has fallen because both the conditions are now relieved surgically.

Bolus-enhanced computed tomography shows retrograde hepatic venous opacification on the early scans and a dif-fusely mottled pattern of hepatic enhancement during the vascular phase of contrast administration.[23]

BIOCHEMICAL CHANGES

In congestive heart failure, the serum bilirubin level usually exceeds 1 mg/dL, and in about one third it is more than 2 mg/dL.[29] The jaundice may be deep, exceeding 5 mg/dL and even up to 26.9 mg/dL.[9,29] The serum bilirubin level corresponds to the degree of heart failure.

The serum alkaline phosphatase value usually is normal or slightly increased. Serum albumin values may be mildly reduced and globulin raised.[29] Protein loss from the intestine may contribute.

Serum transaminase levels are higher in acute than chronic failure and are proportional to the degree of shock and to the extent of zone 3 necrosis. The association of very high values with jaundice may simulate acute viral hepatitis.[4]

The urine shows excess urobilinogen; rarely, gray stools accompany deep icterus.

PROGNOSIS

The prognosis is that of the underlying heart disease. Cardiac jaundice, particularly if deep, is always a bad omen.

Cardiac cirrhosis per se does not carry a bad prognosis, and if the heart failure responds to treatment, the cirrhosis can be expected to become compensated.

Hepatic Dysfunction and Cardiovascular Abnormalities in Pediatric Patients

Infants and children with heart failure and cyanotic heart disease show liver dysfunction.[20] Hypoxemia, systemic venous congestion, and a low cardiac output are associated with increased prothrombin time, serum bilirubin, and transaminase values. The most severe changes are found with a low cardiac output. Liver function correlates with cardiac status.

The Liver in Constrictive Pericarditis

The clinical picture and hepatic changes in constrictive pericarditis are those of the Budd-Chiari syndrome. Cardiac cirrhosis is frequent and marked thickening of the liver capsule simulates sugar icing (*Zuckergussleber*). Microscopically, the picture is of cardiac cirrhosis. Jaundice is absent, and the liver is enlarged and hard. Ascites is gross.

Diagnosis must be made from ascites due to cirrhosis or to hepatic venous obstruction. This is done by determination of the paradoxic pulse and the venous pulse, radiology showing the calcified pericardium, echocardiography, electrocardiography, and cardiac catheterization.

Treatment is that of the cardiac condition. If pericardectomy is possible, liver prognosis is good, although recovery may be slow. Within 6 months of a successful operation, results of liver function tests improve and the liver shrinks. The cardiac cirrhosis cannot be expected to resolve completely, but fibrous bands become narrower and avascular.

Thoracoabdominal Aneurysm

A large thoracoabdominal aneurysm can cause congestive hepatomegaly by compressing the confluence of hepatic veins and the inferior vena cava.[31]

References

1. Anderson MD, Gabrieli E, Zizzi JA. Chronic hemolysis in patients with ball valve prosthesis. J Thorac Cardiovasc Surg 50:510, 1981
2. Arcidi JM Jr, Moore GW, Hutchins P. Hepatic morphology in cardiac dysfunction: a clinicopathologic study of 1000 subjects at autopsy. Am J Pathol 104:159, 1965
3. Berger ML, Reynolds RC, Hagler HK, et al. Anoxic hepatocyte injury: a role of reversible changes in elemental content and distribution. Hepatology 9:219, 1989
4. Carrico JC, Meakins JL, Marshall JC, et al. Multiple organ-failure syndrome. Arch Surg 121:196, 1986
5. Collins JD, Bassendine MR, Ferner R, et al. Incidence and prognostic importance of jaundice after cardiopulmonary bypass surgery. Lancet 1:1119, 1983
6. De La Monte SM, Arcidi JM, Moore GW, et al. Midzonal necrosis as a pattern of hepatocellular injury after shock. Gastroenterology 86:627, 1984
7. Duerinckx AJ, Grant EG, Perrella RR, et al. The pulsatile portal vein in cases of congestive heart failure: correlation of duplex Doppler findings with right atrial pressure. Radiology 176:655, 1990
8. Dunn GD, Hayes P, Breen KJ, et al. The liver in congestive heart failure: a review. Am J Med Sci 265:174, 1973
9. Gadeholt H, Haugen J. Centrilobular hepatic necrosis in cardiac failure: one case with severe acute jaundice. Acta Med Scand 176:525, 1964
10. Gibson PR, Dudley FJ. Ischemic hepatitis: clinical features, diagnosis and prognosis. Aust N Z J Med 14:822, 1984
11. Gourley GR, Chesney PJ, Davis JP, et al. Acute cholestasis in patients with toxic-shock syndrome. Gastroenterology 81:928, 1981
12. Gumucio JJ, Miller DL. Functional implications of liver cell heterogeneity. Gastroenterology 80:393, 1981
13. Hampton WW, Townsend MC, Schirmer WJ, et al. Effective hepatic blood flow during cardiopulmonary bypass. Arch Surg 124:458, 1989
14. Hickman PE, Potter JM. Mortality associated with ischaemic hepatitis. Aust N Z J Med 20:32, 1990
15. Hosoki T, Arisawa J, Marukawa T, et al. Portal blood flow in congestive heart failure: pulsed duplex sonographic findings. Radiology 174:733, 1990
16. Ischaemic hepatitis. Lancet 1:1019, 1985
17. Kantrowitz PA, Jones WA, Greenberger NJ, et al. Postoperative hyperbilirubinemia simulating obstructive jaundice. N Engl J Med 276:591, 1967
18. Klatt EC, Koss, Young TS, et al. Hepatic hyaline globules associated with passive congestion. Arch Pathol Lab Med 112:510, 1988
19. Lockey E, McIntyre N, Ross DN, et al. Early jaundice after open heart surgery. Thorax 22:165, 1967
20. Mace S, Borkat G, Liebman J. Hepatic dysfunction and cardiovascular abnormalities: occurrence in infants, children, and young adults. Am J Dis Child 139:60, 1985
21. Maisel AS, Atwood JE, Goldberger AL. Hepatojugular reflux: useful in the bedside diagnosis of tricuspid regurgitation. Ann Intern Med 101:78, 1984
22. Marotto ME, Thurman RG, Lemasters JJ. Early midzonal cell death during low-flow hypoxia in the isolated, perfused rat liver: protection by allopurinol. Hepatology 8:585, 1988
23. Moulton JS, Miller BL, Dodd GD III, Vu DN. Passive hepatic congestion in heart failure: CT abnormalities. Am J Radiol 151:939, 1988
24. Moussavian SN, Dincsoy HP, Goodman S, et al. Severe hyperbilirubinemia and coma in chronic congestive heart failure. Dig Dis Sci 27:175, 1982
25. Novel O, Henrion J, Bernuau J, et al. Fulminant hepatic failure due to transient circulatory failure in patients with chronic heart disease. Dig Dis Sci 25:49, 1980
26. Nunes G, Blaisdell FW, Margaretten W. Mechanism of hepatic dysfunction following shock and trauma. Arch Surg 100:646, 1970
27. Runyon BA. Cardiac ascites: a characterization. J Clin Gastroenterol 10:410, 1988
28. Schmid M, Hefti ML, Gattiker R, et al. Benign post-operative intrahepatic cholestasis. N Engl J Med 272:545, 1965
29. Sherlock S. The liver in heart failure: relation of anatomical, functional and circulatory changes. Br Heart J 13:273, 1951
30. Shibuya A, Unuma T, Sugimoto M, et al. Diffuse hepatic calcification as a sequela to shock liver. Gastroenterology 89:196, 1985
31. Sigal E, Pogany A, Goldman IS. Marked hepatic congestion

caused by a thoracoabdominal aneurysm. Gastroenterology 87:1367, 1984

32. Te Boekhorst T, Urlus M, Doesburg W, et al. Etiologic factors of jaundice in severely ill patients: a retrospective study in patients admitted to an intensive care unit with severe trauma or with septic intra-abdominal complications following surgery and without evidence of bile duct obstruction. J Hepatol 77:111, 1988

33. Weisiger RA. Oxygen radicals and ischemic tissue injury. Gastroenterology 90;494:1986

Diseases of the Liver, Seventh Edition, edited by Leon Schiff and Eugene R. Schiff. J.B. Lippincott Company, Philadelphia © 1993.

53

The Porphyrias

Joseph R. Bloomer

James G. Straka

Jeffrey M. Rank

The porphyrias are metabolic disorders in which abnormalities in heme biosynthesis cause the excessive accumulation and excretion of porphyrins and porphyrin precursors. The porphyrias have diverse clinical and laboratory findings, and they are encountered in several different areas of medicine. The first clinical reports of these disorders occurred during the latter part of the 19th century.[273] Elucidation of their biochemical features followed the characterization of the heme biosynthesis pathway during the first part of this century.[217] This demonstrated that the porphyrins and their reduced counterparts (porphyrinogens) are the precursors of heme (Fig. 53-1). In 1970, it was shown that the pattern of porphyrin excretion that occurs in a specific type of porphyria reflects an abnormality of one of the enzymatic steps in the heme biosynthesis pathway[235] (Fig. 53-2). In recent years, molecular techniques have been used to define the gene defects that cause these enzyme abnormalities.[254]

The liver has an important role in several of the porphyrias because it is a major site of heme biosynthesis. When the hepatic mixed function oxidase system is induced during the administration of drugs, the amount of heme synthesized in the liver may increase significantly, and the rate of formation of porphyrins and porphyrin precursors thereby increases. The liver's critical role in heme and porphyrin metabolism provides the basis for the classification of several of the porphyrias as hepatic.[210]

The liver also has a role in the excretion of porphyrins.[194] This causes the liver to be susceptible to the toxic effect of porphyrin accumulation in certain types of the porphyrias. Conversely, hepatobiliary disease may cause an increase in urinary excretion of porphyrins, a condition called *secondary porphyrinuria*, when excretion of these compounds is diverted from bile to urine.

In this chapter, the hepatic aspects of the porphyrias are highlighted.

Hepatic Heme Metabolism

Heme is a member of a group of compounds called *tetrapyrroles*. As the name implies, these are composed of four pyrrole rings arranged into a larger ring by one-carbon bridges (see Fig. 53-1). The four pyrrole nitrogen atoms are directed toward the center of the ring. Because of the size of the central cavity and the chemical properties of the central nitrogen atoms, tetrapyrroles have excellent metal-binding characteristics. In nature, tetrapyrrole complexes with iron (hemes),

magnesium (chlorophylls), and cobalt (corrins, or vitamin B_{12}) are involved in many processes crucial to living organisms.

The iron of heme (iron protoporphyrin IX); has four of its six coordination positions occupied by the four nitrogen atoms of the porphyrin. The remaining two coordination positions may be occupied by heteroatoms on the side chains of proteins or by solvent or solute molecules, which in turn affects the chemical properties of the central iron. The chemistry of the heme moiety is thus dictated by its protein microenvironment and the chemistry of the fifth and sixth ligand. Thus, hemoproteins show a wide variety of chemistry, including oxidation–reduction, oxygen activation, and ligand binding (eg, oxygen transport). Hepatic hemoproteins include mixed function oxidases (eg, cytochromes P-450, squalene-2,3-epoxide synthase), dioxygenases (eg, prostaglandin cyclooxygenase), catalase, peroxidases, and tryptophan pyrrolase, all of which are involved in the modification or catabolism of endogenous substrates or potentially toxic compounds. In addition, heme serves as the oxidation–reduction center for the cytochromes of mitochondrial electron transport and of the smooth endoplasmic reticulum.

The liver has been estimated to synthesize 15% to 20% of total body heme, and well over half of that is used in the cytochromes P-450.[117] Estimates based on the activity of the first enzyme of the heme biosynthetic pathway[118,247] or the rate of appearance of heme breakdown products[114] suggest that normal liver synthesizes between 50 and 100 µmol/d of heme (0.8 to 1.4 µmol/d/kg). The daily synthesis of heme is affected by diet, exposure to toxic compounds, physiologic status of the person, or existence of liver pathology or hereditary disease. Thus, these values may increase under certain physiologic or pathologic conditions.

HEME BIOSYNTHESIS PATHWAY

Heme is synthesized in all mammalian tissues in eight enzymatically controlled steps (see Fig. 53-2). The pathway and some of the relevant enzyme mechanisms have been discussed in detail elsewhere[32,117,234] and therefore are discussed only briefly here.

The first and controlling step of hepatic heme biosynthesis is the synthesis of δ-aminolevulinic acid (5-amino-4-oxopentanoic acid; ALA). ALA is synthesized by the condensation of the citric acid cycle intermediate succinyl coenzyme A (CoA) with glycine, followed by spontaneous loss of the glycine-derived carboxylate from the enzyme-bound inter-

δ-**AMINOLEVULINIC ACID (ALA)**   **PORPHOBILINOGEN (PBG)**

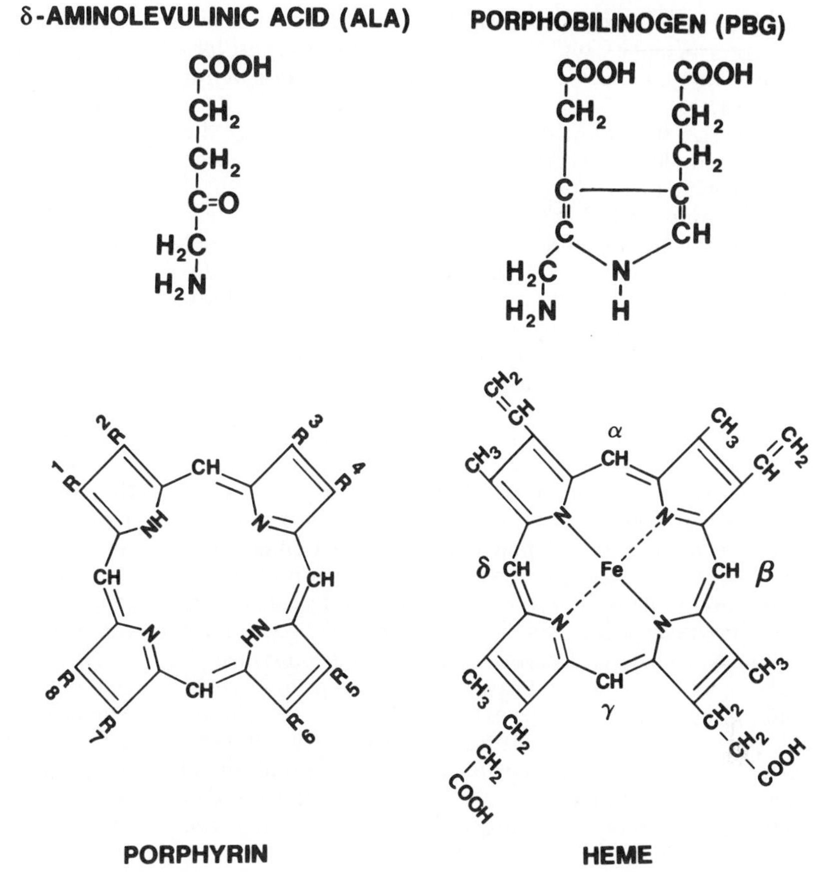

FIGURE 53-1 Structures of the porphyrin precursors δ-aminolevulinic acid, porphobilinogen, porphyrin, and heme. All porphyrins have the same tetrapyrrole ring structure, but they differ in the composition of side chains (R1–8) attached to the ring. Uroporphyrin has eight carboxylic acid side chains, coproporphyrin has four, and protoporphyrin has two. Porphyrinogens are the reduced forms of the porphyrins in which the methene bridges linking the four pyrrole groups are replaced by methylene groups.

PORPHYRIN   **HEME**

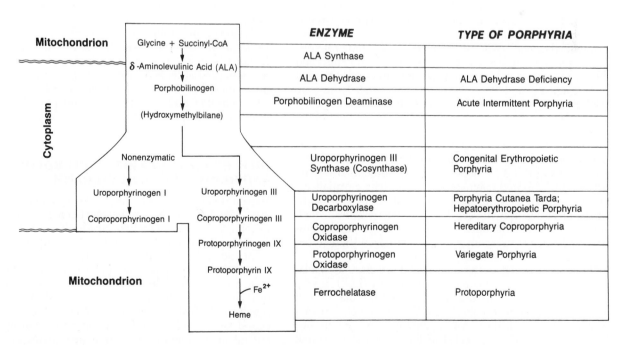

	ENZYME	TYPE OF PORPHYRIA
Mitochondrion Glycine + Succinyl-CoA		
δ-Aminolevulinic Acid (ALA)	ALA Synthase	
Porphobilinogen	ALA Dehydrase	ALA Dehydrase Deficiency
(Hydroxymethylbilane)	Porphobilinogen Deaminase	Acute Intermittent Porphyria
Nonenzymatic	Uroporphyrinogen III Synthase (Cosynthase)	Congenital Erythropoietic Porphyria
Uroporphyrinogen I / Uroporphyrinogen III	Uroporphyrinogen Decarboxylase	Porphyria Cutanea Tarda; Hepatoerythropoietic Porphyria
Coproporphyrinogen I / Coproporphyrinogen III	Coproporphyrinogen Oxidase	Hereditary Coproporphyria
Protoporphyrinogen IX	Protoporphyrinogen Oxidase	Variegate Porphyria
Protoporphyrin IX / Fe²⁺ / Heme	Ferrochelatase	Protoporphyria

FIGURE 53-2 Heme biosynthesis pathway, illustrating the enzyme abnormalities that characterize the different types of porphyria. Heme biosynthesis is distributed between the mitochondria and cytoplasm of the cell as shown.

mediate.[1,2,277] The reaction is catalyzed by the enzyme ALA synthase (succinyl CoA: glycine C-succinyl transferase [decarboxylating]; EC 2.3.1.37), and occurs in the matrix of mitochondria.

The ALA thus formed diffuses into the cytoplasm of the cell. Two molecules of ALA are condensed in a side-to-side manner with loss of two molecules water by the action of ALA dehydrase, EC 4.2.1.24.[117] The product of the condensation is the monopyrrole porphobilinogen (PBG; see Fig. 53-1). Note in Figure 53-1 that PBG has an acetate substituent at position 3 and a propionate at position 4. Four PBG molecules are then joined head to tail with the displacement of the four amino groups from the aminomethyl substituent, a reaction catalyzed by PBG deaminase (PBG ammonia lyase [polymerizing], EC 4.3.1.8), forming the linear tetrapyrrole hydroxymethylbilane.[6,15,48] Hydroxymethylbilane spontaneously cyclizes to form uroporphyrinogen I. (Porphyrinogens are structures comprising four pyrrole units joined by methylene [-CH$_2$-] groups; porphyrinogen molecules are nonplanar and nonaromatic.) This isomer has a four-fold axis of symmetry due to the distribution of substituents around its periphery; each pyrrole unit has an acetate and a propionate substituent, and in uroporphyrinogen I, these are strictly alternating. Enzymic cyclization of hydroxymethylbilane is region-specific and catalyzed by uroporphyrinogen III synthase (also called cosynthase; EC 4.2.1.75).[81,137,244] The result of this reaction is the destruction of the four-fold symmetry by reversing the sense of the fourth pyrrole unit (the D ring). Referring to Figure 53-1, the order of substituents after enzymic cyclization, beginning with group R1 through R8, is acetate-propionate (A ring), acetate-propionate (B ring), acetate-propionate (C ring), propionate-acetate (D ring).

Uroporphyrinogen decarboxylase (uroporphyrinogen carboxylase; EC 4.1.1.37) is a cytosolic enzyme that catalyzes the stepwise decarboxylation of each of the acetate substituents of uroporphyrinogen, leaving methyl substituents.[117,233,257] It is a unique decarboxylating enzyme in that no cofactors or coenzymes are involved.[233] The enzyme is active with both uroporphyrinogen I and III[110] but is not active with the oxidized form of the substrate, uroporphyrin. Uroporphyrinogen has eight carboxylate substituents, and during the course of the decarboxylation, intermediates that have seven, six, and five carboxylates are generated; these are referred to as heptacarboxylate, hexacarboxylate, and pentacarboxylate porphyrinogens, respectively. The product of the reaction is the tetracarboxylate coproporphyrinogen.

The next step in the pathway is catalyzed by coproporphyrinogen oxidase (coproporphyrinogen decarboxylase [oxidizing]; EC 1.3.3.3). The propionate substituents at R2 and R4 (see Fig. 53-1) of coproporphyrinogen III are oxidatively decarboxylated, forming the vinyl ($-CH = CH_2$) substituents of protoporphyrinogen IX.[109,202] The enzyme, which is located between the outer and inner mitochondrial membranes,[74] is active only with coproporphyrinogen III; no other isomer can serve as substrate.

Protoporphyrinogen IX undergoes a six-electron oxidation, catalyzed by protoporphyrinogen oxidase (EC 1.3.3.4). In mammalian liver, the reaction requires molecular oxygen as the final electron acceptor,[184] but the primary electron acceptor and, indeed, the electron pathway to oxygen are unknown. The enzyme is located in the inner mitochondrial membrane.

The final biochemical transformation in heme biosynthesis involves the insertion of divalent (ferrous) iron into pro-

toporphyrin IX, forming heme; the reaction is catalyzed by ferrochelatase (protoheme ferrolyase; EC 4.99.1.1). The enzyme is an integral protein of the inner mitochondrial membrane.[115] The enzyme is active with other dicarboxylic porphyrin substrates of the isomer IX series (eg, meso- and deuteroporphyrin IX) and with other divalent metal ions, such as Co(II) and Zn(II); it is not active with trivalent metals (eg, Fe[III] or Co[III]).[117,237] The enzyme has a monomeric molecular weight of about 40,000 but appears to function as a dimer in situ.[29,57,232]

HEME CATABOLISM

Heme biosynthesis is a metabolically expensive process. A single mole of heme requires 8 mol of succinyl-CoA, which costs the cell up to 64 mol of adenosine triphosphate (ATP) per mole of heme had the succinyl-CoA been metabolized through the citric acid cycle and normal electron transport. Little is known about the extent to which hepatic heme is recycled. Because heme, as well as uncomplexed iron, has been implicated in the production of reduced and highly toxic forms of oxygen, it is likely that most spent heme is catabolized rather than rerouted or reutilized.

Heme is catabolized in hepatocytes, granulocytes, and cells of the reticuloendothelial system in essentially two steps. The first step, catalyzed by heme oxygenase (EC 1.14.99.3), is the oxidative scission of the porphyrin ring.[238] Molecular oxygen bound to the heme iron oxidizes the α-carbon of the heme (ie, the bridge carbon between the A and B rings). That carbon is released as carbon monoxide and is the only naturally occurring reaction in mammalian systems in which carbon monoxide is formed. This release may be used as a measure of heme turnover in biologic systems. The iron is released, and the linear tetrapyrrole biliverdin IX-α is produced. In mammalian tissue, biliverdin undergoes a two-electron reduction catalyzed by biliverdin reductase (EC 1.3.1.24) at the central bridge carbon, producing bilirubin IX-α.[239]

Although biliverdin is water soluble, the configurational isomer of bilirubin produced by the action of biliverdin reductase (the Z,Z isomer) is water insoluble.[44] Bilirubin must be conjugated at its two carboxylate groups generally as the glucuronide before it can be excreted in bile.[258] Unconjugated bilirubin and bilirubin monoglucuronide and diglucuronide concentrations in serum may become altered in pathologic states.

DIFFERENCES BETWEEN ERYTHROPOIETIC AND HEPATIC HEME METABOLISM

Hepatic and erythropoietic heme biosynthesis are directed toward different ends. Where hepatic heme is destined primarily for cytochrome production, nearly all erythropoietic heme is incorporated into hemoglobin. Not surprisingly, overall heme biosynthesis is different in these two tissues. Besides a distinct difference in the ratios of the enzymes of the pathway, there appear to be different control mechanisms. Where hepatic heme biosynthesis is normally controlled by the level of activity of the first enzyme of the pathway, ALA synthase (discussed later), there is evidence that other steps may be important in the control of erythropoietic heme biosynthesis. Several of the enzymes of the pathway appear to be induced during erythroid differentiation.[203] It has been suggested from studies of erythroid cells in culture that ferrochelatase may have a rate-determining role in heme biosynthesis.[199] Heme is known to be a required cofactor in the protein elongation factor in reticulocyte systems,[64] so that the activation effect ascribed to heme on heme and hemoglobin biosynthesis in these cell cultures may be less direct than suggested.

CONTROL OF HEPATIC HEME BIOSYNTHESIS

The overall rate and therefore extent of hepatic heme biosynthesis is controlled primarily by the expression of ALA synthase activity (Fig. 53-3). Heme directly inhibits the enzyme allosterically.[211,264] Because the inhibition constant for heme is relatively high (about 10 μmol), however, this mode of control is probably not primary in controlling the rate of ALA synthesis.

ALA synthase exists as two tissue-specific enzymes.[52,191] One form is found in all tissues examined (ie, the housekeeping enzyme).[26] Hepatic ALA synthase is a dimer with mature subunit molecular weight between 50,000 and 65,000, the native molecular weight being about 110,000.[26] The gene encoding this enzyme has been mapped to the short arm of chromosome 3, most likely region 3p21.[26] Transcription of this gene in hepatic tissue is negatively controlled by heme.[151,152,220,227,272] In addition, posttranscriptional processing and transport of the gene product into the mitochondrion is inhibited by heme.[105,274] These two mechanisms appear to be the most important in controlling the level of ALA synthase activity and hence the rate of hepatic heme biosynthesis.

The second ALA synthase isoenzyme is expressed only in erythropoietic tissues.[26,52,191] It has been mapped to the X chromosome between Xp21 and Xq21, the most likely location on band Xp11.2.[52] X-linked sideroblastic anemia has been attributed to a hereditary defect in the production of the erythroid isoenzyme.[52] During erythroid differentiation, the tissue level of ALA synthase increases, but the control mechanism is unknown.

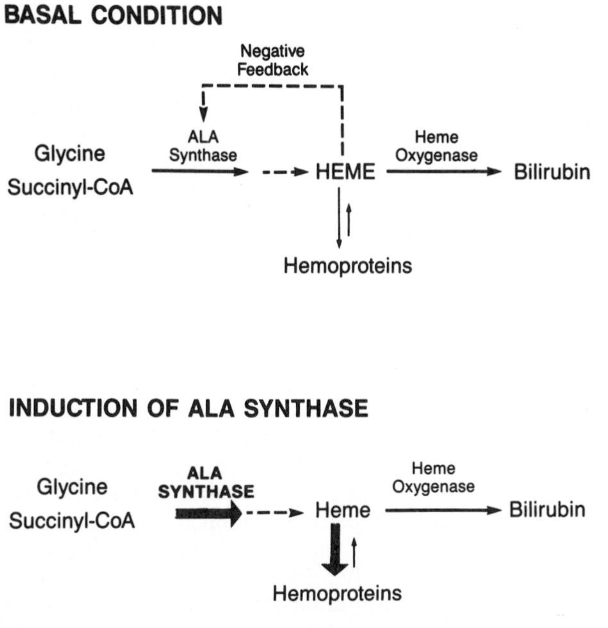

PBG deaminase, the second cytosolic enzyme of heme biosynthesis, is present at low levels in hepatic tissues.[117] The level of PBG deaminase activity is not affected by tissue heme concentrations.[117] Under conditions in which ALA synthase activity is increased (ie, low tissue heme concentration), the activity of PBG deaminase may become the rate-limiting enzyme of heme biosynthesis. Thus, drugs or toxins that place a strain on heme biosynthesis by inducing the synthesis of cytochrome P-450, thereby reducing the tissue concentration of heme, have been shown to result in increased hepatic ALA synthase activity.[117,151] If ALA synthase activity is sufficiently increased, PBG deaminase may not be present in sufficient quantity to keep up, resulting in accumulation of the two preceding substrates, PBG and ALA.

The only other enzyme present in relatively low concentrations is ferrochelatase. Ferrochelatase may become rate limiting in the liver under the influence of certain toxic compounds, such as allylisopropyl acetamide, griseofulvin, or diethyldihydrocollidine.[151,152] These compounds interact with the heme of cytochrome P-450, alkylating a central nitrogen atom of the heme, displacing the iron, and producing N-alkylated protoporphyrin IX species.[152] N-alkyl protoporphyrins are potent competitive inhibitors of ferrochelatase.[57,152]

Biochemical Features of the Porphyrias

The porphyrias are a family of inborn errors of metabolism, each caused by a decrease in the expressed activity of one of the enzymes of heme biosynthesis. The importance of this pathway for life is suggested by the fact that the normal activities of the enzymes of the pathway are at sufficiently high levels that nonlethal deficiency diseases may exist at each step.

ENZYME ABNORMALITIES IN THE PORPHYRIAS

An enzyme deficiency at a particular step in heme biosynthesis results in the predictable accumulation of biochemical intermediates proximal to that step (Table 53-1; see Fig. 53-2), whereas net heme biosynthesis appears to remain adequate in most cases. For example, a deficiency of uroporphyrinogen decarboxylase leads to an accumulation of uroporphyrinogen and partially decarboxylated intermediates (heptacarboxylate through pentacarboxylate porphyrinogens) as well as the abnormal isomer form of these intermediates. People with PCT, however, are not anemic and are still capable of nearly normal liver function.

Certain of the porphyrias, notably acute intermittent porphyria (AIP), ALA dehydrase deficiency, hereditary coproporphyria (HCP), and variegate porphyria (VP), result in an increase in the level of hepatic ALA synthase activity.[32,117] As an example, AIP results from a deficiency in PBG deaminase activity[117] (Fig. 53-4). As noted, this enzyme is present at relatively low levels under normal circumstances. Thus, a genetically derived depression of this enzyme level would presumably lead to decreased heme production and an in-

BASAL CONDITION

INDUCTION OF ALA SYNTHASE

FIGURE 53-3 Control of hepatic heme biosynthesis. Under basal conditions, the rate-limiting enzyme in the pathway, δ-aminolevulinic acid (ALA) synthase, is under negative feedback control by a putative regulatory heme pool. An increased demand for hepatic heme biosyntheses, such as occurs when there is formation of more cytochrome P-450 or other hemoproteins, may deplete this pool. This removes the negative feedback control, which causes induction of ALA synthase and thereby increases the synthesis of porphyrins and porphyrin precursors.

TABLE 53-1   *Major Clinical and Biochemical Features of the Porphyrias*

Type of Porphyria	Inheritance	Neurologic Dysfunction	Photocutaneous Lesions	Major Site of Biochemical Abnormality	Principal Biochemical Features
Protoporphyria	Autosomal dominant	−	+	Bone marrow (liver variable)	Protoporphyrin in red cells, bile, and feces
Porphyria cutanea tarda	Autosomal dominant	−	+	Liver	Uroporphyrin in urine; isocoproporphyrin in feces
Hepatoerythropoietic porphyria	Autosomal recessive	−	+	Bone marrow and liver	Zn-protoporphyrin in red cells; uroporphyrin in urine; isocoproporphyrin in feces
Congenital erythropoietic porphyria	Autosomal recessive	−	+	Bone marrow	Uroporphyrin in urine; uroporphyrin and coproporphyrin in feces
Acute intermittent porphyria	Autosomal dominant	+	−	Liver	ALA and PBG in urine
Variegate porphyria	Autosomal dominant	+	+	Liver	ALA, PBG, and coproporphyrin in urine; protoporphyrin in bile and feces
Hereditary coproporphyria	Autosomal dominant	+	+	Liver	ALA, PBG, and coproporphyrin in urine; coproporphyrin in feces
ALA dehydrase deficiency	Autosomal recessive	+	−	Liver	ALA in urine

crease in the activity of ALA synthase. The increase in ALA synthase activity has two significant results. First, overproduction of ALA leads to maintenance of excessive concentrations of the substrate PBG, which by mass action drives the production of sufficient hydroxymethylbilane to support adequate heme synthesis for normal cell metabolism. Second, the precursors ALA and PBG accumulate behind the blocked step. The acute attack abates when sufficient heme is produced (or exogenous heme is administered) to reduce ALA synthase activity to normal levels, and production of ALA and PBG returns toward normal levels.[43]

Similar arguments may be made for any of the porphyrias that exhibit neurologic symptoms. In the case of VP, it has been shown that protoporphyrinogen IX, which accumulates behind defective protoporphyrinogen oxidase, appears to inhibit PBG deaminase.[47,155] As might be predicted, this also leads, during an acute attack of VP, to neurologic symptoms similar to those seen in AIP.[32]

GENETIC DEFECTS IN THE PORPHYRIAS

Specific protein and genetic defects have been demonstrated in several of the porphyrias (Table 53-2). Of the diseases thus far studied, all have shown genetic polymorphism in the nature of genetic defects. Insufficient studies have been conducted to determine the extent to which genetic polymorphism exists in the normally expressed forms of these enzymes.

AIP results from a decrease in the activity of PBG deaminase. The gene for PBG deaminase has been described.[50,99,198] It comprises 15 exons and has been shown to possess two promoter sites separated by about 3 kb. The upstream site is active in nonerythroid tissues; the downstream site is active only in erythroid tissues and codes for a protein that has 17 fewer amino acids at the amino terminus than that coded by the upstream promoter.[99,198]

At least four types of AIP have been described on the basis of the ratio of cross-reactive immunologic material (CRIM) to enzyme activity found in tissues of people with AIP.[66] For the purposes of this discussion, normal CRIM/enzyme activity ratio is defined as unity. A CRIM-positive mutation is one in which CRIM is found at normal or increased levels while enzyme activity is reduced; that is, CRIM/activity ratios are significantly greater than 1. A CRIM-negative mutation is one in which CRIM is reduced roughly in proportion to the decrease in enzyme level; CRIM/activity ratio remains about 1. In AIP, two CRIM-positive and two CRIM-negative patterns have been described.

In AIP, CRIM-negative type 1, enzyme activity and CRIM are both reduced to about half of normal in all tissues, including erythrocytes. Major gene deletions had been ruled out in most cases by investigation of the Msp I restriction fragment length polymorphism.[145] Although this is the most common form of AIP, the gene defect has been characterized in only one family. A point mutation (C to T) in exon 9 resulted in conversion of a glutamine codon to a stop codon, resulting in a prematurely truncated peptide that had neither enzyme activity nor immunoreactivity.[214] This mutation was found in only 1 of 43 unrelated patients studied; thus, the CRIM-negative type 1 form of this disease presumably has more extensive polymorphism.

The CRIM-negative type 2 form of AIP is curious in that normal levels of both enzyme activity and CRIM are expressed in red blood cells (RBCs).[66,97] The gene defect in this form of the disease is a single base (G to A) substitution in the canonical 5′-splice donor site of intron 1.[98] The result

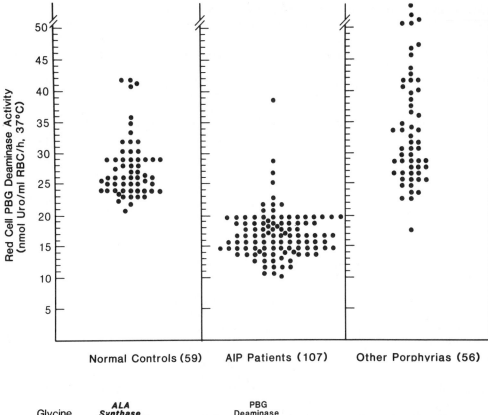

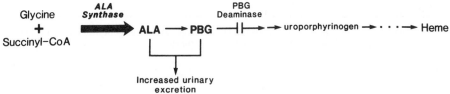

FIGURE 53-4 Enzyme defect in acute intermittent porphyria (AIP). (**Top**) Porphobilinogen (PBG) deaminase activity is deficient in tissues of patients with AIP compared with normal controls and patients with other types of porphyria. (**Bottom**) As a consequence of the deficient PBG deaminase activity, patients with AIP excrete increased amounts of δ-aminolevulinic acid (ALA) and PBG in their urine, particularly when ALA synthase is induced. (Pierach CA, Weimer MK, Cardinal RA, Bossenmaier IC, Bloomer JR. Red blood cell porphobilinogen deaminase in the evaluation of acute intermittent porphyria. JAMA 257:60–61, 1987; copyright 1987, American Medical Association)

is that nonerythroid PBG deaminase is not expressed by the mutant allele. Because the erythroid (downstream) promoter is below the mutation site, erythroid expression of the enzyme is unaffected, leading to the observed phenotype.

The CRIM-positive type 1 form of AIP is characterized by a CRIM/activity ratio of about 2. It was identified with an abnormal protein that possessed either increased substrate affinity or low rate of conversion of bound intermediate forms.[66] Based on CRIM/activity ratios reported, three gene defects thus far have been identified corresponding to this form. In one patient, a G-to-A mutation in exon 12 resulted in the skipping of exon 12 during transcription; the gene product of exon 11 is followed immediately by the product of exon 13.[96] The result was a protein that had no enzyme activity but that was stable and immunologically cross-reactive. A second study[65] found two distinct G to A substitutions in exon 10, one at base position 500 (resulting in arginine-[167]

to glutamate), the other at position 518 (arginine-[173] to glutamate). Both mutations resulted in proteins with significantly decreased (less than 1% of normal) enzyme activity, when measured at the normal pH of 8.0; the protein expressed by the 500-position mutation had a shift in pH optimum to between 6.5 and 7.0, where the activity was increased about three-fold over that when measured at a pH of 8.0. Of eight unrelated CRIM-positive patients studied, four had the mutation at position 500, two at 518, and two at neither site.

A retrospective study of a compound heterozygosity at the PBG deaminase locus has been described, which led to a lethal form of AIP.[22,172] The propositus had died 20 years previously at the age of 7. Each parent was found to have a different G-to-A point mutation, the father at position 500 and the mother at position 518. The affected child presumably inherited two distinct mutant alleles, yielding a homozygous phenotype.

TABLE 53-2   *Gene and Protein Defects in the Porphyrias*

Porphyria	Enzyme Abnormality		Gene Defect	CRIM	Protein Defect
ALA dehydrase deficiency	ALA dehydrase		Compound heterozygosity A [820] to G and C[168] to T	—	ala [274] to thr and ?
Acute intermittent porphyria	PBG deaminase	(a)	C[412] to T in exon 9	Negative, type 1	gln [138], erythroid } gln [155], housekeeping } truncated protein
		(b)	G to A, splice donor site, intron 1	Negative, type 2	Nonerythroid enzyme (allele) not expressed, but erythroid enzyme expressed
		(c)	G[500] to A } G[518] to A } in exon 10	Positive, type 1	arg [167] to glu } Decreased enzyme activity arg [173] to glu } Normal immunoreactivity
		(d)	?	Positive, type 2	?; Enzyme-substrate complex(es) stabilize protein against proteolysis
Congenital erythropoietic porphyria	Uroporphyrinogen III synthase	(a)	Homozygous, C[158] to T	—	pro [53] to leu
		(b)	Compound heterozygosity, C[158] to T and T[216] to C	—	pro [53] to leu: cys [73] to arg
Porphyria cutanea tarda	Uroporphyrinogen decarboxylase	(a)	G to C, splice site intron 6: transcription of exon 6 skipped	Negative	Shortened protein: decreased half-life
		(b)	G[860] to T	Negative	gly [281] to val: decreased half-life
Hepatoerythropoietic porphyria	Uroporphyrinogen decarboxylase		G[860] to A	Negative	gly (281) to glu: decreased half-life

CRIM, cross-reacting immunologic material detected by antibody made against normal enzyme protein; A, adenine; G, guanine; C, cytosine; T, thymidine; ala, alanine; thr, threonine; gln, glutamine; arg, arginine; glu, glutamate; pro, proline; leu, leucine; cys, cysteine; gly, glycine; val, valine

The final CRIM-positive type 2 mutation leads to a CRIM/activity ratio of about 5.[66] The resulting protein has a high affinity for enzyme-bound intermediate products or defective product release. These intermediate forms render the protein more resistant to proteolytic digestion, in turn leading to the markedly high CRIM/activity ratio. No gene studies have been described that correspond to this form of the disease.

Porphyria cutanea tarda (PCT) and hepatoerythropoietic porphyria (HEP) are both results of decreased uroporphyrinogen decarboxylase activity. The former exists as familial PCT, which is inherited as an autosomal dominant trait, and as sporadic PCT, in which no inheritance patterns are seen.[256] HEP results from an apparent homozygous defect in the enzyme and is inherited as an autosomal recessive trait.[77] Exposure to certain toxic chemicals, such as hexachlorobenzene, pentachlorophenol, and certain polyhalogenated biphenyls, may lead to chemical PCT (also called toxic porphyria), similar to the other PCT syndromes in biochemical and pathophysiologic expression.[117]

The gene for uroporphyrinogen decarboxylase comprises 10 exons and extends over about 3 kb.[197] There appears to be considerable genetic polymorphism for the normal gene[87] as well as for mutations that lead to familial PCT and HEP.

A mutation has been described that has been found in 5 of 22 unrelated families with PCT.[88] This is a point G-to-C mutation at the 5' end of intron 6, leading to skipping the 162 bases of exon 6 during transcription. The protein encoded by the mutant gene lacks only those amino acids encoded by exon 6. The mutant protein was found to have no catalytic activity with either urocarboxylate or pentacarboxylate porphyrinogen, and appeared to have a short half-life in vivo. This combination leads to the observed CRIM-negative phenotype of the patients.

Two point mutations in the structural gene encoding amino acid 281 have been found. One was found in two of five unrelated families with HEP.[254,255] The glycine-281–to–glutamate substitution resulted in a protein with a greatly shortened in vivo half-life. The second was found in a single kindred with PCT.[87] In this case, a glycine-281–to–valine substitution again encoded a protein with a half-life that was about 10% of normal. The shortened half-life of these proteins leads to the predicted CRIM-negative phenotype of the affected patients.

Although all other reports of HEP describe a CRIM-negative phenotype, a report of a single patient with a CRIM-positive form of HEP has been reported.[126] Enzyme activity was reduced to about 24% of normal, but the CRIM was found at a level comparable to normal controls. No further genetic studies have been done on this patient.

Congenital erythropoietic porphyria (CEP; Günther's disease) is the result of decreased uroporphyrinogen III synthase activity. Two patients with CEP have been studied at the gene level.[67] One patient had two coexistent point mutations leading to cysteine-[73]–to–arginine and proline-[53]–to–leucine substitutions. The second patient was found to be homozygous for the proline-[53]–to–leucine substitution. Either of these mutations would be predicted to lead to major changes in protein conformation, as well as to changes in catalytic activity or substrate affinity and to the observed low level of enzyme activity.

A single case of ALA dehydrase deficiency porphyria has been studied at the gene level.[108] This patient showed compound heterozygosity for point mutations at the ALA dehydrase locus. One was identified with an alanine-[274]–to–threonine substitution; the second had not yet been characterized.

SECONDARY ABNORMALITIES IN THE PORPHYRIAS

Besides the primary effect of the genetic lesion, certain of the porphyrias have secondary biochemical and pathophysiologic effects. For example, PCT shows altered iron metabolism.[82]

Studies of chemical PCT induced in rodents have shown that excess hepatic iron exacerbates the porphyric effect of the toxins. The role of excess iron in the pathology of either the familial or sporadic form of PCT is not entirely clear. Although some direct inhibition of the enzyme is demonstrable,[129] the degree of inhibition is far too low to account solely for the diminution of enzyme activity seen.[233] One study suggested that iron promotes oxidation of both substrate and enzyme, the effects synergistically decreasing enzyme activity.[161]

Studies of chemically induced porphyria have demonstrated that the P-450 IA2 isoenzyme inducible by methylcholanthrene,[111] polychlorinated or polybrominated biphenyls, or hexachlorobenzene[223] interacts with uroporphyrinogen, producing oxidized uroporphyrin as well as a heat-stable inhibitor of uroporphyrinogen decarboxylase, possibly an oxidation product of uroporphyrin.[85,221] Iron loading the animals exacerbates chemically induced porphyria[221,236] and induces hepatocellular carcinoma in susceptible strains.[222] Furthermore, the cytochrome P-450 mediated oxidation of uroporphyrinogen was increased in the presence of iron–EDTA complex.[112]

In vitro studies have demonstrated oxidation of unsaturated lipid in systems composed of uroporphyrinogen, iron (III), and lecithin liposomes.[147] Porphyrinogens readily undergo spontaneous 6-electron oxidations, passing electrons to molecular oxygen. The reduced oxygen species in the presence of iron undergo Haber-Weiss and Fenton chemistry,[163] the products of which are potent oxidizing agents for unsaturated fatty acids. These studies demonstrated that uroporphyrinogen oxidation was accelerated in the presence of all components of the system, with concomitant formation of lipid oxidation products.

Rat hepatic microsomes can also catalyze a one-electron reduction of uroporphyrin I.[159] The reduced porphyrin may disproportionate or react with oxygen to produce reduced oxygen species, which may in turn oxidize lipids, as noted previously.

The complicated interactions of uroporphyrinogen, hepatic microsomes, lipids, and iron complexes are likely to be responsible for some of the biochemical and physiologic abnormalities seen in PCT. The exact nature of these interactions requires further careful and methodical study of these systems.

EXCRETORY ROUTES OF PORPHYRINS AND PORPHYRIN PRECURSORS

Excretion of intermediates of the heme pathway follows the routes predicted on the basis of their solubility: water-soluble compounds are excreted in the urine, water-insoluble compounds in feces through the biliary system. The first two intermediates, ALA and PBG, both of which are highly water soluble, are excreted in urine, and urinary levels of these compounds are diagnostic for ALA dehydrase deficiency and acute attacks of AIP, HCP, and VP.[138,234] Uroporphyrin, with eight carboxylate substituents around the periphery of the tetrapyrrole nucleus, is the most soluble tetrapyrrole; coproporphyrin, with four carboxylates, is intermediate, and protoporphyrin, with two, is insoluble in water. As predicted, uroporphyrin is excreted mostly in urine; intermediates with seven through five carboxylates and coproporphyrin progressively segregate from urine toward bile (feces), and protoporphyrin is excreted exclusively in bile.[33,146,234] Unlike other compounds excreted in bile, the porphyrins are not conjugated with glucuronate, sulfate, and so forth before excretion. An exception may be the protoporphyrinogen accumulated in VP, where a porphyrin X is found in serum and urine.[146,195] This was shown in an early study to be convertible to protoporphyrin by treatment with silver,[18] suggesting a thioether-linked (proto)porphyrin peptide. Thus, protoporphyrinogen may be handled differently from its oxidized congener.

DIAGNOSIS OF PORPHYRIAS

The excretion pattern of heme biosynthesis intermediates in conjunction with clinical symptoms is used for diagnosis of the porphyrias. Accumulation of intermediates in body fluids and excreta are predictable from knowledge of the pathway and excretion patterns. In some cases (discussed previously), genetic screening tests may soon be available; although with the considerable polymorphisms thus far found, measurement of enzyme activity may be the most sound means for definitive diagnosis.

Protoporphyria

The first case of protoporphyria was reported by Magnus and coworkers in 1961.[150] They described a 35-year-old man who had had intense itching and swelling of his skin on exposure to sunlight since childhood. The patient's urinary excretion of porphyrins and porphyrin precursors was normal, but his RBCs and feces contained excessive amounts of protoporphyrin, and the authors proposed the name *erythropoietic protoporphyria* for his condition. Because subsequent reports indicated that the liver contributes to the increased amount of protoporphyrin excreted in feces, the term *erythrohepatic protoporphyria* has also been used to describe this condition. Protoporphyria is preferred by many authors because it avoids controversy about the sources of the excess protoporphyrin.

Protoporphyria occurs in all ethnic groups. Although the precise incidence and prevalence has not been determined for any group, it is generally believed that protoporphyria is a relatively common type of porphyria, probably having a frequency that is second only to PCT. A reasonable estimate of the prevalence is 1 in 5000 to 10,000 people.

The pattern of inheritance is considered to be that of an autosomal dominant disorder with variable expression.[103] Indeed, some people who are putative carriers of the gene defect may have no clinical manifestations of the disease, and their porphyrin levels may be normal. One study, however, has postulated on the basis of family studies that the inheritance is better described as autosomal recessive with a three allele system.[271] There is no difference in the frequency of the disorder between sexes, either for the gene defect or clinically expressed disease.

BIOCHEMICAL FEATURES

The biochemical hallmark of protoporphyria is an increased level of protoporphyrin in RBCs and feces. The excess protoporphyrin is not complexed with any metal, unlike iron deficiency and lead poisoning, where the excess RBC protoporphyrin is chelated to zinc.[131] The diagnosis of protoporphyria is established by demonstrating an elevated RBC protoporphyrin level in a patient who has the typical clinical features.

The excess accumulation and excretion of protoporphyrin reflects a deficiency of ferrochelatase activity in heme-forming tissues of the patient[37,45,63] (Figs. 53-2 and 53-5). This deficiency is found in liver tissue, bone marrow cells, peripheral blood cells, mitogen-stimulated lymphocytes, and cultured skin fibroblasts. It is transmitted as an autosomal dom-

inant trait in families with protoporphyria.[28] A notable, and as yet unexplained, feature of the enzyme abnormality is that most studies have found the level of ferrochelatase activity to be decreased to 20% to 30% of normal.

Patients with protoporphyria do not excrete increased amounts of PBG and ALA. This implies that hepatic ALA synthase activity is not increased, although in vitro measurements have shown otherwise in some instances.[174] Most patients appear to make normal amounts of heme in both liver tissue and bone marrow, but about 25% have a mild anemia characterized by microcytic indices.[153] Iron metabolism is normal,[249] and iron deficiency can exacerbate the accumulation of protoporphyrin in RBCs.[95] Once the RBC enters the circulation, protoporphyrin is released into the plasma within a few days, unless liver disease is present, and is cleared by the liver for excretion in bile.[177] Thus, the excess protoporphyrin in circulating blood is found predominantly in young RBCs.

The bone marrow is the major source of excess protoporphyrin in most patients with protoporphyria since the daily fecal excretion of protoporphyrin can often be accounted for on the basis of protoporphyrin released from young RBCs. Studies using radiolabeled precursors of protoporphyrin have indicated that the liver may also contribute to excess protoporphyrin production,[164,212] although the interpretation of those studies has been controversial.[213] In addition, metabolic balance studies that have compared fecal protopor-

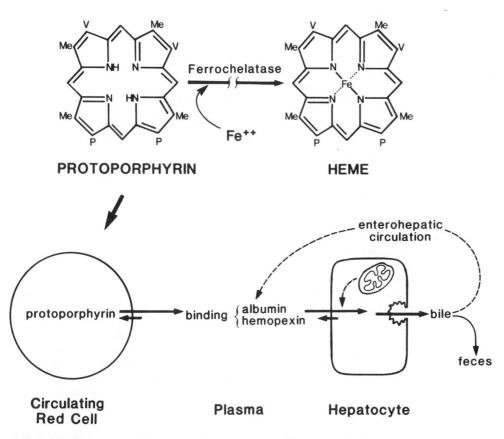

FIGURE 53-5 Protoporphyrin metabolism in protoporphyria. As a consequence of deficient ferrochelatase activity, protoporphyrin accumulates in heme-forming tissues—primarily the bone marrow, with a variable contribution from the liver. This excess protoporphyrin undergoes biliary excretion. An enterohepatic circulation of protoporphyrin contributes to the amount that the liver must excrete in bile. (Bloomer JR. The liver in protoporphyria. Hepatology 8:402–407, 1988)

phyrin excretion to the total mass of RBC protoporphyrin have occasionally demonstrated a significant discrepancy, indicating a hepatic contribution.[179] The amount of excess protoporphyrin produced by the liver may be different among patients because of the variable presence of factors that modulate hepatic ferrochelatase activity.[122]

PHOTOSENSITIVITY

The principal clinical manifestation in protoporphyria is photosensitivity. This is usually lifelong, often first experienced in infancy. Rarely, the photosensitivity has its onset in adulthood. Patients usually describe the photosensitivity as burning or stinging of the skin on exposure to sunlight.[178] Window glass does not prevent the reaction, since the wavelength of light that produces the symptoms (400 to 410 nm) is not filtered by window glass. Some patients also have photosensitivity caused by light emitted from fluorescent fixtures. Erythema and edema of the skin subsequently develop and may persist for several days. Unlike the skin lesions in PCT, the development of vesicles and erosions is rare, perhaps because patients avoid the duration of sun exposure that would cause significant tissue damage. Chronic skin changes, however, are frequently noted in patients who have repeated sun exposure. These are characterized by thickening and lichenification of the skin over the nose and the dorsum of the hand, with the presence of shallow scars.[178] Microscopic examination of the skin demonstrates the deposition of material seen by periodic acid–Schiff staining around the walls of capillaries in the dermis.[80]

Photosensitivity is caused by the excess protoporphyrin that is circulating in blood or is deposited in skin tissue, or by a combination of the two. Experimental studies have shown that cells may be damaged when they are incubated with protoporphyrin and exposed to light with wavelengths of 400 to 410 nm[80] (Fig. 53-6). Absorption of light energy by the porphyrin molecule raises the molecule to an excited state, which can then react with molecular oxygen to produce reactive oxygen species. Cell membranes and mitochondria appear to be the principal targets for protoporphyrin-induced damage.[201] The photoinduced damage is attributed to cross-linking of membrane proteins and peroxidation of membrane lipids.[92,94] A role for the activation of complement in the pathogenesis of skin lesions has also been proposed since complement is depleted in serum containing protoporphyrin when the serum is exposed to light.[91] Mast cells have been shown to release serotonin and arachidonic acid when incubated with protoporphyrin and exposed to ultraviolet light,[139] which would contribute to the photosensitivity as well.

HEPATOBILIARY DISEASE

In 1963, two years after the first clinical report of protoporphyria, a 6-year-old boy with the biochemical features of protoporphyria, hepatosplenomegaly, and abnormal liver chemistries was reported.[183] At the time of subsequent splenectomy, he was found to have a cirrhotic liver. It was not until 1968, however, that it was appreciated that patients with protoporphyria may develop liver disease that progresses to liver failure.[14] Since then, there have been several reports of this occurrence. The frequency remains uncertain, but less than 10% of all patients with protoporphyria appear to develop this complication.

Liver failure has occurred in both men and women. The patients generally have been adults, with only a few cases described in children.[54] The synergistic effect of alcohol has been reported in one case,[40] but liver disease usually has not been associated with other causes of liver damage and thus

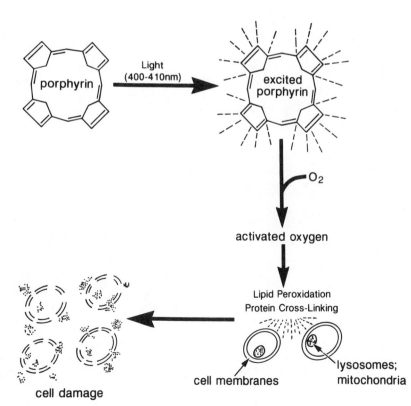

FIGURE 53-6 Sequence by which damage to skin and other tissues may be produced when porphyrins are exposed to light in the presence of molecular oxygen. Uroporphyrin preferentially causes injury to lysosomes in cells, whereas cell membranes and mitochondria appear to be the principal targets in protoporphyrin-induced damage.

appears to be a feature of protoporphyria itself. Laboratory studies in patients with this complication have been nonspecific, showing variable hyperbilirubinemia with mild to moderate increases in the serum transaminase and alkaline phosphatase levels. RBC protoporphyrin levels have been significantly higher than occurs in the usual patient with protoporphyria, ranging from 1404 to 36,800 μg/dL.[40] Along with signs and symptoms of hepatic decompensation, these patients have experienced severe abdominal pain located in the upper abdomen and often radiating into the back. Once jaundice has developed in a patient with protoporphyria, prognosis is poor, and death usually occurs within a few months.

The livers of patients who have died in hepatic failure, or who have come to liver transplantation, have been black in color. The appearance is due to massive deposits of protoporphyrin pigment in hepatocytes, macrophages, Kupffer cells, and biliary structures. The pigment deposits are birefringent when examined by polarization microscopy[30,121] due to the fact that they are composed of crystals[160] (Fig. 53-7).

The liver damage in protoporphyria appears to be caused by the progressive accumulation of protoporphyrin in the liver. Regardless of the tissue source of the excess protoporphyrin, the only means for its excretion is by hepatic clearance and secretion into bile[194] (see Fig. 53-5). During this process, protoporphyrin is kept in solution through protein binding since it is a poorly water-soluble compound that aggregates in aqueous solution. In plasma, most of the protoporphyrin is bound to albumin, with some bound to hemopexin.[130] Within the hepatocyte, it is associated with several proteins, among which is the Z class of liver cytosolic proteins.[259] Protoporphyrin may aggregate and form solid deposits within hepatocytes and small biliary radicles when the solubilizing capacity of the liver and bile for the compound is exceeded. These deposits cause obstruction to bile flow and

damage hepatocytes. Experimental studies have demonstrated that protoporphyrin is also toxic to the liver when it remains in solution. Perfusion of the isolated rat liver with protoporphyrin causes a significant reduction in bile flow.[9] Histologic examination of these livers shows canalicular dilation and distortion, and membrane ATPase activity is reduced.[8] Membrane dysfunction is presumably caused when the lipophilic protoporphyrin molecule intercalates into the membrane and alters the physical chemical properties of the membrane.[78,230]

Because protoporphyrin accumulation in the liver appears to be responsible for liver damage in protoporphyria, it is likely that patients at risk for this complication have a greater abnormality in protoporphyrin metabolism than usual. Indeed, RBC and plasma protoporphyrin levels are significantly higher in patients with liver disease than in normal patients, and the distribution of protoporphyrin according to RBC age changes.[31,133] The ratio of fecal protoporphyrin excretion to the total RBC protoporphyrin content is decreased. Patients with liver disease have a ratio that is less than 0.05, whereas the ratio in patients without liver disease exceeds 0.1.[133] Finally, the ratio of the concentration of protoporphyrin to bile acids in bile of patients with liver disease is significantly higher than in normal patients.[160] These abnormalities, however, have been documented only in patients who already had advanced liver disease. It has not been determined whether these measurements identify patients who are likely to develop liver damage.

Although the frequency of clinical liver disease is not high in patients with protoporphyria, a much greater number of patients have histologic abnormalities in liver biopsy specimens.[55,158] These consist of focal deposits of protoporphyrin pigment, along with portal fibrosis and inflammation. Changes in bile canalicular ultrastructure occur early in hepatic involvement.[186] Patients also appear to have an in-

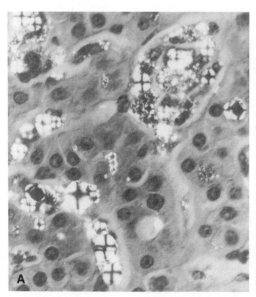 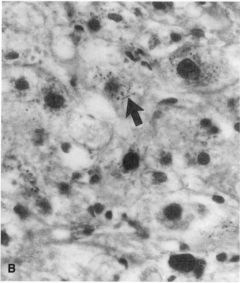

FIGURE 53-7 Hepatic crystals in protoporphyria and porphyria cutanea tarda. (**A**) Polarization microscopy of a liver biopsy specimen from a patient with protoporphyria shows that protoporphyrin pigment deposits are birefringent because they contain crystals. Some deposits have the appearance of a Maltese cross. (**B**) Light microscopy shows needle-like crystals (*arrow*) in a liver biopsy specimen of a patient with porphyria cutanea tarda. (Snover DC. Biopsy diagnosis of liver disease. Baltimore, Williams & Wilkins, 1991)

creased frequency of gallstones, which contain protoporphyrin as one of their substituents.

MANAGEMENT

Photosensitivity in protoporphyria is prevented by having patients avoid sunlight and wear protective clothing. Sunscreens that block the long ultraviolet spectrum (most do not) can also be applied. Oral administration of β-carotene may be effective in some patients; the usual adult dose is 60 to 180 mg/d.

No definitive means has been established to identify patients who are susceptible to serious hepatic disease or to follow the progression of hepatic damage. Any patient with abnormalities in routine tests of liver function or with a higher than usual concentration of RBC protoporphyrin (greater than 1500 μg/dL) should be observed closely, and liver biopsy should be considered to define the patient's status better.

Several options are available to alter the abnormal protoporphyrin metabolism responsible for liver disease in protoporphyria. Since the excess protoporphyrin comes mainly from bone marrow, transfusion therapy has been used to suppress erythropoiesis and thereby lower blood protoporphyrin levels.[70] Exchange transfusion has been used for the same effect,[226] as has the administration of hematin.[31] Iron deficiency may exacerbate the excessive accumulation of protoporphyrin, and iron therapy has successfully reduced protoporphyrin levels and improved hepatic function in some patients.[95] Because other patients have had their clinical and biochemical features worsened by iron therapy,[156] careful monitoring of porphyrin levels is advised.

In addition to measures to decrease the formation of excess protoporphyrin, therapy to facilitate its excretion can be attempted. Based on experimental studies, bile acids should enhance the biliary excretion of protoporphyrin.[7,182] Unexpectedly, RBC and bile levels diminished when chenodeoxycholic acid was administered to patients,[251] suggesting that this bile acid may reduce the synthesis of protoporphyrin or facilitate its conversion to heme, rather than just promoting its excretion in bile. Ursodeoxycholic acid has not received clinical trails, but experimental studies indicate that it is not as efficacious as cholic acid and chenodeoxycholic acid in promoting biliary excretion and may enhance the precipitation of protoporphyrin in bile canaliculi.[21] Because protoporphyrin undergoes an enterohepatic circulation,[107] cholestyramine administration can be used to bind it in the intestine and thereby diminish the amount presented to the liver.[154]

The more definitive therapy for the patient with significant complications of protoporphyria is bone marrow transplantation to replace the affected tissue with normal tissue. Unfortunately, this could be hazardous to the patient who already has liver damage if graft-versus-host disease develops. As mentioned previously, there is no precise means by which to identify in advance the patient who is likely to develop liver failure, which would be the ideal situation for bone marrow transplantation. Thus, liver transplantation has become the major option for patients in whom liver disease is so advanced that other therapeutic options are not beneficial. Several patients with protoporphyria and liver failure have undergone successful liver transplantation. These patients present unique problems during the transplantation and post-transplantation periods due to their abnormal protoporphyrin metabolism. In particular, they are susceptible to photodamage of their tissues from operating room lights.[34] Their tissues should be protected from light as much as possible during the operation, and the use of filters that screen out light with wavelengths less than 450 nm should be considered. After transplantation, the new liver also remains susceptible to damage since the bone marrow production of excess protoporphyrin continues.

Porphyria Cutanea Tarda

The history of PCT is traced to Günther's description of three patients who had the late onset of cutaneous lesions but lacked abdominal pain and paresis.[100,101] Günther called the disease haematoporphyria chronica. The label *porphyria cutanea tarda* was first used by Waldenström in the late 1930s to distinguish this disorder from the porphyrias with cutaneous lesions in which attacks of neurologic dysfunction also occurred.[261] The term was given because the disorder occurred late, commonly in the fourth decade of life or later. The familial form of PCT, however, may have its onset in childhood.[58,72,185]

PCT is the most common porphyria with overt clinical expression in the United States, but the exact prevalence is unknown. It is strongly associated with ethanol use and is thus seen more frequently in societies where alcohol intake is high. Among the Bantu of South Africa, a strikingly high prevalence is seen. This has been attributed to the ingestion of a local beer brewed in iron pots.[13,61] The disorder is more common in men, but the proportion of women with PCT has been increasing. This reflects the use of oral contraceptives and estrogen preparations, which can precipitate PCT.[17]

Although most cases are sporadic and related to ethanol or estrogen use, several kindreds have been described in which there is autosomal dominant inheritance with variable penetrance.[75,83,128,205] In contrast to the sporadic cases in which the enzyme defect is restricted to the liver, the familial cases additionally have a defect in RBC uroporphyrinogen decarboxylase.[76] PCT can also be acquired. In the late 1950s, an epidemic occurred in Turkey after the widespread ingestion of seed grain that had been treated with the fungicide hexachlorobenzene, which is a polyhalogenated aromatic hydrocarbon.[60,208] Experimental porphyria mimicking PCT has been induced with a number of related compounds, including polychlorinated and polybrominated biphenyl and dioxin compounds.[218]

Many disorders have been associated with the development of PCT, including systemic lupus erythematous, rheumatoid arthritis, and Sjögren's syndrome.[53,167,187] Recent reports of an association with acquired immunodeficiency syndrome have begun to appear. Elevations of porphyrin levels in dialysate, plasma, and urine of patients on chronic hemodialysis have been reported.[3,125,181,216] These changes could be seen whether or not cutaneous lesions develop.[216] Treatment of hemodialysis-related PCT with erythropoietin, plasma exchange, and desferoxamine has been reported to be beneficial.[4,69]

BIOCHEMICAL FEATURES

The diagnosis of PCT is generally made on a clinical basis, but biochemical conformation is necessary to differentiate PCT from the other cutaneous porphyrias.[27] Classically, there is an increase in urinary uroporphyrin as the type I isomer. Urinary hexacarboxyl and heptacarboxyl porphyrins are also elevated, mainly as the type III isomer. Coproporphyrin and pentacarboxyl porphyrins are elevated to a lesser degree in the urine and have a more equal distribution between the I and III isomers. Urinary PBG is not elevated, but slight elevations in ALA are common. Fecal porphyrin excretion is increased, with several porphyrin compounds represented, many in the form of isocoproporphyrins.[27]

PHOTOCUTANEOUS LESIONS

The presenting clinical manifestation of PCT is almost invariably the development of bullous lesions in areas of sunlight exposure (Fig. 53-8). The lesions occur after minor trauma due to increased skin fragility. They do not represent acute photoreactions. The dorsum of the hand is the most frequent site of involvement because trauma and sun exposure are common to this area. Other sites of involvement include the forehead, the neck, and the ears. The bullae may become infected, causing prolonged healing that produces scarring and the development of pigment changes. Hypertrichosis, especially in the periorbital area, occurs. This feature was prominent in the Turkish epidemic.[60,208] Sclerodermoid changes may also develop.

The skin lesions in PCT are indistinguishable from those in VP and HCP. Unlike those disorders, PCT is not associated with acute neurologic attacks. The rare disorder HEP also features skin lesions like those in PCT. In contrast to PCT, however, the skin lesions present in infancy and tend to diminish with maturity.

Porphyrins are produced in excess and accumulate in the skin of patients with the cutaneous porphyrias. In the disorders in which bullous lesions occur, there is accumulation of hydrophilic porphyrins within lysosomes of cells.[201] The severe lesions in PCT may be due to the release of proteolytic enzymes from lysosomes into the cytoplasm.[260]

Complement activation has also been proposed as a factor in the pathogenesis of the cutaneous lesions in PCT. Deposition of complement components has been observed at the dermal–epidermal junction near bullae.[140] Elevated levels of complement components and cleavage products have been observed in the fluid contained in these lesions.[140] Complement levels have been shown in vitro to decline in sera containing excess porphyrin after ultraviolet irradiation.[140] Uroporphyrin has also been shown to have a stimulatory effect on collagen biosynthesis by fibroblasts, which may contribute to the fibrotic and sclerodermoid skin changes in PCT.

LIVER DAMAGE IN PCT

Patients with clinically overt PCT usually have liver damage. Chemistries are abnormal in about 65% of patients at the time of diagnosis, with the most common abnormality being a two- to four-fold elevation in serum transaminases.[51,136,149,250] Because PCT is often associated with the use of or exposure to compounds that are hepatotoxins, it has been difficult to determine if liver damage is due to the disorder itself.[189] There are, however, some characteristic hepatic findings.[189]

The liver may have a patchy, slate-gray discoloration when viewed grossly at laparotomy or laparoscopy.[51,225] Liver biopsy specimens from patients with overt disease exhibit a red fluorescence when exposed to ultraviolet light.[79] If water-free preparation of tissue is used, there is a cytoplasmic distribution of fluorescence.[79] Needle-like inclusions within the cytoplasm may be seen in specimens from untreated patients[51,113,263] (see Fig. 53-7). They have also been seen in tissue from patients with subclinical disease.[51] These inclusions, which probably are uroporphyrin crystals, are water soluble and will be lost with tissue processing unless water-free fixation is done.[51]

Common to patients with PCT is some degree of hepatic iron overload, and hemosiderosis is often easily demonstrated with iron stains.[23,136,250] The accumulation of iron cannot be attributed solely to ethanol abuse since it also occurs in familial and estrogen-induced PCT.[23,51]

Fatty liver is common in PCT, having been reported in most biopsy specimens.[23,51,136,250] Although some authors have suggested this may be related to underlying ethanol

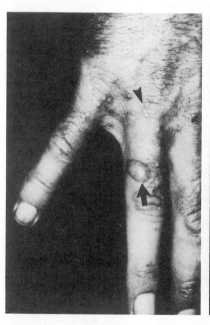
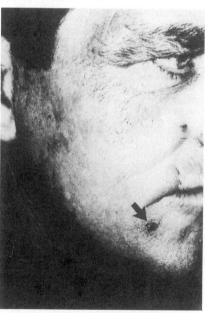

FIGURE 53-8 Skin lesions in porphyria cutanea tarda. Erosions and bullae (*arrows*) occur in sun-exposed areas after minor trauma. Milia (*arrowhead*) are small, whitish papules found on the dorsal aspects of the hands. There is increased facial hair in the periorbital region. Similar skin changes are found in variegate porphyria, hereditary coproporphyria and hepatoerythropoietic porphyria. (Bloomer JR. The hepatic porphyrias. Gastroenterology 71:689–701, 1976)

abuse or diabetes, Cortes and colleagues[51] found no difference in the prevalence of fatty liver in alcohol and nonalcoholic patients with PCT. In most cases, the fatty changes are mild.[136,250]

A granuloma-like lesion consisting of mononuclear cells, Kupffer cells, hemosiderin, and ceroid was described in patients by Lefkowitz and Grossman.[136] They called the nodules lobular lesions of PCT. Other authors[51,250] described similar lesions but found them to be less common. The lesions are present throughout the lobule. They may represent a reaction to collections of iron and uroporphyrin since these are eliminated after phlebotomy therapy.

Another finding is lymphocyte aggregates near terminal bile ducts. The significance of this finding is unknown. Hepatocyte hyperplasia with double cell plates is noted. The cause of this feature of regeneration is also unclear.[51,136]

The extent of hepatic damage is extremely variable, ranging from limited necrosis to cirrhosis. The degree of damage appears to be related in part to the duration of time since diagnosis.[51,123] A correlation between the severity of liver abnormalities and advancing age has also been noted.[51,123,200,240] No definite relation has been established between ethanol abuse and progression of liver damage. In addition, alcoholic hepatitis is infrequent in PCT.[51,250] Although hepatic iron overload may contribute to the liver damage, there is poor correlation between the degree of siderosis and the severity of liver damage. An additional factor is the high prevalence of hepatitis B in the countries from which most data have come regarding liver damage in PCT.[49,51,196,200]

With phlebotomy, there is improvement in some of the abnormalities. Not surprisingly, hemosiderosis disappears as total iron stores are depleted. There is disappearance of fluorescence and the crystalline material as well as the granuloma-like lesions. The liver enzyme abnormalities return toward normal.[49,149] The improvement occurs whether or not ethanol use is decreased or discontinued, again suggesting that liver damage is not explained solely by ethanol use in these patients.

PCT occasionally has been caused by hepatocellular carcinoma. The first report of this relation was in 1957, when Tio[241] noted apparent PCT in a patient with a tumor that fluoresced when exposed to Wood's lamp. After surgical removal of the tumor, the patient's skin lesions improved, and porphyrin excretion returned to normal. There have been other reports of porphyrin-excreting tumors, but they are extremely rare. The pattern of porphyrin excretion is somewhat different than in usual PCT, with excess excretion of several porphyrin compounds besides uroporphyrin.[241]

The more common association is for hepatocellular carcinoma to develop in patients with long-standing PCT. In 1959, Braun and Berman[46] reported the incidence of cirrhosis to be 63% and of hepatocellular carcinoma to be 53% in an autopsy series of patients with PCT. The diagnosis of PCT had been made years before death in all cases, ruling out the possibility that the tumor was responsible for the excess production of uroporphyrin. An autopsy series of PCT patients in Czechoslovakia was reported in 1972 by Kordac,[123] who found cirrhosis in 64% and carcinoma in 47% of patients. Kordac noted that the severity of liver disease and the development of carcinoma correlated with the duration of time since the diagnosis of PCT. Specifically, he found that noncirrhotic patients had a duration of 3.7 years, those with cirrhosis but no carcinoma 6.3 years, and those with carcinoma

11.7 years. Cirrhosis was present in all cases where carcinoma was found. Ethanol use was not universal in the patients, and the degree of hepatic hemosiderosis was variable.[123] Unfortunately, no information was given about the frequency of hepatitis B. Kordac argued that there may be a natural progression of liver damage with development of carcinoma in PCT, which may be independent of precipitating agents.

Studies reported since these publications have been conflicting. In a series of 96 randomly selected patients, Topi and coworkers[243] screened for hepatocellular carcinoma using radionuclide liver scan and measurement of serum α-fetoprotein. There was no evidence of tumor in any of the patients studied; however, the average duration from the time of diagnosis of PCT was only 5.6 years, about half that of the group with carcinoma in Kordac's series. Solis and colleagues[224] found a significant increase of hepatocellular carcinoma in cirrhotic patients with PCT as compared with patients in whom cirrhosis was not associated with PCT. Salata and colleagues[200] also found an increased incidence of carcinoma in PCT. They found that carcinoma correlated with male sex, duration of time since the diagnosis of PCT, and presence of cirrhosis. They found no correlation with ethanol use or hepatitis B serology.

These studies suggest that there is an increased risk for developing cirrhosis and hepatocellular carcinoma in patients with long-standing PCT. It may therefore be prudent to screen patients who have long-standing PCT, particularly those with cirrhosis, for hepatocellular carcinoma with serum α-fetoprotein measurement and hepatic ultrasonography.

MANAGEMENT

The patient with active PCT should avoid light that may excite porphyrins. This occurs maximally at wavelengths of 400 to 410 nm. Light of this wavelength is not filtered by window glass, and the patient should also take precautions when driving a car. Fluorescent lights should also be avoided.

The use of ethanol and estrogens should be eliminated in patients when they have been a factor in causing the disease. If urinary excretion of uroporphyrin is greater than 2000 μg/d, the response provided by just eliminating the precipitating agent will be slow, and phlebotomy therapy should be initiated. Typically 3 to 5 g of iron (6 to 10 L of blood) must be removed to see improvement. An alternate therapy is to use chloroquine or related compounds. These agents appear to mobilize uroporphyrin and promote its urinary excretion by forming a water-soluble complex with the compound. They should be used with some caution because liver necrosis may be caused by massive uroporphyrin mobilization if the dose of chloroquine is too high.

Hepatoerythropoietic Porphyria

Hepatoerythropoietic porphyria is an extremely rare disorder characterized by excretion of high levels of uroporphyrin isomers I and III. Additionally, erythrocyte protoporphyrin levels are elevated, mainly as the zinc chelate. The disorder is clinically similar to CEP. The disease manifests itself early in infancy with discolored urine, photosensitivity, and skin fragility. Hemolytic anemia and splenomegaly may be present.[56,106,175] The first description of this disorder was by

Günther in 1967, with the present name given in 1975.[102,175] As the name implies, significant amounts of porphyrins are produced in both the liver and the bone marrow, and fluorescence of normoblasts may be seen in bone marrow aspirates. Interestingly, as these patients reach adulthood, the skin manifestations may abate.[56,175]

Biochemically, the disorder is characterized by a marked decrease in uroporphyrinogen decarboxylase activity.[77,135,141,219,253] Studies of kindreds of some of these patients support the idea that a homozygous defect in the gene coding for this enzyme is responsible.[242,253] This is in contrast to familial PCT, in which a heterozygous state exists.[19,135] Although a defect in uroporphyrin decarboxylase would explain the elevations of uroporphyrin excretion, the elevated zinc protoporphyrin levels remain unexplained.

Although the defective enzyme is apparently the same in PCT and HEP, the liver damage seen in the two disorders is substantially different. A mild, nonspecific hepatitis has been reported in HEP, and mild increases in transaminases are common. Siderosis has not been reported in HEP, and fibrosis or cirrhosis is uncommon. Serum iron studies are normal in HEP. As in PCT, hepatic fluorescence is seen when appropriate illumination is provided.

Few data are available on therapies for this disorder. Treatment is aimed at avoidance of offending wavelengths of light. One report has been made of transient decreases in urine and RBC porphyrins after phlebotomy therapy.

Congenital Erythropoietic Porphyria

The first description of any porphyria occurred in 1874 when Schultz reported a patient who had urine of port wine color and fragile skin since infancy.[61] This was later recognized as a case of CEP. Less than 200 cases of this disorder have subsequently been described. It is an autosomal recessive disorder and is most commonly diagnosed in infancy.[209] Only six cases of adult onset have been reported.[190] Skin lesions are indistinguishable from those in PCT. The bone marrow of the patients is filled with RBC precursors that fluoresce with ultraviolet irradiation.[209,210] Unlike PCT, the liver shows little or no fluorescence. The disorder is associated with chronic hemolysis, and splenomegaly is common.[252,265] The cause of hemolysis is not well understood but may be related to the toxic effect of porphyrin in the erythroid cells. Neurologic symptoms do not occur.

Treatment is difficult. Therapy has usually been aimed at decreasing the underlying hemolysis in hopes of decreasing heme turnover. Splenectomy has been associated with a variable response, ranging from no effect to long-term remission of overt disease.[166] RBC transfusions decrease porphyrin excretion and improve clinical symptoms but may cause iron overload.[265] Intravenous administration of hematin has also been shown to decrease uroporphyrin excretion, but this has not yet been used as chronic therapy.[190,265]

Inducible (Acute) Porphyrias

The first case of an inducible (acute) porphyria was reported by Stokvis[231] in 1888, when he described a patient who developed paralysis and dark urine after taking sulfonate, a hypnotic agent. The patient eventually died. A similar episode was described in a patient taking barbiturates in 1906.

Waldenström[261] used the term *acute porphyria* to describe a disorder in 103 Swedish patients with episodic neurologic crises. He noted that all the patients had a substance in their urine that reacted with Ehrlich's aldehyde reagent (*p*-dimethylaminobenzaldehyde) to form a red color. This substance was later recognized to be PBG.

Further characterization of the acute porphyrias evolved with the recognition of clinical distinctions and the identification of the various porphyrins and porphyrin precursors that are selectively increased in each. The neurologic manifestations are the same in all (Table 53-3) and are discussed separately after a brief description of each of the disorders.

ACUTE INTERMITTENT PORPHYRIA

Acute intermittent porphyria represented most of the cases of "Swedish porphyria" described by Waldenström. The disorder is inherited in an autosomal dominant manner. There is variable penetrance, and most patients with the gene defect do not have clinically overt manifestations. It is the most common of the inducible porphyrias in the United States, and the prevalence of the gene is about 1 in 10,000 to 20,000 people.[35] AIP is somewhat more common among people of Scandinavian, British, and Irish descent. The incidence may be as high as 3 per 10,000 hospitalized psychiatric patients.[168]

Because only porphyrin precursors, and not porphyrins, are produced in excess, there are no cutaneous manifestations. During acute attacks of AIP, there is a marked increase in the urinary excretion of PBG and ALA. Between episodes, the urinary excretion of the compounds decreases but usually does not return to normal. Like the other acute porphyrias, it is rare for AIP to manifest itself before puberty despite the fact that the gene defect is present at birth.

VARIEGATE PORPHYRIA

A porphyria distinct from Swedish porphyria was described by Barnes[12] in the 1940s. He observed patients who had both acute attacks of neurologic symptoms and a chronic derma-

TABLE 53-3   *Signs and Symptoms of Neurologic Dysfunction During Acute Attacks of Porphyria*

Sign or Symptom	Occurrence (%)
Abdominal pain	95
Sinus tachycardia	80
Peripheral motor weakness or paresis	60
Extremity pain	50
Constipation	48
Bulbar impairment	46
Nausea and vomiting	43
Mental confusion or hallucinations	40
Hypertension	36
Back pain	29
Absent reflexes	29
Peripheral sensory deficit	26
Postural hypotension	21
Seizures	20

(Stein JA, Tschudy DP. Acute intermittent porphyria: a clinical and biochemical study of 46 patients. Medicine 49:1, 1970)

tologic disorder similar to that seen in PCT. Dean[59] observed that "South African porphyria" could present with acute neurologic symptoms, cutaneous symptoms, or both. In the mid-1950s, Dean[62] suggested the name *porphyria variegata* for this disorder because of its diverse presentations. The prevalence of the disorder is dependent on the population studied. The disorder is uncommon in the United States but is estimated at 3 per 1000 in white South Africans.[61] Most of these cases can be traced to a single Boer emigrant from the Netherlands who arrived in South Africa in 1688. The disorder is transmitted in an autosomal dominant manner and, like the other acute porphyrias, rarely manifests itself clinically until the second or third decade of life. During acute attacks, moderate elevations of urinary ALA and PBG excretion are noted, but these return to normal during asymptomatic periods. Excess fecal protoporphyrin excretion occurs chronically in the patients, and fecal porphyrin measurement is helpful in confirming the diagnosis. Bile porphyrin analysis and detection of a characteristic plasma fluorescence marker may also be used for this purpose.[146]

HEREDITARY COPROPORPHYRIA

In 1949, Watson described a series of cases in which patients experienced acute episodes of neurologic dysfunction accompanied by elevation of urinary ALA and PBG.[266] Unlike previously described porphyrias, these patients were also noted to have increased excretion of urinary and fecal coproporphyrin. The patients also had dermatologic lesions similar to those in PCT. Family studies demonstrated an autosomal dominant transmission. The disorder is much less common than AIP, but the prevalence is unknown.

δ-AMINOLEVULINIC ACID DEHYDRASE DEFICIENCY

This is an extremely rare disorder that is characterized by acute episodes of neurologic dysfunction and excess urinary excretion of ALA, but not PBG.[25] There are no cutaneous manifestations. It appears to be an autosomal recessive disorder.

NEUROLOGIC DYSFUNCTION IN THE ACUTE PORPHYRIAS

Clinical Features

The clinical course of the neurologic crises in the acute porphyrias is variable. The attack can be exacerbated by medications that are commonly used in other conditions. It is, therefore, crucial that the diagnosis be made early in the course. The severity of an episode depends on how much damage has occurred before appropriate intervention is instituted. Women more frequently manifest the neurologic episodes and appear to have more severe episodes. This may be due to hormonal induction of ALA synthase activity.[5,204,215] The episodes are often precipitated by the use of medications (Table 53-4) but can also be induced near the end of the menstrual cycle and by fasting.

Abdominal pain is nearly always present during an attack (see Table 53-3). The pain is due to autonomic nerve dysfunction. It is colicky in nature and often localized to the lower quadrants. Abdominal examination reveals decreased or absent bowel sounds, and abdominal radiographs show alternating areas of spasm and dilation. The pain has been relieved by ganglionic blockade, and autopsy examination has revealed destruction of visceral nerve myelin sheaths.[90,269] The patients also complain of constipation or, rarely, diarrhea. Nausea and vomiting are common. Because there is often an associated leukocytosis, the patient may undergo laparotomy for presumed intraabdominal infection before the diagnosis is established.[229]

Other signs and symptoms associated with autonomic dysfunction are seen. Tachycardia is common, and labile hypertension can occur. When these are present, the patient should be monitored carefully because sudden death has been reported.[192,228] Unexplained fevers, bladder distention, dyshidrosis, and postural hypotension may also be seen.[93,229,262]

The peripheral nervous system is also involved, with both motor and sensory dysfunction noted. The motor damage tends to involve proximal muscle groups early, and unlike the Guillain-Barré syndrome, it tends to involve the upper extremities before the lower.[93,229] Respiratory paralysis can be life-threatening and may require intubation with respirator support. Fortunately, this complication usually occurs late in an attack. Diffuse pains involving the extremities, chest, and back due to peripheral sensory nerve involvement are common and may precede the onset of the overt crisis by days.[90,229] Patients may complain of dysesthesia and paresthesia. Deep tendon reflexes are usually normal early but are progressively lost in prolonged attacks. The ankle reflexes may be selectively preserved.

Central nervous system involvement is common.[93,229,262] A complaint of increased irritability may be the first indication of an impending attack. Insomnia, anxiety, and behavioral changes may develop as the attack continues. The patient may become violent and be improperly labeled as hysterical, leading to the use of medications that exacerbate the attack. Psychiatric evaluation may reveal severe depression or paranoia. Frank psychosis with hallucinations may be seen. After resolution of the acute attack, chronic psychiatric disorders, especially depression, occur with an increased frequency compared with the general population.

Seizures are seen in about 20% of acute attacks and present a difficult clinical problem.[24,41,134,170,229] All the common anticonvulsants have demonstrated or theoretic potential for exacerbation of the attack (see Table 53-4). Inappropriate secretion of antidiuretic hormone has been observed, with concomitant hyponatremia. Indeed, hypothalamic lesions have been found at necropsy in patients with AIP.[165,171] Abnormalities in electroencephalograms may occur in the absence of seizure activity, with nonspecific slowing the most common. An organic brain syndrome frequently develops if the attack progresses. If there is no intervention, progressive somnolence and eventual coma may occur.

Diagnosis of Acute Porphyric Attack

The hallmark of diagnosis of the acute porphyric attack is the presence of excess ALA and, with rare exception, PBG in the urine. During an acute attack, levels of these porphyrin precursors are elevated from 20- to 200-fold. The Watson-Schwartz and related tests exploit this fact to give a rapid result when faced with a potential case of acute porphyria. In the Watson-Schwartz test, the patient's urine is mixed with Erlich's reagent (*p*-dimethylaminobenzaldehyde in HCl), titered to pH 4.0 with sodium acetate, and extracted in butanol. A red pigment forms due to reaction of Erlich's reagent with PBG and remains in the aqueous fraction.[267,268] Al-

TABLE 53-4 *Drugs and the Porphyrias*

	Unsafe	**Safe**
Analgesics	Oxycodone, phenacetin	Codeine, fentanyl, meperidine, methadone, morphine
Anesthetics	Fluroxene, mepivacaine, methoxyflurane	Cyclopropane, ether, nitrous oxide, procaine, succinylcholine, tubocurarine
Anticonvulsants	Barbiturates, carbamazepine, hydantoins, phenytoin, valproate	Bromides, magnesium sulfate
Antiinflammatory agents	Danazol, phenylbutazone	Aspirin, ibuprofen, naproxen
Antimicrobials	Chloramphenicol, dapsone, doxycycline, griseofulvin, metronidazole, miconazole, rifampin, sulfonamides, trimethoprim	Acyclovir, aminoglycosides, amoxicillin, amphotericin, ampicillin, ethambutol, flucytosine, gentamicin, penicillin, quinine, streptomycin, tetracycline
Cardiovascular drugs	Amiodarone, nifedipine, verapamil	Adrenaline, atropine, digoxin, procainamide, quinidine
Diuretics and antihypertensives	α-Methyldopa, captopril, clonidine, furosemide, hydralazine, spironolactone, thiazides	Acetazolamide, amiloride, atenolol, ethacrynic acid, propanolol, reserpine, triamterene
Sedatives and tranquilizers	Alprazolam, chlordiazepoxide, diazepam, flurazepam, meprobamate	Chloral hydrate, chlorpromazine, haloperidol, paraldehyde, promazine
Other	Aminophylline, ergot compounds, danazol, estrogens, hydroxyzine, imipramine, sulfonylureas, theophylline, tolbutamide	Beclomethasone, chlorpheniramine, colchicine, corticosteroids, coumarin, heparin, insulin, loperamide, phenformin, promazine, vitamins

(Hift RJ, Meissner PN, Meissner DM. Porphyria. Cape Town, South Africa, MRC/UCT Liver Research Centre, 1991)

though this is a good screening test for acute attacks of porphyria, several caveats exist. Urinary PBG concentrations less than 6 to 8 mg/L are not detected.[36] Therefore, the test may not be effective in screening asymptomatic patients. Additionally, PBG is not elevated in ALA dehydrase deficiency. If acute porphyria is strongly suspected in the face of a negative Watson-Schwartz test, ALA and PBG levels should be quantitated. Any positive test should be followed by quantitation of porphyrins and porphyrin precursors to define the underlying defect better.

Pathogenesis of the Neurologic Dysfunction

A central role for ALA in the development of the acute attack has been postulated (Fig. 53-9). This compound is elevated in all the acute porphyrias during attacks and is normal in the porphyrias without neurologic crises. Also, in hereditary tyrosinemia and lead intoxication, there is a marked elevation in ALA associated with neurologic symptoms that are indistinguishable from those in the acute porphyrias.[16,89,120,142]

Structurally, ALA is similar to γ-aminobutyric acid (GABA), the major inhibitory neurotransmitter in the central nervous system.[275] ALA is a potent GABA receptor agonist,[39,127] and the interaction of ALA with this receptor may be partly responsible for some of the symptoms in the acute attack. Intraventricular injection of ALA in experimental animals results in demonstrable neurotoxicity; and at high concentrations, ALA inhibits neural Na$^+$-K$^+$-ATPase with breakdown of membrane anion gradients.[127]

Although it is intriguing to implicate ALA as a major toxin involved in the neurologic dysfunction in the acute porphyrias, it may not be the sole cause. The severity of any attack does not correlate well with serum ALA levels.[229] Indeed,

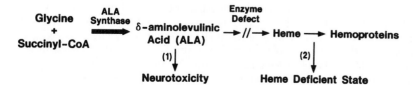

FIGURE 53-9 Schematic showing that neurologic dysfunction in the inducible porphyrias is linked to the biochemical abnormalities. It may be caused by the neurotoxic effect of ALA, a heme-deficient state, or a combination of both.

high serum levels with increased urinary excretion occur in patients without demonstrable neurologic deficits.[170] The cerebrospinal fluid may be devoid of ALA during an acute attack, but the significance of this is questionable since cerebrospinal fluid levels do not correlate well with intracellular neural levels.[170]

An alternate possibility to explain neurologic dysfunction in the acute porphyrias is that impaired heme synthesis causes a decrease in intracellular hemoproteins, leading to depressed cellular respiration in nerve tissue. Another consequence of abnormal heme synthesis is impairment of hepatic metabolism. A deficiency of the heme-containing enzyme, tryptophan pyrrolase, which catalyses the first committed reaction in tryptophan degradation, may cause an elevation of 5-hydroxytryptophan (serotonin).[144] Increased excretion of serotonin has been reported in a few patients with acute porphyria, although the frequency and significance of this finding is unknown.[144]

Autopsy specimen findings depend on the duration of the attack. If the attack was of short duration, no discernible damage may be seen. With prolonged duration, progressive axonal damage and eventual demyelinization of autonomic, motor, and sensory nerves may be seen.[90] This correlates with the clinical picture in that early therapeutic intervention, before neuronal death, is associated with complete and rapid recovery.[90,229] Once paralysis is present, recovery is dependent on axonal regeneration, with recovery of proximal muscle groups taking place earlier than the distal groups, which are innervated with longer axons.

Management of Neurologic Crises

Because of the unpredictable nature of an acute porphyric attack, it is generally necessary to hospitalize the patient early in an episode. Recognition of the nature of the attack and avoidance of exacerbating drug therapy are critical. Any medication that stimulates hepatic heme synthesis is potentially harmful. These medications may directly stimulate heme synthesis or increase heme demand by stimulating the mixed-function oxidase system. Infections also precipitate acute attacks and should be treated promptly.

Narcotic analgesics are safe and effective in treating abdominal pain and pain due to sensory neuropathy. Chloral hydrate may be used for agitation and insomnia. Phenothiazines can be safely used to treat nausea and vomiting as well as psychotic behavior. β-Adrenergic blockers have been used to control tachycardia and hypertension. These agents should be used cautiously, however, since many patients are volume-depleted from gastrointestinal fluid loss.[228] When tachycardia and labile hypertension are present, cardiac monitoring is advised because sudden death has been reported.[192] Intubation and respiratory assistance may be needed if thoracic muscles are compromised or if coma or frequent seizures occur. Electrolytes should be monitored closely because of gastrointestinal fluid losses and because inappropriate secretion of antidiuretic hormone has been reported.[171,228]

Treatment of seizure activity poses a particularly difficult problem. Nearly all known anticonvulsants have been implicated in exacerbations of acute attacks.[24,41,134,207,276] If a search for correctable causes of seizure activity, such as electrolyte abnormalities, has proved unsuccessful, then some pharmacologic intervention will likely be necessary. The hydantoins and barbiturates are known to induce microsomal cytochromes and are contraindicated.[73,193,229] The benzodiazepines are all potentially dangerous in the patient with indu-

cible porphyria, but clonazepam and diazepam have been used without ill effect.[41,134] These agents probably should be reserved for the treatment of status epilepticus. Sodium valproate has been used safely but induces ALA synthesis experimentally.[41,86] The only agents without the potential for exacerbating an attack are the bromides. These agents are difficult to use because their therapeutic window is small, and overdosage is difficult to avoid.

Two therapeutic interventions can be used to diminish ALA production—intravenous glucose administration and hematin administration. These interventions are maximally effective only if done before neuronal destruction takes place, and they should be instituted early in the course of an attack.

Intravenous glucose should be given at the rate of 20 g/h.[173] Experimentally, glucose administration has been shown to suppress the activity of ALA synthase.[42] This may be an indirect effect, with glucose stabilizing the heme pool and thereby decreasing the need for further heme synthesis.[42] Because starvation has been shown to increase hepatic heme turnover and to precipitate acute attacks,[84,270] one effect of glucose administration may be simply that of caloric replenishment.

If a decrease in ALA and PBG excretion, as well as improvement in clinical parameters, is not seen within 48 hours after beginning glucose administration, then hematin therapy should be started. If there is any deterioration in the clinical condition before this time, hematin should be begun immediately. Administration of exogenous heme to a patient with AIP was done for the first time in 1971.[43] The compound, ferriheme hydroxide (hematin), was administered late in the course of the acute attack after the failure of other therapeutic interventions. Biochemical improvement was shown, with rapid reduction in serum ALA and PBG; however, the patient did not show clinical improvement and eventually died. Since then, the experience with hematin in the treatment of the acute porphyrias has been extensive, and it is clear that if the compound is administered early in an attack, there is clinical as well as biochemical improvement.[162,173]

The reason for hematin's effect is at least in part the suppression of hepatic ALA synthase activity.[220,227,274] Hematin is supplied in a lyophilized form that is reconstituted in water before use. It should be administered immediately after hydration because the compound is unstable in solution, and the breakdown products have been implicated in adverse effects.[173] The most common complication is local phlebitis. This can be overcome by using a fresh preparation delivered slowly through a freely flowing intravenous line.[173] Coagulation abnormalities have been noted, but clinically significant bleeding is rare.[162] The use of fresh preparations greatly decreases the potential for significant coagulopathy.[162] The dosage most commonly used is 3 to 5 mg/kg every 12 hours.[173] One report of renal failure followed the administration of 1000 mg.[68] Heme arginate, a stable and water-soluble preparation of heme, is available in Europe.[162] This compound is as effective as hematin and appears to be safer (Fig. 53-10). It has not yet been approved in the United States.

Prevention of Neurologic Crises

Once the diagnosis of acute porphyria has been made, the prevention of further attacks becomes imperative. Elimination of all potentially hazardous medications, abstinence from ethanol, and avoidance of prolonged fasting is recommended. Infections should be treated promptly. If the epi-

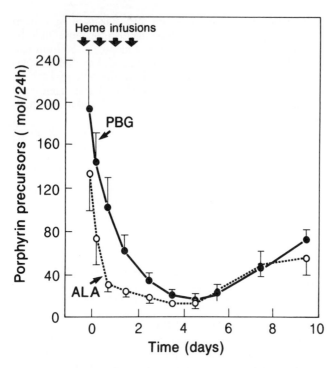

FIGURE 53-10 Effect of intravenous infusion of heme arginate (3 mg/kg) on the excretion of δ-aminolevulinic acid (ALA) and porphobilinogen (PBG) in six patients with acute intermittent porphyria (mean ± SE). (Mustajoki P. Acute intermittent porphyria. Semin Dermatol 5:155–160, 1986)

sodes are related to the menstrual cycle, then endocrine manipulation by administration of a gonadotrophin-releasing hormone analogue, or by cycling with oral contraceptives, may be considered.[5,215]

LIVER DAMAGE IN THE ACUTE PORPHYRIAS

Relatively little information is available regarding structural liver changes in the acute porphyrias. Increased hepatic fat and siderosis, together with a mild, nonspecific inflammatory process, have been seen in biopsy specimens.[169] Ultrastructural mitochondrial changes have been reported, with crystalline material seen within the mitochondria.[23,169] Functional studies have revealed abnormalities in bile salt handling and in aminopyrine breath tests in a high percentage of patients, suggesting dysfunction of microsomal cytochrome systems.[169] The significance of these observations has yet to be defined, and a long-term prospective examination of liver damage in this group of patients is needed.

Two recent studies have suggested an association between the acute porphyrias and hepatocellular carcinoma.[119,143] One study found 11 hepatomas in a group of 206 patients with AIP.[143] A second study found the relative risk of developing hepatocellular carcinoma in AIP and VP to be 61 times that in the general population.[119] As in PCT, the presence of carcinoma correlated with increasing age and the presence of cirrhosis.[119,143] The studies were from Scandinavian countries where the prevalence of hepatitis B is low. No information regarding alcoholism in these patients was given, but it is expected that alcoholic liver disease would be rare in this population.

Secondary Porphyrinurias

Several different disorders are associated with a mild to moderate increase in the urinary excretion of porphyrins, particularly coproporphyrin, a condition termed *secondary porphyrinuria* (Table 53-5). Since patients with these disorders occasionally have abdominal pain or other symptoms suggestive of the genetic porphyrias, this may present a diagnostic dilemma to the clinician. Usually, a careful history and physical examination indicates that a genetic type of porphyria is unlikely to be the cause of the excess urinary porphyrin excretion. As an additional means of avoiding a misdiagnosis, it is important to remember that the genetic porphyrias in which abdominal pain is a prominent symptom have increased urinary excretion of ALA and PBG. With the exception of lead poisoning and hereditary tyrosinemia, the conditions associated with secondary porphyrinuria do not have increased urinary excretion of these compounds. A few of the types of secondary porphyrinuria that are more likely to be encountered by the gastroenterologist or hepatologist are described next.

LEAD POISONING

Lead poisoning is associated with several abnormalities in porphyrin metabolism because lead affects the heme biosynthesis pathway at more than one site. A common feature of the affected sites may be enzymes containing sulfhydryl groups. Erythrocyte levels of zinc protoporphyrin are elevated in patients with lead poisoning,[131] and this measurement has become a method for screening large populations for the disorder.[176] Lead poisoning is also associated with increased urinary excretion of coproporphyrin and ALA. Since abdominal pain is a prominent clinical feature of the condition, and since patients may also have peripheral neuropathies, it is possible that the mechanism for neurologic dysfunction in lead poisoning is the same as in the genetic porphyrias. Indeed, hematin has been used as adjunctive therapy in lead poisoning,[132] with a significant diminution in urinary ALA excretion.

TABLE 53-5   *Causes of Secondary Porphyrinuria*

Hepatobiliary Disorders
Acute and chronic hepatitis
Alcoholic liver disease
Cirrhosis (alcoholic and nonalcoholic)
Cholestatic disorders

Hematologic Disorders
Aplastic anemia, hemolytic anemia, pernicious anemia
Leukemias
Hodgkin's disease

Toxins
Heavy-metal poisoning (lead, arsenic, gold, iron)
Benzene and benzene congeners
Haloalkanes and haloaromatic compounds

Miscellaneous
Hereditary conjugated hyperbilirubinemias (Dubin-Johnson and Rotor's syndromes)
Bronze-baby syndrome
Diabetes

HEREDITARY TYROSINEMIA

Hereditary tyrosinemia type I is a metabolic disorder in which patients have liver damage in infancy that may progress rapidly to cirrhosis, with the subsequent development of hepatocellular carcinoma. Patients with this disorder accumulate succinylacetone (4,6-dioxoheptanoic acid) and succinylacetoacetate due to a block in tyrosine metabolism at the level of the fumarylacetoacetase reaction.[142] Succinylacetone is a potent inhibitor of the enzyme ALA dehydrase[206,245] (see Fig. 53-2), resulting in increased urinary excretion of ALA in the urine. Some patients also have neurologic manifestations that resemble those in the acute porphyrias.[157] It is tempting to consider that the mechanism of neurologic dysfunction is the same since patients with tyrosinemia may respond to the intravenous administration of hematin.[188] The biochemical abnormalities are corrected by liver transplantation, although minor defects persist that are thought to be of renal origin.[248]

DUBIN-JOHNSON SYNDROME

Dubin-Johnson syndrome is an inherited disorder characterized by conjugated hyperbilirubinemia and the accumulation of lipomelanin pigment in hepatocytes. Other tests of liver function are normal, and liver biopsy specimens show no abnormalities other than the pigment accumulation. A characteristic pattern of urinary coproporphyrin excretion has been found in patients.[20,124] The total amount of coproporphyrin in urine is normal or only slightly increased, whereas the proportion of coproporphyrin present as the type I isomer is significantly increased. Thus, the total coproporphyrin in the urine present as the type I isomer exceeds 90%, in contrast to the 33% that is present in normal urine. The abnormality in urinary coproporphyrin may reflect the fact that patients with the Dubin-Johnson syndrome have a defect in the biliary excretion of coproporphyrin as well as conjugated bilirubin. There does not appear to be an abnormality in the hepatic formation of heme in the condition.

MISCELLANEOUS HEPATOBILIARY DISEASES

Since the bile is a route of porphyrin excretion, any hepatobiliary disease in which bile formation is impaired may cause a diversion of porphyrins to the urine.[10,71] Urinary excretion of coproporphyrin increases the most in hepatobiliary diseases. Uroporphyrin may also increase, but protoporphyrin is not excreted in the urine even in the face of severe cholestasis due to its poor water solubility.

When there is extrahepatic biliary obstruction causing cholestasis, the increase in urinary coproporphyrin excretion is accompanied by a higher proportion of the type I isomer than normally occurs. This is due to the fact that the type I isomer is normally excreted preferentially in bile over the type III isomer.[116] Two patterns have been observed in parenchymal liver diseases. In alcoholic cirrhosis, the increased excretion of urinary coproporphyrin is associated with a proportion of coproporphyrin I in urine that is similar to that in normal people, whereas the pattern in other types of parenchymal disease is more like that in biliary obstruction. Due to significant overlap among these conditions, however, the urinary coproporphyrin isomer distribution cannot be used in the differential diagnosis of hepatobiliary disorders. Acute ingestion of alcohol may also cause a significant increase in the urinary excretion of coproporphyrin, usually beginning 2 to 4 days after intoxication.

Although impaired biliary excretion is probably the main factor responsible for increased urinary porphyrin excretion in hepatobiliary disorders, there also may be alterations in synthesis. Hepatic ALA synthase activity is increased in homogenates of cirrhotic livers,[38] suggesting that there may be an increased rate of porphyrin production. Experimentally, it has been shown that acute ethanol administration can also increase hepatic ALA synthase activity.[11]

Summary

The porphyrias are genetic disorders in which abnormalities in the pathway of heme biosynthesis cause the excessive accumulation and excretion of porphyrins and porphyrin precursors, which are intermediates of the pathway. The liver has a prominent role in heme biosynthesis and is the principal site of overproduction of porphyrins and porphyrin precursors in several of the porphyrias.

A defect in a specific enzymatic step of the heme biosynthesis pathway has been described for each of the porphyrias. These enzyme defects are placed at points in the pathway that explain the patterns of excessive excretion of porphyrins and porphyrin precursors characteristic of the porphyrias. The nature of the enzyme defects has been examined by comparing the amount of immunoreactive enzyme protein with the catalytic activity of the enzyme and, more recently, by sequencing the genes for the enzyme proteins. These studies have demonstrated genetic heterogeneity in the porphyrias; that is, more than one gene defect can lead to the phenotypic expression characteristic of the porphyria.

Although the clinical features of the porphyrias are diverse, encompassing many areas of medicine, the two principal manifestations are photocutaneous lesions and neurologic dysfunction. Cutaneous lesions in the porphyrias are caused by the photosensitizing effects of porphyrins that are deposited in the skin or that are circulating in dermal blood vessels. The photosensitizing effects of the porphyrins result from their ability to absorb light. This excites the porphyrin to an elevated energy state, which can then react with molecular oxygen to form activated oxygen species that damage cell membranes and organelles through peroxidation of membrane lipids and cross-linking of membrane proteins. Other mechanisms that may also be important in the development of photocutaneous lesions are activation of the complement system and the release of vasoactive substances from mast cells.

Neurologic dysfunction occurs in those porphyrias that are characterized by acute attacks, the paradigm of which is AIP. Any portion of the nervous system may be involved, leading to a wide variety of symptoms, the most frequent of which is abdominal pain. The excretion of ALA is increased in all the porphyrias characterized by acute attacks of neurologic dysfunction, and experimental evidence indicates that ALA may act as a neurotoxin. Alternatively, a heme deficiency state may arise and lead to neurologic dysfunction, or a combination of the two may be responsible.

Structural liver damage occurs in two types of porphyria: PCT and protoporphyria. Patients with long-standing PCT may develop cirrhosis and hepatocellular carcinoma. A small percentage of patients with protoporphyria have developed fatal liver disease due to massive deposition of protoporphyrin pigment in liver tissue.

Therapy in the porphyrias is directed toward modifying the biochemical abnormalities since the clinical manifestations of the porphyrias are linked to them. Perhaps the most important advance has been the recognition that the intravenous administration of hematin may be used to abort life-threatening attacks of neurologic dysfunction in the porphyrias. This therapy was developed because of experimental data showing that heme exerts negative feedback control over hepatic ALA synthase, the rate-limiting enzyme in hepatic heme biosynthesis. Prevention also remains important in the management of patients with porphyria. Patients who carry the gene defect should be counseled to avoid situations that may precipitate acute attacks of neurologic dysfunction, such as the ingestion of certain drugs.

The clinician must also recognize that several other diseases, particularly those disorders that affect the liver, may be associated with an increase in urinary porphyrin excretion, particularly coproporphyrin. This condition, secondary porphyrinuria, should not be confused with the genetic porphyrias. Careful attention to the history and physical findings, as well as measurement of both porphyrins and porphyrin precursors, allows the secondary porphyrinurias to be distinguished from the genetic types of porphyria.

Acknowledgments

We wish to thank Tamika Jeter for her outstanding organizational and typing skills and for always being available to run another copy. We thank Elaine Johnson for her participation during fluoroscopy sessions at BIMC. Our heartfelt thanks are extended to Ruth Fregon, RN, and to Alma Mattison, who gave unselfishly of their time so that we could add another case to their already busy schedules.

References

1. Abboud MM, Jordan PM, Akhtar M. Biosynthesis of 5-aminolevulinic acid: involvement of a retention-inversion mechanism. J Chem Soc Chem Comm 643, 1974.
2. Akhtar M, Abboud MM, Barnard G, Jordan PM, Zaman Z. Mechanism and stereochemistry of enzymic reactions involved in porphyrin biosynthesis. Philos Trans R Soc Lond [Biol] 273:117, 1973
3. Anderson CD, Rossi E, Garcia-Webb P. Porphyrin studies in chronic renal failure patients on maintenance hemodialysis. Photodermatology 4:14, 1987
4. Anderson KE, Goeger DE, Carson RW, Lee SK, Stead RB. Erythropoietin for the treatment of porphyria cutanea tarda in a patient on long-term hemodialysis. Med Intell 322:315, 1990
5. Anderson KE, Spitz IM, Sassa S, Bardin CW, Kappas A. Prevention of cyclical attacks of acute intermittent porphyria with a long-acting agonist of luteinizing hormone-releasing hormone. N Engl J Med 311:643, 1984
6. Anderson PM, Desnick RJ. Purification properties of uroporphyrinogen I synthase from human erythrocytes: identification of stable enzyme-substrate intermediates. J Biol Chem 255: 1993, 1980
7. Avner DL, Berenson MM. Effect of choleretics on canalicular transport of protoporphyrin in the rat liver. Am J Physiol 242:G347, 1982
8. Avner DL, Larsen R, Berenson MM. Inhibition of liver surface membrane, Na, K-adenosine triphosphatase, Mg-adenosine triphosphatase and 5'-nucleotidase activities by protoporphyrin: observations in vitro and in the perfused rat liver. Gastroenterology 85:700, 1983
9. Avner DL, Lee RG, Berenson MM. Protoporphyrin-induced cholestasis in the isolated in situ perfused rat liver. J Clin Invest 67:385, 1981
10. Aziz MA, Schwartz S, Watson CJ. Studies of coproporphyrin. VIII. Reinvestigation of the isomer distribution in jaundice and liver disease. J Lab Clin Med 63:596, 1964
11. Badawy AAB, Morgan CJ, Davis NR. Effects of acute ethanol administration on rat liver 5-aminolevulinate synthase activity. Biochem J 262:491, 1989
12. Barnes HD. A note on porphyrinuria with a resume of eleven South African cases. Clin Proceed 5:269, 1945
13. Barnes HD. Porphyria in the Bantu races on the Witwatersrand. S Afr Med J 29:781, 1955
14. Barnes HD, Hurworth E, Millar JHD. Erythropoietic porphyrin hepatitis. J Clin Pathol 21:157, 1968
15. Battersby AR, Fookes CJR, Hart G, Matcham GWJ, George WJ, Pandey PS. Biosynthesis of porphyrins and related mactocycles: 21. the interaction of deaminase and its product (hydroxymethylbilane) and the relationship between deaminase and cosynthetase. J Chem Soc Perkin Trans I:3042, 1983
16. Baxter CS, Ivey HE, Cardin AD. Evidence for specific lead-δ-aminolevulinate complex formation by carbon-13 nuclear magnetic resonance spectroscopy. Toxicol Appl Pharmacol 47:477, 1979
17. Behm AR, Unger WP. Oral contraceptives and porphyria cutanea tarda. Can Med Assoc J 110:1052, 1974
18. Belcher RV, Smith SG, Mahler R. Biliary protein-bound porphyrins in porphyria variegata. Clin Chem Acta 25:45, 1969
19. Benedetto AV, Kushner JP, Taylor JS. Porphyria cutanea tarda in three generations of a single family. N Engl J Med 298:358, 1978
20. Ben-Ezzer J, Rimington C, Shani M, Seligsohn V, Sheba C, Szeinberg A. Abnormal excretion of the isomers of urinary coproporphyrin by patients with Dubin-Johnson syndrome in Israel. Clin Sci 40:17, 1971
21. Berenson MM, Günther C, Samowitz WS, Bjorkman DJ. Formation of biliary thrombi in protoporphyrin-induced cholestasis in perfused rat liver. Hepatology 11:757, 1990
22. Beukeveld GJJ, Wolthers BG, Nordmann Y, Deybach JC, Grandchamp B, Wadman SK. A retrospective study of a patient with homozygous form of acute intermittent porphyria. J Inherit Metab Dis 13:673, 1990
23. Biempica L, Kosower N, Ma M H, Goldfischer S. Hepatic porphyrias: cytochemical and ultrastructural studies of liver in acute intermittent porphyria and porphyria cutanea tarda. Arch Pathol 98:336, 1974
24. Birchfield RI, Cowger ML. Acute intermittent porphyria with seizures: anticonvulsant medication-induced metabolic changes. Am J Dis Child 112:561, 1966
25. Bird TD, Hamernyik P, Nutter JY, et al. Inherited deficiency of delta-aminolevulinic acid dehydratase. Am J Hum Genet 31:662, 1979
26. Bishop DF, Henderson AS, Astrin KH. Human δ-aminolevulinate synthase: assignment of the housekeeping gene to 3p21 and the erythroid-specific gene to the X chromosome. Genomics 7:207, 1990
27. Bloomer JR, Bonkovsky HL. The porphyrias. Dis Mon 35:1, 1989
28. Bloomer JR, Bonkovsky HL, Ebert PS, Mahoney MJ. Inheritance in protoporphyria: comparison of heme synthetase activity in skin fibroblasts with clinical features. Lancet 2:226, 1976
29. Bloomer JR, Hill HD, Morton KO, Anderson-Burnham LA, Straka JG. The enzyme defect in bovine protoporphyria: studies with purified ferrochelatase. J Biol Chem 262:667, 1986
30. Bloomer JR, Phillips MJ, Davidson DL, Klatskin G. Hepatic

disease in erythropoietic protoporphyria. Am J Med 58:869, 1975

31. Bloomer JR, Pierach CA. Effect of hematin administration to patients with protoporphyria and liver disease. Hepatology 2:817, 1982

32. Bloomer JR, Straka JG. Porphyrin metabolism. In: Arias IM, Jakoby WB, Popper H, Schachter D, Shafritz DA, eds. The liver: biology and pathobiology, ed 2. New York, Raven Press, 1988, p 451

33. Bloomer JR, Straka JG, Hill HD, Weimer MK, Ruth GR. Comparison of bile porphyrin concentrations in cattle and human beings with protoporphyria. J Am Vet Med Assoc 51:1144, 1990

34. Bloomer JR, Weimer MK, Bossenmaier IC, Snover DC, Payne WD, Ascher NL. Liver transplantation in a patient with protoporphyria. Gastroenterology 97:188, 1989

35. Bonkovsky HL. Porphyrin and heme metabolism and the porphyrias. In: Zakim D, Boyer TD, eds. Hepatology: a textbook of liver diseases. Philadelphia, WB Saunders, 1982, p 351

36. Bonkovsky HL. The porphyrias. In: Conn RB, ed. Current diagnosis, ed 7. Philadelphia, WB Saunders, 1985, p 799

37. Bonkovsky HL, Bloomer JR, Ebert PS, Mahoney MJ. Heme synthetase deficiency in human protoporphyria: demonstration of the defect in liver and cultured skin fibroblasts. J Clin Invest 56:1139, 1975

38. Bonkovsky HL, Pomeroy JS. Human hepatic δ-aminolevulinate synthase: requirement of an exogenous system for succinyl-coenzyme A generation to demonstrate increased activity in cirrhotic and anti-convulsant-treated subjects. Clin Sci J Med 52:509, 1977

39. Bonkovsky HL, Schady W. Neurologic manifestations of acute porphyria. Semin Liver Dis 2:108, 1982

40. Bonkovsky HL, Schned AR. Fatal liver failure in protoporphyria: synergism between ethanol excess and the genetic defect. Gastroenterology 90:191, 1986

41. Bonkovsky HL, Sinclair PR, Scott E, Sinclair JF. Seizure management in acute hepatic porphyria: risks of valproate and clonazepam. Neurology 30:588, 1980

42. Bonkovsky HL, Sinclair PR, Sinclair JF. Hepatic heme metabolism and its control. Yale J Biol Med 52:13, 1979

43. Bonkovsky HL, Tschudy DP, Collins A, et al. Repression of the overproduction of porphyrin precursors in acute intermittent porphyria by intravenous infusions of hematin. Proc Natl Acad Sci USA 68:2725, 1971

44. Bonnett R, Davies JE, Hursthouse MB. Structure of bilirubin. Nature 262:326, 1976

45. Bottomley SS, Tanaka M, Everett MA. Diminished erythroid ferrochelatase activity in protoporphyria. J Lab Clin Med 86:126, 1975

46. Braun A, Berman J. Pathological anatomy in porphyria cutanea tarda. Acta Univ Carol 8:597, 1959

47. Brenner DA, Bloomer JR. The enzymatic defect in variegate porphyria: studies with human cultured skin fibroblasts. N Engl J Med 302:765, 1980

48. Burton G, Fagerness PE, Hosozawa S, Jordan PM, Scott AI. C-13 NMR Evidence for a new intermediate, pre-uroporphyrinogen, in the enzymic transformation of porphobilinogen into uroporphyrinogen I and uroporphyrinogen II. J Chem Soc Chem Commun 202, 1979

49. Chlumska A, Chlumsky J, Malina L. Liver changes in porphyria cutanea tarda patients treated with chloroquine. Br J Dermatol 102:261, 1980

50. Chretien S, Dubart A, Beaupain D, et al. Alternative transcription and splicing of the human porphobilinogen deaminase gene result either in tissue-specific or in housekeeping gene. Proc Natl Acad Sci USA 85:6, 1988

51. Cortes JM, Oliva H, Paradinas FJ, Hernando-Guio C. The pathology of the liver in porphyria cutanea tarda. Histopathology 4:471, 1980

52. Cox TM, Bawden MJ, Abraham NG, et al. Erythroid 5-ami-

nolevulinate synthase is located on the X-chromosome. Am J Hum Genet 46:107, 1990

53. Cram DL, Epstein JH, Tuffanelli DL. Lupus erythematosus and porphyria. Arch Dermatol 108:779, 1973

54. Cripps DJ, Gilbert LA, Goldfarb S. Erythropoietic protoporphyria: juvenile protoporphyrin hepatopathy, cirrhosis and death. J Pediatr 91:744, 1977

55. Cripps DJ, Scheuer PJ. Hepatobiliary changes in erythropoietic protoporphyria. Arch Pathol 80:500, 1965

56. Czarnecki DB. Hepatoerythropoietic porphyria. Arch Dermatol 116:307, 1980

57. Dailey HA, Fleming JE. Bovine ferrochelatase: kinetic analysis of inhibition by N-methylprotoporphyrin, manganese and heme. J Biol Chem 258:11453, 1983

58. Day RS, Eales L, Pimstone NR. Familial symptomatic porphyria in South Africa. S Afr Med J 56:909, 1979

59. Dean G. Porphyria. Br Med J 12:1291, 1953

60. Dean G. The Turkish epidemic of porphyria. S Afr Med J 35:509, 1961

61. Dean G. The porphyrias: a study of inheritance and environment, ed 2. London, Pitman Medical, 1971

62. Dean G, Barnes HD. The inheritance of porphyria. Br Med J 9:89, 1955

63. DeGoeij AFPM, Christianse K, Van Steveninck I. Decreased haem synthetase activity in blood cells of patients with erythropoietic protoporphyria. Eur J Clin Invest 5:397, 1975

64. Delaunay J, Ranu RS, Levin DH, Ernst V, London IM. Characterization of a rat liver factor that inhibits initiation of protein synthesis in rabbit reticulocyte lysates. Proc Natl Acad Sci USA 74:2265, 1977

65. Delfau MH, Picat C, de Rooij FWM, et al. Two different point G to A mutations in exon 10 of the porphobilinogen deaminase gene are responsible for acute intermittent porphyria. J Clin Invest 86:1511, 1990

66. Desnick RJ, Ostasiewicz LT, Tishler PA, Mustajoki P. Acute intermittent porphyria: characterization of a novel mutation in the structural gene for porphobiliogen deaminase: demonstration of noncatalytic enzyme intermediates stabilized by bound substrate. J Clin Invest 76:865, 1985

67. Deybach J-C, Verneuil H de, Boulechfar S, Grandchamp B, Nordmann Y. Point mutations in the uroporphyrinogen III synthase gene in congenital erythropoietic porphyria (Günther's disease) Blood 75:1763, 1990

68. Dhar GJ, Bossenmaier I, Cardinal R, et al. Transitory renal failure following rapid administration of a relatively large amount of hematin in a patient with acute intermittent porphyria in clinical remission. Acta Med Scand 203:437, 1978

69. Disler P, Day R, Burman N, Blekkenhorst G, Eales L. Treatment of hemodialysis-related porphyria cutanea tarda with plasma exchange. Am J Med 72:989, 1982

70. Dobozy A, Csato M, Siklosi C, Simon N. Transfusion therapy for erythropoietic protoporphyria. Br J Dermatol 109:571, 1983

71. Doss M. Pathobiochemical transition of secondary coproporphyrinuria to chronic hepatic porphyria in humans. Klin Wochenschr 58:141, 1980

72. Doutre MS, Beylot C, Beylot J, Nordmann Y, De Verneuil H, Bioulac P. Porphyrie cutanee tardive de l'enfant: une observation avec etude enzymatique familiale. Nouv Presse Med 10:1502, 1981

73. Eales L. Porphyria and the dangerous life-threatening drugs. S Afr Med J 56:914, 1979

74. Elder GH, Evans JO. Evidence that coproporphyrinogen oxidase activity of rat liver is situated in the intermembrane space of mitochondria. Biochem J 172:345, 1978

75. Elder GH, Sheppard DM, de Salamanca RE, et al. Identification of two types of porphyria cutanea tarda by measurement of erythrocyte uroporphyrinogen decarboxylase. Clin Sci 58:477, 1980

76. Elder GH, Sheppard DM, Tovey JA, Urquhart AJ. Immu-

noreactive uroporphyrinogen decarboxylase in porphyria cutanea tarda. Lancet 1:1301, 1983

77. Elder GH, Smith SG, Herrero C, et al. Hepatoerythropoietic porphyria: a new uroporphyrinogen decarboxylase defect or homozygous porphyria cutanea tarda? Lancet 1:916, 1981

78. Emiliani C, Delmelle M. The lipid solubility of porphyrins modulates their phototoxicity in membrane models. Photochem Photobiol 37:487, 1983

79. Enerback L, Lundvall O. Properties and distribution of liver fluorescence in porphyria cutanea tarda (PCT). Virchows Arch [A] 350:293, 1970

80. Epstein JH, Tuffanelli DL, Epstein WL. Cutaneous changes in the porphyrias: a microscopic study. Arch Dermatol 107:689, 1973

81. Evans JN, Davies RC, Boyd AS, et al. Biosynthesis of porphyrins and corrins. 1. 1H and 13C NMR spectra of (hydroxymethyl)bilane and uroporphyrinogens I and III. Biochemistry 25:894, 1986

82. Felsher BF, Kushner JP. Hepatic siderosis and porphyria cutanea tarda: relation of iron excess to the metabolic defect. Semin Hematol 14:243, 1977

83. Felsher BF, Norris ME, Shih JC. Red-cell uroporphyrinogen decarboxylase activity in porphyria cutanea tarda and other forms of porphyria. N Engl J Med 299:1095, 1978

84. Felsher BF, Redeker AG. Acute intermittent porphyria: effect of diet and griseofulvin. Medicine 46:217, 1967

85. Francis JE, Smith AG. Oxidation of uroporphyrinogens by hydroxyl radicals: evidence for nonporphyrin products as potential inhibitors of uroporphyrinogen decarboxylase. FEBS Lett 233:311, 1988

86. Garcia-Merino JA, Lopez-Lozano JJ. Risks of valproate in porphyria. Lancet 2:856, 1980

87. Garey JR, Hansen JL, Harrison LM, Kennedy JB, Kushner JP. A point mutation in the coding region of uroporphyrinogen decarboxylase associated with familial porphyria cutanea tarda. Blood 73:892, 1989

88. Garey JR, Harrison LM, Franklin KF, Metcalf KM, Radisky ES, Kushner JP. Uroporphyrinogen decarboxylase: a splice site mutation causes the deletion of exon 6 in multiple families with porphyria cutanea tarda. J Clin Invest 86:1416, 1990

89. Gentz J, Johansson S, Lindblad B, et al. Excretion of δ-aminolevulinic acid in hereditary tyrosinemia. Clin Chim Acta 23:257, 1969

90. Gibson JB, Goldberg A. The neuropathy of acute porphyria. J Pathol Bacteriol 71:495, 1956

91. Gigli I, Schothorst AA, Soter NA, Pathak MA. Erythropoietic protoporphyria: photoactivation of the complement system. J Clin Invest 66:517, 1980

92. Girotti AW. Photodynamic action of protoporphyrin IX on human erythrocytes: cross-linking of membrane proteins. Biochem Biophys Res Comm 72:1367, 1976

93. Goldberg A. Acute intermittent porphyria: a study of 50 cases. Q J Med 28:183, 1959

94. Goldstein BD, Harber LC. Erythropoietic protoporphyria: lipid peroxidation and red cell membrane damage associated with photohemolysis. J Clin Invest 51:892, 1972

95. Gordeuk VR, Brittenham GM, Hawkins CW, Mukhtar H, Bickers DR. Iron therapy for hepatic dysfunction in erythropoietic protoporphyria. Ann Intern Med 105:27, 1986

96. Grandchamp B, Picat C, de Rooij F, et al. A point mutation G–A in exon 12 of the porphobilinogen deaminase gene results in exon skipping and is responsible for acute intermittent porphyria. Nucleic Acids Res 17:6637, 1989

97. Grandchamp B, Picat C, Kauppinen R, et al. Molecular analysis of acute intermittent porphyria in a Finnsh family with normal erythrocyte porphobilinogen deaminase. Eur J Clin Invest 19:415, 1989

98. Grandchamp B, Picat C, Mignotte V, et al. Tissue-specific splicing mutation in acute intermittent porphyria. Proc Natl Acad Sci USA 86:661, 1989

99. Grandchamp B, Verneuil H de, Beaumont C, Chretien S, Walter O, Nordmann Y. Tissue-specific expression of porphobilinogen deaminase: two isoenzymes from a single gene. Eur J Biochem 162:105, 1987

100. Günther H. Die bedeutung der haematoporphyrine in physiologie und pathologie. Ergeb Allg Path Anat 20:608, 1922

101. Günther H. Die haematoporphyrie. Dtsch Archiv Klin Med 105:89, 1911

102. Günther WW. The porphyrias and erythropoietic protoporphyria: an unusual case. Australas J Dermatol 9:23, 1967

103. Haeger-Aronsen B. Erythropoietic protoporphyria: a new type of inborn error of metabolism. Am J Med 35:450, 1963

104. Harbin BM, Dailey HA. Orientation of ferrochelatase in bovine liver mitochondria. Biochemistry 24:366, 1985

105. Hayashi N, Kurashima Y, Kikuchi G. Mechanism of allylisopropylacetamide-induced increase of [delta]-aminolevulinate synthetase in liver mitochondria. Arch Biochem Biophys 148:10, 1972

106. Hofstad F, Seip M, Eriksen L. Congenital erythropoietic porphyria with a hitherto undescribed porphyrin pattern. Acta Paediatr Scand 62:380, 1973

107. Ibrahim GW, Watson CJ. Enterohepatic circulation and conversion of protoporphyrin to bile pigment in man. Proc Soc Exp Biol Med 127:890, 1968

108. Ishida N, Fujita H, Noguchi T, Doss M, Kappas A, Sassa S. Message amplification phenotyping of an inherited [delta]-aminolevulinate dehydratase deficiency in a family with acute hepatic porphyria. Biochem Biophys Res Commun 172:237, 1990

109. Jackson AH, Elder GH, Smith SG. The metabolism of coproporphyrinogen III into protoporphyrinogen IX. Int J Biochem 9:877, 1978

110. Jackson AH, Sancovich HA, Ferramola AM, et al. Macrocyclic intermediates in the biosynthesis of porphyrins. Phil Trans R Soc Lond 273:191, 1976

111. Jacobs JM, Sinclair PR, Lambrecht RW, Sinclair JF, Jacobs NJ. Role of inducer binding in cytochrome P-450 IA2 mediated uroporphyrinogen oxidation. J Biochem Toxicol 5:193, 1990

112. Jacobs JM, Sinclair PR, Lambrecht RW, Sinclair JF. Effects of iron-EDTA on uroporphyrinogen oxidation by liver microsomes. FEBS Lett 250:349, 1989

113. James KR, Cortez JM, Paradinas FJ. Demonstration of intracytoplasmic needle-like inclusions in hepatocytes of patients with porphyria cutanea tarda. Tech Meth 3:899, 1980

114. Jones EA, Bloomer JR, Berlin NI. The measurement of the synthetic rate of bilirubin from hepatic hemes in patients with acute intermittent porphyria. J Clin Invest 50:2259, 1971

115. Jones MS, Jones OTG. The structural organization of haem synthesis in rat liver mitochondria. Biochem J 113:507, 1969

116. Kaplowitz N, Javitt N, Kappas A. Coproporphyrin I and III excretion in bile and urine. J Clin Invest 51:2895, 1972

117. Kappas A, Sassa S, Galbraith RA, Nordmann Y. The porphyrias. In: Scriver CR, Beaudet AL, Sly WS, Valle, D, eds. The metabolic basis of inherited disease, ed 6. New York, McGraw Hill, 1989, p 1305

118. Kaufman L, Marver HS. Biochemical defects in two types of human hepatic porphyria. N Engl J Med 283:954, 1970

119. Kauppinen R, Mustajoki P. Acute hepatic porphyria and hepatocellular carcinoma. Br J Cancer 57:117, 1988

120. King ES, Gerald PS. Hereditary tyrosinemia and abnormal pyrrole metabolism. J Pediatr 77:397, 1970

121. Klatskin G, Bloomer JR. Birefringence of hepatic pigment deposits in erythropoietic protoporphyria: specificity and sensitivity of polarization microscopy in the identification of hepatic porphyrin deposits. Gastroenterology 67:294, 1974

122. Kools AM, Straka JG, Hill HD, Whitmer DI, Holman RT, Bloomer JR. Modulation of hepatic ferrochelatase activity by dietary manipulation of mitochondrial phospholipid fatty acyl groups. Hepatology 9:557, 1989

123. Kordac V. Frequency of occurrence of hepatocellular carcinoma in patients with porphyria cutanea tarda in long-term follow-up. Neoplasma 19:135, 1972

124. Koskelo P, Toironen I, Adelcreutz H. Urinary coproporphyrin isomer distribution in the Dubin-Johnson syndrome. Clin Chem 13:1006, 1967

125. Kostler VE, Heinicke HJ. Porphyria cutanea tarda: Pseudoporphyrie und Hamodialyse chronisch Niereninsuffizienter. Z Gesamte Inn Med, Jahrg Heft 2:41, 1986

126. Koszo F, Elder GH, Roberts A, Simon N. Uroporphyrinogen decarboxylase deficiency in hepatoerythropoietic porphyria: further evidence for genetic heterogeneity. Br J Dermatol 122:365, 1990

127. Kramer S, Viljoen D, Becker D, et al. A possible explanation for the neurological disturbances in the porphyrias. S Afr J Lab Clin Med 17:103, 1971

128. Kushner JP, Barbuto AJ, Lee GR. An inherited enzymatic defect in porphyria cutanea tarda: decreased uroporphyrinogen decarboxylase activity. J Clin Invest 58:1089, 1976

129. Kushner JP, Lee GR, Nacht S. The role of iron in the pathogenesis of porphyria cutanea tarda: an in vitro model. J Clin Invest 51:3044, 1972

130. Lamola AA, Asher I, Muller-Eberhard U, Poh-Fitzpatrick M. Fluorimetric study of the binding of protoporphyrin to haemopexin and albumin. Biochem J 196:693, 1981

131. Lamola AA, Yamane T. Zinc protoporphyrin in the erythrocytes of patients with lead intoxication and iron deficiency anemia. Science 186:936, 1974

132. Lamon JM, Frykholm BC, Tschudy DP. Hematin administration to an adult with lead intoxication. Blood 53:1007, 1979

133. Lamon JM, Poh-Fitzpatrick MB, Lamola AA. Hepatic protoporphyrin production in human protoporphyria: effects of intravenous hematin and analysis of erythrocyte protoporphyrin distribution. Gastroenterology 79:115, 1980

134. Larson AW, Wasserström WR, Felsher BF, Shih JC. Posttraumatic epilepsy and acute intermittent porphyria: effects of phenytoin, carbamazepine and clonazepam. Neurology 28:824, 1978

135. Lazaro P, De Salamanca RE, Elder GH, Villaseca ML, Chinarro S, Jaqueti G. Is hepatoerythropoietic porphyria a homozygous form of porphyria cutanea tarda? Inheritance of uroporphyrinogen decarboxylase deficiency in a Spanish family. Br J Dermatol 110:613, 1984

136. Lefkowitch JH, Grossman ME. Hepatic pathology in porphyria cutanea tarda. Liver 3:19, 1983

137. Levin EY. Uroporphyrinogen cosynthetase from mouse spleen. Biochemistry (USA) 7:3781, 1968

138. Lim CK, Peters TJ. Urine and faecal prophyrin profiles by reversed-phase high performance liquid chromatography in the porphyrias. Clin Chim Acta 139:55, 1984

139. Lim HW, Gigli I, Wasserman SI. Differential effects of protoporphyrin and uroporphyrin on murine mast cells. J Invest Dermatol 88:281, 1987

140. Lim HW, Gigli I. Role of complement in porphyrin-induced photosensitivity. J Invest Dermatol 76:4, 1981

141. Lim HW, Poh-Fitzpatrick MB. Hepatoerythropoietic porphyria: a variant of childhood-onset porphyria cutanea tarda. J Am Acad Dermatol 11:1103, 1984

142. Lindblad B, Lindstedt S, Stein G. On the enzymatic defects in hereditary tyrosinemia. Proc Natl Acad Sci USA 74:4641, 1977

143. Lithner F, Westerberg L. Hepatocellular carcinoma in patients with acute intermittent porphyria. Acta Med Scand 215:271, 1984

144. Litman DA, Correia MA. Elevated brain tryptophan and enhanced 5-hydroxytryptamine turnover in acute hepatic heme deficiency: clinical implications. J Pharmacol Exp Ther 232:337, 1985

145. Llewellyn DH, Elder GH, Kalsheker NA, et al. DNA polymorphism of human porphobilinogen deaminase gene in acute intermittent porphyria. Lancet II:706, 1987

146. Logan GM, Weimer MK, Ellefson M, Pierach CA, Bloomer JR. Bile porphyrin analysis in the evaluation of variegate porphyria. N Engl J Med 324:1408, 1991

147. Loveless MD, Straka JG, Bloomer JR. On the mechanism of liver damage in porphyria cutanea tarda. (Abstract) Hepatology 6:1160, 1986

148. Ludwig GD, Epstein IS. A genetic study of two families having the acute intermittent type of porphyria. Ann Intern Med 55:81, 1961

149. Lundvall O, Weinfeld A. Studies of the clinical and metabolic effects of phlebotomy treatment in porphyria cutanea tarda. Acta Medica Scand 184:191, 1968

150. Magnus IA, Jarrett A, Prankerd TAJ, Rimington C. Erythropoietic protoporphyria: a new porphyria syndrome with solar urticaria due to protoporphyrinaemia. Lancet 2:448, 1961

151. Marks GS, McClusky SA, Mackie JE, Riddick DS, James CA. Disruption of hepatic heme biosynthesis after interaction of xenobiotics with cytochrome P-450. FASEB J 2:2774, 1988

152. Marks GS, McClusky SA, Mackie JE, Riddick DS, James CA. Interaction of chemicals with cytochrome P-450: implication for the porphyrinogenicity of drugs. Clin Biochem 22:169, 1989

153. Mathews-Roth M. Anemia in erythropoietic protoporphyria. JAMA 230:824, 1974

154. McCullough AJ, Barron D, Mullen KD, et al. Fecal protoporphyrin excretion in erythropoietic protoporphyria: effect of cholestyramine and bile acid feeding. Gastroenterology 94:177, 1988

155. Meissner PN, Adams P, Kirsch RE. Inhibition of porphobilinogen deaminase by heme precursors: a possible mechanism for the acute attack of variegate porphyria. Mol Aspects Med 11:51, 1990

156. Milligan A, Graham-Brown RAC, Sarkany I, Baker H. Erythropoietic protoporphyria exacerbated by oral iron therapy. Br J Dermatol 119:63, 1988

157. Mitchell G, Larochelle J, Lambert M, et al. Neurologic crises in hereditary tyrosinemia. N Engl J Med 322:432, 1988

158. Mooyaart BR, de Jang GM Th, van der Veen S, Driessen LHHM, Beukeveld GJJ, Grand J, et al. Hepatic disease in erythropoietic protoporphyria. Dermatalogica 173:120, 1986

159. Morehouse K, Moreno SNJ, Mason RP. The one-electron reduction of uroporphyrin I by rat hepatic microsomes. Arch Biochem Biophys 257:276, 1987

160. Morton KO, Schneider F, Weimer MK, Straka JG, Bloomer JR. Hepatic and bile porphyrins in patients with protoporphyria and liver failure. Gastroenterology 94:1488, 1988

161. Mukerji SK, Pimstone NR, Burns M. Dual mechanism of inhibition of rat liver uroporphyrinogen decarboxylase activity by ferrous iron: its potential role in the genesis of porphyria cutanea tarda. Gastroenterology 87:1248, 1984

162. Mustajoki P, Tenhunen R, Pierach C, Volin L. Heme in the treatment of porphyrias and hematological disorders. Semin Hematol 26:1, 1989

163. Naqui A, Chance B, Cadenas E. Reactive oxygen intermediates in biochemistry. Annu Rev Biochem 55:137, 1986

164. Nicholson DC, Cowger ML, Kalivas J, Thompson RDH, Gray CH. Isotope studies of the erythropoietic and hepatic components of congenital porphyria and erythropoietic protoporphyria. Clin Sci 44:135, 1973

165. Nielsen B, Thorn NA. Transient excess urinary excretion of antidiuretic material in acute intermittent porphyria with hyponatremia and hypomagnesemia. Am J Med 38:345, 1965

166. Nordmann Y, Deybach JC. Congenital erythropoietic porphyria. Semin Liver Dis 2:154, 1982

167. Nyman CR. Porphyria cutanea tarda, carcinoma of the lung, rheumatoid arthritis, right hydronephrosis. Proc R Soc Med 65:688, 1972

168. O'Connor JA, Tishler PV, Gordon BJ, et al. Prevalence of

intermittent acute porphyria (IAP) in psychiatric and normal populations. Biochem Genet 16:37A, 1978

169. Ostrowshi J, Kostrzewska EWA, Michalak T, Zawirska B, Medrzejewski W, Gregor A. Abnormalities in liver function and morphology and impaired aminopyrine metabolism in hereditary hepatic porphyrias. Gastroenterology 85:1131, 1983

170. Percy VA, Shanley RC. Porphyrin precursors in blood, urine and cerebrospinal fluid in acute porphyria. S Afr Med J 52:219, 1977

171. Perlroth MG, Tschudy DP, Marver HS, et al. Acute intermittent porphyria: new morphologic and biochemical findings. Am J Med 41:149, 1966

172. Picat C, Delfau MH, de Rooij FWM, et al. Identification of the mutations in the parents of a patient with a putative compound heterozygosity for acute intermittent porphyria. J Inherited Metab Dis 13:684, 1990

173. Pierach CA. Hematin therapy for the porphyric attack. Semin Liver Dis 2:125, 1982

174. Pimstone NR, Webber BL, Blekkenhorst GH, Eales L. The hepatic lesion in protoporphyria (PP): preliminary studies of haem metabolism, liver structure and ultrastructure. Ann Clin Res 8(Suppl 17):122, 1976

175. Pinol Aquade J, Herrero C, Almeida J, et al. Porphyrie hepatoerythrocytaire, une nouvelle forme de porphyrie. Ann Dermatol Syphilol 102:129, 1975

176. Piomelli S. The diagnostic utility of measurements of erythrocyte porphyrins. Hematol Oncol Clin North Am 1:419, 1987

177. Piomelli S, Lamola AA, Poh-Fitzpatrick MB, Seaman C, Harber LL. Erythropoietic protoporphyria and lead intoxication: the molecular basis for difference in cutaneous photosensitivity. 1. Different rates of disappearance of protoporphyrin from the erythrocytes, both in vivo and in vitro. J Clin Invest 56:1519, 1975

178. Poh-Fitzpatrick MB. Pathogenesis and treatment of photocutaneous manifestations of the porphyrias. Semin Liver Dis 2:164, 1982

179. Poh-Fitzpatrick MB. Protoporphyrin metabolic balance in human protoporphyria. Gastroenterology 88:1239, 1985

180. Poh-Fitzpatrick MB, Bellet N, DeLeo VA, Grossman ME, Bickers DB. Porphyria cutanea tarda in two patients treated with hemodialysis for chronic renal failure. N Engl J Med 299:292, 1978

181. Poh-Fitzpatrick MB, Masullo AS, Grossman ME. Porphyria cutanea tarda associated with chronic renal disease and hemodialysis. Arch Dermatol 116:191, 1980

182. Poh-Fitzpatrick MB, Sklar JA, Goldsman C, Lefkowitch JH. Protoporphyrin hepatopathy: effects of cholic acid ingestion in murine griseofulvin-induced protoporphyria. J Clin Invest 72:1449, 1983

183. Porter FS, Lowe BA. Congenital erythropoietic protoporphyria. I. Case reports, clinical studies and porphyrin analyses in two brothers. Blood 22:521, 1963

184. Poulson R. The enzymic conversion of protoporphyrinogen IX to protoporphyrin IX in mammalian mitochondria. J Biol Chem 251:3730, 1976

185. Prado MJC, De Salamanca RE, Hernando MV, Payero MLP, Beltran TC, Aguilar AR. Two cases of infantile and familial porphyria cutanea tarda. Dermatologica 161:205, 1980

186. Rademakers LHPM, Cleton MI, Kooijman C, Baart de la Faille H, van Hattum J. Early involvement of hepatic parenchymal cells in erythrohepatic protoporphyria: an ultrastructural study of patients with and without overt liver disease and the effect of chenodeoxycholic acid treatment. Hepatology 11:449, 1990

187. Ramasamy R, Kubik MM. Porphyria cutanea tarda in association with Sjogren's syndrome. Practitioner 226:1297, 1982

188. Rank JM, Pascual-Leone A, Payne W, et al. Hematin therapy for the neurologic crisis of tyrosinemia. J Pediatr 118:136, 1991

189. Rank JM, Straka JG, Bloomer JR. Liver in disorders of porphyrin metabolism. J Gastroenterol Hepatol 5:573, 1990

190. Rank JM, Straka JG, Weimer MK, Bossenmaier I, Taddeini L, Bloomer JR. Hematin therapy in late onset congenital erythropoietic porphyria. Br J Haematol 75:617, 1990

191. Riddle RD, Yamamoto M, Engle JO. Expression of 5-aminolevulinate synthase in avian cells: separate genes encode erythroid specific and non-specific isozymes. Proc Natl Acad Sci (USA) 86:792, 1989

192. Ridley A. Porphyric neuropathy. In: Dyck PJ, Thomas PK, Lambert EH, eds. Peripheral neuropathy, vol 2. Philadelphia, WB Saunders, 1975. p 942

193. Rifkind AB, Gillette PN, Song CS, Kappas A. Drug stimulation of a-aminolevulinic acid synthetase and cytochrome P-450 in vivo in chick embryo liver. J Pharmacol Exp Ther 185:214, 1973

194. Rimington C. Biliary secretion of porphyrins and hepatogenous photosensitization. In: Taylor W, ed. The biliary system. Philadelphia, FA Davis, 1965, p 325

195. Rimington C, Lockwood WH, Belcher RV. The excretion of porphyrinpeptide conjugates in porphyria variegata. Clin Sci 35:211, 1968

196. Rocchi E, Gibertini P, Cassanelli M, Pietrangelo A, Jensen J, Ventura E. Hepatitis B virus infection in porphyria cutanea tarda. Liver 6:153, 1986

197. Romana M, Dubart A, Beaupain D, Chabret C, Goossens M, Romeo PH. Structure of the gene for human uroporphyrinogen decarboxylase. Nucl Acids Res 15:7347, 1987

198. Romeo PH, Chretien S, Dubart A, et al. Erythroid specific promoter of an housekeeping gene. Prog Clin Biol Res 251:55, 1987

199. Rutherford T, Thompson GG, Moore MR. Heme biosynthesis in Friend erythroleukemia cells: control by ferrochelatase. Proc Natl Acad Sci USA 76:833, 1979

200. Salata H, Cortes JM, De Dalamanca RE, et al. Porphyria cutanea tarda and hepatocellular carcinoma: frequency of occurrence and related factors. J Hepatol 1:477, 1985

201. Sandberg S, Romslo I, Hovding G, Bjorndal T. Porphyrin-induced photodamage as related to the subcellular localization of the porphyrins. Acta Derm Venereol (Suppl) 100:75, 1982

202. Sano S, Granick S. Mitochondrial coproporphyrinogen oxidase and protoporphyin formation. J Biol Chem 236:1173, 1961

203. Sassa S. Sequential induction of heme pathway enzymes during erythroid differentiation of mouse Friend leukemia virus–infected cells. J Exp Med 143:305, 1976

204. Sassa S, Bradlow HL, Kappas A. Steroid induction of d-aminolevulinic acid synthase and porphyrins in liver: structure-activity studies on the permissive effects of hormones on the induction process. J Biol Chem 254:10011, 1979

205. Sassa S, de Verneuil H, Anderson KE, et al. Purification and properties of human erythrocyte uroporphyrinogen decarboxylase: immunological demonstration of the enzyme defect in porphyria cutanea tarda. Trans Assoc Am Physicians 46:65, 1983

206. Sassa S, Kappas A. Hereditary tyrosinemia and the heme biosynthesis pathway: profound inhibition of d-aminolevulinic acid dehydratase activity by succinylacetone. J Clin Invest 73:625, 1983

207. Scane AC, Wight JP, Godwin-Austen RB. Acute intermittent porphyria presenting as epilepsy. Br Med J 292:946, 1986

208. Schmid R. Cutaneous porphyria in Turkey. Med Intell 263:397, 1960

209. Schmid R, Schwartz S, Sundberg HD. Erythropoietic (congenital) porphyria: a rare abnormality of the normoblasts. Blood 10:416, 1955

210. Schmid R, Schwartz S, Watson CJ. Porphyrin content of bone marrow and liver in the various forms of porphyria. Arch Intern Med 93:167, 1954

211. Scholnick PL, Hammaker LE, Marver HS. Soluble hepatic

ALA synthase: end product inhibition of the partially purified enzyme. Proc Natl Acad Sci USA 63:65, 1969

212. Scholnick P, Marver HS, Schmid R. Erythropoietic protoporphyria: evidence for multiple sites of excess protoporphyrin formation. J Clin Invest 50:203, 1971

213. Schwartz S, Johnson JA, Stephenson BD, Anderson AS, Edmondson PR, Fusaro RM. Erythropoietic defects in protoporphyria: a study of factors involved in labelling of porphyrins and bile pigments from ALA-³H and glycine-¹⁴C. J Lab Clin Med 78:411, 1971

214. Scobie GA, Llewellyn DH, Urquhart AJ, et al. Acute intermittent porphyria caused by a C→T mutation that produces a stop codon in the porphobilinogen deaminase gene. Hum Genet 85:631, 1990

215. Semon C, Dupond JL, Mallet H, Grandmottet-Cambefort G, Humbert P. Traitement d-une porphyrie aigue intermittente avec attaques cycliques par un agoniste LH-RH adminstre par voie nasale. Ann Endocrinol (Paris) 47:399, 1986

216. Seubert S, Seubert A, Rumpf KW, Kiffe H. A porphyria cutanea tarda-like distribution pattern of porphyrins in plasma, hemodialysate, hemofiltrate, and urine of patients on chronic hemodialysis. J Invest Dermatol 85:107, 1985

217. Shemin D, Rittenberg D. The biological utilization of glycine for the synthesis of the protoporphyrin of hemoglobin. J Biol Chem 166:621, 1946

218. Silbergeld EK, Fowler BA. Mechanisms of chemical-induced porphyrinopathies. NY Acad Sci 514:1, 1987

219. Simon N, Berko GY, Schneider I. Hepato-erythropoietic porphyria presenting as scleroderma and acrosclerosis in a sibling pair. Br J Dermatol 96:663, 1977

220. Sinclair PR, Granick S. Heme control on the synthesis of [delta]-aminolevulinic acid synthetase in cultured chick embryo liver cells. Ann NY Acad Sci 244:509, 1975

221. Smith AG, De Matteis F. Oxidative injury mediated by the hepatic cytochrome P-450 system in conjunction with cellular iron: effects on the pathway of haem biosynthesis. Xenobiotica 20:865, 1990

222. Smith AG, Francis JE, Carthew P. Iron as a synergist for hepatocellular carcinoma induced by polychlorinated biphenyls in Ah-responsive C57BL/10ScSn mice. Carcinogenesis 11:437, 1990

223. Smith AG, Francis JE, Green JA, Grieg JB, Wolf CR, Manson MM. Sex-linked hepatic uroporphyria and the induction of cytochromes P-450 IA2 in rats caused by hexachlorobenzene and polyhalogenated biphenyls. Biochem Pharmacol 40:2059, 1990

224. Solis JA, Betancor P, Campos R, et al. Association of porphyria cutanea tarda and primary liver cancer. J Dermatol 9:131, 1982

225. Solis-Herruzo JA, Nunoz-Yague MT, Enriquez De Salamance R. Algunas investigaciones sobre la significacion de la imagen laparoscopica del higado en las porfiria hepatica cronica. Gastroenterol Hepatol 1:155, 1978

226. Spiva DA, Lewis CE. Erythropoietic protoporphyria: therapeutic response to combined erythrocyte exchange and plasmapheresis. Photodermatology 5:211, 1984

227. Srivastava G, Borthwick IA, Maguire DJ, et al. Regulation of 5-aminolevulinate synthase mRNA in different rat tissues. J Biol Chem 263:5202, 1988

228. Stein JA, Curl FD, Valsamis M, Tschudy DP. Abnormal iron and water metabolism in acute intermittent porphyria with new morphologic findings. Am J Med 53:784, 1972

229. Stein JA, Tschudy DP. Acute intermittent porphyria: a clinical and biochemical study of 46 patients. Medicine 49:1, 1970

230. Stenhagen E, Rideal EK. The interaction between porphyrins and lipoid and protein monolayers. Biochem J 33:1591, 1939

231. Stokvis BJ. Concerning two unusual pigments in the urine of patients. Ned Tijdschr Geneeskd 25:409, 1889

232. Straka JG, Bloomer JR, Kempner ES. The functional size of

233. Straka JG, Kushner JP. Purification and characterization of bovine hepatic uroporphyrinogen decarboxylase. Biochemistry (USA) 22:4664, 1983

234. Straka JG, Rank JM, Bloomer JR. Porphyria and porphyrin metabolism. Annu Rev Med 41:457, 1990

235. Strand LJ, Felsher BF, Redeker AG, Marver HS. Heme biosynthesis in intermittent acute porphyria: decreased hepatic conversion of porphobilinogen to porphyrins and increased d-aminolevulinic acid synthetase activity. Proc Natl Acad Sci USA 67:1315, 1970

236. Sweeney GD, Jones KD, Cole FM, Basford D, Krestynski F. Iron deficiency prevents liver toxicity of 2,3,7,8-tetrachlorodibenzo-p-dioxin. Science 204:332, 1979

237. Taketani S, Tokunaga R. Purification and substrate specificity of bovine liver ferrochelatase. J Biochem 127:443, 1982

238. Tenhunen R, Marver HS, Schmid R. Microsomal heme oxygenase: characterization of the enzyme. J Biol Chem 244:6388, 1969

239. Tenhunen R, Ross ME, Marver HS, Schmid R. Reduced nicotinamide adenine dinucleotide phosphate dependent biliverdin reductase: partial purification and characterization. Biochemistry (USA) 9:298, 1970

240. Timme AH, Dowdle EB, Eales L. Symptomatic porphyria: 1. the pathology of the liver in human symptomatic porphyria. S Afr Med J 48:1803, 1974

241. Tio TH, Leijnes B, Jerret A, Rimington C. Acquired porphyria from a liver tumour. Clin Sci 16:517, 1957

242. Toback AC, Sassa S, Poh-Fitzpatrick MB, et al. Hepatoerythropoietic porphyria: clinical, biochemical and enzymatic studies in a three-generation family lineage. N Engl J Med 316:645, 1987

243. Topi GC, Gandolfo LD, Griso D, Morini S. Porphyria cutanea tarda and hepatocellular carcinoma. Int J Biochem 12:883, 1980

244. Tsai S-F, Bishop DF, Desnick RJ. Purification and properties of uroporphyrinogen III synthase from human erythrocytes. J Biol Chem 262:1268, 1987

245. Tschudy DP, Hess RA, Frykholm BC. Inhibition of δ-aminolevulinic acid dehydrase by 4,6-dioxoheptanoic acid. J Biol Chem 256:9915, 1980

246. Tschudy DP, Lamon JP. Porphyrin metabolism and the porphyrias. In: Bondy PK, Rosenberg LE, eds. Metabolic control and disease. Philadelphia, WB Saunders, 1980, p 939

247. Tschudy DP, Perlroth MG, Marver HS, Collins A, Hunter G Jr, Rechcigl M Jr. Acute intermittent porphyria: the first "overproduction disease" localized to a specific enzyme. Proc Natl Acad Sci USA 53:841, 1965

248. Tuchman M, Freese DK, Sharp HL, Ramnaraine ML. Ascher N, Bloomer JR. Contribution of extrahepatic tissues to biochemical abnormalities in hereditary tyrosinemia type 1: study of three patients after liver transplantation. J Pediatr 110:399, 1987

249. Turnbull A, Baker H, Vernon-Roberts B, Magnus IA. Iron metabolism in porphyria cutanea tarda and in erythropoietic protoporphyria. Q J Med 42:341, 1973

250. Uys CJ, Eales L. The histopathology of the liver in acquired (symptomatic) porphyria. S Afr J Lab Clin Med 9:190, 1963

251. Van Hattum J, Baart de la Faille H, Van den Berg JWO, Edixhoven-Bosdijk A, Wilson JHP. Chenodeoxycholic acid therapy in erythrohepatic protoporphyria. J Hepatol 3:407, 1986

252. Varadi S. Haematological aspects in a case of erythropoietic porphyria. Br J Haematol 4:270, 1958

253. Verneuil H de, Beaumont C, Deybach JC, et al. Enzymatic and immunological studies of uroporphyrinogen decarboxylase in familial porphyria cutanea tarda and hepatoerythropoietic porphyria. Am J Hum Genet 36:613, 1984

254. Verneuil H de, Grandchamp B, Beaumont C, Picat C, Nord-

mann Y. Uroporphyrinogen decarboxylase structural mutant (Gly[281]→Glu) in a case of porphyria. Science 234:732, 1986

255. Verneuil H de, Hansen J, Picat C, et al. Prevalence of the 281 (Gly→Glu) mutation in hepatoerythropoietic porphyria and porphyria cutanea tarda. Hum Genet 78:101, 1988

256. Verneuil H de, Nordmann Y, Phung N, et al. Familial and sporadic porphyria cutanea tarda: two different diseases. Eur J Biochem 9:927, 1978

257. Verneuil H de, Sassa S, Kappas A. Purification and properties of uroporphyrinogen decarboxylase from human erythrocytes: a single enzyme catalyzing the four sequential decarboxylations of uroporphyringens I and III. J Biol Chem 258:2454, 1983

258. Vessey DA, Goldenberg J, Zakim D. Differentiation of homologous forms of hepatic microsomal UDP-glucuronyltransferase. II. Characterization of the bilirubin conjugating form. Biochim Biophys Acta 309:75, 1973

259. Vincent SH, Muller-Eberhard U. A protein of the Z class of liver cytosolic proteins in the rat that preferentially binds heme. J Biol Chem 260:14521, 1985

260. Volden G, Thune P. Photosensitivity and cutaneous acid hydrolases in porphyria cutanea tarda. Ann Clin Res 11:129, 1979

261. Waldenström J. Some observations on acute porphyria and other conditions with a change in the excretion of porphyrins. Acta Med Scand 83:281, 1934

262. Waldenstrom J. The porphyrias as inborn errors of metabolism. Am J Med 22:758, 1957

263. Waldo ED, Tobias H. Needle-like cytoplasmic inclusions in the liver in porphyria cutanea tarda. Arch Pathol 96:368, 1973

264. Warnick GR, Burnham BF. Regulation of porphyrin biosynthesis: purification and characterization of 5-aminolevulinic acid synthase. J Biol Chem 246:6880, 1971

265. Watson CJ, Bossenmaier I, Cardinal R, Petryka ZJ. Repression by hematin of porphyrin biosynthesis in erythrocyte precursors in congenital erythropoietic porphyria. Proc Natl Acad Sci USA 71:278, 1974

266. Watson CJ, Schwartz S, Schulze W, Jacobson LO, Zagaria R. Studies of coproporphyrin. III. Idiopathic coproporphyrinuria: a hitherto unrecognized form characterized by lack of symptoms in spite of the excretion of large amounts of coproporphyrin. J Clin Invest 28:465, 1965

267. Watson CJ, Schwartz S. Simple test for urinary porphobilinogen. Proc Soc Exp Biol Med 47:393, 1941

268. Watson CJ, Taddeini L, Bossenmaier I. Present status of the Ehrlich aldehyde reaction for urinary porphobilinogen. JAMA 190:501, 1964

269. Wehrmacher WH. New symptomatic treatment for acute intermittent porphyria. Arch Intern Med 89:111, 1952

270. Welland FH, Hellman ES, Gaddis EM, Collins A, Hunter GW, Tschudy DP. Factors affecting the excretion of porphyrin precursors by patients with acute intermittent porphyria. I. Effects of diet. Metabolism 13:232, 1964

271. Went LN, Klasen EC. Genetic aspects of erythropoietic protoporphyria. Ann Hum Genet 48:105, 1984

272. Whiting MJ. Synthesis of δ-aminolevulinate synthase by isolated liver polyribosomes. Biochem J 158:391, 1976

273. With TK. A short history of porphyrins and the porphyrias. Int J Biochem 11:189, 1980

274. Yamamoto M, Hayashi N, Kikuchi G. Regulation of synthesis and intracellular translocation of delta-aminolevulinate synthase by heme and its relation to the heme saturation of tryptophan pyrrolase in rat liver. Arch Biochem Biophys 209:451, 1981

275. Yeung AC, Moore MR, Goldberg A. Pathogenesis of acute porphyria. Q J Med 63:377, 1987

276. Yeung Laiwah AC, Thompson GG, Philip MF, et al. Carbamazepine-induced non-hereditary acute porphyria. Lancet 1:790, 1983

277. Zaman Z, Jordan PM, Akhtar M. Mechanism and stereochemistry of the 5-aminolevulinate synthetase reaction. Biochem J 135:257, 1973

Diseases of the Liver, Seventh Edition, edited by Leon Schiff and Eugene R. Schiff. J.B. Lippincott Company, Philadelphia © 1993.

54

Amyloidosis of the Liver

Alan S. Cohen

Martha Skinner

Background

In the early 19th century, Rokitansky[112] and others observed a unique disorder causing a waxy, enlarged liver and, occasionally, similar changes in the spleen. Virchow subsequently observed that the "lardaceous" liver and spleen stained with iodine and sulfuric acid and, because of his belief that it had a certain similarity to cellulose, named it amyloid.[25,27] This substance was studied for about 60 years at the autopsy table and in experimental animals until direct biopsy procedures (1928) and the Congo red test and stain were introduced in the 1920s.[9,151] In the subsequent 30 years, a wide variety of studies, both clinical and experimental, were carried out on what was then considered an extremely rare degenerative condition. It has become apparent, however, that amyloidosis is far more common than had been thought, that it often is of great clinical significance, that it is associated with an extraordinarily wide variety of diseases, and, in the past several decades, that a number of genetically determined amyloidoses exist.[29]

Amyloidosis may be defined as the extracellular deposition of the fibrous protein amyloid in one or more sites of the body. A more modern definition would include the fact that this protein shows green birefringence on polarization microscopy after Congo red staining, 70- to 100-nm fibrils on electron microscopy, and a cross-β pattern on x-ray diffraction analysis. The substance may be local and isolated with no clinical consequences; may grossly involve virtually any organ system of the body, leading to severe pathophysiologic changes; or may fall between these two extremes. The natural history is poorly understood, and the clinical diagnosis is often not made until the disease is far advanced.

Although early studies showed that amyloid was often an accompaniment of chronic suppuration, it became apparent over 100 years ago that amyloidosis could also occur without predisposing disease. This led to a variety of classifications of amyloidosis, starting with that of Lubarsch[93] (typical, common, or secondary variety versus atypical, uncommon, or primary variety) and leading to the popular classification proposed by Reimann and coworkers[111] of primary amyloidosis (no antecedent or coexisting disease; mesodermal tissue involvement; variability of staining; tendency to nodular deposits), secondary amyloidosis (chronic disease-associated; liver, spleen, kidney, adrenal involvement; constant staining properties), tumor-forming amyloidosis (single or multiple masses of amyloid in eye, genitourinary or respiratory tract), and amyloidosis associated with multiple myeloma. King[78] subsequently commented on the overlap in organ involvement and staining properties and proposed that amyloid be called

typical (one or many focal deposits) with or without associated disease. Dahlin[45] returned to the use of primary (systemic or focal), secondary (systemic or focal), and myeloma-related disease. Symmers[141] emphasized the overlap in the many parameters and suggested division into generalized amyloidosis associated with a recognizable predisposing disease (generalized secondary amyloidosis), generalized amyloidosis without a recognized predisposing disease (generalized primary amyloidosis), and localized amyloidosis.

CLASSIFICATION

In recent years, it has become apparent that the heredofamilial amyloidoses, with their varying clinical manifestations, are not accommodated in the above schemes. A new system of classification has therefore been devised based on the polarization optical properties of amyloid as defined by Missmahl and Hartwig.[100] These investigators, who reaffirmed the green birefringence of amyloid after Congo red staining, believed that amyloid is laid down along either reticulin fibers or collagen fibers and classified it accordingly.[68,70]

As information has accrued regarding the basic chemical and immunologic properties of amyloid, it has seemed reasonable and clinically useful to classify the various types according to these new data. Thus, a nomenclature has been established that uses the letter A to designate amyloid fibril proteins.[39] This is modified by a second letter indicating the nature of the protein and the tissue, organ system, or disorder with which it is associated (Table 54-1). Primary and multiple myeloma-associated amyloid, which has an N-terminal sequence homologous with a portion of the variable part of immunoglobulin light chains, is designated AL. Secondary amyloidosis has a unique N-terminal sequence termed A-protein and is called AA. Many heredofamilial types of amyloid with polyneuropathy are classified ATTR and formed from the protein transthyretin. The serum counterpart of some of these tissue proteins is identified by addition of the letter S as a prefix, for example, SAA for the serum component related to AA.

INCIDENCE

The incidence of amyloidosis in the population at large is not known. The only data available are those based on postmortem studies, which, for the most part, give a falsely low indication of the autopsy incidence (because special stains that identify many cases of amyloid are not routinely carried out). There are a few studies on selected populations (patients with known leprosy, chronic tuberculosis, and so on) in which an

TABLE 54-1   *1990 Guidelines for Nomenclature and Classification of Amyloid and Amyloidosis*

Amyloid Protein*	Protein Precursor	Protein Type of Variant	Clinical
AA	Apo SAA		Reactive (secondary) Familial Mediterranean fever Familial amyloid nephropathy with urticaria and deafness (Muckle-Wells syndrome)
AL	κ, λ (eg, κ-III)	Aκ, Aλ (eg, Aκ-III)	Idiopathic (primary), myeloma, or macroglobulinemia-associated
AH	IgG-1 (γ1)	Aγl	
ATTR	Transthyretin	(eg, Met 30[†]) (eg, Met 111) TTR or Ile 122	Familial amyloid polyneuropathy, Portuguese Familial amyloid cardiomyopathy, Danish Systemic senile amyloidosis
AApoAI	Apo AI	Arg 26	Familial amyloid polyneuropathy, Iowa
AGel	Gelsolin	Asn 187[‡] (15)	Familial amyloidosis, Finnish
ACys	Cystatin C	Gln 68	Hereditary cerebral hemorrhage with amyloidosis, Icelandic
Aβ	β-protein precursor (eg, BPP$_{695}$)		Alzheimer's disease Down's syndrome
		Gln 618 (22)	Hereditary cerebral hemorrhage with amyloidosis, Dutch
Aβ$_2$M	β$_2$-microglobulin		Associated with chronic dialysis
AScr	Scrapie protein precursor 33–35[‖] cellular form	Scrapie protein 27–30 (eg, Leu 102)	Creutzfeldt-Jakob disease; Gerstmann-Straussler-Scheinker syndrome
ACal	(Pro)calcitonin	(Pro)calcitonin	In medullary carcinomas of the thyroid
AANF	Atrial natriuretic factor		Isolated atrial amyloid
AIAPP	Islet amyloid polypeptide		In islets of Langerhans; diabetes type II, insulinoma

AA, amyloid A protein; SAA, serum amyloid A protein; L, immunoglobulin light chain; H, immunoglobulin heavy chain
*Nonfibrillar proteins such as protein AP (amyloid P component) excluded
[†]ATTR Met 30 when used in text.
[‡]Amino acid positions in the mature precursor protein; the position in the amyloid fibril protein is given in parentheses.
[§]Number of amino acid residues.
[‖]Molecular mass (kilodaltons).
(Modified from Husby G, Araki S, Benditt EP, et al. The 1990 guidelines for nomenclature and classification of amyloid and amyloidosis. In: Natvig JB, Forre O, Husby G et al, eds. Amyloid Amyloidosis. Dordrecht, Kluwer, 1990)

exceedingly high incidence (up to 50%) of amyloid disease has been observed at postmortem examination. In the heredofamilial form of amyloid associated with familial Mediterranean fever, for which clinical and postmortem data have been carefully assessed, evidence of amyloidosis has been obtained in 26.5% of 470 patients.[134]

AMYLOID OF THE LIVER

Because the liver was possibly the first organ in which amyloid was described, the association has been well known to pathologists and clinicians alike. It has, however, attracted remarkably little detailed attention because (1) many reports were isolated case histories, (2) many cases undoubtedly went undetected, and (3) even when involved, hepatic amyloid was believed to be seldom of great clinical consequence. Until the 1920s, the diagnosis of hepatic amyloid disease was rarely, if ever, made while the patient was alive.

In 1928, Waldenström[151] demonstrated the value of biopsy when he performed the procedure on a patient with hepatomegaly and demonstrated the presence of amyloid. The role of the liver in the general pathophysiology of amyloid disease

remained minor, and in one review in 1936, it was stated that jaundice never occurred in amyloidosis.[101] Despite the fact that amyloid was usually secondary in origin when classified as parenchymal (kidney, spleen, liver, lymph node distribution) and was usually regarded as primary when classified as mesenchymal (heart, blood vessels, gastrointestinal tract), the literature suggested that there was little diffuse parenchymal liver involvement in secondary amyloid. Indeed, one group in 1941[147] studied 30 cases of secondary amyloid and found the liver function tests to be virtually normal in all. Before that, Rosenblatt[113] had reviewed 100 cases of amyloidosis without finding a single case of jaundice.

In 1933, one of the earliest cases of amyloidosis associated with hepatomegaly and severe ascites was reported by Bannick and coworkers.[2] Although jaundice was not initially present, it developed 1 week after the patient's hospitalization; the bilirubin rose to 9.4 mg/dL; and the patient died in hepatic coma. At autopsy, the liver weight was 3187 g. In 1941, Tiber and associates[147] noted that, although the 30 patients they studied had no jaundice, a review of 100 records of patients with amyloid who came to autopsy indicated one instance of clinical jaundice. In 1944, Spain and Riley[137] reported a case of jaundice in a patient with amyloidosis secondary to tuberculosis. They found that of the previous 12,000 autopsies at Bellevue Hospital, there were 78 recorded cases of amyloidosis, 50 with liver disease and none with jaundice. Orloff and Felder[105] in 1946 described a patient with primary amyloidosis with jaundice who at autopsy was found to have a liver weighing 5900 g. Their review of 2260 autopsy cases at Montefiore Hospital recorded 102 cases of amyloid disease, none with jaundice.

Over the next few years, it became clear that, although severe liver dysfunction leading to jaundice was an unusual accompaniment of amyloidosis, it was not as rare as had been previously thought. Jaundice with evidence of portal hypertension (ascites and esophageal varices) was found in a patient with massive amyloid hepatomegaly (liver weight, 5540 g)[1]; a similar case (liver weight, 3200 g) was reported in 1947,[157] and severe jaundice and hemorrhage were found in another patient in 1949 (liver weight, 3250 g).[13]

In some cases in which hepatomegaly was associated with evidence of portal hypertension, classic cirrhosis was mimicked, and only when tissue was obtained was the issue clarified.[66] Hepatomegaly and evidence of portal hypertension were reported in a number of other series.[19,42,67,77,108,153] In more recent studies, jaundice has not been as rare. For example, Levine[85] reported it in 3 of 13 patients (23%) with primary hepatic amyloid and in 1 of 34 patients (3%) with secondary amyloid. In our reported series of 42 patients, ascites was found in 4 and portal hypertension in 1.[17] Levy and coworkers[87] reported clinical ascites in 14% of 21 patients with amyloidosis but in 47% of these patients at autopsy. In 1978, we reviewed our experience and found that of 78 patients with primary amyloidosis, 4 (5.3%) developed severe intrahepatic cholestasis.[114] More recent analysis of the histopathology has led to a clearer understanding of the distribution and overlap of the various types of systemic amyloidosis.[24] More recently, in examining the survival of 82 patients, we found that 32% of them had liver disease as a major clinical feature, although it was a cause of death in only 3 of the patients.

Pathology

GENERAL CHARACTERISTICS

Gross Appearance

Amyloid is an amorphous, eosinophilic, glassy, hyaline, extracellular substance that is ubiquitous in its distribution. Grossly, it may be identified by the classic iodine and diluted sulfuric acid stain first used by Virchow. When successful, this stain imparts a blue-purple color to the amyloid. It is inconstant, however, and only of historical interest. When small amounts of amyloid are present, no gross organ abnormalities are demonstrable. With larger amounts, the involved organs take on a rubbery, firm consistency. They may have a waxy pink or gray appearance. Organ enlargement (especially liver, kidney, spleen, and heart) may be prominent when the deposits are large. In patients with long-standing renal involvement, however, the kidneys may become small and pale. Gastrointestinal ulcerations are not uncommon. The heart, in addition to being enlarged because of interstitial myocardial involvement, may have nodular elevations on its pericardial and endocardial surfaces as well as lesions on the valves. Nerves are often normal, even when involved, but at times are described as thickened and nodular. Other gross findings are variable and depend on the presence of local nodular deposits of amyloid.

Tinctorial Properties

Microscopically, amyloid is pink with the hematoxylin-eosin stain and shows crystal-violet or methyl-violet metachromasia, although it is orthochromatic when stained with toluidine blue. The van Gieson stain for collagen stains the latter red and most of the background yellow but imparts a khaki color to amyloid. The periodic acid–Schiff stain gives amyloid a violaceous hue.

Congo red remains the most widely used stain. It is not completely specific because it stains elastic tissue and, unless carefully decolorized, stains dense bundles of collagen. However, when formalin-fixed Congo red–stained sections are viewed in the polarizing microscope, a unique green birefringence is present. *This is the single most useful procedure for establishing the presence of amyloid.* Amyloid has also been stained with fluorochromes to produce a secondary fluorescence, and thioflavine dyes in particular have been found to be sensitive indicators of amyloid. The lack of specificity of these dyes, however, makes it mandatory for them to be employed primarily for screening and to be followed by more specific stains. Cotton dyes, especially Sirius red, have also been found to be useful and specific. A comparative evaluation of these stains has borne out the high degree of sensitivity and specificity of the green birefringence after Congo red or Sirius red staining.[41]

Light and Electron Microscopic Appearance

Under the light microscope, amyloid is almost invariably extracellular in the connective tissue. The deposits may be focal in almost any area of the body, but most often, perivascular amyloid is present. The amyloid may involve bone marrow, spleen, capillaries, venules, veins, arterioles, or arteries. The heart may have focal or diffuse interstitial deposits in the myocardium, endocardium, or pericardium. In the kidney, the glomerulus is primarily affected, although interstitial, peritubular, and vascular amyloid may be prominent. In early lesions, small nodular or diffuse deposits near the basement membrane appear, and as the disease progresses, the glomerulus may be massively laden with apparent occlusion of the capillary bed. Atrophic glomeruli laden with amyloid may show marked thickening in the area of Bowman's capsule, and rarely, the glomerulus may be almost replaced by connective tissue. Tubular dilation, casts, and interstitial amyloid deposits may be found in the medulla.

In the gastrointestinal tract, there may be perivascular deposits only, or irregular or diffuse deposits may be found in the submucosa, muscularis mucosa, or subserosa. The amyloid may appear at any level or portion of the gastrointestinal tract, including gallbladder and pancreas. Hepatic deposits may be perivascular only; more commonly, diffuse amyloid is found between the Kupffer and parenchymal cells (see section on liver pathology). In the nervous system, amyloid has been described along peripheral nerves and in autonomic ganglia, senile plaques, and vessels of the central nervous system. It may be found in any portion of the orbit, including the vitreous humor and cornea.

The bronchopulmonary tract may be involved focally or extensively. The unique aspect of pulmonary or pleural involvement is that, whereas amyloid in virtually all areas of the body remains without any evidence of resorption or foreign-body reaction, pulmonary amyloid deposits may be accompanied by large numbers of macrophages about and within the lesions. These deposits may also contain islets of cartilage and ossification. Thus, virtually no area of the body is spared. This ubiquitous distribution elicits a wide variety of clinical symptoms and signs.

In 1959, Cohen and Calkins[30] found, on direct examination of amyloid tissues in the electron microscope, that the amyloid itself consists of fine fibrils. This has been amply confirmed, and it is now known that all types of human amyloid—primary, secondary, heredofamilial—[27,36] no matter how classified, consist of these fine, nonbranching rigid fibrils measuring in tissue sections about 100 nm in diameter. They are usually arranged randomly when distal to the cell; proximally, however, they may be parallel or perpendicular to the plasmalemma, with which they occasionally appear to merge. Intracellular fibrils with dimensions comparable to those outside the cell are also occasionally observed. Their precise nature has not yet been established.

In the kidney, amyloid fibrils are usually first seen closest to mesangial cells[120]; as deposits enlarge, they appear closer to endothelial and, finally, epithelial cells. In the liver, they first border the Kupffer cells but finally fill the space of Disse and abut the hepatic cells as well. In many other locations, they have been found close to blood vessels, pericytes, and endothelial cells. Thus, although the cells that form amyloid fibrils appear in many instances to be in the reticuloendothelial or macrophage family, it is possible that, under some circumstances or in advanced disease, the ability to produce these fibrils may be a more ubiquitous phenomenon. The probable production of amyloid fibrils by reticuloendothelial cells in isolated spleen explants[37] and cultures[3] has been suggested by autoradiographic techniques at the light and electron microscopic levels. It is now clear that secondary amyloid (AA) has as its precursor SAA, which is produced in the liver as an acute-phase reactant in response to the monokines interleukin-1 and interleukin-6.[10,143]

The amyloid fibrils thus visualized can be extracted from amyloid-laden tissues in a variety of ways for more definitive ultrastructural, chemical, and immunologic study. When isolated, they can be specially stained (positively or negatively with phosphotungstic acid) and their delicate, thin, nonbranching fibrous character illustrated. The individual fibril has a diameter of about 70 nm, and the fibrils tend to aggregate laterally. Each fibril is made up of filaments, and subunit protofibrils (about 30 to 35 nm in diameter) have been defined. The protofibril is beaded, may consist of two subunits, and exists in spirals of five protofibrils or multiples of two such subunits.[119]

A second protein, P component (AP), which has a pentagonal ultrastructure and unique chemical characteristics, has been isolated from amyloid and shown to be identical to a circulating α-globulin present at a level of 5 to 7 mg/dL in all sera.[126,129] Protein AP is bound to all forms of amyloid thus far investigated by a calcium-dependent ligand.[106] It was originally thought to be present in only minute amounts but recently has been measured and found in varying amounts averaging 5% of fibril weight; however, it is not responsible for the characteristic tinctorial properties or ultrastructure of amyloid.[130] It has been shown to have many similarities to C-reactive protein (CRP) in that both are pentagonal in appearance and have some sequence homology. AP is antigenically distinct from CRP, however, and is of unknown signif-

icance in the pathogenesis of amyloid. Its molecular weight is twice that of CRP, and it appears as doublets in the electron microscope.

LIVER PATHOLOGY

The incidence of amyloid of the liver in association with generalized primary and secondary amyloidosis has undergone reassessment in recent years as better staining techniques have become available. In our opinion, the most sensitive and specific method is the properly used Congo red stain on formalin-fixed tissues (with appropriate controls) and the assessment of such tissues by means of polarization microscopy. The green birefringence observed under such conditions is characteristic of amyloid.[35]

In 1949, Dahlin[44] found parenchymal amyloid infiltration in two of six cases of primary disease leading to severe atrophy of the hepatic cords. The amyloid was laid down between the sinusoids and cords of liver cells. Two additional patients had lesser amounts, and two showed no parenchymal amyloid. All six, however, had small vessel infiltration of amyloid, especially in the arteries of the portal triads. The livers with moderate or severe amyloid were firm and rubbery and had an average weight of 2880 g. In his study of 30 cases of secondary amyloid, Dahlin[43] found that 26 demonstrated liver involvement, one with massive amyloid (liver weight, 2900 g). As with primary amyloid, the substance was deposited between the hepatic cords and sinusoids and was present in artery and vein wells.

Eisen[53] collected 48 cases of primary amyloid from the literature up to 1945 and found 8 with hepatic involvement. Subsequently, Mathews[95] updated his review to 1954 and found hepatic amyloid in 27 of 50 cases. In 1957, Bero[12] stated that liver involvement was almost universal in secondary amyloidosis and that it occurred in 30% to 40% of cases of primary disease. In his series, 8 of 9 livers (in 12 cases) whose weights were recorded were enlarged, many massively so; one weight was recorded as 5900 g. Symmers[140] found amyloid in all 5 cases of primary amyloid studied, although the deposits were small and solely vascular in most. Briggs[18] noted that the liver was most commonly involved in secondary amyloidosis (52 of 53 cases positive), although hepatic involvement in primary amyloid was also common (17 of 20 cases). In 3 of his cases, liver weights of over 4000 g were recorded. Six previous cases of amyloid liver weights from 5000 to 9000 g have been reported.[115] Levine[85] found the liver to be the third most commonly involved organ in 84 patients affected (ie, 47 of 84, or 56%, had hepatic amyloid). Kuhlback and Wegelius[81] found amyloid in 17 of 20 patients with the secondary type, and Hallen and Rudin[68] found it in all but 3 of 15 cases of primary amyloidosis.

In our earlier study of 42 patients with biopsy-proved amyloid disease,[17] tissue was available from 17 patients with hepatomegaly and from 6 with no liver enlargement. All specimens had amyloid present in either parenchyma or blood vessels, or in both. In our more recent analysis of liver tissue from 54 amyloidotic patients,[34] amyloid deposits were again found to be a universal phenomenon, although the distribution and magnitude varied. Two of our hepatic amyloid specimens were massive and weighed 7200 and 8200 g, respectively. Both were from patients with primary amyloidosis. Other isolated instances of massive hepatomegaly have been reported with liver weights of 3050, 6125, and 8500 g.[74,98,109]

In a more recent study, we analyzed the histopathology of the liver to evaluate the spectrum of morphologic changes in primary (AL) and secondary (AA) amyloidosis and to determine whether these two forms are distinguishable based on such analysis.[24] Thirty-eight patients with systemic amyloid (25 primary or myeloma and 13 secondary, reactive [AA]) were evaluated. Overall architectural distortion, alterations of portal triads, and predilection for topographic deposition in the parenchyma or blood vessel walls were noted. Significant histopathologic differences in AL or AA amyloid liver involvement included (1) portal fibrosis, seen in 7 of 25 (28%) AL patients and 8 of 13 (62%) AA patients; (2) parenchymal amyloid deposition, seen in 25 of 25 AL patients and 10 of 13 (77%) AA patients; and (3) vascular amyloid deposition, found in 17 of 25 patients (68%) with AL amyloid and 13 of 13 patients with AA amyloid. These data varied from the widely held concept that deposition of amyloid is predominantly vascular in the AL form and parenchymal in amyloid AA. Clearly, however, in individual cases, significant overlap occurred, and characterization of amyloid types based on morphologic distribution of amyloid deposits may be possible in only a minority of cases. In most cases, differentiation of amyloid AL and amyloid AA forms requires clinical, histochemical, immunochemical, and sometimes more elaborate laboratory amino acid sequence studies for accurate identification. In 1988, Looi and Sumithran[92] confirmed our observations; that is, in 19 patients with AA amyloidosis, amyloid was found in portal tract vessels, while in 12 AL patients, the deposits had a sinusoidal as well as vessel wall pattern. We do not believe, however, that the differences are as specific as these authors state.

Thus, amyloid of the liver is extremely common whether the patient has primary or secondary disease. Postmortem, the involved organ is found to be enlarged, smooth, and of a waxy, rubber consistency. It may be massive. Microscopic study of the amyloid shows that it is close to the Kupffer cells and that it lies between the sinusoids and the parenchymal cells (Figs. 54-1 and 54-2). Vascular deposits around arteries and veins, especially in the portal area, are common (Figs. 54-3 and 54-4). Periportal and pericentral area distribution has been described. Sasaki and colleagues[118] reported in 1990 on the intrahepatic biliary tree amyloid pattern in 19 autopsies (13 AL and 6 AA). Amyloid was seen under the lining epithelium of the intrahepatic large bile duct in 10 of 19 and around the peribiliary glandular acini in 7 of 19 cases. These deposits correlated with the amount of hepatic amyloid but not with the type. The progress of the hepatic amyloid is unpredictable and has on serial biopsy appeared to be stable in some cases and rapidly progressive in others.[85] Experience with hepatic amyloid in the French literature was reviewed by Dao and coworkers in 1990.[46]

Hepatic amyloid has also been studied by electron microscopy. Thiery and Caroli[146] reported on the fibrous ultrastructure of human hepatic amyloid in 1961. Manitz and Themann[94] in 1962 analyzed the ultrastructure of several amyloid liver biopsy specimens. The fine fibrils were found

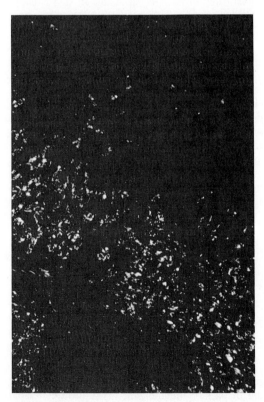

FIGURE 54-1 Amyloidosis of the liver secondary to rheumatoid arthritis. Although the amyloid is diffusely present, its concentration is more marked in the periportal area. Deposits are localized between the Kupffer cells and parenchymal cells when the lesions are small, whereas diffuse distortion of the architecture occurs when the lesions are more massive (Congo red stain, × 120).

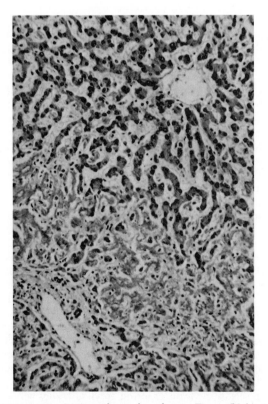

FIGURE 54-2 Section identical to that in Figure 54-1, viewed through the polarizing microscope, demonstrating the birefringence of the amyloid deposits. In color, the birefringence has a clearcut green appearance (× 120).

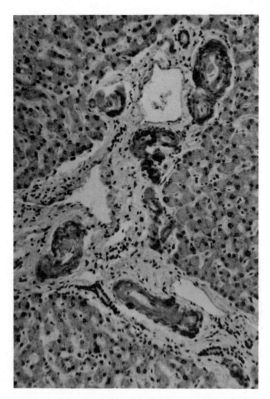

FIGURE 54-3   Primary amyloidosis of the liver. Pattern of massive amounts of amyloid in the blood vessel walls and virtually none in the hepatic parenchyma (Congo red stain, × 120).

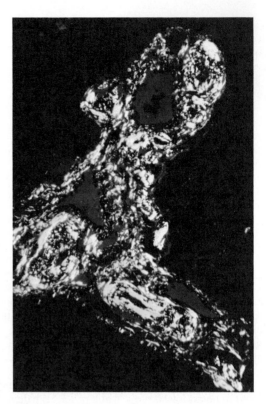

FIGURE 54-4   Section identical to that in Figure 54-3 but viewed in the polarizing microscope. Again, the striking birefringence of the amyloid is noted (× 120).

within but not completely confined to the space of Disse. Amyloid extended between seemingly normal parenchymal cells. Skinner and coworkers[133] reported on the fine structure of hepatic amyloid associated with multiple myeloma. They found fine fibrils filling and distending the spaces of Disse. The fibrils frequently were oriented at right angles to the plasma membrane of the hepatic parenchymal cells and the adjacent sinusoidal lining cells. These findings are comparable to those seen in experimental animals in which the ultrastructure of hepatic amyloidosis has been extensively studied.[4,20,31,59,135,136,140] Representative electron microscopy of hepatic amyloid demonstrates the fine rigid fibrils and close relation to Kupffer cells as well as to parenchymal cells (Figs. 54-5 and 54-6). In one study,[107] a liver biopsy from a patient with primary amyloidosis was found to show degenerative changes in the cytoplasmic periphery of hepatocytes. These were interpreted as indicating shedding of peripheral parts of the cytoplasm with (1) protrusion and sequestration of hernia-like blebs of cytoplasm and (2) shedding of vesicles derived from degenerated endoplasmic reticulum. This resulted in an increased fractional volume of mitochondria (which were retained in the cell) and was thought to represent the mechanism by which the cell adapts to the unfavorable environment created by the amyloid.[107] The perisinusoidal functional unit in amyloid was described in more detail in 1987.[47]

Deposits in the form of round amyloid bodies between or within hepatocytes have been reported and are thought to be of benign nature.[58,91] A more extensive study of 14 cases with globular hepatic amyloid suggested that it is not clinically distinguishable from other forms of classic hepatic amyloid,

and in 7 patients on whom autopsy was performed, extensive systemic (nonglobular) amyloid was found.[76] The globular form of hepatic amyloid was recently described in a goat.[55]

A freeze-etched liver specimen of mice with casein-induced amyloid showed the felt-like structure of the amyloid fibrils, amyloid bundles, and globular profiles among amyloid fibrils. Amyloid bundles enveloped by the cytoplasmic membrane of Kupffer cells projected from the concave surface of the cytoplasmic membrane into Disse's space and had a stone column-like appearance. The amyloid bundles projecting from the invaginated cytoplasmic membrane were in close contact with it and deeply rooted in the Kupffer cell cytoplasm.[73] Scanning electron microscopy of the mouse amyloid liver showed amyloid bundles in close contact with the Kupffer cell cytoplasm and projecting from the cell into the space of Disse on three-dimensional figures.[142]

Pathogenesis

The cause of amyloidosis is not known. Throughout the years, however, amyloid has been regarded as (1) a disorder of serum proteins with associated hyperglobulinemia, (2) a disorder of protein metabolism, (3) a disorder related to an abnormality of the reticuloendothelial system, (4) the result of chronic immunologic stimulation leading to excessive antibody production and the deposition of antibody or antibody–antigen complexes as amyloid, (5) a disorder of delayed hypersensitivity, or (6) a combination of the above-mentioned disorders. These hypotheses are not mutually exclu-

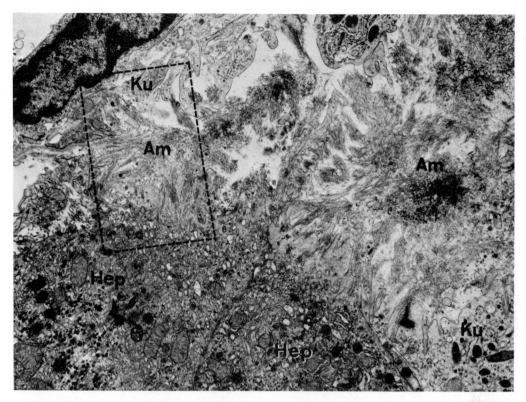

FIGURE 54-5 Low-power electron micrograph of mouse liver with amyloidosis induced by repeated casein injections. Amyloid (Am) deposits in two areas surrounded by Kupffer cells (Ku) and hepatocytes (Hep). Amyloid fibrils deposit densely and in random array in the central portion of the amyloid mass, whereas in the peripheral portion, they form bundles of amyloid fibrils well oriented perpendicularly to the cell border. This area appears stellar under the light microscope, the so-called amyloid star. The area surrounded by dotted lines is seen at higher magnification in Figure 54-6 ($\times$ 7000).

sive, and because the cause is unknown, it is difficult to be certain as to when a specific abnormality is present and whether it is of primary significance or represents a secondary phenomenon.[31]

Early observations suggested to many that amyloid might be related to a specific serum protein because of its association with multiple myeloma and its known plasma protein aberrations and because of the potential for intense antigenic stimulation in the many inflammatory disorders complicated by amyloid. The pendulum of scientific opinion swung away from this hypothesis when several studies showed the lack of identity of serum proteins with whole amyloid fibrils and when increasing numbers of patients with primary amyloid and no form of other disease and no M components were apparent.

Extracts of amyloid that were prepared in a number of laboratories demonstrated the absence of γ-globulin and other serum constituents even in purified preparations. Thus, until several years ago, amyloid was regarded as a unique fibrous protein immunologically distinct from γ-globulin. Chemical studies showed it to have a high nitrogen content and no unique amino acids and to lack the components of both collagen and elastin (hydroxyproline, hydroxylysine, desmosine, isodesmosine, lysinonorleucine).[26,28]

Neutral sugars are present in small amounts; whether glycosaminoglycans are present as part of the molecule or in the milieu in which the fibril is embedded is not known. X-ray diffraction studies have demonstrated that the amyloid fibril has a cross-β pattern, suggesting the pleated sheet morphology of Corey and Pauling.[15,52]

The interesting observation that primary amyloid fibrils are predominantly immunoglobulin light chains or the variable segments thereof is consistent with the clinical observation of an abnormal serum protein or M component in these patients.[14,51,63,64,89,123] In addition, patients may have Bence Jones proteinuria and increased bone marrow mature plasma cells (15% to 20%) but no overt myeloma. Extensive deposits of amyloid are frequently present in the spleen, liver, heart, intestines, tongue, blood vessels, and other organs.

Also, a proportion of patients with clearcut multiple myeloma manifested by sheets of immature plasma cells in the bone marrow and lytic lesions in bones develop amyloidosis. For reasons yet unknown, only a limited number of such patients do so. Although this type of amyloid is biochemically indistinguishable from primary amyloid, the mean survival is much shorter and clinically separates these forms of disease from each other.

Biochemically, various sizes of light-chain fragments make up the major portion of the amyloid fibril; N-terminal sequence studies suggest that it is always the variable portion of the light chain with or without part or all of the constant segment. Various types of light chains have been identified thus far, including κ chains I, II, and III and λ chains I, II, III, IV, and VI.[51,56,110,145] One unique type of light chain, a λ-VI with an aspartic amino terminus, has been found only in association with amyloid and may be implicated etiologi-

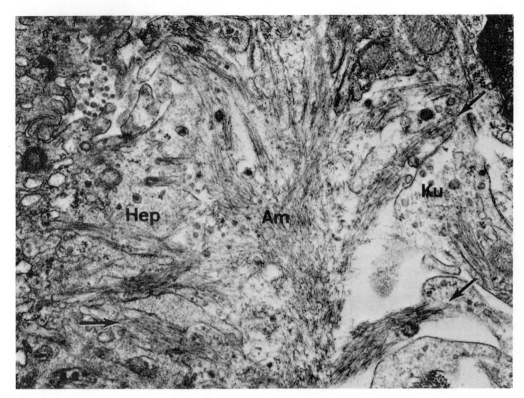

FIGURE 54-6   Higher-power micrograph of the area outlined in Figure 54-5. Kupffer cell (Ku) and the hepatocyte (Hep) form many deep invaginations that contain bundles of well-oriented amyloid fibrils (Am). At the amyloid–cell border, especially at the bottom of the invagination containing the bundle of amyloid fibrils, the plasmalemma appears indistinct (*arrows*; × 24,000).

cally.[111] λ Amyloid proteins outnumber κ by about 2:1, a reversal of the ratio seen in multiple myeloma. The serum or urinary M component and the amyloid protein from the same patient are identical.

Not all amyloid, however, is related to immunoglobulin. Protein AA and its serum counterpart SAA have been associated with the type of amyloidosis known to be secondary to chronic inflammatory or infectious disease. Protein AA is the main constituent of the amyloid fibrils in secondary amyloidosis in humans as well as in animals and has been identified in tissue extracts from the amyloid of patients with rheumatoid arthritis, bronchiectasis, and tuberculosis as well as the amyloid associated with familial Mediterranean fever. It is about 8600 daltons in size and has a unique 76-residue sequence.[6,84]

SAA is an acute-phase reactant induced by interleukin-1 that is the putative precursor of protein AA and is found in the blood plasma as a polypeptide of about 12,500 daltons. It has been found to be one of the apoproteins of the high-density lipoproteins.[7,8] Studies have shown a marked increase in the liver content of SAA after stimulation with casein or lipopolysaccharide in the mouse model. It is speculated that the liver may be one site of synthesis of this apoprotein.[10,143] SAA is polymorphic, and serum contains a mixture of two gene products, SAA 1 and SAA 2.[5,139] Genetic analyses reveal four human genetic loci, similar to the description of murine SAA genes. In the murine model, one gene product, SAA 2, has sequence identity with amyloid protein AA, suggesting selective deposition.[54,71,128]

The AP, a separate protein found in association with amyloid, is completely distinctive from the amyloid fibril components (both the AL and the AA proteins) and has distinctive morphologic, tinctorial, immunologic, and biochemical properties.[126] It is made up of a parallel pair of pentagonal units with a subunit size of about 23,000 daltons. It shares several characteristics with CRP, including its ultrastructure, calcium-dependent binding properties, and a 60% sequence homology.[104,130] AP is synthesized by the liver, has a relatively short half-life of 7 to 8 hours, and is maintained at a stable serum concentration of about 5 mg/dL.[132,143] The hamster female protein (FP) has structural similarities to AP and CRP, giving the name *pentraxins* to the three proteins.

The amyloid fibrils in the dominantly inherited familial amyloid polyneuropathies (FAP) have been found to be composed of the protein transthyretin (prealbumin) with variant molecular structures.[11] In the FAP type I kinships of Swedish, Portuguese, and Japanese origins, a methionine is substituted for valine at position 30.[50,117,124,144] Other substitutions have recently been found in amino acids 30, 33, 36, 42, 50, 58, 60, 77, 84, 90, 111, and 114. Other mutant proteins forming amyloid fibrils include gelsolin in the Finnish variety and apolipoprotein AI in a lower limb neuropathy.[96,102] Apolipoprotein AI amyloidosis is of particular interest because it has been associated with hepatomegaly as well as nephropathy and neuropathy. The disease has been described in two families, and a mutation of arginine for glycine occurs at position 26 in Apo AI.[75,103]

The actual pathogenesis of the various types of amyloidosis is probably complex. Specific mutations in transthyretin, gelsolin, and Apo AI clearly lead to amyloidogenility of these proteins. It is likely that a mutant amino acid structure of the light-chain protein in AL disease accounts for its propensity to form fibrils.

Recent studies have shown variations in the ability of monocytes and polymorphonuclear leukocytes to degrade the SAA protein, suggesting genetic differences.[83,122] Neutrophilic serine proteases have been found closely associated with amyloid fibrils of all types and may play a role in the proteolytic processing of amyloid fibrils.[125]

Clinical Features

Whether a patient has primary, secondary, or heredofamilial amyloidosis, the clinical manifestations depend on the anatomic site of the deposit and the degree of interference with normal organ function.[27] The genetically determined forms, in which clinical patterns are usually recognizable, are the subject of another report.[11,29] Renal involvement is potentially the most serious manifestation of the disease and the major cause of death in most series. Despite this, renal amyloid may be present and asymptomatic for many years, and the disorder does not inevitably progress rapidly. Most patients, however, exhibit proteinuria, possibly massive, and a classic nephrotic syndrome may be the presenting manifestation or may develop. Patients with renal amyloid may also have hematuria. Radiologically, the kidneys may be large, but with increased duration of disease, small, shrunken kidneys develop. Hypertension is rare early in the course, but as patients with renal amyloid survive longer, the incidence of hypertension increases.

When present, cardiac amyloid also may be asymptomatic but on occasion may be severe enough to cause congestive heart failure. Electrocardiographic abnormalities include a wide variety of conduction abnormalities, especially heart block, but with flutter and fibrillation. Patients with cardiac amyloid may have arrhythmia precipitated by digitalis and calcium-channel blockers, and these drugs should be used with caution. The electrocardiogram in cardiac amyloid may indicate coronary artery disease without clinical symptoms. The reading is usually that of anterior or anteroseptal infarction and often shows decreased voltage. The use of two-dimensional echocardiography with Doppler has led to a more precise definition of the extent of amyloid cardiomyopathy.

Gastrointestinal symptoms in amyloidosis are common. They may result from direct involvement of the gastrointestinal tract at any level or from infiltration of the autonomic nervous system with amyloid. The symptoms include those of obstruction, ulceration, malabsorption, hemorrhage, protein loss, and diarrhea. Whereas hepatic involvement is common, liver function abnormalities are unusual and occur late in the disease. The test most frequently abnormal in hepatic amyloid is the level of serum alkaline phosphatase activity. Signs of portal hypertension occur but are uncommon. Because amyloidosis can involve any level of the respiratory tract, symptoms vary widely and include hoarseness, hemoptysis, epistaxis, and dysphagia. Neurologic symptoms are especially prominent in several of the heredofamilial amyloidoses, and a patient may show an asymmetric or symmetric sensory or motor neuropathy, severe autonomic nervous dysfunction, or even isolated cranial nerve lesions. Amyloid of

the eye or orbit may cause proptosis, decreased visual acuity, muscle weakness, or ptosis. Thus, virtually any organ of the body may be involved, and the symptoms depend on the site and size of the deposit.

No laboratory abnormalities are specific to or unique for amyloid. Routine blood studies (hematocrit, white cell count, and differential) are within normal limits unless there is blood loss or complicating disease. The erythrocyte sedimentation rate (ESR) and other nonspecific indices of inflammation may or may not be elevated. The ESR may be markedly elevated in primary amyloidosis with the nephrotic syndrome. Occasionally, the fibrinogen level is nonspecifically elevated (especially in familial Mediterranean fever). No uniform changes in serum complement have been found. There are no specific changes in serum proteins. Urinary abnormalities include mild or severe proteinuria, hematuria, and the occasional presence of granular casts. Levels of cerebrospinal fluid proteins may be elevated in certain heredofamilial forms. Serum transthyretin (prealbumin) levels appear to be decreased in FAP.[40]

The occasional bleeding reported is usually due to injury to amyloid-infiltrated blood vessels, although disseminated intravascular coagulation has been observed. In severe hepatic amyloid, however, the prothrombin time may be slightly elevated, and the literature has documented an acquired selective factor X (Stuart factor) deficiency.[60] Although selective factor X deficiency is most common, multiple clotting factor deficiencies may exist in patients with a rapidly progressing form of primary amyloidosis. Our in vitro experimentation has shown that when clotting factors are incubated with amyloid fibrils and calcium, a clotting factor activity can subsequently be eluted from the fibrils with citrate.[131] It is presumed that such calcium-dependent binding can occur in vivo and that clinical deficiencies of clotting factors in amyloidosis are not due to decreased hepatic synthesis of clotting factors but rather to their calcium-dependent adsorption to the amyloid fibrils.

Diagnosis

The diagnosis of amyloidosis rests first on one's clinical acumen, that is, the recognition of a patient with a predisposing disorder such as rheumatoid arthritis in whom proteinuria and hepatomegaly develop, or the recognition of a typical pattern of symptoms and signs attributed to a heredofamilial amyloid syndrome. Inevitably, however, the diagnosis depends largely on biopsy, use of the appropriate stain (Congo red), and observation of such stained tissue in the polarizing microscope for the characteristic green birefringence.[35]

Biopsy has been shown to be safe if an accessible site (gingiva, rectum, abdominal fat) is used and simple precautions taken.[61,149] In general, to cope with the potential problem of bleeding, it is preferable to perform biopsy on sites that can be seen directly. The abdominal fat aspiration technique is the method of choice because of its sensitivity (80% of patients known to have amyloid are positive) and because it is a procedure easily performed at the bedside.[48,49,90,152] Amyloid deposits lend a tissue a certain amount of rubbery rigidity, which makes it prone to hemorrhage. This is seen with the ecchymoses associated with amyloid of the skin, the hematuria seen in renal amyloid, and the startling gastrointestinal bleeding that may occur when amyloid is present in the intestinal tract. With appropriate precautions, however, and with knowledge of the platelet count, prothrombin time, and bleeding and clotting times, closed biopsies can be undertaken with relative impunity. Renal biopsy has been successfully performed in many cases of suspected or known amyloid of the kidney. Hepatic biopsy is usually safe, although the procedure should be approached with caution in patients with massive hepatomegaly (discussed later). Peroral small intestinal biopsy has been performed as well as splenic biopsy. In patients with respiratory tract masses, direct biopsy of laryngeal or bronchial lesions may determine the diagnosis. Nerve biopsy is indicated whenever amyloid neuropathy is suspected.

Treatment and Prognosis

No specific treatment has proved successful for any variety of amyloidosis. Eradication of the predisposing disease apparently slows the progress of secondary amyloidosis, and, in rare cases, serial biopsy in some organs suggests that reabsorption takes place. The cure of the underlying disease does not guarantee freedom from amyloid; however, there are a number of recorded cases of its appearance many years after activity of the primary disorder has ceased. In most of the reported cures of amyloid, direct biopsy proof is lacking, and judgment is made on the basis of a clinical diagnosis (ie, hepatomegaly). In some of these cases, however, the circumstantial evidence for amyloid and its regression is strong. In one series of four cases of massive hepatic amyloid (liver weights, 4200, 3600, 2300, and 2000 g), two showed clinical hepatomegaly without cholestasis and the other two less pronounced hepatomegaly but severe and progressive intrahepatic cholestasis.[97]

Various agents that have been used or recommended include whole liver extract, adrenocortical steroids, ascorbic acid, and immunosuppressive agents. None has caused clear improvement. With conservative supportive measures (ie, treatment of complicating infections), however, the prognosis is far better than was once thought.[17] We have followed patients with renal amyloid for over 12 years. In selected instances, renal transplantation has been performed with surprisingly good results.[38] Ten-year survival has been reported after such transplantation. Colchicine has been shown to be effective in preventing acute febrile attacks in familial Mediterranean fever and the amyloid associated with it. In the casein-induced amyloid model in the mouse, inhibition of amyloid development has been reported,[121] and it is possible that colchicine may be effective in preventing new amyloid deposits. Clinical studies demonstrate that daily colchicine appears to prolong life in AL primary amyloid as does cyclic use of melphalan and prednisone.[32,82] Studies are in progress to evaluate the combined use of these two modalities.

Hepatic Amyloid

Amyloidosis of the liver is one of the most common manifestations of the disease. It can occur at any age and has been reported in children as a complication of juvenile rheumatoid arthritis and de novo in a child of 9 years.[65] In most modern series, as already noted, amyloid is present at least in the blood vessels in most cases, whether primary, secondary,

or myeloma related. In all 54 cases of our series from which tissue was available, amyloid was present, occasionally in massive amounts, occasionally as a minor finding near blood vessel walls. Liver weights of up to 9000 g have been reported.

The clinical presentation of amyloid liver disease may be nonspecific, and often the patient appears with vague abdominal complaints. In many of these patients, hepatomegaly is the only positive physical finding. Clinical signs such as spider angiomas, clubbing, gynecomastia, and alopecia are rare. Several series recorded no such findings.[79,87] Levine found that although 29 of 47 patients (62%) had symptoms or physical findings suggesting hepatic involvement, none showed peripheral stigmata of cirrhosis (ie, spider angiomas, abdominal collaterals, palmar erythema, or testicular atrophy).[85] Presenting complaints were referable to the liver in only three patients, one with ascites and two with an abdominal mass. One of Levine's patients developed signs of hepatic coma (with stupor and flapping). Death was attributed to hepatic amyloid in that case and in two others, both with intractable ascites unassociated with renal failure.

In our previous report[17] of 42 patients, spider angiomas were found in only 1 patient, Dupuytren's contractures (longstanding) were found in 1, and clubbing was present in 2 (1 with associated bronchiectasis and 1 with granulomatous ileitis). Unilateral gynecomastia developed in one patient. Palmar erythema, asterixis, and alopecia were not observed. Jaundice was present in one, ascites in 4 (2 of whom also had congestive heart failure), and portal hypertension in 1. The multiple case reports of patients with jaundice and the increasing longevity of patients with amyloid suggest that jaundice, while not a common presenting sign, may be observed more frequently in the future.

One reviewer[86] noted an incidence of jaundice of 4.7% in 490 patients with hepatic amyloid, although serum bilirubin rarely exceeded 5 mg/dL. Severe obstructive jaundice is rarer; a limited number of patients with such cholestatic jaundice has been reported.[99,114] All these patients had a poor prognosis and died within months of the diagnosis. Konikoff and coworkers[80] recently reported a patient with λ AL amyloid with severe intrahepatic cholestasis leading to terminal liver failure.

The more serious complications secondary to portal hypertension, fortunately, are late manifestations, but they do occur and, in our experience, are seen progressively more frequently. An unusual association, congenital dilation of the intrahepatic bile ducts and amyloidosis, has recently been reported in two cases.[57] Focal intrahepatic mass lesions, comprising extensive amyloid infiltration of the liver, and spontaneous rupture of the liver are the most rarely reported manifestations.[72,88,148]

Laboratory abnormalities in amyloidosis of the liver are surprisingly sparse. Levine[85] assessed the value of 10 liver function tests in 47 cases and found the most common abnormalities to be hypoalbuminemia, elevated bromsulphalein (BSP) retention, alkaline phosphatase, cholesterol, and thymol turbidity. These tests were thought to be of little value, however, because they did not clearly distinguish those patients with from those without hepatic amyloid or differentiate one type of amyloid from another. Furthermore, no correlation was found between the degree of functional abnormality and the extent of hepatic amyloid infiltration. Some patients with massive amounts of amyloid had normal liver function tests, whereas others with minimal vascular deposits had abnormal tests. In 1988, Gertz and Kyle[62] reviewed the natural history of 80 patients with hepatic amyloid of the AL primary type. They found that liver function tests were not sensitive or specific and that hepatomegaly was frequently seen with normal levels of alkaline phosphatase, aspartate aminotransferase, and bilirubin.

Our previous study[17] and those of others[87] are in general agreement with the detailed analyses of Levine.[85] We noted occasional mild hypoprothrombinemia, rare elevations in serum lactic acid dehydrogenase and glutamic-oxaloacetic transaminase levels, and rare mild elevations in bilirubin. Abnormal BSP excretion and elevated serum alkaline phosphatase levels proved to be useful, but even these did not correlate well with the true extent of the disease.

Although liver biopsy in the diagnosis of amyloid liver disease was introduced in 1928,[151] it did not receive extensive use until the 1950s.[153] In a detailed review, Volwiler and Jones[150] reported one death from hemorrhage after amyloid liver biopsy. This tended to temper the use of liver biopsy as a diagnostic procedure; however, although this precaution is reasonable, it is our experience that the procedure is more than routinely dangerous only in patients with massive hepatomegaly, who often are in the terminal stages of the illness. A second death after liver biopsy in a patient with extensive hepatic amyloid was also reported.[22] At about the same time, another patient with jaundice and liver disease of unknown cause was reported to have been subjected to an open liver biopsy. The patient died 48 hours postoperatively, and although there was widespread amyloid and diffuse focal hemorrhage throughout the body, there also occurred extensive retroperitoneal hemorrhage, with 450 mL of free blood in the peritoneal cavity.[116]

In 1961, Stauffer and coworkers[138] reported a series of 18 needle biopsies of the liver in patients with amyloid liver disease. No difficulties were encountered in 17, but in 1 patient, intraperitoneal bleeding probably occurred, requiring one transfusion. They concluded that the procedure was important in reaching the conclusive diagnosis of amyloidosis. Certainly, if the diagnosis has already been established in other organs (eg, by rectal biopsy), one would have to have a special indication for doing a liver biopsy in addition. In a patient with hepatomegaly of unknown cause, liver biopsy is a reasonable procedure to consider for the diagnosis of amyloidosis, in conjunction with measures noted previously. Several case reports in letters from India[16] and Spain[155] have testified recently as to its utility.

Liver scans have been performed on a number of patients with amyloid and produced variable results. No diagnostic pattern is demonstrated, and the appearance varies from normal scan with patchy cold spots to cirrhotic liver with decreased liver and increased splenic and bone marrow uptake. Peritoneoscopy is said to be of help when it reveals a light-colored liver with a rosy violet appearance.[21]

We evaluated the bone-scanning radionuclides technetium-99m pyrophosphate and methylene diphosphonate to delineate soft tissue amyloidosis. Of 23 patients, 6 had abnormal soft tissue uptake of radionuclide. The most common soft tissue abnormality observed was diffuse hepatic uptake, which occurred in 3 of 8 patients with biopsy-proven hepatic amyloidosis (Fig. 54-7). It was concluded that this procedure is not sensitive enough for definitive diagnosis but that amyloidosis should be considered in patients with diffuse hepatic or other soft tissue uptake of bone-seeking radionuclides.[156] Angiographic findings in a case of hepatic amyloid included

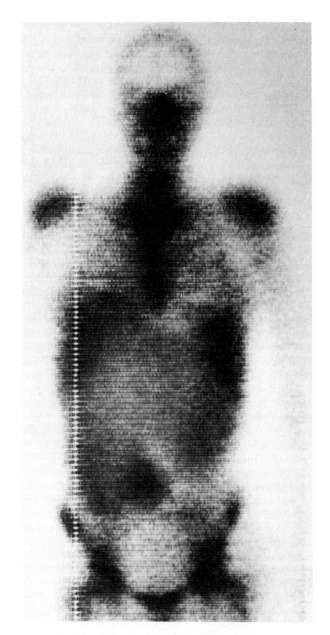

FIGURE 54-7 ^{99m}Tc-pyrophosphate bone scan (anterior view) of a 47-year-old woman with primary amyloidosis. Note the intense diffuse hepatic, as well as splenic, cardiac, and shoulder joint, uptake of radionuclide.

narrowing of the intrahepatic vessels, mimicking an intrahepatic mass.[154]

Recently, radiolabeled SAP has been shown to localize in amyloid-laden tissues, including liver, spleen, kidneys and adrenals, and scintigraphy after its injection may prove useful for diagnosis and evaluation of extent of disease.[33,69]

Personal Observations

Between 1965 and 1975, 80 patients with biopsy-proven systemic amyloidosis have been studied by the members of the Boston University Arthritis Center at the University Hospital and in the Thorndike Memorial Laboratory of the Boston City Hospital. Data on some of these patients have already been reported, with emphasis on clinical presentation and prognosis in 42 cases[17]; immunoglobulin abnormalities in 62 cases[23]; and therapeutic trial of colchicine in 82 cases.[32]

Data on some patients were reported to us by other institutions, and because liver disease occasionally was not suspected, liver function studies are not available in these cases. A number of patients are alive and have not had liver biopsies. Several patients were brought to our attention only on the basis of an autopsy diagnosis, so that, again, clinical information is lacking. In 73 patients with biopsy-proven amyloidosis (any site), some data concerning the liver were available. This information included (1) histologic material from a biopsy or postmortem examination, (2) adequate clinical evaluation of liver size or postmortem liver weight, and (3) two or more laboratory studies of liver functions (from alkaline phosphatase, BSP extraction, serum glutamic-oxaloacetic acid level, lactic acid dehydrogenase level, bilirubin, prothrombin time, and serum albumin).

Several preliminary conclusions can be drawn from these data. In 54 patients, tissue was available for examination. All 54 had some amyloid present either in the parenchyma or around blood vessels. Information on clinical estimation of liver size was available in 42 patients, and in 39, hepatomegaly was believed to be present. Among the remaining 19 patients in whom no tissue was available, hepatomegaly was present in only 12.

Clinical stigmata of liver disease were unusual in this series of patients. Palmar erythema occurred in two cases, jaundice in four, and spider angiomas in six. Ascites was present in eight patients but was associated with generalized anasarca and renal failure. Two patients with primary amyloid who had markedly infiltrated livers histologically developed esophageal varices with bleeding. In one of these, the condition was terminal. Hepatic coma occurred and was the cause of death in only one patient.

As has been noted in other series, elevated alkaline phosphatase levels and increased BSP extraction appear to be among the earliest and most useful chemical determinations. The remarkable degree to which the liver parenchyma can be replaced by amyloid is indicated by one patient who had a liver that was palpable below the iliac crest and that weighed 7200 g at postmortem examination; his liver function tests showed a BSP of 17% with only moderately elevated alkaline phosphatase level. Others with significant liver involvement had normal liver function tests in all respects.

One patient with amyloid (small amounts) proved by biopsy had a normal liver scan, whereas six others were abnormal. The scans generally showed a diffuse decrease in uptake, but there was some variation.

Despite the previous comments, detailed liver function tests showed mild abnormalities in 75% of cases. Most frequent were elevation of alkaline phosphatase level and prolongation of the prothrombin time. Occasionally, there was minor elevation in the levels of serum glutamic-oxaloacetic transaminase, lactic dehydrogenase, and bilirubin. Serum albumin was often low (in 75% of the patients tested); however, this was nearly always associated with elevated levels of serum cholesterol and renal failure. We found in a more recent analysis that 4 of 78 patients (5.3%) had severe intrahepatic cholestasis.[98] Data were reviewed on an additional eight patients recorded in the literature. Criteria for inclusion were a tissue diagnosis of amyloidosis, a serum bilirubin level greater than 5 mg/dL, histopathologic evidence of cholestasis, and no extrahepatic biliary obstruction. Hepatomegaly was present in 12 patients (100%), ascites in 9 (75%), and pruritus in 8 (67%). Serum bilirubin ranged from 9 to 44 mg/dL; serum alkaline phosphatase was markedly increased in 10 patients (83%); and hypercholesterolemia occurred in 7 (58%). Microscopic examination of the liver revealed diffuse amyloid deposition and compression atrophy in 12 patients (100%). The amyloid was prominent in the periportal regions, and some sparing of the centrilobular areas was observed. Bile thrombi and bilirubin staining of hepatocytes were predominantly in the centrilobular zones. Liver cell necrosis, fibrosis, and nodularity were uncommon.

The pathogenesis of intrahepatic cholestasis in these patients was probably related to the deposition of amyloid in a manner that interferes with the passage of bile from the canaliculi or the small intrahepatic bile ducts to the septal bile ducts. Obstructive jaundice carried a poor prognosis. Of 12 patients, 9 (75%) died of renal failure 3 weeks to 2 months after the onset of jaundice. Amyloidosis should be considered in the patient with unexplained intrahepatic cholestasis, and liver tissue should be stained with Congo red and viewed under polarized microscopy.

In the group of patients in whom tissue histology was available, only a rough correlation could be made between the degree of liver involvement with amyloid and the liver function test abnormalities. Elevated BSP and alkaline phosphatase levels and slightly prolonged prothrombin time occurred in half of the patients in whom only blood vessels were involved with amyloid. More of the patients with marked parenchymal infiltration had the same abnormalities (80% to 90% of those tested). Patients with either primary or secondary disease had patterns of parenchymal or blood vessel involvement that were indistinguishable from each other except for the previously noted rare intrahepatic cholestasis.

References

1. Atkinson AJ. Clinical pathological conference. Gastroenterology 7:477, 1946
2. Bannick EG, et al. Diffuse amyloidosis—three unusual cases: a clinical and pathologic study. Arch Intern Med 51:978, 1933
3. Bari WA, et al. Electron microscopy and electron microscopic autoradiography of splenic cell cultures from mice with amyloidosis. Lab Invest 20:234, 1969
4. Battaglia S. Elektronenoptische Untersuchungen am Leberamyloid in der Maus. Beitr Pathol Anat 126:300, 1962
5. Bausserman LL, et al. Heterogeneity of human serum amyloid A proteins. J Exp Med 152:641, 1980
6. Benditt EP, et al. The major proteins of human and monkey amyloid substance: common properties including unusual N-terminal amino acid sequences. FEBS Lett 19:169, 1971
7. Benditt EP, et al. Amyloid protein SAA is associated with high density lipoprotein from human serum. Proc Natl Acad Sci USA 74:4025, 1977
8. Benditt EP, et al. Amyloid protein SAA is an apoprotein of mouse plasma high density lipoprotein. Proc Natl Acad Sci USA 76:4092, 1979
9. Bennhold H. Eine spezifische Amyloidfarbung mit Kongorot. Munchen Med Wochenschr 69:1537, 1922
10. Benson MD, et al. Synthesis and secretion of serum amyloid protein A (SAA) by hepatocytes in mice treated with casein. J Immunol 124:495, 1980
11. Benson MD, Wallace MR. Amyloidosis. In: Scriver CR,

in liver trauma instead of the atrial caval shunt. The inferior vena cava can be accessed by cannulating the femoral vein in the groin. The inflow cannulation site is approached by cutdown on the axillary vein. A centrifugal pump is used to assist flow. Hepatic vascular inflow occlusion can then be accomplished by clamping the suprahepatic vena cava at the diaphragm, suprarenal vena cava, and porta hepatis. This method eliminates the need to open the chest and avoids the risk of placing the atrial caval shunt while still maintaining venous return from the inferior vena cava.

Hepatic Resection and Debridement

Hepatic resection is indicated in 2% to 4% of cases.[14,35,37,42] Even in experienced centers, mortality associated with resection for trauma approaches 50%.[41] Absolute indications for liver resection and debridement include dead or devitalized tissue, intraparenchymal injury to large bile ducts, and inaccessible bleeding. Debridement is usually nonanatomic removal of devitalized tissue with the injury. Although the liver is composed of eight functional segments, anatomic resection in trauma is usually limited to right lobectomy, left lobectomy, and left lateral segmentectomy. The anatomic features of the liver are extremely variable, and the surgeon must be aware of the various anatomic anomalies that may be present. The type and extent of resection is usually determined by the nature of the injury.

To carry out hepatic resection, the surgeon must first mobilize the liver by dividing its ligamentous attachments. For a right lobectomy, both leaves of the coronary ligament need to be divided. Access for left lobe resection is enhanced by division of the triangular ligament. Useful techniques have been developed for all forms of resectional debridement. After the capsule of the liver is incised, the liver parenchyma is readily dissected with the blunt end of a scalpel handle. Blood loss is minimized by compression of the liver between the assistant's hands. As vessels and bile ducts are encountered, they can be ligated individually (Fig. 55-5). Small vessels and parenchymal ooze can be controlled with electrocautery on the argon beam coagulator.

Nonanatomic resection should be carried out for debridement of devitalized tissue that does not fall within a standard anatomic region. Resection should be limited only to devitalized tissue. Bleeding vessels should be controlled with clips or suture ligation. Care should be taken to avoid injury to large vascular structures during nonanatomic resection. Raw surfaces left after resection can be covered with omentum to facilitate hemostasis.

Left lateral segmentectomy consists of resection of the liver that lies to the left of the falciform ligament. Care should be taken not to ligate vessels that may be supplying the medial segment of the left lobe. Hemostasis during resection can be maintained by compression of the medial segment. After resection, the raw surface can be covered by mobilizing the falciform ligament and reflecting it over the raw area.

If the medial segment of the left lobe of the liver is severely damaged, left hepatic lobectomy is indicated. Medial segmentectomy, although a viable option in an elective setting, is time-consuming, and associated injuries make this a poor choice in the trauma patient. The line of resection for a left lobectomy should be carried out to the left of the gallbladder fossa. It is absolutely necessary to identify the middle hepatic vein during resection since it drains the superior segment of the right lobe and commonly drains into the left hepatic vein. The left hepatic vein should be ligated and divided distal to the junction with the middle hepatic vein. The left portal vein should not be ligated until it is well exposed within the hilum because it might give off a branch to the anterior segment of the right lobe. Care also should be taken when dividing the left hepatic duct because a segmental hepatic duct from the right frequently crosses the segmental fissure to drain into the left hepatic duct. The left hepatic artery supplies only the left side and can be readily ligated.

In performing a right hepatic lobectomy, the line of resection should be carried to the left of the gallbladder fissure. The middle hepatic vein should be divided early and proximally to avoid injury to the left hepatic vein. The dissection

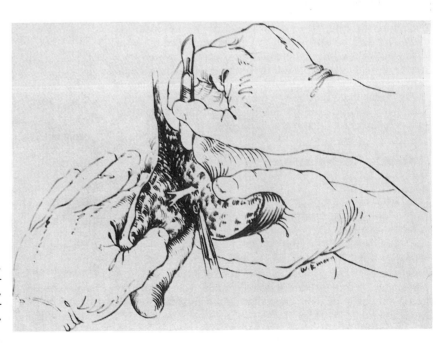

FIGURE 55-5 Technique of liver resection. Liver is compressed manually, while the surgeon proceeds with the dissection. (Blaisdell W, Trunkey DD. Trauma management, vol 1. Abdominal trauma. New York, Thieme-Stratton, 1982, p 141)

should then be carried toward the vena cava to the right of the middle hepatic vein. The right hepatic artery and portal vein can be dissected early in the resection and ligated to decrease blood loss. Care should be taken to avoid damage to the occasional branch of the hepatic artery, which may supply the medial segment of the left lobe. Division of hepatic parenchyma and ligation of small vessels and bile ducts are done as previously described.

Packing

The initial poor results obtained with packing the liver with gauze rolls led Madding and Kennedy[29] to recommend avoiding this treatment after the World War II experience. More recent reports[12,13] demonstrated great success with packing the liver injury with multiple laparotomy sponges. This technique is particularly effective when coagulopathy or hypothermia develops during repair or resection of the liver. Massive bleeding, transfusion, and hypothermia all contribute to severe coagulopathy, which can make meticulous hemostasis in the severely injured liver impossible. In 2% to 5% of patients with unrelenting hemorrhage, packing of the liver stops the hemorrhage and should be performed. The abdomen is closed, and the patient is further resuscitated in the intensive care unit by rewarming and administrating directed blood transfusion products to reverse the coagulopathy. Pack removal is then accomplished at 24 to 72 hours when the coagulopathy is corrected. Patients undergoing packing of their liver have a 40% mortality rate and suffer multiple complications due to the severity of their injuries. The sepsis rate associated with this technique can approach 25%.[40] Proper packing does not involve simply stuffing laparotomy sponges around the liver. Although some have advocated placement of plastic between the gauze and the liver, use of plain gauze is equally effective. For large lacerations of the liver, the goal is to pack the perihepatic region so that closure and compression of the injury are accomplished. Packs can be placed in the right retrohepatic space to roll the right lobe of the liver anteriorly and close any laceration. Packs can also be placed between the liver and the rib cage to provide posterior compression of the injury to control retrohepatic caval or posterior liver injuries. The key is to compress the liver without occluding the inferior vena cava. Return to the operating room can then be undertaken in a more controlled environment and with a full complement of personnel, which may not be available in the acute trauma setting. The surgical team should be prepared for atrial caval shunt or venovenous bypass to facilitate hepatic vascular isolation for repair of injuries. It is also possible after packing to transport the patient to a different center that has additional resources.

Hepatic Transplantation

If trauma to the liver has resulted in massive parenchymal destruction, hepatic transplantation may be required. Three cases have been reported of transplantation after severe hepatic trauma, with two successes.[2,9] The indication for hepatic transplantation secondary to trauma is severe nonreconstructible injuries to the porta hepatis. Concomitant intraabdominal injuries and head injuries are relative contraindications. The availability of an appropriate donor is unpredictable, and every effort should be made to consult a liver transplant center as soon as possible so the anhepatic period is minimized.

Drainage

Whether or not to drain a liver injury is controversial, especially when dealing with class I and II injuries (see Table 55-1). There is little evidence to support drainage of livers with class I and class II injuries, and the drain may contribute to infection and abscess formation.[38] More severe injuries should be drained with closed suction drains to diminish fluid collection and control biliary leak. Drains should be placed not only in the region of the injury but also posterior to the injury to provide dependent drainage of fluid collections.

Repair of Injuries to the Porta Hepatis

Injuries to the porta hepatis are difficult to manage and carry significant morbidity and mortality rates (about 50%). These injuries are formidable and usually are associated with massive hemorrhage. Control of hemorrhage is the first priority. The key to successful management is wide exposure. We favor an extended Kocher maneuver, which entails taking down the entire right colon and mobilizing it toward the midline along with the duodenum. This exposes the portal vein and a significant portion of the inferior vena cava and the aorta, which may also be injured. In certain instances, it may be necessary to expose the most proximal portion of the portal vein at the junction of the splenic vein and superior mesenteric vein by dividing the neck of the pancreas. After the portal injury has been treated, a distal pancreatectomy can be performed. Although ligation can be carried out with reportedly few sequelae, every attempt should be made to repair the portal vein injury. Repair can be carried out by direct suture repair or lateral repair.[43] In instances in which vein has been lost or destroyed, it may be necessary to place a patch or interposition graft of saphenous vein or internal jugular vein to reestablish flow. In the case of associated splenic injury, the splenic vein may be used for the repair after splenectomy.

Injuries to the hepatic artery also create difficult management problems. Although the hepatic artery carries only one quarter of blood flow to the liver, it carries half of the oxygen supply. Many authors advocate direct ligation of the hepatic artery when the injury is to the common hepatic artery. We prefer to perform repair of the hepatic artery whenever possible. The artery can be dissected free, the damaged area resected, and primary anastomosis performed. When necessary, a saphenous vein interposition graft can be used to provide repair without tension. We make a special effort to repair injuries of the hepatic artery rather than using ligation.

Injuries to the extrahepatic biliary tree are usually associated with penetrating trauma, although blunt trauma can cause stretch or avulsion injuries. Gallbladder injuries are uncommon. The treatment of choice is cholecystectomy for most of these injuries.

When the injury is to the bile ducts, repair can be tedious. The bile ducts should be meticulously dissected and exposed. Small lacerations can be directly sutured. For moderate injuries, the ducts must be debrided before suture repair. Repair should be performed over a T-tube to provide drainage. The most common site of disruption is at the junction of the pancreas and the common bile duct. For proximal common bile duct injuries, biliary drainage can be accomplished using a Roux-en-Y procedure to either the common hepatic duct or the gallbladder. The Roux-en-Y choledochojejunostomy can be difficult to perform with a normal-sized common bile duct, as is the case in most trauma patients. To make this anastomosis technically easier, a modification of the vascular Carrel patch has been described.[30] A 1-cm length of cystic duct is preserved after cholecystectomy and the side wall opened onto the common bile duct remnant. This patch of bile duct is then used to anastomose in an end-to-side fashion to the Roux limb. A Roux-en-Y can also be brought to the right or left hepatic duct to provide drainage. In the unstable patient, biliary drainage can be accomplished by placing catheters into the right and left hepatic ducts or the common bile duct, which are then brought out of the abdomen laterally. Delayed reconstruction of the biliary system can be accomplished after the patient recovers from other injuries.

POSTOPERATIVE MANAGEMENT AND COMPLICATIONS

Massive blood loss, transfusion, tissue trauma, shock, hypothermia, and liver dysfunction contribute to coagulopathy, both intraoperatively and postoperatively. Treatment of the coagulopathy requires rewarming of the patient as well as replenishment of clotting factors using transfusion of either fresh whole blood or fresh frozen plasma in conjunction with cryoprecipitate and platelets. Hematocrits, platelet counts, and prothrombin times should be measured frequently as a guide to therapy for coagulopathy. If the coagulopathy has been corrected and the patient continues to hemorrhage, reexploration is indicated. For complex liver injuries (classes IV and V), we advocate second-look reoperation at 24 to 48 hours.

Postoperative pulmonary failure is frequent after major trauma. Tissue trauma, large-volume fluid resuscitation, and associated injuries (eg, rib fracture) contribute to pulmonary failure. The patient should be managed with endotracheal intubation and positive pressure ventilation until hemodynamically stable. The patient should be extubated as soon as possible, but with the knowledge that reintubation may be necessary.

Jaundice occurs frequently after liver trauma. This may be a sign of severe hepatic dysfunction but usually is related to resorption of hematomas, breakdown of transfused red cells, and mild hepatic dysfunction from central lobular necrosis secondary to shock. Hepatic function returns to normal promptly, although elevated bilirubin levels in the serum may persist for weeks.

Bile leaks and fistulas can usually be detected when the perihepatic area has been drained. Unless these leaks are from a major bile duct, they usually close spontaneously.

Hematobilia is an uncommon complication, occurring in 1% of complex injuries. The typical presentation is days to weeks after the injury and can be manifest by melena, upper gastrointestinal bleeding, hypotension, or biliary colic. The diagnosis is confirmed by visualizing blood coming from the ampulla during upper gastrointestinal endoscopy. Treatment is preferentially by percutaneous transvascular selective embolization of the involved artery.

Sepsis after hepatic trauma occurs in 7% to 12% of patients and is related to intraabdominal abscess, pneumonia, acalculous cholecystitis, and ischemic bowel. Risk factors associated with intraabdominal abscess postoperatively include associated splenectomy, liver packing to control hemorrhage, class IV or V injury, large transfusion requirement, and colon injury. Subphrenic and subhepatic abscesses are usually marked by fever 4 to 7 days after operation. Pleural effusion may be noted on chest radiograph. Diagnosis can be made by ultrasound or CT scan. Treatment includes percutaneous or surgical drainage and intravenous antibiotics. Prophylactic antibiotics are not recommended postoperatively unless there is an associated bowel injury.

References

1. Aaron WS, Fulton RL, Mays ET. Selective ligation of the hepatic artery for trauma of the liver. Surg Gynecol Obstet 141:187, 1975
2. Angstadt J, Jarrell B, Moritz M, et al. Surgical management of severe liver trauma: a role for liver transplantation. J Trauma 29:606–608, 1989
3. Bismuth H. Surgical anatomy and anatomical surgery of the liver. World J Surg 6:3–9, 1982
4. Bivins BA, Sachatello SR, Daugherty ME, Ernst GB, Griffen WO. Diagnostic peritoneal lavage is superior to clinical evaluation in blunt abdominal trauma. Am Surg 44:637–644, 1978
5. Burch JM, Feliciano DV, Mattox KL. The atriocaval shunt: facts and fiction. Ann Surg 207:555–568, 1988
6. Clagett GP, Olsen WR. Non-mechanical hemorrhage in severe liver injury. Ann Surg 187:369–374, 1978
7. Cogbill TH, Moore EE, Jurkovich GJ, Feliciano DV, Morris JA, Mucha P. Severe hepatic trauma: a multi-center experience with 1,335 liver injuries. J Trauma 28:1433–1438, 1988
8. Elerding SC, Aragon GE, Moore EE. Fatal hepatic hemorrhage after trauma. Am J Surg 138:883–888, 1979
9. Esquivel CD, Bernardas A, Makowka L, Imatsuki S, Grodon RD, Starzl TE. Liver replacement after massive hepatic trauma. J Trauma 27:800–802, 1987
10. Fabian TC, Stone HH. Arrest of severe liver hemorrhage by an omental pack. South Med J 73:1487, 1980
11. Federle MP, Goldberg HI, Kaiser JA, Moss AA, Jeffrey RB Jr, Mall JC. Evaluation of abdominal trauma by computed tomography. Radiology 138:637–644, 1981
12. Feliciano DB, Mattox KL, Birch JM. Packing for control of hepatic hemorrhage: 58 consecutive patients. J Trauma 26:738, 1986
13. Feliciano DB, Mattox KL, Jordan GL Jr. Intraabdominal packing for control of hepatic hemorrhage: a reappraisal. J Trauma 21:285, 1981
14. Feliciano DB, Mattox KL, Jordan GL Jr, et al. Management of 1000 consecutive cases of hepatic trauma (1979–1984). Ann Surg 204:438, 1986
15. Furnival CM, Mackenzie RJ, Blumgart LH. The mechanism of impaired coagulation after partial hepatectomy in the dog. Surg Gynecol Obstet 143:81–86, 1976
16. Garre C. Contribution to surgery of the liver. Bruns Beitr Klin Chir 4:181, 1888
17. Griffith BP, Shaw BW Jr, Hardesty RL, Iwatsuki S, Bahnson HT, Starzl TE. Venovenous bypass without systemic anticoagulation for transplantation of the human liver. Surg Gynecol Obstet 160:270–272, 1985
18. Heaney J, Scanton W, Halbert D, et al. An improved technique for vascular isolation at the liver: experimental study and case reports. Ann Surg 163:237–241, 1966
19. Huguet C, Nordlinger B, Bloch P. Tolerance of the human liver to prolonged normothermic ischemia. Arch Surg 113:1448, 1978
20. Kaku N. Short term and long-term changes in hepatic function in 60 patients with blunt liver injury. J Trauma 27:607–609, 1987
21. Karp MP, Cooney DR, Pros GA, et al. The nonoperative management of pediatric hepatic trauma. J Pediatr Surg 18:512–518, 1983

22. Knudson MM, Lim RC, Oakes DD, Jeffrey RB. Nonoperative management of blunt liver injuries in adults: the need for continued surveillance. J Trauma 30:1494–1499, 1990
23. Kudsk KA, Sheldon FG, Lim RC Jr. Atrial caval shunting (ACS) after trauma. J Trauma 22:81–85, 1982
24. Larrey DJ (translated by JC Mercer). Surgical memoirs of the Campaigns of Rurrid, Germany, and France. Philadelphia, Carey & Lea, 1832, p 166
25. Lennon RL, Hosking MP, Gray JR. The effects of intraoperative blood salvage and induced hypotension on transfusion requirements during spinal surgical procedures. Mayo Clin Proc 62:1090–1094, 1987
26. Lim RC Jr. Injuries to the liver and extrahepatic ducts in trauma management. In: Blaisdell FW, Trunkey DD, eds. Trauma management, vol 1. New York, Thieme-Stratton, 1982
27. Luna GK, Dellinger EP. Nonoperative observation therapy for splenic injuries: a safe therapeutic option? Am J Surg 153:462–468, 1987
28. Madding GF, Kennedy PA. Trauma to the liver. Philadelphia, WB Saunders, 1971
29. Madding GF, Lawrence KB, Kennedy PA. Forward surgery of the severely injured. Second Auxiliary Surgical Group 1:307, 1942–1945
30. Mavroudis C, Trunkey DD. Choledochoplasty for choledochojejunostomy: variations on a theme by Carrel. Am J Surg 142:305, 1987
31. McDougal EG, Mandel SR. Traumatic hemobilia: successful nonoperative treatment in two cases. Am Surg 50:169–172, 1984
32. Meade, RH. An introduction to the history of general surgery. Philadelphia, WB Saunders, 1968
33. Michels NA. Newer anatomy of the liver and variant blood supply and collateral circulation. Am J Surg 112:337, 1966
34. Moon KL, Federle MP. Computed tomography in hepatic trauma. AJR 141:309–314, 1983
35. Moore EE. Critical decisions in the management of hepatic trauma. Am J Surg 148:712–716, 1984
36. Moore EE, Eiseman B, Dunn EL. Current management of hepatic trauma. Contemp Surg 15:91, 1979
37. Moore FA, Moore EE, Seagraves A. Nonresectional management of major hepatic trauma. Am J Surg 150:725, 1985
38. Mullins RJ, Stone HH, Dunlop WE, et al. Hepatic trauma: evaluation of routine drainage. South Med J 78:259, 1985
39. Olsen WR, Hildreth DH. Abdominal paracentesis and peritoneal lavage in blunt abdominal trauma. J Trauma 11:824–829, 1971
40. Pachter HL, Liang HG, Hofstetter SR, Mattox KL. Injury to the liver and biliary tract. In: Moore EE, Feliciano DV, eds. Trauma. Norwalk, CT, Appleton & Lange, 1988
41. Pachter HL, Spencer FC. The management of complex hepatic trauma. Controv Surg 2:241–249, 1983
42. Pachter HL, Spencer FC, Hofstetter SR, et al. Experience with the finger fracture technique to achieve intra-hepatic hemostasis in 75 patients with severe injuries of the liver. Ann Surg 197:771, 1983
43. Peterson SR, Sheldon GJ, Lim RC Jr. Management of portal vein injuries. J Trauma 19:616–620, 1979
44. Phillips TF, Soulier G, Wilson RF. Outcome of massive transfusion exceeding two blood volumes in trauma and emergency surgery. J Trauma 27:903–910, 1987
45. Pringle JH, Notes on the arrest of hepatic hemorrhage due to trauma. Ann Surg 48:541–549, 1908
46. Schrock T, Blaisdell FW, Mathewson C Jr. Management of blunt trauma to the liver and hepatic veins. Arch Surg 96:698–704, 1968
47. Shaw BW, Martin DJ, Marquez JM, et al. Venous bypass in clinical liver transplantation. Ann Surg 200:524–534, 1984
48. Stone HH, Lamb JM. Use of pedicled omentum as an autogenous pack for control of hemorrhage in major injuries of the liver. Surg Gynecol Obstet 141:92, 1975
49. Suzuki T, Nakayasu A, Kavabe K, Takeda H, Honjo J. Surgical significance of anatomic variations of the hepatic artery. Am J Surg 122:505, 1971
50. Vandamme JP, Bonte J. The branches of the celiac trunk. Acta Anat 122:110, 1985
51. Walker, K. The story of medicine. London, Hutchinson, 1954

Diseases of the Liver, Seventh Edition, edited by
Leon Schiff and Eugene R. Schiff. J.B. Lippincott Company, Philadelphia © 1993.

56

Hemobilia

Philip Sandblom

Hemobilia, or bleeding into the biliary tract, occurs when disease or trauma produces an abnormal communication between blood vessels and bile ducts. It corresponds to hematuria in urinary tract disease but is probably less common, or at least less often recognized. If the urine becomes bloody, it is noticed immediately; but if blood enters the intestine through the papilla of Vater, it only comes to light as hematemesis or melena, and its origin may well be mistaken or unidentified. Therefore, hemobilia is a problem of differential diagnosis with regard to other and more common sources of bleeding in the gastrointestinal tract, rather than a diagnostic sign of liver or biliary tract disease.

Because of its apparent rarity, hemobilia was late in becoming an acknowledged entity. It was repeatedly discovered only to be forgotten again. As early as 1654, Francis Glisson,[9] in the first detailed description of the anatomy of the liver, discussed the possibility of hemorrhage through the biliary tract in the following words:

> I believe that if the liver is injured by a contusion, it may lead to blood leaving the body by way of vomit or the stool for there is no doubt that the biliary duct takes unto itself (to the great good of the patient) some of the blood issuing into the liver and leads it down to the intestines. From there, it is either impelled upwards through reverse peristalsis or downwards the usual way.

Glisson's observations sank into oblivion, and a whole century was to elapse before the subject of hemorrhage into the biliary tract was brought up again. In Morgagni's epistles (1765), the founder of clinical pathology noted, in the section on the causes of dilation of the biliary tract, that both abscesses in the liver and the voiding of sharp gallstones could lead to bleeding through the biliary ducts.

A little later, in 1777, Antoine Portal[21] gave an admirable presentation of a case where he made the diagnosis before the death of the patient and confirmed it at autopsy. In this early treatise, Portal drew attention to the difficulty of finding the source of hemorrhages in the biliary tract, "when they are slight in quantity and occur but seldom," and to the risk of mistakenly tracing them to a healthy organ, a mistake that has been made repeatedly in the history of hemobilia.

The first case on the American continent was published by a Boston surgeon, Jackson[10] (1834), who gave a careful clinical and pathologic report of an "Aneurysm of the Hepatic Artery Bursting Into the Hepatic Duct," the first direct observation of an abnormal communication between the blood vessels and biliary ducts. Finally, in 1871, the German surgeon Quincke[22] gave a masterly account of the course of events in biliary tract hemorrhage and established it's three cardinal symptoms—gastrointestinal hemorrhage, biliary colic, and jaundice.

Incidence and Clinical Features

Hemobilia was formerly regarded as a medical curiosity. With better knowledge of the syndrome and with improved diagnostic methods, it is recognized with increasing frequency. There is, in addition, an absolute increase in incidence partly because of the rising number of traffic accidents, which often result in liver injury, and partly because of more invasive diagnostic and therapeutic procedures, which may cause iatrogenic hemobilia.[4,5] *Index Medicus* did not add the term *hemobilia* until 1980 and now has about 25 references per year, whereas *hematuria* was adopted from the beginning in 1880 and has three times as many references yearly.

Bleeding in hemobilia can be of varying degree, from exsanguinating hemorrhage, leading rapidly to the death of the patient, to occult bleeding, which, if it continues, may result in chronic secondary anemia.

Profuse hemobilia is rare, but when it occurs, it is not only an essential symptom but also a dangerous, sometimes life-threatening complication of liver or biliary tract disease, which may constitute the main reason for treatment. Minor or occult hemobilia is frequent but generally overlooked or neglected because it is rarely of clinical significance.[27]

Most hemorrhage of consequence is arterial in origin. When only veins are injured, the bleeding is often slight, but it may be significant if the portal pressure is increased. In minor hemobilia, the blood does not mix with the bile (Fig. 56-1). It either remains fluid and flows unobtrusively into the intestine or coagulates to form a cast of the duct when trapped above the closed sphincter of Oddi[30] (Fig. 56-2).

The clot acts like a calculus, causing biliary colic when passed or obstructive jaundice when retained. It generally has an ephemeral existence, given that it is promptly lysed through the fibrinolytic property of the bile (Fig. 56-3A and B). Through this activity, the bile plays the same role as urine and saliva in clearing fibrin deposits from their respective ducts. When protected from the bile stream, clots may escape this lytic action and remain solid; they are then easily mistaken for gallstones[26] (Fig. 56-4). This can occur when the bile flow is diverted through a T-tube above the clot (see Fig. 56-3C) or when it is totally obstructed by the clot itself (see Fig. 56-2). An excluded gallbladder can offer a hiding place, where the clots can remain for long periods and cause

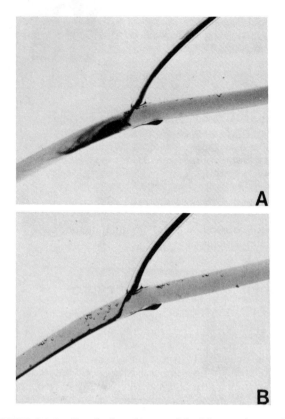

FIGURE 56-1 Detail of a tubing model of the extrahepatic bile ducts. Blood is injected into bile streaming through the system. (**A**) When injected forcefully to imitate major hemobilia, the blood causes turbulence and mixes with the bile. (**B**) When injected gently to imitate minor hemobilia, it flows immiscibly to the lower portion and forms a pure coagulum. (Sandblom P, Mirkovitch V. Minor hemobilia. Ann Surg 190:254, 1979)

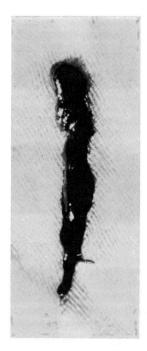

FIGURE 56-2 An obstructing blood clot extracted from the common duct in a case of traumatic hemobilia. Note the protuberance, probably a cast of the distal end of the pancreatic duct. (Sandblom P, Mirkovitch V. Minor hemobilia. Ann Surg 190:254, 1979)

cholecystitis[23] or turn into stones. Their role in the formation of so-called primary duct stones is uncertain.

The clots that are produced by hemobilia have certain characteristics that allow their recognition and differentiation from calculi (see Fig. 56-3). Generally, they are casts of the lumen where they are produced. When formed in the common duct, they are thus cylindric (see Fig. 56-3C); on the casts from the lower periampullary duct, one may recognize the impressions of the sphincter, and even the pancreatic duct may show up (see Fig. 56-2). When formed in the ampulla, the clots are rounded with one flat surface that was horizontal at the time of coagulation (see Fig. 56-3G and *H*). Clotting of blood flowing with the bile stream makes band-like structures, and clotting in the smaller ducts produces long, branched strings. Solid clots may be expelled into the gastrointestinal tract and have sometimes appeared in vomit after an attack of biliary colic. The surface of the clots is often shaggy with fibrin threads; this has also been noticed at choledochoscopy. The color, red at the start, soon becomes dark brown. The consistency varies from mushy and fragile to tenacious and firm.

The qualities described have induced surgeons who are unaware of hemobilia to give these clots a variety of names— *inspissated bile, bile plugs, tissue debris,* and so forth. Most of the features that characterize the clots on direct inspection,

especially their form, can be recognized in the cholangiogram. A fresh clot, especially when it is mixed with bile, presents an indistinct surface (see Fig. 56-3A). Because of their affinity to the mucosa, clots are often attached to the wall, sometimes in a string-like fashion (see Fig. 56-3E).

These clinical and experimental observations show how important it is for the surgeon to remember that a free body in the biliary tract is not always a stone. Even if no hemobilia has been observed, it may be a fibrin deposit or a blood clot. If this is the case, operation is not necessary, since the fibrinolytic effect of the bile generally suffices to clear the biliary tract.[26] The surgeon must avoid measures that prevent the bile from exerting this action. If a suspected clot still remains, perfusion or washouts with bile or a fibrinolytic agent, such as streptokinase, may be tried. If a clot continues to cause a total obstruction that helps it to escape fibrinolysis, it eventually will have to be extracted.

Bearing in mind the fibrinolytic effect of bile, reports of successful dissolution of "retained stones" through perfusion with various media should be critically assessed. Apparent dissolution may occasionally represent only fibrinolysis and expulsion of clots (see Fig. 56-3G and *H*).

The natural history of hemobilia includes gastrointestinal bleeding in 90%, biliary colic in 70% and jaundice in 60% of the cases. These constitute the pathognomonic symptom triad of hemobilia. The biliary colic caused by passage of coagula corresponds to the colic in gallstone disease. Such pain may also be produced by an arterial aneurysm bursting into a duct; this event causes violent pain from the sudden increase in intraluminal pressure. The jaundice is usually temporary and recedes when an obstructive clot is lysed or expelled into the intestine, usually followed by a large gush

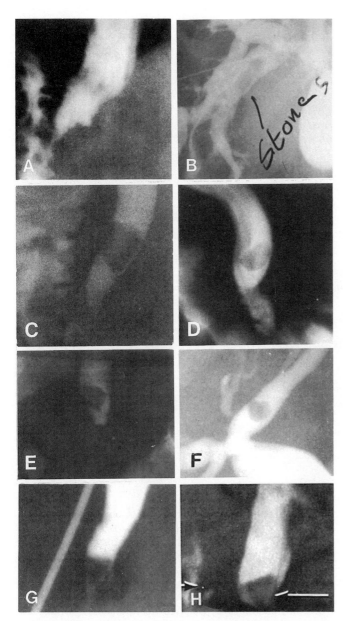

FIGURE 56-3 Characteristics of cholangiographic defects caused by clots, which often are misinterpreted as calculi. (**A**) This defect with indistinct borders was caused by a blood clot that appeared in connection with choledocholithotomy. The common duct was reopened to ascertain that the defect was not due to a remaining stone. (**B**) A fresh, multilobular coagulum in an intrahepatic duct immediately after a liver puncture, diagnosed as stones. At operation the next day, only some small fringes remained. (**C**) A solid, cylindric clot formed postoperatively during 3 weeks of total bile drainage after choledocholithotomy. (**D**) The remaining resistant fragment of a large, dissolved clot looks like a cast of the ampulla. (**E**) A clot resulting from minor hemobilia in an otherwise normal biliary tract during excessive anticoagulant therapy. Note the attachments to the ductal mucosa. (**F**) A pure fibrin clot adhering to the duct wall. (**G**) A contrast defect reported to be caused by a stone, which dissolved during 7 days of treatment with saline solution. It looks like, and probably was, a blood clot. (**H**) This defect in a postoperative cholangiogram disappeared within a week in spite of continuous bile drainage. It looks like a cast of the ampulla and was probably due to a clot.

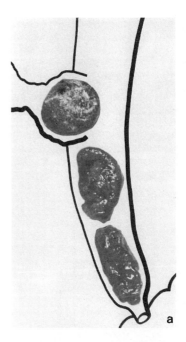

FIGURE 56-4 The resemblance between stone and clots. Drawing of an operative finding with photographs of a stone penetrating into the common duct and two occluding firm clots distally. Their resemblance explains why they so often are misinterpreted.

of blood with hematemesis and melena. Occasionally, it has to be removed surgically.

Secondary symptoms are hemorrhagic shock, if the bleeding is substantial, and anemia, if it is prolonged.

Diagnosis

Because of the characteristic and consistent symptom triad, the diagnosis of major hemobilia is easy to establish, provided the physician is aware of the syndrome. It should always be suspected when gastrointestinal hemorrhage is combined with biliary tract symptoms.

Until recently, far too many cases of hemobilia have been diagnosed too late—at autopsy—or with undue delay after one or more inappropriate or inadequate operations, such as blind gastric resection.

When hemorrhage into the biliary tract is suspected, the following diagnostic procedures should be undertaken in turn. The first measure should be gastrointestinal endoscopy to rule out other bleeding sources. Direct observation of blood flowing from the papilla of Vater is not uncommon in hemobilia.[2] Endoscopy may be combined with retrograde cholangiopancreatography, which sometimes reveals clots in the ducts.

Ultrasonography or computed tomographic scanning[13] often demonstrates even small traumatic lesions if a hematoma is produced, but not if there is only an arteriobiliary fistula. Clotted blood in the biliary tract produces less distinctive shadows (or defects) than stones; these shadows often are interpreted as being due to gravel or inspissated bile (Fig. 56-5).

The best way to verify the diagnosis is by selective arteriography, which reveals the source of bleeding in a high per-

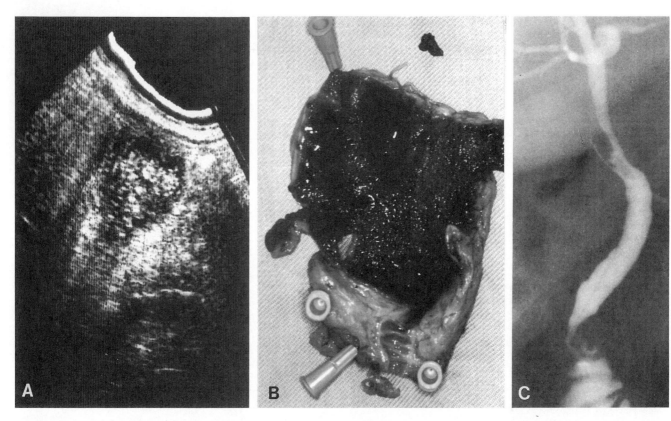

FIGURE 56-5   Hemobilia caused by clotting defect during anticoagulation therapy. (**A**) Sonogram indicates dense material in the gallbladder, interpreted as microcalculi or inspissated bile. (**B**) In the gallbladder, there was clotted blood firmly attached to the wall. (**C**) Defects in the peroperative cholangiogram caused by clots, the large proximal one attached to the wall, the distal one band-like.

centage of cases by displacement of the vessels around a liver mass or by filling an aneurysm (Fig. 56-6). When caught at the right moment, contrast material may be seen traveling down the hepatic duct, thus establishing the existence of a communication with the biliary tract (see Fig. 56-6). In some cases, the artery opens into the portal system as well.[32] The arteriographic catheter should not be withdrawn until it has been decided whether embolization of the feeding artery should be considered as treatment. This procedure is of special value in discovering central liver lesions, which may be difficult or impossible to localize, even at exploratory laparotomy. Cholangiography, either preoperatively or postoperatively, may reveal a lesion by contrast-filling of a cavity or by dislocation of the ducts (Fig. 56-7).

Treatment

The treatment of hemobilia depends on the cause of the hemorrhage; cholecystectomy is done for gallstones, resection for tumor, embolization or vascular repair for aneurysms. In general, there is a choice between resection of the liver and obstruction of the feeding artery though ligature, temporary balloon tamponade, or definitive embolization.[11] This decision depends on the location of the bleeding source. For peripheral and well-localized lesions, resection may be preferred because a minimum of liver parenchyma is sacrificed.

Ligature of the hepatic artery or of one of its branches, first done by Kehr in 1903 (Fig. 56-8), is now reserved for cases in which the abdomen has been opened for exploration or repair and in which embolization is not possible or has been unsuccessful. A condition for ligature of the main artery is a free flow through the portal vein that adequately nourishes the hepatic parenchyma. Arterial embolization (see Fig. 56-6) has become the preferred treatment. Abnormal communications between the branches of the hepatic artery and the biliary tract can be selectively occluded by large particulate material of different kinds. The first successful treatment of hemobilia by this method was reported by Walter and colleagues[35] in 1976.

Several advantages make embolization preferable to surgery in the treatment of hemobilia. The risk of hepatic necrosis exists but should be minimal since the obstruction can be limited to a segmental branch of the hepatic artery. In addition, embolization may be repeated easily if hemobilia recurs.

Since embolization techniques have been popularized, the overall picture of the therapeutic management of hemobilia patients has changed. Formerly, resection and arterial ligature were performed with equal frequency and with comparable results as to cure, morbidity, and mortality.[25] During the past decade, liver resection has decreased to about 10% of the treated cases, whereas operative ligature is performed in about 30% and embolization in no less than 60% with an overall success rate of about 95%.

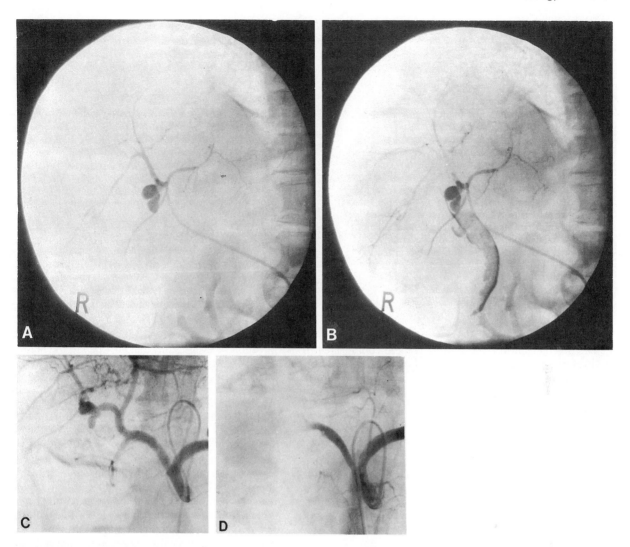

FIGURE 56-6 After complicated cholecystectomy, an iatrogenic pseudoaneurysm developed. It ruptured into the biliary tract and caused exsanguinating hemobilia, diagnosed by duodenal endoscopy and then treated successfully with embolization. (**A**) Selective arteriogram demonstrates a pseudoaneurysm of the hepatic artery located at the liver hilium. (**B**) A few seconds later, the contrast material is seen flowing down the hepatic duct displaying the arteriobiliary fistula. (**C** and **D**) The same aneurysm before and after obliteration of the feeding artery with artificial embolus. (Kelley CJ, Hemingway AP, McPherson GA, et al. Non-surgical management of post-cholecystectomy haemobilia. Br J Surg 70:502, 1981)

Etiology

The bleeding in hemobilia may originate in the liver parenchyma or in the intrahepatic or extrahepatic biliary tract, including the gallbladder. The pancreas is a rare source.[24]

Common causes of the abnormal communication between blood vessels and the biliary tract that give rise to hemobilia are trauma (due to accident, operation, or liver puncture), inflammation, gallstones, tumors, and vascular disorders. There are many conditions that occasionally give rise to hemobilia, such as echinococci, choledochal cysts, pancreatitis, portal hypertension, and blood coagulation defects. Their relative frequencies are shown in Figure 56-9. The proportion noted in the diagram relates to massive hemobilia. If cases of minor hemobilia were considered, gallstones would be the most frequent cause since biliary tract operations and colic from gallstones nearly always are accompanied by minute bleeding from the injured biliary tract mucosa. In the era before cholecystography, the occurrence of microscopic melena after attacks of biliary colic was one of the main diagnostic signs of gallstone disease.[19]

Accidental Trauma

The most common cause of hemobilia in the western world is trauma—accidental or iatrogenic. The mechanism in penetrating trauma is evident. The first case of hemobilia in the literature, described by Glisson,[9] was that of a young nobleman who bled to death through the biliary tract after having been pierced by a sword through his liver when fighting a duel. A common "weapon" today in penetrating trauma is the physician's punch needle.[36]

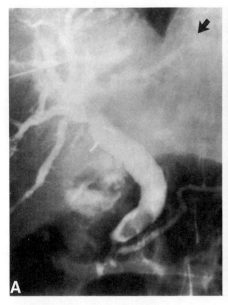
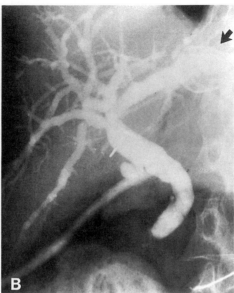

FIGURE 56-7 Lesion during transhepatic cholangiography, producing a blood clot in the common duct. (**A**) The transhepatic catheter points toward a lesion in the left hepatic duct (*arrow*). A multilobular filling defect in the common duct was caused by a bile plug, probably a blood clot, which was removed at operation. (**B**) A postoperative cholangiogram clearly shows the extravasation from the ductal lesion. The filling defect is gone. (Sandblom P, Saegesser F, Mirkovitch V. Hepatic hemobilia: hemorrhage from the intrahepatic biliary tract, a review. World J Surg 8:41, 1984)

The mechanism in blunt trauma is more complicated. If the liver is compressed, the fragile and inelastic parenchyma tears easily. The disrupting force is greatest in the center of the organ, which explains the high frequency of subcapsular liver rupture. This is often combined with smaller superficial rifts caused by direct force. When these rifts are seen at emergency exploration, the surgeon is apt to be satisfied with repairing them and may miss the central cavity, which is not directly visible. The surgeon may even create a defect when performing a superficial suture of a deep laceration.[16] The surgeon should not expect hemobilia to be a common complication of liver lesions that are open to the peritoneal cavity and in which intraabdominal bleeding is the predominant and alarming factor. Traumatic hemobilia is found in central liver ruptures caused by blunt trauma and has more obscure and less acute symptoms. If a hepatic vein tears, bile may be sucked into the circulation, causing bilirubinemia, so-called bilhemia.[3]

Central liver ruptures can be of different sizes, from large cavities extending into both lobes to simple arteriobiliary fistulas. Occasionally, no bleeding or only temporary bleeding occurs, but most of the time, there is long-standing, often repeated hemobilia.[25] The rupture tears bile ducts, arteries, and veins, which fill the cavity with bile and blood. If a large artery is torn, exsanguinating gastrointestinal hemorrhage may occur, necessitating emergency surgery to save the patient's life. Usually, the cavity fills slowly, and the escape of bloody bile is delayed by coagulation in the cavity or in the diverting duct, assisted by a contracting sphincter of Oddi. Finally, after days or weeks, the pressure in the cavity suddenly forces the clot down the tract into the intestine, followed by a large gush of blood and bile.

During these events, the patient first experiences an increasing, dull pain over the area of the liver. Sometimes, enlargement of the liver can be detected, and there may be signs of obstructive jaundice. Finally, the patient experiences intense biliary colic followed by hematemesis and melena. This classic triad of biliary colic, gastrointestinal hemorrhage, and jaundice should always arouse the suspicion of hemobilia. The patient feels relieved after evacuation of the cavity; the liver size diminishes; and the jaundice subsides. A favorable prognosis may mistakenly be given. Unfortunately, relief usually is only temporary since the course is repeated over months and years. The syndrome is thus characterized by a distinct periodicity. There is little hope for spontaneous healing (Fig. 56-10).

The explanation for the curious course of traumatic hemobilia is that although the liver regenerates quickly, local lesions heal slowly. During the first few hours after liver trauma, the parenchymal cells prepare for growth, and in a few days, regeneration is in full swing. In contradistinction, the healing of localized lesions is retarded, even prevented,

FIGURE 56-8 A case of true aneurysm in the right hepatic artery, rupturing into the gallbladder. This original drawing by Hans Kehr in 1903 shows the pathologic picture in the first case of hemobilia, which was successfully treated by ligature of the hepatic artery proper.

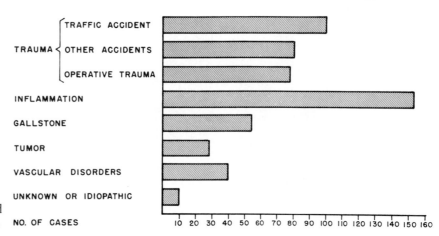

FIGURE 56-9 Distribution of 545 published cases of major hemobilia with respect to cause.

by a fibrinolytic effect of the bile. There is a striking difference in healing rate between liver wounds open to the peritoneal cavity and liver wounds that heal in the presence of bile (Fig. 56-11). In the latter, there is diminished production of fibrinous exudate, granulating tissue, and fibrous scar.[29] As a result, a central cavity is lined by easily damaged parenchymal cells rather than by sturdy granulation tissue. Because spontaneous healing is rare, the only hope for cure is adequate operative treatment. This active surgical approach has considerably lowered mortality.

The surgical treatment may be prophylactic. Adequate handling of a liver lesion at the primary emergency laparotomy can prevent later hemobilia. The operation should include careful exploration of cavities and meticulous hemostasis and suturing of open bile ducts before drainage and closure.[16] If this does not suffice, or if hemobilia occurs in spite of these efforts, a more radical course of action is necessary.

IATROGENIC INJURY

Iatrogenic hemobilia from operative trauma is encountered as frequently as hemobilia from traffic accidents. During biliary tract surgery, the hepatic artery may be damaged by a suture or by the dissection, which can result in an arteriobiliary fistula or a false aneurysm leaking or eroding into the extrahepatic bile ducts (see Fig. 56-6). Intrahepatic lesions are caused more commonly by instrumentation of the biliary tree. Not all surgeons are aware of the vulnerability of this region, and efforts to extract intrahepatic calculi may exceed the resistance of the ductal wall. Because the hepatic arteries are in proximity, there is a potential risk of intrahepatic hematoma due to arterial injury. The result can be profuse hemobilia, often through a T-tube.

Diagnostic liver puncture is a rapidly increasing source of hemobilia. Occult bleeding is reported to occur in 3%[36] to 10%[1] of patients. Macroscopic hemobilia is rare, especially if

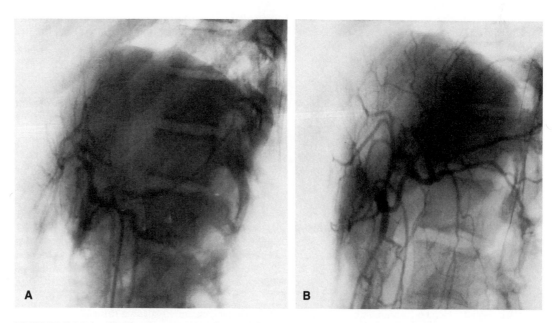

FIGURE 56-10 The healing process of a central liver hematoma treated conservatively was followed with serial angiograms. (**A**) The arteriogram shows the arteries separated, surrounding what was probably a hematoma. Because no further hemobilia occurred, no operation was performed. Repeated angiograms indicated progressive healing. (**B**) An angiogram 2 years later demonstrated the growth of new vessels.

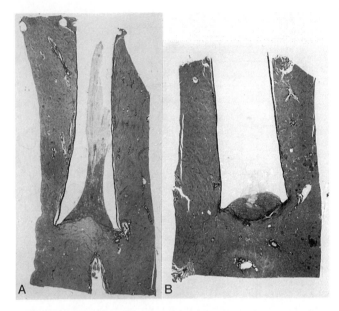

FIGURE 56-11 Three months after injury to the liver, there is a marked difference in healing between lesions open to the peritoneal cavity (**A**), where healing is normal, and lesions open to the gallbladder (**B**), where there is striking diminution of fibrinous exudate, granulation tissue, and fibrous scar. (Sandblum P, et al. The healing of liver wounds. Ann Surg 183:679, 1976)

fine-caliber needles are used, but there are still cases reported with exsanguinating hemobilia occurring as late as 6 to 10 days after biopsy.[15b]

Transhepatic cholangiography carries an even greater risk because of the close relation between bile ducts and blood vessels.[36] The difficulty of finding a bile duct, especially if of normal caliber, may require repeated puncture. The production of clots in this form of minor hemobilia often causes diagnostic problems; because abnormal findings are expected, the clot often is mistaken for stones and thus treated inadequately.

If the catheter used for cholangiography is left in place to drain the biliary tree (a procedure of questionable value because of the high complication rate), the risk of hemorrhage increases considerably.[20] In a series of 94 patients, hemobilia occurred in 13 patients; 6 patients had severe hemorrhage, and 1 patient died.[18]

Endobiliary prostheses are used with increasing frequency for temporary relief of obstructive jaundice due to malignancy. In one series of 300 patients, 9 developed profuse hemobilia related to a transhepatic biliary catheter; 8 of them were successfully treated with hepatic artery embolization, and the bleeding was ultimately fatal in 1 patient.[32]

Hemobilia caused by operations and liver punctures may cease spontaneously, but active intervention, usually obstruction of the damaged artery, often is necessary.

NEMATODES

Many cases of inflammatory hemobilia are caused by nematodes, particularly *Ascaris*, with most of them originating in China, Vietnam, or Korea. These organisms tend to invade the bile ducts, where they frequently produce bleeding lesions (Fig. 56-12). This so-called tropic hemobilia is said to be an everyday problem in surgical departments in Asia.[33]

GALLSTONE DISEASE

In gallstone disease, microscopic hemorrhage is frequent and can be proved in every third case. The bleeding occurs when the stones injure the mucosa, especially in connection with biliary colic. Macroscopic hemobilia is rare, with only 50 cases reported in the literature. It generally occurs when a large stone erodes the cystic artery or penetrates into an adjacent viscus.

TUMORS

As has been mentioned, tumors play an insignificant role as a source of bleeding in the biliary tract. This is especially striking when compared with the urinary tract, where tumors

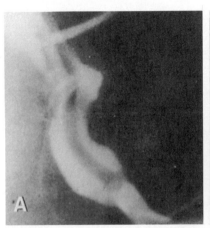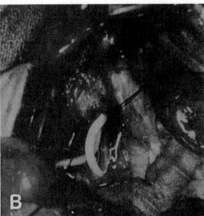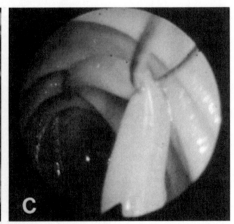

FIGURE 56-12 Hemobilia from an ascaris. (**A**) The T-tube cholangiogram visualizes a string-like filling defect. (Courtesy of J. Sawyer, Vanderbilt University) (**B**) Operative extraction of an ascaris through a choledochectomy. (Courtesy of G.B. Ong, University of Hong Kong) (**C**) Endoscopic extraction of an ascaris, protruding through the papilla. (Courtesy of R. Cavin, Lausanne, Switzerland)

constitute a major cause of hematuria. Tumors are as rare in the gallbladder as they are frequent in the urinary bladder.

The common tumors of the liver are not likely to bleed into the ducts. The hepatomas that cause hemobilia are of the more unusual kind that arise from the ductal epithelium. Benign hemangioma has been the source of bleeding in a few cases. Metastatic tumors in the liver hardly ever bleed (only two cases have been reported[12b]) but hemobilia has been described from metastases in such rare locations as the gallbladder wall.

VASCULAR DISEASE

Vascular disease, formerly a common cause, is now responsible for only 10% of cases of gross hemobilia. True aneurysms of the hepatic artery rupturing into the biliary tract are diminishing with the disappearance of the mycotic aneurysm, leaving only those of atherosclerotic origin or those associated with arteriopathy (eg, polyarteritis nodosa). When an aneurysm only leaks, it might give rise to inconspicuous hemobilia, but if it ruptures into the biliary tract, the symptoms generally are stormy, with exsanguinating hemorrhage and intense biliary colic (see Fig. 56-8). An arterial angiogram should then precede an emergency operation or embolization. When the aneurysm is surgically accessible, it might be resected and even replaced by a graft; most frequently, however, and especially if it is located within the liver, embolization is the intervention of choice.

Sometimes vascular lesions associated with arterial hypertension give rise to hemobilia. The structure usually affected is the gallbladder, and the disorder is then designated *apoplexy of the gallbladder* or *hemocholecyst*. In a few cases of portal hypertension, the general congestion in the mucosa of the digestive tract caused rupture of dilated veins, with profuse bleeding into the biliary tract.

COAGULOPATHY

Like hematuria and epistaxis, hemobilia may result from coagulopathy with or without minimal trauma[7] or from anticoagulant therapy. The increasing frequency of the latter probably will result in a number of cases of minor hemobilia with the formation of clots, imitating stones. Knowledge of this risk may prevent unnecessary surgery.[26]

Summary

Hemobilia has become a generally recognized syndrome. It is not as rare as was once thought. Surgical treatment is often necessary when the hemorrhage is substantial or repeated. When an adequate operation is performed with the aid of angiography, the mortality rate is below 20%. Minor hemobilia is frequent, and resulting clots have often been mistaken for gallstones and erroneously treated as such.

More than 200 years ago, Portal[21] complained that many physicians mistake hemorrhage through the biliary tract for bleeding from other sources and hence prescribe the wrong treatment. With increasing knowledge of the diagnosis and treatment of hemobilia, the number of misinterpreted or mistreated cases should diminish.

"The light which experience gives us," said Coleridge, "is a lantern on the stern which shines only on the waves behind us." With a syndrome as comparatively rare as hemobilia, experience, therefore, has to be replaced by knowledge: a lantern on the bow to enlighten us so that we can both recognize and treat the syndrome when we encounter it.

References

1. Adolph K. Gallungangs- und Pankreas-diagnostik. Stuttgart, Enke Verlag, 1968, p 153
2. Carr-Locke DL, Westwood CA. Endoscopy and endoscopic retrograde cholangiopancreatography finding in traumatic liver injury and hemobilia. Am J Gastroenterol 73:162, 1980
3. Clemens M, Wittrin G. Bilhämie and Hämobilie nach Reitunfall. Taglich Nordw Dtsch Chirurg Vortrag:116, 1975
4. Cox EF. Hemobilia following percutaneous needle biopsy of the liver. Arch Surg 95:198, 1967
5. Curet P, Baumer R, Roche A, et al. Hepatic hemobilia of traumatic or iatrogenic origin: recent advances in diagnosis and therapy, review of the literature from 1976–1981. World Surg 8:1, 1984
6. Czerniac A, et al. Hemobilia: a disease in evolution. Arch Surg 129:718, 1988
7. Elte P, et al. Hemobilia after liver biopsy. Early detection in a patient with mild hemophilia A. Arch Intern Med 140:839, 1980
8. Enge I, et al. Central rupture of the liver with traumatic haemobilia: a pre- and post-operative angiographic study. Br J Radiol 41:789, 1968
9. Glisson F. Anatomia hepatis. Amsterdam, 1654
10. Jackson JBS. Aneurysm of the hepatic artery bursting into the hepatic duct. Med Mag 3:115, 1834
11. Keller FS, et al. Percutaneous angiographic embolization: a procedure of increasing usefulness: review of a decade of experience. Am J Surg 149:5, 1981
12. Kelley CJ, Hemingway AP, McPherson GA, et al. Non-surgical management of post-cholecystectomy haemobilia. Br J Surg 70:502, 1983
12b. Kolok K, et al. Successful control of hemobilia secondary to metastatic liver cancer. Am J Gastroenteral 86:1642, 1991
13. Krudy AG, Doppman JL, Bissonette MB, et al. Hemobilia: computed tomographic diagnosis. Radiology 148:785, 1983
14. Lackgren G, et al. Hemobilia in childhood. J Pediatr Surg 29:105, 1988
15. Laffey PA. Ultrasound of hemobilia: a clinical and experimental study. JCU 16:167, 1988
15b. Lichtenstein DR, et al. Delayed massive hemobilia following percutaneous liver biopsy. Am J Gastroenteral 87:1832, 1992
16. Madding GF, Kennedy JA. Trauma to the liver. Philadelphia, WB Saunders, 1971
17. Mays ET. Lobar dearterialization for exsanguinating wounds of the liver. J Trauma 12:39, 1972
18. Monden M, et al. Hemobilia after percutaneous transhepatic biliary drainage. Arch Surg 115:161, 1980
18b. Morgagni S. Opera omnia. Liber III, epistle XXXVII. 1765, p 82
19. Naunyn B. Klinik der Cholelithiasis. Leipzig, 1882
20. Nilsson U, et al. Percutaneous transhepatic cholangiography and drainage: risks and complications. Acta Radiol 24:433, 1982
21. Portal A. Sur quelques maladies du foie. Hist Acad R 1777: 601, 1790
22. Quincke H. Ein Fall von Aneurysma der Leberarterie. Berl Clin Wochenschr 8:349, 1871
23. Sandblom P. Hemorrhage into the biliary tract following trauma: "traumatic hemobilia." Surgery 24:571, 1948

24. Sandblom P. Gastrointestinal hemorrhage through the pancreatic duct. Ann Surg 171:61, 1970
25. Sandblom P. Hemobilia. Springfield, IL, Charles C Thomas, 1972
26. Sandblom P. Stones or clots in the biliary tract. Acta Chir Scand 147:673, 1981
27. Sandblom P, Mirkovitch V. Minor hemobilia. Ann Surg 190:254, 1979
28. Sandblom P, Saegesser F, Mirkovitch V. Hepatic hemobilia: hemorrhage from the intrahepatic biliary tract—a review. World J Surg 8:41, 1984
29. Sandblom P, et al. The healing of liver wounds. Ann Surg 183:679, 1976
30. Sandblom P, et al. Formation and fate of fibrin clots in the biliary tract. Ann Surg 185:356, 1977
31. Sandblom P. Iatrogenic hemobilia. Am J Surg 151:754, 1986
32. Sarr MG, Kaufmann SL, Zuidema GD, et al. Management of hemobilia associated with transhepatic internal biliary drainage catheters. Surgery 95:603, 1984
33. Ton-Than-Tung. Les hémobilies tropicales. Chirurgie 98:43, 1972
34. Uflacker R, et al. Hemobilia: transcatheter occlusive therapy and long-term follow-up. Cardiovasc Intervent Radiol 12:136, 1989
35. Walter JF, Paaso BT, Cannon WB. Successful transcatheter embolic control of massive hematobilia secondary to liver biopsy. AJR 127:847, 1976
36. Wiechel KL. Percutaneous transhepatic cholangiography. Acta Chir Scand (Suppl) 330:35, 1964

Diseases of the Liver, Seventh Edition, edited by
Leon Schiff and Eugene R. Schiff. J.B. Lippincott Company, Philadelphia © 1993.

57

Granulomatous Liver Disease

D. Geraint James

There is no longer any part of the alimentary tract that cannot provide histologic biopsy material by an aspirating needle or peritoneoscopy with the guidance of computed tomography. This means that we are frequently confronted by granulomas in various organs. Aspiration liver biopsy is undertaken in the investigation of many systemic disorders or even fever of unknown origin. Because the hepatic granuloma often is featureless and nonspecific, there needs to be a clinico-pathologic synthesis of data by clinician, histologist, micro-biologist, and, occasionally, immunologist to provide a di-agnosis or prognosis or for the management of the disorder. The causes of hepatic granulomas (Table 57-1) should be viewed within the framework of a large family of granuloma-tous disorders.[13,21]

Pathogenesis

Granuloma formation is the end result of a complex interplay between invading antigen, prolonged antigenemia, macro-phage presentation, T4-helper response, B-cell overactivity, circulating immune complexes, and numerous biologic me-diators. Activated macrophages present antigen to CD4 T4 lymphocytes by way of interleukin 1, and in turn, the T cells cause interferon to increase the expression of major histo-compatibility class II molecules on the surface of macro-phages. Thereafter, a cascade of chemical mediators contrib-ute to granuloma formation and, ultimately, fibrosis[5,6,9] (Fig. 57-1).

Persistent and poorly degradeable antigens, chemicals, or other irritants provide the nidus for a spider's web granuloma. The center of the granuloma is composed of epithelioid and giant cells and CD4 helper cells. The periphery contains a large number of antigen-presenting interdigitating macro-phages associated with CD8 suppressor–cytotoxic lympho-cytes. This architectural arrangement of a well-organized granuloma is presumably efficient. It is noted in tuberculoid leprosy, in which few bacilli are found, contrasting with the haphazard, slovenly granuloma of lepromatous leprosy, in which bacilli are profuse.[10,12]

Granuloma formation gives rise to a damaged battlefield, and subsequent fibrosis represents a process of reparation.

Granulomas are infiltrated by fibroblasts, and increased deposition of intracellular reticulin is gradually replaced by formed, banded collagen. Thereafter, collagen is transformed into structureless eosinophilic hyaline material. This pro-gression is advanced by a chemical cascade of mediators (see Fig. 57-1).

Etiology

Sarcoidosis, tuberculosis, schistosomiasis, and liver disease are the most common causes, but about 10% of granulomas remain undiagnosed. A comparison of series investigated in London and New Haven is surprisingly similar[8] (Table 57-2).

INFECTIOUS CAUSES

There are numerous causes of hepatic granulomas, which may be due to infections, immunologic aberrations, enzyme defects, drugs and other chemicals, and neoplasia. The most frequent infections are tuberculosis, brucellosis, toxoplas-mosis, atypical mycobacteriosis, deep-seated fungal diseases, syphilis, leishmaniasis,[11] and the infestations schistosomiasis and toxocariasis.

Tuberculosis is still a frequent worldwide cause, and the incidence is increasing as a result of the acquired immuno-deficiency syndrome (AIDS). Acid-fast bacilli are only dem-onstrated in one tenth of patients. It is always suspected in the Asian, particularly if there is fever, sweating, respiratory symptoms, splenomegaly, and a strongly positive tuberculin skin test. Bacillus Calmette-Guérin vaccine gives rise to liver granulomas, a fact that should be remembered not only when it is used in the prophylaxis of tuberculosis but also in the treatment of bladder cancer.[7] Schistosomiasis caused by *Schistosoma mansoni* should not be overlooked in endemic areas. The ova are readily recognized in the center of the sarcoid granuloma and may also be found by rectal biopsy. Likewise, in other endemic areas, *histoplasmosis, blastomy-cosis,* and *coccidioidomycosis* may be responsible. Eosinophils may be a pointer to parasite granulomas. They were con-stantly noted in Saudi Arabia, together with dark brown Perls-negative pigment and angiomatoids in portal tracts.[15,16]

Q Fever

The hepatic granuloma in Q fever is surrounded by fibrin, producing a halo effect surrounding the necrosis. Sometimes it is described as a doughnut or fibrin-ring granuloma. Sim-ilar fibrin-ring granulomas are seen in boutonneuse fever caused by *Rickettsia conorii,*[4] visceral leishmaniasis, cyto-megalovirus infection, Hodgkin's disease, and allopurinol hy-persensitivity.[11,16,20]

Acquired Immunodeficiency Syndrome

The acquired immunodeficiency syndrome provides an impoverished terrain that allows many different organisms—bacteria, viruses, fungi—to flourish in addition to the caus-

1499

TABLE 57-1   *Causes of Hepatic Granulomas*

Infections	*Chemicals*
	Beryllium
Mycobacteria	Drugs
Tuberculosis	
Leprosy	*Immunologic Upset*
Atypical	Sarcoidosis
	Crohn's disease
Bacteria	Ulcerative colitis
Brucella	Primary biliary cirrhosis
Francisella tularense	Hypogammaglobulinemia
Yersinia	Systemic lupus erythematosus
Propioni	Immune complexes
Pseudomonas pseudomallei	Hepatic granulomatous
(melioidosis)	(granulomatous hepatitis)
Cat scratch disease	Whipple's disease
	AIDS
Spirochetes	
Treponema	*Enzyme Defect*
	Chronic granulomatous disease
Fungi	of children
Blastomyces	
Coccidioides	*Neoplasia*
Histoplasma	Reticulosis
Cryptococcus	Carcinoma
Protozoa	*Miscellaneous*
Leishmania	BCG vaccine
Toxoplasma	Cholestasis
	Polymyalgia rheumatica
Metazoa	
Schistosoma	*Drugs*
Rickettsia	
Q fever	
Boutonneuse fever	
Viruses	
Epstein-Barr virus	
Cytomegalovirus	
HIV	
Helminths	

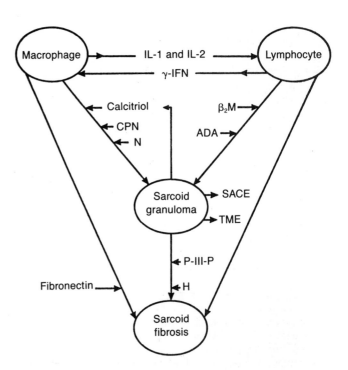

FIGURE 57-1 Chemical mediator interplay between macrophages, lymphocytes, and granuloma formation. IL-1, interleukin 1; IL-2, interleukin 2; γ-IFN, γ-interferon; CPN, carboxypeptidase; N, neopterin; β_2M, β_2-microglobulin; ADA, adenosine deaminase; SACE, serum angiotensin-converting enzyme; TME, metallopeptidase; P-III-P, type III procollagen; N, terminal peptide; H, hyaluronic acid.

ative virus. Granulomas are found in various organs, including the liver, often as a result of disseminated *Mycobacterium avium-intracellulare*, visualized by diatase–periodic acid–Schiff or the Ziehl-Neelsen stain. All aspiration liver biopsy samples should be subjected to special stains and culture. Hepatic granuloma formation is an optimistic sign and a ray of hope for the wretched victim. It indicates that impoverished defenses are at least attempting to fight the invasion of opportunistic infections to which he might otherwise succumb. Granulomas are not only caused by infections but also by drugs (including talc) or complicating lymphoma, both of which lead to granuloma formation in AIDS patients.

NONINFECTIOUS CAUSES

Sarcoidosis

Hepatic granulomas are found in two thirds of aspiration liver biopsies of sarcoidosis patients.[5,6,8,13] They are evident in portal tracts, often in well-defined clusters with multinucleated

giant cells that contain inclusions. There are associated inflammatory cells, including plasma cells and eosinophils. Central necrosis is less conspicuous than in tuberculosis, and the reticulin network is well preserved. Older lesions display dense hyalinized collagen, and the granuloma becomes converted into an acellular mass of hyaline material. Whereas pulmonary sarcoidosis may heal with troublesome complicating fibrosis, this is an extremely rare complication in the liver. The two complications, presinusoidal portal hypertension and cholestasis, are virtually restricted to black men aged 40 to 50 years with extensive fibrotic sarcoidosis in lungs and eyes (Table 57-3). Portal hypertension and intrahepatic cholestasis[3,14] are rare complications of hepatic sarcoidosis, occurring in only 1 of 300 patients with sarcoidosis in Europe.[1,5] It seems to be a more common problem in the United States. Liver disease in sarcoidosis has recently been reviewed in the Armed Forces Institute of Pathology, based on the liver biopsies of 100 patients referred since 1975.[3] The histologic features fell into four categories—cholestasis and necroinflammatory, vascular, and mass space-occupying lesions; granulomas were also universally noted. A portal-periportal distribution was most frequent. Chronic cholestasis was so frequent that it was recommended that sarcoidosis should be considered in the differential diagnosis of any cholestatic liver disease. This is a reflection of sarcoidosis in black Americans and would probably also hold true for sarcoidosis in the West Indies, but it is less frequently seen in sarcoidosis in Europe. Nonetheless, sarcoidosis should be considered in the differential diagnosis of nonsuppurative destructive cholangitis caused by primary biliary cirrhosis (PBC)

TABLE 57-2 *Comparison of Hepatic Granulomas Investigated at Yale and London*

	Yale*		London†	
Causes	Cases	Percentage	Cases	Percentage
Sarcoidosis	217		75	
Liver disease	174		41	
Tuberculosis	70	85	3	88
Schistosomiasis	19		1	
Undiagnosed	37	7	14	10
Positive Kveim test	109	69	95	72
TOTAL	565	100	138	100

*Data from Klatskin G. Hepatic granulomata: problems in interpretation. Ann NY Acad Sci 278:427, 1976.
†Data from Neville E, Pyasena KHG, James DG. Granulomas of the liver. Postgrad Med J 51:3651, 1975.

and the periductal fibrosis of primary sclerosing cholangitis. Hepatitis-like necroinflammatory lesions and vascular lesions such as sinusoidal dilatation or nodular regenerative hyperplasia were frequently observed. They used the term *hepatic sarcoidoma* for confluent granulomas forming space-occupying lesions.

Primary Biliary Cirrhosis
Primary biliary cirrhosis must always be considered as a close second to sarcoidosis as a cause of noninfective hepatic granulomas. The granulomatous battlefield between antigen and antibody often is adjacent to bile ducts. Whereas the granu-lomas in sarcoidosis are abundant and well formed with rare inconspicuous bile duct damage, the granulomas in PBC are few and poor and bile duct damage is extensive. The clinical picture usually is distinctive. The Kveim test and serum mitochondrial antibodies are helpful in distinguishing these two granulomatous disorders.[16-18]

Lymphoma
It is most important that hepatic granulomas caused by Hodgkin's disease are not confused with sarcoidosis because the consequences of managing the wrong disease may be catastrophic.

TABLE 57-3 *Comparison of Hepatic Granulomas Associated With Intrahepatic Cholestasis and Primary Biliary Cirrhosis*

Features	**Intrahepatic Cholestasis**	**Primary Biliary Cirrhosis**
Ethnic group	Black	White
Sex	Male	Female
Age (y)	20–50	40–50
Jaundice	+	+
Pruritus	+	+
Hepatomegaly	+	+
Splenomegaly	+	+
Clubbing	±	+
Keloids	+	−
Uveitis	+	−
Chest radiograph	Abnormal	Normal
Portal hypertension	+	+
Bilirubin	↑	↑
IgG	↑	−
IgM	−	↑
SACE	↑	±
Positive Kveim test	+	−
Mitochondrial antibodies	−	+
Granulomas	Abundant, well-formed	Few poor
Bile duct damage	Inconspicuous	Damaged
Duration (y)	20	10–20

Chronic Granulomatous Disease of Childhood

The killing of bacteria depends on a burst of respiratory enzyme activity, which leads to the production of hydrogen peroxide and superoxide in phagocytes. Neutrophils in chronic granulomatous disease of children are unable to kill some ingested bacteria because they are deficient in enzymes needed for this superoxide respiratory burst.

The classic X-linked disorder occurs in boys aged about 5 years, presenting with hepatosplenomegaly, generalized lymphadenopathy, weeping granulomatous skin lesions, and diffuse miliary lung infiltration. Neutrophil leukocytes from normal patients with bacterial infections reduce nitroblue tetrazolium from colorless to form blue-black formazan granules in the cytoplasm. This fails to occur in the leukocytes of children with chronic granulomatous disease or in the mothers of the X-linked variety.[5]

Crohn's Regional Enteritis

Sarcoid granulomas are found in the intestine, perineum, penis, and other paragenital areas and occasionally in the liver. The clinical picture usually is clearcut, and there are several differences between sarcoidosis and Crohn's regional enteritis.

Immune Complex Disease

Immune complexes are large molecular aggregates composed of antigen, antibody, and complement. They are constantly being formed in the circulation as a means of removing offending antigen. When antigen is in excess of antibodies immunoglobulin G and immunoglobulin M, the complex remains soluble and may persist in the circulation. When antibody is in excess, immune complexes tend to be insoluble and are rapidly removed by the reticuloendothelial system. Immune complex tissue injury includes vasculitis, hemorrhage, thrombosis, ischemic necrosis, and, sometimes, granuloma formation. Granulomas may also be found in liver and lymph nodes in patients with hypogammaglobulinemia and with selective immunoglobulin A deficiency.

Hepatic Granulomatous Disease

Hepatic granulomatous disease is also called granulomatous hepatitis—a misnomer because there is no hepatitis but just clusters of hepatic granulomas in the portal tracts that resemble sarcoidosis. This diagnosis is only contemplated when all other causes of hepatic granulomas have been excluded; in this sense, it may be regarded as an idiopathic ragbag. It has certain features that give it some character. The patient typically is a middle-aged man with recurrent fever, vague abdominal pain, and malaise. He has been extensively investigated, and the only abnormality is the presence of hepatic granulomas, pointing to sarcoidosis. All tests for sarcoidosis are negative. There are no symptoms or signs of liver disease, except for possible cholestasis and raised levels of alkaline phosphatase. Sooner or later, he is treated with steroids, which reduce the temperature to normal. Colchicine and prostaglandin inhibitors, such as indomethacin, are also effective in controlling the fever. We remain ignorant of its cause.[5,21]

Whipple's Disease

Whipple's disease is not a common disease, but it does cause widespread alimentary tract granulomas, including hepatic granulomas. It has been confused with both sarcoidosis and Crohn's regional enteritis.[2] The management is different, so it is important to recognize the differences. Think of Whipple's disease when the older patient has polyarthritis, steatorrhoea, and widespread alimentary tract granulomas. At first, the patient is suspected of having tuberculosis or a lymphoma, but in due course, its benign behavior suggests sarcoidosis. Intestinal biopsy with the appropriate staining is definitive.

Drugs

Not only the disorder injuring the liver but drugs indicated for the treatment of the disorder may cause hypersensitivity liver granulomas as well as considerable confusion in the

TABLE 57-4   *Drugs Causing Hepatic Granulomas*

Allopurinol	Oxyphenbutazone
Beryllium	Paraaminosalicylic acid
Carbamazepine	Perhexilene maleate
Chlorpromazine	Phenylbutazone
Chlorpropamide	Phenytoin
Clofibrate	Procainamide
Contraceptive steroids	Quinidine
Diazepam	Quinine
Diphenylhydantoin	Silicon
Halothane	Starch
Hydralazine	Sulfonamides
Hydrochlorothiazide	Sulfonylureas
Methyldopa	Talc
Nitrofurantoin	Tolbutamide

TABLE 57-5   *Investigative Routine for Liver Granulomas*

Investigation	For
Polarized light	Talc in drug abusers
Special stains	Tuberculosis
	Q fever
	Whipple's disease
	AIDS
Drug history	See Table 57-4
Chest radiograph	Tuberculosis
	Sarcoidosis
	Schistosomiasis
	Lymphoma
	Q fever
Skin tests	Tuberculosis
	Sarcoidosis
	Histoplasmosis
Serum antibodies	Brucella
	Treponema
	Protozoa
	Metazoa
	Rickettsia
	Viruses
Mitochondrial antibody	Primary biliary cirrhosis
Serum globulins	Hypogammaglobulinemia
Immune complexes	Immune complex disease

TABLE 57-6 *Management of Some Alimentary Tract Granulomas*

Cause	Site	Helpful Investigations (Other Than Histology)	Treatment
Sarcoidosis	All tissues except pancreas and adrenals	Chest radiograph Siltzbach-Kveim test Slit lamp of eyes Hypercalcemia Hypercalciuria Serum angiotensin-converting enzyme	Corticosteroids Chloroquine Methotrexate
Primary biliary cirrhosis	Liver, spleen, lymph nodes	Serum mitochondrial antibodies Cholesterol Alkaline phosphatase Liver, copper	Parenteral replacement of vitamins Calcium Ursodeoxycholic acid Cyclosporine
Tuberculosis	Liver, spleen, adrenals, intestine, peritoneum	Strongly positive tuberculin test Isolate organism	Isoniazid Rifampin Ethambutol Pyrazinamide Streptomycin
Hodgkin's disease	Liver, spleen, intestine, lymph nodes	Abdominal CT scan Lymphangiography Splenectomy	Quadruple chemotherapy Radiotherapy
Crohn's regional ileitis	Intestine, liver, perineum	Radiography	Corticosteroids Azathioprine Salazopyrine Metronidazole Cyclosporine
Brucellosis	Liver, spleen	Occupational exposure Skin test Serum antibodies	Tetracycline
Toxocara infestation	Liver, lungs, brain	Skin test Eosinophilia Examine fundi	Thiabendazole
Hepatic granulomatous disease	Liver, spleen		
Childhood		Nitroblue tetrazolum	Antibiotics Levamisole
Adult febrile		Exclusion of all else	Colchicine Indomethacin Prednisolone

practical management of the original disease. Many drugs are hepatotoxic, and several produce eosinophil-rich granulomas; drugs should always be suspected, even if they are not included in the current list (Table 57-4). Cholestasis and disturbances of the hepatocyte may be additional pointers.

Investigative Routine

The management of granulomatous diseases depends on their cause, so investigation must be thorough. Liver histology is supplemented whenever possible by histologic examination of other tissues, bacteriology of part of the submitted specimen, and radiology. The routine includes a drug history, geographic origins, chest radiograph, slit lamp examination of the eyes, skin tests, and serum antibodies. It may be nec-essary to perform computed tomographic scanning and gallium uptake (Tables 57-5 and 57-6).

References

1. Bass NM, Burroughs AK, Scheuer PJ, James DG, Sherlock S. Chronic intrahepatic cholestasis due to sarcoidosis. Gut 23: 417, 1982
2. Cho C, Linscheer WG, Hirschkorn MA, Ashutosh K. Sarcoid like granulomas as an early manifestation of Whipple's disease. Gastroenterology 87:941, 1984
3. Epstein MS, Devaney KO, Goodman ZD, Zimmerman HJ, Ishak KG. Liver disease in sarcoidosis. Hepatology 12:839A, 1990
4. Guardia J, Martinez-Vazquez, Moragas A, Rey C, Vilaseca J, Tornos J, Beltran M, Bacardia R. The liver in boutonneuse fever. Gut 15:549, 1974

5. James DG, Jones Williams W. Sarcoidosis and other granulomatous disorders. Philadelphia, WB Saunders, 1985

6. James DG, Studdy PR. A color atlas of respiratory diseases. St. Louis, CV Mosby, 1992

7. Kesten S, Title L, Mullen B, Grossman R. Pulmonary disease following intravesical BCG treatment. Thorax 45:709, 1990

8. Klatskin G. Hepatic granulomata: problems in interpretation. Ann NY Acad Sci 278:427, 1976

9. Mishra BB, Poulter LW, Janossy G, James DG. The distribution of lymphoid and macrophage-like cell subsets of sarcoid and Kveim granulomata; possible mechanism of negative PPD reaction in sarcoidosis. Clin Exp Immunol 54:705, 1983

10. Modlin RL, Hofman FM, Meyer PR, Sharma OP, Taylor CR, Rea TH. In situ demonstration of T lymphocyte subsets in granulomatous inflammations: leprosy, rhinoscleroma and sarcoidosis. Clin Exp Immunol 51:430, 1983

11. Moreno A, Marazuela M, Yebra M, Hernandez MJ, Hellin T, Montalban C, Vargas JA. Hepatic fibrin-ring granulomas in visceral leishmaniasis. Gastroenterology 95:1123, 1988

12. Naryanan RB, Bhutani LK, Sharma AK, Nath I. T cell subsets in leprosy lesions: in situ characterisation using monoclonal antibodies. Clin Exp Immunol 51:421, 1983

13. Neville E, Pyasena KHG, James DG. Granulomas of the liver. Postgrad Med J 51:361, 1975

14. Rudzki C, Ishak KG, Zimmerman HJ. Chronic intrahepatic cholestasis due to sarcoidosis. Am J Med 59:373, 1975

15. Satti MB, Al-Freihi H, Ibrahim EM, et al. Hepatic granulomas in Saudi Arabia: a clinicopathological study of 59 cases. Am J Gastroenterol 85:669, 1990

16. Scheuer PJ. Liver biopsy interpretation, ed 4. London, Bailliere Tindal, 1988

17. Sherlock S, Dooley J. Diseases of the liver and biliary system, ed 9. Oxford, UK, Blackwell Scientific Publications, 1992

18. Stanley NN, Fox RA, Whimster WF, Sherlock S, James DG. Primary biliary cirrhosis or sarcoidosis or both. N Engl J Med 287:1282, 1972

19. Valla D, Pessegueiro-Miranda H, Degott C, Lebrec D, Rueff B, Benhamon J-P. Hepatic sarcoidosis with portal hypertension: a report of seven cases with a review of the literature. Q J Med 242:531, 1987

20. Vanderstigel M, Zafrani ES, Lejonc JL, Schaeffer F, Portos JL. Allopurinol hypersensitivity syndrome as a cause of hepatic fibrin-ring granulomas. Gastroenterology 90:188, 1986

21. Vella M, James DG. Alimentary tract granulomas. Sarcoidosis 2:142, 1985

Diseases of the Liver, Seventh Edition, edited by
Leon Schiff and Eugene R. Schiff. J.B. Lippincott Company, Philadelphia © 1993.

58

Total Parenteral Nutrition and the Liver

Samuel Klein

The technique of total parenteral nutrition (TPN), first introduced in the late 1960s,[29,30,145] has proved to be one of the major advances in medical care in this century. Although the use of TPN may cause infection, catheter-related problems, and metabolic abnormalities, improvements in insertion techniques, catheter materials, use of nutrient formulas, and patient care have decreased the incidence of complications. Hepatic abnormalities associated with TPN, however, still occur frequently and involve both pediatric and adult patients. The first suggestion of TPN-associated liver disease was reported in 1971 by Peden and colleagues,[102] who described a case of cholestatic jaundice, bile duct proliferation, and cirrhosis in a premature infant who had received TPN for 71 days. Subsequent studies have shown that cholestasis is the most frequent hepatic complication in TPN-fed infants and correlates directly with decreased gestational age, decreased birth weight, and increased duration of TPN therapy.[11,104] Hepatic abnormalities in infants usually are more severe than those in adults. Liver disease associated with TPN in children has been the subject of several detailed reviews[9,87,144] and will not be discussed here.

In adults, the relationship between TPN and liver disease has been evaluated in more than 1700 patients who have been described in more than 40 different publications.[1,8,13,16,23,34,35,38,65,117,120,146] Few studies, however, have been performed in a prospective, randomized, controlled fashion. Four prospective studies compared patients receiving different types of TPN formulations,[32,85,118,138] one evaluated the use of concomitant antibiotics,[21] and only two compared patients receiving parenteral nutrition with those receiving enteral nutrition.[1,92] The paucity of prospective, randomized trials raises concern that liver abnormalities found in TPN-fed patients could have been caused by factors unrelated to the use of TPN itself. Patients who require TPN often have such illnesses as inflammatory bowel disease, sepsis, or cancer, which can cause liver abnormalities. Many patients may have received hepatotoxic drug therapy or blood transfusions. Most studies did not exclude or document these potentially confounding variables in their patient populations. Interpretation of the available literature also is complicated because patient heterogeneity, differences in nutritional formulas, and differences in presentation of the study data make comparisons between studies difficult. The timing of obtaining liver function tests (LFTs), the specific tests reported, and the criteria used to define increased values differed among studies. Evaluation of histologic abnormalities associated with TPN is limited because liver biopsies were obtained in only a small percentage of patients. Therefore, it is difficult to establish firmly a cause-and-effect relationship between the use of TPN and many of the reported liver abnormalities.

Several hepatic complications have been associated with the use of TPN in adults (Table 58-1). These abnormalities usually are benign and transient. A small subset of patients with more serious and progressive liver disease, however, have been reported. Most complications occur early, within a month of starting TPN therapy. Fewer, but often more severe complications, occur late, usually after 4 months of TPN therapy. The complications can be divided into biochemical and histologic abnormalities (see Table 58-1), although both may occur in any given patient. This chapter will review the relationship between TPN and liver disease in adult humans and discuss the potential factors involved in the pathogenesis of these abnormalities (Table 58-2).

Biochemical Abnormalities

Biochemical abnormalities associated with liver disease have been observed often in patients receiving TPN (Table 58-3). The most commonly measured of these LFTs include those that are markers of hepatocellular disease, aspartate aminotransferase (AST) and alanine aminotransferase (ALT), and those that are markers of cholestasis, serum alkaline phosphatase, and bilirubin. Most studies did not evaluate γ-glutamyl transpeptidase (GGT), but a limited number of reports suggest that it often may be affected in patients receiving TPN.[1,26,32,95] LFT results themselves, however, do not necessarily reflect true liver function,[84] and abnormal findings may indicate liver injury without any deterioration in liver function. Functional tests of liver status, such as the hepatic clearance tests or hepatic protein synthetic ability, rarely are reported in studies of patients receiving TPN. It also is difficult to determine the relationship between LFT result abnormalities and liver morphology because liver biopsies have been obtained infrequently.

A true cause-and-effect relation between TPN and abnormal LFT results has not been proved. The only two prospective, randomized, controlled trials report different results.[1,92] In the first study,[92] 15 heterogeneous postoperative patients were randomized to receive either TPN or enteral feeding by needle catheter jejunostomy for 7 to 10 days. Mean serum transaminase levels increased slightly in both groups, alkaline phosphatase increased in the enterally fed group and decreased in the TPN group, and GGT increased in both groups. Statistical comparisons were not made, but it is unlikely that statistically significant differences were present be-

TABLE 58-1   *Hepatic Abnormalities in Adult Patients Receiving Total Parenteral Nutrition*

Biochemical Abnormalities

Histologic Abnormalities
Steatosis
Lipidosis and phospholipidosis
Cholestasis
 Intrahepatic
 Extrahepatic
Severe liver disease
 Steatohepatitis
 Fibrosis
 Cirrhosis

tween groups because of the small number of patients and the variability in the measured values. In the second study,[1] 29 patients with inflammatory bowel disease were randomized to receive TPN or enteral feeding for 2 to 3 weeks. The percentage of patients who had at least one abnormal LFT value was much greater in those who received TPN (62%) than in those who received enteral feeding (6%). GGT was most frequently elevated, being abnormal in 46% of the patients receiving TPN but in none of the enterally fed patients. If this liver enzyme was not measured, there would have been no statistically significant differences in LFT values between the two groups.

Different patterns of LFT value abnormalities have been observed in adult patients receiving TPN (see Table 58-3). Increased levels of transaminases are most common, usually

TABLE 58-2   *Potential Factors Involved in the Pathogenesis of Hepatic Complications in Adult Patients Receiving Total Parenteral Nutrition (TPN)*

Clinical Factors
Primary illness
Preexisting liver disease
Hepatotoxic medical therapy
Blood transfusions

TPN Administration
Excessive glucose calories
Excessive lipid infusion
Amino acid degradation products
Aluminum toxicity

Nutritional Deficiencies
Essential fatty acid deficiency
Carnitine deficiency
Inadequate glutamine administration

Gut Factors
Translocation of intestinal bacteria or endotoxin
Bacterial overgrowth
Bacterial metabolism of bile acids

Biliary Tract Disease
Gallbladder stasis, sludge, and stones

occurring between 1 and 2 weeks after starting TPN and often normalizing without the stopping or changing of the TPN infusion.[12,42,49,74] Increases in plasma alkaline phosphatase and bilirubin occur less often and later, after 2 to 3 weeks of TPN.[121,143]

The caloric content and composition of the TPN formula seems to be related to the frequency of finding abnormal LFT results. High-calorie infusions of glucose-based TPN are associated with a greater incidence of abnormal LFT results[72,74] than are lower-calorie infusions that provide a portion of calories as fat.[22,26,85] In most studies reported before 1980, glucose-based TPN was infused at high rates, providing 3 to 4 L of solution daily. Lipid emulsions were used either sparingly or not at all.

The first report of an association between liver disease and TPN in adults was described in 1972 in patients receiving glucose-based TPN.[49] In 6 of 19 patients (32%) with normal baseline values, LFT abnormalities developed between the 5th and 10th days of TPN therapy. All 6 of the patients had a 3-fold increase in AST, 4 had a 2-fold increase in alkaline phosphatase, and 3 had a 20-fold increase in ALT levels. The LFT abnormalities resolved despite continued TPN. In later studies, LFT abnormalities were found in 68% to 93% of patients receiving glucose-based TPN for more than 7 days. The largest and most frequent increase in LFT values usually was seen in serum transaminases. Sheldon and colleagues,[121] however, described increases in alkaline phosphatase and bilirubin in 26 patients receiving glucose-based TPN for 2 to 91 days. One possible explanation for this different experience may be related to differences in underlying disease in the patient populations. Many patients Sheldon and associates[121] studied had clinical complications that could cause cholestasis and were severely ill, as manifested by a 73% mortality rate.

Most studies reported in the 1980s provided a portion of the infused calories as a lipid emulsion. In some studies, a lipid-based formula was compared with glucose-based TPN.[2,26,118,138,143] In general, the frequency and magnitude of LFT abnormalities were less in patients receiving at least 20% of their nonprotein calories in the form of lipids than in those receiving a glucose-based formula. Tulikoura and Huikuri[138] found that LFT results did not change at all in patients receiving TPN with 55% of nonprotein calories as lipid, but mean transaminase levels increased after 8 to 10 days of TPN in patients receiving an equicaloric solution with all nonprotein calories as glucose. Meguid and colleagues[85] studied 88 patients in a prospective, randomized fashion in which glucose-based TPN was given to one group and one third of the glucose calories were replaced by a fat emulsion in the other. Mean AST and ALT levels increased 2.5-fold and 5-fold, respectively, after 7 to 14 days in the glucose group. Mean AST levels did not change and mean ALT levels increased only 2.5-fold in the lipid group. In a retrospective analysis of 40 patients, Wagner and associates[143] found that the incidence of LFT abnormalities in 25 patients who received 70% of their nonprotein calories as lipid was about half that of 15 patients who received all of their nonprotein calories as glucose.

In contrast to most of the reported studies, some have found that high-lipid infusions were associated with cholestasis. In a series of three studies involving a total of 19 patients, Allardyce and coworkers[2,3,118] reported that serum alkaline phosphatase and bilirubin values increased in 50% to 75% of patients receiving lipid-based TPN, in which 60% to 70% of

TABLE 58-3   *Studies Evaluating Biochemical Tests in Adult Patients Receiving Total Parenteral Nutrition (TPN)*

First Author, Year	Patients	Approximate TPN Formula			Patients With Biochemical Alterations (%)	Specific Biochemical Changes	Approximate Onset of Change (Days on TPN)
		Protein (g/kg/d)	Glucose*	Lipid*			
Host, 1972[49]	19	1.3	100	0	32	AST, ALT	5–10
					21	AP	5–10
Jeejeebhoy, 1976[54]	12	1	15	85	50	AST	10–43
					25	AP	10–43
Jeejeebhoy, 1976[55]	12	1.1	65	35	42	AST, AP	>120
Grant, 1977[42]	100	NR	100	0	93	AST	3–10
					89	ALT	3–10
					26	B	8
					16	AP	32
Sheldon, 1978[121]	26	NR	100	0	100[†]	AP, B	10–30
Allardyce, 1978[3]	32	2	40	60	75	AP, AST	10–40
					60	B	20–63
Lindor, 1979[72]	48	NR	100	0	68	AST	9–12
					54	AP	9–12
					21	B	9–12
MacFayden, 1979[76]	42	NR	100	0	NR	AST	7–14
					NR	AP	28
					NR	B	35
Lowry, 1979[74]	40	1.4	100	0	83	AST, ALT, AP	14
Salvian, 1980[118]	32	NR	30	70	NR	AP, B	20–25
		NR	90	10	0		
Greenlaw, 1980[45]	23	NR	100	0	9	AST, ALT, AP	6–8
Carpentier, 1981[22]	36	1.4	50	50	14	AP	11–19
					11	AST	11–26
Fouin-Fortunet, 1981[36]	17	1.6	60	40	65	AST, ALT, AP	>7
Allardyce, 1982[2]	35	1.2	30	70	56	AP, B	>20
		1.2	70	30	6	AP, B	NR
Fouin-Fortunet, 1982[37]	15	1.7	60	40	47	AP	21
					33	AST, ALT	14
Messing, 1982[90]	27	1.6	50	50	74	ALT	>14
					63	AP	>14
					26	B	>14
Wagman, 1982[142]	143	1.8	>80	<20	NR	AST, ALT	7
					NR	AP	14
Toulikoura, 1982[138]	28	1.1	100	0	NR	AST, ALT	8–10
		1.1	45	55	0		
		3.1	100	0	NR	AST, ALT, AP	NR
Pallares, 1983[100]	27	1.6	50	50	NR	ALT, AP, B, GGT	14
Wagner, 1983[143]	40	NR	100	0	87	AST, ALT	11–13
					64	AP	14
					33	B	18
		NR	30	70	60	AST	12
					36	ALT	14
					33	AP	15
					13	B	18
Capron, 1983[21]	16	NR	NR	NR	NR	ALT, AP, B	30
Nanji, 1984[94]	59	NR	60	40	53	AST	5–10
Meguid, 1984[85]	88	1.9	100	0	NR	AST, ALT	7
		1.9	70	30	NR	AST, ALT	7
Nanji, 1985[95]	59	NR	90	10	71	GGT	7–48
					51	AP	7–48
Bengoa, 1985[12]	92	1.2	75	25	25	AST, ALT, AP, B	7–14
Bowyer, 1985[18]	60	1–2	75–90	10–25	15	AST, AP, B	>120
Muggia-Sullam, 1985[92]	8	NR	NR	NR	NR	AST, ALT, GGT	7–10

(continued)

TABLE 58-3 *(continued)*

First Author, Year	Patients	Approximate TPN Formula			Patients With Biochemical Alterations (%)	Specific Biochemical Changes	Approximate Onset of Change (Days on TPN)
		Protein (g/kg/d)	Glucose*	Lipid*			
Robertson, 1986[113]	26	NR	65	35	89	AST, ALT, AP, GGT	7–21
Stanko, 1987[130]	18	1	75	25	22	AST, ALT, AP, B	>30
Fabri, 1987[32]	20	NR	90	10	NR	GGT	7
DeGott, 1988[26]	9	1.5	90	10	80	AP, GGT	>120
					60	AST, ALT	>120
		1.5	70	30	25	ALT, GGT	75–150
Abad-Lacruz, 1990[1]	13	2.3	60	40	46	GGT	16–18
					23	B	16–18
					15	ALT, AP	16–18
					8	AST	16–18
Tayek, 1990[135]	25	1.5	80	20	56	GGT	7
					36	AP	7
					32	AST	7
					12	B	7
Berner, 1990[13]	16	1–1.3	80	20	81	AP	>120
					53	AST	>120
					6	B	>120
Clarke, 1991[23]	420	NR	50	50	32	AP	28
					31	B	28
					27	AST	28

NR, not reported; AST, aspartate aminotransferase; ALT, alanine aminotransferase; AP, alkaline phosphatase; B, bilirubin; GGT, γ-glutamyl transpeptidase.
*Percentage of nonprotein calories.
†Only patients with abnormal liver function test results were reported.

nonprotein calories were provided as lipid (3 g/kg/d). Patients randomized to receive glucose-based TPN, in which 10% to 30% of nonprotein calories were provided as lipid, rarely had abnormal LFT values. The highest rate of lipid infusion was reported by Jeejeebhoy and colleagues,[54] who gave patients 83% of nonprotein calories as lipid (3.5 g/kg/d). Bilirubin concentrations did not increase and alkaline phosphatase levels increased in only 25% of patients. The reason for the differences in these studies is not clear but could be related to the longer duration of TPN therapy in the patients studied by Allardyce and coworkers[2,3,118] or to differences in patient population between studies.

Little information is available on LFT results in patients receiving long-term (more than 4 months) TPN. In the earliest series, Jeejeebhoy and colleagues[55] reported their experience with 12 patients who had received TPN for 4 to 60 months. Five patients (42%) had slightly high AST and alkaline phosphatase levels. Bowyer and colleagues[18] found that 51 of 60 (85%) patients receiving TPN for 4 to 122 months had either no abnormalities or mild and transient elevations of AST, alkaline phosphatase, or bilirubin. Nine (15%) patients had more severe and persistent elevations in AST, alkaline phosphatase, or bilirubin levels for 8 to 95 months. Berner and associates[13] found that many of their patients who had received home TPN for 12 to 157 months and who did not have known liver disease had abnormal LFT results. Thirteen of 16 (81%) had increased levels of alkaline phosphatase; 9 of 16 (56%), AST; and 1 of 16 (6%), bilirubin. In most patients, however, LFT abnormalities were mild.

Histologic Abnormalities

Several morphologic abnormalities have been observed in liver biopsy specimens taken from patients receiving TPN. Although biopsy results from more than 200 patients have been reported, this represents less than 15% of the total number of patients in whom LFT results were measured. Because liver biopsies were performed in only a small percentage of patients, the precise relation between histologic liver findings and LFT values is not known. Results obtained from a small subset of patients, however, suggest that liver structure is usually normal when LFT values are normal. Biopsies performed in 24 patients with normal LFT values[26,36,42,49,138] showed that liver structure was normal in 21 patients,[36,42,49,138] but phospholipidosis, steatosis, portal fibrosis, or cholestasis were found in the other 3 patients.[26] In most studies, liver biopsies were performed when LFT levels were elevated, and histologic examination always showed some abnormality. These abnormalities can be divided into four categories: steatosis, lipidosis and phospholipidosis, cholestasis, and severe liver disease with steatohepatitis, fibrosis, or cirrhosis. One or more of these abnormalities can coexist in any patient.

The importance of TPN in the genesis of histologic abnormalities has been questioned.[53,146] In a retrospective analysis of 93 patients receiving TPN and 35 control subjects not receiving TPN, Wolfe and coworkers[146] found that histologic abnormalities in liver correlated with clinical factors, such as preexisting liver disease, abdominal sepsis, renal failure, and blood transfusion, but not with the administration of TPN. The results of other clinical studies and experimental data suggest that steatosis and lipidosis may be caused by TPN, but the relationship between TPN and other liver lesions is less clear.

STEATOSIS

Steatosis is the histologic abnormality most frequently associated with administration of TPN. The increase in hepatic fat usually is macrovesicular, but microvesicular changes have also been described.[17] The composition of the fat consists almost entirely of triglyceride.[57] Most commonly, fatty infiltration involves the periportal areas,[42,49] but it also has been found more centrally[18,138] and throughout the liver lobule.[26,72] The presence of even extensive steatosis does not predict further liver disease, and complete resolution to normal has been reported.[79]

Steatosis is caused by an imbalance between the rate of triglyceride synthesis and the rate of triglyceride breakdown or very low density lipoprotein secretion. In patients receiving TPN, the development of fatty infiltration may be related to administration of excessive glucose calories. Steatosis often is the major liver abnormality in patients receiving all of their nonprotein calories as glucose,[42,49,72,118,38] and is less predominant or absent when a portion of nonprotein calories is supplied as lipid.[2,3,12,118,138] In a dramatic prospective study, liver biopsy specimens were obtained in 28 surgical patients before and after 11 to 13 days of either glucose- or lipid-based TPN.[138] The amount of total calories infused was similar in both groups. Hepatic fat content increased significantly in the group receiving glucose-based TPN but did not change in the group receiving lipid-based TPN.

Experimental studies in humans and animals have clarified the role of glucose infusion on the genesis of steatosis. At relatively low rates of glucose infusion, less than half of infused glucose is oxidized in humans.[147] When the rate of glucose infusion is increased to more than 5 mg/kg/min (about 2000 kcal/d for a patient weighing 70 kg), the percentage of infused glucose oxidized further decreases. Certainly, part of the infused glucose that is not oxidized is stored in the liver as fat. Increases in total body fat have been observed when glucose infusion exceeds 7 mg/kg/min in patients with gastrointestinal disease.[77] Inadequate protein intake may further increase hepatic lipid content during hypercaloric glucose-based TPN infusions.[59] Providing a portion of TPN calories as lipid has been shown to attenuate the TPN-related increase in hepatic fat in rats,[20,131] and isocaloric exchange of lipid for part of glucose calories has reversed fatty liver in patients receiving long-term TPN.[55,83] Cycling glucose calories, by stopping the infusion of glucose for 8 to 10 hours each day, enhances the mobilization of stored triglycerides and may reverse steatosis.[79] The specific mechanism responsible for glucose-induced steatosis has been studied in rats. Glucose-based TPN both decreases hepatic triglyceride secretion,[46,59] and enhances fat synthesis by increasing the ratio of insulin to glucagon in the portal vein[69,70] and stimulating hepatic acetyl coenzyme A carboxylase (the regulatory enzyme for fatty acid synthesis) activity.[46,57]

Other factors related to the use of TPN may cause steatosis, including hepatotoxic components of TPN such as tryptophan degradation products, and the absence of specific nutrients in TPN, such as essential fatty acids, carnitine, choline, or glutamine. These factors, however, probably are of little importance in the pathogenesis of steatosis in most patients.

Degradation products of tryptophan and possibly other amino acids, produced when TPN is exposed to light, have been found to cause periportal fatty change in rats.[14,42] The quantity of tryptophan degradation products present in standard TPN and its contribution to liver disease are unknown.

Essential fatty acid deficiency can limit the secretion of hepatic lipoproteins, thereby causing accumulation of fat in the liver. Deficiency in essential fatty acids can occur within weeks in patients receiving continuous infusion of lipid-free TPN formulas because of both the absence of infused essential fatty acids and the inhibition of essential fatty acid release from stored fat.[10,66,111] The proportion of patients receiving TPN who have steatosis caused by essential fatty acid deficiency is not known. Although fatty liver has been normalized in patients after they have received intravenous lipids,[55,56,83,110] it is not known whether this effect was caused by the provision of essential fatty acids present in the lipid emulsion, a decrease in glucose calories, or some other factor.

Carnitine, a quarternary amine, is essential for oxidation of long-chain fatty acids.[134] Although carnitine can be synthesized from amino acids present in TPN (lysine and methionine), carnitine itself is not a component of TPN formulas. Low carnitine levels in blood and liver have been found in patients receiving long-term TPN.[17,101,148] The observation that primary carnitine deficiency causes hepatic steatosis[58] led to the hypothesis that carnitine deficiency may contribute to steatosis in TPN-fed patients. Although some case reports have found that LFT results improved after carnitine administration in carnitine-deficient patients receiving home TPN,[101] normalizing blood and hepatic carnitine with carnitine supplementation for 1 month has not been shown to change hepatic fat content.[19]

Choline deficiency has been documented to cause fatty liver in rats.[73,125] Choline is necessary for hepatic lipoprotein production and thus is important for triglyceride packaging and secretion from the liver.[75] In theory, TPN-induced stimulation of hepatic triglyceride synthesis in malnourished patients who have depleted choline stores could cause fatty liver. Although both oral and intravenous choline have been found to prevent fat accumulation in rats receiving high-calorie, glucose-based TPN,[57] the possibility that choline deficiency causes steatosis in parenterally fed humans has not been evaluated carefully.

Inadequate glutamine administration has been proposed as a cause of fatty liver. Standard, commercially available amino acid solutions used in TPN do not contain glutamine because of its potential instability. Studies in rats by Grant and Snyder[44] found that infusion of glutamine-supplemented TPN decreased fatty infiltration of the liver. A subsequent study by these researchers,[43] however, found that differences in amino acid formulation, not the absence or presence of glutamine, were associated with the development of steatosis.

Patients who require TPN may be at increased risk for steatosis and other liver abnormalities because of translocation of intestinal bacteria or endotoxin across the gut wall into the portal circulation. Studies in parenterally fed animals suggest that the absence of both enteral nutrients and intravenous glutamine causes intestinal atrophy and decreased mucosal defense.[5,68,98] The diminution in gut barrier purportedly leads to the translocation of hepatotoxic bacteria or endotoxins.[96,137] Data from animal studies support the potential importance of the intestine in causing liver dysfunction.

Liver triglycerides increase rapidly after endotoxin injection in rabbits.[47] Freund and associates[40] found that antibiotic therapy (and presumed decrease in gut flora) decreased TPN-induced steatosis in rats. Others have demonstrated that experimentally induced small bowel overgrowth in rats caused bacterial translocation and hepatic injury.[71] Abnormalities in LFT values and liver structure were prevented or resolved with antibiotic therapy. Although bacteria translocation has been documented in humans with gastrointestinal diseases,[6,25,141] its relationship to the development of fatty liver and other liver abnormalities is not known.

Clinical factors that affect hepatic triglyceride synthesis and secretion may be important contributors to fat accumulation in patients receiving TPN (see Chap. 31). Starvation, malnutrition, inflammatory bowel disease, diabetes, and sepsis often cause fatty liver and are common diagnoses in patients who require TPN. For example, mean hepatic lipid content in patients with chronic infection who were receiving TPN was found to be more than double that found in noninfected patients receiving TPN.[57]

LIPIDOSIS AND PHOSPHOLIPIDOSIS

Administering large amounts of commercially prepared lipid emulsions can cause hepatic lipid accumulation, known as lipidosis. The distribution of hepatic fat in lipidosis differs from that of typical steatosis and occurs when infused lipid accumulates in hepatic lysosomes and Kupffer cells.[15,39,81,91,136]

Phospholipidosis was first observed in patients receiving TPN in 1988.[26] This liver abnormality is characterized by the presence of cytoplasmic phospholipid deposits and large multilamellar lysosomes in hepatocytes. In more severe cases, abnormal lysosomes also are found in Kupffer cells and portal macrophages. Degott and colleagues[26] found phospholipidosis in eight of nine patients who had been receiving home TPN that contained 5% to 35% nonprotein calories as lipid. The severity of the abnormality was directly proportional to the duration of TPN. It is presumed that phospholipidosis is caused by accumulation of phospholipids provided by the intravenous infusion of lipid emulsions. Typically, phospholipid accumulation occurs only in patients who have inherited lysosomal storage disease or who have been exposed to certain drugs. Because the diagnosis of phospholipidosis requires histochemical staining and ultrastructural evaluation not routinely performed on liver biopsy specimens, the prevalence of this abnormality may be underestimated in patients receiving TPN. Earlier reports of lipidosis may, in fact, have included patients with unrecognized phospholipidosis.

CHOLESTASIS

Cholestasis is the predominant liver abnormality reported after 2 to 3 weeks of TPN therapy.[2,3,118,121] The diagnosis usually is based on blood tests because histologic evaluation of the liver has been obtained infrequently. Usually, LFT results return to normal with discontinuation of TPN.[3,22,85,138] Biopsies, when performed, demonstrate a mixed (granulocytic and lymphocytic) portal and periportal inflammatory infiltrate, periportal canalicular bile plugs, and bile duct proliferation.[2,3,49,72,118,121] The highest incidence of cholestasis was reported by Allardyce and coworkers,[3] who found an increase in alkaline phosphatase in 75% and an increase in bilirubin

in 60% of their patients after a mean of 19 and 30 days of TPN therapy, respectively. Unfortunately, in most studies, diagnostic evaluations to exclude either the presence of extrahepatic obstruction or nonliver sources of alkaline phosphatase and bilirubin were not performed. Therefore, the true incidence of intrahepatic cholestasis is impossible to determine, particularly because patients receiving TPN are at high risk for developing biliary tract disease,[27,88,90,106,107] which can cause extrahepatic obstruction, and metabolic bone disease,[64,99,123] which can cause increased alkaline phosphatase.

Many factors may be involved in the pathogenesis of intrahepatic and extrahepatic cholestasis in patients receiving TPN. These factors can be divided into those related to the patient's clinical condition and those directly related to the use of TPN itself. Because many patients who require TPN are seriously ill or have gastrointestinal disease, or both, the incidence of cholestasis may have been influenced by factors other than the use of TPN itself. These clinical factors could explain differences in the frequency of cholestasis observed between studies.

The most important clinical factors involved in cholestasis are those associated with bacteria or endotoxin, such as systemic and abdominal infections, translocation of intestinal bacteria or endotoxins into portal blood, and intestinal bacterial metabolism of bile salts. Bacterial infection is a known cause of cholestasis[149] and may increase the frequency of cholestasis in TPN-fed patients. The incidence of hyperbilirubinemia in septic patients receiving TPN has been reported to be two- to three-fold greater than that in nonseptic patients.[113,127] Portal endotoxemia alone can cause cholestasis in the absence of systemic infection.[139] The translocation of intestinal endotoxins into the portal system can occur when the mucosal barrier is disrupted or is overwhelmed by bacterial overgrowth. The potential importance of intestinal bacteria in the pathogenesis of cholestasis is supported by studies that showed that antibiotic therapy with metronidazole in patients receiving long-term TPN both prevented cholestasis[21] and returned elevated LFT values to normal.[31] Latham and colleagues[67] found that a specific factor in serum, presumably endotoxin, from a patient receiving long-term TPN could induce cholestasis when perfused into rat liver. Cholestasis was blocked when antiserum to *Escherichia coli* endotoxin also was given and was reproduced with infusion of *E coli* endotoxin. The absence of enteral feeding may predispose patients receiving TPN to gut bacteria or endotoxin translocation. Bowel rest impairs gut barrier function by causing intestinal atrophy[68] and impaired immune defense,[5] and enhances bacterial overgrowth by decreasing intestinal motility.[105,140] Relatively small amounts of enteral intake might be beneficial. Pallares and associates[100] found that mean LFT values did not change in patients receiving TPN plus hypocaloric (less than 500 kcal/d) oral feedings, compared with an increased incidence of cholestasis in patients receiving TPN alone.

The presence of bacterial overgrowth in the small intestine or delivery of unabsorbed bile acids to the colon in patients with intestinal resection can result in the production of hepatotoxic bile salts. Lithocholic acid, a secondary bile acid, formed after bacterial dehydroxylation of chenodeoxycholic acid,[80] has been implicated in the pathogenesis of cholestasis. This relation was first suspected when it was noticed that cholestatic changes in liver biopsy specimens during TPN therapy were similar to those in animals treated with lithocholic acid.[33,51] Fouin-Fortunet and colleagues[37] further demonstrated that increased LFT values occurred in patients receiving TPN who had an increase in biliary lithocholic acid concentration from 7% to 15% of total biliary bile acids, but not in those in whom the concentration of lithocholic acid remained normal at 1% of total biliary bile acids. Therefore, the beneficial effect of metronidazole therapy in preventing and treating cholestasis could be a result of its action on bile salt metabolism in addition to potential effects on endotoxin translocation referred to earlier.

Several components of TPN may be toxic to the liver. Allardyce and coworkers[2,3,118] reported that providing more than 60% of calories as lipid (3 g/kg/d) caused cholestatic changes in LFT results. The infusion of amino acids has been implicated in increasing serum bile acids,[112] decreasing bile acid secretion,[103] and causing cholestasis in infants.[11] Aluminum contaminants in TPN solutions have been found to accumulate in the liver, thereby causing a decrease in bile flow and an increase in serum bile acids.[60–63] It also has been suggested that the high osmolality of TPN solutions decreases bile flow.[82] There is no conclusive evidence that any of these TPN components are clinically important in the genesis of cholestasis in adult patients.

Patients receiving long-term TPN are prone to the development of cholelithiasis, which could lead to extrahepatic obstruction and cholestasis. In two large series, cholelithiasis developed in 23% to 35% of patients without preexisting gallstones while they were receiving long-term TPN, and was more prevalent in patients with ileal disorders.[107,116] Most TPN-related gallstones are pigment stones containing large amounts of calcium bilirubinate.[88,93,97,108]

Much animal and human research has demonstrated that parenteral feeding in the absence of enteral nutrients causes gallbladder stasis, resulting in gallbladder sludge formation and subsequently the development of pigment gallstones. Animal studies, using the prairie dog model, have documented that TPN feeding causes gallbladder stasis, sludge, increased calcium and bilirubin concentration in bile, and pigment stones.[27,106] Manipulations that increase gallbladder emptying by stimulating gallbladder contraction with either cholecystokinin injections[28,114] or enteral nutrition,[115] or by decreasing resistance to bile flow with sphincterotomy,[52] have prevented gallstone formation in the prairie dog. Similar results have been documented in human studies. In one such study, the incidence of gallbladder disease in patients receiving TPN with little or no enteral feeding was twice that in patients given TPN and additional enteral feeding.[116] Other factors that contribute to gallbladder stasis in parenterally fed patients, such as narcotic use, anticholinergic therapy, and truncal vagotomy, have been correlated with increased gallstone formation.[116,119] By performing serial biliary ultrasonography, Messing and colleagues[88] found that gallbladder sludge developed in 14 of 23 (61%) patients receiving prolonged courses of TPN; stones developed in 6 of the 14 patients with sludge (26% of all study patients); none were observed in patients without sludge. Sludge formation also correlated with the duration of TPN. Gallbladder sludge developed in 6% of patients in the first 3 weeks, in 50% between 4 and 6 weeks, and in 100% after 6 weeks of TPN therapy. All sludge had cleared in patients who were examined 4 weeks after TPN was stopped and oral feeding restarted. Calcium bilirubinate crystals, a precursor to pigment stones, have been found in bile of patients receiving TPN who have gallbladder sludge.[4] In a randomized, double-

blind, controlled trial in patients receiving TPN for more than 21 days, daily injections of cholecystokinin stimulated normal gallbladder contraction and completely prevented sludge formation, which occurred in 63% of saline-injected control subjects.[126] Gallbladder function, however, may be impaired in some patients, making therapy with cholecystokinin less effective. Apelgren and associates[7] could elicit gallbladder contractions in only 2 of 14 patients given intravenous cholecystokinin after 8 days of TPN.

The presence of biliary tract infection also may be related to the development of pigment stones.[128,129] Analysis of gallstones from 85 patients after cholecystectomy found that 25 of 32 pigmented stones had evidence of bacterial microcolonies in the interior of the stones.[124] In contrast, none of 35 cholesterol gallstones contained bacteria. Thus, infectious complications may be far more common in patients with pigment gallstones than in those with cholesterol stones,[48,132] and could explain the higher incidence of acute cholecystitis in patients with TPN-induced stones compared with the large number of patients with asymptomatic gallstones in the general population.

SEVERE LIVER DISEASE

Hepatic abnormalities usually are transient in patients receiving TPN. When elevated LFT values do occur, they often return to normal after reduction or cessation of TPN or even during continued TPN administration. The speculation that TPN use causes permanent liver damage is based on reports of chronic liver disease and cirrhosis in some patients.[18,24,109] As noted, patients who require TPN are at high risk for developing liver disease because of their illness, medical therapy, or blood transfusions. It therefore is impossible to separate the contribution of other clinical factors from that of TPN alone in the development of liver disease. For example, in a group of 18 patients receiving TPN for at least 6 months, severe liver abnormalities were found only in patients with massive intestinal resection (entire jejunum and right hemicolon), and not in others with modest (30 to 100 cm of terminal ileum and ascending colon) or no resection.[130] In addition to greater gut loss, patients with massive intestinal resection presumably were sicker and had a greater likelihood of having received hepatotoxic therapy.

Severe and progressive liver disease has been found only in patients receiving TPN for at least 4 months. The first adult patient reported to have progressive liver disease had received TPN for 30 months after massive intestinal resection.[24] Serial liver biopsies showed progression of liver disease from mild steatosis after 3 months of TPN to foci of liver cell necrosis and fibrosis and giant mitochondria at 16 months, to more severe disease with an alcoholic hepatitis-like lesion, progressive cholestasis, fibrosis, and cirrhosis. A second report described a patient with short bowel syndrome who died of liver failure after 5 years of home TPN.[109] The LFT values were normal during the first 4 years of TPN therapy, when bilirubin and alkaline phosphatase increased. Subsequent liver biopsies showed increasing cholestasis, fibrosis, and proliferation of Kupffer cells with foamy cytoplasm containing neutral lipids and periodic acid–Schiff–, diastase-positive material. Later, Bowyer and colleagues[18] found that progressive liver disease developed in 9 of 60 (15%) patients receiving long-term home TPN (mean duration, 29 months; range, 4 to 122 months). These patients had persistently high LFT levels for 8 to 95 months that led to at least one liver biopsy in each patient. The liver lesions found in this series were similar to those observed in the previous case reports. The most frequent abnormality was the presence of ceroid pigment in Kupffer cells, and portal macrophages found in all 9 patients. Eight patients had steatohepatitis, characterized by centrilobular and midzonal fatty change, focal necrosis, and mixed inflammatory infiltrates. Three patients had cholestasis; 3, centrilobular fibrosis; and 1, early cirrhosis. In 6 patients, the liver abnormalities were not associated with clinical symptoms, whereas progressive and severe clinical liver disease developed in the other three. Two of these 3 patients died—1 of hepatic encephalopathy and hepatorenal syndrome and 1 after biliary tract exploration for protracted intrahepatic cholestasis. Messing and coworkers[89] reported that chronic liver disease developed in 4 of 22 (22%) patients receiving home TPN for 4 to 59 months. Liver biopsies showed that three patients had cholestasis with bridging fibrosis and one had cirrhosis.

Data from large national registries of patients receiving home TPN suggest that the number of patients with severe liver disease is small. Of the 945 patients entered in the United States National Home TPN Registry, only 11 (1%) were admitted to the hospital in 1983 because of organ dysfunction.[50] The number of these hospitalizations related to liver disease was not given. From 1977 to 1987, 3 of 228 (1%) patients entered into the United Kingdom Home Parenteral Nutrition Register manifested cholestatic jaundice and died of liver failure.[123] The number of patients still alive with serious liver disease was not reported.

Clinical Management

Appropriate clinical management of TPN-fed patients involves both prevention and treatment of hepatic complications (Table 58-4). The following guidelines may be useful in preventing hepatic complications: administer adequate nutrients, particularly amino acids and essential fatty acids; provide a portion (20% to 50%) of nonprotein calories as fat; consider cyclic TPN in which the glucose infusion is stopped for at least 8 to 10 hours a day[41,78,79]; encourage enteral intake when possible; and avoid excessive glucose (more than 6 g/kg/d) or lipid (more than 2 g/kg/d or 0.1 g/kg/h) calories.

TABLE 58-4   *Clinical Approach to Adult Patients Receiving Total Parenteral Nutrition*

Considerations for Preventing Hepatic Complications
Administer adequate nutrients
Provide a portion (20%–50%) of nonprotein calories as fat
Cycle glucose calories
Encourage enteral feedings if possible
Avoid excessive glucose or lipid calories
Stimulate gallbladder contraction with cholecystokinin injection, bolus amino acid infusion, or lipid–protein meals
Prophylactic cholecystectomy

Considerations for Patients in Whom Liver Abnormalities Develop
Evaluate for possible causes of liver disease and treat as indicated
Institute preventive measures listed above
Limit copper and manganese if cholestasis is present
Trial of oral metronidazole therapy

If abnormal LFT values or other evidence of liver damage does occur, careful clinical assessment is needed to rule out other possible causes of liver disease. TPN does not need to be discontinued, but the same principles used in preventing hepatic complications can be applied therapeutically. When the pattern of LFT results suggests cholestasis, copper and manganese should be decreased or deleted from the TPN formula because these trace minerals are secreted in bile and can accumulate in the liver and basal ganglia, respectively.[86,122,124] In addition, a trial of metronidazole or stimulating bile flow with small lipid and protein meals or cholecystokinin may be helpful. The development of cirrhosis or liver failure are the most worrisome of TPN-associated liver abnormalities. Usually, TPN has been administered for long periods of time in these patients and cannot be discontinued because it is required for survival. The manipulations listed here can be tried, but their usefulness is unproved.

The known course of gallstones in patients receiving TPN makes it important to be alert for biliary complications in patients fed parenterally for more than 3 to 4 weeks. Preventive measures should be targeted for those patients who are at high risk for developing gallstones—those who have had ileal resections, who have no enteral intake, and who have been receiving TPN for more than 3 weeks. The simplest approach is aimed at preventing gallbladder stasis. Small amounts of lipid and protein meals given enterally, injections of cholecystokinin, and intermittent infusions of large quantities of crystalline amino acids can be used to stimulate gallbladder contraction. Prophylactic cholecystectomy may be a reasonable consideration in certain patients. In those patients shown to have gallbladder sludge already present, both oral refeeding and cholecystokinin injection are effective in clearing the gallbladder. Because sludge seems to be a precursor for gallstones, routine serial imaging of the gallbladder in high-risk patients may help identify those who might benefit from choleretic therapy. Stimulating gallbladder contraction, however, could be hazardous and has been shown to cause right upper quadrant pain, fever, leukocytosis, and elevated LFT values in patients who have small stones in addition to sludge.[8]

Summary

The use of TPN is associated with biochemical and histologic abnormalities of the liver. Although these abnormalities usually are benign and transient, the development of progressive and severe liver disease in patients receiving prolonged courses of TPN is worrisome. Prospective, randomized, controlled trials comparing parenteral with enteral feeding are needed to establish the true relation between TPN and liver disease. Confounding factors may have influenced results in most reported studies, because patients who require TPN often have illnesses or have received medical therapy that can cause hepatic injury. The most judicious course is to try to prevent hepatic complications by providing appropriate nutrients, avoiding excessive glucose or lipid calories, and encouraging enteral feedings.

References

1. Abad-Lacruz A, Gonzalez-Huix F, Esteve M, Fernandez-Banares F, Cabre E, Boix J, Acero D, Humbert P, Gassull

Index

Note: Page numbers followed by f indicate figures;
page numbers followed by t indicate tables; CF indicates a color figure.

ISBN 0-397-51363-1

90000

9 780397 513635